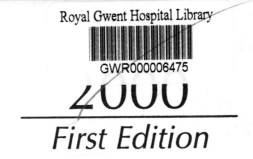
2000
First Edition

Complete Directory
for
Pediatric Disorders

- Disorder Descriptions
- Body Systems Descriptions
- National & State Associations
- Libraries & Resource Centers
- Support Groups & Hotlines
- Books & Periodicals
- Research Centers
- Web Sites

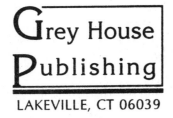

Grey House
Publishing

LAKEVILLE, CT 06039

i

PUBLISHER: Leslie Mackenzie
EDITORIAL DIRECTOR: Laura Mars
MEDICAL EDITOR: Alan H. Freidman, M.D., Yale University, School of Medicine
CONTRIBUTING MEDICAL WRITERS: Joy E. Bartnett, BS, AMIA, AMWA, ASAE
Debra L. Madden, BA, AMWA, ASAE
ASSOCIATE MEDICAL EDITORS: Karen Goldberg, M.D. Dyan Griffin, M.D., Sanand Menon, M.D.
Erin Springhorn, M.D., Mark Vincent, M.D., Michael Wilhelm, M.D.
PRODUCTION MANAGER: Anita DeMarco
EDITORIAL ASSISTANT: Robin Williams
MARKET RESEARCH: Jessica Moody
COPY EDITOR: Elaine Alibrandi
GRAPHIC DESIGN: Deb Fletcher
PRODUCTION: Tami Barilli, Yvonne Coburn, Stacey Curtis
Nancy McNamara, Sharon Moskiewicz, Fridai Regenhardt

Grey House Publishing, Inc.
Pocket Knife Square
Lakeville, CT 06039
860.435.0868
FAX 860.435.6613
http://www.greyhouse.com

ONLINE DATABASE

You can have immediate access to the thousands of resources for Pediatric Disorders, Diseases, Diasbilities and Conditions listed in this directory with *The Complete Directory for Pediatric Disorders – Online Database*. This Online Database will be available for subscription via the Internet in Summer 2000.

With *The Complete Directory for Pediatric Disorders – Online Database*, you will have direct access to Disorder Descriptions, National & State Agencies, Support Groups, Hotlines and much more with hotlinks to listee's websites and email address. Finding information sources for Pediatric Disorders has never been easier and now it's only a click away. For more information, call 800-562-2139.

MAILING LIST INFORMATION

This directory is available in mailing list form on mailing labels or diskettes. Please call 800-562-2139 to place an order or inquire about counts. There are a number of ways we can segment the database to meet your mailing list requirements.

DATABASE ON DISK

The database of this directory is available on diskette in an ASCII text file, delimited or fixed fielded. Call 800-562-2139 for details.

---

www.greyhouse.com

Clicking on www.greyhouse.com takes you through our complete line of directories providing business, health and education information. The site is fully illustrated and provides comprehensive descriptions of each book along with easy ordering capability.

Grey House Publishing Health Directories

The Complete Mental Health Directory, 2000

This is the first comprehensive resource covering the field of behavioral health, with critical information for both the layman and the mental health professional. For the layman, this directory offers understandable descriptions of 24 Mental Health disorders as well as detailed information on Associations, Media, Support Groups and Mental Health Facilities. For the professional, *The Complete Mental Health Directory* offers critical and comprehensive information on Managed Care Organizations, Information Systems, Government Agencies and Provider Organizations. This comprehensive volume of needed information will be widely used in any reference collection.

ISBN 0-939300-85-0	*559 pages*	*softcover*	*$165.00*
ISBN 0-939300-94-X	*559 pages*	*hardcover*	*$190.00*

The Complete Directory for People with Rare Disorders, 2000/01

This outstanding resource is produced in conjunction with the National Organization for Rare Disorders, with information never before available in one directory. It provides comprehensive and needed access to important information on over 1,000 rare disorders, including Cancers, Muscular, Genetic and Blood Disorders, and more. Each description is followed by information on Organizations, Publications and Government Agencies involved with the disorder. For quick, easy access to information, this directory contains two indexes: Entry Name Index and Acronym/Keyword Index.

> *"Quick access to information... public libraries and hospital patient libraries will find this a useful resource in directing users to support groups or agencies dealing with a rare disorder."*
> *– Booklist*

> *"A worthy addition to health collections."*
> *– Library Journal*

ISBN 1-891482-86-6	*800 pages*	*softcover*	*$165.00*
ISBN 1-891482-87-4	*800 pages*	*hardcover*	*$190.00*

The Complete Directory for People with Chronic Illness, 2000/01

The widely hailed *Complete Directory for People with Chronic Illness*, updated for 2000 is structured around the 85 most prevalent chronic illnesses – from Asthma to Cancer to Wilson's Disease, providing a comprehensive overview of the support services and information resources available for people diagnosed with a chronic illness. Each chronic condition contains a brief description of the illness in layman's language followed by National and Local Organizations, State Agencies, Newsletters, Research Centers, Hotlines, Books and Periodicals. New to this edition are sections on General Resources, both Associations and Media, as well as a chapter on Death and Bereavement.

> *"This is the place to start for general information on chronic illness... it contains the kind of information any public library would use regularly."*
> *– Booklist*

ISBN 1-891482-98-X	*1,100 pages*	*softcover*	*$165.00*
ISBN 1-891482-99-8	*1,100 pages*	*hardcover*	*$190.00*

The Complete Directory for People with Disabilities, 2000

A wealth of information, now in one comprehensive sourcebook. Completely updated for 2000, with thousands of new entries and enhancements to existing entries, this Eighth Edition is the most comprehensive resource available for people with disabilities, detailing Independent Living Centers, Rehabilitation Facilities, State and Federal Agencies, Associations and Support Groups. This one-stop resource provides immediate access to the latest products and services for people with disabilities, such as Periodicals and Books, Assistive Devices, Employment and Education Programs, and Camps and Travel Groups. Each year, more libraries, schools, colleges, hospitals, rehabilitation centers and individuals add *The Complete Directory for People with Disabilities* to their collections, making sure that this information is readily available to the families, individuals and professionals who can benefit most from the amazing wealth of resources catalogued here.

"No other reference tool exists to meet the special needs
of the disabled in one convenient resource for information."
– Library Journal

ISBN 1-891482-22-X	*928 pages*	*softcover*	*$165.00*
ISBN 1-891482-23-8	*928 pages*	*hardcover*	*$190.00*

Older Americans Information Directory, 1999/2000

This Second Edition is a comprehensive guide to resources for and about Older Americans, detailing National and State Organizations, Government Agencies, Health, Research Centers, Libraries and Information Centers, Legal Resources, Discount Travel Information and Continuing Education Programs. The first edition was published by Gale Research in 1994. *Older Americans Information Directory* includes about 4,000 new listings and two new chapters on Disability Aids & Assistive Devices and Health: Associations, Support Groups and Hotlines, which provides important information on 16 conditions, including Alzheimer's Disease, Arthritis, Heart Disease and Stroke. This Second Edition also contains two new indexes, including a Geographic Index and a Website Section. This comprehensive resource is a highly useful source of information for Older Americans searching for information and for those who care for and support them.

"A useful purchase for libraries serving seniors and programs for and about them."
– Choice

"Recommended for general collections with an interest in aging."
– Library Journal

ISBN 1-891482-36-X	*956 pages*	*softcover*	*$165.00*
ISBN 1-891482-37-8	*956 pages*	*hardcover*	*$190.00*

The Complete Women's Health Directory, 2000

This exciting, brand new reference work focuses on the health concerns of women. *The Complete Women's Health Directory* not only provides important information on Women's Health, but also on all aspects of Women's Life, including Emotional Concerns and Life Changes. You'll find necessary and detailed resources on important Women's Health Concerns, including Breast Cancer, Child Birth, Contraception, Depression, Eating Disorders, Fertility, Heart Disease, Menopause, Menstruation, Pregnancy, SExually Transmitted Diseases, Weight and much more. *The Complete Women's Health Directory* includes understandable descriptions of common disorders and health issues and thousands of resources for support, including National Associations and Agencies, Support Groups, Hotlines, Books, Magazines and Websites. For easy access to information, this directory has three indexes: Entry Name Index, Subject Index and Geographic Index. Never before has such a broad range of resources for Women's Health issues been brought together.

ISBN 1-891482-45-9	*800 pages*	*softcover*	*$165.00*
ISBN 1-891482-46-7	*928 pages*	*hardcover*	*$190.00*

To preview any of our Directories for 30 days, please call toll-free (800) 562-2139 or fax to (860) 435-3004

Introduction

Welcome to *The Complete Directory for Pediatric Disorders*. This first edition is published to fulfill three important purposes:

- To meet the growing consumer demand for current, understandable medical information on pediatric disorders, conditions, and diseases.

- To provide an extensive overview of the educational resources and support services available for parents of children with such conditions.

- To serve as a comprehensive resource for physician assistants, case workers, social workers, genetic counselors, medical librarians, and other professionals who are dedicated to providing concerned parents and other caregivers with vital supportive services.

The *Directory* is a "one-stop" resource, enabling professionals and the families they serve to obtain immediate, important information from one comprehensive source. It is organized in the following six sections:

Section I – Disorders

This section includes *descriptions* of 228 pediatric disorders, diseases, or conditions, from achondroplasia to XYY Syndrome, written in understandable language with appropriate medical terms cited for future reference. Each description includes the following:

- Disorder name and synonyms
- Related disorders
- Disorder Type and Bodily System affected
- Primary symptoms and physical findings
- Cause
- Standard treatment measures

Following each description are *disorder-specific resources*, including Associations, State Agencies, Support Groups, Libraries, Resource Centers, Research Centers, Web sites and Media Resources. These resource listings include contact information, such as mailing address, phone, toll free, and fax numbers, e-mail and Web site addresses, contact name and brief description.

The amount of medical data available on the Internet continues to grow. Hospitals, medical organizations and agencies, and advocacy groups continue to create Web sites that offer not only specific information on disorders, such as descriptions, symptoms, and treatments, but also helpful resources and current media information. We have included many of these Web sites in the hope of providing, combined with all the resources listed, the most comprehensive coverage available of the pediatric disorders covered in this *Directory*.

Section II – General Resources

This section includes resources such as Support Groups, Newsletters, Books and Magazines that are not limited to a specific disorder, but offer information and support for a wide range of issues and pediatric disorders.

These general resources, combined with disorder-specific resources, provide readers with almost 5,400 listings that create a comprehensive information network critical to the successful management of a pediatric disorder.

Section III – The Human Body

This section provides a comprehensive overview of the human body, beginning with the structure and function of human cells and tissues, continuing on to bodily systems, and then to prenatal and postnatal growth and development. This information enables the reader to broaden his or her understanding of how the disorders relate to the body. The descriptions in Section I reference those bodily systems that are affected by a particular disorder.

Section IV - Glossary

This guide to medical terminology provides important navigational tips and more than 200 commonly used medical prefixes, roots, and suffixes to help readers decipher terms they may encounter in the disorder descriptions.

Section V - Guidelines for Obtaining Additional Information and Resources

These guidelines may assist parents and caregivers who are interested in obtaining more information on such diverse topoics as physicians who specialize in certain pediatric disorders, accredited hospitals, approved drugs or medical devices for certain pediatric conditions, or current clinical trials that are investigating possible new therapies for particular diseases.

Sections VI - Indexes

The Complete Directory for Pediatric Disorders contains three indexes to help readers access the information from several places:

Entry Index is an alphabetical listing of all entry names.

Geographic Index groups listings by state.

Subject Index includes an alphabetical list of pediatric disorders, condition names, synonyms, and related disorders.

Table of Contents

The Complete Directory for Pediatric Disorders

First Edition

Introduction

Each disorder chapter includes a description and all or some of the following:

National Associations & Support Groups	Conferences
State Agencies & Support Groups	Media Resources
Libraries & Resource Centers	Camps
Research Centers	Web Sites

Each disorder chapter includes a description and all or some of the following:

National Associations & Support Groups	Conferences
State Agencies & Support Groups	Media Resources
Libraries & Resource Centers	Camps
Research Centers	Web Sites

Each disorder chapter includes a description and all or some of the following:

National Associations & Support Groups	Conferences
State Agencies & Support Groups	Media Resources
Libraries & Resource Centers	Camps
Research Centers	Web Sites

Each disorder chapter includes a description and all or some of the following:

National Associations & Support Groups   Conferences
State Agencies & Support Groups   Media Resources
Libraries & Resource Centers   Camps
Research Centers   Web Sites

Each disorder chapter includes a description and all or some of the following:

National Associations & Support Groups	Conferences
State Agencies & Support Groups	Media Resources
Libraries & Resource Centers	Camps
Research Centers	Web Sites

Each disorder chapter includes a description and all or some of the following:

National Associations & Support Groups	Conferences
State Agencies & Support Groups	Media Resources
Libraries & Resource Centers	Camps
Research Centers	Web Sites

DESCRIPTION

1   **ACHONDROPLASIA**
Synonyms: Chondrodystrophy, Fetal rickets
Disorder Type: Genetic Disorder
May involve these systems in the body (see Section III):
Skeletal System

Achondroplasia is an inherited autosomal dominant disorder of the skeletal system that belongs to a group of diseases known as chondrodystrophies. These disorders involve a disturbance in the development of cartilage of the long bones (e.g., arms and legs). In achondroplasia, there is an abnormality in the conversion of cartilage into bone. The arms and legs are usually affected; bone growth is delayed and ceases at a relatively early age. Symptoms and characteristic findings include a disproportionately large head with protruding or prominent forehead (frontal bossing); a flattened nasal bridge; an underdeveloped upper jaw and prominent lower jaw (prognathism); a well-developed, shortened trunk; and short, bowed arms and legs. The upper portion of the arms and legs are proportionately shorter than other parts of the limbs; the elbows may have a limited range of motion. In addition, the fingers and toes are usually short with a v-shaped space or gap between the third and fourth fingers; however, the hands are relatively wide. As children with achondroplasia grow, the pelvis tilts forward, resulting in a pronounced spinal curvature (lumbar lordosis) characterized by a prominent abdomen and buttocks.

Achondroplasia may be inherited as an autosomal dominant trait or occur as the result of a spontaneous change in a gene (mutation). Achondroplasia occurs in approximately three to 15 out of every 100,000 births.

The physical findings associated with achondroplasia occur as the result of the premature conversion of cartilage into bone at the growing ends (epiphyses) of the long bones, particularly of the arms and legs. This process prevents the bones from further growth, thus resulting in the characteristic findings of this disorder. Complications associated with achondroplasia may include dental problems such as malocclusion as well as chronic and severe middle ear infections (otitis media) that may lead to conductive hearing loss. Potentially life-threatening complications include the temporary cessation of breathing during sleep (sleep apnea) due to obstruction of the airway as a result of certain craniofacial abnormalities or compression of the spinal cord at its entrance to the vertebral column (foramen magnum). In addition, hydrocephalus, which is a condition characterized by an abnormal accumulation of cerebrospinal fluid within the brain, may also have life-threatening implications. Hydrocephalus may result from obstruction of the foramen magnum.

Treatment for achondroplasia is directed toward identification, evaluation, and prevention or correction of complications. Monitoring head growth during infancy to ensure that it is within established guidelines is effective to determine the presence of hydrocephalus and the need for surgical intervention or other measures.

To avoid further complications, dental irregularities, ear infections, and some skeletal irregularities may respond to physiotherapy as well as the use of orthopedic appliances such as braces. In addition, emotional and psychologic support may be provided through appropriate counseling.

The following organizations in the General Resources Section can provide additional information: National Organization for Rare Disorders, Inc. (NORD), NIH/Office of Rare Diseases, Genetic Alliance, NIH/National Institute of Arthritis and Musculoskeletal, and Skin Diseases, Online Mendelian Inheritance in Man: www3.ncbi.nlm.nih/gov/Omim/searchomim.html

National Associations & Support Groups

2   **Human Growth Foundation**
7777 Leesburg Pike, Ste 202
South Falls Church, VA 22043   703-883-1773
                                                            800-451-6434
                                      e-mail: kim@genetic.org

3 Little People of America, Inc.
PO Box 9897
Washington, DC 20016   301-589-0730
    800-243-9273
e-mail: LPADataBase@juno.com
www.lpaonline.org

Helps people with height deficiencies deal with everyday problems and questions that may arise.

4 Little People of America, National Headquarters
PO Box 745
Lubbock, TX 79408   806-797-8830
    888-572-2001
Fax: 806-797-8830
e-mail: LPADataBase@Juno.com

Helps people with height deficiencies deal with everyday problems and questions that may arise.

Monica Pratt

5 MAGIC Foundation for Children's Growth
1327 North Harlem Avenue
Oak Park, IL 60302   708-383-0808
    800-362-4423
Fax: 708-383-0899
e-mail: mary@magicfoundation.org
www.magicfoundation.org

Support and education provided to families of children with growth related disorders. Specialty divisions include: Growth Hormone Deficiency; Precocious Puberty; Congenital Adrenal Hyperplasia; McCune Albright Syndrome; Congenital Hypothyroidism; Russell-Silver Syndrome; Tuners Syndrome; Sepo Optic Dysplasia.
10,000 members

Mary Andrews, Executive Director

6 Short Stature Foundation
4521 Campus Dr. #130
Irvine, CA 92715   714-258-1833
    800-243-9273

Improves everyday life through the dispersion of information for commonly asked questions and problems of these with growth-related disorders.

Research Centers

7 Little People's Research
80 Sister Pierre Dr
Towson, MD 21201   410-494-0055
    800-232-5773
Fax: 410-494-0062

Helps people with height deficiencies deal with everyday problems and questions that may arise.

Web Sites

8 Cliniweb
www.ohsu.ed/cliniweb/C5/C5.116.99.343.

9 Dysmorphic Syndromes
www.hgmp.mrc.ac.uk/dhmhd-bin/hum-look-up

10 Human Growth Foundation
www.genetic.org/hgf/index.shtml

11 Little People of America, Inc.
www.lpaonline.org

12 Magic Foundation for Children's Growth
www.magicfoundation.org

13 Medical College of Wisconsin
www.chorus.rad.mcw.edu/doc/01026.html

14 PedBase
www.icondata.com/health/pedbase/files

Pamphlets

15 Achondroplasia
Human Growth Foundation
7777 Leesburg Pike Suite 202 South
Falls Church, VA 22043   703-883-1773
    800-451-6434

Signs, causes, and prevention of achondroplasia.

DESCRIPTION

16   ACUTE INFECTIOUS DIARRHEA

Disorder Type: Infectious Disease
May involve these systems in the body (see Section III):
Digestive System

Acute infectious diarrhea refers to a condition characterized by the frequent passage of loose, watery feces most commonly resulting from a viral or bacterial infection. Infection by either agent may be transmitted in a variety of ways. For example, contaminants may be present in infants' food, on their bottles, or on the hands of their caregivers; and airborne pathogens may be introduced into the body through inhalation.

Symptoms associated with acute infectious diarrhea may include vomiting, fever, lethargy, poor feeding, and blood in the feces. In addition, a temporary inability to properly digest milk may result as a consequence of a viral infection that damages the mucosal lining of the small intestine, thereby interfering with the production of lactase, the enzyme needed to absorb sugar (lactose) from milk. Untreated or severe diarrhea may result in excessive loss of fluid from the body (dehydration) and an imbalance of certain vital substances in the fluid portion of the blood (electrolytes such as sodium, chloride, and potassium). Dehydration and electrolyte imbalance may lead to potentially life-threatening complications. Symptoms and findings associated with dehydration in infants may include flushed, dry, loose skin; glazed-over eyes; a coated tongue; protracted crying; sleepiness; a decrease in urine output (oliguria); confusion; increased irritability; unresponsiveness; and an alarming drop in blood pressure. Other signs of dehydration in infants may include sunken eyes and a depression in the soft spot (fontanelle) toward the front of the head.

Treatment of acute infectious diarrhea is geared toward the prevention or correction of dehydration. Such treatment involves replacement of fluids and electrolytes either orally or intravenously, depending upon such factors as degree of severity. Once dehydration is corrected, nursing infants may resume breast-feeding at the earliest opportunity, while other infants may resume feedings with a lactose-free formula, gradually followed by their regular formula. Although some cases of acute infectious diarrhea will resolve spontaneously, other treatment may be directed toward the underlying cause. In addition, because transmission of pathogens that cause diarrhea are so often passed on through fecal-oral contamination, prevention of this potentially severe condition may often be accomplished by attention to good hygiene.

The following organizations in the General Resources Section can provide additional information: NIH/National Institute of Allergy and Infectious Diseases, NIH/National Digestive Diseases Information Clearinghouse, World Health Organization, Centers for Disease Control (CDC), WHO/Child Health and Development (CHD) www.who.int/chd/

National Associations & Support Groups

17   Digestive Disease National Coalition
507 Capital Court, Suite 200
Washington, DC 20002   202-544-7497
                             Fax: 202-546-7105

Objective is to inform the public about technology improvements through several media forms.

18   International Foundation for Functional Gastrointestinal Disorders
P.O. Box 17864
Milwaukee, WI 53217   414-964-1799
                             888-964-2001
                             Fax: 414-964-7176
                             e-mail: iffgd@execpc.com
                             www.execpc.com/iffgd

The organization offers responses to those commonly asked questions for families and individuals who's lives have been touched with the disorder.

19   Intestinal Disease Foundation
1323 Forbes Avenue, Suite 200
Pittsburgh, PA 15219   412-261-5888
                             Fax: 412-471-2722

Encourages the individuals who have been diagnosed to have a posotive outlook through several support groups and reading materials.

Web Sites

20 **American Gastroenterological Association**
www.gastro.org/brochure.html

21 **Child Health Research Project**
http://ih.jsph.edu/chr/chr.htm

DESCRIPTION

22 ACUTE LYMPHOBLASTIC LEUKEMIA
Synonyms: Acute lymphocytic leukemia, ALL
Disorder Type: Neoplasm: Benign or Malignant
Tumor

Acute lymphoblastic leukemia (ALL) is a malignant disease characterized by excessive production of immature white blood cells known as lymphoblasts in the blood, bone marrow, and other tissues of the body. ALL is the most common type of childhood cancer with a slightly higher predominance in boys. Although this type of leukemia may develop in adolescents or occasionally in adults, ALL occurs most commonly in children from the ages of two to five years.

Lymphoblasts normally develop into lymphocytes, a type of white blood cell that is found in the circulating blood system; however, uncontrolled lymphoblast production associated with ALL results in their accumulation in the bone marrow, thus impairing the ability of the bone marrow to produce mature blood cells. In addition, lymphoblasts are released into the general blood circulation and carried to other organs where they continue to reproduce, sometimes resulting in damage to the individual organs. Symptoms and characteristic findings associated with this type of leukemia often appear suddenly and may include loss of appetite (anorexia) and a generalized feeling of ill health followed by fatigue, and weakness resulting from decreased levels of circulating red blood cells (anemia); bleeding from the gums or nose resulting from decreased levels of blood platelets; and infection and fever resulting from decreased levels of mature white blood cells. In addition, children with ALL may appear pale, bruise easily, develop relatively small red or purple spots on the skin (petechiae), vomit, or experience headache and bone or joint pain. Other findings may include swollen lymph glands and an enlarged spleen (splenomegaly).

Acute lymphoblastic leukemia is believed to result from a chromosomal change or mutation in the genetic material of white blood cells resulting in uncontrolled cell division and subsequent overproduction of leukemic blood cells. Certain factors may place children at increased risk for developing ALL including Down's syndrome, certain genetic disorders such as Fanconi's anemia, certain blood disorders, and exposure to radiation, some chemotherapy drugs, and certain chemicals such as benzene.

The diagnosis of ALL may be established through blood testing demonstrating the presence of lymphoblasts in the blood, as well as microscopic examination of a bone marrow sample obtained through biopsy. Treatment for this type of leukemia is directed toward the destruction of leukemic cells through the administration of chemotherapy. Treatment for the presence of leukemic cells in the brain or the membranes surrounding the brain and spinal cord (meninges) may require the direct injection of the chemotherapy agent methotrexate through the spinal cord (intrathecal injection) into the cerebrospinal fluid. In addition, radiation may sometimes be administered to the brain. Additional treatment may include blood transfusions to alleviate anemia and bleeding irregularities, as well as the administration of antibiotics to offset the effects of increased susceptibility to infection resulting from chemotherapy. Relapse after successful remission of ALL usually involves the bone marrow, brain, or testes and may necessitate the administration of an additional chemotherapeutic regimen and bone marrow transplantation. In addition, boys with recurring leukemic cells in the testes may require radiation therapy in addition to systemic chemotherapy. Other treatment is symptomatic and supportive.

The following organizations in the General Resources Section can provide additional information: Candlelighters Childhood Cancer Foundation, Candlelighters Childhood Cancer Foundation Canada, National Childhood Cancer Foundation, NIH/National Cancer Institute, NIH/National Heart, Lung and Blood Institute

National Associations & Support Groups

23 B.A.S.E. Camp Children's Cancer Foundation
7501 Glenmoor Lane
Winter Park, FL 32792   407-673-5060
                              Fax: 407-673-5095
                    e-mail: basecampcf@aol.com

Does not grant wishes, but does help obtain free
or reduced price tickets to Walt Disney World,
Universal Studios, and other central Florida attractions, for children with a hematology/oncol-
ogy disease and their immediate family. The
child with cancer must be on treatment when
tickets are used. B.A.S.E. needs to receive a
written request and doctor's statement (containing child's name, disease, and whether he/she is
medically able to visit any central Florida attraction) 2-3 weeks prior to.

24 Cancer Care, Inc.
1180 Avenue of the Americas
New York, NY 10036   212-302-2400
                            800-813-4673
                       Fax: 212-719-0263

Free telephone service that provides immediate
psychological support to cancer patients and
their families in Florida, Delaware, Pennsylvania, and New Jersey. The line is staffed by professional social workers who offer counseling,
support, education, information, and referral.
This organization also provides some funds to
help with chemotherapy, transportation, or radiation.

25 Cancer Cured Kids
P.O. Box 189
Old Westbury, NY 11568   516-484-8160
                                800-225-7525
                           Fax: 516-484-8160

Organization dedicated to the quality of life of
kids who have survived cancer. Cancer Cured
Kids supplies information about the educational
and psychosocial needs of survivors.

26 Cancer Fund of America
2901 Breezewood Lane
Knoxville, TN 37921
                            800-578-5284
                       Fax: 615-938-2968

Helps defray cancer-related expenses not covered by insurance.

27 ChemoCare
2 North Road Suite A
Chester, NJ 07930   908-233-1103
                           800-552-4366
                      Fax: 908-233-0228

Provides one-to-one emotional support to cancer
patients (children or adults) and their families
undergoing chemotherapy, radiation, and/or surgery, from trained and certified volunteers who
have undergone the treatments themselves.

28 Children's Blood Foundation, Inc.
333 East 38th Street, Room 830
New York, NY 10016   212-297-4336
                           Fax: 212-297-4340
              e-mail: cbf@nyh.med.cornell.edu

Devoted to supplying families and friends of children diagnosed, with the knowledge and facts
that they require.

29 Dreams Come True, Inc. Emery Clinic-Peds
1365 Clfton Road NE
Atlanta, GA 30322   778-248-3496

Serves any child with cancer or chronic blood
disease treated at Emory University Homo/Onc
Clinic. Dreams submitted by children.

30 Grant A Wish Foundation
P.O. Box 21211
Baltimore, MD 21228   410-242-1549
                             800-933-5470
                        Fax: 410-242-8818
        e-mail: grant-a-wish@worldnet.att.net

Provides a variety of special services and programs (such as beach and mountain retreats, attending Orioles games) to any child up to 18
years of age who is being treated for cancer.
Services are provided free to charge and are
available on an ongoing basis throughout treatment.

31 Hair Club for Kids: Hair Club for Men
270 Farmington Avenue
Farmington, CT 06032
                            800-888-4236
                       Fax: 860-676-0805

If your child expresses an interest in wearing a
wig, send pictures prior to hair loss with snip-
pets of hair for a good match of original color
and texture. The cost of the wig may be covered
by insurance.

32 Just In Time
P.O. Box 27693
Philadelphia, PA   215-247-8777

Contact us to order several styles of reversible, all cotton headwear for girls 7 to 12 and women who have experienced hair loss.

33 Leukemia Society of America, Inc.
600 Third Avenue, 4th Floor
New York, NY 10016   212-573-8484
                            800-955-4572
                       Fax: 212-856-9686
e-mail: infocenter@leukemia.org
                       www.leukemia.org

The Leukemia Society will give the caller the address and phone number for the nearest local chapter. Application for financial aid is made to the local chapter. It is important to apply as soon as possible after diagnosis.

34 Leukemia and Lymphoma Society
600 Third Ave, 4th Floor
New York, NY 10013   212-573-8484
                            800-955-4572
                       Fax: 212-856-9686
www.leukemia-lymphoma.org

Provides information, education and support to people living with Leukemia, Lymphoma and other blood related cancers.

35 National Bone Marrow Transplant Link
29209 Northwestern Highway #624
Southfield, MI 48034   810-932-8483
                              800-546-5268

Human service agency that encourages contact by families and health professionals. It operates a hot line, and provides peer support, a library, clearinghouse, and suggestions for financial assistance.

36 National Coalition for Cancer Survivorship
1010 Wayne Road, Fifth Floor
Silver Spring, MD 20910   301-650-8868
                                 800-422-6237
                            Fax: 301-565-9670

Furnishes information about legal rights and advocacy services for cancer survivors of all ages. Publications include: Health Insurance and Cancer: What You Need to Know; Working It Out: Your Employment Rights As a Cancer Survivor; and Charting the Journey: An Almanac of Practical Resources for Cancer Survivors.

37 National Leukemia Association
585 Stewart Avenue Suite 536
Garden City, NJ 11530   516-222-1944

State Agencies & Support Groups

38 BMT Family Support Network
P.O. Box 845
Avon, CT 06001
                            800-826-9376

Links families involved in bone marrow transplants for telephone assistance. Also provides information and resources. Serves grieving families.

39 Parents Caring and Sharing
c/o Chumie Bodek, 109 Rutledge St
Brooklyn, NY 11211   718-596-1542

Provides outreach and support network and writes a newsletter for Jewish Orthodox families with children with cancer. Holds monthly meetings and links families of children with similar diseases.

Research Centers

40 International Bone Marrow Transplant Registry
Medical College of Wisconsin
P.O. Box 26509,8701 Watertown Plank R
Milwaukee, WI 53226   414-456-8325

This research organization collects and analyzes data on transplants from over 250 institutions in 30 countries. It studies factors that affect the success of transplants, but does not make donor matches. It publishes a newsletter, and will supply a publication list upon request.

41 National Leukemia Research Association,Inc
585 Stewart Avenue, Suite 536
Garden City, NY 11530   516-222-1944
                          Fax: 516-222-0457

Provides families with emotional and financial support, when requested, through these difficult times.

Audio Video

42 Childhood Cancer: Today's Crisis
Children's Hospital Medical Center
Hematology-Oncology Div,Elland Ave
Cincinnati, OH 45229   513-559-4266

How one family coped with their son's diagnosis of leukemia.

43 **Family Portrait: Coping with Childhood Cancer**
Films for the Humanities and Sciences
P.O. Box 253
Princeton, NJ 08543

800-257-5126

Videotape of five family portraits covering issues such as guilt, sibling rivalry, divorce, the adopted child, and involvement of other family members in the care of the child. Introduction and closing by Bob Keeshan (Captain Kangaroo).

25 minutes

44 **My Hair's Falling Out...Am I Still Pretty?**
Necessary Pictures
7 West 20th Street, Suite 2-F
New York, NY 10011

212-675-1809
800-221-3170

Moving film about two children with cancer who are hospital roommates. Using dance, animation, and music, the video explores the feelings of the patients, families, and friends while it sensitively informs and educates the viewers about the emotional and physical aspects of childhood cancer. The child with leukemia grows up to become a doctor, while her roommate with a tumor dies. For school-age children and their families. Purchase is $25 for families and $79 for professionals.

Web Sites

45 **ALL Kids**
www.all-kids.org/

46 **ALL Message Board**
www.healthboards.com/leukemia/39.html

47 **Cancer Care**
www.cancercare.org/faq/cancer_faq.html

48 **CancerNet**
31 Center Drive, MSC 2580
Bethesda, MD 20892

800-422-6237
Fax: 301-402-5874
TTY: 800-332-8615
e-mail: cancermail@icicc.nci.nih.gov
cancernet.nci.nih.gov

A part of the National Cancer Institute, CancerNet is a website offering comprehensive information on cancer. The site offers a children's page with stories, poems, games and more for young patients with cancer.

Books

49 **Child Life Council**
Child Life Council
11820 Parklawn Drive #202
Rockville, MD 20852

301-881-7090
Fax: 301-881-7092
e-mail: clcstaff@childlife.org
www.childlife.org

Child Life Council is a professional association of child life specialists. The Council seeks to promote the well-being of children and families in healthcare settings by supporting the development and practice of the child life profession. The Council provides training, conferences, publications, and information to the membership and the public that is germane to the Child Life profession.

Deborah Brouse, Executive Director

50 **Childhood Leukemia: A Guide for Families, Friends & Caregivers**
Nancy Keene, author

O'Reilly & Associates, Inc.
101 Morris Street
Sebastopol, CA 95472

800-998-9938
Fax: 707-829-0104
e-mail: patientguides@oreilly.com
www.patientcenters.com

Features a wealth of tools to help parents become strong advocates for their child, detailed and precise medical information, and day-to-day practical advice to help cope with procedures, hospitalization, family and friends, schools, social, emotional and financial issues.

528 pages Softcover
ISBN: I-565926-32-3

51 **Having Leukemia Isn't So Bad, of Course, It Wouldn't Be My First Choice**
Cynthia Krumme, author

Sargasso Enterprises, 1993
14 Wildwood Street
Winchester, MA 01890

781-729-9037
Fax: 781-729-2726
e-mail: cak@sargasso.ne.mediaone.net

Personal story of Catherine Krumme, diagnosed with leukemia at age 4, relapsed at age 7, finished treatment at age 10. Catherine graduated from college in 1998 and is a graduate student. The book is a supportive resource for families with cancer, for their friends, and for teachers working with children with health issues.

149 pages Softcover
ISBN: 0-963555-44-8

Ann Combs

52 Late Effects of Treatment for Childhood Cancer
D.M. Green, G. D'Angio, author

John Wiley & Sons, Inc.
1 Wiley Drive
Somerset, NJ 08875   732-469-4400
                          Fax: 732-302-2300
                 e-mail: custserv@wiley.com
                          www.wiley.com

Medical text for oncologists, radiologists, students.

200 pages
ISBN: 0-471561-66-5

53 Non-Chew Cookbook
J. Randy Wilson, author

Wilson Publishing, Inc.
P.O. Box 2190
Glenwood Springs, CO 81602   970-945-5600
                          Fax: 970-945-5600
                 e-mail: randyw@rof.net
                 www//.rof.net/yp/randyw

Contains recipes for patients unable to chew due to the side effects of chemotherapy and/or radiation.

200 pages

Children's Books

54 Draw Me a Picture
Nessim, Susan, and Barbara Wyman, author

Cancervive
6500 Wilshire Blvd., #500
Los Angeles, CA 90048

A fun coloring book for children with cancer (ages 3 to 6). Marty Bunny talks about how it was when he was in the hospital for cancer and invites readers to draw about their experiences.

55 Going to the Hospital
Child Life Council
11820 Parklawn Drive #202
Rockville, MD 20852   301-881-7090

Booklet for children describing hospitalization. Provides simple, honest information illustrated by photographs of children.

56 Kathy's Hats: A Story of Hope
Trudy Krisher, author

Albert Whitman Co.
6340 Oakton Street
Morton Grove, IL 60053
                          800-255-7675

A charming book for ages 5 to 10 about a girl whose love of hats comes in handy when chemo makes her hair fall out.

Magazines

57 Coping Magazine
P.O. Box 682268
Franklin, TN 37068   615-790-2400
                          Fax: 615-794-0179

A bi-monthly publication devoted to people whose lives have been touched by cancer.

Newsletters

58 Friends Network
P.O. Box 4545, ATTN:Kenon Neal
Santa Barbara, CA 93140   805-693-1017
             e-mail: info@cancerfunletter.com
                   www.cancerfunletter.com

A national nonprofit organization which distributes an activities newsletter printed in color, called The Funletter, to children with cancer. We service all major cancer treatment centers throughout the United States.

Pamphlets

59 Children's Cancer Pain Can be Relieved
Wisconsin Cancer Pain Initiative
1300 University Avenue, Room 4720
Madison, WI 53706   608-262-0978
                          Fax: 608-265-4014
                 e-mail: wcpi@facstaff.wisc.edu

A booklet that helps parents determine if their child is in pain and provides methods to manage the pain. Single copy - free. Also, there is a Handbook of Cancer Pain Management, 4th edition.

12 pages

DESCRIPTION

60   ACUTE MYELOID LEUKEMIA
Synonyms: Acute granulocytic leukemia, Acute myeloblastic leukemia, Acute myelocytic leukemia, Acute myelogenous leukemia, Acute myelomonocytic leukemia, AML
Disorder Type: Neoplasm: Benign or Malignant Tumor

Acute myeloid leukemia (AML) is a malignant disease characterized by excessive production and increases in the numbers of certain cells called myelocytes in the bone marrow. Myelocytes are the forerunners of certain white blood cells called granular leukocytes. Although AML is more common in adults, this disease accounts for approximately 20 percent of all childhood leukemias.

The symptoms and characteristic findings associated with acute myeloid leukemia result from the accumulation of myelocytes in the bone marrow, eventually impairing the bone marrow's ability to produce mature blood cells. In addition, myelocytes are released into the general blood circulation and carried to other organs where they continue to grow at a rapid rate. Early symptoms may include shortness of breath, bleeding, infection, headache, fever, vomiting, pale skin coloration, and bone or joint pain. Other findings may include enlargement of the liver and spleen (hepatosplenomegaly) and swollen lymph glands. Some children may also exhibit swollen gums as well as swelling of the salivary glands in front of the ears. In addition, small leukemic cell tumors (chloromas) may develop under the skin or on the membranes surrounding the brain and spinal cord leading to inflammation of these membranes (meningitis). Most children with AML develop blood irregularities such as abnormally low levels of circulating red blood cells (anemia) and platelets (thrombocytopenia), although the white blood cell count may range from low to high.

Acute myeloid leukemia is thought to result from a chromosomal change or mutation in the genetic material of white blood cells. This mutation is thought to cause uncontrolled cell division and subsequent rapid increase in numbers of leukemic blood cells. Certain factors may place children and adults at increased risk for developing AML. Such factors include genetic disorders such as trisomy 21, Bloom syndrome, Fanconi anemia, and certain other inherited disorders as well as a history of chemotherapy or radiation for earlier malignancies.

The diagnosis of AML is confirmed through the evaluation of a bone marrow sample obtained through biopsy. Treatment for this type of leukemia is directed toward the destruction of leukemic cells through the administration of combinations of chemotherapeutic drugs. However, these potent drugs also suppress white blood cell production, thus increasing susceptibility to infection; therefore, antibiotic therapy is often indicated. In some patients, transfusions of red blood cells and platelets may also be indicated to alleviate anemia and bleeding irregularities. Additional chemotherapy may be initiated to destroy leukemic cells affecting the central nervous system or to prevent their recurrence. This type of treatment requires direct injection of medication into the spinal canal (intrathecal injection). In addition, radiation may sometimes be administered directly to the central nervous system. Further treatment may include bone marrow transplantation. Other treatment is symptomatic and supportive.

The following organizations in the General Resources Section can provide additional information: Candlelighters Childhood Cancer Foundation, Candlelighters Childhood Cancer Foundation Canada, National Childhood Cancer Foundation, NIH/National Cancer Institute, NIH/National Heart, Lung and Blood Institute

---

National Associations & Support Groups

61   B.A.S.E. Camp Children's Cancer Foundation
7501 Glenmoor Lane
Winter Park, FL 32792   407-673-5060
                                   Fax: 407-673-5095
                           e-mail: basecampcf@aol.com

Does not grant wishes, but does help obtain free or reduced price tickets to Walt Disney World, Universal Studios, and other central Florida attractions, for children with a hematology/oncology disease and their immediate family. The child with cancer must be on treatment when tickets are used. B.A.S.E. needs to receive a written request and doctor's statement (containing child's name, disease, and whether he/she is medically able to visit any central Florida attraction) 2-3 weeks prior to.

62 Cancer Cured Kids
P.O. Box 189
Old Westbury, NY 11568   516-484-8160
                             800-225-7525
                        Fax: 516-484-8160

Organization dedicated to the quality of life of kids who have survived cancer. Cancer Cured Kids supplies information about the educational and psychosocial needs of survivors.

63 Cancer Fund of America
2901 Breezewood Lane
Knoxville, TN 37921
                             800-578-5284
                        Fax: 615-938-2968

Helps defray cancer-related expenses not covered by insurance.

64 Children's Blood Foundation, Inc.
333 East 38th Street, Room 830
New York, NY 10016   212-297-4336
                        Fax: 212-297-4340
              e-mail: cbf@nyh.med.cornell.edu

Devoted to supplying families and friends of children diagnosed, with the knowledge and facts that they require.

65 Leukemia Society of America, Inc.
600 Third Avenue, 4th Floor
New York, NY 10016   212-573-8484
                             800-955-4572
                        Fax: 212-856-9686
              e-mail: infocenter@leukemia.org
                         www.leukemia.org

The Leukemia Society will give the caller the address and phone number for the nearest local chapter. Application for financial aid is made to the local chapter. It is important to apply as soon as possible after diagnosis.

66 Leukemia and Lymphoma Society
600 Third Ave, 4th Floor
New York, NY 10013   212-573-8484
                             800-955-4572
                        Fax: 212-856-9686
                 www.leukemia-lymphoma.org

Provides information, education and support to people living with Leukemia, Lymphoma and other blood related cancers.

67 National Leukemia Research Association,Inc
585 Stewart Avenue, Suite 536
Garden City, NY 11530   516-222-1944
                        Fax: 516-222-0457

Provides families with emotional and financial support, when requested, through these difficult times.

Web Sites

68 CancerCare:
www.cancercare.org/faq/cancer_faq.html

69 CancerOnline:
www.stonecottage.com/canceronline/

70 ICARE
www.icare.com

71 Mediconsult.com
www.mediconsult.com/mc/mcsite.nsf/condition-nav/

Pamphlets

72 Acute Myelogenous Leukemia
Leukemia and Lymphoma Society

                             800-955-4572

Explanation of the disease, its symptoms, diagnosis, prognosis and treatment, psychological responses to a confirmed diagnosis and current research.

16 pages

DESCRIPTION

73 ALBINISM

Disorder Type: Genetic Disorder, Metabolism
May involve these systems in the body (see Section III):
Dermatologic System

Albinism refers to a condition that is present at birth (congenital) and results from inborn errors in the production and distribution of the pigment melanin. This pigment is responsible for the coloration of the hair, skin, and eyes. Albinism may be inherited as an autosomal recessive, autosomal dominant, or X-linked trait. In addition, several genetic mutations have been identified. Although there are many different types of albinism, two major forms known as tyrosinase negative and tyrosinase positive oculocutaneous albinisms have been identified. The term oculocutaneous refers to both the eyes and the skin. Albinism occurs in about one in 20,000 individuals worldwide.

Tyrosinase negative (type I or IA) albinism, the most severe form of generalized oculocutaneous albinism, results from the reduced or absent activity of the enzyme tyrosinase. This enzyme is essential to the proper metabolism of the pigment melanin. Type I albinism is characterized by the absence of melanin in the hair, skin, and eyes. Characteristic findings include white hair, pink or white skin, and eyes that may appear pink or bluish-gray. In addition, individuals with type I albinism often have other eye irregularities such as involuntary, flickering-type movements of the eyes (nystagmus), nearsightedness (myopia), sensitivity or intolerance to bright light (photophobia), or other visual abnormalities. Tyrosinase negative oculocutaneous albinism is inherited as an autosomal recessive trait. The gene for this form of albinism is located on the long arm (q) of chromosome 11. A specific mutation of this gene is thought to cause a milder form of this type of albinism (type IB) that is prevalent among Amish communities in the United States. Individuals

with type IB albinism have similar characteristics to those of type IA at birth; however, the hair, skin, and eyes tend to darken somewhat with age. In addition, eye irregularities are usually less severe.

Tyrosinase positive (type II) albinism is more common and less severe than type I. This type of albinism is thought to result from an inborn error in the transport of tyrosine, a chemical forerunner of melanin. Newborns with this disorder may have little to no melanin at birth, but pigment may accumulate as these children grow, thus darkening the skin color during the course of childhood. In addition, visual improvements may become apparent as individuals mature. Tyrosinase positive albinism is inherited as an autosomal recessive trait. The gene for this type of albinism is located on chromosome 15. Several other types of tyrosinase positive albinism are thought to be caused by mutations of this gene. In addition, tyrosinase positive albinism may be present in association with several other disorders such as Hermansky-Pudlak syndrome, Chediak-Higashi syndrome, and Cross-McKusick-Breen syndrome.

Other forms of albinism may include ocular albinism that mainly affects the pigment of the eyes and is characterized by sensitivity to light (photophobia); involuntary, rhythmic-type eye movements (nystagmus); and decreased visual clarity. The hair and eyes may be light in color, but not excessively light. Ocular albinism may be inherited as an X-linked trait as in Nettleship-Falls type ocular albinism and Forsius-Eriksson syndrome, or as an autosomal dominant or autosomal recessive trait. In addition, some individuals may have partial albinism, sometimes called piebaldism, that is characterized by the appearance of patchy, unpigmented areas of hair or skin. In some individuals, this type of albinism may be characterized simply by a lock of white hair near the forhead. Piebaldism is inherited as an autosomal dominant trait.

Treatment for albinism is dependent upon the severity of the physical findings. People with albinism are at increased risk for skin cancer resulting from sun exposure; therefore, appropriate sunscreen or avoidance of direct sunlight on the skin is indicated. In addition, lack of pigment in the eyes may indicate the need for tinted or dark glasses to help reduce light sensitivity. Also, early evaluation and treatment for other visual irregularities is necessary so that affected children may overcome potential difficulties in school. Other treatment is symptomatic and supportive.

The following organizations in the General Resources Section can provide additional information: National Organization for Rare Disorders, Inc. (NORD), Genetic Alliance, March of Dimes Birth Defects Foundation, NIH/Office of Rare Diseases, NIH/National Institute of Child Health and Human Development

National Associations & Support Groups

74 **National Organization for Albinism and Hypopigmentation**
1530 Locust Street, #29
Philadelphia, PA 19102
215-545-2322
800-473-2310
Fax: 609-858-4337
e-mail: noah@albinism.org
www.albinism.org/

Presents data for individuals and their families for the commonly asked questions through several media options.

Web Sites

75 **American Council of the Blind**
www.acb.org/

76 **American Foundation for the Blind**
www.afb.org

77 **Assistive Media**
www.assistivemedia.org/

78 **Foundation Fighting Blindness**
www.blindness.org/

79 **International Albinism Center**
www.cbc.umn.edu/iac/

Books

80 **Student with Albinism in the Regular Classroom**
N.A.P.V.I.
P.O. Box 317
Watertown, MA 02272

800-562-6265

DESCRIPTION

81 ALOPECIA AREATA

Synonyms: Alopecia circumscripta, Androgenetic alopecia, Pelade

May involve these systems in the body (see Section III):

Dermatologic System

Alopecia areata is a disease of unknown origin characterized by the sudden, localized loss of patches of scalp hair and other areas of hair growth, such as the eyelashes and eyebrows. These patches are usually well-defined, round or oval in shape, and most often appear on the scalp or beard area. On rare occasions, progression of hair loss may result in the total loss of scalp hair in a condition called alopecia totalis. If the disease progresses to include the total loss of both scalp and body hair, the condition is called alopecia universalis. Another uncommon form of alopecia areata called ophiasis involves the loss of hair in a continuous band around the head. If hair loss associated with alopecia areata is not widespread, the condition is usually reversible, with most patients exhibiting new hair growth within a few months to a year; however, recurrences are quite common. Children who develop this condition at a very young age, patients who experience recurring episodes, and those who have extensive involvement are less likely to experience spontaneous remission. Although this disease occurs most commonly in the adult population, approximately 20 percent of those affected develop the disorder between birth and 20 years of age.

Although the skin in the area of hair loss may appear unremarkable, microscopic examination may reveal the presence of inflammation. In addition, some individual hairs that appear at the margins of the bald, patchy areas may be easily removed and, upon microscopic examination, reveal a lightly-pigmented, tapered hair shaft that ends in a hair root that is reduced in size (exclamation hairs). Symptoms or characteristic findings sometimes associated with alopecia areata include the development of irregularities such as nail pitting and ridging, allergic or hypersensitivity reactions, and opacities of the lenses of the eye (cataracts). Alopecia areata may also be associated with certain autoimmune diseases such as Addison disease, Hashimoto thyroiditis, vitiligo, and others. In addition, approximately seven percent of children with Down's syndrome exhibit the symptoms associated with alopecia areata.

The exact cause of alopecia areata is not known; however, approximately 25 percent of those affected are believed to inherit the disease through autosomal dominant transmission. In dominant disorders, only one copy of the disease gene is inherited; however, it masks the other normal gene and the disease is usually obvious. Other suggested causes include autoimmune responses or emotional factors related to stress. Because alopecia areata so often resolves spontaneously, treatment for this disease in young children may simply include ongoing observation. Other treatment may include the local, topical application of certain fluorinated corticosteroids, minoxidil, or other medications. Injections of certain steroids under the skin may be effective for moderate hair loss; however, this treatment may not be advisable for some children. Other treatments are available, but are more often used for adult patients. Other treatment is supportive. For example, the use of hairpieces and other cosmetic considerations may be beneficial to the emotional well-being of children, especially adolescents, with alopecia areata.

The following organizations in the General Resources Section can provide additional information: National Organization for Rare Disorders, Inc. (NORD), NIH/Office of Rare Diseases, Genetic Alliance, American Autoimmune Related Diseases Association, Inc., NIH/National Institute of Arthritis and Musculoskeletal and Skin Diseases, Online Mendelian Inheritance in Man: www3.ncbi.nlm.nih.gov/Omim/searchomim.html

National Associations & Support Groups

82 **National Alopecia Areata Foundation**
710 C St, Ste 11
San Rafael, CA 94901 415-456-4644
Fax: 415-456-4274
e-mail: 4301.1642@compuserve.com

Extensive examination into the disorder makes
hard to ask questions simpler to answer, and
easy to understand.

Web Sites

83 **Alopecia Areata Page**
anglefire.com/wa/Victor2/alopecia.html

84 **Alopecia Areata Research Foundation**
nhic-nt.health.org/Script/En-
try.cfm?HRCode=HR2250

DESCRIPTION

85 ALPHA-1-ANTITRYPSIN DEFICIENCY

Disorder Type: Genetic Disorder, Metabolism

Alpha-1-antitrypsin deficiency is a hereditary metabolic disorder characterized by deficiency of alpha-1-antitrypsin, an enzyme that is produced by the liver and inhibits the actions of other enzymes that break down certain proteins. Deficiency of alpha-1-antitrypsin may result in progressive destructive changes in the lungs. In addition, some patients may experience liver disease that is thought to result from abnormal retention of the alpha-1-antitrypsin enzyme in liver cells. Alpha-1-antitrypsin deficiency is caused by certain changes (mutations) of a gene known as Pi (protease inhibitor) located on the long arm of chromosome 14 (14q32.1). Although alternative forms of the Pi gene have been identified, only a small number of mutations are associated with deficiency of the enzyme (e.g., PiZZ genotype). Alpha-1-antitrypsin deficiency is typically inherited as an autosomal recessive trait due to inheritance of two deficiency-causing genes (homozygosity). However, in some cases, inheriting one copy of a particular form of the Pi gene (heterozygosity) may predispose some individuals to certain conditions associated with the disorder (e.g., panacinar emphysema).

The specific symptoms associated with alpha-1-antitrypsin deficiency as well as the age of onset vary from patient to patient. Shortly after birth, a small percentage of affected children may develop suppression or cessation of the flow of bile (neonatal cholestasis). Bile, a liquid secreted by the liver, carries waste products away from the liver and assists in the digestion of fats in the small intestine. During the first week of life, affected infants may have yellowish discoloration of the skin, whites of the eyes, and mucous membranes (jaundice); abnormal enlargement of the liver (hepatomegaly); and the presence of unabsorbed fat in the feces. Jaundice often spontaneously re-

solves within two to four months after birth. Affected infants and children may appear to have no further associated symptoms (asymptomatic), may have chronic liver disease, or, in the most severe cases, may experience scarring of the liver and gradual impairment of liver function (cirrhosis). Older children may develop chronic liver disease or cirrhosis and associated high blood pressure within veins from the spleen and intestines to the liver (portal hypertension). In some patients with portal hypertension, there may be a diversion of portal circulation to veins in the walls of the stomach and esophagus, causing abnormal widening of such blood vessels (esophageal varices). Without treatment, some patients with liver disease may experience potentially life-threatening complications.

Alpha-1-antitrypsin deficiency also may cause progressive degeneration of and destructive changes in the air sacs (alveoli) of the lungs (panacinar emphysema). Panacinar emphysema usually becomes apparent in adults during the thrd or fourth decade of life, and most patients have little or no lung disease during childhood.

In children with alpha-1-antitrypsin deficiency, the treatment of associated liver disease is primarily symptomatic and supportive. In some patients, liver transplantation may be effective. The treatment of lung disease associated with alpha-1-antitrypsin deficiency typically includes symptomatic and supportive measures, including prompt, aggressive treatment of respiratory infections and oxygen therapy. In addition, patients should avoid exposure to tobacco smoke, the use of aerosol sprays, and exposure to lung irritants. Alpha-1-antitrypsin enzyme replacement therapy (e.g., prolastin therapy) is available for patients with associated emphysema.

The following organizations in the General Resources Section can provide additional information: National Organization for Rare Disorders, Inc. (NORD), NIH/Office of Rare Diseases, March of Dimes Birth Defects Foundation, Genetic Alliance, Online Mendelian Inheritance in Man:
www3.ncbi.nlm.nih.gov/Omim/searchomim.html

National Associations & Support Groups

86 Alpha-1 National Association
220 Old Shakeopee Red, Ste 101
Minneapolis, MN 55437   612-703-9979
                                    Fax: 612-885-0133
                     e-mail: brandley@slpha1.org
                                    www.alpha1.org

Organized to disclose the knowledge and facts
that individuals need to be emotiomally successful while fighting the disorder.

87 American Liver Foundation
75 Maiden Lane Suite 603
New York, NY 10038   212-668-1000
                                    800-465-4837
                          Fax: 212-483-8179
              e-mail: info@liverfoundation.org
                          www.liverfoundation.org

Organization provides several differant medias
for answering questions and to help clarify any
uncertainties the individual may be experiencing.

88 Children's Liver Alliance
3835 Richmond Ave, Ste 190
Staten Island, NY 10312   718-987-6200
                                    Fax: 718-987-6200
            e-mail: livers4kids@earthlink.net
                                    livertx.org

Aides in easing the physical and emotional
strains that the child is experiencing, so they can
better deal with the disorder through differant
media resources that are also available to both
family and friends.

International

89 Children's Liver Disease Foundation
AXA Equity & Law House
35-37 Great Charles St Queensway
Birmingham Intl,
United Kingdom

                     www.childliverdisease.org

Devoted to caring for individuals and their loved
ones who's lives have been touched by this disease.

Research Centers

90 Research Trust for Metabolic Diseases in Children
Goldengates Lodge Weston Rd., Crewe
Cheshire,
United Kingdom

Dedicated to providing the most up-to-date medical knowledge for the families and friends of people suffering from this and related diseases.

Web Sites

91 Alphalink.org
www.alphalink.org/

92 American Lung Association
www.lungusa.org

Newsletters

93 Alpha-1 Support Group Newsletter
819 Bayview Road
Neenah, WI 54956   414-727-4576

17

DESCRIPTION

94   AMNIOTIC BAND SYNDROME
Synonyms: Amnion rupture sequence, Amniotic band disruption complex, Amniotic band sequence (ABS), Congenital constricting bands
Disorder Type: Birth Defect
May involve these systems in the body (see Section III):
Prenatal & Postnatal Growth & Development

Amniotic band syndrome is a condition characterized by the disturbance of fetal development by strands or bands of tissue that originate from the amniotic sac, the fluid-filled sac that surrounds the fetus. These strands or fibrous bands may encircle and eventually tighten around the developing fetus, resulting in tissue damage. Such tightening or constriction may result in complete amputation or ring-like constrictions of developing arms or legs (limbs), malformations of the fingers and toes, and constriction of the umbilical cord. In addition, confinement or tethering of certain limbs by amniotic bands or decreased levels of amniotic fluid due to leakage (oligohydramnios) may result in abnormally decreased fetal movements, potentially causing additional deformities. Amniotic band syndrome is thought to affect approximately one in 10,000 to 45,000 newborns.

During fetal development, amniotic bands may cause abnormal fluid accumulation in body tissues (edema), bleeding (hemorrhage), and localized loss of tissue (i.e., resorptive necrosis). In affected newborns, associated structural deformities are extremely variable. No specific malformation is consistently associated with the condition. However, in many newborns, there is underdevelopment (hypoplasia) or absence of certain limbs; deep, residual, ring-shaped grooves surrounding certain limbs; incomplete separation of the fingers or toes (digits) with apparent webbing (pseudosyndactyly). Affected newborns may also develop abnormal curvature of the spine (scoliosis) as well as a deformity in which the feet are abnormally twisted out of position or shape (clubfeet or tali-

pes). In addition, severely decreased levels of amniotic fluid surrounding the developing fetus may be associated with incomplete development of the lungs (e.g., pulmonary hypoplasia), leading to breathing difficulties or respiratory insufficiency. Associated symptoms may include abnormally rapid breathing (tachypnea), grunting upon exhalation, drawing in of the chest wall during inhalation, and a bluish discoloration of the skin and mucous membranes (cyanosis).

Amniotic band syndrome appears to occur randomly for unknown reasons (sporadically). Some researchers indicate that, in rare instances, the development of constrictive amniotic bands may be associated with abdominal trauma, certain genetic disorders such as Ehlers-Danlos syndrome, or a procedure during which amniotic fluid is removed from the uterus and used for laboratory analysis (amniocentesis).

Treatment of infants with amniotic band syndrome is symptomatic and supportive. These measures may include plastic surgery techniques to remove deep residual grooves encircling the arms or legs. In addition, in infants with respiratory insufficiency, treatment includes appropriate oxygenation therapy and other supportive measures.

The following organizations in the General Resources Section can provide additional information: National Organization for Rare Disorders, Inc. (NORD), Genetic Alliance, March of Dimes Birth Defects Foundation, NIH/National Institute of Child Health and Human Development, NIH/National Institute of Arthritis and Musculoskeletal and Skin Diseases

National Associations & Support Groups

95   CHERUB—Association of Families and Friends of Children with Limb Disorders
936 Deleware Ave
Buffalo, NY 14209

Answers the questions and problems that families of juveniles diagnosed with a disorder may be experiencing.

96 Children's Craniofacial Association
P.O. Box 280297
Dallas, TX 75243
972-994-9902
800-535-3643
Fax: 972-240-7607
e-mail: DNKM90A@prodigy.com
www.masterlink.com/children

Devoted to the dispersion of medical knowledge of this and similar disorders, along with providing emotional support for the sufferers and their families.

97 Craniofacial Foundation of America
975 E Third St
Chattanooga, TN 37403
423-778-9192
800-418-3223
Fax: 423-778-8172
e-mail: dnkm90@prodigy.com
www.pages.prodigy.com/cranio/facial/htm

Organization assists families with both the physical and emotional aspects, trying to make the everyday events a little easier.

98 FACES: National Association for the Craniofacially Handicapped
P.O. Box 11082
Chattanooga, TN 37401
615-266-1632
800-332-2373

Disperses information to the public on the medical professionals specializing in this field.

99 Forward Face: The Charity for Children with Craniofacial Conditions
Institute of Reconstructive Plastic Surgery
317 34th St, Rm 901A
New York, NY 10016
212-684-5860
800-393-3223
Fax: 212-684-5864

Provision of data and emotional assistance to both sufferers and medical professionals.

100 Let's Face It
P.O. Box 29972
Bellingham, WA 98228
360-676-7325
e-mail: letsfaceit@faceit.org
www.faceit.org/@faceit/

Devoted to disseminating the information to people suffering from facial abnormalities.

101 National Foundation for Facial Reconstruction
317 E 34th St, Rm 901
New York, NY 10016
212-263-6656
800-422-3233
Fax: 212-263-7534

Devoted to assisting individuals and their families with the difficulties associated with the disorder.

Web Sites

102 Association for Children with Hand or Arm Deficiency
www.reach.org.uk/

103 ICAN (International Child Amputee Network)
www.amp-info.net/childamp.htm

104 Mayo Clinic Health Oasis
www.mayohealth.org/mayo/ask-phys/qacur_29.htm

105 Wide Smiles
www.widesmiles.org/syndrom/amniobnd.html

Newsletters

106 Superkids, Inc.
60 Clyde St
Newton, MA 02160

Newsletter for families and friends of children with limb difficulties.

DESCRIPTION

107 ANENCEPHALY

Disorder Type: Birth Defect, Genetic Disorder
May involve these systems in the body (see Section III):
Central Nervous System

Anencephaly is an abnormality that is present at birth (congenital) and belongs to a group of birth defects known as neural tube defects. This condition is characterized by the absence of certain bones of the skull (cranial vault) as well as absence or severe underdevelopment of the brain. Approximately one of 1,000 infants is born with anencephaly. There is a higher-than-average incidence of this birth defect in Ireland and Wales.

During the early stages of pregnancy, a specialized layer of tissue extends along the back portion of the developing embryo. As the embryo grows, this tissue, known as the neural plate, forms a groove that is bordered by folds. This groove eventually deepens and closes to form the neural tube. Later in development, the neural tube gives rise to tissue that later forms the brain and spinal cord. The neural tube is surrounded and protected by the bones of the back (vertebrae). Failure in this sequence of developmental events results in a neural tube defect.

Anencephaly represents a type of neural tube defect that is incompatible with life. Additional physical findings sometimes associated with this abnormality include folded ears, incomplete closure of the palate (cleft palate), and congenital heart defects. Anencephaly is thought to occur as the result of many genetic or environmental factors (multifactorial), alone or in combination. Vitamin deficiencies, nutritional deficiencies, toxic factors, and socioeconomic factors may contribute to the development of anencephaly. In addition, the theory of a genetic predisposition to anencephaly is supported by the fact that the risk of additional children being born with this defect rises with each pregnancy.

Supplementation with folic acid, initiated before pregnancy, may reduce the risk of neural tube defects. Women, especially those who have previously given birth to an infant with a neural tube defect, are encouraged to consult their physicians regarding supplementation with folic acid.

The following organizations in the General Resources Section can provide additional information: Online Mendelian Inheritance in Man: www3.ncbi.nlm.nih.gov/Omim/searchomim.html, Genetic Alliance, March of Dimes Birth Defects Foundation, NIH/National Institute of Child Health and Human Development, NIH/National Institute of Neurological Disorders and Stroke

National Associations & Support Groups

108 Anencephaly Support Foundation
30827 Sifton
Spring, TX 77386
281-364-9222
e-mail: asf@asfhelp.com
www.asfhelp.com

This support group is run by families who have had a baby born with anencephaly. Provides links to personal stories, support group information, medical and causation information, pictures and other information.

109 Association of Birth Defect Children, Inc.
930 Woodcock Road, Suite 225
Orlando, FL 32803
407-245-7035
800-313-2223
Fax: 407-895-0824
e-mail: abdc@birthdefects.org
www.birthdefects.org

Organization devoted to dissemination of data pertaining to birth related malformations.

110 Fighters for Encephaly Support Group
332 Brereton Street
Pittsburgh, PA 15219
412-687-6437

111 National Information Center for Children & Youth with Disabilities
P.O. Box 1492
Washington, DC 20013
202-884-8200
800-695-0285

Web Sites

112 Pedbase
www.icondata.com/health/ped-
base/files/ANENCEPH.HTM

113 Rare Genetic Diseases in Children (NYU)
http://mcrcr2.med.nyu.edu/murphp01/home-
new.nth

DESCRIPTION

114 ANGIOKERATOMAS
Synonyms: Angiokeratosis, Telangiectatic wart
May involve these systems in the body (see Section III):
Dermatologic System

Angiokeratomas are thickened skin growths that are characterized by warty clusters and dilated blood vessels. These individual lesions vary in color and may appear as pink, red, purple, or black, roughly-surfaced lesions. Although angiokeratomas may be present in many different forms, only a few types significantly affect infants, children, and adolescents.

Solitary angiokeratoma refers to the formation of a small, singular, bluish-black, wart-like pimple or papule that appears most commonly on the legs. Solitary angiokeratomas usually develop during childhood or adolescence.

Angiokeratoma circumscriptum is a relatively rare condition that most often occurs during infancy or early childhood and is characterized by the formation of individual, wart-like, bluish-red pimples (papules) and nodules. These solitary lesions often come together to form larger clusters or patches, usually on the leg or trunk. If untreated, these patches often enlarge during adolescence. Treatment is directed toward the eradication of the patches and may include such procedures as surgical excision, electrodessication during which the growths are burned away using electricity, and cryotherapy during which the clusters are frozen using solid carbon dioxide or liquid nitrogen.

Angiokeratoma diffusum, or Fabry disease, is a rare inherited disorder that is transmitted as an X-linked recessive trait. Fabry disease is a metabolic disorder that is manifested by the development of red or bluish-black callused pimples over the lower portion of the body from the naval and hip area to the thighs. Other findings include fever, pain, numbness of the hands and feet, re-tarded growth, and irregularities related to the blood vessels and heart, the kidneys, the blood, and other organs. The skin abnormalities associated with Fabry disease usually develop before adolescence.

Angiokeratoma of Mibelli usually occurs in children or young adults and is thought to be transmitted as an autosomal dominant trait. This disorder is characterized by the formation of soft, red, purple, or black pimples and nodules that become scaly, warty, and sometimes crusted. Although the ears, palms, and soles may sometimes be affected, the growths usually develop on the undersurface of the fingers, toes, elbows, and knees. In addition, the growths may be solitary, amassed, or convergent. This condition often develops subsequent to frostbite or overexposure to the cold that results in redness and swelling of the skin.

The following organizations in the General Resources Section can provide additional information: NIH/National Institute of Arthritis and Musculoskeletal and Skin Diseases

National Associations & Support Groups

115 American Academy of Dermatology
930 North Meacham Road, P.O.Box 4014
Schaumburg, IL 60168   708-330-0230
                              www.aad.org

Largest, most influential and most representative of all dermatologic associations. Committed to the highest quality standards in continuing medical education. Developed a platform to promote and advance the science and art of medicine and surgery related to the skin; promote the highest possible standards in clinical practice, education and research in dermatology and related disciplines; and support and enhance patient care and promote the public interest relating to dermatology.

116 American Skin Assocation
150 East 58th Street, 33rd Floor
New York, NY 10155   212-753-8260
                            800-499-7546
                        Fax: 212-688-6547
        e-mail: AmericanSkin@compuserve.com

DESCRIPTION

117 ANIRIDIA

Synonym: Hypoplasia of iris with rudimentary

Disorder Type: Birth Defect, Genetic Disorder, Vision

Aniridia is a birth defect characterized by absence of all or a portion of the colored area of the eye (iris) at birth. Both eyes are typically affected (bilateral aniridia). According to many reports in the literature, the term aniridia may be a misnomer, since an undeveloped (vestigial) portion of the iris is usually present (i.e., apparent upon slit-lamp examination or gonioscopy). The iris is an involuntary circular muscle that is visible through the transparent, front portion of the eye (cornea). When certain fibers in the iris contract, the hole in the center of the iris (pupil) either widens or constricts, allowing in additional or less light.

In some infants with aniridia, the corneas of the eyes are also abnormally small. In addition, many affected infants and children experience loss of transparency of the lenses of the eyes (cataracts) or displacement of the lenses, which are located behind the pupils. Aniridia is often associated with underdevelopment (hypoplasia) of the macula, the central portion of the retina that distinguishes detail in the central field of vision.

Additional eye abnormalities often associated with aniridia include rapid, involuntary movements of the eyes (nystagmus); reduced fields of vision; abnormally increased sensitivity to light (photophobia); and progressively increased fluid pressure within the eyes (glaucoma). In most cases, glaucoma is not apparent during the first month of life (neonatal period).

Depending upon the range and severity of associated eye abnormalities, children with aniridia may have varying levels of visual impairment. However, in most cases, affected children may have visual acuity of approximately 20/200 or even further reductions in vision. The clearness or sharpness of vision (i.e., visual acuity) is typically measured on a scale comparing a patient's vision at 20 feet with that of an unaffected individual with full visual acuity. Thus, a person with 20/200 vision sees at 20 feet what someone with full visual acuity sees at 200 feet.

Aniridia may be an isolated condition or may occur in association with certain syndromes, such as WAGR syndrome, a rare disorder characterized by kidney tumors (Wilms tumor), abnormalities of the reproductive and urinary tracts (genitourinary anomalies), due to spontaneous genetic changes (mutations). Other cases may be inherited as an autosomal dominant trait (e.g., WAGR syndrome) or, in very rare cases, as an autosomal recessive trait (e.g., aniridia-cerebellar ataxia-mental deficiency). Treatment of aniridia includes symptomatic and supportive measures, such as removal of cataracts, monitoring for and appropriate supportive treatments for glaucoma, and possible visual aids (e.g., artificial pupil contact lenses).

The following organizations in the General Resources Section can provide additional information: National Organization for Rare Disorders, Inc., (NORD), March of Dimes Birth Defects Foundation, NIH/Office of Rare Diseases, Genetic Alliance, Online Mendelian Inheritance in Man: www3.ncbi.nlm.nih.gov/Omim/searchomim.html

National Associations & Support Groups

118 NIH/National Eye Institute (NEI)
9000 Rockville Pike
Bethesda, MD 20892   301-496-5248
                                      www.nei.nih.gov/

119 National Eye Research Foundation
910 Skokie Boulevard
Northbrook, IL 60062

Devoted to the enhancement of care and study of eye related diseases.

Web Sites

120 Aniridia Network
www.clubs.yahoo.com/clubs/aniridianetwork

121 Aniridia Web Site
www.aniridia.org

122 National Association for Visually Handicapped
www.navh.org/

DESCRIPTION

123 ANKYLOSING SPONDYLITIS
Synonyms: AS, Marie-Strumpell spondylitis
Disorder Type: Genetic Disorder
May involve these systems in the body (see Section III):
Muscular System, Skeletal System

Ankylosing spondylitis (AS) is a chronic, progressive, inflammatory disease that affects joints of the spine and results in pain, stiffness, and possible loss of spinal mobility. In most patients, the joints between the spine and the hipbones (sacroiliac joints) are affected. In addition, joints in the spinal column of the upper and lower back (lumbodorsal spine) and the neck (cervical spine) may be involved to varying degrees. Although the disease usually becomes apparent during young adulthood or middle age, it may also begin during childhood at approximately eight years of age or older. Males are more commonly affected than females.

In most cases, affected children initially have periodic inflammation and discomfort in the joints of the arms and legs (transient peripheral arthritis), particularly the large joints of the legs. Many also experience arthritis in the shoulders, the lower jaw bone (i.e., temporomandibular joints), and the feet. Such inflammation results in associated swelling, pain, abnormal warmth, and possible limited movement of affected joints. In children with AS, involvement of the sacroiliac joints may be apparent at the disorder's onset or may develop over several months or years. The different regions of the spine may then be progressively affected, usually beginning in the spinal column of the lower back (lumbar spine) and eventually involving the upper back (thoracic spine) and neck (cervical spine). Children with the disease experience periodic pain and stiffness that may be alleviated by movement. Many have hip, thigh, and lower back pain that is often more severe at night and experience stiffness of affected areas in the mornings. In addition, some affected children have involvement of the joints that con-

nect the ribs to the spine (costovertebral joints). Resulting inflammation, pain, and stiffness may lead to a limited ability to expand the chest to take deep breaths. Disease progression may spontaneously cease at any stage; however, in some cases, all regions of the spine may gradually be affected, potentially resulting in severely impaired spinal mobility.

In some cases, additional symptoms and findings may be associated with ankylosing spondylitis. For example, some affected children may experience fatigue, low-grade fever, lack of appetite (anorexia), low levels of circulating red blood cells (anemia), growth retardation, and repeated inflammation of the colored region of the eye (iris) and its muscle (iridocyclitis). Inflammation of the major artery of the body (aoritis), a finding that is often seen in adults with ankylosing spondylitis, is rarely seen in affected children.

Research has shown that approximately 95 percent of affected individuals have a specific human leukocyte antigen or HLA. Antigens are proteins that stimulate the body to produce certain antibodies in response to invading microorganisms or foreign tissues. Most individuals with ankylosing spondylitis have a specific genetically determined HLA known as HLA-B27. The possible role of HLA-B27 in potentially predisposing an individual to the disorder has not been determined. Ankylosing spondylitis is thought to be an autosomal dominant disorder. In some cases, individuals with a defective gene for AS may not experience symptoms and findings associated with the disorder (reduced penetrance). AS is thought to have a higher penetrance among males.

Although HLA-B27 is present in most individuals with ankylosing spondylitis, it is not considered diagnostic for the disorder. AS is typically diagnosed based upon a complete patient and family history, characteristic physical findings, and specialized x-ray techniques. Treatment of children is primarily directed toward relieving pain and ensuring proper posture to help preserve spinal mobility. Certain medications may be prescribed to help alleviate or manage pain (e.g., indomethacin or other nonsteroidal antiinflammatory medications [NSAIDs]). Special exercises may be recommended to help strengthen back muscles and maintain proper posture. In addition, certain lifestyle changes may be suggested, including avoiding thick pillows and using a firm mattress. Additional treatment is usually symptomatic and supportive.

The following organizations in the General Resources Section can provide additional information: March of Dimes Birth Defects Foundation, National Organization for Rare Disorders, Inc., (NORD), NIH/Office of Rare Diseases, NIH/National Institute of Arthritis and Musculoskeletal & Skin Diseases Clearinghouse, Online Mendelian Inheritance in Man: www3.ncbi.nlm.nih.gov/Omim/searchomim.html

National Associations & Support Groups

124 **American Autoimmune Related Diseases Association, Inc.**
15475 Gratiot Avenue
Detroit, MI 48205   313-371-8600
e-mail: aarda@aol.com
www.aarda.org

Focused on the dissemination of information to a wide public base of similar diseases.

125 **American Juvenile Arthritis Organization**
1330 West Peachtree Street
Atlanta, GA 30309   404-872-7100
e-mail: help@arthritis.org
www.arthritis.org

Caters to the necessity of young arthritic sufferers by providing them with the much-needed ata through a variety of both audio and visual mediums.

126 **Arthritis Foundation**
1330 West Peachtree Street
Atlanta, GA 30309   404-872-7100
e-mail: info@arthritis.org
www.arthiritis.org

Group offers an array of information and important facts for individuals and their families pertaining to their difficulty.

127 **Back Pain Association of America, Inc.**
P.O. Box 135
Pasadena, MD 21123   410-255-3633
e-mail: backpainassoc@MSN.COM

Provides assistance and education materials to individuals suffering from spinal and neck discomfort.

128 **Spondylitis Association of America**
P.O. Box 5872
Sherman Oaks, CA 91413   818-981-1616
800-777-8189
e-mail: Information@spondylitis.org
www.spondylitis.org

Supports research and dissemination and familiarization for medical professionals of the disorder.

International

129 **National Anklosing Spondylitis Society**
P.O. Box 179, Mayfield
East Sussex TN20 6ZL,
United Kingdom
e-mail: nasslon@aol.com
web.ukonline.co.uk/nass

Web Sites

130 **AS Web**
www.asweb.com/home.html

131 **AS Webcenter**
www.jps.net/cwlove/asweb.html

132 **EnAble Center**
www.goodnet.com/~ee72478/enable/Facts1.htm

Pamphlets

133 **Ankylosing Spondylitis**
Arthritis Foundation
P.O. Box 7669
Atlanta, GA 30357   404-872-7100
800-283-7800
Fax: 404-872-0457

DESCRIPTION

134 ANODONTIA

Disorder Type: Birth Defect, Teeth

Anodontia refers to a condition in which some or all of the teeth are missing as the result of a congenital defect or of damage sustained from disease. Certain genetic influences may sometimes result in complete absence of the teeth (total anodontia). For example, ectodermal dysplasias are a group of congenital disorders characterized by abnormalities of the teeth, hair, nails, skin glands, the skin, nervous system, ears and eyes, and the delicate mucous membranes that line the anus and the mouth. Partial anodontia may also result from a common birth defect such as cleft palate. In infants with cleft palate, the roof of the mouth does not close completely. In addition, there are usually abnormalities in the development of the teeth, including malformed, absent, or extra (supernumerary) teeth. Partial anodontia is often a component of certain disorders or syndromes including pseudohypoparathyroidism (a hereditary condition characterized by the inability to respond to the hormone secreted by the parathyroid gland); cleidocranial dysplasia (an autosomal dominant genetic disease characterized by defective formation of the bones of the face); and other disorders affecting the face and skull (craniofacial disorders). The absence of some teeth may result in malocclusion or misalignment of the upper and lower teeth. In some patients, malocclusion sometimes interferes with chewing and grinding of food (mastication).

Treatment of anodontia may include the use of full or partial dentures or other dental prosthetics (e.g., bridgework). In some patients, dental implants may be considered when appropriate. These approaches to treatment may be delayed until underlying structural deficits (e.g., cleft palate) are surgically corrected. In addition, the use of orthodontic appliances may be used to modify the position of the teeth, thus aiding in correction of malocclusion.

The following organizations in the General Resources Section can provide additional information: NIH/National Institute of Child Health and Human Development

National Associations & Support Groups

135 American Academy of Pediatric Dentistry
211 East Chicago Avenue, #700
Chicago, IL 60611   312-337-2169
                          Fax: 312-337-6329
                 e-mail: ajohnson@aapd.org
                          www.aapd.org

The professional organization whose dentist members are specifically trained to provide both primary and comprehensive preventive and therapeutic oral health care for infants, children, adolescents, and patients with special health care needs. The site is for parents, teachers, nurses, media and dentists

4500 members

John S. Rutkauskes, Executive Director
C. Scott Litch, Deputy Executive Director

136 American Association of Orthodontics
401 North Lindbergh Blvd
St. Louis, MO 63141   314-993-1700
                            Fax: 314-997-1745
                    e-mail: info@aaotho.org
                          www.aaortho.org/

A professional association of educationally qualified orthodontic specialists dedicated to advancing the art and science of orthodontics and dentofacial orthopedics, improving the health of the public by promoting quality othodontic care, and supporting the successful practice of orthodontics.

137 American Dental Association
211 East Chicago Avenue
Chicago, IL 60611   312-440-2500
                          www.ada.org

Professional assocation of dentists dedicated to serving both the public and the profession of dentistry. Promotes the profession by enhancing the integrity and ethics of the profession and strengthening the patient/dentist relationship. Fulfills its mission by providing services and through its initiatives in education, research, advocacy and the development of standards.

138 National Institute of Dental Research
31 Ctr Dr Msc 2290, Bldg 31 Rm 2C39
Bethesda, MD 20892   301-496-3571
                                    Fax: 301-402-2185
                e-mail: slavkinh@od31.nidcr.nih.gov
                www.nidr.nih.gov/discover/welcome.htm

The National Institute of Dental Research promotes the general   health of the American people by improving their oral, dental and
craniofacial health. The NIDCR aims to promote health, to prevent diseases and conditions,
and to develop new diagonistics and therapeutics.

Harold Slavkin, DDS

Web Sites

139 Dental Consumer Advisory
www.toothinfo.com/

140 Dental Resources on the Web
www.dental-resources.com
        e-mail: webmaster@dental-resources.com
                www.dental-resources.com

Dental sites for education, practices, laboratories, office supplies, dental care and associations.

141 Straight Talk about Orthodontics
www.aoa.on.ca/faq.htm   416-490-8414
                e-mail: mikeyt@idirect.com
                www.aoa.on.ca/faq.htm

Provides information about various othodontic
treatments.

DESCRIPTION

142 ANORECTAL MALFORMATIONS

Disorder Type: Birth Defect
Covers these related disorders: Anal atresia, Anal fistula, Anal stenosis, Ectopic anus, Imperforate anus
May involve these systems in the body (see Section III):
Digestive System

Anorectal malformations are a group of birth defects affecting the rectum, the anus, or both. The rectum is a muscular tube that forms the lower region of the large intestine. The end of the rectum terminates at an external opening known as the anus. Anorectal malformations vary in severity. For example, the anal opening may be in its normal location but may be unusually small or narrow (e.g., anal stenosis or imperforate anus). Some anorectal malformations may not be apparent upon physical examination (e.g., imperforate anus or anal atresia). In addition, some forms of the condition involve the location of the anus in an unusual (ectopic) area (anal fistula). In infants with imperforate anus, the anal opening is partially or completely closed due to the presence of a thin membrane (i.e., cloacal membrane). In anal atresia, the rectum may end blindly due to absence (atresia) of the anal canal. In addition, in many affected infants, an abnormal channel (fistula) may be present between the rectum and certain other unusual locations. Anorectal malformations affect approximately one in 4,000 newborns.

Most newborns with anorectal malformations experience lower intestinal obstruction within 24 hours after birth due to incomplete passage of meconium, the thick, darkish green material that accumulates in the fetal intestines and forms a newborn's first stool. Newborns normally pass meconium during the first 24 to 48 hours after birth. Affected infants with an unusuallening may also have incomplete or infrequent bowel movements or experience difficulty passing stools (constipation) within days or weeks after birth.

Associated findings may include rectal bleeding; periodic episodes of diarrhea following constipation and associated abrasions of the skin (e.g., of the perineum and the buttocks); and abnormal enlargement of a segment of the large intestine (megacolon). In affected males with a channel between the rectum and the urinary tract, there is typically passage of gas (pneumaturia) and meconium in the urine.

When newborns are diagnosed with anorectal malformations, physicians may consider surgical measures to prevent intestinal or urinary obstruction. Therapies for affected newborns or infants depend upon the nature and location of the anorectal malformation and, in some cases, other associated birth defects that may be present. Treatment measures, which may be conducted during the newborn period or later during infancy, may include surgical correction of anorectal malformations (e.g., anoplasty) and widening (dilatation) of the anal opening or other supportive measures; a colostomy is often needed.

Anorectal malformations are thought to result from abnormalities in the development of certain embryonic structures (e.g., cloaca) that form the rectum and portions of the urinary tract. In cases in which anorectal malformations occur as isolated findings, such malformations are thought to result from abnormal changes (mutations) of one or several different genes, possibly in association with certain environmental factors (multifactorial). However, familial cases have also been reported that appear to have autosomal dominant, autosomal recessive, X-linked, or multifactorial inheritance. In approximately 50 percent of affected infants, anorectal malformations occur in association with other birth defects or underlying malformation syndromes, such as VACTERL association, a rare disorder that may be characterized by (V)ertebral abnormalities, (A)nal atresia, (C)ardiac defects, (T)racheo(E)sophageal fistula, (R)enal malformations, and (L)imb defects. Therefore, it is essential that newborns diagnosed with anorectal malformations are thoroughly examined and carefully monitored to ensure the detection and appropriate treatment of associated abnormalities.

National Associations & Support Groups

143 **Pull-Thru Network**
4 Woody Ln
Westport, CT 06880   203-221-7350
                                 Fax: 203-221-9212
                           e-mail: pullthrunw@aol.com
                           www.members.aol.com/pullthrunw/

Offers information on this and similar disorders, and provides emotional assistance for sufferers and their families.

DESCRIPTION

144 AORTIC VALVE STENOSIS
Synonym: Aortic stenosis
Disorder Type: Birth Defect, Heart

Aortic valve stenosis is an abnormal condition characterized by a narrowing (stenosis) of the valve through which blood flows from the left ventricle of the heart to the aorta. This condition may be present as a single finding, in association with other congenital heart defects or other disorders (e.g., Turner syndrome), or may occur as the result of other disorders such as rheumatic fever or thickening of the heart muscle (cardiomyopathy). In adults, aortic valve stenosis may result from scarring or the accumulation of calcium on the aortic valve. The normal aortic valve comprises three leaflets that permit the flow of blood into the aorta. In infants with aortic valve stenosis, only two leaflets may be present instead of three. In some patients, the leaflets may be fused together or may form an unusual funnel shape. This results in narrowing of the valve and inhibiting of the normal rate and pressure of blood flow. In addition, an irregular valve may not grow as the heart grows with advancing age. In these patients, the opening is not large enough to accommodate the larger volumes of blood pumped by the heart. The heart muscle may eventually sustain damage (e.g., thickened walls), further decreasing its ability to pump sufficiently.

Symptoms of aortic valve stenosis depend upon the severity of the abnormality. Valve obstruction that occurs in early infancy may be characterized by enlargement of the heart (cardiomegaly), congestive heart failure, abnormal accumulation of fluid in the lungs (pulmonary edema), weak pulses, and a low output of urine. Children with less severe irregularities may have no symptoms, while those with more severe involvement may experience fatigue, dizziness, chest pain, and loss of consciousness. Some severe cases of aortic valve stenosis may become life-threatening.

Treatment for aortic valve stenosis is dependent upon the age of the patient and the severity of the obstruction. In some patients, treatment may include surgery to repair or replace the valve or catheterization (valvuloplasty), a procedure in which a thin hollow tube (catheter) with a small balloon attached at its tip is threaded into the valve. Once in place, the balloon is inflated, thus increasing the size of the valve's opening. Recurrence of the valve obstruction is common and usually requires further treatment.

The following organizations in the General Resources Section can provide additional information: Genetic Alliance, March of Dimes Birth Defects Foundation, NIH/National Heart, Lung and Blood Institute, NIH/National Institute of Child Health and Human Development

National Associations & Support Groups

145 American Heart Association
7272 Greenville Avenue
Dallas, TX 75231
                          214-373-6300
                          800-242-8721
                    Fax: 214-706-1341
          e-mail: inquire@amhrt.org
                        www.amhrt.org

Supports research, education and community service programs with the objective of reducing premature death and disability from cardiovascular diseases and stroke; coordinates the efforts of health professionals, and other engaged in the fight against heart and circulatory disease.

146 National Heart, Lung and Blood Institute
National Institute of Health
31 Center Drive Building 31, Room 5A52
Baltimore, MD 20892
                          301-496-4236
                        www.nhlbi.nih.gov

Primary responsibility of this organization is the scientific investigation of heart, blood vessel, lung and blood disorders. Oversees research, demonstration, prevention, education, control and training activities in these fields and emphasizes the prevention and control of heart diseases.

Dr. Claude Lenfant, M.M., Director

Web Sites

147 CliniWeb: Congenital Heart Defects
www.ohsu.edu/cliniweb/C14/C14.240.400.

148 Congenital Heart Disease Resource

www.csun.edu/~hcmth011/heart/

e-mail: sheri.berger@csun.edu

www.csun.edu/~hcmth011/heart/

A place for parents to find more information about specific diseases and other support resources. First established in June 1995 the site is continuously updated by parents and health professionals.

149 Southern Illinois University School of Medicine

www.siumed.edu/peds/teaching/patient%20education.htm

Children's Books

150 Heart Disease

Caroline Arnold, author

Franklin Watts c/o Grolier
90 Old Sherman Turnpyke
Danburry, CT 06816

203-797-3500
800-621-1115
Fax: 203-797-3197
www.grolier.com

Using diagrams, this book discusses strokes and other bloodvessel disorders, as well as their treatment and prevention.

112 pages Grades 7-12
ISBN: 0-531108-84-8

151 Living with Heart Disease

Steve Parker, author

Franklin Watts c/o Grolier
90 Old Sherman Turnpyke
Danbury, CT 06816

203-797-3500
800-621-1115
Fax: 203-797-3197
www.grolier.com

Shows how persons with heart disease can overcome their illness and lead productive lives.

32 pages Grades 5-7
ISBN: 0-531108-45-7

DESCRIPTION

152 APNEA OF PREMATURITY

Synonym: Idiopathic apnea of prematurity
May involve these systems in the body (see Section III):
Respiratory System

Apnea is a condition characterized by a temporary cessation of breathing. Newborns may experience episodes of apnea due to several underlying disorders or conditions, including certain respiratory, neurologic, digestive, cardiovascular, metabolic, or infectious diseases. However, in newborns with apnea of prematurity, apneic episodes occur in the absence of identifiable, underlying disorders (idiopathic). The condition primarily affects premature infants who are born before 34 weeks of pregnancy (gestation). In general, the greater the degree of prematurity, the greater the frequency of the condition.

Apnea of prematurity is thought to occur due to immaturity of the region of the brain that controls breathing (respiratory centers of the medulla), causing failed stimulation of respiratory muscles. Resulting episodes of apnea, which are referred to as central apnea, are characterized by an absence of airflow as well as of chest wall movements. Apnea of prematurity may also be caused by obstruction of the upper airways due to improper coordination of the tongue and upper airway muscles, instability of the throat (pharynx), or other factors. Resulting episodes of apnea, known as obstructive apnea, are characterized by absence of airflow but ongoing chest wall movements. Most infants with apnea of prematurity experience both central and obstructive apnea.

In premature infants with the condition, initial episodes of apnea typically occur on the second to the seventh day of life. Such episodes are defined as serious if breathing spontaneously ceases for more than 15 to 20 seconds or if they result in decreased levels of oxygen in the blood and associated bluish discoloration of the skin and mucous membranes (cyanosis) and slowing of the heart rate (bradycardia).

The frequency of apnea episodes typically increases during the cycle of sleep that is associated with rapid eye movements (REMs), dreaming, increased levels of brain activity, and involuntary muscle jerks. During REM sleep, infants are more likely to experience abnormal chest wall movements during breathing, such as relaxation of the chest muscles while inhaling rather than exhaling. Abnormal chest wall movements as well as inhibition of muscle tone (particularly of the throat) during REM sleep contribute to the increased frequency of apneic episodes.

Infants at risk for episodes of apnea should be monitored with devices that detect abnormal changes in chest wall movements, heart rate, and respiratory activity and sound an alarm when spontaneous breathing temporarily ceases (apnea monitors). In infants who experience mild, occasional episodes of apnea, supportive measures may be sufficient, such as gentle skin stimulation and massage. In patients with severe, prolonged, and recurrent apnea, treatment should include immediate measures to assist breathing (e.g., bag and mask ventilation) and oxygen therapy to ensure sufficient oxygen supply to bodily tissues. Additional measures may include the administration of certain medications, such as theophylline or caffeine.

The following organizations in the General Resources Section can provide additional information: National Organization for Rare Disorders, Inc. (NORD), NIH/Office of Rare Diseases, NIH/National Institute of Neurological Disorders & Stroke, NIH/National Institute of Child Health and Human Development

National Associations & Support Groups

153 American Sleep Apnea Association
1424 K St NW, Ste 302
Washington, DC 20005   202-293-3656
e-mail: asaa@nicom.com
www.sleepanea.org

Devoted to the dissemination to the deterrence of this disorder and related complications.

154 Center for Research in Sleep Disorders
1275 E. Kemper Road
Cincinnati, OH 45246   513-671-3101
                    e-mail: sleepsat1@aol.com

Martin Scharf, PhD

155 National Sleep Foundation
729 15th Street NW 4th Floor
Washington, DC 20005   202-347-3471
                    Fax: 202-347-3472
                    e-mail: natsleep@erols.com
                    www.sleepfoundation.org

Works to improve the quality of life for millions
of Americans who suffer from sleep disorders,
and to prevent the catastrophic accidents that
are related to poor or disordered sleep through
research, education and the dissemination of information towards the cause of Narcolepsy Project. Seeks patients to aid new research project
targeting the cause of the disorder.

Allan I. Pack, M.D., Ph.D., Medical Director

156 Sleep/Wake Disorders Canada
3080 Yonge Street Suite 5055
Toronto, Ontario, M4N
Canada   416-483-9654
                    800-387-9253
                    Fax: 416-483-7081
                    e-mail: swdc@globalserve.net
                    www.geocities.com/~sleepwake/

Web Sites

157 Sleep Home Page
bisleep.medsch.ucla.edu

DESCRIPTION

158 ARNOLD-CHIARI MALFORMATION
Synonyms: ACM, Arnold-Chiari deformity,
Arnold-Chiari syndrome, Chiari malformation
Disorder Type: Birth Defect
Covers these related disorders: Arnold-Chiari
malformation type I, Arnold-Chiari malformation
type II
May involve these systems in the body (see Section III):
Nervous System

Arnold-Chiari malformation is a developmental abnormality characterized by malformations at the base of the brain that are present at birth (congenital). Such deformities typically include abnormal elongation of a portion of the cerebellum (cerebellar tonsils) and the lowest region of the brain stem (medulla oblongata), resulting in protrusion of these regions through the large opening (foramen magnum) in the base of the skull into the upper spinal canal (cervical canal). The cerebellum is a region of the brain that plays an essential role in coordinating voluntary movement and maintaining posture and balance. The brain stem, which is the lowest section of the brain, helps to relay motor and sensory impulses between other regions of the brain and the spinal cord and connects with most of the cranial nerve pairs, which send impulses involved in such functions as taste, vision, swallowing, facial expressions, and tongue, head, and shoulder movements.

In some affected newborns, Arnold-Chiari malformation occurs in association with myelomeningocele, a developmental abnormality characterized by protrusion (herniation) of a portion of the spinal cord and its protective membrane (meninges) through an abnormal opening in the spinal column. The occurrence of Arnold-Chiari malformation without myelomeningocele are said to have Arnold-Chiari malformation type I. Patients who also have a myelomeningocele are said to have Arnold-Chiari malformation type II. In both types, the opening in the base of the skull (foramen magnum) is abnormally enlarged and the base of the skull is also flattened and may appear pushed upward by the upper vertebrae (cervical vertebrae) of the spinal column (basilar impression).

Affected infants and children with Arnold-Chiari malformation type II experience progressive hydrocephalus, a condition characterized by abnormal accumulation of cerebrospinal fluid (CSF) in the brain. In infants and children with hydrocephalus, obstruction or impaired absorption of the CSF causes it to abnormally accumulate and results in an increase in pressure within cavities (ventricles) of the brain. Other findings may include abnormal enlargement of the ventricles, potential enlargement of the head, and other associated symptoms and findings. Some infants with Arnold-Chiari malformation type II may also experience abnormalities due to impairment of lower cranial nerves. Such abnormalities, which may vary in range and severity, may include uncontrollable twitching (fasciculations) of the tongue, a high-pitched sound upon inhalation (i.e., laryngeal stridor), facial weakness, hearing impairment, lagging of the head (sternomastoid paralysis), or weakness or impaired control of muscles that turn the eyes outward (bilateral abducens palsies). Later during childhood, some patients may experience increased stiffness (rigidity), causing restriction of movement (spasticity); abnormalities in walking (abnormal gait); and progressive lack of coordination. During later childhood or adolescence, affected individuals may also experience symptoms and findings often associated with Arnold-Chiari malformation type I.

In patients with Arnold-Chiari malformation type I, associated symptoms may not develop until adolescence or adulthood and often do not include hydrocephalus. Associated symptoms and findings may include recurrent headaches; neck pain; impaired control of voluntary movements (ataxia); or progressive muscle weakness, degeneration (atrophy), spasticity, and potential sensory loss affecting the lower and, in some cases, the upper limbs.

Treatment of individuals with Arnold-Chiari malformation may depend upon the severity of the malformation and associated symptoms and findings. If associated symptoms are considered mild, treatment may include regular monitoring and symptomatic and supportive measures as required. When associated symptoms are more severe and result in functional disability leading to physical handicap, treatment may include surgery (e.g., upper cervical laminectomy). Additional treatment is symptomatic and supportive. Although the exact cause of Arnold-Chiari malformation is unknown, researchers have suggested that it may result from the interaction of several genes, environmental influences, or both (multifactorial inheritance).

The following organizations in the General Resources Section can provide additional information: Genetic Alliance, March of Dimes Birth Defects Foundation, NIH/National Institute of Child Health and Human Development, NIH/National Institute of Neurological Disorders and Stroke, Online Mendelian Inheritance in Man: www3.ncbi.nlm.nih.gov/Omim/searchomim.html

National Associations & Support Groups

159 Arnold-Chiari Family Network
c/o Maureen & Kevin Walsh
67 Spring St
Weymouth, MA 02188   614-334-2368

160 World Arnold-Chiari Malformation Association
31 Newtown Woods Road
Newtown Square, PA 19073   610-353-4737
e-mail: interautbhm@worldnet.att.net
www.pressenter.com

Web Sites

161 National Institute of Health NINDS Information Page
www.ninds.nih.gov

162 Rare Genetic Diseases in Children (NYU)
http://mcrcr2.med.nyu.edu/murphp01/home-new.htm

DESCRIPTION

163 ARTHROGRYPOSIS MULTIPLEX CONGENITA
Synonym: AMC
Disorder Type: Birth Defect
Covers these related disorders: Amyoplasia
May involve these systems in the body (see Section III):
N/S, Skeletal System

Arthrogryposis multiplex congenita (AMC) refers to a group of disorders present at birth (congenital) that are characterized by limited movement or immobility of multiple joints and partial or complete replacement of involved muscle with fibrous or fatty tissue. Affected joints may be permanently flexed or extended in various fixed postures (joint contractures). Approximately 150 syndromes have been identified that are characterized by the presence of multiple contractures at birth. The most common form of arthrogryposis multiplex congenita is known as amyoplasia. This classic form of AMC affects approximately one in 10,000 newborns.

In newborns with amyoplasia, multiple congenital contractions are present that typically affect the upper and lower extremities. In most affected newborns, such contractures include abnormal flexion or extension of the elbows; flexion of the wrists toward the thumb side or pinky side of the hands (radial or ulnar deviation); cupping of the hands; and internal rotation of the shoulders. Many newborns with amyoplasia also have severe deformities of the feet (clubfoot or talipes equinovarus) in which the heels are turned inward and the soles of the feet are flexed (plantar flexion). Additional musculoskeletal deformities are also typically present including abnormal rigidity of the joints between bones of the thumbs and other fingers (interphalangeal joints); deformities of the palms of the hands; fixed flexion or extension of the knees; and abnormal flexion, extension, rotation, and possible dislocation of the hips. These abnormalities are usually similar from one side of the body to the other (symmetric). Amyoplasia is

also characterized by a susceptibility to bone fractures (i.e., perinatal fractures) and progressive abnormal sideways curvature of the spine (scoliosis) that may vary in severity and in age at onset from case to case. Most newborns with amyoplasia also have distinctive facial abnormalities including short, upturned (anteverted) nostrils; a rounded face; a slightly small jaw (mild micrognathia); and a benign, reddish, purple growth in the midportion of the face (midline frontal hemangioma). Amyoplasia appears to occur randomly for unknown reasons (sporadically), and the underlying causes of amyoplasia and other forms of AMC are not fully understood.

All newborns with multiple congenital joint contractures should receive a thorough neuromuscular evaluation to help detect, confirm, or rule out potential underlying muscular or neurologic abnormalities. The treatment of infants and children with amyoplasia includes symptomatic and supportive measures. The presence of fractures should be ruled out or confirmed (e.g., with x-ray studies) and treated as necessary (e.g., with appropriate immobilization) before physical therapy is begun. Treatment measures for congenital contractures and associated abnormalities may include physical therapy (e.g., passive range of motion exercises) and splinting of extremities to improve the range of motion; the use of casts or other orthopedic appliances; and possible surgical interventions. In addition, orthopedic appliances may be used to help slow the progression of scoliosis. In most patients with severe scoliosis, surgical measures may also be required.

The following organizations in the General Resources Section can provide additional information: Genetic Alliance, March of Dimes Birth Defects Foundation, National Organization for Rare Disorders, Inc. (NORD), NIH/National Institute of Arthritis and Musculoskeletel and Skin Diseases, Online Mendelian Inheritance in Man: www3.ncbi.nlm.nih.gov/Omim/searchomim.html

National Associations & Support Groups

164 Human Growth Foundation
7777 Leesburg Pike, Ste 202 S.
Falls Church, VA 22043   703-883-1773
                                800-451-6434

Devoted to the dispersion of medical knowledge of this and similar disorders, along with providing support for the sufferers and their families.

165 Magic Foundation for Children's Growth
1327 N. Harlem Ave
Oak Park, IL 60302   708-383-0808
                            800-362-4423
                            www.magicfoundation.org/

Provides assistance and education for individuals with growth related diseases through several helpful medians.

166 National Support Group for Athrogryposis
P.O. Box 5192
Sonora, CA 95370   209-928-3688

A national support group for people with Arthrogryposis Multiplex Congenita, a rare congenital disease characterized by the presence of multiple joint contractures. Provides a variety of educationaal and support materials including a director of families interested in corresponding with other affected families, a directory of medical professionals with a special interest in Arthrogryposis, a pen pal list for young correspondents, an annotated bibliography on Arthrogryposis, and a newsletter.

167 Short Stature Foundation
4521 Campus Dr., #130
Irvine, CA 92715   714-258-1833
                          800-243-9273

Improves everyday life through the dispersion of information for the commonly asked questions and problems.

State Agencies & Support Groups

International

168 Arthrogryposis Support Group
1 The Oaks
Chesterfield, Derbyshire,
United Kingdom

Support group that gives information to individuals, families and health care professionals interested in the disorder. Educational materials include a directory of medical professionals, pen pal list, newsletter, pamphlets and brochures.

169 Canadian Arthrogryposis Support Team
c/o Medium Chain Acyl-CoA Dehydrogenase
(MCAD)
Family Support Group, 2345 Young St, 9th Floor
Toronto Canada, M4P

Web Sites

170 AMC Bulletin Board
209.101.89.81/cgi-bin/sg/get_links?amc

171 AMC Home Page
members.aol.com/amcchat/amcinfo.htm

172 AMC Online Chat
members.aol.com/amcchat/chat.html

173 Wheelies' Textbook of Orthopaedics
www.medmedia.com/o12/110.htm

DESCRIPTION

174 ASPERGER SYNDROME

Disorder Type: Developmental Milestones, Mental, Emotional or Behavioral Disorder

Asperger syndrome is a condition that many researchers consider a high-functioning form of autism. However, others indicate that the disorder is more appropriately considered a nonverbal learning disability. According to those who classify the condition as a higher functioning form of autism, Asperger syndrome may be differentiated from autistic disorder by a later age at onset and lack of major language delays. The symptoms associated with Asperger syndrome typically become apparent after the age of 30 months and may vary in range and severity from case to case.

Children with Asperger syndrome typically have a normal intelligence quotient (I.Q.), deficient communication and social skills, and autistic-like behaviors. Many affected children appear to have normal language development and develop rich vocabularies. However, they often experience difficulties with the subtitlies of language, such as the slight variations in rhythm and pitch that help to communicate different shades of meaning (prosody). In addition, many children with the disorder have poor motor skills and clumsiness, avoid eye contact, experience varying levels of difficulty processing information, and have impairments in the use and comprehension of certain nonverbal cues and behaviors (e.g., facial expressions, gestures, etc.). Affected children also typically adopt certain routines or rituals; have difficulties with change; may be abnormally preoccupied with one or more areas of interest; and have deficient social skills. For example, many children with Asperger syndrome are socially withdrawn; lack awareness of others' thoughts or feelings; and are unusually sensitive to certain sights, sounds, or tastes. Some affected children may possess an extraordinary talent or skill in a particular area.

The management and treatment of children with Asperger syndrome may include integrated, multidisciplinary techniques, such as therapy to teach practical and social skills, and, in some cases, medication to help treat anxiety that may lead to behavioral inflexibility. The cause of Asperger syndrome is unknown. However, as is the case with autistic disorder, researchers indicate that genetic factors may play some role in causing or resulting in susceptibility for the disorder.

The following organizations in the General Resources Section can provide additional information: National Organization for Rare Disorders, Inc. (NORD), NIH/Office of Rare Diseases, National Mental Health Consumer Self-Help Clearinghouse, NIH/National Institute of Mental Health, NIH/National Institute of Neurological Disorders & Stroke

National Associations & Support Groups

175 National Autistic Society
276 Willesden Lane
London, NW2- 5RB   UK,   181-451-1114
e-mail: nas@nas.org.uk
www.oneworld.org/autism_uk/

Promotes the well being of affected persons through the assistance of fellow sufferers and families.

Web Sites

176 AS Support Network
www.vicnet.net.au/vicnet/community/asperger.htm

177 Autism Resources
http://web.syr.edu/~jmwobus/autism/

178 Family Village
www.familyvillage.wisc.edu/lib_aspe.htm#Mail

179 Online Asperger Syndrome Information and Support
www.udel.edu/bkirby/asperger/
e-mail: bkirby@udel.edu
www.udel.edu/bkirby/asperger/

180 **University Students with Autism and Asperger's Syndrome Web Site**

www.users.dircon.co.uk/~cns/index.html

e-mail: cns@dircon.co.uk

www.users.dircon.co.uk/~cns/index.html

Books

---

181 **Asperger Syndrome: A Guide for Educators and Parents**

Brenda Smith Myles, Richard L. Simpson, author

Pro-Ed
8700 Shoal Creek Boulevard
Austin, TX 78757   512-451-3246
                                                           800-897-3202
                                             Fax: 512-451-8542
                                             www.proedinc.com

A ground-breaking resource on Asperger Syndrome, this text outlines, in lay terms, the characteristics of the syndrome sometimes referred to as higher-functioning autism.

140 pages
ISBN: 0-890797-27-7

182 **Autism and Asperger Syndrome**

Uta Frith, author

Autism Society of North Carolina Bookstore
505 Oberlin Road, Suite 230
Raleigh, NC 27605   919-743-0204
                                                           800-442-2762
                                             Fax: 919-743-0208
                                       e-mail: ASNC@aol.com
                                       www.autismsociety-nc.org

Chapters include topics such as the relationship of autism and asperger syndrome, living with the syndrome and asperger syndrome in adulthood.

1991

DESCRIPTION

183 ASTHMA

Synonym: Bronchial asthma

May involve these systems in the body (see Section III):

Respiratory System

Asthma is a chronic respiratory disorder in which abnormal sensitivity (hyperresponsiveness) to certain stimuli causes inflammation and associated narrowing of the lungs' large and small airways, resulting in shortness of breath and other symptoms. This disorder is the primary cause of chronic illness in children. Up to 10 percent of girls and 15 percent of boys are affected by asthma at some point during childhood. Several factors are thought to play some role in causing the disorder, including immune, infectious, endocrine, and psychologic factors. In addition, many children with asthma have an affected parent or parents, suggesting possible genetic mechanisms. Researchers suggest that asthma is usually caused by the interactions of several genes (polygenic inheritance) in association with environmental factors (multifactorial).

In most patients, asthma becomes apparent during childhood. Initial symptoms occur during the first year of life in about 30 percent of patients and before the age of four to five years in approximately 80 to 90 percent.

Episodes may be triggered by exposure to many different stimuli, such as certain foreign substances (allergens) including pollen, mold, house dust, or animal hair. Asthma attacks may also be triggered by respiratory infections or exposure to smoke, certain chemicals or medications, strong odors, cold air, vigorous exercise, or stress. Exposure to such stimuli or precipitating factors may prompt certain cells within the lungs' airways (e.g., mast cells) to release particular substances that may cause spasms of the smooth muscles lining the airways, inflammation and swelling of the airway walls, excessive secretion of mucus, and associated airway narrowing (bronchoconstriction) and obstruction.

Asthma episodes may vary greatly in frequency, severity, and duration. For example, attacks may subside after minutes or have a duration of hours or even days. Some patients may have only occasional, mild episodes of shortness of breath. Others may regularly cough and produce a high-pitched whistling sound while breathing (wheezing) and experience severe asthma episodes upon exposure to certain triggering stimuli. Most children with asthma have only periodic episodes that are mild to moderate in severity. However, a small percentage of children have severe asthma that interferes with regular daily functioning. Most patients become relatively free of symptoms within 10 to 20 years after disease onset; however, many may have recurrences at some time during adulthood. Children with severe asthma may experience chronic disease through adulthood.

Asthma episodes may begin suddenly or gradually and are initially characterized by signs of air hunger, such as sighing, yawning, wheezing that may be most apparent while exhaling, shortness of breath, and a hacking, nonproductive cough. As mucus secretions increase, exhaling may become abnormally prolonged; however, this finding may not be a obvious in infants and young children. Shortness of breath may become so severe that patients have difficulty walking and become unable to speak other than in a panting manner. These patients may assume a hunched over position in an attempt to make breathing easier. Additional symptoms may include tightness of the chest, profuse sweating due to exertion and anxiety, nausea, and vomiting. During extremely severe episodes, wheezing may diminish due to lack of airflow in the airways; breathing may become irregular and shallow; and patients may become listless (lethargic), appear confused, and develop abnormal bluish discoloration of the skin and mucous membranes (cyanosis) due to abnormally diminished oxygen levels in the blood. Without immediate treatment, such patients may experience life-threatening complications.

The management of asthma may include measures to minimize exposure to possible precipitating factors, such as avoiding rapid changes in humidity or temperature and reducing exposure to tobacco smoke, pollen, strong odors, fumes, or other possible irritants. In some cases, specialized tests may help to determine specific triggering stimuli that should be avoided. In addition, the administration of certain medications, such as cromolyn, may be beneficial in helping to prevent attacks.

Certain medications are also typically prescribed to help alleviate symptoms during asthma episodes. Treatment should be administered as quickly as possible to open the airways and restore normal breathing and proper oxygen levels in the blood. Drug therapy may include medications that relax and widen the airways (bronchodilators), such as albuterol. Depending upon the specific drugs prescribed or the severity of an episode, such medications may be administered by mouth (orally); via a hand-held inhaler; by a nebulizer, which produces a mist for inhalation; or intravenously. Therapies to alleviate symptoms may also include corticosteroid medications by mouth or injection. Other medications may be prescribed, depending upon the severity of a particular episode or other factors. If a severe attack fails to respond to medical therapies, emergency treatment may be required including IV corticosteroids, IV bronchodilators, continuous nebulizer treatments and, in the most severe cases, possibly intubation with mechanical ventilation.

The following organizations in the General Resources Section can provide additional information: Genetic Alliance, American Lung Association, NIH/National Heart, Lung and Blood Institute Information Clearinghouse, Online Mendelian Inheritance in Man.: www3.ncbi.nlm.nih.gov/Omim/searchomim.html, NIH/National Institute of Allergy and Infectious Diseases

---

National Associations & Support Groups

184 Allergy and Asthma Network/Mothers of Asthmatics, Inc.
2751 Prosperity Ave, Ste 150
Fairfax, VA 22031   703-385-4403
                                       800-878-4403
                                  Fax: 703-573-7794
                           e-mail: aanma@aol.com
                                      www.aanma.org

A nonprofit association dedicated to educating families with asthma and allergies. Facilitates communication of accurate information among patients, parents, physicians and industry. Provides an important communication link among the home, school, physician and pharmaceutical industry in an effort to help families create a management program for those with asthma and allergies. Provides accurate guidance and clearly written resources on asthma and allergies.

Nancy Sander, President & Founder

185 American Academy of Allergy and Immunology
611 East Wells Street
Milwaukee, WI 53202

                                       800-822-2762

Allergies can have a profound effect on children's health and learning abilities. The American Academy of Allergy and Immunology can send free literature on various allergies, such as asthma, hay fever, eczema, food allergies, and hives. Referrals to specialists also available.

186 American Lung Association
1740 Broadway
New York, NY 10019   212-315-8700
                                       800-586-4872
                                     www.lungusa.org

A voluntary organization interested in the prevention and control of lung disease. Promotes and distributes public awareness information on a variety of lung disorders, including allergies.

187 Asthma Society of Canada
425-130 Bridgeland Avenue
Toronto, Ontariio, M6A
Canada   416-787-4050
                                       800-787-3880
                                  Fax: 416-787-5807
                          e-mail: asthma@myna.com
                               www.asthmasociety.com

188 Asthma and Allergy Foundation of America
1233 20th St, NW, Ste 402
Washington, DC 20036
202-466-7643
800-727-8462
Fax: 202-466-8940
e-mail: info@aaf.org
www.aafa.org

AAFA is a not-for-profit, voluntary health organization dedicated to improving the quality of life for people with asthma and allergies and their caregivers through education, research and advocacy. The foundation delivers quality asthma and allergy programs, information and services nationally through its network affilated chapters and educational support groups. The foundation also publishes educational pamphlets and a bimonthly patient newsletter with timely asthma and allergy information.

189 National Advisory Allergic and Infectious Disease Council
9000 Rockville Pike
Bethesda, MD 20892
301-496-5717

The principal advisory board of the NIAID. The council is composed of physicians, scientists and representatives of the public and advises on the conduct and support or research, training and dissemination of health information regarding allergies and infectious diseases.

190 Support for Asthmatic Youth (SAY)
Asthma and Allergy Foundation of America
1080 Glen Cove Avenue
Glen Head, NY 11545
516-625-5735
Fax: 516-625-2976

A network of educational/support groups for adolescents between the ages of 9 and 17. All meetings are free and feature guest speakers, informational programs, games and other fun activities.

Renee Theodorakis, M.A., Adolescent Services

State Agencies & Support Groups

Alabama

191 Alabama Chapter of Asthma and Allergy Foundation of America
PMB #307, 150 Inverness Corners
Birmingham, AL 35242
205-408-9077
800-727-8462
Fax: 205-408-4377
e-mail: aafaal@aol.com
www.aafa.org

AAFA is a not-for-profit, voluntary health organization dedicated to improving the quality of life for people with asthma and allergies and their caregivers through education, research and advocacy. The foundation delivers quality asthma and allergy programs, information and services nationally through its network affilated chapters and educational support groups. The foundation also publishes educational pamphlets and a bimonthly patient newsletter with timely asthma and allergy information.

Karen Brennan, Executive Director

California

192 Northern California Chapter of Asthma and Allergy Foundation of America
2269 Chestnut St, Ste 481
San Francisco, CA 94123
415-339-8880
800-727-8462
Fax: 415-339-8881
www.aafa.org

AAFA is a not-for-profit, voluntary health organization dedicated to improving the quality of life for people with asthma and allergies and their caregivers through education, research and advocacy. The foundation delivers quality asthma and allergy programs, information and services nationally through its network affilated chapters and educational support groups. The foundation also publishes educational pamphlets and a bimonthly patient newsletter with timely asthma and allergy information.

Linda Christopher, Executive Director

193 Southern California Chapter of Asthma and Allergy Foundation of America
5900 Wilshire Blvd, Ste 2330
Los Angeles, CA 90036
323-937-7859
800-624-0044
Fax: 323-937-7815
e-mail: aafasocal@aol.com
www.aafasocal.com

AAFA is a not-for-profit, voluntary health organization dedicated to improving the quality of life for people with asthma and allergies and their caregivers through education, research and advocacy. The foundation delivers quality asthma and allergy programs, information and services nationally through its network affilated chapters and educational support groups. The foundation also publishes educational pamphlets and a bimonthly patient newsletter with timely asthma and allergy information.

Francene Lifson, Executive Director

Florida

194 Florida Chapter of Asthma and Allergy Foundation of America
11700 N 58th St., Ste J
Tampa, FL 33617   813-983-0244
                                    800-727-8462
                               Fax: 813-983-9057
                   e-mail: leomatti@aafaflorida.org
                               www.aafaflorida.org

AAFA is a not-for-profit, voluntary health organization dedicated to improving the quality of life for people with asthma and allergies and their caregivers through education, research and advocacy. The foundation delivers quality asthma and allergy programs, information and services nationally through its network affilated chapters and educational support groups. The foundation also publishes educational pamphlets and a bimonthly patient newsletter with timely asthma and allergy information.

Leo Matti, Executive Director

Kansas

195 Greater Kansas City Chapter of Asthma and Allergy Foundation of America
PMB #307, 150 Inverness Corners
Birmingham, AL 35242   205-408-9077
                                    800-727-8462
                               Fax: 205-408-4377
                      e-mail: aafaal@aol.com
                               www.aafa.org

AAFA is a not-for-profit, voluntary health organization dedicated to improving the quality of life for people with asthma and allergies and their caregivers through education, research and advocacy. The foundation delivers quality asthma and allergy programs, information and services nationally through its network affilated chapters and educational support groups. The foundation also publishes educational pamphlets and a bimonthly patient newsletter with timely asthma and allergy information.

Karen Brennan, Executive Director

Maryland

196 Maryland-Greater Washington, DC Chapter of Asthma and Allergy Foundation of America
8600 LaSalle Rd
Towson, MD 21286   410-321-4710
                                    800-727-8462
                               Fax: 410-321-0137
                      e-mail: aafamd@bcpl.net
                               www.aafa-md.org

AAFA is a not-for-profit, voluntary health organization dedicated to improving the quality of life for people with asthma and allergies and their caregivers through education, research and advocacy. The foundation delivers quality asthma and allergy programs, information and services nationally through its network affilated chapters and educational support groups. The foundation also publishes educational pamphlets and a bimonthly patient newsletter with timely asthma and allergy information.

Maryanne Ellis, Executive Director

Massachusetts

197 New England Chapter of Asthma and Allergy Foundation of America
220 Boylston St
Chestnut Hill, MA 02467   617-965-7771
                                    800-727-8462
                               Fax: 617-965-8886
                      e-mail: aafane@aol.com
                               www.aafa.org

AAFA is a not-for-profit, voluntary health organization dedicated to improving the quality of life for people with asthma and allergies and their caregivers through education, research and advocacy. The foundation delivers quality asthma and allergy programs, information and services nationally through its network affilated chapters and educational support groups. The foundation also publishes educational pamphlets and a bimonthly patient newsletter with timely asthma and allergy information.

Patricia Goldman, Executive Director

Michigan

198 Michigan Chapter of Allergy and Asthma Foundation of America
17520 W 12 Mile Rd, Ste 102
Southfield, MI 48076   248-557-8050
                                    888-444-0333
                               Fax: 248-557-8768
                      e-mail: aafamich@aol.com
                               www.aafa.org

AAFA is a not-for-profit, voluntary health organization dedicated to improving the quality of life for people with asthma and allergies and their caregivers through education, research and advocacy. The foundation delivers quality asthma and allergy programs, information and services nationally through its network affiliated chapters and educational support groups. The foundation also publishes educational pamphlets and a bimonthly patient newsletter with timely asthma and allergy information.

Bruce R. Frandsen, Sr., Executive Director

Missouri

199 **St. Louis Chapter of Asthma and Allergy Foundation of America**
9378 Olive Street Rd, Ste 206
St. Louis, MO 63132   314-692-4244
                                         800-727-8462
                                    Fax: 314-692-2822
                           e-mail: aafa@inlink.com
                                         www.aafa.org

AAFA is a not-for-profit, voluntary health organization dedicated to improving the quality of life for people with asthma and allergies and their caregivers through education, research and advocacy. The foundation delivers quality asthma and allergy programs, information and services nationally through its network affiliated chapters and educational support groups. The foundation also publishes educational pamphlets and a bimonthly patient newsletter with timely asthma and allergy information.

Patricia Williams, Executive Director

New York

200 **New York Chapter of Asthma and Allergy Foundation of America**
984 N Village Ave
Rockville Center, NY 11570   540-370-0016
                                         800-727-8462
                                    Fax: 540-370-0015
                           e-mail: aafany@aol.com
                                         www.aafa.org

AAFA is a not-for-profit, voluntary health organization dedicated to improving the quality of life for people with asthma and allergies and their caregivers through education, research and advocacy. The foundation delivers quality asthma and allergy programs, information and services nationally through its network affiliated chapters and educational support groups. The foundation also publishes educational pamphlets and a bimonthly patient newsletter with timely asthma and allergy information.

Peggy McElgunn, Executive Director

Pennsylvania

201 **S.E. Pennsylvania Chapter of Asthma and Allergy Foundation of America**
PO Box 115
Gibbstown, NJ 08027   856-224-9547
                                         800-727-8462
                                    Fax: 856-224-9547
                        e-mail: aafasepa@prodigy.net
                                         www.aafa.org

AAFA is a not-for-profit, voluntary health organization dedicated to improving the quality of life for people with asthma and allergies and their caregivers through education, research and advocacy. The foundation delivers quality asthma and allergy programs, information and services nationally through its network affiliated chapters and educational support groups. The foundation also publishes educational pamphlets and a bimonthly patient newsletter with timely asthma and allergy information.

Debi Maines, Executive Director

Texas

202 **North Texas Chapter of Allergy and Allergy Foundation of America**
PO Box 270819 Ave
Flower Mound, TX 75027   817-430-9737
                                         888-933-2232
                                    Fax: 817-430-9738
                        e-mail: info@aafa-ntx.org
                                         www.aafa.org

AAFA is a not-for-profit, voluntary health organization dedicated to improving the quality of life for people with asthma and allergies and their caregivers through education, research and advocacy. The foundation delivers quality asthma and allergy programs, information and services nationally through its network affiliated chapters and educational support groups. The foundation also publishes educational pamphlets and a bimonthly patient newsletter with timely asthma and allergy information.

Cyndy Scoggin, Executive Director

Washington

203 Washington State Chapter of Asthma and Allergy Foundation of America
108 S Jackson St, Ste 205330
Seattle, WA 98104   206-368-2866
                                     800-778-2232
                                Fax: 206-368-2941
                          e-mail: aafawa@aafawa.org
                                    www.aafawa.org

AAFA is a not-for-profit, voluntary health organization dedicated to improving the quality of life for people with asthma and allergies and their caregivers through education, research and advocacy. The foundation delivers quality asthma and allergy programs, information and services nationally through its network affilated chapters and educational support groups. The foundation also publishes educational pamphlets and a bimonthly patient newsletter with timely asthma and allergy information.

Penny Nelson, Executive Director

Research Centers

204 Center for Interdisciplinary Research on Immunologic Diseases
Children's Hospital Medical Center
300 Longwood Avenue
Boston, MA 02115   617-355-6000

Organizational research unit of the Children's Hospital that focuses on the causes, prevention and treatments of asthma, infections and allergies.

Fred S. Rosen, MD

205 National Jewish Medical & Research Center Denver
1400 Jackson
Denver, CO 80206   303-388-4461
                                     800-222-5864
                                Fax: 303-270-2162

A world reowned institute devoted to the treatment and study of respiratory and allergic diseases.

Rosalind F. Dudden, Health Sciences Librarian

Audio Video

206 A Regular Kid
American Lung Association
1740 Broadway
New York, NY 10017   212-315-8700

This film shows how families and children cope with asthma problems. Proven asthma management strategies are presented through the experiences of four children with asthma, ranging in age from toddler to teenager.

Film

207 Allergy Control Begins at Home: House Dust Allergy
Allergy Control Products Inc.
96 Danbury Rd.
Ridgefield, CT 06877
                                     800-422-3878
                          e-mail: info@allergycontrol.com
                                    www.allergycontrol.com

1993 35min pages

208 Asthma: What You Need to Know
Allergy and Asthma Network/Mothers of Asthmatics
3554 Chain Bridge Road Suite 200
Fairfax, VA 22030   703-385-4403
                                     800-878-4403
                                Fax: 703-352-4354

Basic asthma information for families, schools or physicians' offices. 14 minutes.
Video

209 Breathe Easy Young People's Guide to Asthma
Jonathan H. Weiss, PhD, author

Magination Press
3554 Chain Bridge Road Suite 200
Fairfax, VA 22030   703-385-4403
                                     800-878-4403
                                Fax: 703-352-4354

Practical, personal guide for those up to age 13 with asthma. They will learn how to control their asthma with techniques that will bring increased self-confidence.

1994 Video

210 Free to Breathe
Allergy and Asthma Network/Mothers of Asthmatics
3554 Chain Bridge Road Suite 200
Fairfax, VA 22030
703-385-4403
800-878-4403
Fax: 703-352-4354
TTY: 123-019-99

Characters rap, joke, and learn different ways to use inhalers. Kids are encouraged to talk to their parents and doctor about their choices. 8 minutes.

Video

211 It Only Takes One Bite Food Allergy and Anaphylaxis
Food Allergy Network
1400 Eaton Place, Suite 107
Fairfax, VA 22030
800-929-4040

Explains food induced anaphylaxis and how to live with it, also excellant for training parents, teachers, caregivers and patients.

18 mins.

212 Managing Asthma in School: An Action Plan
Asthma and Allergy Foundation of America
1125 15th Street N.W.-Suite 502
Washington, DC 20005
202-466-7643
Fax: 202-466-8940
TTY: 123-019-99
www.aafa.org

Gives the basics of asthma and a plan for school nurses, parents and physicians to work together.

14 minutes

213 Managing Childhood Asthma
Allergy and Asthma Network/Mothers of Asthmatics
3554 Chain Bridge Road Suite 200
Fairfax, VA 22030
703-385-4403
800-878-4403
Fax: 703-352-4354
TTY: 123-019-99

What parents need to know to manage asthma. 22 minutes.

Video

214 Pharmacologic Therapy of Pediatric Asthma
American Lung Association
1740 Broadway
New York, NY 10017
212-315-8700
TTY: 123-019-99

A Learning Resource Program developed by a joint committee of the American Thoracic Society and the ALA.

Film

215 Power Over Eczema A Guide for Parents
National Eczema Assn. for Science and Education
1220 SW Morrison, Suite 433
Portland, OR 97205
503-228-4430

Discusses the treatment of Eczema or atopic dermatitis.

18 mins.

216 So You Have Asthma Too!
Nancy Sander, author

Allergy and Asthma Network/Mothers of Asthmatics
3554 Chain Bridge Road Suite 200
Fairfax, VA 22030
703-385-4403
800-878-4403
Fax: 703-352-4354
TTY: 123-019-99

Offers a clear description and understanding of childhood asthma. Also see companion book, So You Have Asthma Too! (separately listed), available as a set for $12.00.

Video

217 Super Asthma Kids: We Take Control
Association for the Care of Children's Health
8701 Hartsdale Avenue
Bethesda, MD 20817
301-493-5113

The latest video from the acclaimed Mount Sinai Medical Center production shop, young people with asthma talk about how, despite having asthma, they enjoy life to the fullest.

1997 26 minutes

218 What School Personnel Should Know About Asthma
American Lung Association
1740 Broadway
New York, NY 10017
212-315-8700
TTY: 123-019-99

Professionally produced videotape discussing the triggers, symptoms and management of childhood asthma.

Videotape

219 Wheeze World
Allergy and Asthma Network/Mothers of Asthmatics
3554 Chain Bridge Road Suite 200
Fairfax, VA 22030   703-385-4403
                          800-878-4403
                     Fax: 703-352-4354
                     TTY: 123-019-99

Based on Wayne's World, kids will love this
zany video about asthma. 11 minutes.

Video

220 You're in Charge: Teens with Asthma
Asthma and Allergy Foundation of America
1125 15th Street N.W.-Suite 502
Washington, DC 20005   202-466-7643
                         Fax: 202-466-8940
                         TTY: 123-019-99
                         www.aafa.org

Designed for young adults dealing with the daily
challenges of asthma management. Teens share
their experiences and use of peak flow meters
and prescribed medications.

10 minutes

Web Sites

**221 Allergy and Asthma Network Mothers of
Asthmatics, Inc.**
www.aanma.org

          e-mail: aanma@aol.com
          www.aanma.org

A nonprofit association dedicated to educating
families with asthma and allergies. Facilitates
communication of accurate information among
patients, parents, physicians and industry. Provides an important communication link among
the home, school, physician and pharmaceutical
industry in an effort to help families create a
management program for those with asthma and
allergies. Provides accurate guidance and
clearly written resources on asthma and allergies.

Nancy Sander, President & Founder

**222 American Academy of Allergy Asthma and
Immunology**
www.aaaai.org

Physican refferal database, Patient Public Infro-
mation Center, support resources and children's
materials.

223 American Lung Association
www.lungusa.org

A voluntary organization interested in the prevention and control of lung disease. Promotes
and distributes public awareness information on
a variety of lung disorders, including allergies.

224 Asthma Information Center
www.mdnet.de/asthma/

225 Asthma and Allergy FAQs
www.cs.unc.edu/~kupstas/FAQ.html

226 Asthma and Allergy Foundation of America
www.aafa.org

Issues on current drug alerts, chapters and support groups, educational materials, newsletters
and fequently asked questions.

227 Food Allergy Network
www.foodallergy.org

Information to increase public awareness, education, support and strategies for those with food
allergies.

228 JAMA's Asthma Information Center
www.ama-assn.org/special/asthma

**229 National Eczema Association for Science and
Education**
www.eczema-assn.org

Provides information on coping with eczema,
lists brochures and videos for sale, and presents
a building board for patients to post questions
and full-text versions of its newsletter.

**230 National Heart, Lung, and Blood Institute Lung
Information for Patients and Public**
NHLBI Information Center
P.O. Box 30105
Bethesda, MD 20824   301-592-8573
                         www.nhlbi.nih.gov

Features down-loadable online pamphlets on
asthma (some also in spanish)

231 National Insitute of Allergy and Infectious Diseases
www.niaid.nih.gov/

232 National Jewish Medical and Research Center
www.nationaljewish.org

          800-222-5864
          e-mail: lungline@njc.org
          www.nationaljewish.org

Only U.S. medical facility that is devoted entirely to respiratory and immune disorders.
Staffed by nurses who answer clinical questions
and send helpful brochures and fact sheets.

233 Pedbase
www.icondata.com/health/ped-
base/files/ASTHMA-C.HTM

Books

234 A Parent's Guide to Allergies and Asthma
Marion Steinmann, author

National Allergy and Asthma Network
3554 Chain Bridge Road, Suite 200
Fairfax, VA 22030   703-385-4403
Fax: 703-352-4354
TTY: 123-019-99

A up-to-date, easy-to-read resource offering essential information on asthma and allergies.

**235 Allergy, Asthma & Immunology from Infancy To
Adulthood**
Warren Bieman, et al., author

W.B. Saunders Company
Independence Square West
Philadelphia, PA 19106   215-238-7800
TTY: 123-019-99

1995 (3rd) 784 pages
ISBN: 0-721655-87-4

236 Asthma Care Training for Kids
Asthma and Allergy Foundation of America
1125 15th Street NW, Suite 502
Washington, DC 20005   202-466-7643
Fax: 202-466-8940
TTY: 123-019-99
www.aafa.org

Designed to help children ages 7 to 12 and their
parents take charge of their asthma. In a series
of three action-filled sessions, children and their
parents meet separately with their peers to learn
about asthma management.

**237 Asthma In the School: Improving Control With
Peak Flow Monitoring**
Guillermo Mendoza, MD, author

National Allergy and Asthma Network
3554 Chain Bridge Road, Suite 200
Fairfax, VA 22030   703-385-4403
Fax: 703-352-4354
TTY: 123-019-99

Comprehensive and practical guide to help the
school nurse monitor and assist students with
asthma.

238 Asthma Self Help Book
Paul J. Hannaway, M.D., author

Allerfy Control Products
P.O. Box 793
Ridgefield, CT 06877   203-438-9580
800-422-3878
Fax: 203-431-8963
TTY: 123-019-99
www.allergycontrol.com

A comprehensive manual on the management of
asthma for parents of asthmatic children, adult
asthmatics, and for health professionals.
Softcover

239 Asthma and Exercise
Nancy Hogshead and Gerald S. Couzens, author

Henry Holt and Company
3554 Chain Bridge Road Suite 200
Fairfax, VA 22030   703-385-4403
Fax: 703-352-4354
TTY: 123-019-99

This book offers clear and detailed advice on
how adults and children with asthma can participate in exercise and sports activities.
1990

240 Breathing Easy with Day Care
Nancy Sander, author

Allergy and Asthma Network/Mothers of Asthmatics
3554 Chain Bridge Road Suite 200
Fairfax, VA 22030   703-385-4403
800-878-4403
Fax: 703-352-4354
TTY: 123-019-99

An informative guide and medical health record
for parents and day care providers of children
with asthma and allergies. Endorsed and spon-
sored by the American Academy of Allergy
Asthma and Immunology.

241 Children with Asthma: A Manual for Parents
Thomas E. Plaut, MD, author

Allergy Control Products
P.O. Box 793
Ridgefield, CT 06877   203-438-9580
800-422-3878
Fax: 203-431-8963
TTY: 123-019-99
www.allergycontrol.com

Known as the asthma bible, this second edition
is sprinkled with anecdotes by patients and their
parents.
296 pages Softcover

242 Consumer Update on Asthma

Nancy Sander, author

Allergy and Asthma Network/Mothers of Asthmatics
3554 Chain Bridge Road Suite 200
Fairfax, VA 22030   703-385-4403
                            800-878-4403
                    Fax: 703-352-4354
                    TTY: 123-019-99

Addresses the diagnosis and treatment of all levels of asthma severity in people from infancy to elder years. Includes information on pregnancy, occupational asthma, and environmental control.

243 Infant Formulas for Allergic Infants and Dietetic Concerns for Toddlers

American Allergy Association
P.O. Box 7273
Menlo Park, CA 94026   650-322-1663
                    TTY: 123-019-99

Offers information on reliable food labels, evaluations of infant formulas, FDA labeling requirements under the new law and more.

244 National Asthma Education and Prevention Program Expert Panel Report

National Heart, Lung, and Blood Inst, Info. Center
P.O. Box 30105
Bethesda, MD 20824   301-592-8573

Guidelines for management and diagnosis of asthma. Outlines clinical practice guidelines, treatment and diagnosis, written for physicians, however should be in every health collection.

146 pages

245 School Information Packet

Allergy and Asthma Network/Mothers of Asthmatics
3554 Chain Bridge Road Suite 200
Fairfax, VA 22030   703-385-4403
                            800-878-4403
                    Fax: 703-352-4354
                    TTY: 123-019-99

Practical, medical, and legal information for school administrators and parents of students with asthma.

246 Understanding Asthma

Phil Lieberman, M.D., author

University Press of Mississippi
3825 Ridgewood Road
Jackson, MS 39211   601-432-6205
                            800-737-7788
                    Fax: 601-432-6217
            e-mail: press@ihl.state.ms.us
            www.upress.state.ms.us

Noting that understanding and education are key to halting the rise in numbers of asthma cases, Dr. Phil Lieberman has written this book for families and the individual sufferer. Subjects include lungs of an asthmatic, allergies which trigger the disease, and measures used to control asthma.

120 pages Hardcover
ISBN: 1-578061-41-5

Miriam Bloom, Ph.D, Editor

Children's Books

247 All About Asthma

William Ostrow & Vivian Ostrow, author

Asthma and Allergy Foundation of America
1125 15th Street NW Suite 200
Washington, DC 20005   202-466-7643
                    Fax: 202-466-8940
                    TTY: 123-019-99
                    www.aafa.org

Written by a 10-year-old with asthma, this cleverly illustrated book explains causes and symptoms, and ways to control asthma to lead a normal life.

39 pages Softcover

248 Asthma

Mona Kerby, author

Franklin Watts c/o Grolier
90 Old Sherman Tpke
Danbury, CT 06816   203-797-3500
                            800-621-1115
                    Fax: 203-797-3197
                    www.grolier.com

This book offers vital information on causes and treatments, plus advice on how to prevent flare-ups.

96 pages Grades 7-12
ISBN: 0-531106-97-7

249 Best of Superstuff Activity Booklet

American Lung Association
1740 Broadway
New York, NY 10017   212-315-8700

For young children with asthma featuring a series of activities designed to help youngsters cope with asthma.

32 pages Ages 6-8

250 Childhood Asthma, Learning To Manage
Asthma and Allergy Foundation of America
1125 15th Street NW, Suite 502
Washington, DC 20005   202-466-7643
Fax: 202-466-8940
www.aafa.org

Self-paced, entertaining activity books for home use featuring practical guidelines for managing childhood asthma with a focus on using peak flow meters.

251 Clubhouse Kids Learn About Asthma
Asthma and Allergy Foundation of America
1125 15th Street N.W. Suite 502
Washington, DC 20005   202-466-7643
Fax: 202-466-8940
www.aafa.org

Interactive CD-ROM helps children ages 4-12 learn about asthma at their own pace. Sound, animation and game-like features draw players into the life of Janie, who has just been diagnosed with asthma.

252 Determined to Win: Children Living with Allergies & Asthma
Thomas Bergman, author
Gareth Stevens, Inc.
1555 North River Center Drive
Milwaukee, WI 53212   414-225-0333
Fax: 414-225-0377
www.gsinc.com

1994 48 pages
ISBN: 0-836810-75-9

253 I'm Tougher Than Asthma!
Siri M. Carter & Alden R. Carter, author
Albert Whitman & Company
6340 Oakton Street
Morton Grove, IL 60053   847-581-0033
800-255-7675
Fax: 847-581-0039
www.awhitmanco.com

Eight-year-old Siri loves to sing, play baseball, and catch toads. She won't let her asthma stop her! In her own words (with a little help from Dad), she tells how she was first diagnosed with asthma at age three and how she is learning to understand and manage her disease.

32 pages Hard/Softcover
ISBN: 0-807534-74-9

Abby Levine, Editor
Joseph Boyd, President

254 Let's Talk About Having Asthma
Elizabeth Weitzman, author
Rosen Publishing Group's PowerKids Press
29 East 21st Street
New York, NY 10010   212-777-3017
800-237-9932
Fax: 212-436-4643
TTY: 123-019-99
e-mail: rosenpub@tribeca.ios.com

This book talks about the cause and treatments for asthma as well as the precautions sufferers should take. Recommended for grades K-4.

ISBN: 0-823950-32-8

255 Lion Who Had Asthma
Jonathan London, author
Asthma and Allergy Foundation of America
1125 15th Street NW Suite 502
Washington, DC 20005   202-466-7643
Fax: 202-466-8940
www.aafa.org

A beautifully illustrated book that encourages preschoolers to use their imaginations and take their asthma medications.
24 pages Hardcover

256 Living with Asthma
Margaret O. Hyde & Elizabeth Forsythe, author
Walker & Company
720 Fifth Avenue
New York, NY 10019   212-265-3632

1995 112 pages
ISBN: 0-802782-86-8

257 Luke Has Asthma Too
Alison Rogers, author
Allergy Control Products
P.O. Box 793
Ridgefield, CT 06877
800-422-3878
Fax: 203-431-8963

This gentle book will make for good reading with children, whether they have asthma or not.

258 So You Have Asthma Too!

Nancy Sander, author

Allergy and Asthma Network/Mothers of Asthmatics
3554 Chain Bridge Road Suite 200
Fairfax, VA 22030   703-385-4403
800-878-4403
Fax: 703-352-4354

A children's illustrated book, offering a clear description and understanding of childhood asthma. Available in Spanish. Also see companion video, (listed separately), available as a set for $12.00.

259 Winning Over Asthma

Eileen Dolan Savage, author

Asthma and Allergy Foundation of America
1125 15th Street NW Suite 502
Washington, DC 20005   202-466-7643
Fax: 202-466-8940
www.aafa.org

Simple coloring book explains asthma through a story about five-year-old Graham.

30 pages Softcover

260 You Can Control Asthma

Asthma and Allergy Foundation of America
1125 15th Street NW Suite 502
Washington, DC 20005   202-466-7643
Fax: 202-466-8940
www.aafa.org

A set of low-literacy asthma education books for children ages 6-12 and their families. Developed at Georgetown University and pre-tested with urban families to ensure comprehension and appropriateness.

1995

Magazines

261 Controlling Asthma

American Lung Association
1740 Broadway
New York, NY 10017   212-315-8700

For parents of children with asthma, this newsmagazine tells how parents can help their child deal with the many problems presented by asthma.

16 pages

Newsletters

262 Advance

Asthma and Allergy Foundation of America
1125 15th Street NW Suite 502
Washington, DC 20005   202-466-7643
Fax: 202-466-8940
www.aafa.org

Newsletter for members will increase the patients understanding and ability to control asthma and allergies. Topics include food allergies, exercising and asthma, ragweed and allergies and asthma and pregnancy. Also keeps parents up to date with the key facts for keeping their asthmatic child as healthy as possible.

Bi-Monthly

263 Asthma and Allergy Advance

Asthma and Allergy Fdn. of America
1233 20th St NW, Ste 402
Washington, DC 20036
800-727-8462
info@aafa.org

Contains a variety of authoritative articles on the latest treatments, drugs, and research.

264 Asthma and Allergy Health

Allergy and Asthma Network/ Mothers of Asthmatics
2751 Prosperity Ave, Ste 150
Fairfax, VA 22031   800-878-4403
e-mail: aanma@aol.com

Provides an in-depth reporting on new products, medications, and complementary and alternative therapies.

1999

265 Food Allergy News

Food Allergy Network
10400 Eaton Place, Ste 107
Fairfax, VA 22030
800-929-4040
e-mail: fan@worldweb.net
samples@foodallergy.org

Contains tips for parents, including notices on ingrediants in various foods, and recipes are published annually.

bi-monthly

266 MA Report

Allergy and Asthma Network/Mothers of Asthmatics
2751 Prosperity Ave, Ste 150
Fairfax, VA 22031
800-878-4403
e-mail: aanma@aol.com

free w/member

Pamphlets

267 Asthma and the School Child
American Academy of Allergy, Asthma and Immunology
611 East Wells Street
Milwaukee, WI 53202   414-272-6071
                                   800-822-2762
                                   Fax: 414-272-6070
                                   www.aaaai.org

268 Childhood Asthma
American Academy of Allergy, Asthma and Immunology
611 East Wells Street
Milwaukee, WI 53202   414-272-6071
                                   800-822-2762
                                   Fax: 414-272-6070
                                   www.aaaai.org

269 Childhood Asthma: A Guide for Parents

P.A. Eggleston, MD, author

Asthma and Allergy Foundation of America
1125 15th Street N.W. Suite 502
Washington, DC 20005   202-466-7643
                                   Fax: 202-466-8940
                                   www.aafa.org

This colorful booklet helps parents learn all about asthma in children.

32 pages

270 Childhood Asthma: A Matter of Control
American Lung Association
1740 Broadway
New York, NY 10017   212-315-8700

A guide for parents of children with asthma, this booklet covers topics such as identifying asthma signs and symptoms as well as controlling the condition.

28 pages

271 Superstuff
American Lung Association
1740 Broadway
New York, NY 10017   212-315-8700

Kit specifically designed to help the elementary school child with asthma learn how to manage the condition. The kit contains teaching tools, puzzles, riddles, stories and games.

272 Teens Talk to Teens About Asthma
Asthma and Allergy Foundation of America
1125 15th Street N.W.-Suite 502
Washington, DC 20005   202-466-7643
                                   Fax: 202-466-8940
                                   www.aafa.org

Quotes and thoughts from teens capture the essence of what it feels like to have asthma.

273 There Are Solutions for the Student with Asthma
American Lung Association
1740 Broadway
New York, NY 10017   212-315-8700

Leaflet telling how parents and school personnel can work together to make life easier for children with asthma.

4 pages

274 Your Child and Asthma
National Jewish Center for Immunology
1400 Jackson Street
Denver, CO 80206   303-388-4461

A booklet offerring information to parents and family about their child with asthma. Offers information on diagnosis, treatments, triggers and family concerns.

DESCRIPTION

275 ATAXIA

Disorder Type: Neuromuscular
May involve these systems in the body (see Section III):
Nervous System

Ataxia is a neuromuscular condition characterized by an impaired ability to coordinate voluntary movements. The condition is caused by abnormalities of or damage to the region of the brain known as the cerebellum, nerve pathways that transmit messages to and from the cerebbellum, or certain regions of the spinal cord. The cerebellum plays an essential role in regulating the maintenance of normal postures, sustaining balance, and producing smooth and coordinated movements. The spinal cord conducts sensory and motor impulses to and from the brain. The symptoms associated with ataxia may vary, depending upon the specific regions of the brain that are affected; however, symptoms may often include imbalance and an abnormal staggering manner of walking (gait). Ataxia may be the result of certain infection, malformations of the cerebellum of spinal cord that are present at birth (congenial), head injury, brain tumors, exposure to pacticular medications, or certain genetic disorders. The primary infectious causes of ataxia during childhood include the formation of pus-filled pockets of infection in the cerebellum (cerebellar abscesses); sudden, servere inflammation of the passages within the inner ear (acute labyrinthitis): or acute cerebellar ataxia. Certain severe infections may cause inflammation of the brain and asssociated cerebellar abscesses. Acute labyrinthitis typically occurs due to middle ear infections and may be characterized by vomiting and a sense that one's body or environment is spinning (vertigo). Acute cerebellar ataxia occurs subsequent to certain viral infections, such as chicken pox, and is thought to result from an abnormal immune response causing inflammation of the brain and cerebellar ataxia. Acute cerebellar ataxia typically occurs

suddenly and may be characterized by impaired control of voluntary movements of the torso (truncal ataxia) and difficulties sitting of standing; involuntary, rapid eye movements (nystagmus); and sevarc slurring of speech or an inability to speak. Although the condition typically improves within a few weeks, it sometimes is present for up to two months. Most children have a complete recovery; however, some may have residual speech abnormalities and lack of coordination.

Abnormalities present at birth (congenital) that may cause ataxia include absence of the region of the brain between the two sides or hemispheres of the cerebellum (agensis of cerebellar vermis); protrusion of part of the brain through an opening in the skull (cncephalocele); or protrusion of certain, malformed regions of the brain through the opening at the base of the skull (foramon magnum) into the upper spinal canal (Arnold-Chiari malformation). Infants and children with such birth defects develop ataxia due to malformation of or damage to certain regions of the cerebellum.

Ataxia may also be an intial symptom associated with certain brain tumors, including tumors affecting the cerebellum or a particular area of the cerebrum where it joins with the cerebellum (i.e., frontal lobe). In addition, brain tumors known as neuroblastomas may result in progressive ataxia. Neuroblastomas are solid, malignant tumors that may originate in any part of the sympathetic nervous system, which is that part of the nervous system that regulates certain involuntary activites during times of stress, such as raising blood pressure and increasing the heart rate.

In some children, ataxia may result from the administration of certain drugs, such as anticonvulsant medications, particularly phenytoin. In addition, the condition may be caused by exposure to a household pesticide that is commonly used as a rat poison (thallium).

Ataxia may also occur in association with certain inborn errors of metabolism and is a primary feature of many hereditay degenerative disorders of the brain and spinal cord. These degenerative disorders, which may be referred to as hereditay ataxias, include ataxia-telangiectasia and Friedreich's ataxia.

Ataxia-tolangiectasia (AT) is a multisystem disorder that is inherited as an autosomal recessive trait. Affected children typically develop ataxia at approximately two years of age, eventually leading to an inability to walk. Friedreich's ataxia is a genetic disorder that is usually inherited as an autosomal recessive trait. The disorder is characterized by degenerative changes of certain regions of the spinal cord and is catagorized as a spinocerebellar ataxia. Children with Friedreich's ataxia typically develop ataxia before age 10. The ataxia is slowly progressive and usually affects the legs and feet more severely than the arms and hands. Patients develop unusual high arching and severe muscle weakness of the feet and progressive difficulties walking, typically leading to use of a wheelchair. Additional hereditary spinocerebellar ataxia of childhood, such as Roussy-Levy syndrome, cause symptoms and findings similar to those associated with Friedreich's ataxia. Roussy-Levy syndrome often becomes apparent during infancy and is characterized by loss of joint position sensation (sensory ataxia), causing poorly judged, uncoordinated movements. Such ataxia initially affects the lower legs, causing difficulty walking, and later progresses to affect the hands. Roussy-Levy syndrome is transmitted as an autosomal dominant trait.

Another group of hereditary disorders, known as the olivopontocerebellar atrophics (OPCAs) are associated with ataxia. These disorders are characterized by progressive degeneration of the cerebellum as well as other areas of the brain. Although associated symptoms of most forms of OPCA become apparent during adolescence or adulthood, one form of the disorder is known to occur during infancy (OPCA of neonatal onset). Symptoms may include severely diminished muscle tone; rapidly progressive ataxia; involuntary, rapid eye movements; episodes of abormally increased electrical activity in the brain (seizures); failure to grow and gain weight at the expected rate (failure to thrive); abnormalities in the structure and function of heart muscle (hypertrophic cardiomyopathy); and other symptoms and find-

ings. Methods used in the management of ataxia may vary and depend upon the condition's unerlying cause, the specific form of ataxia present, and other factors. Such measures are typically symptomatic and supportive.

National Associations & Support Groups

276 National Ataxia Foundation
2600 Fernbrook Lane, Suite 119
Minneapolis, MN 55447   612-553-0020
                              Fax: 612-553-0167
                              e-mail: naf@mr.net
                              www.ataxia.org

Objectives of this organization are to make an early diagnosis of ataxia by encouraging all potential victims to be examined. Offers public information and professional education materials and basic research on the disease. Publishes quarterly newsletter, Generations.

277 National Institute of Neurological Disorders & Stroke
31 Center Dr MSC 2540, Bldg 31, Rm 8806
Bethesda, MD 20892   301-496-5751
                            800-352-9424
                            Fax: 301-402-2186
                            www.ninds.nih.gov

Information and advocacy resources for families and professionals. Includes listings of organizations providing general information and organizations focusing on more specific areas of concern to families and young adults who have disabilities.

State Agencies & Support Groups

Alabama

278 Birmingham Support Group National Ataxia Foundation
16 The Oaks Circle
Birmingham, AL 35244   205-987-2883

Fred & Becky Donnelly

Arizona

279 Arizona Ataxia Support Group National Ataxia Foundation
8056 East Nido Avenue
Mesa, AZ 85208   480-984-1660

Mary Lee & George Thyden

California

**280 Central California Support Group National Ataxia
Foundation**
28767 Sequoia Court
Coarsegold, CA 93614   559-658-8675

Ree Howell

**281 Costa Mesa Support Group National Ataxia
Foundation**
The Double Tree Hotel
Orange County Airport
Costa Mesa, CA   612-553-0020
                             www.ataxia.org

**282 Los Angeles Ataxia Support Group National Ataxia
Foundation**
339 W. Palmer Apt. A
Glendale, CA 91204   818-246-5758
                     e-mail: cynlewin@aol.com

Sid Luther, President

**283 Narthern California Support Group National Ataxia
Foundation**
4335 Bordeaux Drive
Oakley, CA 94561   925-625-0738
                  e-mail: fernande@pacbell.net
          www.geocities.com/hotsprings/resort/4177

Mike Fernandes

**284 Orange County Support Group National Ataxia
Foundation**
16162 Windemeier Lane
Huntington Beach, CA 92647   714-842-6401
                  e-mail: mmfb01a@prodigy.com

Kay Bell

285 Pacific Southwest Regional Genetics Group
2151 Berkeley Way, Annex Four
Berkeley, CA 94704   510-540-2696
                             Fax: 510-540-2966

George C. Cunningham, Director

**286 San Diego Support Group National Ataxia
Foundation**
2087 Granlte Hills Drive
El Cajon, CA 92019   619-447-3753
                  e-mail: earllogo@flash.net
          www.geocities.com/enchantedforest/meadow

Earl McLaughlin

Colorado

**287 Denver Colorado Support Group National Ataxia
Foundation**
1771 S. Quebec Way, Apt. V102
Denver, CO 80231   303-369-9874
                  e-mail: MWhite7794@aol.com

Michael A. White

288 Iowa Support Group National Ataxia Foundation
Finley Hospital
350 N. Grandview Ave.
Dubeque, IA 52001   319-589-2372
                  e-mail: theraspeecher@MWCI.net

Elizabeth Burke

289 Mountain States Regional Genetics Services Network
Mountain States Regional Genetics Service Network
4300 Cherry Creek Drive South
Denver, CO 80222   303-692-2423
                             Fax: 303-782-5576

**290 Northern Colorado Area Support Group National
Ataxia Foundation**
1416 Antero Drive
Loveland, CO 80538   970-898-4390
                  e-mail: kittel@webaccess.net
                  www.fortnet.org/ncsg

Joe Kittel

**291 Pike's Peak Area Support Group National Ataxia
Foundation**
730 Elkgen Court
Colorado Springs, CO 80906   719-576-4772

Jacqule Gray

Connecticut

292 Connecticut Area Support Group National Ataxia Foundation
23 Cobb's Mill Lane
Glastonbury, CT 06033   203-659-8855
                    e-mail: pstrong@prodigy.net

Peter Strong

Florida

293 Broward County Support Group National Ataxia Foundation
10603 NW 49th Place
Coral Springs, FL 33076   954-341-8565
                    Fax: 954-753-6761
                    e-mail: pathamilto@aol.com
              www.hometown.aol.com/pathamilto/mypage

Support group provides a friendly, positive and compassionate atmosphere where people with Ataxia, their families and friends can share personal feelings and experiences.

20 members

Patricia B. Hamilton

294 Clearwater, FL Support Group National Ataxia Foundation
2363 Mary Lane
Clearwater, FL 33763   727-799-2852
                    e-mail: joyous7@mciworld.com

Joyce Robbins

295 Littleton Florida Area Support Group National Ataxia Foundation
6374 Fagen Lane
Littleton, FL 32683

Charlotte Prewitt

296 Palm Beach Florida Support Group National Ataxia Foundation
4881 B Adler Drive
West Palm Beach, FL 33417   561-640-5481

Sally Ross

297 Sarasota Florida Support Group National Ataxia Foundation

                    941-383-0275
              e-mail: cynlewin@aol.com

Cynthia Lewin

298 Tampa Support Group National Ataxia Foundation
2363 Mary Lane
Clearwater, FL 33763   813-799-2852
                    e-mail: joyous7@juno.com

Joyce Robbins

Georgia

299 Georgia Ataxia Support Group National Ataxia Foundation
218 Dykes Drive
Savannah, GA   912-927-3744
                    e-mail: jnovikoff1@juno.com

John Novikoff

300 Southeast Regional Genetics Group
2040 Ridgewood Drive
Atlanta, GA 30322   404-727-5844

Louis Elsas, MD, Chairman

Illinois

301 Chicago, IL Area Ataxia Support Group National Ataxia Foundation
2618 Burr Oak Avenue
Blue Island, IL 60406   708-389-3958
                    Fax: 708-389-9348
                    e-mail: WeebleDude@aol.com

Jonas Cepkauskas

302 Southern, IL Support Group National Ataxia Foundation
36 Lindorf Drive
Belleville, IL 62223   618-397-3259

Elaine Darte

Indiana

303 Central Indiana Support Group National Ataxia Foundation
5716 North 225 West
West Lafayette, IN 47906   765-463-3973
                                 Fax: 765-463-3972
                                 e-mail: turtle@laf.cioe.com

Judy Marten

304 NE Indiana Cerebellar Ataxia Support Group
4522 Shenandoah Circle West
Ft. Wayne, IN 46835   219-485-0965

Don & Jenny Roemke

Iowa

305 Great Plains Genetic Service Network
University of Iowa
Division of Medical Genetics
Iowa City, IA 52242   319-356-2674
                             Fax: 319-356-3347

Dolores Nesbitt, PhD, Coordinator

306 Sioux County Iowa Chapter National Ataxia Foundation
209 Second Street NE
Orange City, IA 51041

Joan Vande Brake, President

Kansas

307 Kansas City, MO Support Group National Ataxia Foundation
2704 Swift
North Kansas City, MO 64116   816-471-1840

Anna Lee Wyant

Kentucky

308 Cincinnati Ohio Area Support Group National Ataxia Foundation
619 Overton
Newport, KY 41071   561-640-5481
                           e-mail: prncssk16@aol.com

Mike and Kimberly Price

Louisiana

309 E-NAF (Electric NAF) Support Group National Ataxia Foundation

Baton Rouge, LA
                    e-mail: HBISHOP3@prodigy.net

Helen Bishop

310 Louisiana Chapter National Ataxia Foundation
3113 Roosevelt Blvd
Kenner, LA 70065   504-464-8633
                          e-mail: DD3@peodigy.net
                          www.angelfire.com/la/ataxiachapter/index

Provides information and group meetings for those interested in Hereditary Ataxia. Also sponsors Ataxia Clinics

Denise Drake, President

Maine

311 Maine Support Groups National Ataxia Foundation
56 Ten Penny Street
Freport, ME 04032   207-865-4969

June West

312 New England Regional Genetics Group
RR1 P.O. Box 2630
Turner, ME 04282   207-225-2722
                          Fax: 207-225-3883

Joseph Robinson

Maryland

313 Chesapeake Chapter National Ataxia Foundation
5938 Rossmore Drive
Bethesda, MD 20814   301-530-4989
                           Fax: 301-530-2480
                           e-mail: carljlauter@erols.com
                           www.geocities.com/Hotsprings/Oasis/4988/

A non-profit, charitable organization, whose mission is to combat all types of hereditary Ataxia. The objectives of NAF are to locate patients and persons at risk, increase awareness about the hereditary disorders through educational publications and meetings, and to provide funding for research. We are one of many support groups or chapters located throughout the United States, and publish a newsletter prior to their bi-monthly meetings.

Carl J. Lauter, President

Massachusetts

314 Boston Area Support Group National Ataxia Foundation
17 Highland Street
Lexington, MA 02173   781-862-1979

Michael Martignetti

315 Marshfield, MA Support Group National Ataxia Foundation
100 Hancock Street
Marshfield, MA 02050   617-834-7374

Joan C. Terra

316 New England Support Group National Ataxia Foundation
17 Highland Avenue
Lexington, MA 02421   781-862-1979

Michael Martignetti

Michigan

317 Detroit Michigian Ataxia Support Group National Ataxia Foundation
2050 Hyde Park Drive
Detroit, MI 48207   313-393-0106
e-mail: babcockj@assess.cl.detroit.mi.us

Jill Babcock

Minnesota

318 Chicago County, MN Support Group National Ataxia Foundation
10600 282 Street, Apt. 5
Chicago City, MN 55013   612-257-6014

Roxanne Hippe

319 Minneapolis, MN Support Group National Ataxia Foundation
6309 Cavell Court
Minneapolis, MN 55443   612-504-0909

Joe & Ginny Cain

320 Rochester Minnesota Support Group National Ataxia Foundation
2230 18th Place
Coral Springs, FL 33076   954-341-8565

Ellen Moetsch

321 Southwestern Minnesota Support Group National Ataxia Foundation
412 West Main
Luverne, MN 56156

Julie Schuur

Mississippi

322 Mississippi Chapter National Ataxia Foundation
P.O. Box 17005
Hattlesburg, MS 39404

Camille Daglio, President

Missouri

323 Central Area, Missouri Support Group National Ataxia Foundation
12 Jackson
Jefferson City, MO 65101   573-659-4759
e-mail: dr-susie@plnet.net
www.geocities.com/hotsprings/resort/2999

Dr. Susie Strode, PhD

324 St. Louis, MO Support Group National Ataxia Foundation
1306 Cypress
Pacific, MO 63069   314-271-6432
e-mail: Mbel140@aol.com
www.geocities.com/hotsprings/resort/9241

Mark Bellamy

Montana

325 Central Missouri Area Support Group National Ataxia Foundation
2209 Hillsdale Drive
Jefferson City, MO 65109   573-659-7573
e-mail: dwgl32b@prodigy.com

Cecilia Russell

326 Kansas City Support Group National Ataxia Foundation
2704 Swift
N. Kansas City, MO 64116   816-483-9433

Anna Lee Wyant

327 Springfield, MO Area Support Group National Ataxia Foundation
2012 Air Park Road # 7B
Ozark, MO 65721   417-581-8697

Patty Humbert

Nebraska

328 Omaha, NE Support Group National Ataxia Foundation
5904 Henninger Drive # 104
Omaha, NE 68104   402-573-5838

Lavonne Randolph

New Jersey

329 Belmar, New Jersey Support Group National Ataxia Foundation
68 Avondale Avenue
Neptune, NJ 07753   732-869-1780

Helen Bennett

330 Fairlawn, NJ Support Group National Ataxia Foundation
31-04 Heywood Avenue
Fairlawn, NJ 07410   201-797-6657

Hortense Oberndorf

New York

331 New York City Area Support Group National Ataxia Foundation
150 East 61st Street
New York City, NY 10021   212-355-4083

Karen Chernoff

332 Western New York Area Support Group National Ataxia Foundation
210 East Utica Street
Buffalo, NY 14208   716-881-0677

Diane P. Hall

North Carolina

333 Winston-Salem, NC Support Groups National Ataxia Foundation
455 Salem Vista Court
Winston-Salem, NC 27101   336-777-0442

Ruth Price

Ohio

334 Ohio Support Group National Ataxia Foundation
Box 148
Mesopotamia, OH 44439   440-693-4454

Joe Miller

Oklahoma

335 North Central Oklahoma Support Group National Ataxia Foundation
1704 Surrey Lane
Enid, OK 73703   580-233-1837

Jeannie Howard

Oregon

336 Pacific Northwest Regional Genetics Group
P.O. Box 574
Portland, OR 97207   503-494-8342
                                          Fax: 503-494-4447

Jonathan Zonana, MD, Director

337 Willamette Valley Ataxia Support Group National Ataxia Foundation
Albany General Hospital
1046 6th Ave SW
Albany, OR 97321   541-812-4162
                                          Fax: 541-812-4614
                              e-mail: MalindaOR@aol.com

Melinda Moore, CCC-SLP

Pennsylvania

338 Central Pennsylvania Area Support Group National Ataxia Foundation
51/12 Nichols Street
Weilsboro, PA 16901
                              e-mail: bronson1@epix.net
              www.geocities.com/hotsprings/sauna/7081

Susan Bronson

339 Mid-Atlantic Regional Human Genetics Network
5501 Old York Rd
Philadelphia, PA 19141   215-456-6730
                                          Fax: 215-456-7911

Deborah Eunpu, MS, President

340 Southeast Pennsylvania Support Group National Ataxia Foundation
220 Beechwood Road
Norristown, PA 19401   610-277-7722
                              e-mail: lizout@aol.com
              www.geocities/hotsprings/sauna/1533/

Liz Nussear

Rhode Island

341 Rhode Island Support Group National Ataxia Foundation
11 Orchard Avenue
Warren, RI 02885   401-245-8587

Geraldine DeBlois

South Carolina

342 Carolinas Support Group National Ataxia Foundation
520 Lewellen Drive
Hartsville, SC 29550   843-332-0876
                              e-mail: rutherford@prodigy.net

Tom Rutherford

Texas

343 Golden Triangle Area Support Group National Ataxia Foundation
2801 West Sunset #59H
Orange, TX 77630   409-883-5570
                              members.tripod.com/~ebs_2/main.html

Dana Leblanc

344 North Texas Support Group National Ataxia Foundation
2160 Graham Street
Paris, TX 75460   903-785-7058
                              e-mail: ballard@1starnet.com
              www.geocities.com/hotsprings/resort/5685

David Ballard

345 San Antonio Support Group National Ataxia Foundation
16023 Deer Crest
San Antonio, TX 78248   210-493-2238

Donna Conti

346 Texas Regional Genetics Network
110 West 49th Street
Austin, TX 78756   512-458-7700
                                          Fax: 512-458-7421

William Moore, Coordinator

Utah

347 Utah Support Group National Ataxia Foundation
261 Park Lane
Centerville, UT 84014   801-295-9518
                              e-mail: marlene@ctrutah.com

Marlene Canfield

Washington

348 Seattle, WA Area Support Group National Ataxia Foundation
14342 126th Avenue NE # A101
Kirkland, WA 98034   425-814-8412
                    e-mail: trinanddave@msn.com

Trinity Falk

Wisconsin

349 GLaRGG BLuRBB
Great Lakes Regional Genetics Group
1500 Highland Avenue
Madison, WI 53705   608-265-2907
                    Fax: 608-263-3496
                    NMCHC@circsol.com

Louise Elbaum, Coordinator

350 Madison, WI Area Support Group National Ataxia Foundation
1404 Marthys Road
Monona, WI 53716   608-221-1742
                    e-mail: pflast@itis.com

Carolyn Pflasterer

International

351 Canada Support Group National Ataxia Foundation
#13-1110 Odlum Drive
Vancouver, BC,
Canada   604-255-4590
                    e-mail: queen@istar.ca

Fiona Buss, Information Contact

352 South Central Ontario National Ataxia Foundation
35 Rosewood Avenue
Belleville, Ontario,
Canada   613-962-9623

Cathy Chamberlain

Web Sites

353 Ataxia Classification
www.neuro.wustl.edu/neuromuscular/ataxia

354 Gene Clinics
www.geneclinics.org/profiles/ataxias

355 International Network of Ataxia Friends
http://internaf.merseyside.org/

356 MHG Neurology Web Forums
http://neuro-www.mgh.harvard.edu/forum

Books

357 A Balancing Act Living with Spinal Cerebellar Ataxia
10603 NW 49th Place
Coral Springs, FL 33076   954-341-8565
                    Fax: 954-753-6761
                    e-mail: pathamilto@aol.com
                    www.hometown.aol.com/pathamilto/mypage

Describes living with Spinocerebellar Ataxia.

ISBN: 1-889826-00-6

Patricia B. Hamilton

358 Directory of National Genetic Voluntary Organizations
Alliance of Genetic Support Groups
4301 Connecticut Ave. NW # 404
Washington, DC 20008   202-966-5557
                    800-336-4363
                    Fax: 202-966-8553
                    e-mail: info@geneticalliance.org
                    www.geneticalliance.org

Lists all organizations and associations dealing with genetic disorders.

Lois E. Landon, Helpline and Resources Coordinator

359 Hereditary Ataxia: A Guidebook for Managing Speech & Swallowing
Douglas Fox, author

National Ataxia Foundation
2600 Fernbrook Lane-Suite 119
Minneapolis, MN 55447   612-553-0020
                    Fax: 612-553-0167
                    e-mail: naf@mr.net
                    www.ataxia.org

360 Living with Ataxia

Martha Nance, M.D., author

National Ataxia Foundation
2600 Fernbrook Lane-Suite 119
Minneapolis, MN 55447   612-553-0020
Fax: 612-553-0167
e-mail: naf@mr.net
www.ataxia.org

A compassionate resource for people who have or may be at risk of having ataxia, and for their families. This book explains the nature and causes of ataxia, the basic genetics that underlie many kinds of ataxia, discusses medical management of ataxia, provides practical advice for everyday living, and points the way to many useful resources to help live a good life with ataxia.

112 pages
ISBN: 0-943218-09-8

361 Ten Years to Live

Henry Schut, author

National Ataxia Foundation
2600 Fernbrook Lane-Suite 119
Minneapolis, MN 55447   612-553-0020
Fax: 612-553-0167
e-mail: naf@mr.net
www.ataxia.org

Struggles of the Schut family with hereditary ataxia.

162 pages Softcover
ISBN: 0-962716-31-6

Newsletters

362 Alert
Alliance of Genetic Support Groups
4301 Connecticut Ave. NW #404
Washington, DC 20008   202-966-5557
800-336-4363
Fax: 202-966-8553
e-mail: info@geneticalliance.org
www.geneticalliance.org

Functions as a vehicle of communication between the Alliance and its constituency. Provides timely and useful information on genetics research.

Monthly

Tracy Gilris, Membership Coordinator

363 GENES Information Services
Genetic Network of the Empire State
Empire State Plaza
Albany, NY 12201   518-474-7148
Fax: 518-474-8590

364 Generations
National Ataxia Foundation
2600 Fernbrook Lane-Suite 119
Minneapolis, MN 55447   612-553-0020
Fax: 612-553-0167
e-mail: naf@mr.net
www.ataxia.org

Contains reports on the organization and its chapters, offers research, advice and guides to other resources available. Articles on current research, genetics, and coping/living with ataxia. Membership is $25/ - newsletter free with membership.

48 pages Quarterly

Donna Gruetznx, Editor

365 Genetically Speaking
Pacific Southwest Regional Genetics Network
2151 Berkeley Way, Annex 4
Berkeley, CA 94704   510-540-2696
Fax: 510-540-2966
www.psrgn.org

A genetics newsletter for California, Hawaii, and Nevada.

366 Genetics Northwest
PacNoRGG Office
901, E. 18th Ave.
Eugene, OR 97403   541-346-2610
Fax: 541-346-2624
e-mail: kerrysilvey@ccmail.uoregon.edu

367 Genexus
Great Plains Genetic Service Network
The University of Iowa
Iowa City, IA 52242   319-356-2674
Fax: 319-356-3347

368 Great Lakes Genetic News
Great Lakes Regional Genetics Group
1500 Highland Avenue
Madison, WI 53705   608-266-2907
Fax: 608-263-3496

369 MARGIN
Mid-Atlantic Regional Human Genetics Network
260 S. Broad Street, Ste. 1900
Philadelphia, PA 19102   215-456-7910
Fax: 215-456-7911

370 MSRGSN Newsletter
Mountain States Regional Genetics Service Network
4300 Cherry Creek Drive South
Denver, CO 80222   303-692-2423
                         Fax: 303-782-5576

Joyce Hooker, Coordinator

371 NERG News
New England Regional Genetics Group
P.O. Box 670
Mt. Desert, ME 04660   207-839-5324
                         Fax: 207-839-8637

372 SERGG
Southeast Regional Genetics Group
2040 Ridgewood Drive
Atlanta, GA 30322   404-727-5844

Pamphlets

373 A Fragile X Planation
Louise Elbaum, author

National Maternal and Child Health Clearinghouse
2070 Chain Bridge Road, Suite 450
Vienna, VA 22182   703-356-1964
                         Fax: 703-821-2098

An explanation of fragile X syndrome intended
to be used, in conjunction with genetic counseling, as an aid for family members who are considering molecular testing for the fragile X
syndrome.

374 Alliance Brochure
Alliance of Genetic Support Groups
4301 Connecticut Ave. NW #404
Washington, DC 20008   202-966-5557
                         800-336-4363
                         Fax: 202-966-8553
                e-mail: info@geneticalliance.org
                         www.geneticalliance.or

Explains the services and programs offered by
the Alliance.

Lois E. Landen, Helpline and Resources Coordinator

375 Ataxia Fact Sheet
National Ataxia Foundation
2600 Fernbrook Lane-Suite 119
Minneapolis, MN 55447   612-553-0020
                         Fax: 612-553-0167
                         e-mail: naf@mr.net
                         www.ataxia.org

Describes ataxia as a symptom and its association with other medical problems as well as the
hereditary types. Membership is $25/year

376 Consumer Indicators of Quality Genetic Services
Alliance of Genetic Support Groups
4301 Connecticut Ave. NW #404
Washington, DC 20008   202-966-5557
                         800-336-4363
                         Fax: 202-966-8553
                e-mail: info@geneticalliance.org
                         www.geneticalliance.org

Describes the Alliance of Genetic Support
Groups Partnership Program, which strives to
increase provider awareness of the unique needs
and resources of genetic consumers, improve
provider access to quality, consumer-oriented
support group resources, and develop replaca-
ble educational materials for other programs.

Nachama Wilker, Director of Partnership Program

377 Facts About Friedreich's Ataxia
Muscular Dystrophy Association
3300 E. Sunrise Drive
Tucson, AZ 85718   520-529-2000
                         Fax: 520-529-5300

Explains Friedreich's ataxia in layman's terms
and answers commonly asked questions about
the disease.

378 Familial Spastic Paraplegia
National Ataxia Foundation
2600 Fernbrook Lane-Suite 119
Minneapolis, MN 55447   612-553-0020
                         Fax: 612-553-0167
                         e-mail: naf@mr.net
                         www.ataxia.org

Defines this disorder and notes symptoms,
causes and treatments. Membership is $25/year

379 Frenkel's Exercises
National Ataxia Foundation
2600 Fernbrook Lane-Suite 119
Minneapolis, MN 55447   612-553-0020
                         Fax: 612-553-0167
                         e-mail: naf@mr.net
                         www.ataxia.org

Describes an exercise program designed for
those with ataxia. Membership is $25/year

380 Friedrich's Ataxia
National Ataxia Foundation
2600 Fernbrook Lane-Suite 119
Minneapolis, MN 55447   612-553-0020
                         Fax: 612-553-0167
                         e-mail: naf@mr.net
                         www.ataxia.org

Describes symptoms, diagnosis, genetics and hints on coping. Membership is $25/year

381 Gene Testing for Ataxia
National Ataxia Foundation
2600 Fernbrook Lane-Suite 119
Minneapolis, MN 55447   612-553-0020
                                Fax: 612-553-0167
                                e-mail: naf@mr.net
                                www.ataxia.org

Describes the latest information about who should consider it and where to have it done. Membership $25/year

382 Health Insurance
National Ataxia Foundation
2600 Fernbrook Lane-Suite 119
Minneapolis, MN 55447   612-553-0020
                                Fax: 612-553-0167
                                e-mail: naf@mr.net
                                www.ataxia.org

Offers health insurance advice for persons with ataxia.

383 Hereditary Ataxia Brochure
National Ataxia Foundation
2600 Fernbrook Lane-Suite 119
Minneapolis, MN 55447   612-553-0020
                                Fax: 612-553-0167
                                e-mail: naf@mr.net
                                www.ataxia.org

Describes recessive and dominant ataxias, information on how hereditary ataxia is transmitted and explanations of the NAF's role in education, service and prevention.

384 Hereditary Ataxia: The Facts
National Ataxia Foundation
2600 Fernbrook Lane-Suite 119
Minneapolis, MN 55447   612-553-0020
                                Fax: 612-553-0167
                                e-mail: naf@mr.net
                                www.ataxia.org

Briefly describes the characteristics of recessive and dominant forms of ataxia.

385 Informed Consent: Participation in Genetic Research Studies
Alliance of Genetic Support Groups
4301 Connecticut Ave. NW #404
Washington, DC 20008   202-966-5557
                                 800-336-4363
                                 Fax: 202-966-8553
                          e-mail: info@geneticalliance.org
                                 www.geneticalliance.org

This booklet explains the nature of genetic research with its benefits and risks.

Lois O. Lender, Helpline and Resources Coordinator

386 Pen-Pal Directory
National Ataxia Foundation
2600 Fernbrook Lane-Suite 119
Minneapolis, MN 55447   612-553-0020
                                Fax: 612-553-0167
                                e-mail: naf@mr.net
                                www.ataxia.org

National, state and international directory of others who are affected by ataxia. Available to NAF Pen-Pal members only.

387 Students with Friedreich's Ataxia
National Ataxia Foundation
2600 Fernbrook Lane-Suite 119
Minneapolis, MN 55447   612-553-0020
                                Fax: 612-553-0167
                                e-mail: naf@mr.net
                                www.ataxia.org

Worksheet for teachers, parents and others who need to understand the physical constraints of ataxia.

DESCRIPTION

388 ATRIAL SEPTAL DEFECTS
Synonyms: ASD, Atrioseptal defects
Disorder Type: Birth Defect, Heart

The term atrial septal defects, or ASD, refers to a group of congenital abnormalities characterized by the presence of a hole in the wall (septum) that separates the two upper chambers of the heart (atria). Atrial septal defects are classified according to their location and may occur as a single anomaly or in association with other heart (cardiac) defects. These types of abnormalities occur in approximately 200 out of every 100,000 births.

The upper left chamber of the heart (left atrium) receives blood that is rich with oxygen (oxygenated) from the lungs. The blood then passes into the lower left chamber (left ventricle) from which it is then pumped through the arteries of the body into the general circulation. The right atrium receives blood that has been depleted of oxygen (deoxygenated) that then passes into the lower right ventricle and is pumped to the lungs where it once again receives oxygen. Atrial septal defects may allow the passage of some oxygenated blood from the upper left side of the heart into the upper right side of the heart where it mixes with blood that is oxygen depleted. In some patients, this results in a reduced oxygen supply to the body and an increase in blood flow to the lungs. Physical findings associated with ASDs may include enlargement of the right atrium, the right ventricle, or both, and characteristic heart soundsIn some patients, symptoms may be completely absent, especially in early childhood. ASDs are often discovered during routine physical examination. Some affected individuals may experience fatigue upon exertion or exercise. Other findings or symptoms may become apparent after the age of 30 years or when an affected woman becomes pregnant. In these patients, symptoms may include fatigue upon exercise (exercise intolerance), valve insufficiencies, and other, more serious problems such as heart failure.

In some patients, treatment may include surgery or catheter techniques to repair the defect. These surgical procedures are usually recommended during early childhood.

The following organizations in the General Resources Section can provide additional information: Genetic Alliance, March of Dimes Birth Defects Foundation, NIH/National Heart, Lung and Blood Foundation, NIH/National Institute of Child Health and Human Development

National Associations & Support Groups

389 American Heart Association
7272 Greenville Avenue
Dallas, TX 75231
214-373-6300
800-242-8721
Fax: 214-706-1341
e-mail: inquire@amhrt.org
www.amhrt.org

Supports research, education and community service programs with the objective of reducing premature death and disability from cardiovascular diseases and stroke; coordinates the efforts of health professionals, and other engaged in the fight against heart and circulatory disease.

390 National Heart, Lung and Blood Institute
National Institute of Health
31 Center Drive Building 31, Room 5A52
Baltimore, MD 20892
301-496-4236
www.nhlbi.nih.gov

Primary responsibility of this organization is the scientific investigation of heart, blood vessel, lung and blood disorders. Oversees research, demonstration, prevention, education, control and training activities in these fields and emphasizes the prevention and control of heart diseases.

Dr. Claude Lenfant, M.M., Director

Web Sites

391 Children's Health Information Network/ Congenital Heart Defects
www.ohsu.edu/cliniweb/c14/c14.240.400.html

392 Congenital Heart Disease Resource Page
www.csun.edu/~hcmth011/heart/

393 Southern Illinois University School of Medicine
www.siumed.edu/peds/teaching/patient%20education.htm

Children's Books

394 Heart Disease

Caroline Arnold, author

Franklin Watts c/o Grolier
90 Old Sherman Turnpyke
Danburry, CT 06816   203-797-3500
                           800-621-1115
                           Fax: 203-797-3197
                           www.grolier.com

Using diagrams, this book discusses strokes and
other bloodvessel disorders, as well as their
treatment and prevention.

112 pages Grades 7-12
ISBN: 0-531108-84-8

395 Living with Heart Disease

Steve Parker, author

Franklin Watts c/o Grolier
90 Old Sherman Turnpyke
Danbury, CT 06816   203-797-3500
                           800-621-1115
                           Fax: 203-797-3197
                           www.grolier.com

Shows how persons with heart disease can overcome their illness and lead productive lives.

32 pages Grades 5-7
ISBN: 0-531108-45-7

DESCRIPTION

396 ATTENTION DEFICIT HYPERACTIVITY DISORDER

Synonyms: ADHD, Hyperactive child syndrome, Hyperkinetic syndrome

Disorder Type: Mental, Emotional or Behavioral Disorder

Attention deficit hyperactivity disorder, or ADHD, is a syndrome of childhood and adolescence characterized by impulsive behavior, motor-related overactivity (hyperactivity), and inattention. The short attention span results in a decreased ability or inability to complete chores, assignments, or other tasks. ADHD is four to six times more prevalent among boys than it is in girls. In approximately 50 percent of cases, this disorder develops before the age of four years, while in others it appears before seven years of age. Some behavioral symptoms associated with this disorder may be present at times in children with ADHD or in children with certain other disorders (e.g., conduct disorder, learning disabilities, hearing impairment, etc.). Therefore, specialists often base their diagnosis on the frequent presence of eight or more characteristic findings. Among these are restlessness, difficulty in remaining seated, difficulty in waiting for a turn in group activities, inclination to be easily distracted, impulsively answering questions before they are completed, difficulty following instructions, inability to sustain concentration while performing tasks or playing, shifting to other tasks before completing others, talking excessively, poor ability to play quietly, interrupting or butting in on others, not appearing to listen when others speak, losing things, and frequently taking part in dangerous physical activities with no reg, evaluation of a detailed family and medical history, paying careful attention to such things as activity level, behavior, and temperament during the early years of the life of the affected child, may be helpful in determining the extent of the disorder and the presence of additional difficulties (e.g., learning disabilities, anxiety disorders, conduct disorders, etc.).

Although the cause of ADHD is not genetic influences may be a factor in the development of this disorder. In addition, children with neurological disorders and other abnormalities related to the central nervous system may be predisposed to the development of ADHD. Treatment of attention deficit hyperactivity disorder may include an ongoing behavioral and psychosocial therapeutic plan that includes the cooperation of school personnel, the child, and the child's parents or caregivers. In addition, psychostimulant drugs or other medications may be prescribed and carefully monitored. Affected children may also benefit from a structured environment at home and in school. Studies show that, in many phases children who receive multifaceted treatment are better able to cope with ADHD through their adolescent years and into adulthood. Other treatment is supportive.

The following organizations in the General Resources Section can provide additional information: National Organization for Rare Disorders, Inc. (NORD), NIH/Office of Rare Diseases, National Mental Health consumer self-Help Clearinghouse, Genetic Alliance, NIH/National Institute of Neurological Disorders & Stroke, ARC, March of Dimes Birth Defects Foundation, NIH/National Institute of Mental Health, National Alliance for the Mentally Ill, National Mental Health Association

National Associations & Support Groups

397 AD-IN: Attention Deficit Information Network
475 Hillside Ave
Needham, MA 02194   781-455-9895
Fax: 781-444-5466
e-mail: adin@gis.net

398 ADHD Challenge, Inc.
P.O. Box 2277
West Peabody, MA 01910   978-535-3276
800-233-2322
TDD: 508-535-3276
e-mail: koplow@grs.net

Provision of data and emotional assistance to both sufferers and medical professionals.

399 CHADD: Children and Adults with Attention Deficit Disorders
499 NW 70th Ave, Ste 101
Plantation, FL 33317   305-587-3700
                                        800-233-4050
                                   Fax: 305-587-4599
                        e-mail: national@chadd.org
                                     www.chadd.org

Many children and/or adults have a disorder characterized by deficits in attention span and impulse control, which is frequently accompanied by hyperactivity. CH.A.D.D. (Children and Adults with Attention Deficit Disorders) provides parents, professionals and adults diagnosed with ADD information, support adn educational material dealing with this disorder. CH.A.D.D. has over 600 chapters across the country and over 28,000 active members.

400 Council Children with Behavioral Disorders
1920 Association Drive
Reston, VA 20191   703-620-3660
                                        888-232-7733
                                   Fax: 703-264-9494
                                   TTY: 703-264-9446
                                        www.ccbd.net

The Council for Children with Behavorial Disorders is an international professional organization committed to promoting and facilitating the education and general welfare of children/youth with behavorial and emotional disorders, CCBD publishes several resources and research information for the quality education of children/youth with behavorial and emotional disorders.

401 Learning Disabilities Association of America
4156 Library Road
Pittsburgh, PA 15234   412-341-1515
                         e-mail: ldanatl@usaor.net
                                    www.ldanatl.org/

Helps families of the affected individual through up-to-date technology and further advancement of the changes in the medical fields related to this and similar disorders.

402 National Center for Learning Disabilities
381 Park Avenue South #1401
New York, NY 10016   212-545-7510
                                        www.ncld.org

Disperses information to the educational community and the general public regarding the disorder through reading and video materials.

Audio Video

403 ADD, Stepping Out of the Dark
ADD Videos
P.O. Box 622
New Paltz, NY 12561   914-255-3612
                                   Fax: 914-883-6452

A powerful, effective video, ideal for health professionals, educators and parents providing a visual montage designed to promote an understanding and awareness of attention deficit disorder. Based on actual accounts of those who have ADD, including a neurologist, an office worker, and parents of children with ADD. The video allows the viewer to feel the frustration and lack of attention that ADD brings to many.

Video

Lenae Madonna, Producer

404 ADHD in the Classroom: Strategies for Teachers
Russell A. Barkley, author

Active Parenting Publishers
810 Franklin Court, Suite B
Marietta, GA 30067
                                        800-825-0060
                                   Fax: 770-429-0334
                             www.activeparenting.com

A four-step plan for avoiding potential problems with methods and program manual.
42 pages 39 minutes

405 ADHD: What Can We Do?
Russell A. Berkley, author

Guilford Publications
72 Spring Street
New York, NY 10012   212-431-9800
                                        800-365-7006
                                   Fax: 212-966-6708
                       e-mail: info@guilford.com
                                     www.guilford.com

A video program that introduces teachers and parents to a variety of the most effective technologies for managing ADHD in the classroom, at home, and on family outings.

ISBN: 0-898629-72-1

406 ADHD: What Do We Know?

Russell A. Barkley, author

Guilford Publications
72 Spring Street
New York, NY 10012   212-431-9800
                            800-365-7006
                            Fax: 212-966-6708
                            e-mail: info@guilford.com
                            www.guilford.com

An introduction for teachers and special education practitioners, school psychologists and parents of ADHD children. Topics outlined in this video include the causes and prevalence of ADHD, ways children with ADHD behave, other conditions that may accompany ADHD and longterm prospects for children with ADHD.

Video

407 Around the Clock

Joan F. Goodman, author

Guilford Publications
72 Spring Street
New York, NY 10012   212-431-9800
                            800-365-7006
                            Fax: 212-966-6708
                            e-mail: info@guilford.com
                            www.guilford.com

This videotape provides both professionals and parents a helpful look at how the difficulties facing parents of ADHD children can be handled.

408 Concentration Video

Learning disAbilities Resources
P.O. Box 716
Bryn Mawr, PA 19010   610-525-8336
                             800-869-8336
                             Fax: 610-525-8337

An instructional video which provides a perspective about attention problems, possible causes and solutions.

Video

409 Diagnosis & Treatment of Attention Deficit Disorder in Children

Fanlight Productions
47 Halifax St
Boston, MA 01230   617-469-4999
                          Fax: 617-469-3379
                          e-mail: fanlight@fanlight.com
                          www.fanlight.com

Follows several children with ADD, and includes suggestions about ways to restructure home and school environments to support such children. Dartmouth Hitchcock Medical Center Series, The Doctor is In...

28 minutes

410 Educating Inattentive Children

Samuel Goldstein, PhD, & Michael Goldstein, MD, author

Western Psychological Services
12031 Wilshire Boulevard
Los Angeles, CA 90025
                          800-648-8857
                          Fax: 310-478-7838

An excellent resource for teachers who encounter inattention and hyperactivity in the classroom. It helps teachers distinguish deliberate misbehavior from the incompetent, nonpurposeful behavior of the inattentive child.

Video

411 Help! This Kid's Driving Me Crazy!

Lynn Adkins and Janis Cady, author

Pro-Ed
8700 Shoal Creek Boulevard
Austin, TX 78758   512-451-3246
                          Fax: 512-451-8542

Designed for parents and professionals working with children up to five years old, this videotape and booklet offers information about the nature, special needs, and typical behavioral characteristics for young children with attention deficit disorder.

Video

412 Help! This Kid's Driving Me Crazy: The Young Child with Attention Deficit

8700 Shoal Creek Blvd.
Austin, TX 78757
                          800-897-3202
                          Fax: 800-397-7633

The videotape provides information about the behavior and special needs of young children with ADD and offers suggestions on fostering appropriate behaviors. A pamphlet includes the script and suggested questions.

Video Tape

413 It's Just Attention Disorder

Samuel Goldstein, PhD, & Michael Goldstein, MD, author

Western Psychological Services
12031 Wilshire Boulevard
Los Angeles, CA 90025   310-478-2061
                               800-648-8857
                               Fax: 310-478-7838

This ground-breaking videotape takes the critical first steps in treating attention-deficit disorder: it enlists the inattentive or hyperactive child as an active participant in his or her treatment.

Video

414 Understanding Attention Deficit Disorder
Connecticut Association for Children with LD
25 Van Zant Street Suite 15-5
East Norwalk, CT 06855   203-838-5010
                                         Fax: 203-866-6108
                         e-mail: CACLD@juno.com
                         http://www.CACLD.org

A video in an interview format for parents and professionals providing the history, symptoms, methods of diagnosis and three approaches used to ease the effects of attention deficit disorder. The last 15 minutes deal with ADD in adults.

45 minutes

415 Why Can't Michael Pay Attention?
Active Parenting Publishers
810 Franklin Court, Suite B
Marietta, GA 30067
                                         800-825-0060
                                         Fax: 770-429-0334
                         www.activeparenting.com

Watch a first-grade boy receive a thorough assessment for ADHD. See techniques used to help organize Michael's behavior.

19 minutes

416 Why Won't My Child Pay Attention?
Samuel Goldstein, PhD, author

Western Psychological Services
12031 Wilshire Blvd.
Los Angeles, CA 90025   310-478-2061
                                         800-648-8857
                                         Fax: 310-478-7838

Practical and reassuring videotape, noted child psychologist tells parents about two of the most common and complex problems of childhood: inattention and hyperactivity.

Video

Web Sites

417 ADD on AOL
user.aol.com/jimams/addonaol.html

418 ADHD Help
members.aol.com/ADDisorder/4help/index.html

419 ASK Site
www.azstarnet.com/~ask/sled_map.html

420 Attention.Deficit.Disorder
www.stanford.edu/group/dss/Info.by.disab

421 Pedbase
www.icondata.com/health/pedbase/files/ATTEN-TIO.HTM

Books

422 ADD Book
Courage To Change
P.O. Box 1268
Newburgh, NY 12551
                                         800-440-4003
                                         Fax: 800-772-6499

Outlines effective behavior modification techniques to improve your child's cognitive abilities and reduce hyperactivity without drugs. Offers guidelines to help improve attention and motivation in school, handle frustration, develop time management techniques, and make decisions about medications.

64 pages Soft Cover

423 ADD: Helping Your Child
Warren Umansky & Barbara S. Smalley, author

Warner Books
1271 Avenue of the Americas
New York, NY 10020   212-484-2900

1994 224 pages Softcover
ISBN: 0-446670-13-8

424 ADHD - What Can We Do?
Courage To Change
P.O. Box 1268
Newburgh, NY 12551
                                         800-440-4003
                                         Fax: 800-772-6499

Excellent training material for counselors and teachers. This video offers helpful strategies, and the most effective techniques for managing ADHD in the classroom.

Video

425 ADHD - What Do We Know?
Courage To Change
P.O. Box 1268
Newburgh, NY 12551

800-440-4003
Fax: 800-772-6499

Excellent training material for counselors and teachers. This video outlines the causes and prevalence of ADHD, and ways children with ADHD behave. A special education professional describes the problem in schools. Three young people with ADHD talk about coping with the disorder.

Video

426 ADHD Handbook for Families: A Guide to Communicating with Professionals
Paul L. Weingartner, author

Active Parenting Publishers
810 Franklin Court, Suite B
Marietta, GA 30067

800-825-0060
Fax: 770-429-0334
www.activeparenting.com

Written by a man with ADHD, this book offers practical information about real-life strategies and techniques which can be put to use immediately.

132 pages

427 ADHD Parenting Handbook: Practical Advice for Parents from Parents
Colleen Roberts-Alexander, author

Taylor Publishing
1550 W. Mockingbird
Dallas, TX 75235

214-637-2800

1994 224 pages Softcover
ISBN: 0-878338-62-4

428 ADHD in Schools: Assessment and Intervention Strategies
George J. DuPaul and Gary Stoner, author

Guilford Publications
72 Spring Street
New York, NY 10012

212-431-9800
800-365-7006
Fax: 212-966-6708
e-mail: info@guilford.com
www.guilford.com

This landmark volume emphasizes the need for a team effort among parents, community-based professionals, and educators. Provides practical information for educators that is based on empirical findings. Chapters focus on: how to identify and assess students who might have ADHD; the relationship between ADHD and learning disabilities; how to develop and implement classroom-based programs; communication strategies to assist physicians; and the need for community-based treatments.

269 pages Hard/Softcover
ISBN: 0-898622-45-0

429 ADHD/Hyperactivity: A Consumers Guide For Parents and Teachers
Michael Gordon, PhD, author

Connecticut Association for Children with LD
25 Van Zant Street Suite 15-5
East Norwalk, CT 06855

203-838-5010
Fax: 203-866-6108

Works through information about the assessment and treatment of ADHD in children. Stresses need for parents to develop a collaborative relationship with professionals. Chapters for teachers focusing on educational programming.

178 pages

430 ADHD: Handbook for Diagnosis & Treatment
Russell A. Barkley, PhD, author

Western Psychological Services
12031 Wilshire Boulevard
Los Angeles, CA 90025

310-478-2061
800-648-8857
Fax: 310-478-7838

This second edition helps clinicians diagnose and treat Attention Deficit Hyperactivity Disorder. Written by an internationally recognized authority in the field, it covers the history of ADHD, its primary symptoms, associated conditions, developmental course and outcome, and family context. A workbook companion manual is also available.

700 pages

431 Alphabet Soup: A Recipe for Understanding & Treating ADD
James Javorsky, author

Minerva Books, Ltd.
137 W. 14th Street
New York, NY 10011

212-929-2833

1994 50 pages Softcover
ISBN: 0-934695-00-8

432 Attention Defecit Disorder: Children
Aquarius Health Care Videos
5 Powderhouse Lane, P.O. Box 1159
Sherborn, MA 01770

Fax: 508-650-4216
e-mail: aqvideos@tiac.net
www.aquariusproductions.com

Everyone has been impulsive or easily distracted for different periods of time, so these symptoms that are hallmarks of Attention Defecit Disorder (ADD) have also led to criticism that too many people are being diagnosed with this biochemical brain disorder. This program examines who is being diagnosed, and what treatments are working. An innovative private school speciaalizing in alternative education is profiled, and tips on structuring the school and home environment are included.

Video

433 Attention Deficit Disorder ADHD and ADD Syndromes
Dale Jordan, author

8700 Shoal Creek Blvd.
Austin, TX 78757

800-897-3202
Fax: 800-397-7633

Always up-to-date, this book enters its third edition with even more complete explanations of how ADHD and ADD interfere with: classroom learning, behavior at home, job performance, and social skills development. New chapters explain the critical roles that emotions and feelings play in perception, comprehension, and decision making. Plus, this is the first book about ADHD and ADD to describe in detail the shadow syndromes that tend to accompany ADHD and ADD.

216 pages Softcover
ISBN: 0-890797-42-0

434 Attention Deficit Disorder and Learning Disabilities
Barbara D. Ingersoll, PhD, and Sam Goldstein, PhD, author

Connecticut Association for Children with LD
25 Van Zant Street Suite 15-5
East Norwalk, CT 06855

203-838-5010
Fax: 203-866-6108

Realities, myths, and controversial treatments. Section I tries to dispel the myths and discusses proven treatments for ADHD and LD. Section II explains how the scientific community evaluates new treatment methods, and Section III summarizes alternative treatments and discusses scientific evidence pertaining to its usefulness.

246 pages
ISBN: 0-385469-31-4

435 Attention Deficit Disorder in Children and Adolescents
Jack L. Fadely and Virginia N. Hosler, author

Charles C. Thomas Publishing, Ltd.
2600 South First Street
Springfield, IL 62704

217-789-8980
800-258-8980
Fax: 217-789-9130
e-mail: books@ccthomas.com
www.ccthomas.com

Presents an analysis of case studies of children and adolescents with attentional deficits and hyperactivity, demonstrating causal factors in these disorders and suggesting treatment strategies both in psychological and medical practice. Written as a review and summary of twenty years of private practice.

1992 292 pages Softcover
ISBN: 0-398061-12-2

436 Attention Deficit Disorder: Children
Aquarius Health Care Videos
5 Powderhouse Lane, P.O. Box 1159
Sherborn, MA 01770

Fax: 508-650-4216
e-mail: aqvideos@tiac.net
www.aquariusproductions.com

Everyone has been impulsive or easily distracted for different periods of time, so these symptoms that are hallmarks of Attention Defecit Disorder (ADD) have also led to criticism that too many people are being diagnosed with this biochemical brain disorder. This program examines who is being diagnosed, and what treatments are working. An innovative private school specializing in altenate education is profiled, and tips on structuring the school and home environment are included.

Video

437 Attention Deficit Disorders: Assessment & Teaching
Janet W. Lerner, et al., author

Brooks/Cole Publishing Company
511 Forest Lodge
Pacific Grove, CA 93950

408-373-0728
Fax: 408-375-6414
e-mail: bc-info@brookscole.com
www.brookscole.com

A handy resource that offers teachers, school psychologists, counselors, social workers, administrators, and parents practical advice for working with children who have attention deficit disorders.

1995 258 pages Softcover
ISBN: 0-534250-44-0

438 Attention Deficit Hyperactivity Disorder: What Every Parent Wants to Know

David L. Woodrich, author

Paul H. Brookes & Company
Box 10624
Baltimore, MD 21285   301-337-9580

1993 320 pages Softcover
ISBN: 1-557661-41-3

439 Attention Deficit/Hyperactivity Disorder

Paul Cooper and Katherine Ideus, author

David Fulton Publishers
2 Barbon Close, Great Ormond Street
London, WCIN   171-405-5606
                      Fax: 171-831-4840

Resource material for teachers of children aged between five and sixteen, particularly of interest to those in the SEN field and those concerned with EBD in schools. Addresses many of the key questions that teachers raise about AD/HD, and deals with them in a clear and concise manner. Major emphasis on practical guidance for classroom practice. Also helps teachers deal with parents' questions and helps them in their work with professionals.

July 1996 112 pages Softcover
ISBN: 1-853464-31-7

440 Attention Please!

Edna D. Copeland, PhD, and Valerie L. Love, MEd, author

Connecticut Association for Children with LD
25 Van Zant Street Suite 15-5
East Norwalk, CT 06855   203-838-5010
                                Fax: 203-866-6108

A comprehensive guide for successfully parenting children with attention deficit disorders and hyperactivity. Real life experiences of families includes chapter on self-esteem, homework, and using discipline effectively.

352 pages

441 Attention-Deficit Hyperactivity Disorder Second Education

Russell A. Barkley, author

Guilford Publications
72 Spring Street
New York, NY 10012   212-431-9800
                            800-365-7006
                      Fax: 212-966-6708
              e-mail: info@guilford.com
                      www.guilford.com

A second edition that is the handbook on the diagnosis and treatment of ADHD in the 1990s. A companion workbook is also available with forms that may be photocopied.

747 pages Hardcover
ISBN: 0-898624-43-6

442 Attention-Deficit/Hyperactivity Disorder in the Classroom

Dowdy, Patton, Smith, Polloway, author

Pro-Ed
8700 Shoal Creek Boulevard
Austin, TX 78757   512-451-3246
                          800-897-3202
                    Fax: 512-451-8542
                    www.proedinc.com

A practical guide for teachers, provides educators with a complete guide on how to deal effectively with students with attention deficits in their classrooms. The book emphasises practical applications for teachers to use that will facilitate the success of students, both academically and socially.

291 pages Softcover
ISBN: 0-890796-65-3

443 Conners Rating Scale

C. Keith Conners, author

Pro-Ed
8700 Shoal Creek Blvd.
Austin, TX 78757
                          800-897-3202
                    Fax: 800-397-7633
                    www.proedinc.com

An updated version of the set of measurements used to determine the presence of Attention Deficit/Hyperactivity disorder in children. Test is suitable for children and adolescents age 3 to 17. ADHDT kit includes Examiner's Manual and Summary/Response forms.

Long Version

444 Coping with ADD/ADHD

Jaydene Morrison, MS, author

Rosen Publishing Group
29 East 21st Street
New York, NY 10010   212-777-3017
                            800-237-9932
                      Fax: 212-436-4643
              e-mail: rosenpub@tribeca.ios.com

At least 3.5 million American youngsters suffer from attention deficit disorder. This book defines the syndrome and provides specific information about treatment and counseling.

ISBN: 0-823920-70-4

445 Driven to Distraction

Edward Hallowell and John Ratey, author

National Alliance for the Mentally Ill
P.O. Box 753
Waldorf, MD 20604   703-524-7600

A practical book discussing adult as well as child attention deficit disorder (ADD). Non-technical, realistic and optimistic, it is an informative how-to manual for parents and consumers.

1994

446 Handbook of Childhood Impulse Disorders and ADHD: Theory and Practice

Koziol, Stout, Ruben, author

Charles C. Thomas Publishing, Ltd.
2600 South First Street
Springfield, IL 62704   217-789-8980
                               800-258-8980
                        Fax: 217-789-9130
           e-mail: books@ccthomas.com
                      www.ccthomas.com

This handbook responds to the controversy over diagnosis, use and abuse of pharmacology and offers effectively proven practical treatment typically overlooked in traditional medical treatise.

252 pages Softcover
ISBN: 0-398058-44-X

447 Helping Your Hyperactive Attention Deficit Child

John F. Taylor, PhD, author

Active Parenting Publishers
810 Franklin Court, Suite B
Marietta, GA 30067

                           800-825-0060
                      Fax: 770-429-0334
                  www.activeparenting.com

This book takes a multi-dimensional approach on this topic covering areas such as medical, nutritional, drug therapy and a child's self-esteem.

483 pages

448 Hyperactive Child, Adolescent, and Adult: ADD Through the Lifespan

Paul Wender, MD, author

Connecticut Association for Children with LD
25 Van Zant Street Suite 15-5
East Norwalk, CT 06855   203-838-5010
                         Fax: 203-866-6108

Comprehensive general review. Update on previous research by the author, offering a basic text.

162 pages

449 Hyperactivity: Why Won't My Child Pay Attention?

Sam Goldstein and Michael Goldstein, author

John Wiley & Sons, INC.
605 Third Avenue
New York, NY 10158   212-850-6000
                       Fax: 212-850-6088
                           www.wiley.com

224 pages
ISBN: 0-471530-77-8

450 If Your Child is Hyperactive, Inattentive, Impulsive, Distractable...

Stephen and Marianne Garber, Robyn Spitzman, author

Connecticut Association for Children with LD
25 Van Zant Street Suite 15-5
East Norwalk, CT 06855   203-838-5010
                         Fax: 203-866-6108

Introduces ADHD with a lot of information on basic issues. Offers very specific guidance on changing your child's behavior.

235 pages

451 Kids with Incredible Potential

Mary K. Bailey, author

Active Parenting Publishers
810 Franklin Court, Suite B
Marietta, GA 30067

                           800-825-0060
                      Fax: 770-429-0334
                  www.activeparenting.com

A curriculum for parents of ADHD children with pratical and immediate information.

452 LD Child and the ADHD Child

Suzanne H. Stevens, author

John F. Blair, Publisher
1406 Plaza Drive
Winston-Salem, NC 27103   336-768-1374
                                 800-222-9796
                                 Fax: 336-768-9194
                                 blairpub.com

The author recommends other options that can be explored to treat LD and ADHD children without drugs.

Softcover
ISBN: 0-895871-42-4

453 Life on the Edge: Parenting a Child with ADD/ADHD

David Spohn, author

Active Parenting Publishers
810 Franklin Court, Suite B
Marietta, GA 30067
                                 800-825-0060
                                 Fax: 770-429-0334
                                 www.activeparenting.com

Lighthearted and down-to-earth book which helps other parents to make it through the stresses, chaos and heartbreak that come with raising a child with ADD/ADHD.

81 pages

454 Managing Attention Deficit Hyperactivity Disorder in Children

Sam Goldstein and Michael Goldstein, author

John Wiley & Sons, INC.
605 Third Avenue
New York, NY 10158   212-850-6000
                                 Fax: 212-850-6088
                                 www.wiley.com

This book explores symptoms of ADHD, the crossover into adulthood with such a disorder, and the latest and most controversial treatments.

896 pages
ISBN: 0-471121-58-4

455 Managing Attention Disorders in Children: A Guide for Practitioners

Sam Goldstein, Ph.D., author

Books on Special Children
P.O. Box 305
Congers, NY 10920   914-638-1236
                                Fax: 914-638-0847

Offers information about human personality, structure and dynamics, assessment and adjustment.

214 pages

456 Maybe You Know My Kid: A Parent's Guide to Identifying ADHD

M.C. Fowler, author

Birch Lane Press
120 Enterprise Avenue
Secaucus, NJ 07094
                                 800-447-2665

The author writes about her family experiences with their son, David, who has attention deficit disorder. Contains a comprehensive review of important issues plus descriptions of some helpful management techniques.

222 pages

457 Medications for Attention Disorders and Related Medical Problems

Edna D. Copeland, PhD, author

Specialty Press, Inc.

Plantation, FL
                                 800-233-9273

A comprehensive handbook covering the history, characteristics, and causes of ADHD. The equal importance of appropriate academic programming, counseling, and medication are stressed throughout.

415 pages Hardcover

458 Parents Helping Parents: A Directory of Support Groups for ADD

CibaGelgy, Pharmaceuticals Division
External Communications
Summit, NJ 07901   908-277-5000

459 Parents' Hyperactivity Handbook: Helping the Fidgety Child

D.M. Paltin, author

Plenum Press
233 Spring Street
New York, NY 10013   212-620-8000
                                Fax: 212-463-0742
                                e-mail: info@plenum.com

1993 306 pages
ISBN: 0-306444-65-8

460 Rethinking Attention Deficit Disorders

Miriam Cherkes-Julkowski, Susan Sharp, author

Brookline Books/Lumen Editions
P.O. Box 1047
Cambridge, MA 02238   617-868-0360
                             800-666-2665
                        Fax: 617-868-1772
              e-mail: brooklinebks@delphi.com
              www.people.delphi.com/brooklinebks

Gives the classroom teacher useful information that provides ideas and strategies for working with children suffering from ADD.

ISBN: 1-571290-37-0

461 Ritalin is Not the Answer

David B. Stein, author

Jossey-Bass
350 Sansome Street
San Francisco, CA 94104   415-433-1740
                                 800-956-7739
                            Fax: 800-605-2665
                            www.josseybass.com

A healthy, drug-free alternative to Ritalin and an absolute must read for every physician before prescribing it.

224 pages
ISBN: 0-787945-14-5

462 Survival Guide for Teenagers with LD

Rhoda Cummings and Gary Fisher, author

Connecticut Association for Children with LD
25 Van Zant Street Suite 15-5
East Norwalk, CT 06855   203-838-5010
                           Fax: 203-866-6108

463 Taking Charge of ADHD
Courage To Change
P.O. Box 1268
Newburgh, NY 12551
                                800-440-4003
                           Fax: 800-772-6499

Learn positive strategies for meeting the challenges of raising children with Attention Deficit Hyperactivity Disorder. This excellent resource teaches you how to prevent ADHD from becomming a major obstacle in your child's life. Provides techniques for managing behavior, information on the latest medications and much more.

294 pages Soft Cover

464 Teach and Reach Students with Attention Deficit Disorders

Nancy L. Eisenberg & Pamela H. Esser, author

MultiGrowth Resources
12345 Jones Road, #101
Houston, TX 77070   281-890-5334

Handbook and resource guide for parents and educators of ADD students.

1994 200 pages
ISBN: 0-963084-70-4

465 You and Your ADD Child

Paul Warren & Judy Capehart, author

Nelson Publications
One Gateway Plaza
Port Chester, NY 10573   914-937-8400

1995 252 pages Softcover
ISBN: 0-785278-95-8

Children's Books

466 Getting a Grip on ADD: A Kid's Guide to Understanding & Coping with ADD

Kim T. Frank & Susan J. Smith, author

Educational Media Corporation
6021 Wish Avenue
Encino, CA 91316   818-708-0962

1994 64 pages Softcover
ISBN: 0-932796-60-3

467 Jumpin' Johnny Get Back to Work! A Child's Guide To ADHD/Hyperactivity

Michael Gordon, PhD, author

Connecticut Association for Children with LD
25 Van Zant Street Suite 15-5
East Norwalk, CT 06855   203-838-5010
                           Fax: 203-866-6108

Written primarily for elementary age youngsters with ADHD to help them understand their disability. Also valuable as an educational tool for parents, siblings, friends, and classmates. Includes two pages on medication.

24 pages

468 Putting on the Brakes
Courage To Change
P.O. Box 1268
Newburgh, NY 12551
                                800-440-4003
                           Fax: 800-772-6499

This book written for kids ages 8 to 13 tells all they need to know about ADHD. Also available is a companion activity book that teaches organizing, setting priorities, problem solving, maintaining control and other life management skills. The activity book is 88 pages and sells for $14.95

64 pages Softcover

469 Self-Control Games & Workbook

Berthold Berg, PhD, author

Western Psychological Services
12031 Wilshire Boulevard
Los Angeles, CA 90025   310-478-2061
                               800-648-8857
                          Fax: 310-478-7838

This game is designed to teach self-control in academic and social situations. Addresses a total of 24 impulsive, inattentive and hyperactive behaviors. The companion workbook reinforces the use of positive self-statements, and problem-solving techniques, instead of expressing anger.

Game

470 Shelley, the Hyperactive Turtle

Deborah Moss, author

Woodbine House
6510 Bells Mill Road
Bethesda, MD 20817   301-468-8800
                             800-843-7323
                        Fax: 301-897-5838
         e-mail: info@woodbinehouse.com
                 www.woodbinehouse.com

Entertaining picture book for use with very young children. Sensitive text and colorful illustrations help children understand ADHD.

20 pages

Carol Schwartz, Illustrator

Magazines

471 Attention
Children & Adults with Attention Deficit Disorder
499 NW 70th Avenue, Ste. 101
Plantation, FL 33317   954-587-3700
                              800-233-4050
                         Fax: 954-587-4599

Quarterly

Newsletters

472 ADHD Report
Guilford Publications
72 Spring Street
New York, NY 10012   212-431-9800
                              800-365-7006
                         Fax: 212-966-6708
         e-mail: samples@guilford.com
                 www.guilford.com

Presents the most up-to-date information on the evaluation, diagnosis and management of ADHD in children, adolescents and adults. This important newsletter is an invaluable resource for all professionals interested in ADHD.

Bi-monthly
ISBN: 1-065802-5 -

473 Chadder
Children & Adults with Attention Deficit Disorder
499 NW 70th Avenue, Ste. 101
Plantation, FL 33317   954-587-3700
                              800-233-4050
                         Fax: 954-587-4599

Quarterly

Pamphlets

474 ADHD

Larry B. Silver, M.D., author

Learning Disabilities Association of America
4156 Library Road
Pittsburgh, PA 15234   412-341-1515

A booklet for parents offering information on Attention Deficit-Hyperactivity Disorders and learning disabilities.

475 Attention Deficit Disorders and Hyperactivity
ERIC Clearinghouse on Disabled and Gifted Children
1920 Association Drive
Reston, VA 22091   703-620-3660
                              800-328-0272

476 Attention Deficit-Hyperactivity Disorder: Is It a Learning Disability?

Larry Silver, author

Georgetown University, School of Medicine
3800 Reservoir Road NW
Washington, DC 20007   202-687-2000

Offers information on learning disabilities and related disorders.

Larry Silver, M.D.

477 Children with ADD: A Shared Responsibility
Council for Exceptional Children
1920 Association Drive
Reston, VA 22091   703-620-3660
                               800-232-7323

This book represents a consensus of what professionals and parents believe ADD is all about and how children with ADD may best be served. Reviews the evaluation process under IDEA and 504 and presents effective classroom strategies.

35 pages
ISBN: 0-865862-33-8

478 Coping with Your Inattentive Child
Samuel Nichamin, MD, and James Windell, MA, author
Connecticut Association for Children with LD
25 Van Zant Street Suite 15-5
East Norwalk, CT 06855   203-838-5010
                               Fax: 203-866-6108

Lists signs of ADHD and discusses managing the problems of children with ADHD from infancy through elementary school.

13 pages

479 Educational Strategies for Students with Attention Deficit Disorder
Mark A. Sloane, Laurie Assadi, and Linda Linn, author
Connecticut Association for Children with LD
25 Van Zant Street Suite 15-5
East Norwalk, CT 06855   203-838-5010
                               Fax: 203-866-6108

Common problems for students with ADHD are discussed and interventions offered. For use by teachers and knowledgeable parents.

14 pages

480 Helping Your Child with Attention-Deficit Hyperactivity Disorder
Learning Disabilities Association of America
4156 Library Road
Pittsburgh, PA 15234   412-341-1515

481 How to Own and Operate an Attention Deficit Disorder
Learning Disabilities Association of America
4156 Library Road
Pittsburgh, PA 15234   412-341-1515

Clear, informative and sensitive introduction to ADHD. Packed with practical things to do at home and school, the author offers her own insight being a professional and mother of a son with ADHD.

43 pages

482 Hyperactivity, Attention Deficits, and School Failure: Better Ways
Learning Disabilities Association of America
4156 Library Road
Pittsburgh, PA 15234   412-341-1515

483 Identification and Treatment of Attention Deficit Disorders
Nancy Nussbaum, author
Therapro, Inc.
225 Arlington Street
Framingham, MA 01701   508-872-9494
                               800-257-5376
                               Fax: 508-875-2062

This handbook contains information that is based on research and offers practical suggestions for parents, teachers and other professionals.

484 Learning Disability
Dale Brown, author
Connecticut Association for Children with LD
25 Van Zant Street Suite 15-5
East Norwalk, CT 06855   203-838-5010
                               Fax: 203-866-6108

Unsure social behavior means insecure sexual relationships.

4 pages

485 Management of Children and Adolescents with AD-HD
Friedman/Royal, author
Learning Disabilities Association of America
4156 Library Road
Pittsburgh, PA 15234   412-341-1515

486 Out of Darkness

Connecticut Association for Children with LD
25 Van Zant Street Suite 15-5
East Norwalk, CT 06855   203-838-5010
                               Fax: 203-866-6108

Article by an adult who discovers at age 30 that
he has ADD.

4 pages

487 Packet of ADHD Articles

Connecticut Association for Children with LD
25 Van Zant Street Suite 15-5
East Norwalk, CT 06855   203-838-5010
                               Fax: 203-866-6108

Contains reprints of seven newspapers and other
short articles which discuss various aspects of
ADHD including identification, medication and
other forms of therapy.

488 Parenting Attention Deficit Disordered Teens

Patricia C. Landi, LCSW, author

Connecticut Association for Children with LD
25 Van Zant Street Suite 15-5
East Norwalk, CT 06855   203-838-5010
                               Fax: 203-866-6108

Detailed outline of the various problems of adolescents with ADHD.

14 pages

**489 School Based Assessment of Attention Deficit
Disorders**

National Clearinghouse of Rehabilitation Materials
816 W. 6th St., Oklahoma State
Stillwater, OK 74078   405-624-7650
                              800-223-5219
                         Fax: 405-624-0695

The 1992 OSEP ruling, placing more responsibility on schools for the assessment of students who
may have attention deficit disorders, has raised
questions concerning the assessment process.
This guide was developed to help states formu-
late new policies. The paper seeks to: present an
overview of current thoughts concerning ADD
from an educational perspective, contrast traditional assessment strategies with an alternative
model, and describe phases of evaluation.

490 Understanding Hyperactivity

L. Ripley, author

Psychiatric Support Services, Inc.

Houston, TX   281-580-0046

Designed for parents and teachers, a video explaining the symptoms and consequences of attention deficit hyperactivity disorder.

Video

**491 What Every Parent Should Know About Learning
Diabilities**

C.L. Bete Co., author

Connecticut Association for Children with LD
25 Van Zant Street Suite 15-5
East Norwalk, CT 06855   203-838-5010
                               Fax: 203-866-6108

DESCRIPTION

492 AUTISTIC DISORDER
Synonyms: Infantile autism, Kanner's syndrome
Disorder Type: Developmental Milestones, Mental,
Emotional or Behavioral Disorder

Autistic disorder, also known as infantile autism, is a disorder that usually becomes apparent by three years of age. It is thought to affect approximately four in 10,000 children and is about three to four times more common in males than females. Autistic disorder is characterized by deficient verbal and nonverbal communication, impaired social interactions, and a restricted range of interests and activities.

Children with autistic disorder may fail to acquire or have poorly developed verbal and nonverbal communication skills. If children do communicate verbally, abnormal speech patterns are typically present, such as repetition of another's words or phrases (echolalia); reversal of the proper use of pronouns, such as use of the term you rather than I when referring to themselves; and nonsensical rhyming. In addition, affected children may be withdrawn, make little or no eye contact, resist cuddling, lack awareness of others' thoughts or feelings, or fail to seek comfort when distressed. Children also typically engage in solitary play for hours, perform ritualistic behaviors and repeated body movements (e.g., rocking, flicking fingers), also have a strong need for a predictable, consistent environment. Certain behaviors (e.g., rubbing an object or surface) may demonstrate a heightened awareness of particular stimuli, whereas others, such as a lack of reaction to sudden, loud noises, may indicate a lowered sensitivity to other stimuli. In many children with autistic disorder, disruptions of rituals or routines may result in tantrum-like outbursts or rages. In addition, some children may exhibit self-injurious or outwardly aggressive behaviors. Because of impairment of language and socialization skills, it may be difficult to obtain accurate estimates of overall intelligence levels and potential. Although such testing often demonstrates functional retardation, some affected children perform adequately in nonverbal areas, such as spatial and motor skills, and those with speech skills may perform adequately in all test areas.

In most patients, the symptoms and findings associated with autistic disorder continue to affect them throughout life. In severe cases, therapy with certain medications (e.g., neuroleptics, potent opiate antagonists, etc.) may reduce social withdrawal and stereotypical, self-injurious, or aggressive behaviors. In addition, the management and treatment of affected children may include integrated, multidisciplinary techniques, such as language therapy, structured play and interpersonal exercises, and other behavioral therapies. Some patients, particularly those with speech development, may lead somewhat independent lives with proper support. However, other individuals with autistic disorder may require special, ongoing care.

The cause of autistic disorder is unknown. However, according to the medical literature, several underlying neurologic, infectious, and other disorders are known to produce or to increase a predisposition toward autistic-like behaviors in children. Genetic abnormalities are also thought to play some role in causing or resulting in susceptibility for the disorder. For example, some researchers theorize that autistic disorder may result from certain brain abnormalities during infancy (e.g., particular biochemical abnormalities, brain injury, etc.), potentially in combination with a genetic predisposition for the condition (multifactorial).

The following organizations in the General Resources Section can provide additional information: March of Dimes Birth Defects Foundation, National Mental Health Association, NIH/National Insitute of Neurological Disorder & Stroke, Genetic Alliance, Federation of Families for Children's Mental Heatlh, National Mental Health Consumer Self-Help Clearinghouse, Online Mendelian Inheritance in Man.: www3.ncbi.nlm.nih.gov/Omim/searchomim.html

National Associations & Support Groups

493 ARRISE, Inc.
9238 Parklane Ave
Franklin Park, IL 60131   847-451-2740

Provides information about autism.

494 Autism Network International
P.O. Box 448
Syracuse, NY 13210   315-476-2462
e-mail: jisincla#mailbox.syr.edu

Supported by in individuals, who want to make a difference for the sufferes, the foundation provides a variety of support and educational references to inform on the latest changes in the field.

495 Autism Network for Hearing and Visually Impaired Persons
7510 Ocean Front Avenue
Virginia Beach, VA 23451   757-428-9036

496 Autism Research Institute
4182 Adams Avenue
San Diego, CA 92116   619-281-7165
Fax: 619-563-6840
www.autism.com/autism

A resource center for information on autism and related disorders. Conducts research and compiles research findings to provide parents and professionals with the latest research available. Provides information at no cost or low cost. Specialty is evaluation of biomedical and psychoeducational treatment options. Publishes quarterly newsletter.

Dr. Bernard Rimland, Director

497 Autism Services Center
605 9th St., P.O. Box 507
Huntington, WV 25710   304-525-8014
Fax: 304-525-8026

Provides educational information to the public and professional communities on autism, provides case management activities and referrals for persons afflicted with autism and their families.

498 Autism Society of America
7910 Woodmont Avenue, Ste. 650
Bethesda, MD 20814   301-657-0881
800-328-8476
Fax: 301-657-0869
www.autism-society.org/

A national charitable organization with the mission of providing as much information as possible about autism and the various options, approaches, methods and systems available to parents of children with autism, family members and those professionals who work with them.

Veronica Zysk, Executive Director

499 C.A.N.D.L.E.
4414 McCampbell Drive
Montgomery, AL 36106   334-271-3947
Fax: 334-271-3947

500 Center for Study of Autism
P.O. Box 4538
Salem, OR 97005   503-363-9110
Fax: 503-363-9110
e-mail: autism@euphora.com
www.autism.org/

501 Children and Adults with Autism
Autism Society of America
7910 Woodmont Ave, Ste 650
Bethesda, MD 20814   301-657-0881
800-328-8476

The Autism Society of America (ASA) is a charitable organization with the mission of providing as much information as possible about autism and about the various options, approaches, methods and systems available to parents of autistic children, family members, and those professionals who work with them. ASA also advocates for the rights and needs of autistic individuals and their families.

502 Community Services for People with Autism
751 Twinbrook Parkway
Rockville, MD 20851   301-762-1650

503 Facilitated Learning at Syracuse University
307 Huntington Hall
Syracuse, NY 13244   315-443-1870

College offering facilitated learning research into communication with persons who have autism or severe disabilities. Offers books, videos and public awareness information on the research projects.

504 More Advanced Autistic People
P.O. Box 524
Crown Point, IN 46307   219-662-1311
Fax: 219-662-0638
e-mail: chart@netnitco.net

505 National Autism Hotline/Autism Services Center
605 Ninth St, Prichard Bldg
Huntington, WV 25710   304-525-8014
                             Fax: 304-525-8026

506 National Autistic Society
276 Willesden Lane
London, NW2- 5RB   UK,   181-451-1114
                       e-mail: nas@nas.org.uk
                       www.oneworld.org/autism_uk/

Promotes the well being of affected persons
through the assistance of fellow sufferers and
families.

**507 National Institute on Deafness and Other
Communication Disorders Info.**
1 Communication Avenue
Bethesda, MD 20892   301-907-8830
                   e-mail: nidcdinfo@nidcd.nih.gov
                       www.nih.gov/nidcd/

Conducts and supports biomedical research and
research training on normal mechanisms, as
well as diseases and disorders of hearing, balance, smell, taste, voice, speedh and language.

508 Society for Autistic Children
NYS Society for Autistic Children
879 Madison Ave
Albany, NY 12208   518-459-1418

An organization of people concerned about the
welfare of children with severe disorders of communication and behavior. Provides a directory
of services and programs for autistic children.

509 Son-Rise Program
Option Institute
2080 South Undermountain Road
Sheffield, MA 01257   413-229-2100
                            800-714-2779
                       Fax: 413-229-5030
                  e-mail: sonrise@option.org
                          www.son-rise.org

The Son-Rise Program is an effective, loving,
and respectful method for treating children with
autism. It teaches parents and healing professionals how to set up a home based program using the child's motivation to reach their special
child. It is based on the program Barry and
Samahria Kaufman developed to heal their own
once autistic son as described in the book, son-
Rise: The Miracle Continues by Barry Neil Kaufman.

Gretchen Pfuetze, Director

Libraries & Resource Centers

Georgia

510 Emory Autism Resource Center
Emory University
718 Gatewood Road
Atlanta, GA 30322   404-727-3360
                       Fax: 404-727-8350

Offers on-line bulletin boards which are relevant to autism.

Indiana

511 Indiana Resource Center for Autism
Inst. for the Study of Developmental Disabilities
2853 East Tenth Street
Bloomington, IN 47408   812-855-6508

Michigan

512 Burger School for the Autistic
30922 Beechwood Street
Garden City, MI 48135   734-425-5660

Montana

513 Judevine Center for Autism
9455 Rott Road
St. Louis, MO 63127   314-849-4440

New Jersey

**514 New Jersey Center for Outreach and Services for
the Autism Community(COSAC)**
1450 Parkside Avenue-Suite 22
Ewing, NJ 08638   609-883-8100
                            800-428-8476
                       Fax: 609-883-5509
                  e-mail: njautism@aol.com
                  www.members.aol.com/njautism

Purpose is to assist families, individuals and
agencies concerned with the welfare and education of children and adults with autism and pervasive development disorder not otherwise
specified.

Paul A. Potito, Executive Director

New York

515 Institute for Basic Research in Developmental Disabilities
1050 Forest Hill Road
Staten Island, NY 10314   718-494-0600
                                           Fax: 718-494-0837

516 State University of New York Health Sciences Center
450 Clarkson Avenue, Box 32
Brooklyn, NY 11203   718-778-5332
                                          Fax: 718-778-5397

Child psychiatry research programs.

Adolf Christ, Director

North Carolina

517 Autism Society of North Carolina
Autism Society of North Carolina Bookstore
505 Oberlin Road, Suite 230
Raleigh, NC 27605   919-571-0204
                                          800-442-2762
                                          Fax: 919-743-0208
                                          e-mail: ASNC@aol.com

Offers a library that carries one of the largest selections of books about autism.

518 University of North Carolina at Chapel Hill, Brain Research Center
CB 7250
Chapel Hill, NC 27599   919-966-2405
                                          Fax: 919-966-1844

Kunihiko Suzuki, MD, Director

West Virginia

519 Autism Services Center
605 9th Street, P.O. Box 507
Huntington, WV 25710   304-525-8014

Works to improve appropriate and professional training, advocacy, consulting and information by individuals responsible for the welfare and care of autistic individuals and others with developmental disabilities.

Ruth Christ Sullivan, Director

520 Autism Training Center
Marshall University
400 Hal Greer Blvd.
Huntington, WV 25755   304-696-3640
                                          800-344-5115

Research Centers

521 Center for Neurodevelopmental Studies
5430 W Glenn Drive
Glendale, AZ 85301   623-915-0345
                                          Fax: 623-937-5425

Researches effective treatment methods for autism and developmental disabilities.

Lorna Jean King, Director, Emeritus

522 National Alliance for Autism Research
414 Wall Street
Princeton, NJ 08648   609-430-9160
                                          888-777-6227
                                          Fax: 609-430-9163
                                          e-mail: naar@naar.org
                                          www.naar.org

Audio Video

523 Autism
Fanlight Productions
47 Halifax St
Boston, MA 02130   617-469-4911
                                          Fax: 617-469-3379
                                          e-mail: fanlight@fanligt.com
                                          www.fanlight.com

Dartmouth-Hitchcock Medical Center
28 Minutes

524 Autism: A World Apart
Karen Cunninghame, author

Fanlight Productions
47 Halifax St
Boston, MA 02130   617-469-4999
                                          Fax: 617-469-3379
                                          e-mail: fanlight@tiac.net
                                          www.fanlight.com

In this documentary, three families show us what the textbooks and studies cannot, what it's like to live with autism day after day, raise and love children who may be withdrawn and violent and unable to make personal connections with their families.

29 minutes
ISBN: 1-572950-39-0

525 Getting Started with Facilitated Communication
Syracuse University, Institute on Communication
805 South Krouse
Syracuse, NY 13244   315-443-2693

Describes in detail how to help individuals with autism and/or severe communication difficulties to get started with facilitated communication.

Videotape

526 Going to School with Facilitated Communication
D. Biklen, author

Syracuse University, School of Education
805 South Krouse
Syracuse, NY 13244   315-443-2693

A video in which students with autism and/or severe disabilities illustrate the use of facilitated communication focusing on basic principles fostering facilitated communication.

Videotape

527 Understanding Autism
Fanlight Productions
47 Halifax Street
Boston, MA 02131   617-469-4999
                          Fax: 617-524-8838
                          e-mail: fanlight@tiac.net
                          www.fanlight.com

Parents of children with autism discuss the nature and symptoms of this lifelong disability, and outlines a treatment program based on behavior modification principles.

19 Minutes
ISBN: 1-572951-00-1

Web Sites

528 Autism FAQ
web.syr.edu/~jmwobus/autism/autism.faq.html

529 Autism Network for Dietary Intervention
members.aol.com/AutismNDI/PAGES/link.htm

530 Autism Resources
http://web.syr.edu/!jmwobus/autism/

531 Center for the Study of Autism
www.autism.org/

532 University Students with Autism and Asperger's Syndrome Web Site
www.users.dircon.co.uk/~cns/index.html
                e-mail: cns@dircon.co.uk
        www.users.dircon.co.uk/~cns/index.html

Books

533 Activities for Developing Pre-Skill Concepts in Children with Autism
Toni Flowers, author

Autism Society of North Carolina Bookstore
505 Oberlin Road, Suite 230
Raleigh, NC 27605   919-743-0204
                          800-442-2762
                          Fax: 919-743-0208
                          e-mail: ASNC@aol.com
                          www.autismsociety-nc.org

Chapters include auditory development, concept development, social development and visual-motor integration.

1987

534 Aspects of Autism - Biological Research
Lorna Wing, author

Autism Society of North Carolina Bookstore
505 Oberlin Road, Suite 230
Raleigh, NC 27605   919-743-0204
                          800-442-2762
                          Fax: 919-743-0208
                          e-mail: ASNC@aol.com
                          www.autismsociety-nc.org

Reviews the evidence for a physical cause of autism and the roles of genetics, magnesium and vitamin B6.

1988

535 Autism
Richard L. Simpson and Paul Zionts, author

Autism Society of North Carolina Bookstore
505 Oberlin Road, Suite 230
Raleigh, NC 27605   919-743-0204
                          800-442-2762
                          Fax: 919-743-0208
                          e-mail: ASNC@aol.com
                          www.autismsociety-nc.org

In a question-and-answer format, the authors respond to questions about autism asked by countless parents and family members of children and youths with autism.

1992

536 Autism Treatment Guide
Elizabeth K. Gerlach, author

Autism Society of North Carolina Bookstore
505 Oberlin Road, Suite 230
Raleigh, NC 27605   919-743-0204
                          800-442-2762
                          Fax: 919-743-0208
                          e-mail: ASNC@aol.com
                          www.autismsociety-nc.org

A comprehensive book covering treatments and methods used to help individuals with autism.

1993

537 Autism and Learning

Ed. Stuart Powell and Rita Jordan, author

David Fulton Publishers
2 Barbon Close, Great Ormond Street
London, WCIN   171-405-5606
                                Fax: 171-831-4840

This book is about how a cognitive perception on the way in which individuals with autism think and learn may be applied to particular curriculum areas.

March 1997 160 pages Softcover
ISBN: 1-853464-21-X

538 Autism and the Family:Problems, Prospects, and Coping with the Disorder

David E. Gray, author

Charles C. Thomas Publishing, Ltd.
2600 South First Street
Springfield, IL 62704   217-789-8980
                                     800-258-8980
                                Fax: 217-789-9130
               e-mail: books@ccthomas.com
                          www.ccthomas.com

Examination of certain issues such as stress, coping, stigma. Contains 33 interviews with parents whose children attended an autistic treatmet center. An excellent resource text.

210 pages Softcover
ISBN: 0-398068-42-9

539 Autism in Adolescents and Adults

Autism Society of North Carolina Bookstore
505 Oberlin Road, Suite 230
Raleigh, NC 27605   919-743-0204
                                     800-442-2762
                                Fax: 919-743-0208
                  e-mail: ASNC@aol.com
                      www.autismsociety-nc.org

A survey of the needs, problems and services for autistic adolescents and adults.

1983

Eric Schopler, Editor
Schopler Gary, Mesibov

540 Autism in Adolescents and Adults

Plenum Press
233 Spring Street
New York, NY 10013   212-620-8000
                                Fax: 212-463-0742
                  e-mail: info@plenum.com

1983 456 pages
ISBN: 0-306410-57-5

541 Autism...Nature, Diagnosis and Treatment

Geraldine Dawson, author

Autism Society of North Carolina Bookstore
505 Oberlin Road, Suite 230
Raleigh, NC 27605   919-743-0204
                                     800-442-2762
                                Fax: 919-743-0208
                  e-mail: ASNC@aol.com
                      www.autismsociety-nc.org

Covers perspectives, issues, neurobiological issues and new directions in diagnosis and treatment.

1989

542 Autism: A Strange, Silent World

Filmakers Library
124 East 40th Street
New York, NY 10016   212-808-4980

British educators and medical personnel offer insight into autism's characteristics and treatment approaches through the cameos of three children.

543 Autism: Explaining the Enigma

Uta Firth, author

Autism Society of North Carolina Bookstore
505 Oberlin Road, Suite 230
Raleigh, NC 27605   919-743-0204
                                     800-442-2762
                                Fax: 919-743-0208
                  e-mail: ASNC@aol.com
                      www.autismsociety-nc.org

Explains the nature of autism.

544 Autism: From Tragedy to Triumph

Carol Johnson & Julia Crowder, author

Branden Publishing Company, Inc.
17 Station Street Box 843
Brookline Village, MA 02447   617-734-2045
                                Fax: 617-734-2046
               e-mail: branden@branden.com
                          www.branden.com

A new book that deals with the Lovaas method and includes a foreward by Dr. Ivar Lovaas. The book is broken down into two parts — the long road to diagnosis and then treatment.

1994 192 pages
ISBN: 0-828319-65-0

Adolph Caso, Editor

545 Autism: Identification, Education and Treatment

Dianne Berkell, author

Autism Society of North Carolina Bookstore
505 Oberlin Road, Suite 230
Raleigh, NC 27605   919-743-0204
                          800-442-2762
                    Fax: 919-743-0208
                    e-mail: ASNC@aol.com
                    www.autismsociety-nc.org

Chapters include medical treatments, early intervention and communication development in autism.

1992

546 Autism: Information and Resources for Parents, Families, and Professionals

Richard L. Simpson, Paul Zionts, author

Pro-Ed
8700 Shoal Creek Boulevard
Austin, TX 78757   512-451-3246
                          800-897-3202
                    Fax: 512-451-8542
                    www.proedinc.com

Addresses the frustation and concern of parents and family members by answering questions about autism and summarizing what is known.

188 pages Softcover
ISBN: 0-890795-38-X

547 Autism: The Facts

Simon Baron-Cohen, author

Oxford University Press
2001 Evans Road
Cary, NC 27513   212-726-6000
                          800-451-7556
                    Fax: 212-726-6447
                    www.oup-usa.org

Contains valuable information for families and those inflicted with this condition.

1993 128 pages
ISBN: 0-192623-28-1

548 Autistic Children

Lorna Wing, author

Autism Society of North Carolina Bookstore
505 Oberlin Road, Suite 230
Raleigh, NC 27605   919-743-0204
                          800-442-2762
                    Fax: 919-743-0208
                    e-mail: ASNC@aol.com
                    www.autismsociety-nc.org

An excellent publication for new parents and professionals.

Softcover

549 Behavioral Intervention for Young Children with Autism

Pro-Ed
8700 Shoal Creek Boulevard
Austin, TX 78757   512-451-3246
                          800-897-3202
                    Fax: 512-451-8542
                    www.proedinc.com

This manual, inspired by research which shows benefits from early intervention based on the principles of Applied Behavior Analysis gives concrete information on how to differentiate between fads and scientifically validated interventions.

400 pages
ISBN: 0-890796-83-1

Catherine Maurice, Editor
Gina Green, Co-Editor

550 Beyond Gentle Teaching

John J. McGee & Frank J. Manolascino, author

Autism Society of North Carolina Bookstore
505 Oberlin Road, Suite 230
Raleigh, NC 27605   919-743-0204
                          800-442-2762
                    Fax: 919-743-0208
                    e-mail: ASNC@aol.com
                    www.autismsociety-nc.org

A nonaversive approach to helping those in need, caregivers.

1991

551 Biology of the Autistic Syndromes

Christopher Gillberg & Mary Coleman, author

Autism Society of North Carolina Bookstore
505 Oberlin Road, Suite 230
Raleigh, NC 27605   919-743-0204
                          800-442-2762
                    Fax: 919-743-0208
                    e-mail: ASNC@aol.com
                    www.autismsociety-nc.org

A revision of the original, classic text in the light of new developments and current knowledge. This book covers the epidemiological, genetic, biochemical, immunological and neuropsychological literature on autism.

1992

552 Breakthroughs: How to Reach Students with Autism

Karen Sewell, author

Pro-Ed
8700 Shoal Creek Boulevard
Austin, TX 78757   512-451-3246
                                800-897-3202
                        Fax: 512-451-8542
                        www.proedinc.com

Hands-on approach for teachers of students with autism: suggestions, activities, materials, lesson plans and closed captioned video.

243 pages manual & video

553 Children with Autism

Michael D. Powers Ph.D, author

Woodbine House
6510 Bells Mill Road
Bethesda, MD 20817   301-468-8800
                             800-843-7323
                     Fax: 301-897-5838
        e-mail: info@woodbinehouse.com
                www.woodbinehouse.com

Recommended as the first book parents should read, this volume offers information and a complete introduction to autism, while easing the family's fears and concerns as they adjust and cope with their child's disorder. New edition covers early intervention, educational programs, and more, plus provides a look at the years ahead with a chapter on adults with autism.

1989 368 pages Softcover
ISBN: 0-933149-16-6

554 Children with Autism: A Guide for Practitioners and Carers

Patricia Howlin, author

John Wiley & Sons, INC.
605 Third Avenue
New York, NY 10158   212-850-6000
                     Fax: 212-850-6088
                        www.wiley.com

Covers the disorders of autism, understanding the causes and the different approaches of treatment for autistic children.

342 pages
ISBN: 0-471983-28-4

555 Developmental Delay Resources (DDR)
4401 East West Highway, Suite 207
Bethesda, MD 20814   301-652-2263
                        Fax: 301-652-9133
        e-mail: devdelay@mindspring.com
                    www.devdelay.org

Patricia Lemer, Executive Director

556 Developmental Therapy for Young Children with Autistic Characterisics
8700 Shoal Creek Blvd.
Austin, TX 78757
                                800-897-3202
                        Fax: 800-397-7633

This methods book for teachers and parents describes a complete program of developmental therapy for young children with autistic characteristics. It includes samples of techniques and materials, routines and environments, activity periods, learning experiences, and home programs designed specifically for the young child with autism functioning developmentally from birth to 3 years.

185 pages Large Format
ISBN: 0-890795-87-8

557 Diagnosis and Treatment of Autism

Christopher Gillberg, Et Al., author

Autism Society of North Carolina Bookstore
505 Oberlin Road, Suite 230
Raleigh, NC 27605   919-743-0204
                             800-442-2762
                     Fax: 919-743-0208
            e-mail: ASNC@aol.com
                www.autismsociety-nc.org

Various chapters written by professionals working with autistic children and adults.

1989

558 Educating Children and Youth with Autism

Richard L. Smith, Brenda Smith Myles, Editors, author

Pro-Ed
8700 Shoal Creek Boulevard
Austin, TX 78757   512-451-3246
                                800-897-3202
                        Fax: 512-451-8542
                        www.proedinc.com

A best-practices text that explains and critiques a number of approaches to autism in children with information based on current research literature and the authors' personal expertise.

360 pages
ISBN: 0-890797-43-9

559 Effective Teaching Methods for Autistic Children

Rosalind C. Oppenheim, author

Charles C. Thomas Publishing, Ltd.
2600 South First Street
Springfield, IL 62704   217-789-8980
800-258-8980
Fax: 217-789-9130
e-mail: books@ccthomas.com
www.ccthomas.com

124 pages $20.95 paper
ISBN: 0-398028-58-3

560 Facilitated Communication: The Clinical Social Phenomenon

Howard C. Shane, author

Autism Society of North Carolina Bookstore
505 Oberlin Road, Suite 230
Raleigh, NC 27605   919-571-8555
800-442-2762
Fax: 919-743-0208
e-mail: ASNC@aol.com

561 Fragile Success - Nine Autistic Children, Childhood to Adulthood

Virginia Walker Sperry, author

Autism Society of North Carolina Bookstore
505 Oberlin Road, Suite 230
Raleigh, NC 27605   919-743-0204
800-442-2762
Fax: 919-743-0208
e-mail: ASNC@aol.com
www.autismsociety-nc.org

A book about the lives of autistic children, whom the author has followed from their early years at the Elizabeth Ives School in New Haven, CT, through to adulthood.

562 Handbook of Autism and Pervasive Developmental Disorders

Donald J. Cohen, author

Autism Society of North Carolina Bookstore
505 Oberlin Road, Suite 230
Raleigh, NC 27605   919-743-0204
800-442-2762
Fax: 919-743-0208
e-mail: ASNC@aol.com
www.autismsociety-nc.org

A list of contributors address such topics as characteristics of autistic syndromes and interventions.

1987

563 Hidden Child: The Linwood Method for Reaching the Autistic Child

Jeanne Simons and Sabine Oishi, Ph.D, author

Woodbine House
6510 Bells Mill Road
Bethesda, MD 20817   301-468-8800
800-843-7323
Fax: 301-897-5838
e-mail: info@woodbinehouse.com
www.woodbinehouse.com

Chronicle of the Linwood Children's Center's successful treatment program for autistic children.

286 pages Softcover
ISBN: 0-933149-06-9

564 Higher Functioning Adolescents and Young Adults with Autism

Fullerton, Stratton, Coyne, Gray, author

Pro-Ed
8700 Shoal Creek Boulevard
Austin, TX 78757   512-451-3246
800-897-3202
Fax: 512-451-8542
www.proedinc.com

Practical strategies for teaching and supporting higher functioning students with autism, elementary school through college situations.

96 pages
ISBN: 0-890796-81-5

565 How to Teach Autistic & Severely Handicapped Children

Robert L. Koegel, author

Autism Society of North Carolina Bookstore
505 Oberlin Road, Suite 230
Raleigh, NC 27605   919-743-0204
800-442-2762
Fax: 919-743-0208
e-mail: ASNC@aol.com
www.autismsociety-nc.org

Book provides procedures for effectively assessing and teaching autistic and other severely handicapped children.

1981

566 Keys to Parenting the Child with Autism

Marlene Targ Brill, author

Autism Society of North Carolina Bookstore
505 Oberlin Road, Suite 230
Raleigh, NC 27605   919-743-0204
800-442-2762
Fax: 919-743-0208
e-mail: ASNC@aol.com
www.autismsociety-nc.org

This book explains what autism is and how it is diagnosed.

1994

567 Let Me Hear Your Voice

Catherine Maurice, author

Autism Society of North Carolina Bookstore
505 Oberlin Road, Suite 230
Raleigh, NC 27605   919-743-0204
                                 800-442-2762
                            Fax: 919-743-0208
                       e-mail: ASNC@aol.com
                       www.autismsociety-nc.org

The Maurice family's second and third child were diagnosed with autism. This book recounts their experience with a home program using behavior therapy.

1993

568 Management of Autistic Behavior

Richard L. Simpson and Madelyn Regan, author

Pro-Ed
8700 Shoal Creek Boulevard
Austin, TX 78758   512-451-3246
                            Fax: 512-451-8542

Comprehensive and practical book that tells what works best with specific problems.

450 pages Softcover
ISBN: 0-890791-96-1

569 Mindblindness: An Essay on Autism & Theory of Mind

Simon Baron-Cohen, author

MIT Press
55 Hayward Street
Cambridge, MA 02142   617-253-5646
                            Fax: 617-258-6779

1995 300 pages
ISBN: 0-262023-84-9

570 Miracle Continues

Barry Kaufman, author

Option Institute
2080 South Undermountain Road
Sheffield, MA 01257   413-229-2100
                                 800-714-2779
                            Fax: 413-229-5030
                  e-mail: sonrise@option.org
                          www.son-rise.org

Describes an effective, loving, and respectful method for treating children with autism. It teaches parents and healing professionals how to set up a home based program using the child's motivation to reach their special child.

1994 372 pages
ISBN: 0-915811-61-8

571 Mixed Blessings

William Christopher, author

Autism Society of North Carolina Bookstore
505 Oberlin Road, Suite 230
Raleigh, NC 27605   919-743-0204
                                 800-442-2762
                            Fax: 919-743-0208
                       e-mail: ASNC@aol.com
                       www.autismsociety-nc.org

A real-life family discusses the raising of their autistic son.

572 More Laughing and Loving with Autism

R. Wayne Gilpin, author

Autism Society of North Carolina Bookstore
505 Oberlin Road, Suite 230
Raleigh, NC 27605   919-743-0204
                                 800-442-2762
                            Fax: 919-743-0208
                       e-mail: ASNC@aol.com
                       www.autismsociety-nc.org

A collection of warm and humorous parent stories about raising a child with autism.

1994

573 Neurobiology of Autism

M. L. Bauman, MD & T. L. Kemper, MD, Editors, author

Johns Hopkins University Press
2715 North Charles Street
Baltimore, MD 21218   410-516-6936
                                 800-537-5487
                            Fax: 410-516-6998
                          www.press.jhu.edu

This book brings together leading investigators from the field of autism to discuss advances in scientific research that point to a neurobiological basis for autism and to examine the clinical implications of the research.

272 pages
ISBN: 0-801856-80-9

574 News From the Border: A Mother's Memoir of Her Autistic Son

Jane Taylor McDonnell, author

Houghton Mifflin Company/Order Processing
222 Berkeley St
Boston, MA 02116   617-351-3698
                         800-225-3362

A searingly honest account of the author's family experiences with autism. Raising an autistic child is the central, ongoing drama of her married life and this riveting account of acceptance and coping.

1993 384 pages Cloth

575 Parent Survival Manual

Eric Shopler, author

Autism Society of North Carolina Bookstore
505 Oberlin Road, Suite 230
Raleigh, NC 27605   919-743-0204
                          800-442-2762
                    Fax: 919-743-0208
              e-mail: ASNC@aol.com
              www.autismsociety-nc.org

Compiled from 350 anecdotes told by parents of autistic and developmentally disabled children.

576 Parent's Guide to Autism

Charles A. Hart, author

Autism Society of North Carolina Bookstore
505 Oberlin Road, Suite 230
Raleigh, NC 27605   919-743-0204
                          800-442-2762
                    Fax: 919-743-0208
              e-mail: ASNC@aol.com
              www.autismsociety-nc.org

An essential handbook for anyone facing autism.

577 Preschool Education Programs for Children with Autism

8700 Shoal Creek Blvd.
Austin, TX 78757
                          800-897-3202
                    Fax: 800-397-7633

Written for special education teachers, school administrators, child-study team members, psychologists, speech therapists, and advocates and parents who are concerned about the education of preschool-age children with autism. It will be especially helpful to persons who are considering creating a classroom to serve these children or persons interested in ensuring that the services they currently offer meet state-of-the-art criteria.

252 pages Softcover
ISBN: 0-890795-87-8

578 Psychoeducational Profile — Revised Vol.1

Schopler, Reichler, Bashford, Lansing & Marcus, author

Autism Society of North Carolina Bookstore
505 Oberlin Road, Suite 230
Raleigh, NC 27605   919-743-0204
                          800-442-2762
                    Fax: 919-743-0208
              e-mail: ASNC@aol.com
              www.autismsociety-nc.org

The PEP-R is a revision of the popular instrument that has been used for over 20 years to assess skills and behavior of autistic and communication-handicapped children who function between the ages of 6 months and 7 years.

1995

579 Reaching the Autistic Child A Parent Training Program

Martin Kozloff, author

Brookline Books/Lumen Editions
P.O. Box 1047
Cambridge, MA 02238   617-868-0360
                            800-666-2665
                      Fax: 617-868-1772
            e-mail: brooklinebks@delphi.com
            www.people.delphi.com/brooklinebks

Detailed case studies of social and behavioral change in autistic children and their families show parents how to implement the principles for improved socialization and behavior.

Feb 1998 Softcover
ISBN· 1-571290-56-7

580 Record Book for Individuals with Autism

Nancy Dalrymple, author

Autism Society of North Carolina Bookstore
505 Oberlin Road, Suite 230
Raleigh, NC 27605   919-743-0204
                          800-442-2762
                    Fax: 919-743-0208
              e-mail: ASNC@aol.com
              www.autismsociety-nc.org

Developed with parent input to provide one place to keep information about an autistic child.

1990

581 Riddle of Autism: A Psychological Analysis

George Victor, author

Jason Aronson, Inc.
400 Keystone Industrial Park
Dunmore, PA 18512
                          800-782-0015
                    Fax: 201-840-7242
                    www.aronson.com

Dr. Victor examines the myths that cloud an understanding of this disorder and describes the meanings of its specific behavioral symptoms.

356 pages Softcover
ISBN: 1-568215-73-8

582 Siblings of Children with Autism: A Guide for Families

Sandra Harris, author

Autism Society of North Carolina Bookstore
505 Oberlin Road, Suite 230
Raleigh, NC 27605   919-743-0204
                                 800-442-2762
                            Fax: 919-743-0208
                        e-mail: ASNC@aol.com
                        www.autismsociety-nc.org

Offers information on the needs of a child with autism.

1994

583 Teach Me Language

Sabrina Freeman, Ph.D. and Lorelei Dake, B.A., author

Autism Society of North Carolina Bookstore
505 Oberlin Road, Suite 230
Raleigh, NC 27605   919-571-8555
                                 800-442-2762
                            Fax: 919-743-0208
                        e-mail: ASNC@aol.com

584 Teaching Children with Autism

Tobert L. Koegel and Lynn Kern Koegel, author

Books on Special Children
P.O. Box 305
Congers, NY 10920   914-638-1236
                            Fax: 914-638-0847

Contributions from people in the field regarding communication and language use. Support for families, parent education, school placement, IEP process and other topics relating to many levels of abilites of child. Good book to help understand symptoms and intervention for improving skills in autistic children.

1995 236 pages Softcover
ISBN: 4-557661-80-4

585 Teaching Children with Autism - Strategies to Enhance Communication

Kathleen Ann Quill, EdD, author

Autism Society of North Carolina Bookstore
505 Oberlin Road, Suite 230
Raleigh, NC 27605   919-743-0204
                                 800-442-2762
                            Fax: 919-743-0208
                        e-mail: ASNC@aol.com
                        www.autismsociety-nc.org

This valuable new book describes teaching strategies and instructional adaptations which promote communication and socialization in children with autism.

586 Teaching Children with Autism to Mind- Read: A Pratical Guide

Simon Baron-Cohen and Patricia Howlin, author

John Wiley & Sons, INC.
605 Third Avenue
New York, NY 10158   212-850-6000
                            Fax: 212-850-6088
                               www.wiley.com

This book explains the Theory of Mind, which is the ability to infer other's mental states and then interpret their speech and actions based onthis information. The author applies this theory to autistic children to help their social and communicative abnormalities.

336 pages
ISBN: 0-471976-23-7

587 Teaching Spontaneous Communication to Autistic and Developmentally Handicapped

Watson, Lord, Schaffer, Schopler, author

Pro-Ed
8700 Shoal Creek Boulevard
Austin, TX 78757   512-451-3246
                                 800-897-3202
                            Fax: 512-451-8542
                             www.proedinc.com

This book presents a communication curriculum designed to provide methods for assessing and teaching communication skills to students with autism and related disorders and is specially designed for children who have language skills ranging from a few words to simple sentences.

139 pages Lg Format
ISBN: 0-890795-28-2

588 Teaching and Mainstreaming Autistic Children

Peter Knoblock, author

Love Publishing Company
9101 E. Kinyon Avenue
Denver, CO 80237   303-221-7333
                            Fax: 303-221-7444

Dr. Knoblock advocates a highly organized, structured environment for autistic children, with teachers and parents working together. His premise is that the learning and social needs of autistic children must be analyzed and a daily program be designed with interventions that respond to this functional analysis of their behavior.

ISBN: 0-891081-11-9

589 Ultimate Stranger: The Autistic Child

Carl Delacato, author

Autism Society of North Carolina Bookstore
505 Oberlin Road, Suite 230
Raleigh, NC 27605   919-743-0204
        800-442-2762
      Fax: 919-743-0208
      e-mail: ASNC@aol.com
      www.autismsociety-nc.org

Delacato's thesis is that autism is neuro-genic and not psycho-genic in origin.

1974

590 Understanding and Treating Children with Autism

Rita Jordan and Stuart Powell, author

John Wiley & Sons, INC.
695 Third Avenue
New York, NY 10158   212-850-6000
      Fax: 212-850-6088
      www.wiley.com

188 pages
ISBN: 0-471958-88-3

591 Understanding the Nature of Autism

Jan Janzen, M.S. Ph.D. and Lorelei Dake, B.A., author

Autism Society of North Carolina Bookstore
505 Oberlin Road, Suite 230
Raleigh, NC 27605   919-571-0204
      800-442-2762
      Fax: 919-743-0208
      e-mail: ASNC@aol.com

592 Until Tomorrow: A Family Lives with Autism

Dorothy Zietz, author

Autism Society of North Carolina Bookstore
505 Oberlin Road, Suite 230
Raleigh, NC 27605   919-743-0204
      800-442-2762
      Fax: 919-743-0208
      e-mail: ASNC@aol.com
      www.autismsociety-nc.org

The central theme of this book is an effort to show what it is like to live with a child who cannot communicate.

1988

593 Visually Structured Tasks

Autism Society of North Carolina Bookstore
505 Oberlin Road, Suite 230
Raleigh, NC 27605   919-571-8555
      800-442-2762
      Fax: 919-743-0208
      e-mail: ASNC@aol.com

Independent activites for students with autism and other visual learners.

594 Winter's Flower

Ranae Johnson, author

Autism Society of North Carolina Bookstore
505 Oberlin Road, Suite 230
Raleigh, NC 27605   919-743-0204
      800-442-2762
      Fax: 919-743-0208
      e-mail: ASNC@aol.com
      www.autismsociety-nc.org

The story of Ranae Johnson's quest to rescue her son from a world of silence. A story of love, patience and dedication.

1992

595 World of the Autistic Child Autism & Prevention Development

Bryne Siegal, author

Oxford University Press
2001 Evans Road
Cary, NC 27513   212-726-6000
      800-451-7556
      Fax: 212-726-6447
      www.oup-usa.org

1995 320 pages
ISBN: 0-195076-67-2

Children's Books

596 Joey and Sam

Illana Katz and Edward Ritvo, author

Autism Society of North Carolina Bookstore
505 Oberlin Road, Suite 230
Raleigh, NC 27605   919-743-0204
      800-442-2762
      Fax: 919-743-0208
      e-mail: ASNC@aol.com
      www.autismsociety-nc.org

A beautifully illustrated storybook for children, focusing on a family with two sons, one of whom suffers from autism.

1993 Softcover

597 Russell Is Extra Special

Charles Amenta, III, author

Autism Society of North Carolina Bookstore
505 Oberlin Road, Suite 230
Raleigh, NC 27605   919-743-0204
                                            800-442-2762
                                      Fax: 919-743-0208
                                  e-mail: ASNC@aol.com
                                  www.autismsociety-nc.org

A sensitive portrayal of an autistic boy written by his father.

1992 Hardbound

598 Wild Boy of Aveyron

Harlan Lane, author

Autism Society of North Carolina Bookstore
505 Oberlin Road, Suite 230
Raleigh, NC 27605   919-743-0204
                                            800-442-2762
                                      Fax: 919-743-0208
                                  e-mail: ASNC@aol.com
                                  www.autismsociety-nc.org

Journals

599 Focus on Autism and Other Developmental Disabilities

8700 Shoal Creek Blvd.
Austin, TX 78757

                                            800-897-3202
                                      Fax: 800-397-7633

Practical elements of management, treatment, planning, and education for persons with autism or other pervasive developmental disabilities. Published quarterly, Focus publishes articles representing diverse philosophical and theoretical positions and reflecting a wide range of disciplines, including education, psychology, psychiatry, medicine, physical therapy, occupational therapy, speech/language pathology and related areas.

Quarterly

Newsletters

600 Autism - Families of More Able Autistic People, MAAP Newsletter

P.O. Box 524
Crown Point, IN 46307

601 Autism Society of North Carolina News

Autism Society of North Carolina
505 Oberlin Road, Suite 230
Raleigh, NC 27605   919-743-0204
                                            800-442-2762
                                      Fax: 919-743-0208
                                  e-mail: ASNC@aol.com
                                  www.autismsociety-nc.org

Offers information on chapter programs, services, fund-raising events and legislative news for public and professionals interested in autism.

Monthly

Pamphlets

602 Autism Society of America, General Information on Autism

7910 Woodmont Avenue, Suite 650
Bethesada, MD 20814   301-657-0881
                                            800-328-8476
                                      Fax: 301-657-0869

Offers a definition and introduction to autism, offers reading material and suggested resources pertaining to autism and points out the educational implications of students with autism.

603 Avoiding Unfortunate Situations

Dennis Debbaudt, author

Autism Society of North Carolina Bookstore
505 Oberlin Road, Suite 230
Raleigh, NC 27605   919-743-0204
                                            800-442-2762
                                      Fax: 919-743-0208
                                  e-mail: ASNC@aol.com
                                  www.autismsociety-nc.org

A collection of tips and information from and about people with autism and other developmental disabilities.

604 Enhancing Communication in Individuals with Autism Through Pictures/Words

Michelle G. Winner, author

Autism Society of North Carolina Bookstore
505 Oberlin Road, Suite 230
Raleigh, NC 27605   919-743-0204
                                            800-442-2762
                                      Fax: 919-743-0208
                                  e-mail: ASNC@aol.com
                                  www.autismsociety-nc.org

Booklet addressing the description and implementation of visually aided communication.

1989

605 Fact Sheet: Autism

Autism Society of America
7910 Woodmont Avenue, Ste. 300
Bethesda, MD 20814   301-657-0881
                                        800-328-8476
                                   Fax: 301-657-0869
                             www.autism-society.orgl

Offers information on autism. What it is, symptoms, causes, diagnosis, treatments and research.

**606 Parents as Trainers of Legislators, Other Parents
and Researchers**

Ruth Christ Sullivan, author

Autism Services Center
101 Richmond Street
Huntington, WV 25702   304-525-8014

Reprint offering information on parents of autistic children that learn early in their child's life
how little professionals know about autism.

607 Sex Education: Issues for the Person with Autism

Nancy Dalrymple, author

Autism Society of North Carolina Bookstore
505 Oberlin Road, Suite 230
Raleigh, NC 27605   919-743-0204
                                        800-442-2762
                                   Fax: 919-743-0208
                             e-mail: ASNC@aol.com
                             www.autismsociety-nc.org

Discusses issues of sexuality and provides methods of instruction for people with autism.
    1991

DESCRIPTION

608 BELL'S PALSY

May involve these systems in the body (see Section III):

Nervous System

Bell's palsy is the most common form of facial nerve paralysis and may affect children at any age from infancy through adolescence. The facial nerve, also known as the seventh cranial nerve, arises from a certain area of the brain (i.e., brainstem) and divides into several branches that supply (innervate) the forehead, mcalp, eyelids, cheeks, jaws, and muscles of facial expression. The facial nerve also conveys taste sensations from the front two thirds of the tongue. Bell's palsy usually develops suddenly approximately two weeks after a widespread viral infection, such as Epstein-Barr virus, herpesvirus, or mumps virus. It is thought to represent a postinfectious demyelination of the facial nerve (neuritis) due to allergic or immune responses.

Bell's palsy typically affects one side of the face and may involve upper and lower areas on the affected side. Children with the condition may experience weakness or slight paralysis of the upper and lower face; drooping of the corner of the mouth; an inability to close the eye; floss of taste sensations from the front two thirds of the tongue; or abnormal sensitivity to loud sounds (hyperacusis). Because the affected eye may be overexposed to the air, some patients may develop inflammation (exposure keratitis) of the transparent, front region of the eye (cornea). In addition, saliva may dribble from the corner of the mouth and food may tend to collect between the teeth and lips.

The treatment of children with Bell's palsy is supportive, including eye drops to lubricate the cornea, particularly at night. In over 85 percent of affected children, Bell's palsy spontaneously resolves with no remaining facial weakness. About 10 percent may have mild longstanding weakness, and approximately five percent may experience severe, permanent facial weakness.

The following organizations in the General Resources Section can provide additional information: National Organization for Rare Disorders, Inc., (NORD), March of Dimes Birth Defects Foundation, NIH/National Institute of Neurological Disorders and Stroke (NINDS)

National Associations & Support Groups

609 American Academy of Otolaryngology-Head and Neck Surgery
1 Prince Street
Alexandria, VA 22314   703-836-4444
Fax: 703-683-5100
TTY: 703-519-1585
e-mail: webmaster@entnet.org
www.entnet.org

The missions of the AAO-HNS and its foundation are to advance the art and science of otolaryngology-head and neck surgery through state-of-the-art education, research, and learning; and to unite, serve, and represent the interests of its members and their patients to the public, government, other medical specialists, and related organizations. Founded in 1896, the AAI-HNS is the world's largest organization of otolaryngologist-head and neck surgeons.

11,600 Members

Research Centers

610 Bell's Palsy Research Foundation
9121 E Tanque Verde
Tuscon, AZ 85749   520-749-4614
Fax: 520-749-0489
e-mail: bellspalsy@aol.com

Web Sites

611 About.com
disabilities.miningco.com/msub44.htm

612 Bell Palsy Network
www.bellspalsy.net/

613 National Institute of Neurological Disorders and Stroke (NINDS)
www.ninds.nih.gov

614 **University of Chicago**
www.uhs.bsd.uchicago.edu/uhs/top-
ics/bells.html#def

DESCRIPTION

615 BILIARY ATRESIA

Disorder Type: Birth Defect
May involve these systems in the body (see Section III):
Digestive System

Biliary atresia is a rare condition that is present at birth (congenital) and is characterized by the absence of or the abnormal or incomplete development (hypoplasia) of the bile ducts. This duct work carries bile from the liver and gall bladder into the small intestine. Bile, which is secreted by the liver, is a yellowish or greenish fluid that aids in the digestion of fats. Bile passes through the common bile duct and into the upper portion of the small intestine (duodenum). Absence of or underdevelopment of the bile ducts interferes or prevents the passage of bile into the intestine and, as a result, characteristic findings and symptoms may be noticed within the first few weeks of life.

Symptoms may include progressively darkening urine; pale stools (acholic); a persistent yellowing of the skin, eyes, and mucous membranes (jaundice); and enlargement of the liver (hepatomegaly). If untreated, additional symptoms and findings may become apparent within two or three months. These may include growth retardation, increased irritability, and itching (pruritus). A potential complication of biliary atresia involves an increase in pressure in the vein that conveys blood from the spleen, stomach, pancreas, and intestine to the liver (portal hypertension). In addition, untreated biliary atresia may result in a life-threatening condition known as biliary cirrhosis, in which the liver's function is impaired and, eventually, the liver becomes irreversibly damaged.

Treatment for biliary atresia is often determined by the site of the obstruction and includes various surgical procedures. In some infants, surgery may be performed as a means to help postpone cirrhosis and growth retardation until liver transplanta-

tion is feasible. Biliary atresia occurs in approximately one of every 12,500 births.

The following organizations in the General Resources Section can provide additional information: Genetic Alliance, NIH/Office of Rare Diseases, National Organization for Rare Disorders, Inc. (NORD), Online Mendelian Inheritance in Man: www3.ncbi.nlm.nih.gov/Omim/searchomim.html, NIH/National Digestive Diseases Information Clearinghouse

National Associations & Support Groups

616 American Association for the Study of Liver Diseases
1729 King Street, Suite 100
Alexandria, VA 22314   703-299-9766
Fax: 703-299-9622
e-mail: aasld@aasld.org
www.aasld.org

Conducts symposia and educational courses for professionals interested in disease of the liver and biliary tract.

617 Children's Liver Alliance
3835 Richmond Ave. Box 190
Staten Island, NY 10312   718-687-6200
Fax: 718-687-6200

Empowering the hearts and minds of children with liver disease, their families and the medical professionals who care for them.

618 United Liver Association
11646 West Pico Boulevard
Los Angeles, CA 90064   310-445-4204
Fax: 310-575-3871

Offers a health of informational topics in which touch upon and assist in helping individuals confront and deal with their disease.

Research Centers

619 Clinical Research Center, Pediatrics
Children's Hospital Research Foundation
Elland & Bethesda Avenues
Cincinnati, OH 45229   513-559-4412
Fax: 513-559-7431

Studies of pediatric acquired diseases including liver disease and Reyes Syndrome.

Dr. James Heubi, Director

620 Univ. of Texas - Southwestern Med. Ctr. at Dallas - Clinical Ctr. for Liver Disease
5323 Harry Hines Blvd.
Dallas, TX 75235   214-648-3323
                       Fax: 214-648-3715
              e-mail: lee03@utsw.swmed.edu

Conferences

621 CHARGE Syndrome Conference
Sheraton Crown Hotel
Houston, TX
                        800-784-7581

CHARGE (Coloboma, Heart Malformations, Atresia Choanae, Retardation, Genital Abnormalities, Ear Abnormalities)
July 23-25

Web Sites

622 Children's Liver Alliance
www.livertx.org

623 Children's Liver Association for Support Services (C.L.A.S.S.)
www.classkids.org

Books

624 Liver Disease in Children
Frederick J. Suchy, author
Mosby Year Book
11830 Westline Industrial Dr.
St. Louis, MO 63146   314-872-8370
                           800-325-4177

800 pages

625 Liver Disorders in Childhood
Alex P. Mowat, author
Butterworth-Heinemann
225 Wildwood Ave.
Woburn, MA 01801   617-928-2500
                        800-366-2665
                   Fax: 800-446-6520

432 pages
ISBN: 0-750610-39-5

Pamphlets

626 Biliary Atresia
American Liver Foundation
1425 Pompton Avenue
Cedar Grove, NJ 07009   973-857-2626
                           800-223-0179

627 Facts on Liver Transplantation
American Liver Foundation
1425 Pompton Ave.
Cedar Grove, NJ 07009   973-256-2550
                           800-223-0179

DESCRIPTION

628 BIPOLAR DISORDER
Synonyms: Manic-depressive disorder,
Manic-depressive illness, Manic-depressive psychosis
Disorder Type: Genetic Disorder, Mental,
Emotional or Behavioral Disorder

Bipolar disorder, also known as manic-depressive disorder, is a condition characterized by alternating depression and mania or, in rare cases, mania alone. The disorder is thought to affect less than two percent of the general population. Although bipolar disorder usually becomes apparent during the third or fourth decade of life, a significant proportion of individuals are initially affected in childhood, adolescence, or early adulthood. Individuals with bipolar disorder may initially experience either a depressive or a manic episode. In some affected children and adolescents, manic episodes may be more frequent than depressive episodes during the first years of illness. However, as the disease progresses, episodes of depression may become more frequent than manic episodes. Bipolar disorder is often further classified as unipolar in cases in which only depression is experienced and bipolar when mania occurs with or without depression. In addition, mixed affected states are characterized by the occurrence of depressive and manic symptoms during a single episode.

In children and adolescents with bipolar disorder, associated symptoms resemble those seen in affected adults. Depressive states usually emerge gradually and may be characterized by feelings of sadness, despair, hopelessness, and discouragement; loss of self-esteem; physical and emotional exhaustion; and lack of interest of formerly enjoyed activities. In severe cases, affected individuals may have suicidal tendencies, and hospitalization in a pediatric, general, or psychiatric facility may be essential. In such cases, consultation with child psychiatrists may be important for ongoing support and decision-making regarding treatment options.

In affected children and adolescents, many states may be characterized by overactivity (hyperactivity); excessive talking; inability to sleep (insomnia); impulsive behavior and impaired judgment that may result in reckless spending; elation that may quickly change to irritability and anger; personal neglect that may result in poor hygiene; and, in some cases, delusions of grandeur and persecution (paranoid delusions). Initial episodes of depression or mania often last approximately six months without treatment. Although most manic or depressive episodes usually cease in months, some individuals may be affected for longer periods.

Adolescents with bipolar disorder may be misdiagnosed, e.g., with a psychotic disorder characterized by disturbances in behavior, cognition, and emotional reactions (schizophrenia) or a maladjusted reaction to a stressful life event (adjustment disorder). However, most affected individuals are correctly diagnosed with bipolar disorder during adulthood. According to reports in the literature, the earlier the onset of bipolar disorder, the more susceptible affected individuals may be to frequent episodes, rapid cycling between depressive and manic states, and severe episodes that may result in suicidal tendencies. In addition, earlier onset of the disorder is often associated with an increased incidence of depression and bipolar disorder in immediate (first-degree) relatives.

The treatment of children and adolescents with bipolar disorder may include therapy with certain medications (e.g., lithium carbonate, carbamazepine) and integrated, multidisciplinary management (e.g., behavioral therapy; individual, family, or group psychodynamic therapy; etc.). In children and adolescents with the disorder, thorough patient and family histories and specific medical evaluations are typically conducted before medications are prescribed. Pretreatment evaluation for lithium may include assessment of electrolyte levels, kidney (renal) function tests, and thyroid tests. Pretreatment evaluation for tricyclic antidepressants may include a cardiovascular examination. If such medications are prescribed, regular blood levels should be taken until an adequate dose is determined. As mentioned above, in some severe cases (e.g., if suicidal tendencies are present), hospitalization in a pediatric, general, or psychiatric facility may be essential.

The exact cause of bipolar disorder is unknown. However, many researchers agree that genetic abnormalities may play some role in causing or resulting in susceptibility for the disorder. Although a specific pattern of inheritance has not been determined, researchers suggest that the disorder may result from abnormal changes (m) of one of several different genes expressed either alone or together (polygenic). Depending upon the specific disease gene(s), the condition is thought to have autosomal dominant, X-linked, or polygenic inheritance. In addition, many researchers theorize that the underlying cause(s) of bipolar disorder may be due to certain biochemical abnormalities of the brain, such as abnormalities of certain neurotransmitters (e.g., dopamine, serotonin, norepinephrine). Others indicate that psychosocial factors may play a role in causing bipolar disorder, suggesting, for example, that affected individuals may have a genetic trait that causes increased susceptibility and vulnerability to psychosocial stress.

The following organizations in the General Resources Section can provide additional information: Online Mendelian Inheritance in Man: www3.ncbi.nlm.nih.gov/Omim/searchomim.html

---

National Associations & Support Groups

629 Center for Mental Health Services Knowledge Exchange Network
US Dept of Health and Human Services, PO Box 42490
Washington, DC 20015
USA

800-789-2647
Fax: 301-984-8796
e-mail: ken@mentalhealth.org
www.mentalhealth.org

Resuorces, technical assistance, research, training, networks, and other federal clearing houses, and fact sheets and materials. Information specialists refer callers to mental health resources in their communities as well as state, federal and non-profit contacts. After hours, callers may leave messages and an information specialist will return their call.

630 Depressive and Manic-Depressive Assocation of Mount Sinai
100 LaSalle Street, #5A
New York, NY 10027   212-241-8924
www.columbia.edu/~jgg17/DMDA/PAGE_1.html

631 Federation of Families for Children's Mental Health
1021 Prince Street
Alexandria, VA 22314   703-684-7710
Fax: 703-836-1040
e-mail: ffcmh@crosslink.net
www.ffcmh.org

Assists young adults through the change of life with several support and educational tools in which they can use through the years.

632 Lithium Information Center/Obsessive Compulsive Information Center
7617 Mineral Point Road Suite 300
Madison, WI 53717   608-827-2470
e-mail: INFOCTRS@healthtechsys.com
www.healthtechsys.com/mimmain

633 National Alliance for the Mentally Ill
200 North Glebe Road #1015
Arlington, VA 22203   703-524-7600
800-950-6264
TDD: 703-516-7991
e-mail: membership@nami.org
http://www.nami.org

634 National Depressive and Manic-Depressive Association
730 North Franklin Street Suite 501
Chicago, IL 60610
800-826-3632
Fax: 312-642-7243
www.ndmda.org

Informs the public of the severity of the untreated individuals diagnosed with the potentially threatening disorder through various informational avenues.

635 National Institute of Mental Health
5600 Fishers Lane
Rockville, MD 20857   301-443-4513
www.nimh.nih.gov

636 National Mental Health Association
1021 Prince Street
Alexandria, VA 22314   703-684-7722
                              800-969-6642
                         TDD: 800-433-5959
                    e-mail: nmhainfo@aol.com
                              www.nmha.oeg

Notifies the public of the various groups and foundations to answer and assist them with their concerns and questions.

637 National Mental Health Consumer Self-Help Clearinghouse
1211 Chestnut Street
Philadelphia, PA 19107   215-751-1810
                              800-553-4539
                         Fax: 215-636-6310
                   e-mail: info@mhselfhelp.org
                              www.mhselfhelp.org

Offers information, support, and appropriate referrals; and promotes public and professional education. Provides networking for those with special interests related to albinism and promotes and supports research and funding that will improve diagnosis and management of albinism and hypopigmentation.

Research Centers

638 Information Centers for Lithium, Bipolar Disorders Treatment & Obsessive Compuls
Madison Institute of Medicine
7617 Mineral Point Road, Suite 300
Madison, WI 53717   608-827-2470
                         Fax: 608-827-2479
                e-mail: mim@healthtechsys.com
                       www.healthtechsys.com/mim.html

The Information Centers publish information booklets. Authorized by experts on each disorder, these patient guides offer information about various psychiatric disorders and their treatments and address the questions most frequently asked by patients and their families.

639 National Alliance for Research on Schizophrenia & Depression
60 Cutter Mill Road Suite 404
Great Neck, NY 11021   516-829-0091
                              800-829-8289
                    www.mhsource.com/narsad

Audio Video

640 Families Coping with Mental Illness
Mental Illness Education Project, Inc.
P.O. Box 470813
Brookline Village, MA 02247
USA   617-562-1111
                              800-343-5540
                         Fax: 617-779-0061
                     e-mail: miep@tiac.net
                              www.miepvideos.org

Ten family members share their experiences of having a family member with schizophrenia or bipolar disorder. Designed to provide insights and support to other families, the tape also profoundly conveys to professionals the needs of families when mental illness strikes. In two versions: a 22-minute version ideal for short classes and workshops, and a richer 43-minute version with more examples and details. Discounted price for families/consumers.

Video

Web Sites

641 Between a Giggle and a Tear
www.geocities.com/~duxuedikk/manic.html

642 Bipolar Disorders Information Center
http://www.mhsource.com/bipolar
                e-mail: webmaster@mhsource.com
                http://www.mhsource.com/bipolar

643 Bipolar World
http://bipolar.virtualave.net/

644 Cyber Psych
www.cyberpsych.org/

645 Internet Mental Health
www.mentalhealth.com

646 Mental Healthnet
mentalhelp.net/disorders/sx20.htm

647 Planetpsych
www.planetpsych.com

648 Soc. Support Depression Manic
www.soc.support.depression.manic

Books

649 Bipolar Disorders: A Guide to Helping Children & Adolescents

Mitzi Waltz, author

O'Reilly and Associates, Inc.
101 Morris Street
Sebastopol, CA 95472
800-998-9938
Fax: 707-829-0104
e-mail: patientguides@oreilly.com
www.patientcenters.com

A million children and adolescents in the United States may have childhood-onset bipolar disorder, including an estimated 23 percent of those currently diagnosed with ADHD, Bipolar Disorders helps parents and professionals recognize, treat, and cope with bipolar disorders in children and adolescents. It covers diagnosis, family life, medications, talk therapies, other interventions (improving sleep patterns, diet, preventing seasonal mood swings), insurance, and school.

380 pages
ISBN: 1-565926-56-0

650 Bipolar Disorders: Clinical Course and Outcome

Joseph F. Goldbert MD; Martin Harrow PhD, author

American Psychiatric Press, Inc.
1400 K Street NW
Washington, DC 20005
USA
202-682-6262
800-368-5777
Fax: 202-789-2648
e-mail: order@appi.org
www.appi.org

Provides a concise, up-to-date summary of affective relapse, comorbid psychopathalogy, functional disability, and psychocial outcome in contemporary bipolar disorders.

312 pages Hardcover
ISBN: 0-880487-68-2

651 Bipolar Puzzle Solutions

National Alliance for the Mentally Ill
200 N Glebe Road, Suite 1015
Arlington, VA 22203
USA
703-524-7600
800-950-6264
Fax: 703-524-9094
TDD: 703-516-7227
www.nami.org

An informative book on bipolar illness in a question-and-answer format.

652 Combating Distorted Thinking

New Harbinger Publications, Inc.
5674 Shattuck Avenue
Oakland, CA 94609
USA
510-652-2002
800-748-6273
e-mail: customreservice@newharbinger.com
www.newharbinger.com

ISBN: 0-934986-27-4

653 Covert Modeling & Covert Reinforcement

New Harbinger Publications, Inc.
5674 Shattuck Avenue
Oakland, CA 94609
USA
510-652-2002
800-748-6273
e-mail: customreservice@newharbinger.com
www.newharbinger.com

ISBN: 0-934986-29-0

654 Guideline for Treatment of Patients with Bipolar Disorder

American Psychiatric Press, Inc.
1400 K Street NW
Washington, DC 20005
USA
202-682-6262
800-368-5777
Fax: 202-789-2648
e-mail: order@appi.org
www.appi.org

Provides guidance to psychiatrists who treat patients with bipolar I disorder. Summarizes the pharmacologic, somatic, and psychotherapeutic treatments used for patients.

96 pages Softcover
ISBN: 0-890423-02-4

655 Management of Bipolar Disorder -Pocketbook

Stuart A Montgomery, MD; Giovanni B Cassano, MD, author

American Psychiatric Press, Inc.
1400 K Street NW
Washington, DC 20005
USA
202-682-6262
800-368-5777
Fax: 202-789-2648
e-mail: order@appi.org
www.appi.org

Contains the need for treatment, what defines bipolar disorders, spectrum of the disorder, getting the best out of the treatment of mania and bipolar depression, preventing new episodes, special problems in treatment, mood stabilizers, and case studies.

96 pages
ISBN: 1-833172-74-X

656 Manic Depressive Illness
National Alliance for the Mentally Ill
200 N Glebe Road, Suite 1015
Arlington, VA 22203
USA

703-524-7600
800-950-6264
Fax: 703-524-9094
TDD: 703-516-7227
www.nami.org

A definitive overview of bipolar disorder.

657 Touched with Fire - Manic Depressive Illness & the Artistic Temperament

Kay Redfield Jamison, MD, author

Free Press
866 3rd Avenue
New York, NY 10022
USA

212-832-2101
800-323-7445
Fax: 800-943-9831
www.simonsays.com

Describing and discussing the markedly increased rates of sever mood disorders and suicides among the artistically cerative and the reasons why.

370 pages

Pamphlets

658 Bipolar Disorder
National Institutes of Health
5600 Fishers Lane Room 7C-02
Rockville, MD 20857

301-443-3706
Fax: 301-443-6349

A short booklet offering a concise description of this disorder, which is also called manic-depressive illness.

DESCRIPTION

659 BRAIN TUMORS

Disorder Type: Neoplasm: Benign or Malignant Tumor

Brain tumors are abnormal growths in or on the brain that may be cancerous (malignant) or non-cancerous (benign). In addition, these growths may be classified as primary tumors that arise directly from brain tissue or as secondary tumors, which are almost always malignant, that have spread or metastasized to the brain from other parts of the body. Space-occupying benign tumors may also present complications resulting from increasing intracranial pressure. Symptoms and characteristic findings associated with brain tumors depend upon their location as well as their size and growth. However, many symptoms are common to most types of brain tumors and may include recurrent or constant headache, irregularities of vision, difficulties in balance and the coordination of voluntary movements, muscle weakness, speech difficulties, and sometimes seizures. Nausea, vomiting, fever, and fluctuations in pulse rate, breathing rate, and blood pressure may be later manifestations. Although there are many different types of brain tumors, children are most commonly affected by primary tumors, especially those that develop toward the back of the brain (posterior fossa tumor).

The most common of the posterior fossa tumors in children is the cerebellar astrocytoma. This type of tumor may be fluid-filled (cystic) or relatively solid and may often have a low grade of malignancy. However, cerebellar astrocytomas may sometimes invade the fibers on each side of the cerebellum that connect with other areas of the brain as well as the spinal cord (cerebellar peduncles). Symptoms and findings may include an abnormal accumulation of cerebrospinal fluid, often under increased pressure, within the skull (hydrocephalus) that is characterized by an increase in head size in infants as well as irritability, vomit-

ing, lethargy, irregular reflex action, and leg rigidity followed by drowsiness and seizures. Older children may have a headache and may vomit, lose coordination, and exhibit deteriorating mental capabilities. Effective treatment for low-grade cerebellar astrocytoma includes surgical removal. Radiation treatment may be indicated for children with cerebellar astrocytoma of high-grade malignancy or in children who exhibit evidence of tumor growth after surgery.

Medulloblastoma is the second most common of the posterior fossa tumors in children and, in children younger than seven years of age, is the most common brain tumor. This type of malignant tumor usually grows relatively fast and spreads to other parts of the brain, the spinal cord, and sometimes other areas. Symptoms associated with medulloblastoma may include headache, recurrent vomiting, and frequent falling. Diagnosis is achieved through procedures such as magnetic resonance imaging (MRI) or computer tomography (CT scan). Treatment may include surgical excision. In addition, children older than four years of age may receive radiation therapy, especially if the tumor is small and has not yet spread. Children who have evidence of some remaining tumor growth after surgery and those whose tumor has spread may benefit from chemotherapy in addition to surgery and radiation therapy. Due to the possibility of adverse effects on the brain, radiation is delayed in very young children with medulloblastoma.

Craniopharyngioma is a tumor that appears most often in children and adolescents, and arises from the pituitary, an endocrine gland that is located at the base of the skull. This type of tumor may sometimes interfere with pituitary gland and other endocrine functions as well as cause compression resulting in the excessive accumulation of fluid around the brain (hydrocephalus) and its associated symptoms. Other findings may include headache, vomiting, irregularities in vision, and short stature resulting from hormonal irregularities. Treatment for craniopharyngioma includes surgical excision. Additional treatment with radiation may be indicated for those children whose tumor is not able to be completely removed through surgery or who experience a recurrence. Subsequent to surgery, some children may develop such hormonal abnormalities as an underactive thyroid (hypothyroidism), growth hormone deficiency, diabetes insipidus, and other problems. Evaluation for these hormonal disorders is indicated and treatment is dependent upon the particular abnormality.

The following organizations in the General Resources Section can provide additional information: National Organization for Rare Disorders, Inc. (NORD), NIH/Office of Rare Diseases, NIH/National Cancer Institute, Candlelighters Childhood Cancer Foundation Canada, Candlelighters Childhood Cancer Foundation, National Childhood Cancer Foundation, NIH/National Institute of Neurological Disorders & Stroke, Online Mendelian Inheritance in Man.: www3.ncbi.nlm.nih.gov/Omim/searchomim.html

National Associations & Support Groups

660 American Brain Tumor Association
2720 River Road
Des Plaines, IL 60018   847-827-9910
                               800-886-2282
                          Fax: 847-827-9918
                   e-mail: info@abta.org
                               www.abta.org

We are an independent not-for-profit oganization; services include over 20 easy-to-understand publications which address brain tumors, their treatment, and coping with the disease. Materials address brain tumors in all age groups. Provide free social service consultations, mentorship program for new support group leaders, nationwide database of support groups, pen-pal programs, networking with other organizations, and a resource listing of physicians offering investigative treatments.

Naomi Berkowitz, Executive Director

661 American Cancer Society, Inc.
Brain Tumor Support Group
ACS Building, 8900 Carpenter Freeway
Dallas, TX 75260   214-631-3850
                               www.cancer.org

Attacks the support aspect of this disease from every angle including data on lowering risks to dealing with grief.

Maureen Bergmann

662 Brain Tumor Foundation for Children, Inc.
2231 Perimeter Park Road, Suite 9
Atlanta, GA 30341   770-458-5554
                          Fax: 770-458-5467
                   e-mail: eallman1@Juno.com

Disseminates data and support agencies for the family and friends of juveniles diagnosed with a neurological disorder.

663 Brain Tumor Foundation of Canada
650 Waterloo Street, Suite 100
London, ON N6B 2R4,
Canada   519-642-7755
                               800-265-5106
                          Fax: 519-685-8473
                   e-mail: btfc@gtn.net
                               www.btfc.org

664 Brain Tumor Information Line
National Brain Tumor Foundation
785 Market Street-Suite 1600
San Francisco, CA 94103   415-284-0208
                               800-934-2873
                          Fax: 415-284-0209
                               www.braintumor.org

Quickly access brain tumor information and resources.

665 Brain Tumor Society
124 Watertown Street, Suite 3H
Watertown, MA 02472   617-924-9997
                               800-770-8287
                          Fax: 617-924-9998
                   e-mail: info@tbts.org
                               www.tbts.com

Establishment founded for the purpose of dispersing information to concerned families and friends of people with neurological complications.

**666 Brain Tumor Support Group at NovaCare
Rehabilitation Institute of Tucson**
2650 N Wyatt Drive
Tucson, AZ 85726   520-293-8040

Scott Gulbrandsen

667 Brain Tumor Support Group at Phoenix
St. Joseph's Hospital and Medical Center
350 West Thomas Road
Phoenix, AZ 85026   602-873-2757

Steve Westerhoff

668 Childhood Brain Tumor Foundation
20312 Watkins Meadow Dr
Germantown, MD 20876   301-515-2900
Fax: 301-540-8367
e-mail: jpyoung88@aol.com
www.mnsinc.com/cbtf

Provides the Childhood Cancer Ombudsman Program, a free service consisting of volunteers trained in the disiplines of medicine, law, and education who provide assistance in : 1) seeking second opinions, 2) access to healthcare, and 3) combating discrimination.

669 Children's Brain Tumor Foundation
274 Madison Avenue Suite 1301
New York, NY 10016   212-448-9494
www.childrensneuronet.org

670 Heads Up Brain Tumor Support Group
Dominican Hospital Educational Building
B-1
Santa Cruz, CA 95060   408-688-7619

671 Healing Exchange Brain Trust
Kendall Square Box 425743
Cambridge, MA 02142   617-623-0066
Fax: 617-623-2203
e-mail: info@braintrust.org
www.braintrust.org

672 National Brain Tumor Foundation
414 - 13th Street, Suite 700
Oakland, CA 94612   510-839-9777
800-934-2873
Fax: 510-839-9779
e-mail: nbtf@braintumor.org
www.braintumor.org

The National Brain Tumor Foundation (NBTF) ia non-profit health organization founded in 1981 by patients and family members. NBTF raises funds for research and provides information and support to patients, their family, friends, and health professionals. NBTF sponsors national and regional conferences, patient and caregiver programs, support groups, special patient programs including a teleconference series, a newsletter, a medical advice nurse and a wide variety of patient information.

673 Pediatric Brain Tumor Foundation of the U.S.
315 Ridgefield Court
Asheville, NC 28806   828-665-6891
800-253-6530
Fax: 828-655-6894
e-mail: pbtfus@ibm.net
www.ride4kids.org

An organization devoted to raising funds for pediatric brain tumor research. They also help educate the public about brain tumors in children, and can provide additional information on caregiving resources for parents.

674 Preuss Foundation
2223 Avenida de la Playa, Suite 220
La Jolla, CA 92037   619-454-0200
Fax: 619-454-4449
e-mail: preussfd@cerf.net

International

675 Acoustic Neuroma Association of Canada
PO Box 369
Edmonton, AB T5J   403-425-3384
800-561-2622
e-mail: anac@compusmart.ab.ca

676 Brainchild Suppor Group
Hospital for Sick Children
555 University Ave, Ste 1504
Toronto,   905-634-8295

Pam West

677 Pediatric Brain Tumor Support Group
Children's Hospital of Western Ontario
800 Commissioners Rd E
London, Ontario,   519-685-8500

David Rynard, PhD, Psychologist

State Agencies & Support Groups

Alabama

678 Pediatric Brain Tumor Support Group
Children's Hospital
1600 7th Avenue South
Birmingham, AL 35203   205-939-9090

Groups for parents and siblings of brain tumor patients. Related to Children's Hospital of Alabama. Babysitting available.

Paula Teague

California

679 Brain Tumor Patient & Family Support Group
St. Jude Medical Center
101 E. Valencia Mesa Dr Rm 3NA
Fullerton, CA 92634   949-645-3395

Periodic guest presentations.

Robert Merlino

**680 Brain Tumor Support Program Cedars-Sanai
Neurosurgical Inst. & Wellness Community**
8631 West 3rd St., Ste 800 East
Los Angeles, CA 90048   310-855-7900
                                    Fax: 310-423-0777

681 Children Living with Illness
The Center for Attitudinal Healing
19 Main Street
Tiburon, CA   415-331-6161

For children who are ill, have an ill sibling, or
an ill parent. Parent group meets separately at
the same time.

Jimmy Pete

682 Fresno Brain Tumor Support Group
1303 East Herndon
Fresno, CA 93720   559-449-3452
                                    Fax: 559-449-3990

Paula Jordan

683 Inland Empire Brain Tumor Support Group
Kaiser Hospital
Fontana, CA 92324   909-877-4923

Sheri Kyander

684 Neuroscience Institute Brain Tumor Support Group
Hospital of the Good Samaritan
637 South Lucas Avenue, Suite 501
Los Angeles, CA 90052   213-977-2234
                                    800-762-1692

Claudia Perdices, MSW

685 Northridge Hospital: Leavey Cancer Center

Northridge, CA 91324   818-832-5287

David Antelman

686 Palo Alto Brain Tumor Support Group
Palo Alto Medical Foundation Bldg, Urgent Care Ctr
920 Bryant St, 2nd Floor Room B
Palo Alto, CA 94303   415-284-0208

Joanie Taylor, RN

**687 Peninsula Support & Education Group for Parents
of Children with Brain Tumors**
Parents Helping Parents
3041 Olcott
Santa Clara, CA   650-325-4523

Sheri Sobrato, MA, MFC

688 Sacramento Area Brain Tumor Support Group
UC Davis Medical Center, Camellia Cottage
4501 X St, Room 1101-1103
Sacramento, CA 95813   916-734-3658

Karen Smith, RN

689 San Francisco Brain Tumor Support Group
UC San Francisco, Clinical Sciences Building
521 Parnassus Avenue Rm C130
San Francisco, CA 94188   415-284-0208

Contact is National Brain Tumor Foundation.
Holiday potluck with other Bay Area support
groups, lending library (books audio and visual
tapes).

Sharon Lamb, RN

690 Santa Barbara Brain Tumor Support Group
Cancer Foundation of Santa Barbara
300 West Pueblo Conference Room
Santa Barbara, CA 93102   805-682-7300

Carol Spungen, LCSW

691 Santa Cruz County Brain Tumor Support Group
3031 Main Street
Soquel, CA 95073   831-438-8344

Gregory Valki-Tarsy

692 Santa Rosa Brain Tumor Support Group
Santa Rosa/Petaluma

Santa Rosa, CA 95402   415-476-2966

Jane Rabbitt, RN

693 South Bay Brain Tumor Support Group
667 Chapman Street
San Jose, CA 95101   650-725-8630

Genny See-Tho, RN

694 Southern California Pediatric Brain Tumor Network
UCLA Medical Center
10833 LeConte Avenue, Suite 501
Los Angeles, CA   818-362-3428

For parents of children with brain tumors, and
for teenagers with brain tumors.

Kathy Riley

695 Support Group for Caregivers of Brain Tumor Patients
UCLA Medical Center
UCLA Medical Plaza Building
Los Angeles, CA 90052   310-206-6731

Guest speakers on occasion.

Pamela Hoff, LCSW

696 Support Group for Parents of Children with Brain Tumors
Oakland Children's Hospital
747 52nd St Auditorium Sd II
Oakland, CA 94623   510-428-3885

Contact can be reached at extension 2161.

Trish Murphy

697 Vital Options
4419 Coldwater Canyon
Studio City, CA 91604   818-508-5657

Support group for young adult cancer patients.

698 Wellness Community San Francisco/East Bay
3276 McNutt Avenue
Walnut Creek, CA 94596   925-933-0107

Many general support groups, workshops,
classes, etc. offered. Calendar available.

Erika Maslan, MFCC

699 West Los Angeles Brain Tumor Support Group
2716 Icean Park Blvd, Suite 1040
Santa Monica, CA 90406   310-314-2555

Michael States, Program Director

Colorado

700 Brain Tumor Patient Family Group
University of Colorado Cancer Center

Denver, CO 80202   303-315-5652

Deb Hopper, RN

701 Brain Tumor Patient/Family Group
University of Colorado Cancer Center

Denver, CO 80220   303-372-1791

Joint and separate sessions for patients and family members.

Amy Paul-Ebert, Secretary

702 Brain Tumor Resource and Vital Encouragement
Children's Hospital
Denver, CO 80218   303-861-8888

Pediatric focus. Education and support. Retreats for parents of brain tumor patients.

Joanne Pearson, Outpatient Oncology

703 Brain Tumor Support Group
Poudre Valley Hospital
1024 S Lemay, Neuroscience Fl
Ft. Collins, CO 80521   970-490-4134

Shirley Friese
George Knaub

Connecticut

704 Brain Tumor Support Group
Helen and Harry Gray Cancer Center

Hartford, CT 06101   860-545-2776

Marcia Caruso-Bergman, RN, MSN

705 Connecticut Brain Tumor Support Group (Adult)
Yale New Haven Hospital
20 York St, Room 201 Childrens Hospital
New Haven, CT 06050   203-688-7528

Betsy D'Andrea

Delaware
---

706 Pediatric Brain Tumor Support Group
Ronald McDonald House
1901 Rockland Road
Wilmington, DE   302-995-0938

Cathy Francisco

District of Columbia
---

707 Washington DC Metropolitan Area Support Group
George Washington University
2150 Pennsylvania Ave. NW Rm. 7426
Washington, DC 20052

Florida
---

708 Angels in the Sun Brain Tumor Support Group
Health South Rehabilitative Hospital
3251 Proctor Road
Sarasota, FL 34230   941-364-9105

Anna Browder

709 Brain Tumor Support Group
American Cancer Society
1703 West Colonial Drive
Orlando, FL 32862   407-740-0007

Dr. David Cox

710 Brain Tumor Support Group at Miami
Miami Children's Hospital Foundation
3000 SW 62nd Ave Founders
Miami, FL 33152   305-662-8386

Maria Penate, RN
Raquel Pasaron

711 Brain Tumor Support Group at Newport Beach
Hoag Cancer Center Auditorium
4000 Pacific Coast Highway
Newport Beach, CA 92658   949-760-5542

Speakers once a month, education materials available.

Kris O'Neal

712 Brain Tumor Support Group at San Diego
UC San Diego Complex
132 Dickinson St, Camelot Room
San Diego, CA 92199   619-543-5540

Donna Gilpatrick, RN, MS, FNP

713 Brain Tumor Support Group at San Luis Obispo
1911 Johnson Avenue
San Luis Obispo, CA 93401   805-461-3989

Becky Nunez

714 Brain Tumor Support Group at Santa Monica
Wellness Community
2200 Colorado Boulevard
Santa Monica, CA 90406   310-453-2200

Michael Slater, Program Director

715 Brain Tumor Support Group at St Petersburg
St Anthony's Hospital

St Petersburg, FL 33730   727-825-1244

Al Hall

716 Brain Tumor Support Group at St. Petersburg
St. Anthony's Hospital
St. Petersburg, FL 33730   813-825-1100

Contact can be reached at extension 4231.

Karen McGough

717 Brain Tumor Support Group at Tampa
Moffitt Cancer Ctr, Dept. Psychosocial Onocology
12902 Magnolia Drive
Tampa, FL 33630   813-979-7258
                        800-456-3434

Inez Rodriquez

718 Cancer Support Group for Children
Memorial Hospital Children's Center
3501 Johnson St 4th Fl
Hollywood, FL   954-987-2000

Sub-groups for children with brain tumors and
their parents. Contact at ext. 4193.

Suzanne Baxter, RN

719 South Florida Brain Tumor Association
Boca Raton Community Hospital, Ed. Cntr.
800 Meadows Rd Classroom C
Boca Raton, FL 33431   954-755-4307

Neuropsychologist Dr. Laurence Miller and
therapist Marjorie O'Sullivan are present to facilitate the meetings.

Sheryl Shetsky

720 Tampa Bay Area Brain Tumor Support Group
St Joseph's Hospital, Medical Arts Building
3001 Martin Luther King Blvd
Tampa Bay, FL 33630   813-870-4327

Contact is St. Joseph's Hospital. Educational
materials available.

Georgia

721 Brain Tumor Foundation for Children, Inc
P O Box 422471
Atlanta, GA 30342   404-843-3700
                          Fax: 404-256-0039
                          e-mail: eallman1@juno.com

The BFTC provides information and emotional
support for families of children with brain tumors. They also raise funds for brain tumor research and provide a telephone network system
of parents who offer emotional support.

722 Emory Clinic Brain Tumor Support Group
Building B, 4th Floor Library
Atlanta, GA 30304   404-778-5376

Kaye Coker

723 Hearts and Minds
Piedmont Hospital, 1968 Peachtree Rd NW
35 Bdg, Dining Room
Atlanta, GA 30309   404-373-5202

Neal Kuhlhorst

724 SBTF Brain Tumor Support Group
Cathedral of St Philip

Atlanta, GA 30304   404-843-3700

Eve Herman

**725 Support Group for Brain Tumor Patients and
Family Members**
Clairmont Presbytarian Church
Clairmont Road & North Druid Hills
Atlanta, GA 30304   404-712-7711

Susan Herring

Hawaii

726 Brain Tumor Support Group
St. Christopher's Episcopal Church, Choir Room
93 N. Kainalu, Kailu
Oahu, HI   808-254-1989

Chuck Rogers
Kari Rogers

Illinois

727 Brain Tumor Network and Support Group
Chicago Institute of Neurosurgery & Neuroresearch
Columbus Hospital, 2520 North Lakeview, 7th
Floor
Chicago, IL 60607   773-388-7834

Teresa Omert, RN, MS

728 Brain Tumor Resource & Support Group
Central DuPage Hospital
Neuro Spine Unit
Winfield, IL 60190   630-682-1600

Contact can be reached at extension 6955.

Deborah Brunelle, RN

729 Brain Tumor Support Group
Northwestern Memorial Hospital
303 E Superior
Chicago, IL 60607   312-908-8177

Mary Ellen Maher Deleon

**730 Brain Tumor Support Group Lutheran General
Hospital**
Cancer Care Center
1700 Luther Lane, 2nd Floor
Park Ridge, IL 60068   708-696-5475

Syril Gilbert, LCSW

731 Brain Tumor Support Group at Park Ridge
Lutheran General Hospital, Cancer Care Center
1700 Luther Lane 2nd Fl
Park Ridge, IL 60068   847-696-5475

Syril Gilbert, LCSW

**732 Brain Tumor Support Grp Northwestern Memorial
Hospital**
303 E. Superior, Family Conference Room
Passavant Pavilion Room 466
Chicago, IL 60611   312-908-6811

Educational program offered at each meeting by
members of the professional committee.

Kathryn Wirtz, RN

733 Parents of Children with Brain Tumors (PCBT)
Children's Memorial Hospital
707 W. Fullerton Ave
Chicago, IL 60614   773-880-4485

Monthly newsletter. Library available at meetings (at CMH). Educational speakers and family
functions.

Laura Dove, SW

Indiana

734 Brain Tumor Support Group
First Christian Church

Bloomington, IN 47401   812-876-5678

Jean Bauer

735 Brain Tumor Support Group at Indianapolis
Community Hospital
East 1500 N Ritter Avenue
Indianapolis, IN 46206   317-485-6616

Lisa Peters, RN

736 Brain Tumor Support Group of Indiana
Community Hospital East 1500 N. Ritter Ave
Bradley Board Room (1st Fl)
Indianapolis, IN 46219   317-577-3900

Lisa Peters, RN
Marsha Cline

**737 Primary Brain Cancer Support Group Lutheran
Hospital**

Fort Wayne, IN 46802   219-435-7959

Linda Jordan, RN

Iowa

738 Neurological Center of Iowa
1215 Pleasant St. Ste 608
Des Moines, IA 50318   515-241-5760

Networks people in similar situations.

Lu Ann Nunn, RN

739 Quad Cities Brain Tumor Support Group
Genesis Medical Center
1803 E Kimberly, Northgate Shopping Center
Davenport, IA 52802   319-421-1905

Pat Christy, RN

Kansas

740 Headstrong Brain Tumor Support Group
Victory in the Valley
917 N Market
Witchita, KS 67276   316-262-7559

Diana Thomi

Kentucky

741 Kentucky Brain Tumor Support Group
Markley Cancer Center
800 Rose St
Lexington, KY 40511   606-257-4310

Educational materials.

Claire Courtney

Louisiana

742 Greater New Orleans Brain Tumor Support Group
West Jefferson Medical Center
1111 Medical Center Blvd S570
Marrero, LA 70072   504-830-7833

Joanne Mcgee

Maine

743 Brain Tumor Support Group
9 Spring Street
East Millinocket, ME 04430   207-746-5863

Joan Gordon

744 Brain Tumor Support Group of Maine
Maine Medical Center

Portland, ME 04104   207-871-4527

Karen Richards, RNC

745 Brain Tumor Support Grp of Maine
Kennebec Medical Center
6 East Chestnut Street
Augusta, ME 04330   207-283-4027

Mark Estes, RNC

Maryland

746 Brain Tumor Support Group of Maryland
University of Maryland Medical Center
22 S Greene Street, S-12-D
Baltimore, MD 21233   410-328-8621

Amy Yerkes

Massachusetts

747 Brain Center Brain Tumor Support Group
Promontory Point

New Seabury, MA 02536   508-477-5300

Eleanor Grace
Dick Grace

748 Brain Tumor Support Group
Brigham & Women's Hospital
75 St Francis Street
Boston, MA 02155   617-732-6826

Nancy Olson, RN, MBA

749 Brain Tumor Support Group at Burlington
Lahey Clinic
41 Mall Road
Burlington, MA 01803   978-538-4625

Michele Lucas

750 Brain Tumor Support Group at Hampden
Hampden Town House

Hampden, MA 01036   413-566-3959

Donald Dorn
Barbara Dorn

751 Brain Tumor Support Group at Worcester
University of Massachusetts Medical Ctr.
Department of Surgery
55 Lake Avenue North
Worcester, MA 01605   508-856-3611

Informal family meetings, occasional MD speakers.

Dorrie Silver, RN, BSN

752 Headstrong
81 Highland Avenue
Salem, MA 01970

Maryanne Ferry, MSW

753 Long Term Survivors Support Group
Brain Tumor Society

Boston, MA 02105   800-770-8287

Robert D. Calhoun, ACSW, LICSW

754 Massachusetts General Hospital Support Group for Brain Tumor Patients & Family

Boston, MA 02105   617-726-5841

Sarah Murphy, LICSW

755 Neurological Support Group of St. Luke's Hospital
101 Page Street
New Bedford, MA 02741   508-997-1515

Contact can be reached at extension 2764.

Diane Robinson, RN

756 Parent Education/Support Group
Dana Farber Cancer Institute, Smith Family Room
44 Binney Street
Boston, MA   617-632-3319

For parents of children with brain tumors.

Beverly LaValley, RN, MS

Michigan

757 Barbara Ann Karmanos Cancer Institute
Harper Hospital Frankel Center
18831 West Twelve Mile Road
Lathrup Village, MI 48076   313-745-1811
                                    800-527-6266

Marguerite DeBello, RN

758 Brain Tumor Support Group at Ann Arbor
St Joseph Mercy Hospital, Cancer Care Center
5301 E Huron River Drive
Ann Arbor, MA 48106   313-712-3658

Paula Nedela, RN

759 Brain Tumor Support Group at Detroit
Henry Ford Hospital
2799 West Grand Boulevard
Detroit, MI 48233   313-876-7174

Kathy Campbell, RN

760 Brain Tumor Support Group at Grand Rapids
Blodgett Memorial Medical Ctr
1840 Wealthy SE
Grand Rapids, MI 49506   616-774-7449

Guest speaker each month focusing on relevant topics.

Deb Hansen, RN

761 Brain Tumor Support Group for Patients & Families - U. of Michigan Medical Ctr
1500 E. Medical Center Drive Reception Area C
Dept. Neuro-Oncology Library
Ann Arbor, MI   734-936-9071

Michaelyn Page

762 Spectrum Brain Tumor Support Group
Spectrum Health East
1840 Wealthy SE
Grand Rapids, MI 49501   616-774-7278

Nancy Rude

763 West Michigan Cancer Center Support Group
200 North Park St
Kalamazoo, MI 49003   616-349-4460

Morrey Edwards, Ph.D

Minnesota

764 Brain Tumor Support Group at Duluth
St Mary's Medical Center
407 East 3rd Street Michiras Rm
Duluth, MN 55806   218-726-4230

Jan Stevens, RN

765 Brain Tumor Support Group at Robbinside
North Memorial Medical Center North Ed Ctr
3300 Oakdale Ave N
Robbinside, MN 58422   612-520-5594

Facilitated by Radiation RN, social worker, rehab staff, chaplain and physician.

Judy Zak

766 Brain Tumor Support Group at St. Paul Minnesota Neurology Specialists
United Hospital, Ritchie Medical Plaza
310 N Smith Ave Suite 300
St. Paul, MN 55101   612-220-5291

Sharon Mason, MA

767 Brain Tumor Support Group for Benign Tumors - Minneapolis Neuroscience Inst.
Abbott Northwestern Hospital
Sister Kennedy Inst. 800 E 28th St
Minneapolis, MN 55440   612-863-3339

Marva Bohen, RN

768 Brain Tumor Support Group for Malignant Tumors, Minneapolis Neuroscience Inst.
Abbott Northwestern Hospital
Sister Kennedy Institute, 800 E 28th Street
Minneapolis, MN 55440   612-863-3339

Marva Bohen, RN

Mississippi

769 Brain Tumor Support Group
Special Olympics Building
Madison
Jackson, MI 39205   601-957-8517

Tammy Wellington

Missouri

770 AMOR - A Cancer Support Group for Patients & Their Families
Brain Tumor Institute of Kansas City
2316 E Meyers Blvd., 7th Fl Classroom
Kansas City, MO 64141   816-276-3311

Peggy Smith, MS, RN

771 Brain Cancer Support Group Mid-America Cancer Center
St. John's Regional Health Center
2055 South Fremont
Springfield, MO 65801   417-885-3324
                            800-432-2273

Primary and metastatic brain tumors; patients, families, friends welcome.

Connie Zimmerman

772 Brain Tumor Support Group
St. Luke's Hospital of Kansas City
44th & Wornall Rd
Kansas City, MO 64141   816-932-5610

Educational materials, telephone help line, newsletter, lectures, bereavement support group.

Adrienne Williams

773 Brain Tumor Support Network of St. Louis
Missouri Baptist Medical Center
3015 N Ballas Rd, Cancer Waiting Rm., 1st Fl
St. Louis, MO 63155   314-569-5263

Alternates between speakers and support time. Provides literature, lending library of books and audiotapes, newsletters.

Sharon Weissman, MSW

774 Pediatric Brain Tumor Support Network
St. Louis Children's Hospital
1 Children's Place 3rd Fl
St. Louis, MO   314-454-6103

Occasional guest speakers. Affiliated with the Brain Tumor Support Network which produces newsletter.

Sally Koesterer, MSW, LCSW

Montana

775 Brain Tumor Support Group
Deconess Medical Center
2800 Tenth Ave North
Billings, MT 59101   406-657-4165

Lottie Harris, RN

New Hampshire

776 Brain Tumor Support Group
Frisbie Memorial Hospital
Whitehall Rd 1st Fl
Rochester, NH 03867   603-693-4194

Patti Gauvin, RN

777 Portsmouth Regional Home
Health and Hospice Services

Portmouth, NH 03801   603-692-4194
                             888-870-6952

Pam Sollenberger, BSW

New Jersey

778 Brain Tumor Support Group
Saint Barnabas Medical Center

Livingston, NJ 07039   973-322-5854

Valerie Karlin

779 Brain Tumor Support Group at Livingston
Saint Barnabas Medical Center
East Wing Suite 108
Livingston, NJ 07039   973-533-5853

Joanne Hall

**780 Brain Tumor Support Group at North Plainfield,
      Muhlenberg Regional Med. Cnt**
St. Luke's Roman Catholic Church
300 Clinton Ave
North Plainfield, NJ 07060   732-321-7000

Patty Phillips, RN

**781 Brain Tumor Support Group at Plainfield
      Muhlenberg Reg. Med. Cntr., Neuroscience**
St. Luke's Roman Catholic Church
300 Clinton Ave.
North Plainfield, NJ 07060   908-668-0650

Patty Phillips, RN

782 Brain Tumor Support Group of Monmouth County
Hazlet Township Library
251 Middle Rd
Hazlet, NJ 07730   732-739-2657

Darren Eagan

New Mexico

783 NM Alliance for the Neurologically Impaired
531 Harkle Rd., Suite B
Santa Fe, NM 87501   505-986-0600

Resource for brain injured patients.

Sandra Knutson

New York

784 Brain Tumor Support Group
Albany Medical Center
ME 176, Hematology/Oncology waiting room
Albany, NY 12212   518-262-6696

Susan Weaver, MD
Christina Blanchard, CSW, PhD

785 Brain Tumor Support Group at Manhattan
NYU Medical Center
540 First Ave, Skirball Conf. Rm, 3rd Fl
Manhattan, NY 10001   212-263-8002

Dr. Patrick Kelley, MD

786 Brain Tumor Support Group at Schenectady
Sunnyview Hospital and Rehabilitation Center
1270 Belmont Avenue, Room 184A
Schenectady, NY 12301   518-399-9300

Diana Swanker

787 Brain Tumor Support Group of CNY

Syracuse, NY 13220   315-442-7136

Phillip E. Peterson

788 Brain Tumor Support Grp.
Columbia Presbyterian, 8th Fl. (Knuckle Room)
168th St. & Ft. Washington Ave.
Manhattan, NY 10032   212-305-5571

Discounted parking available.

Michael Fetell, MD

789 Brainstormers
Strong Memorial Hospital

Rochester, NY 14692   716-334-4502

Sue Allen

790 Childhood Survivors of Cancer
Strong Memorial Hospital
1000 Elmwood Avenue
Rochester, NY   716-464-3593

Judy Black, RN

791 Goodays Brain Tumor Support Group
Holiday Inn - Henrietta 111 Jefferson Road
Courtyrd Marriott, 33 Corp
Rochester, NY   716-334-4502

For parents/children or caregivers of individuals
with brain tumor/spinal cord tumors.

Sue Allen

**792 Long Island Adult Brain Tumor Support Group -
Nassau Chapter**
Plainview-Old Bethpage Public Library
999 Old Country Rd.
Plainview, NY 11803   516-747-8749

Billie Wilczek

793 Long Island Brain Tumor Support Group
120 Main St, Emma Clark Library
Setauket, NY 11733   516-747-8749

Billie Wilczek

**794 People Treated for Brain Tumors and their
Caregivers**
Memorial Sloan-Kettering Cancer Center
215 E 68th Street Ground Fl
Manhattan, NY   212-717-3527

The Post-Treatment Resource Program (PTRP)
offers support groups, lectures, and open house
meetings. Newsletter, lending library, and special counseling also available.

Melinda Friedrich, CSW

**795 People Treated for Brian Tumors and Their
Caregivers**
Memorial Sloan-Kettering Cancer Center
215 E 68th St, Ground Fl
Manhattan, NY 10001   212-717-3527

Melinda Friedrich, CSW

796 Support for Parents of Children with Brain Tumors
19 East 88 Street Suite 1D
Manhattan, NY   212-534-8877

Marcia Greenleaf, MD

North Carolina

797 Brain Tumor Support Group
Wake Forest University-Baptist Medical Ctr.

Winston-Salem, NC 27102   336-716-4137

Rayetta Johnson, RN, MSN

798 Charlotte Brain Tumor Support Group
Carolina Neurosurgery and Spine Associates

Charlotte, NC 28228   704-384-9429

Karen Carson, RN

799 Duke Brain Tumor Support Group
Duke University Medical Center

Durham, NC 27701   919-684-3608

Bebe Guill, Director

**800 Duke Pediatric Brain Tumor Family Support
Program**
Duke Univ Medical Center
Durham, NC   919-684-3401

Bebe Guill, Director of Family Suppor Program

801 Raleigh Area Brain Tumor Support Group
Raleigh Community Hospital
3400 Wake Forrest Rd.
Raleigh, NC 27626   919-876-1856

Lectures, educational materials, newsletter.
Home and hospital visitation.

Barbara Brookshire

Ohio

802 Brain Tumor Support Group
The Cleveland Clinic Cancer Center
9500 Euclid Ave, Conference Rm T-120
Cleveland, OH 44101   216-445-6910
                                           800-223-2273

Kathy Lupica, RN, MSN

803 Central Ohio Brain Tumor Support Group
Arthur Jaames Cancer Hospital and Research Inst.
300 W 10th Ave, Rm 518
Columbus, OH 43216   614-293-8427

Diana Blue, MSW

804 Cleveland Brain Tumor Patient Network - Adult and Pediatric
University Hospitals of Cleveland
Neurosurgery Conference Rd
Cleveland, OH 44101   216-556-5315

Lynn Szakacs

805 Neuro-Oncology Support Group
Wellness Community of Greater Cincinnati
8044 Montgomery Rd, Ste 385
Cincinnati, OH 45214   513-791-4060

Don Smith
Sherry Wethers

806 Southwest Ohio Brain Tumor Support Group Brain Tumor Support Group
Kettering Hospital
3535 Southern Blvd., Dining Rm 2B
Dayton, OH 45401   937-687-3325

Darlene Carroll

807 Support Group for Parents of Children with a Brain Tumor
Children's Hospital Med Ctr
Cincinnati, OH 45229   513-559-4726

Karen Burkett, CNS
Susan Mcgee, CNS

Oregon

808 Brain Tumor Support Group
Good Samaritan Hospital & Medical Center
1130 NW 22nd Ave, 2nd Fl, Conference Rm.
Portland, OR 97208   503-413-7848

Val Ivey, LCSW

Pennsylvania

809 Braim Tumor Support Group of the Lehigh Valley
St. John's Lutheran Church
5th and Chestnut St.
Emmaus, PA 18049   610-776-2566

Dolores Fioriglio

810 Brain Tumor Family Support Group
West Pennsylvania Hospital, 4800 Friendship Ave.
Consultation Room Unit 4800
Pittsburgh, PA 15224   412-578-5105

Charlene Amato, MSW

811 Brain Tumor Support Group
Bradford Regional Med. Cntr
116 Interstate Pkwy.
Bradford, PA 16701   814-362-8329

Debby Abrams

812 Brain Tumor Support Group at Bradford
Bradford Regional Med Ctr 116 Interstate Parkway
Bradford, PA 16701   814-362-8329

Debby Abrams

813 Brain Tumor Support Group at Lancaster
St. Joseph's Hospital

Lancaster, PA 17064   717-392-4512

Betty Greider

814 Brain Tumor Support Group at Philadelphia
Hospital of University of Pennsylvania Cancer Ctr.
3400 Spruce St., Bridge Level, Penn Town Hotel
Philadelphia, PA 19104   215-662-4485

Nancy O'Connor, RN, MSN
Linda Stevenson

815 Brain Tumor Support Group at Pittsburgh
Cancer Caring Center

Pittsburgh, PA 15219   412-622-1212

Rebecca Whitlinger

816 Brain Tumor Support Group of Philadelphia
Hospital of Univ. of PA Cancer Center
3400 Spruce St. Bdg Level, Penn Tower Hotel
Philadelphia, PA 19104   215-662-4485

Nancy O'Conner, RN, MSN

817 Brain Tumor Support Group of Pittsburgh
Pittsburgh Cancer Institute
Monte Fiore Hospital, 7 Main Lounge
Pittsburgh, PA   412-624-1115
                             800-237-4724

Contact is the Cancer Info and Referral Services.

818 Brain Tumor Support Group of the Lehigh Valley
St. John's Lutheran Church
5th and Chestnut Street
Emmaus, PA   610-776-2566

24 hour phone service for families of, or for, people with questions regarding brain tumors.

Dolores Fioriglio

819 C-Brain (Cranial Base Resource & Information Network)
230 Lothrop St.
Pittsburgh, PA 15219   412-683-4273

Liz Odoroff

820 Pittsburgh Area Brain Tumor Support Group
Allegheny General Hospital
320 E. North Ave. Magoven Conference Ctr. 2nd Fl.
Pittsburgh, PA 15212
                             800-448-0904

Separate meetings for people with advanced disease and benign tumors/post-acute patients.

Stacy Lang

821 Presbyterian Hospital/Pittsburgh Cancer Center
DeSoto At O'Hara Street
Pittsburgh, PA 15213   412-647-3475

Susan Chamberlin-Downie

822 Support Group for Parents & Children with Brain Tumors
Children's Hospital of Philadelphia
34th & Civic Center Boulevard
Philadelphia, PA   609-924-7367

Six newsletters each year, informal meetings alternate with guest speakers.

Marion Roemner

823 Support Group for Parents and Children with Brain Tumors
Children's Hospital of Philadelphia
34th & Civic Center Blvd.
Philadelphia, PA 19104   609-924-7367

Six newsletters each year, informal meetings alternate with guest speakers.

Marion Roemner

824 Wills Eye Brain Tumor Support Group
900 Walnut St
Philadelphia, PA 19104   215-928-7045

Ann Marie DiBona

Rhode Island

825 Brain Tumor Support Group at Providence
Brown University Campus
BioMedical Center
Providence, RI 02940   401-789-0126

Judy Allenson

South Carolina

826 Newbury County Memorial Hospital

Newberry, SC 29106   803-276-5290

Tina Doran

Tennessee

827 Nashville Brain Tumor Support Group
Southern Hills Medical Center
391 Wallace Rd
Nashville, TN 37202   615-781-4190

Ronnie Gammons

828 Regional Brain Tumor Support Group
Medical Education Research Institution

Memphis, TN 38101   901-726-5875

Heidi Bergstrom, RN, BSN

Texas

829 Brain Tumor Support Group at Austin
Health South Rehab Hospital
1215 Red River, Cafeteria
Austin, TX 78710   512-474-5700
                e-mail: buglady999@apl.com

Sue Haley

830 Brain Tumor Support Group at Dallas
ACS Building
8900 Carpenter Freeway
Dallas, TX 75260   214-648-9116

Marilyn Early

831 Brain Tumor Support Group at Plano
Medical Center Plano

Plano, TX 75074   972-596-6848

Marlene Cohen

832 Brain Tumor Support Group for Families of Children with Brain and Spinal Tumors
Methodist Hospital, Hodges Care Center
3615 - 19th Street Conference Room
Lubbock, TX   806-792-1011
                800-687-5437

Jim Powell

833 HOPE (Helping Oncology Parents Endure) Brain Tumor Foundation of the Southwest
Children's Medical Center of Dallas
1935 Motor Street
Dallas, TX   214-640-6139

Deborah Doxey

834 Houston Area Brain Tumor Network
Neuro and Supportive Care Clinic UTMD Anderson

Houston, TX 77001   713-792-0772

Wendy Nes, LMSW/ACP

835 Houston Area Brain Tumor Support Network
Jesse Jones Rotary House International
1600 Holcombe Blvd.
Houston, TX 77001   713-792-0760

Dialogue, sharing and educational programs.

Wendy Nes, LMSW/ACP

836 Shirvers Cancer Center Brain Tumor Support Group
University of Texas Nursing School
1215 Red River, Cafeteria
Austin, TX 78710   512-469-7378

Ann Harris
Karen Martin

837 Shirvers Cancer Center Brain Tumor Support Group
University of Texas Nursing School
1700 Red River Room 5180
Austin, TX 78712   512-469-7378

Ann Harris
Karen Martin

838 We've Just Begun to Live Brain Tumor Support Group
Audie Murphy VA Hospital
7400 Merton Minter, 2nd Fl, Rm 234
San Antonio, TX 78265   210-617-5300

Diane Johnson

839 West Texas Brain Tumor Support Group
Abilene Regional Med. Ctr., 2nd Fl. Room 270
1680 Antilley Rd.
Abilene, TX 79604   915-698-7566

Jana Boss, RN

Utah

840 Peer-Led Brain Tumor Support Group
University of Utah Hospital and Clinics
50 N Medical Dr, 2nd Fl, next to chapel
Salt Lake City, UT 84119   801-581-2584

Karen Elliott

Virginia

841 Brain Tumor Support Group
St. Mary's Hospital
Education Ctr, 5801 Bremo Rd
Richmond, VA 23261   804-828-5712

Cindy Carmack

Washington

842 Adult Brain Tumor Support Group
Virginia Mason Medical Center
1201 Terry St, N Pavillion, 7th Fl, Neurology
Seattle, WA 98109   206-341-0420

Michelle Handler

843 Brain Tumor Support Group University of Washington Medical Center
Cancer Center Conference Room, 1st Fl.
1959 NE Pacific St.
Seattle, WA 98105   206-548-4108

Occasional lectures.

Susan Goedde, MSW

844 Brain Tumor Support Group at Seattle
University of Washington Medical Center
Cancer Ctr Conf. Rm, 1st Fl, 1959 NE Pacific St
Seattle, WA 98109   206-548-4108

Susan Goedde, MSW

845 Northwest Hospital Brain Tumor Support Group
Northwest Hospital
1560 N 115th St., Bldg. 4, Lower G Level
Seattle, WA 98109   206-368-1304

Mark Filler, SW

846 Northwest Hospital Brain Tumor Group Support Hotline
Northwest Hospital, 1560 N. 115th St.
Bldg. 4, Lower G Level Conference Rm.
Seattle, WA 98644   206-368-1606

West Virginia

847 Southern West Virginia Brain Tumor Support Group
First Presbyterian Church
16 Broad St., Room A-204
Charleston, WV 25301   304-744-0393

Jeri McDonald

Wisconsin

848 Brain Tumor Support Group
Luther Hospital
1221 Whipple St., Conference Rms. 2 & 3
Eau Claire, WI 54703   715-838-3258

Julie Brave
Alyce Kneuppel

849 Brain Tumor Support Group at Milwaukee
St Lukes Medical Center
2900 West Oklahoma Avenue
Milwaukee, WI 53201   414-649-5796

Linda Piacentine, RN, MS, CNRN

850 Brain Tumor Support Group at Wauwatosa
Froederdt Memorial Lutheran Hospital
MCW Conference Center A & B
9200 W. Wisconsin Ave.
Wauwatosa, WI   414-259-2629

Celeste Volcesek
Denise Lemke

851 Brain Tuor Support Group at Milwaupee
Radiation Oncology Reception
St. Luke's Medical Center, 2900 W. Oklahoma
Ave.
Milwaupee, WI   414-649-5796

Linda Piacentine, RN, MS, CNRN

852 John Sierzant Brain Tumor Support Group
Lutheran Hospital, Gunderson Clinic
1836 South Avenue, 3rd Floor
LaCrosse, WI 54601   608-782-7300

Polly Davenport-Fortune, Nurse Practioner

853 LODAT (Living One Day at a Time) Brain Tumor
Support Group
Children's Hospital of Wisconsin
Room 888
Milwaukee, WI   414-962-8984

Parent support group for families of chidren
with cancer. Monthly newsletter, informational
meetings, social activities for families, and bereavement support.

Frances Swigart

Libraries & Resource Centers

854 Brain Tissue Resource Center
McLean Hospital
115 Mill Street
Belmont, MA 02178   781-855-2400

Edward D. Bird, Director

Research Centers

855 Brain Research Center
Children's Hospital National Medical Center
111 Michigan Avenue NW
Washington, DC 20010   202-884-2070

Barbara Herman, Chief

856 Brain Research Foundation
208 S LaSalle Street
Chicago, IL 60604   312-782-4311

Nancy W. Hohfeler, Executive Director

857 National Brain Research Association
1439 Rhode Island Avenue NW
Washington, DC 20005   202-483-6272

Also provides support groups for parents

858 University of California, San Francisco Brain Tumor
Research Center
1001 Portero Road
San Francisco, CA 94110   415-206-8313

Research done on brain tumors.

Lawrence H. Pitts, MD
Pitts, MD

Audio Video

859 National Brain Tumor Conference Audiotapes
National Brain Tumor Foundation
785 Market Street, Suite 1600
San Francisco, CA 94103   415-284-0208
                                       800-934-2873
                                  Fax: 415-284-0209
                         e-mail: nbtf@braintumor.org
                                www.braintumor.org

Audiotapes of keynote addresses and conference
workshops from NBTF's biennial National
Brain Tumor Conferences where leading researchers, physicians and health professionals
address a wide range of issues affecting brain tumor survivors, such as new approaches to radiation and surgery, research and coping skills for
families.

Web Sites

860 Cancer Resource List
www.cancercare.org/faq/cancer_faq.html

861 CancerCare:
www.cancercare.org/faq/cancer_faq.html

862 Meningioma Mailing List
www.med.jhu.edu/radiosurgry/trial/mening
e-mail: jw@jhu.edu
www.med.jhu.edu/radiosurgry/trial/mening

Jeffery Williams

863 Starting Point: To Connect with Resources Related to Pediatric Neuro-oncology
www.med.miami.edu/neurosurgery/start_intro.htm
e-mail: jragheb@newssun.med.miami.edu
www.med.miami.edu/neurosurgery/start_intro.htm

Children's Books

864 Alex's Journey: The Story of a Child with a Brain Tumor
American Brain Tumor Association
2720 River Road, Suite 146
Des Plaines, IL 60018
847-827-9910
800-886-2282
Fax: 847-827-9918
e-mail: info@abta.org
www.abta.org

56 pages Booklet
ISBN: 0-944093-29-9

Newsletters

865 Childhood Brain Tumor Foundation Newsletter
12141 Pineneedle Court
Woodbridge, VA 22192
703-492-0045
Fax: 703-492-0045
www.mnsinc.com/cbtf

A major service this organization provides is the CHILDHOOD CANCER OMBUDSMAN PROGRAM, a free service consisting of volunteers trained in the disciplines of medicine, law, and education who provide assistance in: 1) seeking second opinions, 2) access to healthcare, and 3) combating discrimination. They also publish a quarterly newsletter.

866 Message Line
American Brain Tumor Association
2720 River Road, Suite 146
Des Plaines, IL 60018
847-827-9910
800-886-2282
Fax: 847-827-9917
e-mail: info@abta.org
www.abta.org

Describes research advances and announces updates to publications.
Booklet

867 SEARCH
National Brain Tumor Foundation
785 Market Street-Suite 1600
San Francisco, CA 94103
415-284-0208
800-934-2873
Fax: 415-284-0209
e-mail: nbtf@braintumor.org
www.braintumor.org

Newsletter that covers topics of current interest to brain tumor survivors and their families.

Pamphlets

868 A Brain Tumor Sharing Hope
American Brain Tumor Association
2720 River Road, Suite 146
Des Plaines, IL 60018
847-827-9910
800-886-2282
Fax: 847-827-9918
e-mail: info@abta.org
www.abta.org

Also available in Spanish.
Pamphlet

869 A Primer of Brain Tumors
American Brain Tumor Association
2720 River Road, Suite 146
Des Plaines, IL 60018
847-827-9910
800-886-2282
Fax: 847-827-9918
e-mail: info@abta.org
www.abta.org

A patient's reference manual offering information on brain tumors.
Pamphlet
ISBN: 0-944093-35-3

870 About Ependymoma
American Brain Tumor Association
2720 River Road, Suite 146
Des Plaines, IL 60018
847-827-9910
800-886-2282
Fax: 847-827-9918
e-mail: info@abta.org
www.abta.org

Pamphlet
ISBN: 0-944093-40-X

871 About Glioblastoma Multiforme and Anaplastic Astrocytoma
American Brain Tumor Association
2720 River Road, Suite 146
Des Plaines, IL 60018   847-827-9910
                                  800-886-2282
                          Fax: 847-827-9918
                          e-mail: info@abta.org
                                  www.abta.org

Pamphlet
ISBN: 0-944093-36-1

872 About Medulloblastoma/PNET (Medulloblastom a)
American Brain Tumor Association
2720 River Road, Suite 146
Des Plaines, IL 60018   847-827-9910
                                  800-886-2282
                          Fax: 847-827-9918
                          e-mail: info@abta.org
                                  www.abta.org

Pamphlet
ISBN: 0-944093-33-7

873 About Meningioma
American Brain Tumor Association
2720 River Road, Suite 146
Des Plaines, IL 60018   847-827-9910
                                  800-886-2282
                          Fax: 847-827-9918
                          e-mail: info@abta.org
                                  www.abta.org

Pamphlet
ISBN: 0-944093-23-X

874 About Metastatic Tumors to the Brain and S pine
American Brain Tumor Association
2720 River Road, Suite 146
Des Plaines, IL 60018   847-827-9910
                                  800-886-2282
                          Fax: 847-827-9918
                          e-mail: info@abta.org
                                  www.abta.org

Pamphlet
ISBN: 0-944093-26-4

875 About Oligodendroglioma and Mixed Glioma
American Brain Tumor Association
2720 River Road, Suite 146
Des Plaines, IL 60018   847-827-9910
                                  800-886-2282
                          Fax: 847-827-9918
                          e-mail: info@abta.org
                                  www.abta.org

Pamphlet
ISBN: 0-944093-43-4

876 About Pituitary Tumors
American Brain Tumor Association
2720 River Road, Suite 146
Des Plaines, IL 60018   847-827-9910
                                  800-886-2282
                          Fax: 847-827-9918
                          e-mail: info@abta.org
                                  www.abta.org

Pamphlet
ISBN: 0-944093-44-2

877 About the American Brain Tumor Association
American Brain Tumor Association
2720 River Road, Suite 146
Des Plaines, IL 60018   847-827-9910
                                  800-886-2282
                          Fax: 847-827-9918
                          e-mail: info@abta.org
                                  www.abta.org

Pamphlet

878 Brain Tumor Resource Directory
NBTF Publications and Items

                                  800-934-2873

A comprehensive reference for health care providers. The directory contains the names and phone numbers of various organizations that offer services and products of particular interest to brain tumor patients and their families.

879 Brain Tumor Support Groups in North America
NBTF

                                  800-934-2873

A listing of over 170 groups for patients and families.

880 Brain Tumors, A Guide
National Brain Tumor Foundation
785 Market Street-Suite 1600
San Francisco, CA 94103   415-284-0208
                                  800-934-2873
                          Fax: 415-284-0209
                          www.braintumor.org

Published by the National Brain Tumor Foundation, this easy-to-read booklet about brain tumors contains valuable information for newly diagnosed patients, long term survivors, family members and health professionals. Current information on treatment, patient rights, nutrition, research and more. Also contains a glossary of terms, plus information on support groups and other resources.

56 pages

881 Brain Tumors: Understanding Your Care
NBTF Publications and Items

800-934-2873

This publication provides basic information about diagnosis and treatment for the newly diagnosed brain tumor patient. Developed and published by Staywell-Krames Communications.

882 Chemotherapy of Brain Tumors
American Brain Tumor Association
2720 River Rd., Suite146
Des Plaines, IL 60018   847-827-9910
800-886-2282
Fax: 847-827-9918
e-mail: info@abta.org
www.abta.org

Provides information that will help you understand and participate in your chemotherapy treatment.

883 Clinical Trial Information
National Brain Tumor Foundation
785 Market Street, Suite 1600
San Francisco, CA 94103   415-284-0208
800-934-2873
Fax: 415-284-0209
e-mail: nbtf@braintumor.org
www.braintumor.org

Lists of clinical trials by state, tumor type and/or treatment type.

884 Coping with Your Loved One's Brain Tumor
NBTF Publications and Items

800-934-2873

A brochure about how a brain tumor effects the family and practical suggestions to help cope with these changes.

885 Coping with a Brain Tumor Part I: From Diagnosis to Treatment
American Brain Tumor Association
2720 River Rd., Suite 146
Des Plaines, IL 60018   847-827-9910
800-886-2282
Fax: 847-827-9918
e-mail: info@abta.org
www.abta.org

ISBN: 0-990933-02-

886 Coping with a Brain Tumor Part II: During and After Treatment
American Brain Tumor Association
2720 River Rd., Suite 146
Des Plaines, IL 60018   847-827-9910
800-886-2282
Fax: 847-827-9918
e-mail: inffo@abta.org
www.abta.org

ISBN: 0-990933-10-

887 Dictionary for Brain Tumor Patients
American Brain Tumor Association
2720 River Rd., Suite 146
Des Plaines, IL 60018   847-827-9910
800-886-2282
Fax: 847-827-9918
e-mail: info@abta.org
www.abta.org

Offers a dictionary of terms used in the diagnosis and everyday living with brain tumors.

ISBN: 0-944093-27-2

888 National Brain Tumor Foundation Fact Sheets
NBTF

800-934-2873

Titles include: Pilocytic Astrocytoma in Adults, Childhood Brain Tumors Occurring in the Adult, Clinical Trials for Brain Tumors, Issues to Consider When Choosing a Treatment Center, Gene Therapy: A New Experimental Treatment for Brain Tumors, New Chemotherapy Drugs for Brain Tumor Patients, Who Gets Brain Tumors and Why? and Preguntas Sobre Los Tumores Cerebrales (In Spanish.)

889 Organizing a Support Group
American Brain Tumor Association
2720 River Rd., Suite 146
Des Plaines, IL 60018   847-827-9910
                                     800-886-2282
                                Fax: 847-827-9918
                           e-mail: info@abta.org
                                     www.abta.org

**890 Radiation Therapy of Brain Tumors Part I: A Basic
Guide**
American Brain Tumor Association
2720 River Rd., Suite 146
Des Plaines, IL 60018   847-827-9910
                                     800-886-2282
                                Fax: 847-827-9918
                           e-mail: info@abta.org
                                     www.abta.org.

ISBN: 0-944093-28-0

**891 Radiation Therapy of Brain Tumors Part II:
Background and Research Guide**
American Brain Tumor Association
2720 River Rd., Suite 146
Des Plaines, IL 60018   847-827-9910
                                     800-886-2282
                                Fax: 847-827-9918
                           e-mail: info@abta.org
                                     www.abta.org.

892 Stereotactic Radiosurgery
American Brain Tumor Association
2720 River Rd., Suite 146
Des Plaines, IL 60018   847-827-9910
                                     800-886-2282
                                Fax: 847-827-9918
                           e-mail: info@abta.org
                                     www.abta.org.

ISBN: 0-944093-42-6

**893 Understanding Brain Tumors: Glioblastoma
Multiforme**
NBTF Publications and Items

                                     800-934-2873

A 16 page brochure to help patients and caregivers understand more about the diagnosis and
treatment of the glioblastoma multiforme.

**894 Understanding and Coping with Your Child's Brain
Tumor**
National Brain Tumor Foundation
785 Market Street-Suite 1600
San Francisco, CA 94103   415-284-0208
                                     800-934-2873
                                Fax: 415-284-0209
                                     www.braintumor.org

Published by the National Brain Tumor Foundation, this guide for families and resource for
hope contains information for parents of children with brain tumors. Provides information
about diagnosis, tumor types, treatment methods, social and emotional support and more.
Also contains a glossary and listings of organizations and resources.

895 Using a Medical Library
American Brain Tumor Association
2720 River Rd., Suite 146
Des Plaines, IL 60018   847-827-9910
                                     800-886-2282
                                Fax: 847-827-9918
                           e-mail: info@abta.org
                                     www.abta.org.

896 What You Need to Know About Brain Tumors
National Cancer Institute
Building 31, Room 10A24
Bethesda, MD 20892
                                     800-422-6237

Offers factual information about brain tumors,
possible causes, primary and secondary tumors,
symptoms, diagnosis, treatment, side effects, fol-
lowup care, support and medical terms.

897 When Your Child is Ready to Return to School
American Brain Tumor Association
2720 River Road, Ste. 146
Des Plaines, IL 60018   847-827-9910
                                     800-886-2282
                                Fax: 847-827-9918
                           e-mail: info@abta.org
                                     www.abta.org

Guides parents and teachers through a successful return to school when a child has had a brain
tumor.

ISBN: 0-944093-21-3

DESCRIPTION

898 BRONCHOPULMONARY DYSPLASIA
Synonym: BPD

Bronchopulmonary dysplasia (BPD) is a chronic lung disease of infancy that is characterized by injury of the lung's airways, causing abnormal tissue changes, inflammation, and eventual scarring of lung tissue. BPD often affects infants who have become dependent on the long-term use of ventilators to mechanically assist breathing. In infants with BPD, lung injury is thought to result from prolonged breathing of high concentrations of oxygen under abnormally high pressure and volume (oxygen toxicity, barotrauma, and volutrauma). BPD affects infants who are born prior to 37 weeks of pregnancy (premature newborns) and are affected by severe respiratory distress syndrome of the newborn (RDS) that requires long-term mechanical ventilation. RDS is a breathing disorder characterized by insufficient production of a substance that is produced as the lungs mature during fetal development (surfactant). Surfactant reduces the surface tension of fluids lining the air sacs (alveoli) of the lungs, enabling the air sacs to remain open between breaths. Due to insufficient surfactant in newborns with RDS, greater pressure is required to expand the lungs' airways and air sacs. As a result, the air sacs may collapse and the lungs may become unable to properly provide oxygenated blood to the body. Within minutes or hours after birth, newborns with RDS experience increasing difficulty breathing (dyspnea), characterized by rapid, labored, shallow breaths (tachypnea); grunting upon exhalation; drawing in of the chest wall during inhalation; and bluish discoloration of the skin and mucous membranes (cyanosis) due to lack of sufficient oxygen supply to bodily tissues (hypoxia). In infants with severe RDS, treatment typically includes prolonged support with a ventilator (positive pressure ventilator).

Despite receiving increasing concentrations of oxygen and other treatment measures, newborns with RDS and subsequent bronchopulmonary dysplasia continue to experience severe respiratory symptoms rather than improve as expected. These infants have ongoing respiratory distress associated with lack of sufficient oxygen supply to bodily tissues (hypoxia), abnormally high levels of carbon dioxide in the blood (hypercarbia), a reduced ability of the right side of the heart to pump blood efficiently (right-sided heart failure), and continued oxygen dependency. Approximately two to three weeks after continued ventilation support, x-ray examination and other diagnostic techniques may demonstrate the abnormal tissue changes (bronchiolar metaplasia) and scarring of lung tissue associated with bronchopulmonary dysplasia.

The treatment of infants with BPD may include gradual weaning off mechanical ventilation; prescription of corticosteroid medications (e.g., dexamethasone); administration of medications to help expand the airways of the lungs (bronchodilators) and drugs to promote the excretion of fluid from the body (diuretics); restriction of fluid intake; and measur to help prevent or treat certain respiratory infections (e.g., respiratory syncytial virus). Growth of the lungs is the most important treatment and most patients recover by approximately six to 12 months. However, these children may have an increased susceptibility to inflammation of the lungs (pneumonia) due to respiratory infections or other potential complications, such as temporary growth failure. In some patients with severe BPD, prolonged hospitalization may be necessary.

The following organizations in the General Resources Section can provide additional information: March of Dimes Birth Defects Foundation, Genetic Alliance, NIH/National Heart, Lung and Blood Institute Information Center, National Organization for Rare Disorders, Inc. (NORD), NIH/Office for Rare Diseases, NIH/National Institute of Child Health and Human Development

National Associations & Support Groups

899 American Lung Association
1740 Broadway
New York, NY 10019   212-315-8700
                        e-mail: info@lungusa.org
www.lungusa.org/press/report/pedlung/pedbronchfa.h
                                                  tm

Offers research, medical updates, fund-raising,
educational materials and public awareness campaigns relating to lung disease and related disorders. Focuses on asthma, tobacco control, and
environmental issues.

Web Sites

900 University of Ottawa
www.cheo.on.ca/bpd/BPDindex.html

DESCRIPTION

901 BURN INJURIES

May involve these systems in the body (see Section III):
Dermatologic System

Burn injuries account for approximately 6,000 deaths per year in the United States. Among children, it follows only automobile accidents as a leading cause of accidental fatalities. Burns may be caused by heat, chemicals, or electrical current and are classified as first degree burns, second degree burns, or third degree burns, according to the severity and depth of the injury.

First degree burns, the least severe, affect the surface of the skin (superficial) and are characterized by a sensitive or painful reddened area of skin that sometimes swells and, in some cases, peels off. These types of burns affect only the top layer of skin (epidermis), do not blister, and, in most cases, heal spontaneously with no complications.

Second degree burns affect both the upper layer of skin and varying degrees of the underlying layer (dermis). This type of burn causes blistering. Even if the burn is relatively superficial, the pain may be intense as a result of exposed nerve endings. Superficial second degree burns usually heal within one to two weeks with no residual effects. Deeper second degree burns may actually be less painful and, if kept clean and free of infection, also heal with no complications. Second degree burns that cover more than 30 percent of the body surface area are considered critical.

Third degree burns destroy the upper layer of the skin and the underlying tissues; therefore, this type of burn typically requires skin grafting or other special treatment. Third degree burns are usually characterized by either a white or charred appearance; however, the burned area may appear bright red. Third degree burns that cover more than 10 percent of the body surface area or that involve the face or extremities are considered critical.

Hospitalization for first and second degree burn injuries is largely determined by the amount of the body surface area that is affected. As a general rule, if there is less than 10 percent involvement, treatment may be provided at home or on an outpatient basis. Treatment may include thorough cleansing of the wounds and topical application of antibacterial ointments to small burn areas. Blister management may be provided through cream dressings. If blisters break, thorough cleansing to prevent infection (debridement) is indicated. Bandage or gauze dressings may be applied to keep the injured areas clean to avoid infection. Skin grafting may be indicated for extensive second degree burns. Other treatment may include the administration of antibiotics and painkillers, as well as injection of a tetanus booster, if necessary.

Third degree or other severe burns may be life-threatening and usually require hospitalization. Emergency procedures may include the administration of oxygen and establishment of an airway to assist in breathing. Vital signs are routinely checked. To prevent kidney failure and other serious complications such as shock, other treatment usually includes intravenous replacement of proteins, body fluids, and essential elements in the fluid portion of the blood (electrolytes such as sodium, potassium, and calcium) lost as a result of extensive injury. The wounds are meticulously cleaned and dressed, and antibiotics are usually administered intravenously to prevent infection. As with less severe burns, tetanus immunization is updated. Extreme vigilance is observed in order to preserve the integrity of surrounding tissue, sometimes necessitating the surgical removal of crusted dead skin (escharotomy) that may interfere with circulation. If injured, arms or legs are elevated. In order to help avoid the tightening and contracting of skin and muscles, the limbs may be splinted. Temporary skin grafting may be performed until permanent grafting is possible. In addition, nutritional considerations may necessitate the administration of supplements or, in the case of those unable to eat or drink, insertion of a tube through the nose to deliver nutrition directly into the stomach. Burns sustained through chemical and electrical influences may involve other systems of the body and, as such, are treated symptomatically. Psychological support by a team of professionals is an extremely important element in the recovery of individuals with burn injuries. Other treatment is symptomatic and supportive.

Web Sites

902 Burn Institute
www.burninstitute.org

903 Burn Prevention Foundation
www.burnprevention.org

904 Consumer Products Safety Commission
www.cpsc.gov

905 Cool the Burn
www.cooltheburn.com

906 International Society for Burn Injuries
www.worldplasticsurgury.org.isbi.html

907 National Burn Victim Foundation
www.nbvf.org

908 National Fire Programs
www.usfa.fema.gov/nfirs/

909 National Fire Protection Association
www.nfpa.org

910 Northwest Burn Foundation Camp
weber.u.washington.edu/~doitsum/burn.html

911 Trauma Foundation
www.traumafdn.org/injuries/fire5.html

DESCRIPTION

912 CAFE-AU-LAIT SPOTS
Synonym: CAL Spots
May involve these systems in the body (see Section III):
Dermatologic System

Cafe-au-lait spots are pale tan or light brown (i.e., coffee-colored) discolorations of the skin. These areas of discoloration are termed macules, meaning that they are not elevated above the surface of the skin. These macules are often oval in shape and uniform in color, usually have smooth borders, and may vary greatly in size from approximately 0.5 to 12 centimeters in diameter. Cafe-au-lait spots develop due to a localized increase in the number of specialized skin cells (melanocytes) that produce melanin, a pigment that gives coloration to the skin.

In many individuals, the presence of cafe-au-lait spots has no clinical significance. In fact, up to 10 percent of children may have one to three cafe-au-lait spots in the absence of any underlying disorder. The macules may be present at birth or may become apparent during childhood.

In other cases, the presence of multiple or irregular cafe-au-lait spots is a characteristic finding that occurs in association with certain genetic disorders, such as neurofibromatosis type I or McCune-Albright syndrome. Neurofibromatosis type I (NF1) is a genetic disorder that is characterized by the appearance of multiple cafe-au-lait spots and benign, fibrous tumors of nerve and skin tissue (neurofibromas); benign, tumor-like nodules (Lisch nodules) on the pigmented areas of the eyes (irides); associated skeletal abnormalities; and other symptoms and findings. In most children with NF1, several cafe-au-lait spots may develop by approximately one year of age. The macules typically increase in number and size over time, and approximately 80 percent of affected individuals have six or more spots measuring 1.5 centimeters or more in diameter after the onset of puberty. McCune-Albright syndrome is a genetic disorder characterized by multiple areas of abnormal fibrous growth that displaces bone tissue (polyostotic fibrous dysplasia); cafe-au-lait spots; and abnormalities of certain hormone-producing glands that assist in regulating the body's growth, controlling the rate of metabolism, and promoting the development of secondary sexual characteristics (puberty). In children with McCune-Albright syndrome, cafe-au-lait spots may be apparent at birth or during later childhood. The macules are relatively large, tend to be asymmetric with irregular borders, and usually develop most extensively on the side of the body that is most severely affected by polyostotic fibrous dysplasia. In addition, in some cases, cafe-au-lait spots may be associated with other underlying genetic disorders (e.g., tuberous sclerosis, ataxia telangiectasia, and Watson syndrome).

Because cafe-au-lait spots may occur in association with certain underlying disorders, physicians may conduct thorough clinical examinations and regularly monitor affected children to detect characteristic findings associated with such disorders and to ensure early diagnosis and prompt, appropriate treatment.

The following organizations in the General Resources Section can provide additional information: NIH National Institute of Arthritis and Musculoskeletal and Skin Diseases

National Associations & Support Groups

913 American Academy of Dermatology
930 North Meacham Road, P.O. Box4014
Schaumburg, IL 60168   708-330-0230
www.aad.org

Largest, most influential and most representative of all dermatologic associations. Committed to the highest quality standards in continuing medical education. Developed a platform in which to promote and advance the science and art of medicine and surgery related to the skin; promote the highest possible standards in clinical practice, education and research in dermatology and related disciplines; and support and enhance patient care and promote the public interest relating to dermatology.

914 American Skin Association
150 East 58th Street, 33rd Floor
New York, NY 10155   212-753-8260
                                    800-499-7546
                              Fax: 212-688-6547
              e-mail: AmericanSkin@compuserve.com

DESCRIPTION

915 CAMPTODACTYLY
Synonym: Camptodactylia
Disorder Type: Birth Defect, Genetic Disorder

Camptodactyly refers to a condition that is present at birth (congenital) and is characterized by the permanent bending (flexion contracture) of one or more of the joints of the finger(s) (interphalangeal joints). This condition may not be readily apparent in some infants until later in their childhood. Although all the fingers may be involved, the little or pinky finger is most commonly affected, while involvement of the thumb is very rare. In addition, camptodactyly may be manifested evenly on both hands (bilateral) with mild to severe involvement. If camptodactyly involves only the little fingers, the defect may also be called streptomicrodactyly or streblomicrodactyly. Other characteristic findings may include an absence of skin creases on the palm side of the affected site, as well as irregular skin ridge patterns (dermatoglyphics). Some children may also have irregularly bent (flexed) toes. Streblodactyly is a related, but possibly distinct, malformation in which all the fingers are permanently flexed at the joints closest to the hand (proximal interphalangeal joints).

Camptodactyly may occur as an isolated abnormality that is inherited through an autosomal dominant trait with males and females equally affected. This condition may also be a characteristic finding of other inherited syndromes with various modes of transmission.

For example, craniocarpotarsal dystrophy (Freeman-Sheldon syndrome), also an autosomal dominant disorder, is characterized by camptodactyly, a flattened mask-like facial appearance, an abnormally small mouth (microstomia), protruding lips, wide-set eyes (hypertelorism) that are deep-set, deformities of the foot, and other skeletal irregularities.

Treatment for camptodactyly is related to the severity and extent of the deformity. Most children experience only mild loss of function and may benefit from physical therapy, occupational therapy, or such orthopedic measures as splinting or the application of casts. Surgical intervention is only moderately effective in correcting the flexion contractures associated with camptodactyly. Other treatment is symptomatic and supportive.

The following organizations in the General Resources Section can provide additional information: National Organization for Rare Disorders, Inc. (NORD), Genetic Alliance, NIH/National Institute of Child Health and Human Development, March of Dimes Birth Defects Foundation, NIH/National Institute of Arthritis and Musculoskeletal and Skin Diseases

National Associations & Support Groups

916 CHERUB—Association of Families and Friends of Children with Limb Disorders
936 Deleware Ave
Buffalo, NY 14209

Answers the questions and problems that families of juveniles diagnosed with a disorder may be experiencing.

917 Shriners Hospitals for Children
PO Box 31356
Tampa, FL 33613
813-281-0300
800-237-5055
Fax: 813-281-8496
www.shrinershq.org

Web Sites

918 Eaton Hand Link
www.eatonhand.com/thr/thr019.htm

Newsletters

919 Superkids, Inc.
60 Clyde St
Newton, MA 02160

Newsletter for families and friends of children with limb difficulties.

DESCRIPTION

920 CELIAC DISEASE
Synonyms: CD, Celiac sprue, Gluten-sensitive enteropathy, GSE, Nontropical sprue
May involve these systems in the body (see Section III):
Digestive System

Celiac disease (CD) is a digestive disorder in which the lining of the small intestine is damaged by gluten, a protein that is found in wheat, barley, rye, and oats. People with CD are thought to have an abnormal immune response to dietary gluten, causing degeneration (atrophy) and flattening of the tiny projections that line the small intestine (villi). Flattening of the surface area of the intestinal villi seriously impairs their ability to absorb fats and other nutrients from food products (malabsorption). Although the specific underlying cause of CD is unknown, the disorder is thought to result from the interactions of many genes (polygenic) in association with certain environmental factors (multifactorial inheritance). CD may affect young children as well as adults. The frequency of the disorder varies greatly in different countries and among different populations, and more cases occur in Europe than in the United States. Approximately one in 10,000 infants is thought to be affected by CD in the U.S.

The symptoms associated with celiac disease do not become apparent until gluten is introduced into the diet. In most children with the disorder, symptoms begin to occur between the ages of one to five years. Although symptoms and findings may be variable, many children initially have diarrhea, and the stools become abnormally bulky, pale, frothy, and offensive smelling due to an abnormally increased fat content (steatorrhea). Additional abnormalities may include excessive gas (flatulence), a failure to grow and gain weight at the expected rate (failure to thrive), lack of appetite (anorexia) and weight loss, vomiting, and swelling (distension) of the abdomen. Many children also experience muscle wasting, are unusually clingy and irritable, and have abnormally pale skin (pallor). Due to malabsorption of fats and other nutrients, children typically have deficiencies of certain vitamins, and some patients may have abnormally reduced levels of the oxygen-carrying protein of the blood (hemoglobin) due to iron deficiency (iron-deficiency anemia).

The treatment of celiac disease requires the elimination of gluten from the diet. Wheat and rye products must be completely excluded; however, many children with CD may be able to tolerate some barley and oat products. Because gluten is widely used in various food products, parents and children may initially require the assistance and guidance of an experienced dietitian. In addition, specially manufactured, gluten-free food products are available commercially, such as gluten-free pasta, bread, and flour. Treatment may also include iron and vitamin supplementation as required.

The following organizations in the General Resources Section can provide additional information: Genetic Alliance, NIH/Office of Rare Diseases, National Organization for Rare Disorders, Inc. (NORD), Online Mendelian Inheritance in Man: www3.ncbi.nlm.nih.gov/Omim/searchomim.html, NIH/National Digestive Diseases Information Clearinghouse

National Associations & Support Groups

921 American Celiac Society - Dietary Support Coalition
Dietary Support Coalition
58 Musano Court
West Orange, NJ 07052   973-325-8837

A non-profit, tax exempt organization that supports efforts in education, research, and mutual support. Helps to set up support groups, sponsers conferences, seeks funding for education and research, identifies ingredients in foods, and educates the public about problems facing its members.

922 American Celiac Society Hotline
Dietary Support Coalition
59 Crystal Avenue
West Orange, NJ 07052   973-325-8837

Provides practical assistance to members and individuals with celiac disease and information about the disease to the public.

Annette Bentley, President

923 Celiac Disease Foundation
13251 Ventura Blvd, #1 Studio City
Los Angeles, CA 91604   818-990-2354
                              Fax: 808-990-2379
                      e-mail: cdf@primenet.com
                          www.celiac.org/cdf

924 Celiac Sprue Association/USA, Inc.
P.O. Box 31700
Omaha, NE 68131   402-558-0600

National support organization that provides information and referral services for persons with celiac sprue and dermatitis herpetiformis and parents of celiac children. Made up of 6 regions in the U.S., with 42 chapters and 78 resource units.

925 Gluten Intolerance Group of North America
1833 Broadway Avenue
Seattle, WA 98102   206-325-6980
                          Fax: 206-320-1172

Provides instructional and general information materials, as well as counseling and access to ents to persons with celiac sprue and their families; operates telephone information and referral service; conducts educational seminars for health professionals; conducts and supports research; and offers leadership and assistance t

Susan Eliot

Audio Video

926 Adjustment to Long-Term Health Problems
Gluten Intolerance Group of North America
15110 10th Avenue SW, Suite A
Seattle, WA 98166   206-246-6652
                          Fax: 206-246-6531

927 Autoimmune Disorders Genetically Related to Celiac Disease
Gluten Intolerance Group of North America
15110 10th Avenue SW, Suite A
Seattle, WA 98166   206-246-6652
                          Fax: 206-246-6531

928 Celiac Disease in the U.S.A. - Where We Are vs. Where We Need to Be
Gluten Intolerance Group of North America
15110 10th Avenue SW, Suite A
Seattle, WA 98166   206-246-6652
                          Fax: 206-246-6531

Question and answer session.

929 Great Gluten-Free Baking Ideas
Gluten Intolerance Group of North America
15110 10th Avenue SW, Suite A
Seattle, WA 98166   206-246-6652
                          Fax: 206-246-6531

930 Pathologist's View of Celiac Sprue
Gluten Intolerance Group of North America
15110 10th Avenue SW, Suite A
Seattle, WA 98166   206-246-6652
                          Fax: 206-246-6531

931 Taking Charge of Your Life
Gluten Intolerance Group of North America
15110 10th Avenue SW, Suite A
Seattle, WA 98166   206-246-6652
                          Fax: 206-246-6531

932 Well-Plan Foods Demonstration
Gluten Intolerance Group of North America
15110 10th Avenue SW, Suite A
Seattle, WA 98166   206-246-6652
                          Fax: 206-246-6531

Web Sites

933 Celiac Life Discussion Group
www.nowheat.com/bbs.hts

934 Celiac Listserv Cel-Kids News Group
maelstrom.stjohns.edu/archives/cel-kids.html

935 Celiac Listserv News Group
www.fastlane.net/homepages/thodge/archive.htm

936 Celiac Listserv News Group Archives
maelstrom.stjohns.edu/archives/celiac.html

937 Celiac Support Page
www.celiac.com/other.html#listserv

938 Gluten-Free Page
www.panix.com/~donwiss

Books

939 GIG Cookbook
Gluten Intolerance Group of North America
15110 10th Avenue SW, Suite A
Seattle, WA 98166   206-246-6652
Fax: 206-246-6531
e-mail: gig@accessone.com

Newsletters

940 GIG Quarterly
Gluten Intolerance Group of North America
15110 10th Avenue SW, Suite A
Seattle, WA 98166   206-246-6652
Fax: 206-246-6531

Offers updated medical and technological information for patients with celiac sprue, their families and health care professionals.

Quarterly

Pamphlets

941 Celiac Sprue Resource Guide
Gluten Intolerance Group of North America
15110 10th Avenue SW, Suite A
Seattle, WA 98166   206-246-6652
Fax: 206-246-6531

942 Diet Instruction
Gluten Intolerance Group of North America
15110 10th Avenue SW, Suite A
Seattle, WA 98166   206-246-6652
Fax: 206-246-6531

943 Introductory Brochure
Gluten Intolerance Group of North America
15110 10th Avenue SW, Suite A
Seattle, WA 98166   206-246-6652
Fax: 206-246-6531

Offers facts and statistics on celiac sprue and
dermatitis herpetiformis.

944 On the Celiac Condition
Celiac Sprue Association/USA, Inc.
P.O. Box 31700
Omaha, NE 68131   402-558-0600

Handbook with information on celiac sprue and
dermatitis herpetiformis.

945 Patient Packets - Celiac Sprue
Gluten Intolerance Group of North America
15110 10th Avenue SW, Suite A
Seattle, WA 98166   206-246-6652
Fax: 206-246-6531

Includes various brochures and research reports
on celiac sprue, recipes, diet instruction and
more.

DESCRIPTION

946 CEREBRAL PALSY
Synonym: CP
Disorder Type: Neuromuscular
Covers these related disorders: Ataxic cerebral palsy, Choreoathetoid cerebral palsy, Mixed cerebral palsy, Spastic cerebral palsy
May involve these systems in the body (see Section III):
Central Nervous System, Muscular System

Cerebral palsy (CP) is a nonprogressive condition characterized by stiff, rigid, and awkward movements (spasticity); involuntary, slow writhing movements (athetosis); and poor balance and coordination of voluntary movement (ataxia). Approximately two of every 1,000 infants are affected with cerebral palsy. Both premature and low birth weight infants are particularly at risk for this condition. Cerebral palsy may occur as the result of an injury to the brain during pregnancy, birth, or the early childhood years. Such brain injuries may be caused by a decrease in the supply of oxygen to the brain during the birthing period; an infection passed from the mother to the fetus during pregnancy; or an excess of red bile pigment (bilirubin) in the developing fetus, usually arising from a blood incompatibility between mother and child. After birth, cerebral palsy may result from head trauma, an infection of the brain (e.g., encephalitis, etc.), an infection of the membranes surrounding the brain (meningitis), or other insult to the brain or surrounding tissue.

This condition is categorized into four main types including spastic, choreoathetoid, ataxic, and mixed cerebral palsy. Spastic cerebral palsy is the most common type of this condition and is characterized by stiff and weak muscles in the arms and legs on one or both sides of the body. Choreoathetoid cerebral palsy is characterized by poorly controlled, spontaneous slow movements of the muscles and accounts for approximately 20 percent of affected children. Ataxic cerebral palsy affects approximately 10 percent of all those with cerebral palsy and is characterized by poor coordination and shaky movements. Mixed cerebral palsy is a combination of two types of this abnormality and is characterized by the physical characteristics of both types. Although some children with cerebral palsy have below-average intelligence or are mentally retarded, others are of average or above-average intelligence.

There is no cure for cerebral palsy, but effective treatment improves the quality of life of affected children and their families. The type and extent of treatment depends upon the degree and type of disability experienced by the individual child. For example, occupational and physical therapy may aid affected children with walking and muscle coordination and control. Some children may benefit from the use of braces or other orthopedic intervention. Speech therapy may be useful for improvement of speech and eating difficulties. Stimulation and support are very important aspects of treatment and will aid in helping children with cerebral palsy to realize their full potential.

The following organizations in the General Resources Section can provide additional information: March of Dimes Birth Defects Foundation, NIH/National Institute of Child Health and Human Development, NIH/National Institute of Neurological Disorders and Stroke, National Easter Seal Society

National Associations & Support Groups

947 ADA Technical Assistance Program
6959 Old Dominion Drive Ste 250
McLeanChurch, VA 22101
703-448-6155
800-949-4232
Fax: 703-442-9015
TTY: 703-448-3079
e-mail: adata@adata.org
www.adata.org

A federally funded network of grantees which provides information, training, and technical assistance to businesses and agencies with duties and responsibilities under the ADA and to people with disabilities with rights under the ADA (American with Disibilities Act). Materials - the ADA and newsletters are available.

Lyn Sowdon, Project Director

**948 American Academy for Cerebral Palsy and
Developmental Medicine**
6300 North River Road Suite 727
Rosemont, IL 60018   847-698-1635
                                               Fax: 847-823-0536
                                       e-mail: woppenhe@ucla.edu
                                                   149.142.183.10/

**949 National Information Center for Children and
Youths with Disabilities**
PO Box 1492
Washington, DC 20013   202-884-8200
                                                       800-695-0285

950 United Cerebral Palsy Association
1660 L Street N.W., Ste. 700
Washington, DC 20036   202-776-0406
                                                       800-872-5827
                                               Fax: 202-776-0414
                                               TTY: 202-973-7197
                                        e-mail: ucpnatl@ucpa.org
                                                     www.ucpa.org

A network of approximately 180 state and local
voluntary agencies which provide services, conduct public and professional education programs and support research in cerebral palsy.

Jack Schellenger, President
Schellenger John D., Kemp

951 United States Cerebral Palsy Athletic Association
200 Harrison Ave
Newport, RI 02840   401-848-2460
                                               Fax: 401-848-5280
                                  e-mail: uscpaa@mail.bbsnet.com
                                                   www.uscpaa.org

**952 WE MOVE - Worldwide Education and Awareness
for Movement Disorders**
Mt. Sinai Med Ctr.
204 W. 84th Street
New York, NY 10024   212-241-8567
                                                       800-437-6682
                                               Fax: 212-875-8389
                                       e-mail: wemove@wemove.org
                                                   www.wemove.org

WE MOVE provides movement disorder information and educational materials to physicians,
patients, the media, and the public via its comprehensive Web site, training courses, patient
support group guide and more. Its goal is to
make early diagnosis, up-to-date treatment and
patient support a reality for all people living
with movement disorders.

Judith Blazer, Executive Director

Research Centers

953 Orthopaedic Biomechanics Laboratory
Shriners Hospital for Crippled Children
3160 Geneva Street
Las Angeles, CA 90020   213-388-3151
                                               Fax: 213-387-7528

Offers research and studies into cerebral palsy.

Stephen R. Skinner, Clinical Director

**954 United Cerebral Palsy Research and Educational
Foundation**
1660 L St. NW, Suite 700
Washington, DC 20036   202-776-0406
                                                       800-872-5823
                                               Fax: 202-776-0414

Provides research grants to prevent cerebral
palsy and to improve treatment, management
and functioning of persons with cerebral palsy.

Audio Video

955 CP: A Multimedia Tutorial
Children's Medical Center, University of Virginia
www.virginia.edu/docs/cmc/tutorials/cp/

956 I Am Not What You See
Sig Gerber, author

Filmakers Library
124 East 40th Street
New York, NY 10016   212-808-4980

Sondra Diamond was born with cerebral palsy,
resulting in Sondra becoming a quadriplegic
with limited ability to care for herself.
Films

Web Sites

**957 CP: A Multimedia Tutorial Children's Medical
Center**
University of Virginia
www.med.virginia.edu/docs/cmc/tutorials

958 Cerebral Palsy Support Network
www.home.aone.net.au/cpsn/

959 Infinitec
www.infinitec.org/helpyourself.hmtl

960 Scope (UK)
www.scope.org.uk/

961 Usenet
www.alt.support.cerebal-palsy

Books

---

962 A Mother's Touch: The Tiffany Callo Story
Jay Matthews, author

United Cerebral Palsy Associations
1660 L Street NW, Ste. 700
Washington, DC 20005   202-776-0406
                              800-872-5823
                       Fax: 202-776-0414
             e-mail: ucpnatl@ucpa.org
                          www.ucpa.org

A vivid portrayal of a woman with cerebral palsy who faced discrimination because of her disability.

963 After the Tears: Parents Talk About Raising a Child with a Disability
Robin Simons, author

United Cerebral Palsy Associations
1522 L Street NW, Ste. 700
Washington, DC 20036   202-776-0406
                              800-872-5823
                       Fax: 202-776-0414
             e-mail: ucpnatl@ucpa.org
                          www.ucpa.org

Book draws on stories of parents who have struggled, learned and grown in the years since their child was born with a disability.

89 pages Softcover

964 An Introduction to Your Child Who Has Cerebral Palsy
Medic Publishing Company
P.O. Box 89
Redmond, WA 98073   425-881-2883

Information and answers to questions for parents of children with cerebral palsy.

965 Breaking Ground: Ten Families Building Opportunities Through Integration
United Cerebral Palsy Associations
1522 L Street NW, Ste. 700
Washington, DC 20036   202-776-0406
                              800-872-5823
                       Fax: 202-776-0414
             e-mail: ucpnatl@ucpa.org
                          www.ucpa.org

Gives examples of strategies families have used to integrate the children fully into their schools and communities.

75 pages Softcover

966 Children with Cerebral Palsy
Elaine Geralis, author

Woodbine House
6510 Bells Mill Road
Bethesda, MD 20817   301-468-8800
                              800-843-7323
                       Fax: 301-897-5838
        e-mail: info@woodbinehouse.com
                    www.woodbinehouse.com

Explains what cerebral palsy is, and discusses its diagnosis and treatment. Also offers information and advice concerning daily care, early intervention, therapy, educational options and family life.

1991 432 pages Softcover
ISBN: 0-933149-15-8

967 Connecting Students: A Guide to Thoughtful Friendship Facilitation
United Cerebral Palsy Associations
1522 L Street NW, Ste. 700
Washington, DC 20036   202-776-0406
                              800-872-5823
                       Fax: 202-776-0414
             e-mail: ucpnatl@ucpa.org
                          www.ucpa.org

Contains helpful strategies on real-life experiences on building friendships.

48 pages Softcover

968 Coping with Cerebral Palsy
Jay Schleichkorn, author

Pro-Ed
8700 Shoal Creek Boulevard
Austin, TX 78758   512-451-3246
                       Fax: 512-451-8542

This book provides parents of children with cerebral palsy the answers to more than 300 questions that have been carefully researched; it represents 40 years of experience by the author and is presented in a highly readable, jargon-free manner.

196 pages Second Edition
ISBN: 0-936104-95-3

969 Discovery Book
Sky Chaney, author

United Cerebral Palsy Association, Inc.
959 Transport Way, A-1
Petaluma, CA 94952   707-765-6770

Created within a United Cerebral Palsy group for childern with physical disabilities; The Discovery Book is an exploration of social and psychological aspects of childhood disability. Accompanied by their artwork, children speak in their own words about important areas of life such: as What about friends?; Doctors and hospitals; Problems and challenges; and Goals, wishes & dreams.

96 pages

970 Each of Us Remembers: Parents of Children With Cerebral Palsy

Sally Weiss, author

United Cerebral Palsy Associations
1522 L Street NW, Ste. 700
Washington, DC 20036   202-776-0406
                                800-872-5823
                          Fax: 202-776-0414
                e-mail: ucpnatl@ucpa.org
                             www.ucpa.org

Parents of children with cerebral palsy answer questions that people really need to know.

971 Handling the Young Cerebral Palsied Child At Home

Nancie R. Finnie, author

United Cerebral Palsy Associations
1522 L Street NW, Ste. 700
Washington, DC 20036   202-776-0406
                                800-872-5823
                          Fax: 202-776-0414
                e-mail: ucpnatl@ucpa.org
                             www.ucpa.org

Offers chapters on bathing, feeding, dressing and play for parents of children with cerebral palsy.

337 pages Softcover

972 Natural Supports in School/Work/Community for the Severely Disabled

Jan Nisbet, author

United Cerebral Palsy Associations
1522 L Street NW, Ste. 700
Washington, DC 20036   202-776-0406
                                800-872-5823
                          Fax: 202-776-0414
                e-mail: ucpnatl@ucpa.org
                             www.ucpa.org

Promotes the position that assistance must be defined by the needs of individuals rather than the requirements of the service systems.

361 pages Softcover

973 No Time for Jello: One Family's Experience

Berneen Bratt, author

Brookline Books

One family's story of their attempts to remediate and cure the effects of cerebral palsied condition the oldest son was born with. The Bratts traveled traditional routes, through distinguished medical centers in Boston, and nontraditional routes in a search for treatments that would help their son.

Softcover

974 Opening Doors: Strategies for Including All Students in Regular Education

C. Beth Schaffner, author

United Cerebral Palsy Associations
1522 L Street NW, Ste. 700
Washington, DC 20036   202-776-0406
                                800-872-5823
                          Fax: 202-776-0414
                e-mail: ucpnatl@ucpa.org
                             www.ucpa.org

Contains practical information for including and supporting all students in regular classes.

55 pages Softcover

Children's Books

975 Can't You be Still?

Sarah Yates, author

Gemma B. Publishing, Inc.
Box #713-740 Corydon Avenue
Winnipeg, MN, R3M 0Y1, IT
                          Fax: 204-475-9903

This wonderfully written children's book features a heroine with cerebral palsy going to school for the first time.

28 pages Softcover

976 Cerebral Palsy

Nathan Aaseng, author

Franklin Watts c/o Grolier
90 Old Sherman Tpke
Danbury, CT 06816   203-797-3500
                                800-621-1115
                          Fax: 203-797-3197
                             www.grolier.com

A look at the causes, detection, prevention, effects and treatment of cerebral palsy.

112 pages Grades 7-12
ISBN: 0-531125-29-7

977 Karen

Maria Kililea, author

Dell Publishing
666 5th Avenue
New York, NY 10103   212-765-6500
                                   800-223-6834

After seeing many doctors, the family found that
Karen had cerebral palsy. The parents developed many ways to deal with Karen's problems
and figured out simulation activities.

286 pages Softcover
ISBN: 0-440943-76-0

978 Mine for Keeps

Jean Little, author

Little, Brown & Co.
34 Beacon Street
Boston, MA 02108   617-227-0730
                                   800-343-9204

Sarah Jean Copeland was born with cerebral
palsy. She was placed in a school for handicapped children but made such good progress
that she returned home, which meant a new
school, and new adjustments to her parents, two
sisters, and her brother. Sarah was scared and
didn't think she could do all the things she
needed to do, but soon learned her fears were
not well-founded.

186 pages Hardcover

979 My Brother, Matthew

Mary Thompson, author

Woodbine House
6510 Bells Mill Road
Bethesda, MD 20817   301-468-8800
                                   800-843-7323
                          Fax: 301-897-5838
           e-mail: info@woodbinehouse.com
                   www.woodbinehouse.com

A book written from the point of view of David,
the brother of Matthew, who has multiple disabilities. David describes the incidents charac-
terizing how life in his family changes.

28 pages Grades K-5

Sarah Strickler

980 Walk with Me

Eric Grimm, author

United Cerebral Palsy Associations
1522 L Street NW, Ste. 700
Washington, DC 20036   202-776-0406
                                   800-872-5823
                          Fax: 202-776-0414
                e-mail: ucpnatl@ucpa.org
                        www.ucpa.org

A story written by eight-year-old Eric Grimm
covering his thoughts on living with cerebral
palsy.

Newsletters

981 Family Support Bulletin
United Cerebral Palsy Associations
1522 L Street NW, Ste. 700
Washington, DC 20036   202-776-0406
                                   800-872-5823
                          Fax: 202-776-0414
                e-mail: ucpnatl@ucpa.org
                        www.ucpa.org

A detailed quarterly journal that takes a comprehensive look at the latest policies, resources
and legislative information enacted in Washington and state capitals.

Quarterly

982 Networker
United Cerebral Palsy Associations
1522 L Street NW, Ste. 700
Washington, DC 20036   202-776-0406
                                   800-872-5823
                          Fax: 202-776-0414
                e-mail: ucpnatl@ucpa.org
                        www.ucpa.org

Offers the latest information on the newest technology available for persons with cerebral palsy.

Quarterly

Pamphlets

983 Cerebral Palsy - Facts & Figures
United Cerebral Palsy Associations
1522 L Street NW, Ste. 700
Washington, DC 20036   202-776-0406
                                   800-872-5823
                          Fax: 202-776-0414
                e-mail: ucpnatl@ucpa.org
                        www.ucpa.org

Offers information on what cerebral palsy is,
the effects, causes, types, and prevention.

DESCRIPTION

984 CHARCOT-MARIE-TOOTH DISEASE
Synonym: Peroneal muscular atrophy
Disorder Type: Genetic Disorder, Neuromuscular
Covers these related disorders:
Charcot-Marie-Tooth disease type 1A (CMT1A;
hereditary motor and)
May involve these systems in the body (see Section III):
Nervous System

Charcot-Marie-Tooth disease belongs to a group of disorders known as hereditary motor-sensory neuropathies or HMSNs. The HMSNs are progressive disorders of nerves outside of the central nervous system that extend from the brain and spinal cord to particular areas of the body (peripheral nervous system). Symptoms and findings associated with these disorders are primarily the result of involvement of motor nerve fibers. These nerves transmit various nerve impulses away from the brain and spinal cord to their termination (e.g., muscle tissue). As these disorders progress, affected individuals may experience some symptoms due to sensory and autonomic involvement. Sensory nerve fibers carry impulses to the brain and spinal cord. The autonomic nervous system is the portion of the peripheral nervous system that regulates involuntary functioning of particular tissues and organs.

There are different types of Charcot-Marie-Tooth disease that have varying modes of inheritance. Charcot-Marie-Tooth disease (in all its forms) is the most prevalent hereditary peripheral neuropathy, affecting approximately one in 2,500 individuals. The most common form of the disease, known as Charcot-Marie-Tooth disease type 1A or CMT1A, is inherited as an autosomal dominant trait. A disease gene for CMT1A is located on the short arm of chromosome 17 (17p11.2).

Children with Charcot-Marie-Tooth disease type 1A usually do not have associated symptoms until late childhood or early adolescence. However, some may experience abnormalities in their man-ner of walking (gait disturbances) as early as the second year of life. In other, rare instances, associated symptoms may not become apparent until middle adulthood. CMT1A initially affects muscles supplied by nerves of the lower legs (peroneal and tibial nerves), causing muscle degeneration (atrophy) in the lower legs and feet. This is accompanied by muscle weakness and a distinctive stork-like contour of the legs. Bending movements of the ankles become progressively weaker, eventually resulting in footdrop, a condition in which the foot does not flex or bend upward. In addition, the arch of the foot becomes unusually increased in height (pes cavus deformities). An unstable gait may develop, and children may appear clumsy, easily tripping or falling. Although muscles of both legs are affected, disease progression and associated findings usually differ slightly from one side of the body to the other.

As the disorder progresses, individuals with CMT1A also usually develop a loss of muscle tissue mass and weakness in the forearms and hands. These areas seem to be less severely affected than the lower legs. However, patients may eventually develop permanent fixation of certain joints in a bent position. This typically occurs in the fingers and wrists. Some patients also experience gradual sensory involvement, such as abnormal burning or tingling sensations (paresthesias) in the feet. Associated autonomic abnormalities may include unusual paleness (pallor) or blotching of the skin of the feet. In individuals with CMT1A, specialized testing typically reveals a marked reduction in the transmission of motor and sensory nerve signals to affected muscles (reduced conduction velocities).

Although CMT1A is progressive, most affected individuals maintain the ability to walk. However, the use of special orthopedic appliances, such as stiff boots that reach to the midcalf, plastic splints, or light leg braces, are typically necessary to help stabilize the ankles. Surgical measures may be considered, such as surgical fusion of the ankles. In addition, certain medications may help to alleviate burning sensations in the feet (e.g., carbamazepine or phenytoin). Other treatment is symptomatic and supportive.

In addition to Charcot-Marie-Tooth disease type 1A, additional autosomal dominant, autosomal recessive, and X-linked forms of the disease have been identified. Specific symptoms and findings and the nature of disorder progression may vary, depending upon the specific form of the disease that is present.

The following organizations in the General Resources Section can provide additional information: National Organization for Rare Disorders, Inc., (NORD), March of Dimes Birth Defects Foundation, NIH/Office of Rare Diseases, Genetic Alliance, Online Mendelian Inheritance in Man.:
www3.ncbi.nlm.nih.gov/Omim/searchomim.html

National Associations & Support Groups

985 Charcot-Marie-Tooth Association
601 Upland Avenue
Upland, PA 19015   610-499-7486
                          800-606-2682
                   Fax: 610-499-7487
          e-mail: cmtassoc@aol.com
          www.charcot-marie-tooth.org

Works to inform and educate patients and their families, the medical community and the public about medical treatment for CMT. Offers support groups for patients and their families and finances research.

Patrica Dreibelbis, Program Director

986 Charcot-Marie-Tooth Disorder
Charcot-Marie-Tooth International
One Springbank Drive, St. Catherine
Ontario L2S 2K1,
Canada   905-687-3630

Linda Crabtree

987 Charcot-Marie-Tooth International
1 Spring Bank Drive, St. Catherines
Ontario L2S 2K1,
Canada

Web Sites

988 CMT Net
www.ultranet.com/~smith/CMTnet.html

989 Charcot-Marie-Tooth Association
www.charcot-marie-tooth.org/

990 Dr. Koop
www.drkoop.com/adam/peds/top/000727.htm

991 Genetic Clinics
www.geneclinics.org/publications/fa-cmt.

992 Muscular Dystrophy Association
www.mdausa.org/publications/fa-cmt.html

993 PedBase
www.icondata.com/health/pedbase/files/CHARCOT-.HTM

Newsletters

994 CMT Newsletter
CMT International
One Springbank Drive
St. Catharines, Ontario, L2S   905-687-3630
                              Fax: 905-687-8753
                  e-mail: cmtint@vaxxine.com
                             www.cmtint.org

Offers information on all facets of CMT, articles by doctors, research reports, drugs that can make the disorder worse, and many letters and articles from readers who have CMT or HNPP.

32 pages 6X

Linda Crabtree, Founder/Exec. Dir.

995 CMTA Report
CMT Association
601 Upland Avenue
Upland, PA 19015   610-499-7486
                   Fax: 610-499-8872

Contains articles on CMT topics, research news and patient profiles.

Quarterly

Patricia Dreibelbis, Editor

Pamphlets

996 Accepting CMT: The Grieving Process and You
CMT International
One Springbank Drive
St. Catharines, Ontario, L2S   905-687-3630
                              Fax: 905-687-8753
                  e-mail: cmtint@vaxxine.com
                             www.cmtint.org

997 Basics of Charcot-Marie-Tooth Disease
CMT International
One Springbank Drive
St. Catharines, Ontario, L2S   905-687-3630
                                 Fax: 905-687-8753
                        e-mail: cmtint@vaxxine.com
                                    www.cmtint.org

Questions answered and what you need to know to look after yourself (sent out in new member's introductory kit.).

Linda Crabtree, Founder/Exec. Dir.

998 Bracing Available for CMT Feet and Ankles
CMT International
One Springbank Drive
St. Catharines, Ontario, L2S   905-687-3630
                                 Fax: 905-687-8753
                        e-mail: cmtint@vaxxine.com
                                    www.cmtint.org

999 CMT & Exercise
CMT International
One Springbank Drive
St. Catharines, Ontario, L2S   905-687-3630
                                 Fax: 905-687-8753
                        e-mail: 194int@vaxxine.com
                                    www.cmtint.org

Excerpts from the CMT Newsletter plus how to test to see if you are exercising muscles served by CMT affected nerves.

1000 CMT Facts I
Charcot-Marie-Tooth Association
601 Upland Avenue
Upland, PA 19015   215-499-7486
                                     800-606-2682

Offers information on the neurotrophic drugs, genetics and therapies for CMT, surgical options and an overview of the disorder.
16 pages

1001 CMT Facts II
Charcot-Marie-Tooth Association
601 Upland Avenue
Upland, PA 19015   215-499-7486
                                     800-606-2682

Offers information on adaptive devices, feature specialists and the Amercians with Disabilities Act.
24 pages

1002 CMT Facts III
Charcot-Marie-Tooth Association
601 Upland Avenue
Upland, PA 19015   215-499-7486
                                     800-606-2682

Offers information on neurotrophic drugs, neuromuscular disorders, genetic news and doctor's questions and answers.
24 pages

1003 CMT Feet
CMT International
One Springbank Drive
St. Catharines, Ontario, L2S   905-687-3630
                                 Fax: 905-687-8753
                        e-mail: cmtint@vaxxine.com
                                    www.cmtint.org

1004 CMT Hands
CMT International
One Springbank Drive
St. Catharines, Ontario, L2S   905-687-3630
                                 Fax: 905-687-8753
                        e-mail: cmtint@vaxxine.com
                                    www.cmtint.org

1005 CMT and Alternate Therapies
CMT International
One Springbank Drive
St. Catharines, Ontario, L2S   905-687-3630
                                 Fax: 905-687-8753
                        e-mail: cmtint@vaxxine.com
                                    www.cmtint.org

Experiences of members and suggestions for good books.

Linda Crabtree, Founder/Exec. Dir.

1006 CMT and Coping with the Pain
CMT International
One Springbank Drive
St. Catharines, Ontario, L2S   905-687-3630
                                 Fax: 905-687-8753
                        e-mail: cmtint@vaxxine.com
                                    www.cmtint.org

Linda Crabtree, Founder/Exec. Dir.

1007 CMT and Dentistry
CMT International
One Springbank Drive
St. Catharines, Ontario, L2S   905-687-3630
                                 Fax: 905-687-8753
                        e-mail: cmtint@vaxxine.com
                                    www.cmtint.org

1008 CMT, Children and Youth
CMT International
One Springbank Drive
St. Catharines, Ontario, L2S   905-687-3630
                                     Fax: 905-687-8753
                        e-mail: cmtint@vaxxine.com
                                    www.cmtint.org

Linda Crabtree, Founder/Exec. Dir.

1009 Charcot-Marie-Tooth Disease and Anesthetics
CMT International
One Springbank Drive
St. Catharines, Ontario, L2S   905-687-3630
                                     Fax: 905-687-8753
                        e-mail: cmtint@vaxxine.com
                                    www.cmtint.org

Linda Crabtree, Founder/Exec. Dir.

1010 Charcot-Marie-Tooth Disease and Wellness
CMT International
One Springbank Drive
St. Catharines, Ontario, L2S   905-687-3630
                                     Fax: 905-687-8753
                        e-mail: cmtint@vaxxine.com
                                    www.cmtint.org

The signs and symptoms of CMT and how to
keep yourself as well as possible.

Linda Crabtree, Founder/Exec. Dir.

1011 Charcot-Marie-Tooth Disease: A Brief Overview
CMT International
One Springbank Drive
St. Catharines, Ontario, L2S   905-687-3630
                                     Fax: 905-687-8753
                        e-mail: cmtint@vaxxine.com
                                    www.cmtint.org

Profiles of five people who have various degree
of CMT.

17 minutes

Linda Crabtree, Founder/Exec. Dir.

1012 Diagnosing CMT
CMT International
One Springbank Drive
St. Catharines, Ontario, L2S   905-687-3630
                                     Fax: 905-687-8753
                        e-mail: cmtint@vaxxine.com
                                    www.cmtint.org

How a diagnosis is made.

Linda Crabtree, Founder/Exec. Dir.

1013 When You Fall
CMT International
One Springbank Drive
St. Catharines, Ontario, L2S   905-687-3630
                                     Fax: 905-687-8753
                        e-mail: cmtint@vaxxine.com
                                    www.cmtint.org

How to prepare yourself for the inevitable.

DESCRIPTION

1014 CHICKENPOX

Synonym: Varicella

Disorder Type: Infectious Disease

Covers these related disorders: Neonatal chickenpox

Chickenpox is a common, highly contagious viral disease caused by infection with varicella zoster virus (VZV), a member of the herpesvirus family. About 90 to 95 percent of individuals contract this infection during childhood, with most cases occurring before the age of 10. Those who do not contract chickenpox during childhood remain susceptible to the disease during adulthood. Varicella zoster infection is typically more severe in affected adults. There are approximately three million cases of chickenpox in the United States each year. The varicella zoster virus is spread by the inhalation of airborne droplets that contain the virus or through direct contact with fluid from skin blisters. In most patients, associated symptoms occur approximately 14 to 16 days after infection. Some patients, particularly older children, may initially experience generalized symptoms, including fever, headache, mild abdominal pain, lack of appetite, and a general feeling of ill health (malaise). A characteristic rash then develops that consists of masses of small, red, extremely itchy (pruritic) spots that soon become clear, fluid-filled blisters (vesicles). These skin lesions usually initially develop on the chest, abdomen, face, or scalp. As the first lesions begin to dry out and form scabs, new crops of skin lesions typically form on the chest, arms, and legs. In some patients, lesions may develop on the eyelids, inside the mouth, in the windpipe, and within the vagina in girls. As lesions heal, affected areas may have abnormally diminished skin coloration (hypopigmentation) for several days or weeks. However, scarring of affected areas is unusual.

The most common complication of chickenpox is secondary bacterial infection of skin lesions. In rare cases, other complications may include inflammation of the brain (encephalitis) or impaired control of voluntary movements (cerebellar ataxia). Children who have an impaired immune system may develop a severe, progressive form of chickenpox. Such patients may be more likely to develop inflammation of the lungs (pneumonia) or other severe complications of chickenpox.

Newborns may also experience a particularly severe, progressive form of chickenpox (neonatal chickenpox). Infection is usually due to the mother's infection with chickenpox (maternal varicella zoster) during the week prior to delivery. In addition, infants who contract chickenpox during the first year of life may experience severe, progressive chickenpox. Affected newborns and infants may be at an increased risk for the more serious complications that may be associated with varicella zoster infection, such as inflammation of the lungs (pneumonia), the liver (hepatitis), or the brain (encephalitis).

The treatment of children with mild cases of chickenpox usually includes symptomatic and supportive measures. Parents should keep their children's nails clipped short to help prevent scratching of skin lesions that may lead to secondary infection. The use of skin lotions and wet compresses may help to alleviate itching. In more severe cases of chickenpox, therapy may include the administration of the antiviral drug acyclovir.

A vaccine is now available in the United States to help prevent chickenpox. Parents should consult with their child's pediatrician to determine whether such vaccination would be appropriate for their child. In addition, women of child-bearing age who have not previously contracted chickenpox may consider consulting with their physicians to discuss the appropriateness of such vaccination to help prevent neonatal chickenpox due to maternal varicella infection.

The following organizations in the General Resources Section can provide additional information: National Organization for Rare Disorders, Inc. (NORD), March of Dimes Birth Defects Foundation, NIH/National Institute of Allergy and Infectious Disease, World Health Organization (WHO), Centers for Disease Control (CDC)

Web Sites

1015 Be Well
http:bewell.com/hic/chickenpox

1016 Dr. Koop
drkoop.com/adam/peds/top/001592.htm

1017 Kids Health
kidshealth.org/parent/common/chicken_pox.html

1018 LSU Medical Center
lib-sh.lsumc.edu/fammed/pted/chknpox.htm

DESCRIPTION

1019 CHILDHOOD DERMATOMYOSITIS

Synonym: Juvenile dermatomyositis (JDMS)

May involve these systems in the body (see Section III):

Connective Tissue, Dermatologic System, Muscular System

Dermatomyositis is a connective tissue disorder characterized by inflammatory and degenerative changes of the muscles and distinctive lesions of the skin. Although the disorder may become apparent at any time, it most commonly occurs in children between five to 15 years of age or adults between the ages of 40 to 60 years. In children, the average age at onset is eight or nine years. More females than males are affected by dermatomyositis.

The cause of dermatomyositis is unknown. However, immune, genetic, and environmental factors are thought to play some role in causing the disorder. Many researchers suggest that dermatomyositis is an autoimmune disorder resulting from abnormal immune responses directed against the body's own tissues.

The symptoms and findings associated with childhood dermatomyositis are similar to those seen in the adult form of the disease. However, involvement of the gastrointestinal (GI) tract and the development of abnormal calcium deposits (calcifications) within skin and muscle tissues are more frequent and widespread in childhood dermatomyositis. Affected children usually have widespread inflammation of small blood vessels (vasculitis) within connective tissues of the skin, muscles, tissues beneath the skin (subcutaneous tissues), and tissues underlying the nails (nail beds). In addition, although associated, cancerous growths (malignancies) occur in approximately 20 percent of affected adults, malignancies are rarely seen in those with childhood dermatomyositis.

In most patients with childhood dermatomyositis, the onset of symptoms is relatively gradual and subtle. Children initially experience slowly progressive muscle weakness affecting the upper arms, shoulders, hips, and thighs (proximal muscles) as well as the trunk. Involved muscles tend to be sore, stiff, tender, or abnormally hard. Affected children may develop an awkward manner of walking (gait) and gradually lose the ability to perform certain tasks, such as lifting the arms above the shoulders, combing their hair, dressing, climbing stairs, or rising from the floor unassisted (Gowers' sign). Involved muscles may eventually show varying degrees of degeneration (atrophy) and, in severe cases, permanent bending or extension in various fixed postures (joint contractures). Although muscles of the upper arms or legs are typically most severely affected, any muscle may become involved. In severe cases, affected muscles may include those of the roof of the mouth and those involved in respiration, resulting in a nasal quality to the voice; breathing difficulties; hyperventilation; breathing of foreign materials into the respiratory passages (bronchial aspiration); and potentially life-threatening complications. In addition, involvement of muscles of the gastrointestinal tract may cause difficulties swallowing; abdominal pain; passage of dark, tarry stools containing digested blood (melena); and infrequent bowel movements or difficulty passing stools (constipation). In severe cases, gastrointestinal bleeding (hemorrhage) or other associated abnormalities (e.g., perforations) may cause potentially life-threatening symptoms.

Patients with childhood dermatomyositis also develop characteristic skin changes, such as a reddish-purple rash of the upper eyelids (heliotrope rash); an abnormal accumulation of fluid in body tissues surrounding the eyes and in other facial areas (periorbital and facial edema); a reddish rash across the skin of the nose and cheeks (butterfly rash); and reddish-purple, raised, scaling skin lesions (papules) on the surfaces of certain joints, particularly the knuckles (Gottron's sign), elbows, and knees. These scaling lesions develop a central area of tissue loss (atrophy) that lacks color (vitiligo) or has increased pigmentation (hyperpigmentation). Patients may also have a dusky reddish rash covering the upper arms and legs and the upper trunk.

Approximately 20 to 50 percent of affected children also develop abnormal calcium deposits (calcifications) within muscle, skin, and subcutaneous tissues. These deposits may contribute to localized areas of muscle loss or the freezing of joints in permanently bent positions (contractures). Some patients may also experience additional symptoms and findings, such as a low-grade fever, joint inflammation (arthritis), enlargement of the liver and spleen (hepatosplenomegaly), or other abnormalities. In most patients, childhood dermatomyositis gradually becomes inactive over several years.

The treatment of patients with childhood dermatomyositis requires early, aggressive measures to help prevent potentially life-threatening complications. Such measures include evaluation to detect possible involvement of the respiratory or gastrointestinal systems and provision of ongoing nursing care for those with such involvement. Such care may include mechanical suctioning of the throat by way of the nose (nasopharyngeal suction), the creation of a temporary opening in the throat to ease breathing difficulties (tracheostomy), or mechanical breathing support (e.g., endotracheal intubation or respirator). In addition, the treatment of patients typically includes the use of corticosteroids (e.g., prednisone) to help suppress the inflammatory process of the disease. Blood levels of certain muscle enzymes are regularly measured to help gauge the effectiveness of such therapy. Once such enzyme levels are reduced to normal ranges, the steroid dosage may gradually be decreased to the minimum level of effectiveness. After about two years, such treatment may be discontinued without the reemergence of symptoms. In patients who do not respond to steroid therapy, certain immunosuppressant drugs such as methotrexate, azathioprine, or cyclosporine or, in some patients, intravenous immunoglobulin therapy may be beneficial. In addition, treatment may include surgical removal of calcium deposits. Physical therapy (e.g., passive exercises, eventual use of active exercises) is important in helping to rebuild muscle strength and prevent permanent, disabling fixation of joints (contractures). Splints may be required to help ensure proper positioning of certain limbs. Proper skin hygiene is also important in patients with childhood dermatomyositis.

The following organizations in the General Resources Section can provide additional information: National Organization for Rare Disorders, Inc., (NORD), NIH/Office of Rare Diseases, NIH/National Institute of Arthritis and Musculoskeletal and Skin Diseases, Online Mendelian Inheritance in Man.: www3.ncbi.nlm.nih.gov/Omim/searchomim.html

National Associations & Support Groups

1020 American Autoimmune Related Diseases Association, Inc.
15475 Gratiot Avenue
Detroit, MI 48205   313-371-8600
e-mail: aarda@aol.com
www.aarda.org

Focused on the dissemination of information to a wide public base of similar diseases.

1021 American Juvenile Arthritis Organization
1330 West Peachtree Street
Atlanta, GA 30309   404-872-7100
e-mail: help@arthritis.org
www.arthritis.org

Caters to the necessity of young arthritic sufferers by providing them with the much-needed data through a variety of both audio and visual mediums.

1022 Arthritis Foundation
1330 West Peachtree Sreet
Atlanta, GA 30309   404-872-7100
e-mail: info@arthritis.org
www.mdausa.org

Group offers an array of information and important facts for individuals and their families pertaining to their difficulty.

1023 Juvenile Dermatomyositis
Arthritis Foundation
P.O. Box 7669
Atlanta, GA 30357   404-872-7100
800-283-7800
Fax: 404-872-0457
e-mail: info@jdfcure.com
www.jdfcure.com

1024 Myositis Assocaition of America, Inc.
755 Cantrell Avenue Suite C
Harrisonburg, VA 22801   540-433-7686
                              e-mail: maa@mytosis.org
                              www.mytosis.org

1025 New Onset Juvenile Dematomytosis Registry
2300 Children's Plaza Center
Chicago, IL 60614   773-880-3333
                          e-mail: e-mendez@nwu.edu

Registry firm on giving children and their families the proper outlets in which to deal with this disorder.

International

1026 Dermatomyositis and Polymyositis Support Group
146 Newtown Road
Southhampton S02- 9HR,
United Kingdom

DESCRIPTION

1027 CHILDHOOD SCHIZOPHRENIA

Disorder Type: Genetic Disorder, Mental, Emotional or Behavioral Disorder

Childhood schizophrenia is characterized by disturbances in behavior, thought, and emotional reactions. These changes initially become apparent between approximately seven years of age and the onset of adolescence. Affected children may become increasingly withdrawn, have flat or blunted emotions that do not appear to change in response to environmental or external stimuli, experience episodes of unexplained silliness (hebephrenic silliness), exhibit aggressive behaviors, and experience distortions in thinking. For example, some children may regularly repeat the same responses to different questions; experience sudden blockages in thought; perceive sights, sounds, or other sensations in the absence of external stimuli (hallucinations); and hold false beliefs in spite of evidence to the contrary (psychotic delusions), such as delusions of persecution (paranoid delusions). Affected children often appear to be chaotic in their emotions, thought, and behavioral patterns.

The relationship of childhood schizophrenia and adult schizophrenia remains unclear. Because schizophrenia typically becomes apparent during late adolescence or early adulthood and affects approximately one percent of the general population, only a small percentage of children exhibit symptoms that meet the criteria for a diagnosis of schizophrenia. In addition, many children who are diagnosed with schizophrenia before puberty are later diagnosed with mood disorders, such as bipolar disorder, or other conditions, such as mental retardation or a metabolic disorder. Although there is no clear relationship between childhood and adult schizophrenia, childhood symptoms that most likely predict adult psychotic disorders appear to include social withdrawal, disturbed interpersonal relationships, and blunted emotions. Though the specific underlying abnormalities that may contribute to childhood schizoid behaviors are unknown, genetic factors and certain biochemical abnormalities of the brain play some role in their development.

The treatment of children with schizoid behaviors may include therapy with certain medications known as neuroleptics to manage psychotic delusions, hallucinations, and severe agitation. In addition, an integrated, multidisciplinary approach may include individual therapy or parental training to help modify behavior. In severe cases, hospitalization may be required to ensure appropriate medication adjustments, to prevent children from harming themselves, or to prevent them from hurting others if they exhibit aggressive or violent behavior.

Although certain medications may be administered to help treat children with schizoid behaviors, these drugs should be prescribed with great caution due to the potential for side effects. For example, such therapy may result in tardive dyskinesia (TD), a condition characterized by tics or spasms of facial muscles and involuntary, rapid or writhing movements of the limbs (choreoathetoid movements). In other cases, therapy may cause abnormally slow movement (bradykinesis); involuntary hand movements; abnormal twisting of the neck (torticollis); drooling; and other findings. If TD develops, treatment with other medications may be indicated and the neuroleptic medication may be decreased or discontinued. In some cases, TD may not be reversible.

The following organizations in the General Resources Section can provide additional information: Federation of Families for Children's Mental Health, Online Mendelian Inheritance in Man: www3.ncbi.nlm.nih.gov/Omim/searchomim.html, National Insitute of Mental Health

National Associations & Support Groups

1028 American Mental Health Foundation (AMNF)
1049 5th Avenue
New York, NY 10028
USA

212-639-1561
Fax: 212-737-9027

Dedicated to the extensive and intensive research in the theories and techniques of treatment of emotional illness and to the implementation of reforms in the mental health system. Efforts have resulted in development of better and less expensive treatment methods. Findings are disseminated in English and other major languages.

Monroe W. Spero, MD

1029 American Schizophrenia Association
900 N. Federal Hgwy, Ste 300
Boca Raton, FL 33432   561-393-6167

1030 Association for Persons with Mental and Developmental Disabilities
132 Fair Street
Kingston, NY 12401   914-334-4336
                            800-331-5362
                       Fax: 914-331-4569
                    e-mail: nadd@mhv.net

Non-profit organization designed to promote interest of professional and parent development with resources for individuals who have the co-existence of mental illness and mental retardation. Provides conference, educational services and training materials to professionals, parents, concerned citizens and service organizations. Formerly known as the National Association for the Dually Diagnosed.

Robert Fletcher, Executive Director

1031 Center for Family Support
333 7th Ave.
New York, NY 10001   212-629-7939
                       Fax: 212-239-2211
                         www.cfsny.org

Provides simple, in-depth answer to the most commonly asked questions and situation.

Steven Vernickofs, Executive Director

1032 Center for Mental Health Services Knowledge Exchange Program
U.S. Department of Health and Human Services
P.O. Box 42490
Washington, DC 20015
                            800-789-2647
                       Fax: 301-984-8796
                e-mail: ken@mentalhealth.org
                      www.mentalhealth.org

Supplies the public with responses to their commonly asked questions.

1033 Lithium Information Center/Obsessive Compulsive Information Center
7617 Mineral Point Road Suite 300
Madison, WI 53717   608-827-2470
          e-mail: INFOCTRS@Healthtechsys.com
              www.healthtechsys.com/MIMMAIN

1034 Mental Health Clinical Research Center for Schizophrenia/Psychiatry
VA Medical Center
Wilshire and Sawtelle Blvds.
Los Angeles, CA 90073   213-824-6620

Offers research into the various facets of schizophrenia and mental illness.

Dr. Robert Liberman, Director

1035 Mental Illness Foundation
772 W 168th Street
New York, NY 10032   212-682-4699
                       Fax: 212-682-4896

Supports community housing, treatment, research, outreach and public-awareness efforts for people with mental illness. Publications: Mental Illness Foundation, quarterly newsletter. Directory that lists mental illnesses and provides information on how to contact related associations. Annual meeting.

1036 National Alliance for the Mentally Ill
200 North Glebe Road #1015
Arlington, VA 22203   703-524-7600
                            800-950-6264
                       TDD: 703-516-7991
             e-mail: membership@nami.org
                          www.nami.org

Aids families and individuals find the emotional and physical answers to the habitual forming disorders through several media resources.

1037 National Mental Health Association
1021 Prince Street
Alexandria, VA 22314   703-684-7722
                            800-969-6642
                       TDD: 800-433-5959
             e-mail: nmhaininfo@aol.com
                          www.nmha.org

Notifies the public of the various groups and foundations to answer and assist them with their concerns and questions.

1038 National Mental Health Consumer Self-Help Clearinghouse
1211 Chestnut Street
Philadelphia, PA 19107   215-751-1810
                                800-553-4539
                            Fax: 215-636-6310
                   e-mail: info@mhselfhelp.org
                            www.mhselfhelp.org

Disperses information to the families and friends of an individual diagnosed with a mental illness.

1039 Schizophrenia Society of Canada
75 The Donway West Suite 814
Don Mills Ontario Canada, M3C2E 416-445-8204
                                 800-809-4673
                   e-mail: info@schizophrenia.ca
                            www.schizophrenia.ca

1040 World Schizophrenia Fellowship
238 Cavenport Road Box 118
Toronto, Ontario, Canada, M5R1J 416-975-1631
                   e-mail: wsf@origo.com
                            www.orgio.com/wsf/

Libraries & Resource Centers

1041 National Alliance for Research on Schizophrenia & Depression
60 Cutter Mill Road Suite 404
Great Neck, NY 11021   516-829-0091
                                800-829-8289
                         www.mhsource.com/narsad

Research Centers

1042 Families Coping with Mental Illness
Mental Illness Education Project, Inc.
P.O. Box 470813
Brookline Villge, MA 02247   617-562-1111
                                800-343-5540
                            Fax: 617-779-0061
                   e-mail: miep@tiac.net
                            www.miepvideos.org

Ten family members share their experiences of having a family member with schizophrenia or bipolar disorders. Designed to provide insights and support to other families, the tape also profoundly conveys to professionals the needs of families when mental illness strikes.

1997

1043 National Alliance for Research on Schizophrenia & Depression
60 Cutter Mill Road Suite 404
Great Neck, NY 11021   516-829-0091
                                800-829-8289
                         www.mhsource.com/narsad

1044 Schizophrenia Research Branch: Division of Clinical and Treatment Research
Chief, 500 Fishers Lane
Parklawn Bldg Rm 18
Rockville, MD 20857   301-443-4707
                            Fax: 301-443-6000

Plans, supports, and conducts programs of research, research training, and resource development of schizophrenia and related disorders. Reviews and evaluates research developments in the field and recommends new program directors. Collaborates with organizations in and outside of the National Institute of Mental Health to stimulate work in the field through conferences and workshops.

1045 Schizophrenic Biologic Research Center
VA Medical Center
130 W. Kingsbridge Road
Bronx, NY 10468   718-579-1630
                            Fax: 719-933-2121

Focuses on mental illness and schizophrenia

Audio Video

1046 Bonnie Tapes
Mental Illness Education Project, Inc.
P.O. Box 470813
Brookline Village, MA 02447   617-562-1111
                                800-343-5540
                            Fax: 617-779-0061
                   e-mail: miep@tiac.net
                            www.miapvideos.org

Bonnie's account of coping with schizophrenia will be a relevation to people whose view of mental illness has been shaped by the popular media. She and her family provide an intimate view of the frequently feared, often misrepresented, and much stigmatized illness-and the human side of learning to live with a psychiatric disability.

1997 $143.88 for 3

Web Sites

1047 Cyber Psych
www.cyberpsych.org/

1048 Department of Psychiatry and Behavorial Sciences
www.med.jhu.edu/schizophrenia

1049 Internet Mental Health
www.mentalhealth.com

1050 Mental Healthnet
mentalhelp.net/guide/schizo.htm

1051 Mental Wellness
www.mentalwellness.com

1052 Planetpsych
www.planetpsych.com

1053 Psych Central
www.psychcentral.com

1054 Schizophrenia Support
www.alt.support.schizophrenia

Books

1055 Breakthroughs in Antipsychotic Medications A Guide for Consumers, Families, Clinics

Peter J. Weiden, MD and Patricia L. Scheifer, author

National Alliance for the Mentally Ill
200 N. Glebe Rd, Ste 1015
Arlington, VA 22203   703-524-7600
                          800-950-6264
                     Fax: 703-516-7227
                          www.nami.org

Helps consumers and their families weigh the pros and cons of switching from older antipsychotics to newer ones. Answers frequently asked questions about antipsychotics and guides readers through the process of switching. Includes fact sheets on the new medications and their side affects.

1999 200 pages

1056 Contemporary Issues in the Treatment of Schizophrenia
American Psychiatric Press, Inc.
1400 K St., NW
Washington, DC 20005   202-682-6262
                          800-368-5777
                     Fax: 202-789-2648
               e-mail: oder@appi.org
                          www.appi.org

Covers approaches to the patient by investigating biological, pharmacological, and psychological treatments.

1995 960 pages

Christian L. Shriqui, MD, Editor
Henry A. Nasrallah, MD, Editor

1057 Innovations in the Psychological Management of Schizophrenia

Max J. Birchwood and Nicholas Tarrier, author

John Wiley & Sons, Inc.
605 3rd Avenue
New York, NY 10058   212-850-6000
                     Fax: 212-850-6008
               e-mail: info@wiley.com
                          www.wiley.com

Innovations in the Psychological Management of Schizophrenia: Assessment, Treatment and Services.

1992 338 pages

1058 New Pharmacotherapy of Schizophrenia

Richard S. Keefe and Philip D. Harvey, author

American Psychiatric Press, Inc.
1400 K St., NW
Washington, DC 20005   202-682-6262
                          800-368-5777
                     Fax: 202-789-2648
               e-mail: order@appi.org
                          www.appi.org

Discusses the new class of antipsychotic agents that promises superior efficiency and more favorable side-effects; offers an improved understanding of how to employ exsisting pharmachotherapeutic agents.

1996 272 pages

1059 Prenatal Exposures in Schizophrenia
American Psychiatric Press, Inc.
1400 K St., NW
New York, NY 20005   202-682-6262
                          800-368-5777
                     Fax: 202-789-2648
               e-mail: order@appi.org
                          www.appi.org

Considers a range of epigenetic elements thought to interact with abnormal genes to produce the onset of illness. Attention to the evidence implicating obstetric complications, prenatal infection, autoimmunity and prenatal malnutrition in brain disorders.

1999 352 pages Hardcover

1060 Psychoses and Pervasive Development Disorders in Childhood and Adolescence
American Psychiatric Press, Inc.
1400 K St., NW
New York, NY 20005   202-682-6262
                          800-368-5777
                     Fax: 202-789-2648
               e-mail: order@appi.org
                          www.appi.org

Provides a concise summary of currently knowledge of psychosis and pervasive developmental disorders of childhood and adolescence. Discusses recent range changes in aspects of diagnosis and definition of these disorders, advances in knowledge, and aspects of treatment.

1996 368 pages

DESCRIPTION

1061 CHOREA

Disorder Type: Neuromuscular
Covers these related disorders: Benign familial chorea, Drug-induced chorea, Sydenham's chorea
May involve these systems in the body (see Section III):
Nervous System

Chorea is a neuromuscular condition characterized by irregular, rapid, jerky movements that may appear to be well coordinated but actually occur involuntarily. These movements may be simple or highly complex. In addition, the arms and legs may have abnormally diminished muscle tone (hypotonia) and therefore may be abnormally loose or slack. Choreic movements are often subtle. However, if several of these movements are present, they may essentially flow into one another, causing them to appear relatively slow, sinuous, and writhing in nature (athetosis).

The specific underlying cause of chorea is unknown. However, some researchers suspect that it may result due to overactivity of certain neurotransmitters (dopamine) in the brain. Neurotransmitters are naturally produced chemicals that regulate the transmission of messages between certain nerve cells (neurons). In some children, chorea may result from the use of particular drugs, such as certain antiseizure medications, particularly phenytoin, or antipsychotic (neuroleptic) drugs, such as haloperidol or phenothiazines. Chorea may also occur in association with certain underlying disorders, such as systemic lupus erythematosus (lupus) or Wilson disease. In addition, chorea is a primary feature of a rare genetic disorder known as benign familial chorea in which nonprogressive chorea begins in infancy or early childhood in the absence of other neurologic abnormalities. Associated symptoms and findings include delays in obtaining certain motor milestones during childhood and poorly coordinated movements of the arms and legs. Be-

nign familial chorea is likely inherited as an autosomal dominant trait.

In addition, chorea is the dominant feature of a disorder known as Sydenham's chorea. This disorder is the most common cause of acquired chorea during childhood. Sydenham's chorea occurs in association with rheumatic fever, which is an inflammatory disease following throat infection with certain strains of streptococcal bacteria. Patients with rheumatic fever may experience fever, inflammation and swelling of one or more large joints, or inflammation of the heart (carditis), potentially causing thickening, scarring, and associated narrowing of heart valves (mitral stenosis). If rheumatic fever affects the nervous system, Sydenham's chorea may result. Although Sydenham's chorea previously occurred in as many as half of those with rheumatic fever, recent studies suggest that it more likely affects approximately 10 percent of rheumatic patients in the United States.

Sydenham's chorea most commonly occurs in children between ages five and 15. The condition may begin subtly and gradually, sometimes as long as several months after other symptoms associated with rheumatic fever. Patients may initially experience increasing clumsiness. As symptoms progress, involuntary movements may become prominent in the face, trunk, and arms and legs; move from one muscle group to another; and eventually affect all motor movements, particularly arm movements, walking, and speech. In some patients, chorea may be restricted to one side of the body (hemichorea). If children have severe chorea and abnormally diminished muscle tone (hypotonia), they may become unable to dress, feed themselves, or walk. Many children with the condition also experience rapid mood swings and episodes of uncontrollable crying (emotional lability).

Sydenham's chorea is usually a self-limited disorder that subsides in weeks or months. However, in some patients, the condition may persist for up to one to two years. In approximately 20 percent of children, the condition may recur within two years of the initial episode. If patients experience mild symptoms, treatment may include symptomatic and supportive measures, including minimizing stress as much as possible. In children with more severe symptoms, treatment may be attempted with the drug diazepam.

The following organizations in the General Resources Section can provide additional information: National Organization for Rare Disorders, Inc. (NORD), Genetic Alliance, March of Dimes Birth Defects Foundation, NIH/Office of Rare Diseases, Online Mendelian Inheritance in Man: www3.ncbi.nlm.nih.gov/Omim/researchomim.html, NIH/National Institute of Neurological Disorders & Stroke

National Associations & Support Groups

1062 Muscular Dystrophy Association
3300 E Sunrise Dr
Tucson, AZ 85718   520-529-2000
                         Fax: 520-529-5300
                         e-mail: mda@mdausa.org
                         www.mdausa.org

Dedicated to supplying the general public with the knowledge to properly assess and choose their doctors and medical facilities.

1063 National Digestive Diseases Information Clearinghouse
9000 Rockville Pike
Bethesda, MD 20892   301-654-3810
                           800-891-5389
                           Fax: 301-907-8906
                           www.nih.gov

Conducts and supports research and provides leadership for a national program in diabetes, endocrinology and metabolic diseases; digestive diseases and nutrition; and kidney, urologic and hematologic diseases.

1064 Society for Muscular Dystrophy Association
P.O. Box 479
Bridgewater, NS Canada, B4V   902-685-3961
                           Fax: 902-685-3962
                           e-mail: smdi@auracom.com

1065 We Move (Worldwide Education and Advocacy for Movement Disorders)
204 East 84th Street
New York, NY 10024   212-241-8567
                            800-437-6682
                         Fax: 212-987-7363
                         e-mail: wemove@wemove.org
                            www.wemove.org

Gives the general public the knowledge that they desire regarding any disorder involving movement difficulties.

Web Sites

1066 Pedbase (Sydenham chorea)
www.icondata.com/health/pedbase/files/SYDENHAM.HTM

DESCRIPTION

1067 CHRONIC HEPATITIS

Disorder Type: Infectious Disease
Covers these related disorders: Chronic active hepatitis, Chronic persistent hepatitis

Chronic hepatitis refers to a condition associated with prolonged inflammation of the liver that continues for six months or longer. It is characterized by variable symptoms and findings that range from very mild to severe. Chronic hepatitis may occur as the result of a continuing viral infection or an autoimmune response in which the body mistakenly attacks its own healthy tissue. This type of autoimmune response is more common in women than in men. Chronic hepatitis may also result from metabolic irregularities such as Wilson disease or from the use of certain drugs such as isoniazid, nitrofurantoin, methyldopa, sulfonamide drugs, etc. In some patients, the exact cause of the disease is not known. Previous infection with certain types of viruses known to cause hepatitis (i.e., type C and type B, sometimes in conjunction with type D) is the most common cause of chronic hepatitis in the United States. For example, approximately 90 percent of infants who are infected with the hepatitis B virus by the age of 12 months develop chronic hepatitis. This rate is much lower (i.e., five to 10 percent) in older children and adults. In the general population, between 50 and 75 percent of people with acute hepatitis C infection develop chronic disease. Chronic hepatitis may be categorized as persistent or active.

Chronic persistent hepatitis is a nonprogressive form of this disorder that affects only certain areas of the liver and typically produces no significant liver damage. Children with this type of chronic hepatitis often have no symptoms, although some will experience a loss of appetite or generalized fatigue. Diagnosis is confirmed through the study of liver tissue samples (liver biopsy) obtained with the use of a special needle. Chronic persistent hepatitis usually does not result in subsequent liver disease, although adults with this disorder may be at some risk for chronic degeneration of the liver (cirrhosis), liver failure, or cancer of the liver. In rare cases, children with severe chronic persistent hepatitis (caused by previous infection with hepatitis type B or C virus) may benefit from treatment with the antiviral agent interferon-alpha. Other treatment is symptomatic and supportive.

Chronic active hepatitis is a progressive inflammatory liver condition that results in the progressive loss of liver tissue and the formation of scar tissue (fibrosis) in the liver, possibly leading to liver failure. Associated findings are variable and may range from absent or mild symptoms such as fatigue and loss of appetite to more pronounced symptoms such as fever, skin rashes, and abdominal discomfort. Symptoms and findings associated with progressive liver involvement may include an unusual yellowish discoloration of the eyes, skin, and mucous membranes (jaundice); enlargement of the spleen (splenomegaly); accumulation of fluid in the abdomen (ascites); and other irregularities. Other findings, especially among those with chronic active hepatitis resulting from autoimmune influences, may include behavioral changes, eruptions of acne, inflammation of the thyroid (thyroiditis) or blood vessels (vasculitis), kidney inflammation (nephritis), painful swelling of the joints (arthritis), excessive levels of gamma globulins in the blood (hypergammaglobulinemia), and the cessation of menstruation in adolescent females (amenorrhea). Diagnosis of chronic active hepatitis must be confirmed through liver biopsy in order to exclude other disorders and to establish the severity of inflammation, the extent of liver degradation, and the underlying cause. Treatment for chronic active hepatitis caused by hepatitis B or C may include intramuscular administration of interferon-alpha. Disease resulting from autoimmune factors may be treated with carefully controlled regimens of corticosteroid therapy, sometimes in association with low doses of the immunosuppressive agent azathioprine. In addition, liver transplantation may be the treatment of choice for severe, life-threatening liver disease of any cause. Chronic active hepatitis resulting from certain medications may be treated by withdrawal of the offending drug, while disease caused by metabolic irregularities or other influences is dependent upon the underlying cause. Other treatment is symptomatic and supportive.

The following organizations in the General Resources Section can provide additional information: National Organization for Rare Disorders, Inc. (NORD), NIH/National Institute of Allergy and Infectious Disease, World Health Organization (WHO), Centers for Disease Control (CDC)

National Associations & Support Groups

1068 American Liver Foundation
75 Maiden Lane Suite 603
New York, NY 10038   212-668-1000
800-465-4837
Fax: 212-483-8179
e-mail: info@liverfoundation.org
www.liverfoundation.org

Organization provides several different medias for answering questions and to help clarify any uncertainties the individual may be experiencing.

1069 Hepatitis B Coalition
1537 Selby Avenue Suite 229
Saint Paul, MN 55104   612-647-9009

Works to prevent transmission of Hepatisis B in high risk groups, to achieve vaccination of all infants, children and adolescents and to promote education and treatment for Hepatisis B carrier.

1070 Hepatitis B Foundation
101 Greenwood Ave, 570
Jenkintown, PA 19046   215-884-8786
e-mail: info@hepb.org
www.hepb.org

1071 Hepatitis Education Project
P.O. Box 95162
Seattle, WA 98145   206-447-8136
e-mail: hep@scn.org

James Hart-Osborne, President

1072 Hepatitis Foundation International
Thelma King Thiel, author
30 Sunrise Terrace
Cedar Grove, NJ 07009   973-239-1035
800-891-0707
Fax: 973-875-5044
e-mail: hfi@intac.com
www.hepfi.org

The Hepatitis Foundation International seeks to increase awareness of the world-wide problem of viral hepatitis and to educate the public and healthcare providers about its prevention, diagnosis, and treatment.

Thelma King Thiel, Chair and CEO

1073 National Headquarters Hepatitis C Foundation
1502 Russett Dr
Warminster, PA 18974   215-672-2606
Fax: 215-672-1518
e-mail: hepatitis_c_foundation@msn.com
www.hepcfoundation.org

Web Sites

1074 Columbia University
www.cpmcnet.columbia.edu/dept/gi/

1075 Hepatitis United
www.hepu.org/

1076 PedBase
www.icondata.com/health/pedbase/files/HEPATITI.HTM

1077 University of Chicago
www.uhs.bsd.uchicago.edu/uhs/topics/hepatitis.html

Books

1078 Hepatitis
National Institute of Allergy & Infectious Disease
National Institutes of Health
Bethesda, MD 20892   301-496-4000

A pamphlet discussing the cause, symptoms, transmission, diagnosis, tests, prevention and the latest research on hepatitis.

1079 Hepatitis A, B & C; Liver Disease You Should Know About
American Liver Foundation
1425 Pompton Avenue
Cedar Grove, NJ 07009

800-223-0179

Explains viral hepatitis, transmission, symptoms, testing and acute chronic hepatitis.

1080 Hepatitis B Prevention
National Center for Infectious Diseases
Hepatitis Branch
Atlanta, GA 30333   404-332-4555

Explains what hepatitis B is, what behaviors are risky and how to protect oneself against it.

1081 Hepatitis B Prevention: A Resource Guide
National Digestive Diseases Info. Clearinghouse
Box NDDIC, 9000 Rockville Pk
Bethesda, MD 20824   301-468-6344

Designed to assist health care and other professionals who work in planning or administering hepatitis B prevention programs.

252 pages

1082 Hepatitis Fact Sheet
Shering Corporation

Kenilworth, NJ 07033   908-298-4001

Offers information on the causes, symptoms, prevention and treatments for hepatitis.

1083 How Many Times a Day Do You Risk Being Infected with Hepatitis B?
American Liver Foundation
1425 Pompton Avenue
Cedar Grove, NJ 07009   973-256-2550
800-223-0179

A flyer emphasizing the importance of vaccination against hepatitis B.

1084 Liver Disease in Children
Frederick J. Sucky, author

Mosby Year Book
11830 Westline Industrial Drive
St. Louis, MO 63146   314-872-8370
800-325-4177

1993 800 pages
ISBN: 1-556443-77-2

1085 Liver Disoders in Childhood
Alex P. Mowat, author

Butterworth-Helnemann
223 Wildwood Avenue
Woburn, MA 01801   617-928-2500
800-366-2665

1994 432 pages
ISBN: 0-750610-39-5

1086 Q and A: Hepatitis B Prevention
SmithKline Beecham Pharmaceuticals
1 Franklin Plaza, 200 N. 16th St.
Philadelphia, PA 19010   215-751-4000

Informational booklet written for healthcare personnel by the manufacturer of Engerix-B vaccine, reviews hepatitis B prevention.

1087 War Against Hepatitis B
William Muraskin, author

University of Pennsylvania Press
418 Service Drive
Philadelphia, PA 19104   215-898-6261

1995 256 pages
ISBN: 0-812232-67-4

Newsletters

1088 Hepatitis B Coalition News
Hepatitis B Coalition
1573 Selby Avenue-Suite 229
Saint Paul, MN 55104   612-647-9009

Newsletter with brochures, articles, videotapes, audio-cassette tapes and manuals for different ethnic populations.

Pamphlets

1089 What Health Care Workers Should Know About Hepatitis B
Channing L. Bete Company
200 State Road
South Deerfield, MA 01373

800-628-7733

Presents information in easy-to-read, simple English for health care workers about hepatitis B.

15 pages

DESCRIPTION

1090 CLEFT LIP AND CLEFT PALATE

Disorder Type: Birth Defect

Cleft lip and cleft palate are birth defects that may occur together or as isolated conditions. Newborns with cleft lip have a groove in the upper lip that may be a small notch or, in more severe cases, may be deep and extend up to the nose. Cleft palate is characterized by incomplete closure of the roof of the mouth (palate). In affected newborns, an abnormal gap runs along the midline of the soft, fleshy area of the palate (soft palate) and, in some patients, extends into one or both sides of the bony, front region of the palate (hard palate). As a result, the nasal cavity may open into the palate. Cleft lip with or without cleft palate affects approximately one in 600 newborns, whereas cleft palate alone occurs in about one in 1,000 births.

In newborns with cleft lip, the defect may occur on one or both sides of the upper lip and typically affects the bony ridge of the upper jaw (upper alveolar ridge). This ridge contains the sockets in which the roots of the teeth are held (dental alveoli). As a result, affected children often experience improper development of certain teeth, potentially resulting in absent, malformed, improperly positioned, or extra teeth and increased risk of dental decay (dental caries). In addition, infants with cleft lip and cleft palate typically have feeding difficulties associated with poor suckling capability and excessive swallowing of air. Affected children with cleft palate are also prone to repeated infections of the middle ear (otitis media) that, in some cases, may contribute to associated hearing loss. Many children also experience speech defects that may be due to inadequate functioning of certain muscles of the throat and palate (pharyngeal and palatal muscles).

In affected newborns, treatment initially consists of measures to ensure improved feeding and proper intake of nutrients. In many patients, a plastic device (a prosthetic known as an obturator) may be fitted that covers the gap in the palate, thereby improving suction and intake of fluids. The obturator is typically replaced every few weeks due to rapid growth during infancy. In addition, in those with cleft palate, modified artificial nipples may help to improve feeding. In many cases, cleft lip may be surgically closed by approximately two months of age and additional corrective surgery may be performed later during childhood. If affected children do not have associated physical abnormalities, surgical correction of cleft palate may be performed before the age of one year to help improve normal speech development. However, if surgery is delayed until the age of three years or later, a device (such as a contoured speech bulb) may be used to help close off the uppermost portion of the throat (nasopharynx) during the production of certain sounds. This helps children to develop understandable speech. Treatment may also include dental procedures to correct improperly positioned teeth or to replace absent teeth (e.g., with prosthetic devices). Speech therapy may be beneficial for some affected children. Additional treatment for infants and children with cleft lip and cleft palate is symptomatic and supportive.

Cleft lip and cleft palate may occur as isolated conditions or in association with several underlying chromosomal disorders or malformation syndromes. Isolated cleft lip and/or cleft palate may potentially result due to certain environmental factors, occur randomly for unknown reasons (sporadically), or be familial. Many cases have been reported in which several individuals in multigenerational families (kindreds) have been affected by isolated cleft lip and cleft palate. In such cases, the specific modes of inheritance are not understood. The frequent association of cleft lip and cleft palate is thought to result from certain developmental abnormalities during embryonic growth.

The following organizations in the General Resources Section can provide additional information: National Organization for Rare Disorders, Inc. (NORD), NIH/Office of Rare Diseases, March of Dimes Birth Defects Foundation, Genetic Alliance, Online Mendelian Inheritance in Man.: www3.ncbi.nlm.nih.gov/Omim/searchomim.html

National Associations & Support Groups

1091 AboutFace USA
PO Box 737
Warrington, PA 18976   215-491-0602
                                        800-225-3223
                        e-mail: aboutface2000@aol.com
                                www.aboutface2000.org

Provides information, services, emotional support and educational programs for and on behalf of individuals with facial differences and their families. Working to increase understanding through public awareness and education.

3M members

Rickie Anderson, Executive Director

1092 Cleft Palate Foundation
1829 E Franklin St, Ste 1022
Chapel Hill, NC 27514   919-933-9044
                                        800-242-5338
                            Fax: 919-996-9604
                        e-mail: cleftline@aol.com
                                www.cleft.com

Provides the proper instruction information for the family and friends of people suffering from this disorder.

1093 Cleft Palate/Cranofacial Birth Defects Cleft Palate Foundation
104 S Estes Dr, Ste 204
Chapel Hill, NC 27514   919-933-9044
                                        800-242-5338
                            Fax: 919-933-9604

The Cleft Palate Foundation operates a toll-free CLEFTLINE for parents with children born with cleft lip, palate and other craniofacial birth defects. Referrals are made to cleft palate/craniofacial healthcare teams and to parent-support groups. Free information is available to parents.

1094 Craniofacial Foundation of America
Tennessee Craniofacial of America
975 E. Third St
Chattanooga, TN 37403   423-778-9192
                                        800-418-3223
                            Fax: 423-778-8172
                        e-mail: farmertm@erlanger.org
                                www.erlanger.org/cranio

Organization assissts families with both the physical and emotional aspects, trying to make everyday events a little easier.

1095 FACES: National Association for Craniofacially Handicapped
P.O. Box 11082
Chattanooga, TN 37401
                                        888-332-2373

Disperses information to the public on the medical professionals specializing in this field.

1096 Prescription Parents
22 Ingersoll Road
Wellesley, MA 02181   617-965-2946
                        e-mail: seltzer@samizdat.com
                                www.samizdat.com

Organization that gives information and support on children with cleft lip and cleft palate through its educational and support materials, including its directory, newsletter and brochures.

1097 Wide Smiles
P.O. Box 5153
Stockton, CA 95205   209-942-2812
                        e-mail: widesmiles@aol.com
                                www.widesmiles.org

Gathering of concerned people and medical professionals that have put together the educational and media resources to better help the general public.

International

1098 Cleft Lip and Palata Association (CLAPA)
138 Buckingham Palace Road
London,
United Kingdom
                        e-mail: clapa@mcmail.com
                                www.clapa@mcmail.com

Books

1099 A Curriculum for Infants and Toddlers with Cleft Palate

Lynch, Brookshire, Fox, author

Pro-Ed
8700 Shoal Creek Boulevard
Austin, TX 78757   512-451-3246
                         800-897-3202
                    Fax: 512-451-8542
                    www.proedinc.com

This curriculum is a complete revision and expansion of the widely used 'A Parent-Child Cleft Palate Curriculum.

1100 Children with Facial Difference

Hope Charkins, M.S.W., author

Woodbine House
6510 Bells Mill Road
Bethesda, MD 20817   301-468-8800
                           800-843-7323
                      Fax: 301-897-5838
           e-mail: info@woodbinehouse.com
                  www.woodbinehouse.com

The first guide for parents about their child's congenital craniofacial anomaly - a condition that affects the apparance and fuction of the head and face. This accessible book dicusses conditions such as cleft lip, cleft palate, Teacher Collins syndrome, Crouzon syndrome, and more. Parents learn about the diagnostic process, interdisciplinary treatment approach, education, speech and language issues, and how to help their child and family adjust emotionally.

361 pages Softcover
ISBN: 0-933149-61-1

Pamphlets

1101 Cleft Lip & Palate
March of Dimes Resource Center
1275 Mamaroneck Avenue
White Plains, NY 10605   888-663-4637
                          Fax: 914-997-4763

DESCRIPTION

1102 CLUBFOOT

Synonym: Talipes

Disorder Type: Birth Defect

Covers these related disorders: Talipes equinovarus

May involve these systems in the body (see Section III):

Skeletal System

Clubfoot, also known as talipes, is a deformity in which the foot is abnormally twisted out of position at birth (congenital). There are a number of foot deformities that are sometimes loosely classified as clubfoot. These include defects in which the inner portion of the foot is raised with the sole turned inward (metatarsus varus) or the front area of the foot is raised and the heel is turned outward (talipes calcaneovalgus). However, the term clubfoot is most commonly used to refer to a specific deformity in which the heel is turned inward and the sole is flexed with the toes downward (plantar flexion). More specifically, in infants with this condition, which is also known as talipes equinovarus, the forefoot is turned upward and inward toward the body; the heel is inverted; and the arch is high due to plantar flexion. These abnormalities are thought to occur as a result of deformity of the ankle bone (talus) and discoloration of the ankle (i.e., talonavicular joint). Depending upon the severity of the deformity, the affected foot may have varying levels of stiffness and inflexibility. In addition, the foot and lower leg may be unusually small. Muscles of the foot and calf are also typically underdeveloped, which may become more apparent with advancing age.

Talipes equinovarus is approximately twice as common in males than in females. In approximately 50 percent of children with this condition, both feet are affected. When one foot is affected, the right side is most often involved. Talipes equinovarus often occurs an an isolated condition. Such cases occur randomly for unknown reasons (sporadically) or may be familial. In familial cases, the condition is thought to result from the interaction of an abnormal (mutated) gene, possibly in association with the involvement of other genes or certain environmental factors (multifactorial inheritance). Although deformity of the ankle bone was considered the primary abnormality, researchers speculate that a neuromuscular abnormality may be the underlying cause of the talus deformities and associated findings.

In some cases, talipes equinovarus may also occur due to or in association with certain neuromuscular disorders (e.g., arthrogryposis multiplex congenita) or other underlying disorders or syndromes. In addition, some researchers suspect that the deformity may also result from abnormal positioning of the foot during fetal development. Talipes equinovarus may affect up to one in 1,000 newborns.

The treatment of talipes equinovarus usually begins soon after birth. Treatment measures may include repeated, gentle manipulations of the affected foot toward a more normal position and the use of taping, casts, or splints (e.g., malleable splints, serial plaster casts) to hold the foot in a corrected position; casts to maintain proper positioning (e.g., holding casts); and other orthopedic appliances and corrective shoes to assist with walking. If the use of taping, splints, or casts does not result in appropriate correction, surgical methods may be recommended. Physicians may continue to regularly monitor affected children to detect possible recurrence and to ensure ongoing -improvement.

The following organizations in the General Resources Section can provide additional information: March of Dimes Birth Defects Foundation, Easter Seals, NIH/National Institute of Arthritis and Musculoskeletal and Skin Diseases, Online Menedelian Inheritance in Man.: www3.ncbi.nlm.nih.gov/Omim/searchomim.html

Web Sites

1103 Club Foot Resource Page:
members.aol.com/clubft/index.html

1104 Clubfoot.org
www.clubfoot.org/

1105 Wheelies' Textbook of Orthopaedics
www.medmedia.com/o12/110.htm

Pamphlets

1106 Club Foot
March of Dimes Resource Center
1275 Mamaroneck Avenue
White Plains, NY 10605   888-663-4637
                               Fax: 914-997-4763

DESCRIPTION

1107 COARCTATION OF THE AORTA

Disorder Type: Birth Defect
May involve these systems in the body (see Section III):
Cardiovascular System

Coarctation of the aorta is a congenital heart defect characterized by a narrowing or constriction of the body's main artery. This artery, known as the aorta, carries blood away from the heart to nourish the tissues of the body. Most of these defects are located just below the origin of the artery that supplies blood to the left arm, (left subclavian artery) the last of the head vessels. Because this constriction reduces blood flow to the lower portion of the body, affected individuals may have unusually low blood pressure and weak or absent pulses in their legs. In addition, there may be higher blood pressure and strong pulses in the arms.

The severity of associated symptoms relates to the degree of pressure changes resulting from aortic narrowing. Although some children have no symptoms, others may experience dizziness, headache, weakness, fainting, nosebleeds, cold legs, and leg pain or cramps. Some affected infants may develop heart failure within the first few weeks of life. In some newborns, heart failure may result in decreased blood flow and abnormally high levels of acid in the blood (metabolic acidosis), sometimes accompanied by severe diarrhea and kidney (renal) failure. This life-threatening situation will require immediate treatment. As these infants age, the narrowing may recur (restenosis) necessitating dilation or opening of the vessel through a procedure called balloon angioplasty, during which a balloon-tipped tube is inflated inside the aorta, thus helping to expand the narrowed area of the vessel. Treatment of coarctation in a newborn requires surgery. Correction of coarctation of the aorta through surgical or balloon catheter means may be recommended in older children with significant involvement. Because coarctation of the aorta is very often accompanied by other heart defects, early intervention is often warranted. Other cardiac anomalies often associated with this defect include bicuspid aortic valve (i.e., the heart valve between the left ventricle and the aorta is composed of two leaflets, or cusps, instead of the normal three); abnormalities of the mitral valve (located between the left atrium and the left ventricle); and an abnormal opening in the wall between the left and right ventricles (ventricular septal defect).

The cause of coarctation of the aorta is unknown. Some researchers think that it develops in the fetus in association with certain types of cardiac abnormalities. Coarctation of the aorta is more prevalent in males than in females by a ratio of about two to one.

The following organizations in the General Resources Section can provide additional information: March of Dimes Birth Defects Foundation, NIH/National Heart, Lung and Blood Institute, NIH/National Institute of Child Health and Human Development, Genetic Alliance

National Associations & Support Groups

1108 American Heart Association
7272 Greenville Avenue
Dallas, TX 75231

214-373-6300
800-242-8721
Fax: 214-706-1341
e-mail: inquire@amhrt.org
www.amhrt.org

Supports research, education and community service programs with the objective of reducing premature death and disability from cardiovascular diseases and stroke; coordinates the efforts of health professionals, and other engaged in the fight against heart and circulatory disease.

Web Sites

1109 Children's Health Information Network/ Congenital Heart Defects
www.ohsu.edu.cliniweb/c14/c14.240.400.html

1110 Congenital Heart Disease Resource Page
www.csun.edu/~hcmth011/heart/

1111 Southern Illinois University School of Medicine
www.siumed.edu/peds/teaching/patient%20edu-
cation.htm

DESCRIPTION

1112 COLIC

Synonyms: Infantile colic, Three-month colic

May involve these systems in the body (see Section III):

Digestive System

Colic refers to a condition in which infants experience frequent episodes of abdominal pain, accompanied by irritability and intense crying or screaming. These episodes usually begin suddenly and continue for several hours. Symptoms and physical findings of colic may also include flushing of the face, swelling of the abdomen, repeated extending or flexing of the legs, and unusually cold feet.

It is suspected that colic is intestinal in origin; however, its exact cause is not known. Contributing factors may include the excessive swallowing of air during episodes of unceasing crying, overfeeding, hunger, certain foods, intestinal allergy, and environmental stress. Attacks of colic usually commence within the first few weeks of life and occur most often in the afternoon or evening. Colic often resolves spontaneously within three or four months, without residual effects.

Infants with symptoms associated with colic should be evaluated to determine if another, perhaps more serious disorder is causing the pain and discomfort. The treatment of colic may include soothing, comforting gestures such as holding, patting, stroking, rocking, and other repetitive movements. Some affected infants may benefit from white noise or other comforting background sounds; the application of a warm wash cloth, hot water bottle, or warm heating pad under the stomach; or a ride in the car. Some episodes of colic may resolve with the passing of gas or stool. In addition, parents and caregivers may be advised to refrain from overstimulating, overfeeding, or underfeeding babies with colic. Physicians often advise that parents or caregivers try to avoid fatigue, as this may sometimes add to other environmental stress factors that contribute to episodes of colic. Other treatment is supportive.

The following organizations in the General Resources Section can provide additional information: NIH/National Digestive Diseases Information Clearinghouse

National Associations & Support Groups

1113 Center for Digestive Disorders - Central: Dupage Hospital
25 North Winfield Road
Winfield, IL 60190   630-682-1600

1114 Digestive Disease National Coalition
507 Capital Courte, Suite 200
Washington, DC 20002   202-544-7497
          Fax: 202-546-7105

Objective is to inform the public about technology improvements through several media forms.

Web Sites

1115 Colic in Infants Assessment
www.ibionet.com/colicininfants.html

1116 Pediatric Database (Pedbase)
www.icondata.com/health/pedbase/files/COLIC.HTM

DESCRIPTION

1117 CONDUCT DISORDER

Disorder Type: Mental, Emotional or Behavioral Disorder

Covers these related disorders: Group conduct disorder, Solitary aggressive conduct disorder, Undifferentiated conduct disorder

Conduct disorder refers to a group of distinct behavioral abnormalities characterized by the repetition of certain types of disruptive or antisocial behaviors. Children or adolescents with conduct disorder may often lie, steal, skip school, run away from home, use drugs or alcohol, hurt animals, commit arson or vandalism, engage in physical violence, use weapons, and commit other criminal acts. Those affected with solitary aggressive conduct disorder are usually selfish, rarely get along with or relate well to others, and often lack remorse for their behavior. Children and adolescents with group conduct disorder, however, may be attached and faithful to a particular clique, gang, or other group of friends while at the same time violating the rights of or displaying antisocial behavior toward those outside of the group. In some cases, affected individuals may display behavior characteristic of both solitary aggressive and group conduct disorders and, subsequently, may be diagnosed with undifferentiated conduct disorder.

Conduct disorder may be caused by a variety of factors including genetic as well as environmental influences (e.g., childrearing, etc.). In many cases, children with this type of behavioral irregularity have parents or caregivers who display similar patterns of conduct. In addition, parents or caregivers often have inconsistent parenting skills or may be overly aggressive in punishing or disciplining. Some parents or caregivers may be unsupportive of the child, or may lack other basic skills that help the child to develop a sense of self-worth, respect for others, etc. Several factors may influence whether affected children carry these characteristic patterns of behavior into adulthood. Some factors include parental or caregiver influences, the age of onset, the severity and type of behavior, the number of different types of antisocial behaviors exhibited, and whether the episodes of disruptive behavior continue to increase.

Treatment of conduct disorder may include individual, group, and family therapy, as well as parental or caregiver management training. In some cases, children with severe conduct disorder may benefit from hospitalization for psychiatric evaluation and treatment. Medication is, in most cases, not indicated for the treatment of conduct disorder; however, it is sometimes prescribed to treat other underlying disorders (e.g, depression, attention deficit hyperactivity disorder, etc.). Other treatment is supportive.

The following organizations in the General Resources Section can provide additional information: Federation of Families for Children's Mental Health, National Alliance for the Mentally Ill, National Mental Health Association, National Mental Health Consumer Self-Help Clearinghouse, NIH/National Institute of Mental Health, Online Mendelian Inheritance in Man: www3.ncbi.nlm.nih.gov/Omim/searchomim.html

National Associations & Support Groups

1118 American Mental Health Foundation (AMNF)
1049 5th Avenue
New York, NY 10028
USA
212-639-1561
Fax: 212-737-9027

Dedicated to the extensive and intensive research in the theories and techniques of treatment of emotional illness and to the implementation of reforms in the mental health system. Efforts have resulted in development of better and less expensive treatment methods. Findings are disseminated in English and other major languages.

Monroe W. Spero, MD

1119 Association for Persons with Mental and Developmental Disabilities
132 Fair Street
Kingston, NY 12401
USA

914-334-4336
800-331-5362
Fax: 914-331-4569
e-mail: nadd@mhv.net

Non-profit organization designed to promote interest of professional and parent development with resources for individuals who have the co-existence of mental illness and mental retardation. Provides conference, educational services and training materials to professionals, parents, concerned citizens and service organizations. Formerly known as the National Association for the Dually Diagnosed.

Robert Fletcher, Executive Director

1120 Center for Family Support (CFS)
333 7th Avenue
New York, NY 10001
USA

212-629-7939
Fax: 212-239-2211
www.cfsny.org

Service agency devoted to the physical well-being and development of the retarded child and the sound mental health of the parents. Helps families with retarded children with all aspects of home care including counseling, referrals, home aide service and consultation. Offers intervention for parents at the birth of a retarded child with in-home support, guidance and infant stimulation. Pioneered training of nonprofessional women as home aides to provide supportive services in homes.

Steven Vernickofs, Executive Director

1121 Center for Mental Health Services Knowledge Exchange Network
US Dept of Health and Human Services
PO Box 42490
Washington, DC 20015
USA

800-789-2647
Fax: 301-984-8796
e-mail: ken@mentalhealth.org
www.mentalhealth.org

Information about resources, technical assistance, research, training, networks, and other federal clearing houses, and fact sheets and materials. Information specialists refer callers to mental health resources in their communities as well as state, federal and non-profit contacts. Staff available Monday through Friday, 8:30-5:00 EST, excluding federal holidays. After hours, callers may leave messages and an information specialist will return their call.

1122 Mental Illness Foundation
772 W 168th Street
New York, NY 10032

212-682-4699
Fax: 212-682-4896

Supports community housing, treatment, research, outreach and public-awareness efforts for people with mental illness. Publications: Mental Illness Foundation, quarterly newsletter. Directory that lists mental illnesses and provides information on how to contact related associations. Annual meeting.

Research Centers

1123 Child & Family Center
PO Box 829
Topeka, KS 66601

785-380-5000
800-288-3950
Fax: 785-273-8625
www.menninger.edu

The Center's goal is to further develop emerging understanding of the impact of childhood maltreatment and abuse to chart primary prevention strategies that will foster healthy patterns of caregiving and attachment and reduce the prevalence of maltreatment and abuse; to devlop secondary prevention strategies that will promote early detections of attachment-related problems and effective interventions to avert the development of chornic and severe disorders, and to develop more effective treatmen

Web Sites

1124 Internet Mental Health
www.mentalhealth.com

Books

1125 Aggression and Violence Throughout the Life Span

Ray DeV Peters, Rober McMahon, Vernon L
Quinsey, author

Sage Publications, Inc.
2455 Teller Road
Thousand Oaks, CA 91320
USA   805-499-0721
                          Fax: 805-499-0871
                    e-mail: info@sagepub.com
                        www.sagepub.com

A unique life span developmental perspective on
some of society's most perplexing and pernicious
probles, aggressive and violent behaviors. Examines issues in the development of aggressive behaviors in young children, the progression of
these behaviors to older children and adolescents, cause, effect and treatment of aggressive
and violent behaviors in adults. Intergrates empirical research with clinical applications.

360 pages Softcover
ISBN: 0-803945-51-5

**1126 Conduct Disorders in Childhood and Adolescence,
Devlopmental Clinical Psych**

Sage Publications, Inc.
2455 Teller Road
Thousand Oaks, CA 91320
USA   805-499-0721
                          Fax: 805-499-0871
                    e-mail: info@sagepub.com
                        www.sagepub.com

Conduct disorder is a clinical problem among
children and adolescents that includes aggressive acts, theft, vandalism, firesetting, running
away, truancy, defying authority and other antisocial behaviors. This book describes the nature
of conduct disorder and what is currently
known from research and clinical work. Topics
include psychiatric diagnosis, parent psychopathology and child-rearing processes.

160 pages Hardcover

**1127 Conduct Problem/Emotional Problem
Interventions: A Holistic Perspective**

Slosson Educational Publications
P.O. Box 280
East Aurora, NY 14052
USA   716-625-0930
                               800-756-7766
                          Fax: 800-655-3840
                   e-mail: slosson@slosson.com
                        www.slosson.com

This innovative book is broad in scope and addresses the now what sensation that many professionals get when charged with the education
or treatment of individuals with conduct disorders or emotional disturbance. Distinct intervention and screening strategies and patient
involvement strategies are offered in clear and
practical terms.

1128 Difficult Child

Stanley Turecki, MD; Leslis Tonner, Stella Chess,
author

1540 Broadway
New York, NY 10036
USA   212-782-9000
                          Fax: 212-782-9700

1129 Preventing Antisocial Behavior Interventions

Joan McCord, Richard E Tremblay, author

Guiford Publications
72 Spring Street
New York, NY 10012
USA   212-431-9800
                               800-365-7006
                          Fax: 212-966-6708
                    e-mail: info@guilford.com
                        www.guilford.com

Establishes the crucial link between theory,
measurement and intervention. Brings together
a collection of studies that utilize experimental
approaches for evaluating intervention programs, both the feasibility and necessity of independent evaluation. Also shows how the
information obtained in such studies can be
used to test and refine prevailing theories about
human behavior in general and behavior
changes in particular.

391 pages
ISBN: 0-898628-82-2

DESCRIPTION

1130 CONGENITAL CATARACTS

Disorder Type: Genetic Disorder, Vision

Congenital cataracts refers to a condition in which cloudiness or opacities in the lens of the eye or eyes are present at birth. These opacities may vary in severity, with some resolving spontaneously as in cataracts of prematurity. Other congenital cataracts, if left untreated, may result in loss of transparency of the lens and subsequent visual impairment. In addition, in some newborns, remnants of other eye tissues may contribute to the formation of a stationary opacity of the cornea. In most patients, this type of stationary cloudiness does not contribute to visual impairment.

Congenital cataracts may occur as the result of many different factors (multifactorial), including genetic influences, associated metabolic and chromosomal disorders, congenital infections, and toxic influences. If inherited as an isolated event, congenital cataracts are usually transmitted as an autosomal dominant or autosomal recessive trait. Several metabolic disorders are characterized by congenital cataracts, including galactosemia, in which an enzyme deficiency results in the inability to process the simple sugar galactose; oculocerebrorenal syndrome (Lowe's syndrome), an X-linked metabolic disorder that affects many systems of the body; certain metabolic diseases known as lyosomal storage disorders; and several other diseases related to inborn errors of metabolism. Other contributing metabolic factors may include low blood levels of calcium (hypocalcemia) or glucose (hypoglycemia). In addition, cataracts are sometimes diagnosed in newborns whose mothers have diabetes mellitus. Several chromosomal disorders are also characterized by congenital opacities including Down's syndrome, trisomy 13 syndrome, Turner's syndrome, and others. Congenital cataracts are sometimes the result of maternal infections that occur during pregnancy. Such infections may include German measles (ru-

bella), syphilis, measles, influenza, certain herpes infections, and others. Additional contributing factors may include toxic influences from drug substances taken by the mother during pregnancy.

Treatment for congenital cataracts depends upon the extent of the defect and its influence on vision. To restore lost transparency of the lens resulting from cataracts, surgery may be performed in which the cataract and lens are removed. To reestablish the ability of the eye to deflect light that was lost with lens removal, special contact lenses or implants are then fitted to the eye. In some cases, additional surgery may be indicated. Because congenital opacities of the lens are so often associated with other eye irregularities (e.g., amblyopia, glaucoma, strabismus, etc.) and in order to obtain the best outcome, treatment may also be directed toward any associated abnormalities. In addition, patients are followed carefully after surgery in order to prevent, correct, or treat any possible complications.

The following organizations in the General Resources Section can provide additional information: National Organization for Rare Disorders, Inc. (NORD), Genetic Alliance, Online Mendelian Inheritance in Man: www3.ncbi.nlm.nih.gov/Omim/searchomim.html, NIH/National Eye Institute

National Associations & Support Groups

1131 Association for Education & Rehabilitation of the Blind & Visually Impaired
206 North Washington Street Suite 320
Alexandria, VA 22314   703-823-9690
                              Fax: 703-823-9695

The only professional membership organization dedicated to the advancement of education and rehabilitation of the blind and visually impaired children and adults

1132 Council of Families with Visual Impairments
American Council of the Blind
1155 15th Street NW Suite 1004
Washington, DC 20005   202-467-5081
                              800-424-8666
                          Fax: 202-467-5085
                        e-mail: info@acb.org
                                www.acb.org

A network of parents with blind or visually impaired children that offers support and outreach, shares experiences in parent/child relationships, exchanges educational, cultural and medical information about child development and more.

1133 National Association for Parents of the Visually Impaired
National Office
PO Box 317
Watertown, MA 02471

800-562-6265
Fax: 781-972-7444

The only national organization that strives to serve families of children of all ages and ranges with visual loss. It is a community-based organization whose members include parents, parent organizations, agencies and other persons with common objectives - the support and services to the parents of children with visual impairments.

1134 National Association for Visually Handicapped
22 West 21st Street 6th Floor
New York, NY 10010

212-889-3141
Fax: 212-727-2931
e-mail: staff@navh.org
www.navh.org

Serves the parially seeing (not totally blind) with informational literature, newsletters for adults and children, educational outreach, referrals, counsel and guidance. Works with eye care professionals and the buisness community regarding abilities for the partially seeing.

Lorraine Marchi, Founder/CEO

1135 National Eye Research Foundation
910 Skokie Boulevard
Northbrook, IL 60062

Devoted to the enhancement of care and study of eye related diseases.

1136 National Retinoblastoma Parent Group
P.O. Box 317
Watertown, MA 02272

800-562-6265

Dedicated to providing information and support to parents of children with Retinoblastoma, a malonma tumor appearing in one or both eyes. Provides a variety of educational and support materials including a regular newsletter and medical journal article reprints concerning Retinoblastoma.

1137 Parents of Cataract Kids
179 Hunter Lane
Devon, PA 19333   215-293-1917

Web Sites

1138 National Association for Visually Handicapped
www.navh.org

1139 Royal National Institute for the Blind
www.rnib/org.uk/info/eyeimpoi/congen.htm

DESCRIPTION

1140 CONGENITAL DIAPHRAGMATIC HERNIA
Synonym: CDH
Disorder Type: Birth Defect

Congenital diaphragmatic hernia (CDH) is a birth defect characterized by projection or bulging of organs of the abdomen into the chest cavity. This occurs as a result of an abnormal opening in the diaphragm, the dome-shaped muscular organ that separates the abdomen from the chest and plays an essential role in breathing. Approximately one in 5,000 newborns are affected by the condition. CDH is thought to result due to failed closure of a certain area of the embryonic diaphragm (i.e., the foramen of Bochdalek). In some cases, disrupted development in other areas of the growing fetus may also cause CDH. This birth defect may occur as an isolated condition or, in about 20 to 30 percent of patients, in association with other abnormalities or underlying malformation syndromes, such as Down syndrome, trisomy 18 syndrome, or trisomy 13 syndrome. There are reports of several infants with isolated CDH in certain families (kindreds). In such cases, the condition is thought to result from abnormal changes (mutations) of different genes, possibly in association with certain environmental factors (multifactorial inheritance).

In newborns with CDH, the diaphragmatic defect may be small or affect up to half of the diaphragm. The left side of the diaphragm is most commonly involved. The lungs may also be unusually small and underdeveloped (pulmonary hypoplasia), and associated abnormalities of the blood vessels supplying the lungs may also be present. In addition, the intestines may not be positioned properly (intestinal malformation). Most newborns with CDH experience increasing difficulties breathing (respiratory distress) within the first 24 hours after birth. Associated symptoms include labored breathing (dyspnea), grunting upon exhalation, drawing in of the chest wall during inhalation, and a bluish discoloration of the skin and mucous membranes (cyanosis). These findings may potentially result in life-threatening complications. In addition, in some affected newborns, air may collect in the chest cavity, causing the lung(s) to collapse (pneumothorax). In some cases, symptoms associated with CDH may not become apparent until after the first few weeks of life. Such infants may experience mild respiratory symptoms or intestinal obstruction and associated vomiting (emesis).

In newborns with CDH, immediate measures may be necessary to prevent or treat potentially life-threatening complications. Surgery to repair the diaphragmatic defect is deferred until the newborn's respiratory status has been stabilized. Ongoing supportive measures may be employed before surgery, such as use of a device known as an extracorporeal membrane oxygenator (ECMO). This device supplies oxygen to the infant's blood and returns this oxygenated blood to the body. In addition, certain medications may also be used (e.g., surfactant therapy to help improve oxygenation, etc.).

The following organizations in the General Resources Section can provide additional information: National Organization for Rare Disorders, Inc., (NORD), Genetic Alliance, NIH/National Institute of Child Health and Human Development, NIH/Office of Rare Diseases, NIH/National Digestive Diseases Information Clearinghouse

National Associations & Support Groups

1141 CHERUBS - The Association of Congenital Diaphragmatic Hernia Research
Advocacy and Support
P.O. Boc 1150
Creedmore, NC 27522   919-693-8158
e-mail: cherubs@gloryroad.net
www.gloryroad.net/~cherubs

1142 Digestive Disease National Coalition
507 Capitol Court, Ste 200 NE
Washington, DC 20002   202-544-7497
Fax: 202-546-7105

Web Sites

1143 Family Village
www.familyvillage.wisc.edu/lib_cdh.html

DESCRIPTION

1144 CONGENITAL GLAUCOMA

Synonym: Infantile glaucoma

Disorder Type: Birth Defect, Vision

Covers these related disorders: Primary glaucoma, Secondary glaucoma

Glaucoma refers to a condition in which the fluid pressure within the eyes (intraocular pressure) is abnormally elevated. This may occur as a result of the buildup of fluid (aqueous humor) due to obstruction or other problems with the eyes. Glaucoma that develops by the third year of life is referred to as congenital or infantile glaucoma, which is a very rare occurrence. Primary glaucoma refers to the condition as it relates to an irregularity in the mechanism that drains the eye. Secondary glaucoma refers to increased intraocular pressure that results from other types of irregularities that may or may not be accompanied by drainage deficit.

Symptoms associated with congenital glaucoma may include an abnormal sensitivity to light (photophobia), involuntary, repeated squeezing and closing of the eyelids (blepharospasm), abnormal tearing, swelling and enlargement of the cornea, difficulty in seeing, and other ocular irregularities. Affected infants under three months of age are at additional risk of incurring tissue damage due to heightened sensitivity of the cornea to elevated fluid pressure within the eye. Eye irregularities may be observed by a physician upon ophthalmic examination.

Congenital glaucoma may develop subsequent to certain congenital problems such as trauma, bleeding (hemorrhage) within the eye, or tumors and inflammation. Other associated abnormalities may include the lack of transparency (opacity) of the lenses of the eye (cataracts), displacement of the lenses (ectopia lentis), partial absence of the iris (aniridia), and other abnormalities. Disorders often associated with congenital glaucoma include certain chromosomal disorders that may affect various systems of the body such as Sturge-Weber syndrome, oculocerebrorenal syndrome, neurofibromatosis, and Marfan syndrome.

Treatment for congenital glaucoma includes surgery to relieve the pressure within the eye to prevent optic nerve damage and preserve vision. In some cases, more than one surgery may be necessary and follow-up therapy may be required. Additional treatment is directed toward associated irregularities and complications.

The following organizations in the General Resources Section can provide additional information: National Organization for Rare Disorders, Inc. (NORD), Genetic Alliance, Online Mendelian Inheritance in Man: www3/ncbi.nlm.nih.gov/Omim/searchomim.html

National Associations & Support Groups

1145 Glaucoma Support Network
Glaucoma Research Foundation
200 Pine St, Ste 200
San Francisco, CA 94104

415-986-3162
800-826-6693
Fax: 415-986-3763
www.glaucoma.org

A peer support service for glaucoma patients and their families. The Network answers questions of individuals concerned about vision and glaucoma.

1146 NIH/National Eye Institute (NEI)
9000 Rockville Pike
Bethesda, MD 20892

301-496-5248
www.nei.nih.gov/

1147 National Center for Sight
National Society to Prevent Blindness
500 East Remington Road
Schaumburg, IL 60173

847-843-8458
800-331-2020
Fax: 847-843-2020

A toll-free line offering information on a broad range of vision, eye health and safety topics including sports eye safety, lazy eye, diabetic retinopathy, glaucoma, cataracts, children's eye disorders, and more.

1148 National Eye Research Foundation
910 Skokie Blvd
Northbrook, IL 60062

Libraries & Resource Centers

1149 Florida Ophthalmic Institute
7106 NW 11th Place
Gainesville, FL 32605   352-331-2020

Nonprofit organization that understands and treats ocular diseases including glaucoma.

Norman S. Levy, MD, Director

1150 Foundation for Glaucoma Research
200 Pine St, Ste 200
San Francisco, CA 94104   415-986-3162
                                 Fax: 415-986-3763

Clinical and laboratory studies of glaucoma.

Robert N. Shaffer, MD, Chairman

1151 Glaucoma Laser Trabeculoplasty Study
Sinai Hospital of Detroit
29275 Northwestern Highway
Southfield, MI 48034   248-493-5157

Examines the effectiveness and safety of the treatments of glaucoma.

Hugh Beckman, Chairman

Web Sites

1152 CliniWeb
www.ohsu.edu/clini-web/C11/C11.525.html#C11.525.381

1153 Glaucoma Associates
www.glaucoma.net/gany/faq/questions.html

1154 Glaucoma Research Foundation
www.glaucoma.com/

1155 National Association for Visually Handicapped
www.navh.org/

1156 Royal National Institute for the Blind
www.rnib.org.uk/info/eyeimpoi/congen.htm

1157 University of Iowa
htto://mol.ophth.uiowa.edu/MOL_WWW/Glau.html

Books

1158 Childhood Glaucoma - A Reference Guide for Families
N.A.P.V.I.
P.O. Box 317
Watertown, MA 02272
                                 800-562-6265

Pamphlets

1159 Glaucoma
Foundation for Glaucoma Research
200 Pine Street, Suite 200
San Francisco, CA 94104   415-986-3162
                                 Fax: 415-986-3763
                                 www.glaucoma.org

Offers information on what glaucoma is, the causes, treatments, types of glaucoma, eye exams and prevention.

1160 Glaucoma - the Sneak Thief of Sight
National Association for Visually Handicapped
22 West 21st Street, 6th Floor
New York, NY 10010   212-889-3141
                            Fax: 212-727-2931
                            e-mail: staff@navh.org
                            www.navh.org

A pamphlet describing the disease, treatment and medications.

1161 Information on Glaucoma
Foundation for Glaucoma Research
200 Pine Street, Suite 200
San Francisco, CA 94104   415-986-3162
                                 Fax: 415-986-3763
                                 www.glaucoma.org

DESCRIPTION

1162 CONGENITAL RUBELLA

Synonym: Congenital rubella syndrome
Disorder Type: Birth Defect, Infectious Disease
May involve these systems in the body (see Section III):
Prenatal & Postnatal Growth & Development

Congenital rubella refers to a condition in which the virus that causes German measles (rubella) is passed from an affected mother through the placenta to the fetus. Although this viral transmission may take place at any time during the pregnancy, the likelihood of transmission and the potential for miscarriage, stillbirth, or the most severe developmental abnormalities occur during the first three months of pregnancy. Conversely, the later the transmission, the less severe and widespread the abnormalities. Multisystem abnormalities associated with congenital rubella may include generalized growth retardation; heart (cardiac) defects; problems with the eyes such as lens opacities (cataracts) and a severe reduction in the size of the eyes (microphthalmos); an unusually small head (microcephaly); and purplish skin lesions. In addition, many infants with congenital rubella syndrome have inner ear or auditory nerve defects that may result in hearing difficulties.

Additional findings may include mental retardation and delays in motor development. These findings may be the result of inflammation of the brain and its surrounding membranes (meningoencephalitis). Infants with congenital rubella are also at risk for inflammation of the liver (hepatitis); reduced levels of circulating red blood cells (anemia); a decrease in the levels of circulating blood platelets (thromocytopenia); lower respiratory infections (e.g., pneumonia); and bone irregularities.

Prevention of congenital rubella syndrome is directed toward immunization with rubella vaccine during the childhood years. Any unvaccinated women of child-bearing age who have not had German measles should be immunized, but should then wait a minimum of three months before attempting to become pregnant. Also, pregnant women, including those who may have already had German measles or the rubella vaccine, are usually advised to avoid direct exposure to the disease. In addition, newborns with congenital rubella syndrome continue to shed virus for a prolonged period after birth; therefore, pregnant women are cautioned to avoid exposure to these infants. Treatment for congenital rubella syndrome is symptomatic and supportive.

The following organizations in the General Resources Section can provide additional information: Genetic Alliance, March of Dimes Birth Defects Foundation, NIH/National Institute of Allergy and Infectious Disease, NIH/National Institute of Child Health and Human Development, World Health Organization (WHO), National Organization for Rare Disorders, Inc. (NORD)

Web Sites

1163 Canadian Task Force on Preventive Care
www.ctphc.org/Tables.Ch12tab.htm

DESCRIPTION

1164 CONGENITAL SYPHILIS

Disorder Type: Birth Defect, Infectious Disease

Congenital syphilis is a systemic infectious disease, present at birth, caused by the spiral-shaped bacterium (spirochete) Treponema pallidum. This disease is transmitted from mother to fetus through the placenta. Although the fetus is at risk at any time during pregnancy, the risk of transmission depends upon the stage of the mother's disease. The greatest risk of transmission occurs during the early stages of the mother's untreated disease (i.e., primary, secondary, and early latent periods).

Infants born with congenital syphilis may manifest no symptoms at birth but, if left untreated, may soon develop characteristic findings associated with this disease. For example, within the first month or so of life, many affected infants may develop blisters, rashes, and other problems of the skin and mucous membranes. This is followed by shedding (exfoliation) of the skin of the hands and feet. Other findings may include irregular, wart-like growths (condylomatous lesions) on the mucous membranes; yellowing of the skin, eyes, and mucous membranes (jaundice); enlargement of the liver and spleen (hepatosplenomegaly) and other liver abnormalities; and enlarged lymph nodes. Blood tests may reveal irregularities such as anemia resulting from the early or premature destruction of red blood cells (hemolytic anemia) as well as reduced levels of circulating platelets (thrombocytopenia). Inflammation of the specialized connective tissue that covers the bones (periostitis) and painful inflammation of the bones and cartilage (osteochondritis) may also develop. Sometimes these painful conditions result in lack of movement of the affected limb or limbs. Additional abnormalities involving the central nervous system and the kidneys may become apparent with advancing age. Some affected infants develop inflammation of the gastrointestinal tract, pancreas, eyes, and lungs.

Symptoms and findings associated with late-stage congenital syphilis usually develop gradually over the first 20 years of life. These may include the formation of knob-like projections of the bones in the legs and skull as well as other abnormalities associated with changes in the skeleton. For example, involvement of the bones and cartilage in and around the bridge of the nose may cause the nose to appear sunken or depressed (saddle nose). This is sometimes accompanied by a hole or opening in the wall that separates the two nasal cavities (nasal septum). In addition, dental anomalies may include notched, peg-shaped, widely spaced upper incisors (Hutchinson teeth), occasionally accompanied by irregularities in the outermost covering of the teeth (enamel). Other findings may include seizures and changes in behavior and intellect. In addition, some children may develop excessive immune system responses resulting in visual and auditory irregularities that, in some cases, may lead to blindness and loss of hearing.

Prevention of congenital syphilis may be accomplished through penicillin injections administered to the infected mother during pregnancy. However, because the effectiveness of this treatment cannot always be determined, newborns are tested and monitored after birth and, in some cases, given additional penicillin therapy. Other treatment is symptomatic and supportive.

The following organizations in the General Resources Section can provide additional information: Genetic Alliance, March of Dimes Birth Defects Foundation, NIH/National Institute of Child Health and Human Development, World Health Organization (WHO), Centers for Disease Control (CDC)

Web Sites

1165 Cedars-Sinai Medical Center
www.neonatalogy.org

1166 Kid's Health.org
kidshealth.org/parent/common/

1167 Pediatric Behavior and Development
www.dbpeds.org

1168 Vanderbilt University
www.mc.vanderbilt.edu

DESCRIPTION

1169 CONJUNCTIVITIS

Synonym: Pinkeye

Disorder Type: Allergy, Infectious Disease

Covers these related disorders: Infectious conjunctivitis, Noninfectious conjunctivitis

Conjunctivitis refers to a condition characterized by acute inflammation of the delicate mucous membranes that line the inside of the eyelids and the whites of the eyes (sclerae). This condition may be caused by a virus or bacterium. Allergic reactions or exposure to certain chemicals and other environmental factors may also play a role in certain types of conjunctivitis. Neonatal conjunctivitis (also known as neonatal ophthalmia or ophthalmia neonatorum) becomes apparent during the first four weeks of life and is considered an infectious disease resulting from bacterial or viral infections carried by the mother and passed to the child during the birthing process. Bacteria responsible for neonatal conjunctivitis infections may be common disease-causing organisms (pathogens) or may include Chlamydia trachomatis, the bacteria that causes the sexually transmitted disease (STD) chlamydia or Neisseria gonorrhoeae, responsible for the STD gonorrhea. In addition, viral transmission may be caused by herpes simplex type 2 virus, which is responsible for genital herpes. In addition, bacterial contamination may occur in a hospital nursery (Pseudomonas aeruginosa) and may, in some cases, cause severe infection.

The characteristic symptoms associated with infectious neonatal conjunctivitis include redness and severe swelling of the conjunctiva, including the eyelids and whites of the eyes, and a discharge from the eyes that may or may not contain pus (purulent). Symptoms of neonatal infection resulting from transmission during the birthing process may be present at birth or may appear during the second week of life, depending on the bacterium or virus responsible. Any early conjunctival infection should be evaluated as soon as possible to determine its cause and, subsequently, the appropriate course of treatment in order to prevent complications that could potentially lead to impaired vision or blindness.

During the birthing process, silver nitrate, erythromycin, or tetracycline drops or ointment are routinely administered to the eyes of the newborn to prevent gonococcal (gonorrheal) conjunctivitis. Silver nitrate itself, however, may cause a conjunctival inflammation but typically resolves on its own within 48 hours. Other preventive measures are directed toward identification and treatment of pregnant women with gonococcal infection. This combination of preventive therapy has resulted in a dramatic decrease in conjunctivitis and subsequent complications resulting from gonococcal infection.

Treatment for bacteria-caused neonatal conjunctivitis includes the use of particular antibiotics. In addition, washing (irrigating) the eye with a solution containing salt (saline) or direct application of antibiotic ointment to the eyes is often effective in relieving itching and discomfort and clearing up the discharge. Conjunctivitis caused by viral transmission may be treated with antiviral eye drops or ointment. Sometimes the antiviral drug acyclovir may be administered to prevent viral spread.

Additional causes of conjunctivitis in children may include other viruses associated with systemic diseases such as measles, some viruses of the adenovirus family, and intestinal viruses of the enterovirus family. This type of conjunctivitis is usually characterized by a watery discharge from the eyes, is usually self-limited, and treatment is symptomatic. However, one such adenovirus may cause severe itching and burning of the eyes, sensitivity to light (photophobia), and involvement of the cornea. This type of conjunctivitis is known as keratoconjunctivitis and affects the membranes lining the eyelids as well as the corneas. This virus is transmitted by direct contact. Conjunctivitis caused by allergies is usually seasonal and is characterized by swelling, tearing, and itching. Treatment is symptomatic and may include the application of antihistamine eye drops. Certain chemicals or environmental factors may also cause noninfectious, allergic-type conjunctivitis. In addition to silver nitrate used in preventive treatment in newborns, other irritating substances may include cleaning products, different types of sprays, smoke, pollen, and other materials. Treatment is directed toward prevention and relief of symptoms.

In the United States, the occurrence of neonatal conjunctivitis caused by Neisseria gonorrhoeae is extremely rare, while that caused by Chlamydia trachomatis is slightly more than eight out of every 1,000 births.

The following organizations in the General Resources Section can provide additional information: NIH/National Institute of Allergy and Infectious Diseases, NIH/National Eye Institute, World Health Organizations (WHO), Centers for Disease Control (CDC), LSUMC Family Medicine Patient Education: lib-sh.lsumc.edu/fammed/pted/pinkeye.html

Web Sites

1170 American Family Physician
www.aafp.org

1171 Dr. Koop
www.drkoop.com

1172 Harvard
www.immunology.harvard.edu

1173 LSU Medical Center
lib-sh.lsumc.edu

1174 Medicine Net.com
www.medicinenet.com

1175 Virtual Children's Hospital
www.vh.org

DESCRIPTION

1176 CORNELIA DE LANGE SYNDROME

Synonyms: BDLS, Brachmann-de Lange syndrome, CdLS, De Lange syndrome

Cornelia de Lange syndrome is a genetic disorder characterized by growth delays before and after birth (prenatal growth retardation); delays in the acquisition of skills that require the coordination of physical and mental activities (psychomotor retardation), and mild to severe mental retardation. Characteristic physical abnormalities include delays in the maturation of bone; malformations of the head and facial (craniofacial) area that result in a distinctive facial appearance; abnormalities of the arms, legs, hands, and feet (limbs); or other abnormalities. Associated symptoms and findings may vary in range and severity from case to case.

Infants with Cornelia de Lange syndrome often have feeding difficulties (e.g., projectile vomiting, regurgitation, swallowing difficulties); fail to grow and gain weight at the expected rate (failure to thrive); and have a weak, growling cry. Affected infants usually experience breathing problems, such as episodes in which there is temporary cessation of breathing (apnea), inhalation (aspiration) of food into the air passages of the lungs, and increased susceptibility to repeated respiratory infections. Affected infants and children also typically have arched, bushy eyebrows that grow together (synophrys); unusually long, curly eyelashes; a low hair line; and generalized excessive hair growth (hirsutism). Characteristic craniofacial abnormalities may include an abnormally prominent vertical groove in the center of the upper lip (philtrum); thin, downturned lips; and a small jaw (micrognathia). In addition, in many affected children, the teeth may erupt later than expected and are widely spaced.

Many infants and children with Cornelia de Lange syndrome also have malformations of the upper limbs, such as small hands or abnormal positioning of the fifth fingers (clinodactyly) or thumbs. In rare cases, the forearms, hands, and fingers may be absent (phocomelia and oligodactyly). Many affected infants and children also may have abnormally small, short feet with webbing of the second and third toes (syndactyly).

In many cases, additional symptoms and findings are present. For example, in most affected males, the testes may fail to descend into the scrotum (cryptorchidism). Some affected infants may also have digestive abnormalities (e.g., gastroesophageal reflux, pyloric stenosis, bowel obstruction); heart defects (e.g., ventricular septal defects); episodes of uncontrolled electrical activity in the brain (seizures); or other physical abnormalities. In addition, many affected children experience hearing loss and speech delays and may demonstrate behavioral problems, such as self-destructive tendencies.

Treatment of infants and children with Cornelia de Lange syndrome includes symptomatic and supportive measures, such as the prescription of certain medications to help prevent or control seizures (i.e., anticonvulsants); supportive therapies to ensure the proper intake of nutrients and to help prevent or treat respiratory problems; surgical or other appropriate methods to treat heart or digestive defects; etc.

In most cases, Cornelia de Lange syndrome appears to occur randomly for unknown reasons (sporadically). However, in a few reported cases, autosomal dominant inheritance has been suggested. The disorder is thought to affect approximately one in 10,000 newborns.

The following organizations in the General Resources Section can provide additional information: National Organization for Rare Disorders, Inc (NORD), NIH/Office of Rare Diseases, March of Dimes Birth Defects Foundation, Genetic Alliance, Online Mendelian Inheritance in Man: www3.ncbi.nlm.nih.gov/Omim/searchomim.html

National Associations & Support Groups

1177 Cornelia de Lange Syndrome Foundation
302 W Main St #100
Avon, CT 06001   860-676-8166
                                    800-223-8355
                               Fax: 860-676-8337
                        e-mail: cdlsintol@iconn.net
                          www.cdlsoutreach.org

Advocates for people with facial abnormalities
of varying types and degrees, also visual materials to offer knowledge.

Web Sites

1178 Pedbase
www.icondata.com/health/pedbase/files/COR-
NELLA.HTM

DESCRIPTION

1179 CRANIOSYNOSTOSIS

Synonyms: Craniostenosis, Craniostosis

Covers these related disorders: Frontal plagiocephaly, Kleeblattschadel deformity, Scaphocephaly, Trigonocephaly, Turricephaly (oxycephaly or acrocephaly)

Craniosynostosis is a developmental abnormality in which early closure of one or more of the fibrous joints (sutures) between bones of the skull results in deformity of the skull and an abnormally shaped head. The severity of the deformity depends upon which fibrous joint or joints close prematurely as well as the ability of other joints in the skull to expand and compensate for the other closed joint or joints. Craniosynostosis may occur as an isolated condition or in association with certain chromosomal or malformation syndromes. In most instances of isolated craniosynostosis, the condition appears to occur randomly for unknown reasons (sporadically). However, there have been reports of isolated craniosynostosis in members of several multigenerational families (kindreds), indicating autosomal dominant or autosomal recessive inheritance. Many genetic malformation syndromes have been identified in the medical literature that are associated with craniosynostosis. The specific underlying cause of craniosynostosis is not fully understood. Craniosynostosis occurs in approximately one in every 1,000 to 2,000 births and is more prevalent in males than females.

In infants with craniosynostosis, because the skull is unable to enlarge in certain directions relative to the affected fibrous joint in the skull, there is compensatory growth and enlargement in other directions at the sites of open joints. This causes deformity of the skull and an abnormally shaped head. For example, in the most common form of craniosynostosis, there is premature closure of the joint between the upper sides of the skull (sagittal suture), causing the head to appear abnormally long and narrow (scaphocephaly). Affected infants also tend to have a broad forehead and a prominent back portion of the head (occiput). This condition appears to be more common in males than females.

In the form of craniosynostosis known as frontal plagiocephaly, there is early closure of a suture between the upper sides of the head and one of the bones of the forehead (e.g., coronal suture). This results in flattening of one side of the forehead, prominence of the ear, and elevation of the eyebrow and eye on the affected side. Frontal plagiocephaly appears to affect females more commonly than males.

Trigonocephaly, another form of craniosynstosis, is characterized by premature fusion of the suture between the bones forming the forehead (metopic suture). Affected infants have a keel-shaped forehead and closely spaced eyes (hypotelorism). In infants with the form of craniosynostosis known as turricephaly (also called oxycephaly or acrocephaly), premature fusion of coronal and sagittal sutures causes the head to have an abnormally long, narrow, cone-like appearance. In addition, a rare form of craniosynostosis, known as Kleeblattschadel deformity, is characterized by premature closure of multiple cranial sutures, causing the skull to appear cloverleaf-like in shape. Affected infants have a high forehead, marked protrusion of the eyes (proptosis), abnormal prominence of the lower sides of the skull (temporal bones), and other associated abnormalities. Many affected infants also experience hydrocephalus, a condition in which obstruction or impaired absorption of the fluid surrounding the brain and spinal cord (cerebrospinal fluid) causes fluid accumulation under increasing pressure within the brain, resulting in abnormal enlargement of the brain.

In infants with craniosynostosis, premature closure of one suture is rarely associated with increased pressure within the skull or associated neurologic abnormalities, such as mental retardation. In such patients, surgery may be considered for cosmetic purposes. Premature closure of two or more sutures is more likely to cause increased pressure within the skull, potentially resulting in brain damage and associated mental retardation.

Additional findings associated with increased pressure may include vomiting, headaches, and swelling of the area where the optic nerve enters the eye and joints with the nerve-rich membrane at the back of the eye (papilledema). In these infants, surgery is necessary to increase the capacity of the skull in order to prevent excessive pressure within the skull. If craniosynostosis is diagnosed before three months of age, surgery may be conducted to create artificial cranial joints in the skull, allowing skull growth and preventing abnormal shaping of the head.

The following organizations in the General Resources Section can provide additional information: March of Dimes Birth Defects Foundation, Genetic Alliance, NIH/Office of Rare Diseases, National Organization for Rare Disorders, Inc. (NORD)

National Associations & Support Groups

1180 AboutFace USA
1407 N Wells
Chicago, IL 60610

800-665-3223
Fax: 815-444-1943
e-mail: aboutface2000@aol.com
www.aboutface2000.org

Provides information, services, emotional support and educational programs for and on behalf of individuals with facial differences and their families. Working to increase understanding through public awareness and education.

3M members

Rickie Anderson, Executive Director

1181 Children's Craniofacial Association (CCA)
9441 LBJ Freeway, Suite 115
Dallas, TX 75243

214-994-3831
800-535-3643

Devoted to the dispersion of medical knowledge of this and similar disorders, along with providing emotional support for the sufferers and their families.

1182 Craniofacial Family Association
170 Elizabeth Street, Suite 650
Toronto, ON M5G 1X8,

1183 FACES: National Association for the Craniofacially Handicapped
P.O. Box 11082
Chattanooga, TN 37401

423-267-3124
800-332-2373

Disperses information to the public on the medical professionals specializing in this field.

1184 Forward Face
317 East 34th Street, Suite 901
New York, NY 10016

212-684-5860
800-422-3223

Provision of data and emotional assistance to both sufferers and medical professionals.

1185 Guardians of Hydrocephalus Research Foundation
2618 Avenue Z
Brooklyn, NY 11235

718-743-4473
800-458-8655

Provides people with the knowledge regarding the facilities across the nation dedicated to this disorder.

1186 Hydrocephalus Association
870 Market Street, Suite 955
San Francisco, CA 94102

415-776-4713

Supplies both emotional and educational support for the families and friends of children suffering from the disorder.

1187 Hydrocephalus Parent Support Group
225 Dickerson Street, H-893
San Diego, CA 92103

619-695-3139
Fax: 619-726-0507

Determined to provide support to the parent and relatives of the children stricken with the disorder.

1188 Let's Face It
Box 711
Concord, MA 01742

508-371-3186

Devoted to disseminating the information to people suffering from facial abnormalities.

1189 National Craniofacial Foundation
3100 Carlisle Street, Suite 215
Dallas, TX 75204

800-535-1632

1190 National Foundation for Facial Reconstruction
317 East 34th Street
New York, NY 10016   212-340-6656

A nonprofit organization whose major purposes
are to provide facilities for the treatment and assistance of individuals who are unable to afford
private reconstructive surgical care, to train and
educate professionals in this surgery, to encourage research in the field; and to carry on public
education.

1191 National Hydrocephalus Foundation
22427 S River Rd
Joliet, IL 60436   815-467-6548
e-mail: hydrobrat@aol.com

**1192 Society for the Rehabilitation of the Facially
Disfigured, Inc.**
550 First Avenue
New York, NY 10016   212-340-5400

Web Sites

1193 Pediatric Database (PEDBASE)
www.icondata.com/health/pedbase/files/CRA-
NIOSY.HTM

DESCRIPTION

1194 CROHN'S DISEASE

Synonym: Regional enteritis

May involve these systems in the body (see Section III):

Digestive System

Crohn's disease is an inflammatory bowel disease (IBD) characterized by chronic inflammation of any region of the digestive (gastrointestinal) tract from the mouth to the anus. The disease most commonly involves the lower region of the small intestine (ileum) and the major part of the large intestine (colon). Chronic inflammation of these areas causes thickening and scarring of the intestinal wall. The range and severity is extremely variable and depends on the intestinal region affected, the severity of symptoms and findings of inflammation, and associated complications. In children, Crohn's disease usually becomes apparent during the late teens; however, symptoms may begin during early childhood. In developed countries, inflammatory bowel disease, including Crohn's disease, is the most common cause of chronic intestinal inflammation during mid-childhood. Crohn's disease affects males and females in equal numbers and is more common in Jewish individuals. In the U.S., the disease affects approximately 30 to 100 per 100,000 individuals in the general population and occurs more frequently among Caucasians and African-Americans than in Hispanic-Americans and Asian-Americans. Although the exact cause of Crohn's disease is unknown, genetic, immune, and environmental factors are thought to play some role. Some researchers suspect that the disorder may result from an exaggerated immune response to an invading microorganism, such as a particular virus or bacterium.

In most children, Crohn's disease initially involves both the lower region of the small intestine and the major part of the large intestine (ileocolitis). However, initial inflammation may be restricted to the small intestine or the colon. The inflammatory process tends to be segmental in nature, and diseased regions of the intestine are often separated by apparently normal segments (skip lesions). Chronic inflammation causes thickening, ulceration, and scarring of affected areas of the intestinal walls and may lead to the development of abnormal channels (fistulas) between regions of the colon, the intestine and the urinary bladder, or the intestine and the surface of the skin. Additional complications may include the development of pus-filled pockets of infection (abscesses) or intestinal obstruction due to abnormal narrowing of certain intestinal regions.

Many children with Crohn's disease experience episodes of cramping; abdominal discomfort and pain; diarrhea that may contain blood; persistent spasms of the rectum (tenesmus); and a compelling urge to defecate. Additional symptoms and findings typically include fever, chills, easy fatigability, a general feeling of ill health (malaise), lack of appetite (anorexia), weight loss, malnutrition due to impaired intestinal absorption of fats and nutrients (malabsorption) and, in some patients, the development of abnormal channels (fistulas) between segments of the intestine. Many patients also develop abnormal channels (fistulas), pockets of infection (abscesses), or deep grooves or cracks (fissures) in the mucous membranes of the anus. Some children have delayed bone maturation, retarded physical growth, or delayed sexual development as much as one to two years before the onset of other symptoms.

Many patients with Crohn's disease may also develop more generalized, systemic symptoms. These may include joint swelling and inflammation (arthritis); inflammation of the outermost layers of the eye's tough, white, outer coat (episcleritis); eruption of multiple, inflamed, reddish-purplish swellings on the legs and possibly the arms (erythema nodosum); and abnormal concentrations of mineral salts (calcui or stones) in the kidneys or the muscular sac that stores and concentrates bile from the liver (gall bladder). Patients may also be prone to developing ankylosing spondylitis, a chronic, progressive, inflammatory disease that affects joints of the spine and results in pain, stiffness, and possible loss of spinal mobility. In addition, it is suspected that patients who have Crohn's disease for many years may have an increased risk of colon cancer as compared with the general population.

Symptoms typically flare up at irregular intervals throughout life. These episodes may be mild or severe and last for relatively short or prolonged periods. The treatment of Crohn's disease is directed at minimizing symptoms. Therapy may include the use of certain medication, such as prednisone, sulfasalazine, azathioprine, or metronidazole. For example, azathioprine or metronidazole may be helpful in treating anal fistulas, and metronidazole has been beneficial in treating some patients who have not responded to other medications. In many children, treatment may include the administration of nutrients in liquid form (total parenteral nutrition) via a tube through the nose to the stomach (nasogastric tube). Some patients who experience severe, sudden episodes may require hospitalization to ensure proper intake of nutrients and fluids and to receive appropriate medical therapy. In addition, some patients may eventually require surgery to remove diseased portions of the intestine. However, such surgery is reserved for very specific indications, since the recurrence rate is high and the risk of needing additional surgery increases after such a procedure. Additional treatment is symptomatic and supportive.

The following organizations in the General Resources Section can provide additional information: Genetic Alliance, NIH/Office of Rare Diseases, National Organization for Rare Disorders, Inc. (NORD), March of Dimes Birth Defects Foundation

National Associations & Support Groups

1195 Center for Digestive Disorders Central: Dupage Hospital
25 North Winfield Road
Winfield, IL 60190

1196 Crohn's & Colitis Foundation of America
386 Park Avenue South
New York, NY 10016 212-685-3440
800-932-2423
Fax: 212-779-4098

Sources include a helpline for persons with Crohn's Disease.

1197 Crohn's & Collitis Foundation of Canada
21 St. Clair Avenue East, Suite 301
Toronto, On M4T1L9,
Canada 416-920-5035
800-387-1479
Fax: 416-929-0364
e-mail: ccfc@netcom.ca
www.ccfa.ca

1198 Digestive Disease National Coalition
507 Capitol Court, Suite 200
Washington, DC 20002 202-544-7497
Fax: 202-546-7105

Objective is to inform the public about technology improvements through several media forms.

1199 International Foundation for Bowel Dysfunction
P.O. Box 117864
Milwaukee, WI 53217 414-964-1799

1200 Intestinal Disease Foundation
1323 Forbes Avenue Suite 200
Pittsburgh, PA 15219 412-261-5888
Fax: 412-471-2722

Encourages the individuals who have been diagnosed to have a positive outlook through several support groups and reading materials.

Harriet Gibbs, Client Services Manager

1201 Pediatric Crohn's & Colitis Association
P.O. Box 188
Newton, MA 02468 617-489-5854
e-mail: questions@pcca.hypermart.net
www.pcca.hypermart.net

Focuses on all aspects of pediatric and adolescent Crohn's disease and ulcerative colitis, including medical, nutritional, psychological, and social factors. Activities include information sharing, educational forums, newsletters, a hospital outreach program, and support of research.

Crohn's Disease/State Agencies & Support Groups

State Agencies & Support Groups

Alabama

1202 Alabama Chapter of Crohn's & Colitis Foundation of America
244 Goodwin Crest Dr., Suite 120
Birmingham, AL 35209   205-941-9900
Fax: 205-941-1411
e-mail: ccfaal@aol.com
www.ccfa.org

Crohn's and Colitis Foundation of America is a non-profit, voluntary health organization dedicated to improving the quality of life for persons with Crohn's disease or ulcerative colitis.

Arizona

1203 Arizona Chapter of Crohn's & Colitis Foundation of America
1815 W Missouri Ave
Phoenix, AZ   602-947-7233
800-582-7460
Fax: 602-947-0445
e-mail: ccfaal@aol.com
www.ccfa.org

Crohn's and Colitis Foundation of America is a non-profit, voluntayr health organization dedicated to improving the quality of life for persons with Crohn's disease or ulcerative colitis.

California

1204 Greater Bay Area Chapter Crohn's and Colitis Foundation
1730 S. Amphlett Blvd., Suite 230
San Mateo, CA 94402   650-578-6590
800-241-0758
Fax: 650-578-6599
e-mail: cccfagba@pacbell.net
www.ccfa.org

To support basic and clinical scientific research to find the cause of, and cure for Crohn's disease and ulcerative colitis; to provide educational programs for patients, medical professionals and the general public; to offer supportive services for patients, their families and friends including support groups, information packets, education seminars, physician referral hotline and a quarterly newsletter called Rumblings.

Linda Boscono, Development Director

1205 Greater Los Angeles Chapter of Crohn's & Colitis Foundation of America
3731 Wilshire Blvd, #518
Los Angeles, CA 90010   213-380-3800
800-373-3637
Fax: 213-380-6635
e-mail: ccfaal@socalccfa.org
www.ccfa.org

Crohn's and Colitis Foundation of America is a non-profit, voluntary health organization dedicated to improving the quality of life for persons with Crohn's disease or ulcerative colitis.

1206 Long Beach Chapter of Crohn's & Colitis Foundation of America
Long Beach Memorial Medical Center
2801 Atlantic Ave., 5th Fl
Long Beach, CA 90801   310-424-9000
e-mail: ccfaal@aol.com
www.ccfa.org

Crohn's and Colitis Foundation of America is a non-profit, voluntary health organization dedicated to improving the quality of life for persons with Crohn's disease and ulcerative colitis.

1207 Orange County Chapter of Crohn's & Colitis Foundation of America
2030 E Fourth St
Santa Ana, CA 92705   714-547-8500
Fax: 714-547-8585
e-mail: ccfaoc@socalccfa.org
www.ccfa.org

Crohn's and Colitis Foundation of America is a non-profit, voluntary health organization dedicated to improving the quality of life for persons with Crohn's disease or ulcerative colitis.

1208 Sacramento Valley Chapter of Crohn's & Colitis Foundation of America
P.O. Box 19465
Sacramento, CA 95819   530-546-6517
e-mail: vincent@calweb.com
www.ccfa.org

Crohn's and Colitis Foundation of America is a non-profit, voluntary health organization dedicated to improving the quality of life for persons with Crohn's disease or ulcerative colitis.

1209 San Diego Chapter of Crohn's & Colitis Foundation of America
2180 Garnet Ave
San Diego, CA 92109   858-274-8898
Fax: 858-274-8896
e-mail: ccfasd@socalccfa.org
www.ccfa.org

Crohn's and Colitis Foundation of America is a non-profit, voluntary health organization dedicated to improving the quality of life for persons with Crohn's disease or ulcerative colitis.

Colorado

1210 Rocky Mountain Chapter of Crohn's & Colitis Foundation of America
1777 South Bellaire St., Suite 120
Denver, CO 80222 303-639-9163
Fax: 303-693-9166
e-mail: ccfaco.aol.com
www.ccfa.org

Crohn's and Colitis Foundation of America is a non-profit, voluntary health organization dedicated to improving the quality of life for persons with Crohn's disease or ulcerative colitis.

Connecticut

1211 Central Connecticut Chapter of Crohn's & Colitis Foundation of America
Central Connecticut Community Board
P.O. Box 185431
Hamden, CT 06518 203-876-1693
e-mail: ctccfa@aol.com
www.ccfa.org

Crohn's and Colitis Foundation of America is a non-profit, voluntary health organization dedicated to improving the quality of life for persons with Crohn's disease or ulcerative colitis.

1212 Northern Connecticut Chapter of Crohn's & Colitis Foundation of America
P.O. Box 370614
West Hartford, CT 06137 860-677-5150
e-mail: ccfanorthct@aol.com
www.ccfa.org

Crohn's and Colitis Foundation of America is a non-profit, voluntary health organization dedicated to improving the quality of life for persons with Crohn's disease or ulcerative colitis.

Florida

1213 Gold Coast Chapter of Crohn's & Colitis Foundation of America
8177 W Glades Rd, Ste 216
Boca Raton, FL 33434 561-391-2929
800-343-3637
Fax: 561-218-2240
e-mail: goldcoast@ccfa.org
www.ccfa.org

Crohn's and Colitis Foundation of Ameria is non-profit, voluntary health organization dedicated to improving the quality of life for persons with Crohn's disease or ulcerative colitis.

1214 South Florida Chapter of Crohn's & Colitis Foundation of America
1380 N.E. Miami Gardens Drive
Suite 250
North Miami Beach, FL 33179 305-354-2788
Fax: 305-354-7244
e-mail: sfccfa@juno.com
www.ccfa.org

Crohn's and Colitis Foundation of America is a non-profit, voluntary health organization dedicated to improving the quality of life for persons with Crohn's disease or ulcerative colitis.

Georgia

1215 Georgia Chapter of Crohn's & Colitis Foundation of America
2250 N. Druid Hills Rd, Suite 250
Atlanta, GA 30329 404-982-0616
800-472-6795
Fax: 404-982-0656
e-mail: ccfa@mindspring.com
www.ccfa.org

Crohn's and Colitis Foundation of America is a non-profit, voluntary health organization dedicated to improving the quality of life for persons with Crohn's disease or ulcerative colitis.

Illinois

1216 Illinois-Carol Fisher Chapter of Crohn's & Colitis Foundation of America
2250 E Devon Ave, Ste 244
Des Plaines, IL 60018 847-827-0404
Fax: 847-827-6563
e-mail: ccf-16@americatech.net
www.ccfa.org

The Crohn's Colitis Foundation of America is the only non-profit organizaiton dedicated to finding the cause of, and cure for Crohn's disease and ulcerative colitis. The foundation is committed to conquering these devastating diseases.

$25.00 Dues

Kathleen Durkin, Executive Director

Indiana

1217 Indiana Chapter of Crohn's & Colitis Foundation of America
931 East 86th Street #102
Indianapolis, IN 46240 317-259-8071
Fax: 317-259-8091
e-mail: indiana@ccfa.org
www.ccfa.org

Crohn's and Colitis Foundation of America is a non-profit, voluntary health organization dedicated to improving the quality of life for persons with Crohn's disease or ulcerative colitis.

Iowa

1218 Eastern Iowa Chapter of Crohn's & Colitis Foundation of America
3569 Midway Rd
Toddville, IA 52341   319-393-7876
                        e-mail: janetamonk@aol.com
                                www.ccfa.org

Crohn's and Colitis Foundation of America is a non-profit, voluntary health organization dedicated to improving the quality of life for persons with Crohn's disease or ulcerative colitis.

1219 Iowa Chapter of Crohn's & Colitis Foundation of America
P.O. Box 71384
Des Moines, IA 50325   515-252-6179
                                www.ccfa.org

Crohn's and Colitis Foundation of America is a non-profit, voluntary health organization dedicated to improving the quality of life for persons with Crohn's disease or ulcerative colitis.

Kansas

1220 Greater Kansas City Chapter of Crohn's & Colitis Foundation of America
12301 W 106th St
Overland Park, KS 66215   913-307-9320
                                800-945-8722
                        Fax: 913-307-9322
                e-mail: kansascity@ccfa.org
                                www.ccfa.org

Crohn's and Colitis Foundation of America is a non-profit, voluntary health organization dedicated to improving the quality of life for persons with Crohn's disease or ulcerative colitis.

Kentucky

1221 Kentucky Chapter of Crohn's & Colitis Foundation of America
629 S 4th Ave
Louisville, KY 40202   502-582-3891
                        Fax: 502-582-3844
                e-mail: kyccfai@aol.com
                                www.ccfa.org

Crohn's and Colitis Foundation of America is a non-profit, voluntary health organization dedicated to improving the quality of life for persons with Crohn's disease or ulcerative colitis.

Louisiana

1222 Louisiana Chapter of Crohn's & Colitis Foundation of America
4141 Veterans Blvd
Metairie, LA 70002   504-888-1135
                        Fax: 504-888-1132
                e-mail: ccfala@bellsouth.net
                                www.ccfa.org

Crohn's and Colitis Foundation of America is a non-profit, voluntary health organization dedicated to improving the quality of life for persons with Crohn's disease or ulcerative colitis.

Maryland

1223 Maryland Chapter of Crohn's & Colitis Foundation of America
The Village of Cross Keys
332 Center Quadrangle, 2 Hamill Rd
Baltimore, MD 21210   410-435-3300
                                800-618-5583
                        Fax: 410-323-2696
                e-mail: ccfamd@erols.com
                                www.ccfa.org

Our mission is to fund research to find a cure for Crohn's disease and ulcerative colitis and to educate and provide support to patients and families with these diseases.

Edna Ellett, Executive Director

Massachusetts

1224 New England Chapter of Crohn's & Colitis Foundation of America
280 Hillside Avenue
Needham, MA 02494   781-449-0324
                        Fax: 781-449-0325
                e-mail: ne@ccfa.org
                                www.ccfa.org

Crohn's and Colitis Foundation of America is a non-profit, voluntary health organization dedicated to improving the quality of life for persons with Crohn's disease or ulcerative colitis.

Michigan

1225 Grand Rapids Chapter of Crohn's & Colitis Foundation of America
125 Ottawa NW, #350
Grand Rapids, MI 49503   616-774-0805
                        Fax: 616-774-4096
                e-mail: grccfa@iserv.net
                                www.ccfa.org

Crohn's and Colitis Foundation of America is a non-profit, voluntary health organization dedicated to improving the quality of life for persons with Crohn's disease or ulcerative colitis.

1226 Michigan Chapter of Crohn's & Colitis Foundation of America
31313 NW Highway, Ste 209
Farmington Hills, MI 48334   248-737-0900
Fax: 248-737-0904
e-mail: miccfa@aol.com
www.ccfa.org

Crohn's and Colitis Foundation of America is a non-profit, voluntary health organization dedicated to improving the quality of life for persons with Crohn's disease or ulcerative colitis.

Minnesota

1227 Minnesota-Dakotas Chapter of Crohn's & Colitis Foundation of America
1885 University Ave. W., Suite 355
St. Paul, MN 55104   651-917-2424
888-422-3266
Fax: 651-917-2425
e-mail: ccfaminnesota@worldnet.att.net
www.ccfa.org

Voluntary health organization providing education service and support to Crohn's disease and ulcerative colitis patients and the professional community.

Sharon Vangsness, Executive Director

Mississippi

1228 Mississippi Chapter of Crohn's & Colitis Foundation of America
P.O. Box 631
Ridgeland, MS 39158   601-605-1849
e-mail: ccfa@aol.org
www.ccfa.org

Crohn's and Colitis Foundation of America is a non-profit, voluntary health organization dedicated to improving the quality of life for persons with Crohn's disease or ulcerative colitis.

Missouri

1229 St. Louis Chapter of Crohn's & Colitis Foundation of America
8420 Delmar Blvd
St. Louis, MO 63124   314-991-0220
Fax: 314-991-8756
e-mail: missouri@ccfa.org
www.ccfa.org

Crohn's and Colitis Foundation of America is a non-profit, voluntary health organization dedicated to improving the quality of life for persons with Crohn's disease or ulcerative colitis.

New Jersey

1230 Greater New Jersey Chapter of Crohn's & Colitis Foundation of America
241 Forsgate Dr, Ste. #104
Jamesburg, NJ 08831   732-656-1244
e-mail: ccfa@aol.org
www.ccfa.org

Crohn's and Colitis Foundation of America is a non-profit, voluntary health organization dedicated to improving the quality of life for persons with Crohn's disease or ulcerative colitis.

New Mexico

1231 New Mexico Chapter of Crohn's & Colitis Foundation of America

Albuquerque, NM
800-932-2423
e-mail: sskahn@aol.com
www.ccfa.org

Crohn's and Colitis Foundation of America is a non-profit, voluntary health organization dedicated to improving the quality of life for persons with Crohn's disease or ulcerative colitis.

New York

1232 Capital District Chapter of Crohn's & Colitis Foundation of America
4 Normanskill Blvd.
Delmar, NY 12054   518-439-0252
e-mail: ccfacdc@together.net
www.ccfa.org

Crohn's and Colitis Foundation of America is a non-profit, voluntary health organization dedicated to improving the quality of life for persons with Crohn's disease or ulcerative colitis.

1233 Central New York Chapter of Crohn's Colitis Foundation of America
www.ccfa.org   315-463-2219
www.ccfa.org

Crohn's and Colitis Foundation of America is a non-profit, voluntary health organization dedicated to improving the quality of life for persons with Crohn's disease or ulcerative colitis.

1234 Fairfield/Westchester Chapter of Crohn's & Colitis Foundation of America
200 Bloomingdale Rd
White Plains, NY 10605   914-328-2874
e-mail: ccfawestfield.cyburban.com
www.ccfa.org

Crohn's and Colitis Foundation of America is a non-profit, voluntary health organization dedicated to improving the quality of life for persons with Crohn's disease or ulcerative colitis.

1235 Greater New York Chapter of Crohn's & Colitis Foundation of America
386 Park Ave. South, 14th Floor
New York, NY 10016   212-679-1570
Fax: 212-679-3567
e-mail: newyork@ccfa.org
www.ccfa.org

Crohn's and Colitis Foundation of America is a non-profit, voluntary health organization dedicated to improving the quality of life for persons with Crohn's disease or ulcerative colitis.

1236 Long Island Chapter of Crohn's & Colitis Foundation of America
585 Stewart Ave, Ste 414
Garden City, NY 11530   516-222-5530
Fax: 516-222-5535
e-mail: longisland@ccfa.org
www.ccfa.org

Crohn's and Colitis Foundation of America is a non-profit, voluntary health organization dedicated to improving the quality of life for persons with Crohn's disease or ulcerative colitis.

1237 National Headquarters of Crohn' & Colitis Foundation of America
386 Park Ave S
New York, NY 10016

800-932-2423
e-mail: info@ccfa.org
www.ccfa.org

Crohn's and Colitis Foundation of America is a non-profit, voluntary health organization dedicated to improving the quality of life for persons with Crohn's disease or ulcerative colitis.

1238 Rochester Chapter of Crohn's & Colitis Foundation of America
1279 Chili Avenue
Rochester, NY 14624   716-349-4144
e-mail: ccfa@aol.org
www.ccfa.org

Crohn's and Colitis Foundation of America is a non-profit, voluntary health organization dedicated to improving the quality of life for persons with Crohn's disease or ulcerative colitis.

1239 Southern Tier Chapter of Crohn's & Colitis Foundation of America
1159 Vestal Avenue
Binghampton, NY 13903   607-772-0639
www.ccfa.org

Crohn's and Colitis Foundation of America is a non-profit, voluntary health organization dedicated to improving the quality of life for persons with Crohn's disease or ulcerative colitis.

1240 Western New York Chapter of Crohn's & Colitis Foundation of America
P.O. Box 224
Williamsville, NY 14231   716-833-2870
www.ccfa.org

Crohn's and Colitis Foundation of America is a non-profit, voluntary health organization dedicated to improving the quality of life for persons with Crohn's disease or ulcerative colitis.

1241 Western New York Chapter of Crohn's & Colitis Foundation of America
P.O. Box 224
Williamsville, NY 14231   716-833-2870
e-mail: volchapters@ccfa.org
www.ccfa.org

The Crohn's and Colitis Foundation of America sponsors research, educational programs, and support services to those suffering Crohn's disease and ulcerative colitis

North Carolina

1242 North Carolina Chapter of Crohn's & Colitis Foundation of America
6135 Park S
Charlotte, NC 23210   704-945-7171
888-883-2232
Fax: 704-945-7172
e-mail: ccfa@aol.org
www.ccfa.org

Crohn's and Colitis Foundation of America is a non-profit, voluntary health organization dedicated to improving the quality of life for persons with Crohn's disease or ulcerative colitis.

Ohio

1243 Central Ohio Chapter of Crohn's & Colitis Foundation of America
2151 E. Dublin Granville Rd, Ste 218
Columbus, OH 43229   614-781-9970
Fax: 614-781-9972
e-mail: centralohio@ccfa.org
www.ccfa.org

Crohn's and Colitis Foundation of America is a non-profit, voluntary health organization dedicated to improving the quality of life for persons with Crohn's disease or ulcerative colitis.

1244 Greater Cincinnati Chapter of Crohn's & Colitis Foundation of America
2139 Auburn Avenue
Cincinnati, OH 45219   513-585-1775
Fax: 513-585-3071
e-mail: cincinnati@ccfa.org
www.ccfa.org

CCFA is the only national non-profit organization dedicated to finding the cause of and cure for Crohn's disease and ulcerative colitis. We offer support groups as well as educational programs. We also offer a camp for children.

Lisa Raterman, Executive Director

1245 Northeastern Illinois Chapter of Crohn's & Colitis Foundation of America
23366 Commerce Park Road, Suite 203
Beachwood, OH 44122   216-831-2692
Fax: 216-831-2792
e-mail: ccfa@aol.org
www.ccfa.org

Crohn's and Colitis Foundation of America is a non-profit, voluntary health organization dedicated to improving the quality of life for persons with Crohn's disease or ulcerative colitis.

1246 Northeastern Ohio Chapter of Crohn's & Colitis Foundation of America
23366 Commerce Park Rd
Beachwood, OH 44122   213-831-2692
Fax: 213-831-2792
e-mail: ccfaneohio@aol.com
www.ccfa.org

Crohn's and Colitis Foundation of America is a non-profit, voluntary health organization dedicated to improving the quality of life for persons with Crohn's disease or ulcerative colitis.

Oklahoma

1247 Oklahoma Chapter of Crohn's & Colitis Foundation of America
4504 E 67th St, Ste 125
Tulsa, OK 74136   918-523-8540
800-658-1533
Fax: 918-523-8560
e-mail: ccfa@aol.org
www.ccfa.org

Crohn's and Colitis Foundation of America is a non-profit, voluntary health organization dedicated to improving the quality of life for persons with Crohn's disease or ulcerative colitis.

Pennsylvania

1248 Central Pennsylvania Chapter of Crohn's & Colitis Foundation of America
Milton S. Hershey Medical Center, C4808
500 University Drv. P.O. Box 850
Hershey, PA 17033   717-531-8867
800-243-1455
Fax: 717-531-3649
e-mail: ccfa@aol.org
www.ccfa.org

Crohn's and Colitis Foundation of America is a non-profit, voluntary health organization dedicated to improving the quality of life for persons with Crohn's disease and ulcerative colitis.

1249 Philadelphia/Delaware Valley Chapter of Crohn's & Colitis Foundation of America
367 East Street Road
Trevose, PA 19053   215-396-9100
Fax: 215-396-1170
e-mail: ccfaphilly@aol.com
www.ccfa.org

Crohn's and Colitis Foundation of America is a non-profit, voluntary health organization dedicated to improving the quality of life for persons with Crohn's disease or ulcerative colitis.

1250 Western Pennsylvania Chapter of Crohn's & Colitis Foundation of America
580 S Aiken Ave
Pittsburgh, PA 15232   412-687-9775
Fax: 412-687-8544
e-mail: ccfawpa@sgi.net
www.ccfa.org

Crohn's and Colitis Foundation of America is a non-profit, voluntary health organization dedicated to improving the quality of life for persons with Crohn's disease and ulcerative colitis.

1251 Western Pennsylvania Chapter of Crohn's & Colitis Foundation of America
580 S. Aiken Ave, Suite 202
Pittsburgh, PA 15232   412-687-9775
Fax: 412-687-8544
e-mail: ccfawpa@sgi.net
www.ccfa.org

National non-profit research-oriented voluntary health organization dedicated to improving the quality of life for people with Crohn's disease and ulcerative colitis. Our mission: support basic and clinical scientific research to find a cause and cure for Crohn's disease and ulcerative colitis, provide educational programs for patients, medical professioinals, and general public, and offer supportive services for patients, their families and friends.

600+ Members

Joy Jenko, Executive Director
Pat Lehman, Administrative Director

Rhode Island

1252 Rhode Island Chapter of Crohn's & Colitis Foundation of America
P.O. Box 6771
Providence, RI 02940   401-276-5870
e-mail: ccfa@aol.com
www.ccfa.org

Crohn's and Colitis Foundation of America is a non-profit, voluntary health organization dedicated to improving the quality of life for persons with Crohn's disease or ulcerative colitis.

South Carolina

1253 South Carolina Chapter of Crohn's & Colitis Foundation of America
134 McSwain Drive
West Columbia, SC 29169   803-791-3760
e-mail: 250a@aol.com
www.ccfa.org

Crohn's and Colitis Foundation of America is a non-profit, voluntary health organization dedicated to improving the quality of life for persons with Crohn's disease.

Tennessee

1254 East Tennessee Chapter of Crohn's & Colitis Foundation of America
737 Market St
Chattanooga, TN 37402   423-756-7733
Fax: 423-756-7733
e-mail: etnccfa@chatt.net
www.ccfa.org

Crohn's and Colitis Foundation of America is a non-profit, voluntary health organization dedicated to improving the quality of life for persons with Crohn's disease or ulcerative colitis.

1255 West Tennessee Chapter of Crohn's & Colitis Foundation of America
4273 Cherry Center Dr
Memphis, TN 38118   901-365-0101
Fax: 901-365-0113
e-mail: lhduff@hotmail.com
www.ccfa.org

Crohn's and Colitis Foundation of America is a non-profit, voluntary health organization dedicated to improving the quality of life for persons with Crohn's disease or ulcerative colitis.

Texas

1256 Houston-Gulf Coast/South Texas Chapter of Crohn's & Colitis Foundation of America
5102 Woodway
Houston, TX 77056   713-752-2232
800-785-2232
Fax: 713-572-2433
e-mail: ccfa@vl.net
www.ccfa.org

Crohn's and Colitis Foundation of America is a non-profit, voluntary health organization dedicated to improving the quality of life for persons with Crohn's disease or ulcerative colitis.

1257 Illinois/Carol Fisher Chapter of Crohn's & Colitis Foundation of America
2250 E Devon Ave
Des Plaines, IL 60018   847-827-0404
Fax: 847-247-6563
e-mail: ccfail@ameritech.net
www.ccfa.org

Crohn's and Colitis Foundation of America is a non-profit, voluntary health organization dedicated to improving the quality of life for persons with Crohn's disease or ulcerative colitis.

1258 North Texas Chapter of Crohn's & Colitis Foundation of America
2655 Villa Creek Dr, Ste 111
Dallas, TX 75234   972-243-8959
Fax: 972-243-8954
e-mail: ccfa@coserv.net
www.ccfa.org

Crohn's and Colitis Foundation of America is a non-profit, voluntary health organization dedicated to improving the quality of life for persons with Crohn's disease or ulcerative colitis.

Virginia

1259 Greater Washington, D.C. Chapter of Crohn's & Colitis Foundation of America
901 King Street, Ste 101
Alexandria, VA 22314   703-739-2548
e-mail: ccfa@aol.com
www.ccfa.org

Crohn's and Colitis Foundation of America is a non-profit, voluntary health organization dedicated to improving the quality of life for persons with Crohn's disease or ulcerative colitis.

1260 Hampton Roads Chapter of Crohn's & Colitis Foundation of America
624 Clubhouse Rd
Virginia Beach, VA 23452   757-763-7505
e-mail: hrccfa@aol.com
www.ccfa.org

Crohn's and Colitis Foundation of America is a non-profit, voluntary health organization dedicated to improving the quality of life for persons with Crohn's disease or ulcerative colitis.

Washington

1261 Washington State Chapter of Crohn's & Colitis Foundation of America
320 Andover Park E
Seattle, WA 98188   206-574-0698
Fax: 206-574-0869
e-mail: washington@ccfa.org
www.ccfa.org

Crohn's and Colitis Foundation of America is a non-profit, voluntary health organization dedicated to improving the quality of life for persons with Crohn's disease or ulcerative colitis.

Wisconsin

1262 Wisconsin Chapter of Crohn's & Colitis Foundation of America
c/o Sinai Samaritan Medical Center
2401 N Mayfair Rd, Ste 119
Wauwatosa, WI 53226   414-475-5502
877-586-5588
Fax: 414-475-5502
e-mail: wisconsin@ccfa.org
www.ccfa.org

Crohn's and Colitis Foundation of America is a non-profit, voluntary health organization dedicated to improving the quality of life for persons with Crohn's disease or ulcerative colitis.

Research Centers

1263 Crohn's & Colitis Foundation of America, Inc. (CCFA)
National Headquarters
386 Park Avenue South 17th Floor
New York, NY 10016   212-685-3440
800-932-2423
Fax: 212-779-4098
e-mail: info@ccfa.org
www.ccfa.org

Since 1967, CCFA has been the only national voluntary health agency dedicated to funding research to find a cure for Crohn's disease and ulcerative colitis. The Foundation provides educational and patient support services to both the lay and medical communities and plans to provide grants dedicated to pediatric research.

James V. Romano, President & C.E.O.

1264 Krancer Center for Inflammatory Bowel Disease Research
Hahnemann University
Broad & Vine Streets
Philadelphia, PA 19102   215-854-8100
Fax: 215-448-3417

Research into the causes and treatments of ulcerative colitis and Crohn's disease.

Dr. Harris Clearfield, Director

Books

1265 Crohn's Disease and Ulcerative Colitis Fact Book
Crohn's & Colitis Foundation of America
386 Park Avenue South
New York, NY 10016   212-685-3440
800-932-2423
Fax: 212-779-4098

Written in layman's language, this first complete guide is helpful in understanding and coping with inflammatory bowel diseases.

1266 Managing Your Child's Crohn's Disease or Ulcerative Colitis
Crohn's & Colitis Foundation of America, Inc.
386 Park Avenue South, 17th Floor
New York, NY 10016   212-685-3440
800-932-2423
www.ccfa.org

This first full-length book on Crohn's disease and ulcerative colitis specifically targeted for children, teenagers, and their families includes topics on cause and diagnosis, treatment, surgery, hospitalization, diet and nutrition, school and social issues, and resources for the patient.

1267 NEW People...Not Patients: A Source Book for Living with Bowel Disease
Chron's & Colitis Foundation of America, Inc.
386 Park Avenue South, 17th Floor
New York, NY 10016   212-685-3440
800-932-2423
www.ccfa.org

This book contains the essential information you need to help you cope with Chron's disease and ulcerative colitis after you leave the doctor's office.

Newsletters

1268 IBD File
Crohn's & Colitis Foundation of America
386 Park Avenue South
New York, NY 10016

212-685-3440
800-932-2423
Fax: 212-779-4098

Offers updated information and the latest medical news about Crohn's disease and colitis.

Pamphlets

1269 A Guide for Children and Teenagers to Crohn's Disease/Ulcerative Colitis
Crohn's & Colitis Foundation of America
386 Park Avenue South
New York, NY 10016

212-685-3440
800-932-2423
Fax: 212-779-4098

Offers important information on these illnesses to children and teens.

1270 A Teacher's Guide to Crohn's Disease & Ulcerative Colitis
Crohn's & Colitis Foundation of America
386 Park Avenue South
New York, NY 10016

212-665-3440
800-932-2423
Fax: 212-779-4098

1271 ABC's of Pediatric Crohn's Disease
Pediatric Crohn's & Colitis Association
P.O. Box 188
Newton, MA 02468

617-489-5854
e-mail: questions@pcca.hypermart.net
www.pcca.hypermart.net

1272 ABC's of Pediatric Inflammatory Bowel Disease
Pediatric Crohn's & Colitis Association
P.O. Box 188
Newton, MA 02168

617-244-6678

Information pamphlet.

1273 CCFA: A Case for Support
Crohn's & Colitis Foundation of America
386 Park Avenue South
New York, NY 10016

212-685-3440
800-932-2423
Fax: 212-779-4098

Reviews the work of the Crohn's and Colitis Foundation of America, sponsors a nationally recognized research program, which seeks to improve treatment and ultimately find the cure for inflammatory bowel disease.

1274 Coping with Crohn's and Colitis is Tough
Crohn's & Colitis Foundation of America
386 Park Avenue South
New York, NY 10016

212-685-3440
800-932-2423
Fax: 212-779-4098

Offers information on the Crohn's and Colitis Association. Also offers factual information and statistics on the diseases.

1275 Crohn's Disease
NDDIC
2 Information Way
Bethesda, MD 20892

301-654-3810

October 1992

1276 Crohn's Disease, Ulcerative Colitis & Your Child
Crohn's & Colitis Foundation of America
386 Park Avenue South
New York, NY 10016

212-685-3440
800-932-2423
Fax: 212-779-4098

Answers questions about IBD in children, providing information on early signs, growth and developments, treatments and special problems in school.

1277 Crohn's Disease, Ulcerative Colitis and School
Pediatric Crohn's & Colitis Association
P.O. Box 188
Newton, MA 02168

617-244-6678

Information pamphlet.

1278 Questions & Answers About Diet and Nutrition
Crohn's & Colitis Foundation of America
386 Park Avenue South
New York, NY 10016

212-685-3440
800-932-2423
Fax: 212-779-4098

Raises important facts about how diet and nutrition affect persons with Crohn's Disease.

1279 Questions and Answers About Complications
Crohn's & Colitis Foundation of America
386 Park Avenue South
New York, NY 10016   212-685-3440
                                      800-932-2423
                            Fax: 212-779-4098

Medical facts and complications from surgery.

**1280 Questions and Answers About Crohn's Disease &
Ulcerative Colitis**
Crohn's & Colitis Foundation of America
386 Park Avenue South
New York, NY 10016   212-685-3440
                                      800-932-2423
                            Fax: 212-779-4098

Offers information on the illness and answers the most frequently asked questions about Crohn's Disease. Also includes a glossary of IBD terms.

**1281 Questions and Answers About Emotional Factors in
Ileitis and Colitis**
Crohn's & Colitis Foundation of America
386 Park Avenue South
New York, NY 10016   212-685-3440
                                      800-932-2423
                            Fax: 212-779-4098

Answers some of the most commonly asked questions about ileitis and colitis and the role of emotional factors in their cause and course.

**1282 Teacher's Guide to Crohn's Disease and Ulcerative
Colitis**
Crohn's & Colitis Foundation of America
386 Park Avenue South
New York, NY 10016   212-685-3440
                                      800-932-2423
                            Fax: 212-779-4098

The purpose of this brochure is to increase the support and encouragement given to young people with Crohn's disease and ulcerative colitis by teachers who understand their illness.

DESCRIPTION

1283 CRYPTORCHIDISM

Synonyms: Cryptorchidy, Cryptorchism

Covers these related disorders: Ectopic (maldescended) testes, True undescended testes

Cryptorchidism is characterized by failure of one or both testes to descend into the pouch-like structure known as the scrotum. The testes are the paired, oval-shaped glands that produce the male reproductive cells (sperm). Early during male fetal growth, the testes develop within the abdomen near the kidneys. The testes then descend into the scrotum through a tubular canal that passes through lower muscular layers of the abdominal wall (inguinal canal). In males with cryptorchidism, one or both testes fail to complete their descent into the scrotum. Undescended testes that are located along the proper path of descent are known as true undescended testes, whereas those that have completed their descent through the inguinal canal yet have become located in areas other than the scrotum are referred to as ectopic or maldescended testes.

In most cases, one testis is affected (unilateral cryptorchidism); however, both testes may fail to descend (bilateral cryptorchidism) in up to 30 percent of affected male infants. In many cases, undescended testes may move down into the scrotum before one year of age. However, testes that fail to spontaneously descend during the first year of life typically fail to develop properly, may decrease in size, and have decreased numbers of reproductive cells. Without treatment, affected males are at an increased risk of infertility; malignant tumor development in affected testes during the third or fourth decade of life; or pain, swelling, and, in some cases, localized areas of tissue loss (necrosis).

Treatment of cryptorchidism often includes early surgery to relocate undescended testes into the scrotum (i.e., orchiopexy) and to correct inguinal hernias, which typically occur in association with true undescended testes and ectopic testes. Inguinal hernias are characterized by bulging of portions of the intestine into the inguinal canal. Surgical correction of cryptorchidism is typically recommended in the first years of life to help improve proper testicular development and fertility in adulthood.

Cryptorchidism affects about three and a half percent of full-term male newborns and increases in incidence in newborns who are born before 37 weeks of pregnancy (preterm). The condition may occur as an isolated abnormality or, in some cases, due to or in association with a number of different underlying syndromes or conditions.

The following organizations in the General Resources Section can provide additional information: NIH/National Institute of Child Health and Human Development, March of Dimes Birth Defects Foundation, Genetic Alliance, Online Mendelian Inheritance in Man: www3.ncbi.nlm.nih.gov/Omim/searchomim.html, European Society for Paediatric Urology: www.espu.org/

Web Sites

1284 Pediatric Database (PEDBASE)
www.icondata.com/health/pedbase/files/CRYP-TORC.HTM

DESCRIPTION

1285 CUSHING'S SYNDROME

Synonyms: Cushing's basophilism, Hyperadrenocorticism, Pituitary basophilism

Disorder Type: Metabolism

May involve these systems in the body (see Section III):

Endocrine System

Cushing's syndrome refers to a condition characterized by excessive levels of the corticosteroid hormone cortisol in the blood. Cortisol is produced in the outer portion (cortex) of the adrenal glands in response to the secretion of adrenocorticotropic hormone (ACTH; corticotropin). ACTH stimulates the growth of the adrenal cortex and thus the production of cortisol. Cushing's syndrome may be caused by a variety of factors including tumors of the adrenal glands or the pituitary gland, tumors of certain other organs, and excessive intake of corticosteroid drugs. In the very young, Cushing's syndrome occurs in more girls than boys by a ratio of approximately three to one.

Because cortisol assists in the metabolism of fat, protein, and glucose, many characteristic symptoms and findings associated with this disorder are related to the levels and distribution of body fat. For example, children with Cushing's syndrome may be somewhat obese with very full cheeks, a reddish moonface appearance, double chin, and excessive fat deposits on the back of the neck. In addition, the adrenal glands may be stimulated to secrete excessive amounts of other hormones that are converted in the liver to testosterone and estrogen. Overproduction of these androgenic hormones may result in symptoms such as increased amounts of hair on the face and trunk (hypertrichosis), the development of acne, and deepening of the voice as well as other masculine traits. Other findings that may appear over a period of time include elevated blood pressure (hypertension), kidney stones, and increased vulnerability to infection. Children with Cushing's syndrome may also experience growth delays or may not achieve height (short stature). However, those children who develop masculinization symptoms may reach average or above average height. Older children may experience a delay in onset of puberty and develop purplish stretch marks (striae) on the abdomen, breasts, hips, and thighs. In addition, their skin may become thin and fragile, leading to easy bruising. Affected children may develop headaches and weakness, experience increasing difficulty with school work, or become depressed or experience other emotional disturbances.

Treatment of Cushing's syndrome is dependent upon the underlying cause. If the disease results from a benign or malignant tumor or enlargement of the adrenal gland, surgical removal of the tumor or the adrenal gland (adrenalectomy) may be advised. A tumor in the pituitary gland may either be surgically removed or treated with radiation. Subsequent management of surgical or other procedures often includes appropriate hormone replacement therapy. Cushing's syndrome associated with prolonged or excessive intake of corticosteroids may be reversed by a monitored and gradual withdrawal of the medication. Other treatment is symptomatic and supportive.

National Associations & Support Groups

1286 Human Growth Foundation
7777 Leesburg Pike, Suite 202 South
Falls Church, VA 22043   703-883-1773
                                800-451-6434
                                Fax: 703-883-1776
                        e-mail: hgfound@erols.com
                        www.genetic.org/hgf/index.shtml

The Human Growth Foundation is dedicated to helping medical science better understand the process of growth.

1287 National Cushing Syndrome Association
4645 Van Nuys Blvd, Ste 104
Sherman Oaks, CA 91403   818-788-9239

Web Sites

1288 CliniWeb
www.ohsu.edu/cliniweb/C14/C14.907.934

1289 Cushing's Support and Research Foundation
http://world.std.com/~csrf/

1290 Support-Group.com
www.support-group.com/cgi-
bin/sg/get_links?cushings

DESCRIPTION

1291 CYSTIC FIBROSIS

Synonyms: CF, Mucoviscidosis

Disorder Type: Genetic Disorder

May involve these systems in the body (see Section III):

Digestive System, Respiratory System

Cystic fibrosis (CF) is an inherited multisystem disorder that affects several glands of the body (i.e., exocrine glands that release secretions into ducts). Glands of the respiratory and reproductive systems as well as pancreatic glands and sweat glands are affected. CF is considered one of the most common autosomal recessive disorders affecting Caucasians. Cystic fibrosis occurs in approximately one in 2,500 to 3,000 Caucasian infants and about one in 17,000 African-American infants. It is considered extremely rare in other populations. The disorder results from abnormal changes (mutations) of a gene on the long arm (q) of chromosome 7 (7q31.2). More than 400 different mutations of the CF gene have been identified.

In infants, children, and adults with cystic fibrosis, mucus-secreting glands within the air passages of the lungs (bronchi) produce unusually thick secretions, clogging and obstructing the airways and promoting the growth of certain bacteria. As a result, affected individuals may experience chronic obstruction and infection of the airways. In addition, the pancreas lacks sufficient digestive enzymes to break down food materials (malabsorption). Other exocrine gland abnormalities may also be present. For example, the sweat glands produce secretions containing abnormally high levels of salt; glands of the neck of the uterus (cervix) in affected females may produce abnormally increased, thickened secretions of mucus; and certain ducts of the male reproductive system (e.g., epididymis, ductus [vas] deferens, seminal vesicles) may be absent (atretic).

During the first or second day of life, some newborns with cystic fibrosis may experience bloating of the abdomen (abdominal distension), vomiting (emesis), and abnormal blockage of the lower region of the small intestine with meconium (meconium ileus). Meconium is the thick, sticky, darkish green material that accumulates in the fetal intestines and forms a newborn's first stools. Infants with cystic fibrosis also usually fail to grow and gain weight at the expected rate (failure to thrive). Additional symptoms and findings may include abnormally decreased muscle mass; a protruding abdomen; and loose, foul-smelling stools that contain an excessive amount of fat (steatorrhea). Children with cystic fibrosis often have respiratory abnormalities including wheezing; a chronic cough that may be accompanied by gagging and vomiting; recurrent inflammation of the air passages (bronchiolitis); and an increased susceptibility to lower respiratory infections (e.g., pneumonia). Affected adolescents may experience abnormally slow growth and delayed sexual development (i.e., average delay of two years); in addition, affected males may be infertile due to lack of sperm development (azoospermia). As the disease progresses, individuals with cystic fibrosis tend to experience increasingly severe respiratory abnormalities that may result in life-threatening complications.

Cystic fibrosis may be diagnosed based upon characteristic physical findings (e.g., chronic obstructive pulmonary disease, exocrine pancreatic insufficiency), specialized laboratory tests (e.g., sweat testing), and a positive family history (including DNA analysis). The treatment of cystic fibrosis is symptomatic and supportive and includes early intervention, ongoing monitoring, preventive measures, the use of certain medications, and other specialized treatment techniques. Approaches to treatment may include physical therapy, a high protein, high calorie diet, pancreatic enzyme replacement therapy, vitamin supplementation, specialized respiratory therapy, medications to help clean mucus from the airways and prevent or treat respiratory infections (e.g., antibiotic therapy).

The following organizations in the General Resources Section can provide additional information: National Organization for Rare Disorders, Inc (NORD), NIH/Office of Rare Diseases, Genetic Alliance, March of Dimes Birth Defects Foundation, Online Mendelian Inheritance in Man: www3.ncbi.nlm.nih.gov/Omim/searchomim.html, NIH/National Digestive Diseases Information Clearinghouse

National Associations & Support Groups

1292 American Lung Association
1740 Broadway
New York, NY 10019   212-315-8700
e-mail: info@lungusa.org
www.lungusa.com

1293 Cystic Fibrosis Alliance
3443 NW 55th Street, Building 7
Ft. Lauderdale, FL 33309   954-739-5006
800-344-4823
Fax: 954-739-2890
e-mail: florida@cfs.org
www.cfs.org

Cystic Fibrosis Alliance is an all volunteer, non-profit organization, comprised of a group of people with CF, their family members, their friends, and health care providers. The alliance provides resources and referrals to those with CF and provide a liasion between people with CF and their case managers, medical directors and elected officals.

1294 Cystic Fibrosis Foundation
6931 Arlington Road, Ste. 200
Bethesda, MD 20814   301-951-4422
800-344-4823
Fax: 301-951-6378
e-mail: info.cff.org
www.cff.org

Established in 1955 to raise money to fund research to find a cure for cystic fibrosis and to improve the quality of life for the 30,000 children and young adults with the disease. Finances over 111 care centers nationwide and supports 70 chapters and affiliates.

Robert J. Beall, Ph.D., President

1295 Cystic Fibrosis Research, Inc
560 San Antonio Road, Suite 103
Palo Alto, CA 94306   650-856-0546
Fax: 650-856-0554
e-mail: cfri@cfri.org

Cystic Fibrosis Research Inc.'s mission is to alleviate the emotional and physical suffering associated with cystic fibrosis, to offer educational and support programs for people with CF and their families.

1296 International Association of Cystic Fibrosis Adults
82 Ayer Road
Harvard, MA 01451   978-456-8387
Fax: 978-456-8387
e-mail: palys@tiac.net
www.ourworld.compuserve.com

International

1297 Cystic Fibrosis Trust
Alexandria House, 5 Blyth Road
Bromley,
United Kingdom

Primary function is to provide citizens of the United Kingdom with the knowledge and support facilities throughout the country.

State Agencies & Support Groups

1298 Arkansas Cystic Fibrosis Center
Arkansas Children's Hospital
800 Marshall Street
Little Rock, AR 72202   501-320-1018

Robert H. Warren, M.D.

1299 Florida Cystic Fibrosis
4711 N.E. 29th Avenue
Ft. Lauderdale, FL 33308   954-772-1624

Florida Cystic Fibrosis, Inc. is a non-profit organization that began in 1982 to raise funds for patient care, treatment and research in Florida. Wih no administrative costs, all donations go to CF.

Carolyn Shumway, State President

1300 Tucson Cystic Fibrosis Center
Arizona Health Sciences Center
1501 N. Campbell, Rm. 2340
Tucson, AZ 85724   520-626-6121

Wayne J. Morgan, MD

1301 University of South Alabama Cystic Fibrosis Center
USA Children's Medical Center
P.O. Box 40130
Mobile, AL 36640   334-343-6848

Lawrence J. Sindel, MD

Libraries & Resource Centers

Alabama

1302 UAB Cystic Fibrosis Center/Children's Hospital
1600 7th Street South
Birmingham, AL 35233   205-934-6149

Dr. Raymond Lyrene, M.D.

Arizona

1303 Cystic Fibrosis Center - Phoenix Children's Hospital
909 E. Brill Street
Phoenix, AZ 85006   602-239-6925

Peggy Radford, MD, Director

California

1304 Brian Wesley Ray Cystic Fibrosis Center
San Bernadino County Medical Center
780 E. Gilbert Street
San Bernadino, CA 92415   909-387-8111

Gerald Greene, MD

1305 Children's Hospital - Pediatric Pulmonary Center
747 52nd Street
Oakland, CA 94609   510-428-3448

Nancy C. Lewis, M.D.

1306 Children's Hospital of Los Angeles
4650 Sunset Blvd, Stop 83
Los Angeles, CA 90027   213-660-2450

C. Michael Bowman, M.D., Ph.D., Director

1307 Cystic Fibrosis Center
Cedars-Sinai Medical Center
8700 Beverly Blvd.
Los Angeles, CA 90048   310-855-3851
                      Fax: 310-657-1778

C. Michael Bowman, Co-Director
Bowman John, Peters

1308 Cystic Fibrosis Center, University of California at San Francisco
505 Parnassus Ave, Rm M650
San Francisco, CA 94143   415-476-2072

Gert J.A. Cropp, MD, PhD, Director

1309 Cystic Fibrosis and Pediatric Pulmonary Center
Children's Hospital of Orange County
455 S. Main Street
Orange, CA 92668   714-997-3000
                    Fax: 714-289-4672

David Hicks, M.D., Director

1310 Cystic Fibrosis and Pediatric Respiratory Diseases Center
University of California at Davis
2516 Stockton Blvd.
Sacramento, CA 95817   916-734-3691

Ruth McDonald, MD

1311 Miller Children's Hospital Pediatric Pulmonary/Cystic Fibrosis Cent
Memorial Miller Children's Hospital
2801 Atlantic Avenue
Long Beach, CA 90801   562-933-2000
                    Fax: 562-933-8569
      e-mail: enussbaum@memorialcare.org

Offers specialized services for complex pediatric patients, including home ventilator supported patients, tracheostomy care, complex asthma, cystic fibrosis, sleep disorders, bronchopulmonary dysplasia, and a garden variety of pediatric respiratory disorders.

Eliezer Nussbaum, MD, Medical Director

1312 San Diego Cystic Fibrosis and Pediatric Pulmonary Disease Center
University Hospital
200 W Arbor, Mail Code 8448
San Diego, CA 92103   619-294-6125

Michael Light, MD, Director

1313 Stanford CF Center
Packard Children's Hospital at Stanford
725 Welch Road
Palo Alto, CA 94304   650-497-8000

Richard Moss, M.D., Director

Colorado

1314 Denver Children's Hospital
1056 East 19th Avenue
Denver, CO 80218   303-837-2522

Frank Accurso, M.D., Director

Connecticut

1315 University of Connecticut Health Center
263 Farmington Ave, Code 1827
Farmington, CT 06030   860-679-2100

Michelle Cloutier, M.D., Director

1316 Yale University Cystic Fibrosis Research Center
School of Medicine
333 Cedar Street, Fitkin 511
New Haven, CT 06520   203-785-2480

Regina Palazzo, MD, Director

District of Columbia

1317 Metropolitan D.C. Cystic Fibrosis Center
Children's Hospital National Medical Center
111 Michigan Avenue NW
Washington, DC 20010   202-884-2070

Robert J. Fink, MD, Director

Florida

1318 CF & Pediatric Pulmonary Disease Center
University of Florida
P.O. Box 100296
Gainesville, FL 32610   352-392-4061

Mary H. Wagner, M.D., Director

1319 Cystic Fibrosis Center Orlando Regional Medical Center

Orlando, FL   407-237-6327

Joseph J. Chiaro, MD, Director

1320 Cystic Fibrosis Center - All Children's Hospital
880 Sixth Street, South, Ste. 390
St. Petersburg, FL 33731   813-892-4146

Michelle Howenstine, MD, Director

1321 Miami Children's Hospital, Division of Pulmonology
MOB #203, 3200 SW 60th Ct.
Miami, FL 33155   305-666-6511

Moises Simpser, MD

1322 Nemours Children's Clinic-Jacksonville
P.O. Box 5720
Jacksonville, FL 32247   904-390-3600
          800-767-5437
          Fax: 904-390-3498
          www.kidshealth.org

The clinic is an ambulatory care center that provides health care services for children with complex medical or surgical problems.

Erik Kaldor, Public Relations Director

Georgia

1323 Emory University Cystic Fibrosis Center
2040 Ridgewood Drive NE
Atlanta, GA 30322   404-727-3360

Daniel B. Caplan, MD, Director

Idaho

1324 Blank Children's Hospital Cystic Fibrosis Center
1200 Pleasant Street
Des Moines, IA 50309   515-241-5437

Veljko Zivkovich, MD

1325 University of Iowa Hospitals & Clinics
Pediatric Allergy & Pulmonary Division
200 Hawkins Avenue
Iowa City, IA 52242   319-356-1853

Miles Weinberger, M.D., Director

Illinois

1326 Cystic Fibrosis Center Lutheran General Hospital
1775 Dempster Street
Park Ridge, IL 60068   847-923-8409
e-mail: youngran.chung@advocatehealth.com

Youngran Chung, MD, Acting Director

1327 Cystic Fibrosis Center/Children's Memorial Hospital
Northwestern University
2300 Children's Plaza, Box 43
Chicago, IL 60614   773-880-4382

Susanna McColley, MD, Director

1328 Loyola University Medical Center/ Department of Pediatrics
2160 W. First Avenue
Maywood, IL 60153   708-327-9102

Harold Conrad, MD, Director

1329 Saint Francis Medical Center Specialty Clinics, CF Center
Hillcrest Medical Plaza
530 NE Glen Oak Ave, 2nd Fl
Peoria, IL 61637   309-655-3889

Umesh Chatrath, MD, Director

1330 University of Chicago Children's Hospital, Department of Pediatrics
University of Chicago Hospitals and Clinics
5841 S. Maryland Avenue
Chicago, IL 60637   773-702-1000
                          Fax: 773-702-4753
                          www.ucch.org

Provides comprehensive, innovative medical care to children of all social and economic backgrounds. Dedicated to enhancing the health and wellness through patient care, education, and research into the causes and cure of childhood diseases. Immediate access to the full resources of The University of Chicago Hospitals and to faculty of the division of Biological sciences. The hospital sees children from the Chicago area, the Midwest, and around the world who have the most complex medical problems

Joel Schwab, MD, Director Hospitalist Program

Indiana

1331 Cystic Fibrosis and Chronic Pulmonary Disease Clinic
St. Joseph's Medical Center
801 E. LaSalle, P.O. Box 1935
South Bend, IN 46634   219-232-2121
                              800-206-0879

Edward Gergesha, MD

1332 Indiana University Cystic Fibrosis Center
702 Barnhill Drive, Rm. 293
Indianapolis, IN 46202   317-274-8485

Howard Eigen, MD, Director

Kansas

1333 Kansas University Medical Center, Cystic Fibrosis Center
3901 Rainbow Blvd.
Kansas City, KS 66160   913-588-2537

Joseph Kanarek, MD, Director

1334 St. Joseph Medical Center Cystic Fibrosis Care and Teaching Center
3600 E. Harry Street
Wichita, KS 67218   316-685-1111

Leonard Sullivan, M.D., Director

Kentucky

1335 Cystic Fibrosis Center, Kentucky University
760 S. Limestone
Lexington, KY 40536   606-323-8023

Jamshed F. Kanga, MD, Director

1336 Kosair Children's CF Center
233 E. Gray Street, Ste. 201
Louisville, KY 40202   502-629-8830

Nemr Eid, M.D.

Louisiana

1337 Cystic Fibrosis & Pediatric Pulmonary Center
Louisiana State University Medical Center
1501 Kings Hwy, PO Box 33932
Shreveport, LA 71130   318-675-5681

Bettina Hillman, MD, Director

1338 Tulane University Cystic Fibrosis Center
Department of Pediatrics
1430 Tulane Avenue, SL-37
New Orleans, LA 70112   504-587-7625

Scott Davis, M.D., Director

Maine

1339 Central Maine Cystic Fibrosis Center
300 Maine Street
Lewiston, ME 04240   207-795-0111

Ralph V. Harder, MD, Director

1340 Eastern Maine Medical Center, Cystic Fibrosis Clinical Center
489 State Street
Bangor, ME 04401   207-973-7000

Thomas Lever, MD, Director

1341 Maine Medical Center, Cystic Fibrosis Center
22 Bramhall Street
Portland, ME 04102   207-871-0111

Nicholas Fowler, MD, Director

Massachusetts

1342 Children's Hospital, Cystic Fibrosis Center
300 Longwood Avenue
Boston, MA 02115   617-355-6000

Mary Ellen Wohl, MD

Michigan

1343 Cystic Fibrosis Care, Teaching & Resource Center
Children's Hospital of Michigan
3901 Beaubien Blvd.
Detroit, MI 48201   313-745-5437

Debbie Toder, MD, Director

1344 Cystic Fibrosis Center/Pediatric Pulmonary and Sleep Medicine
330 Barclay Avenue NE Suite 200
Grand Rapids, MI 49503   616-391-2125
                                Fax: 616-391-2131

John Schuen, MD, Director
Susan Millard, MD, Director

1345 East Lansing Cystic Fibrosis Center
Michigan State University
401 W. Greenlawn Avenue
Lansing, MI 48910   517-482-4443

Richard Honicky, MD

1346 Kalamazoo Center for Medical Studies
Michigan State University
1000 Oakland Drive
Kalamazoo, MI 49008   616-337-6430

Douglas Homnick, MD, Director

1347 University of Michigan, Cystic Fibrosis Center
1500 E. Medical Center Drive
Ann Arbor, MI 48109   734-936-3236

Samya Nasrimo, Director

Minnesota

1348 University of Minnesota Cystic Fibrosis Center
University of Minnesota Hospital
420 Delaware Street SE
Minneapolis, MN 55455   612-626-5147

Dr. Warren J. Warwick, Director

Mississippi

1349 University of Mississippi Medical Center
2500 N. State Street
Jackson, MS 39216   601-984-5046

Suzanne Miller, MD, Director

Missouri

1350 Children's Mercy Hospital, University of Missouri
Kansas City School of Medicine
24th & Gillham Road
Kansas City, MO 64108   816-231-8895

Michael McCubbin, M.D., Director

1351 Cystic Fibrosis, Pediatric Pulmonary and Pediatric Gastrointestinal Center
Cardinal Glennon Memorial Hospital for Children
1465 S. Grand
St. Louis, MO 63104   314-577-5600

Anthony J. Rejent, MD, Center Director

1352 University of Missouri-Columbia Cystic Fibrosis Center
University of Missouri/Dept. of Child Health
One Hospital Drive
Columbia, MO 65212   573-882-6978

Peter Konig, MD, Director

1353 Washington University Cystic Fibrosis Center
St. Louis Children's Hospital
One Children's Place
St. Louis, MO 63110   314-721-0072

George B. Mallory, M.D., Director

Nebraska

1354 University of Nebraska at Omaha Pediatric Pulmonary/Cystic Fibrosis Center
985190 Nebraska Medical Center
Omaha, NE 68198   402-559-6275
Fax: 402-559-7062

A regional referral site for diagnosis and treatment of infants and children with respiratory disorders. State of the art diagnostic testing and treatment available for all pulmonary diseases and cystic fibrosis.

John L. Colombo, MD, Director

Nevada

1355 Children's Lung Specialists
3838 Meadows Lane
Las Vegas, NV 89107   702-598-4411
Fax: 702-598-1988

Ruben Diaz, MD, Director

New Hampshire

1356 Cystic Fibrosis Care and Teaching Center
Dartmouth Hitchcock Medical Center
1 Medical Center Drive
Lebanon, NH 03756   603-650-5000

William Boyle, Jr., M.D., Director

New Jersey

1357 Monmouth Medical Center, Cystic Fibrosis & Pediatric Pulmonary Center
300 Second Avenue
Long Branch, NJ 07740   732-222-5200

Robert Zanni, MD, Director

1358 New Jersey Medical School Department of Pediatrics
185 S Orange Ave, Rm MSB-F534
Newark, NJ 07103   973-972-4815
888-295-3836
Fax: 973-972-1574
e-mail: turcion1@umdnj.edu

Nelson L. Turcios, MD, Director, Pediatric Pulmonology

New York

1359 Albany Medical College Pediatric Pulmonary & Cystic Fibrosis Center
Department of Pediatrics
47 New Scotland Avenue
Albany, NY 12208   518-262-6880

Robert Kaslovsky, MD, Director

1360 Armond U. Mascia CF Center
NY Medical College
Munger Pavillion, Room 106
Valhalla, NY 10595   914-285-7583

Allen Dozer, M.D., Director

1361 CF & Pediatric Pulmonary Care Center
Mt. Sinai School of Medicine
Fifth Avenue At 100th Street
New York, NY 10029   212-241-7788

Richard J. Bonforte, M.D., Director

1362 CF, Pediatric Pulmonary & GI Center
St. Vincent's Hospital & Medical Center of NY
36 Seventh Avenue, Ste. 509
New York, NY 10011   212-604-8895

Joan DeGelie-Germana, MD, Director

1363 Children's Lung and Cystic Fibrosis Center
Children's Hospital of Buffalo
219 Bryant Street
Buffalo, NY 14222   716-878-7435

Drucy Borowitz, MD, Director

1364 Pediatric Pulmonary Center
Babies Hospital & Columbia Presbyterian
630 West 168th Street
New York, NY 10032   212-305-5122

Lynne M. Quittell, M.D., Director

1365 Schneider Children's Hospital of Long Island
Albert Einstein College of Medicine

New Hyde Park, NY 14040   716-470-3250

Jack D. Gorvoy, MD

North Carolina

1366 UNC CF Center
Department of Pediatrics
509 Burnett-Womack Bldg.
Chapel Hill, NC 27599   919-966-1055

Gerald W. Fernald, M.D., Director

North Dakota

1367 St. Alexius Medical Center/CF Center
311 North 9th Street
Bismarck, ND 58502   701-224-7500

Allan Stillerman, MD, Director

Ohio

1368 Case Western Reserve University Cystic Fibrosis Center
2101 Adelbert Road
Cleveland, OH 44106   216-368-3200

Pamela B. Davis, MD, Director

1369 Columbus Children's Hospital, Cystic Fibrosis Center
700 Children's Drive
Columbus, OH 43205   614-722-6800

Karen S. McCoy, MD, Director

1370 Lewis H. Walker, M.D., CF Center
Children's Hospital Medical Center of Akron
One Perkins Square
Akron, OH 44308   330-379-8200

Robert T. Stone, M.D., Director

1371 Pediatric Pulmonary Center
Children's Medical Center
One Children's Plaza
Dayton, OH 45404   937-226-8300
                          800-228-4055
                     Fax: 937-463-5390

Treats children (birth to 18 years) with cystic fibrosis, reactive airway disease, bronchopulmonary dysplasia, sleep disorders and other chronic lung diseases of childhood. Our physicians are board certified in pediatrics, pediatric pulmonology, internal medicine and sleep medicine.

Dennis Nielson, MD, PhD, Director

1372 University of Cincinnati College of Medicine/Division of Pediatrics
Children's Hospital Medical Center
3333 Burnet Avenue
Cincinnati, OH 45229   513-559-4355

Robert Wilmott, M.D., Director

Oklahoma

1373 University of Oklahoma Cystic Fibrosis Center
940 NW 13th Street
Oklahoma City, OK 73104   405-271-4401

John E. Grunow, M.D., Director

Pennsylvania

1374 CF Center/University of Pennsylvania Medical Center
36th and Spruce Streets
Philadelphia, PA 19104   215-590-3749

James M. Wilson, MD, Director

1375 Cystic Fibrosis Center at Polyclinic Medical Center
Polyclinic Medical Center
2601 N. 3rd Street
Harrisburg, PA 17110   717-782-4101

Muttiah Ganeshananthan, MD, Director

1376 Pediatric Pulmonary and Cystic Fibrosis Center
St. Christopher's Hospital for Children
Erie Avenue at Front Street
Philadelphia, PA 19134   215-427-5000

Daniel Schidlow, M.D., Director

1377 University of Pittsburgh Cystic Fibrosis Center/Children's Hospital
3705 5th Ave at DeSoto St
Pittsburgh, PA 15213   412-648-9670

Raymond A. Frizzell, MD, Director

Rhode Island

1378 Rhode Island Hospital, Cystic Fibrosis Center
CDC-APC
593 Eddy Street, 6th Floor
Providence, RI 02903   401-444-5685

Mary Ann Passero, MD, Director

South Carolina

1379 CF Center/Medical University of South Carolina
171 Ashley Avenue
Charleston, SC 29425   843-792-3561

Robert Baker, M.D., Director

South Dakota

1380 Sioux Valley Hospital, South Dakota Cystic Fibrosis Center
1100 S. Euclid Ave., P.O. Box 5039
Sioux Falls, SD 57117   605-333-1000

Rodney Parry, MD, Director

Tennessee

1381 Memphis Cystic Fibrosis Center
LeBonheur Children's Medical Center
50 N. Dunlap
Memphis, TN 38103   901-572-5222

Robert Schoumacher, M.D., Director

Texas

1382 CF Center, Pulmonary Section
Baylor College of Medicine/Dept. Of Pediatrics
One Baylor Plaza
Houston, TX 77030   713-798-4945

Peter W. Hiatt, MD, Director

1383 Cook-Ft. Worth Medical Center, CF Center
801 7th Avenue
Ft. Worth, TX 76104   254-885-4202

James C. Cunningham, M.D., Director

1384 Cystic Fibrosis Care, Teaching and Research Center
Children's Medical Center
1935 Motor Street, Rm. 316
Dallas, TX 75235   214-640-2000

Claude Prestidge, MD, Director

1385 Cystic Fibrosis-Lung Disease Center Santa Rosa Children's Hospital
519 West Houston Street
San Antonio, TX 78207   210-228-2058

1386 Tri-Services Military CF Center
Brooke Army Medical Center
HSHE-dP (LTC Inscore)
Fort Sam Houston, TX 78234   210-916-3400

Dr. Stephen Inscore, L.T.C., M.C., Director

Utah

1387 University of Utah Intermountain Cystic Fibrosis Center
50 N. Medical Drive
Salt Lake City, UT 84132   801-588-2715
Fax: 801-588-2640
www.med.utah.edu/palm/cf.htm

Multi-disciplinary care center for pediatric and adult patients with Cystic Fibrosis (CF). It is accredited by the North American Cystic Fibrosis Center. Provides care to more than 300 individuals with CF.

Barbara Chatfield, Pediatric Center Director
Bruce Marshall, Adult Center Director

Vermont

1388 Medical Center Hospital of Vermont
Cystic Fibrosis Center
111 Colchester Ave
Burlington, VT 05401   802-862-5529
Fax: 802-847-8742

Donald Swartz, MD, Director

Virginia

1389 CF Center/University of Virginia School of Medicine

Charlottesville, VA 22908   804-924-2250

Robert F. Selden, M.D., Director

1390 Cystic Fibrosis Program of the Medical College of Virginia
P.O. Box 980271
Richmond, VA 23298   804-786-9445

David Draper, MD, Director

1391 Eastern Virginia Medical Center
Children's Hospital of The King's Daughters
601 Children's Lane
Norfolk, VA 23507   757-668-7000

Thomas Rubio, MD, Director

Washington

1392 University of Washington CF Center
4800 Sand Pointway NE, PO Box C5371
Seattle, WA 98105   206-526-2024

Bonnie W. Ramsey, M.D., Director

West Virginia

1393 West Virginia University Mountain State Cystic Fibrosis Center
P.O. Box 9214
Morgantown, WV 26506   304-293-1217
800-982-8242
Fax: 304-293-1216
e-mail: kmoffett@hsc.wvu.edu

Cathryn S. Moffett, M.D., Director

Wisconsin

1394 Medical College of Wisconsin Cystic Fibrosis Center
Children's Hospital of Wisconsin, MS #777A
9000 W. Wisconsin Avenue
Milwaukee, WI 53201   414-266-6730

Mark Splaingard, MD, Director

1395 University of Wisconsin-Madison Cystic Fibrosis/Pulmonary Center
Clinical Science Center H4/430
600 Highland Avenue
Madison, WI 53792   608-263-8555

Michael J. Rock, M.D., Director

Audio Video

1396 Don't Cry for Me
Fanlight Productions
47 Halifax St
Boston, MA 02130   617-469-4999
                                    Fax: 617-469-3379
                                    e-mail: fanlight@tiac.net
                                    www.fanlight.com

Profiles five exceptional young people living with cystic fibrosis. This film is not about death, but about living with the intensity created by the knowledge of a shortened life expectancy.

54 minutes
ISBN: 1-572950-95-1

1397 Embers of the Fire
Mary Kondrat, author

Fanlight Productions
47 Halifax St
Boston, MA 02130   617-469-4999
                                    Fax: 617-469-3379
                                    e-mail: fanlight@tiac.net
                                    www.fanlight.com

Offers a straight-forward explanation of the disease with a primary focus on the stories of several courageous young people with cystic fibrosis during a week at summer camp. Addresses their fears of rejection, isolation, and death while demonstrating the ways they have learned to lead fulfilling lives.

28 minutes
ISBN: 1-572950-98-6

Web Sites

1398 CF Index of Online Resources
vmsb.csd.mu.edu/~541lukasr/cystic.html

1399 CF Web
cf-web.mit.edu

Books

1400 Cystic Fibrosis

Virginia Alvin & Robert Silverstein, author

Franklin Watts c/o Grolier
90 Old Sherman Tpke
Danbury, CT 06816   203-797-3500
                                    800-621-1115
                                    Fax: 203-797-3197
                                    www.grolier.com

1994 128 pages
ISBN: 0-531125-52-1

1401 Cystic Fibrosis: A Guide for Patient and Family
Raven Press
1185 Avenue of the Americas
New York, NY 10036   212-930-9500
                                    800-777-2295

253 pages Softcover
ISBN: 0-397516-53-3

1402 Cystic Fibrosis: The Facts

Ann Harris and Maurice Super, author

Oxford University Press
2001 Evans Road
Cary, NC 27513   212-726-6000
                                    800-451-7556
                                    Fax: 212-726-6447
                                    www.oup-usa.org

1995 128 pages Softcover
ISBN: 0-192625-43-8

1403 Understanding Cystic Fibrosis

Karen Hopken, Ph.D, author

University Press of Mississippi
3825 Ridgewood Road
Jackson, MS 39211   601-982-6205
                                    800-737-7788
                                    Fax: 601-982-6217
                                    e-mail: press@ihl.state.ms.us
                                    www.upress.state.ms.us

A useful guide for families and patients, this book charts the progress that has been made in identifying the mutations that cause cystic fibrosis and understanding how these genetic errors cause a disease whose symptoms range from mild respiratory distress to life threatening lung infections.

128 pages Softcover
ISBN: 0-878059-67-9

Children's Books

1404 Give Me One Wish

Jacquie Gordon, author

Norton Publishers
500 Fifth Avenue
New York, NY 10110   212-354-5500
                           800-233-4830

This book reads like a novel because it re-enacts the author's daughter's bout with cystic fibrosis.

Grades 10-12

1405 Robyn's Book: A True Diary

Robyn Miller, author

Scholastic
P.O. Box 7502
Jefferson City, MO 65102
                           800-325-6149

This book chronicles the life of the author and her battle with cystic fibrosis.

Grades 7-12

1406 Toothpick

Kenneth Ethridge, author

Holiday
40 East 49th Street
New York, NY 10017   212-688-0085

This book uses relationships between two different teenagers to parallel the life of a person with cystic fibrosis.

Grades 6-9

Newsletters

1407 Commitment

Cystic Fibrosis Foundation
6931 Arlington Road
Bethesda, MD 20814   301-951-4422
                           800-344-4823

Offers medical news, fund-raising features, public policy and news from across the nation on cystic fibrosis.

Pamphlets

1408 An Introduction to Cystic Fibrosis for Patients and Families

James C. Cunningham, MD, author

Cystic Fibrosis Foundation
6931 Arlington Road
Bethesda, MD 20814   301-951-4422
                           800-344-4823

Offers up-dated medical information, the latest news on assistive technology and treatments, answers to some frequently asked questions on the illness and more.

94 pages

1409 Consumer Fact Sheet
Cystic Fibrosis Foundation
6931 Arlington Road
Bethesda, MD 20814   301-951-4422

Offers a brief introduction to cystic fibrosis, symptoms, causes, treatments and offers illustrations pertaining to drainage positions.

1410 Cystic Fibrosis: A Guide for Parents
American Lung Association
1740 Broadway
New York, NY 10017   212-315-8700

Comprehensive booklet covering topics such as treatment, social aspects, inheritance, genetics and outlook for the future.

24 pages

1411 Here's Everything You'll Need to Save Money with the CFF Health Services
CFF Home Health & Pharmacy Services
6931 Arlington Road, Ste. T-200
Bethesda, MD 20814
                           800-342-6967
                      Fax: 800-233-3504

Offers information on the Cystic Fibrosis Foundation's home health services.

1412 Home Line
Cystic Fibrosis Foundation
6931 Arlington Road
Bethesda, MD 20814   301-951-4422
                           800-541-4959
            e-mail: comments@CFserv.com
                           www.CFF.org

This bi-monthly newsletter offers valuable information on CFServices pharmacy and its services. It also includes articles written by experts in various fields of cystic fibrosis.

6 pages Bi-monthly

Bill Olmsted, Manager of Business Development

1413 On the Threshold of a Cure...You Can Make the Difference!
Cystic Fibrosis Foundation
6931 Arlington Road
Bethesda, MD 20814   301-951-4422
                           800-344-4823

Offers information on what cystic fibrosis is and what people can do to help support the Foundation's research.

DESCRIPTION

1414 CYTOMEGALOVIRUS

Synonyms: Child care virus, CMV, Cytomegalic inclusion disease

Disorder Type: Infectious Disease

Cytomegalovirus (CMV) is a member of the herpesvirus family. This very common, worldwide viral infection often causes no apparent disease; however, in some patients, CMV infection results in symptoms and physical findings that may range from mild to potentially life-threatening.

Cytomegalovirus may be transmitted from mother to child before birth through the placenta, during birth through genital tract secretions, or after birth through breast milk. CMV is present in the environment; therefore, infection may be acquired at virtually any age. Because this virus may be shed in the urine and saliva for months or years after infection, children and adults who work in child-care settings are especially vulnerable. This is such a common occurrence that CMV infection is sometimes called the child-care virus. CMV may also be excreted in feces or transmitted through blood transfusions and in transplanted organs such as the kidneys, heart, and bone marrow. In the case of transmission through donated organs, CMV symptoms may be particularly severe due to immune suppression that occurs with the use of immune-suppressive drugs used to prevent organ rejection. In this way, these individuals are less capable of mounting a defense against the virus. Other individuals with impaired immune systems such as the elderly and those with acquired immunodeficiency syndrome (AIDS) are also at increased risk of potentially life-threatening complications.

Fetal infection is more common when the mother is infected by CMV for the first time as opposed to recurrent infection. The majority of CMV-infected infants has no symptoms at birth; however, approximately five to 10 percent may exhibit symptoms and physical findings involving different organs of the body. Symptomatic CMV infection in the newborn (congenital CMV) may include such characteristic findings as an unusually small head (microcephaly); accumulations of calcium salts in the tissues of the brain; enlargement of the liver and spleen (hepatosplenomegaly); yellowish discoloration of the skin, eyes, and mucous membranes (jaundice); purplish skin lesions; eye abnormalities (i.e., chorioretinitis); and other irregularities of the central nervous system that may result in loss of sight and hearing, paralysis, and mental retardation. Approximately 10 to 20 percent of asymptomatic newborns later develop similar difficulties associated with the central nervous system. Infants who contract CMV infection after birth may have enlargement of the liver and spleen, inflammation of the liver (hepatitis), or pneumonia. In addition, premature, low birth weight infants who acquire CMV infection through blood transfusion may develop inflammation of the lungs (pneumonitis), jaundice, enlargement of the liver and spleen, grayish skin coloring, and irregularities of the blood. CMV-infected children with acquired immunodeficiency syndrome (AIDS) or transplanted organs may develop potentially life-threatening conditions, including inflammation of the lungs (pneumonitis), inflammation of the retinas of the eyes (retinitis), and gastrointestinal abnormalities. Primary cytomegalovirus infections in children receiving transplants are more likely to have more severe symptoms than those of recurrent infection.

Older affected children and adults with cytomegalovirus infection may develop symptoms and physical findings similar to those of mononucleosis. These findings usually last about two to three weeks and may include fever, rash, headache, fatigue, muscle pain, and enlargement of the liver and spleen (hepatosplenomegaly). In addition, mild CMV infections in many children and adults often subside with no treatment.

In some cases, preventive treatment for CMV infection includes administration of intravenous immunoglobulin. Although this therapy is not usually effective in preventing disease acquired through most types of organ transplantation, it may be beneficial to bone marrow recipients whose compromised immune systems may not be capable of preventing a primary CMV infection. Other preventive measures may include screening of blood and organ donors for cytomegalovirus. In addition, pregnant child-care workers are urged to practice good hygiene, including frequent and thorough handwashing. Certain antiviral drugs (e.g., ganciclovir) are sometimes used to treat symptoms associated with life-threatening disease. However, symptoms tend to recur after treatment is stopped and serious side effects associated with this type of treatment are common. Separate studies on vaccine development and the use of antiviral drugs in the treatment of congenital cytomegalovirus are ongoing. Other treatment is supportive.

The following organizations in the General Resources Section can provide additional information: National Organization for Rare Disorders, Inc. (NORD), March of Dimes Birth Defects Foundation, NIH/National Institute of Allergy and Infectious Diseases, NIH/National Institute of Child Health and Human Development

National Associations & Support Groups

1415 National CMV Disease Registry
Texas Childrens Hospital
6621 Fannin St MC-2371
Houston, TX 77030

713-770-4387
Fax: 713-770-4387
e-mail: cmv@bcm.tmc.edu

Provides copies of pertinent information pieces regarding the disorder along with support facilities.

Web Sites

1416 Kid's Health
www.kidshealth.org

1417 PEDBASE
www.icondata.com/health/ped-base/files/CONGEN02.HTM

DESCRIPTION

1418 DENTAL CARIES
   Synonym: Tooth decay
   Disorder Type: Teeth
   Covers these related disorders: Baby bottle tooth decay

The development of dental caries, also known as tooth decay, is a common condition characterized by the gradual destruction (erosion) of the enamel and, potentially, the dentin and the interior pulp of a tooth. Enamel is the hard, outer, protective covering of the tooth, and dentin is the tissue beneath the enamel that surrounds the pulp. The interior of each tooth contains live pulp, which includes connective tissue, sensory nerves, and blood and lymphatic vessels.

The main cause of dental caries is thought to be plaque, which is a sticky film consisting of food debris and the byproducts of saliva and mucus. Certain bacteria that reside in the mouth break down dietary carbohydrates within plaque, creating acids that gradually wear down (erode) the outer tooth surfaces. Dental caries initially appear as whitish spots on the tooth surfaces. As loss of dental tissue progresses, cavity formation results that gradually destroys the enamel. Without appropriate treatment, the dentin may subsequently erode, allowing bacteria to invade exposed pulp, potentially causing pain, infection, and eventual tooth loss. In affected infants or children, dental caries typically appear on the minute grooves on the grinding surfaces of the back teeth (molars). Additional common sites of decay include the contact surfaces between adjacent teeth.

The frequency of carbohydrate consumption is thought to be a more significant factor in causing dental caries than the overall number of carbohydrates in the diet. For example, infants with baby bottle tooth decay have extensive dental caries due to sleeping with and sampling from nursing bottles that contain milk, fruit juices, or other sugar-containing liquids. In contrast, consumption of the same amount of such liquids during a single meal is considered much less likely to cause dental caries.

Many children may not develop dental caries. However, in those with baby bottle tooth decay, such dental caries typically become apparent between the ages of one to two years. Children with baby bottle tooth decay are more likely to develop future caries than other children. Caries that affect the minute grooves on the grinding surfaces of the molars and the contact surfaces between adjacent teeth usually appear after approximately three years of age.

Advanced dental caries may cause inflammation of the tooth pulp (pulpitis) and associated, potentially severe pain. In severe cases, bacteria may invade areas of the upper or lower jaw bone that surround and support the teeth. Associated symptoms and findings may include localized loss of pulp tissue (pulpal necrosis) and associated tenderness, pain, pus formation, and swelling of surrounding tissues (periapical abscess). In some children, these types of abscesses in a primary tooth may inhibit the normal development of the permanent tooth.

According to estimates in the medical literature, the frequency of dental caries among children has decreased approximately 35 to 50 percent during the past 20 years. These decreases may be the result of advances in preventive measures, such as the addition of the mineral fluoride to the public water supply (fluoridation) and the inclusion of fluoride in toothpaste. Fluoride strengthens the mineral composition of enamel and potentially decreases the acid production associated with bacterial fermentation.

In most cases, dental caries may be treated by removing the decayed area (i.e., through drilling) and filling the cavity with a dental restoration material (e.g., amalgam, composite resin, porcelain filling). If advanced decay causes associated pulp infection, treatment may include removal of the pulp during a procedure known as a root canal, restorative techniques (e.g., crowns for affected molars), or extraction of the tooth. If a tooth must be extracted, treatment also may include measures to prevent abnormal shifting of adjacent teeth and associated poor positioning or failed eruption of permanent teeth. Antibiotic medications may be prescribed for patients with dental infection, particularly patients with impaired immune function or blood clotting abnormalities. Those who are at risk for bacterial infection of the lining of the heart (such as those with certain heart defects) and patients who have infections affecting the upper or lower jaw bone may also be advised to take antibiotic medications. Additional treatment is symptomatic and supportive.

As mentioned above, certain measures may help to prevent the development of dental caries. Such measures include following proper oral hygiene, such as brushing with a fluoride toothpaste and flossing daily (i.e., with parental supervision); decreasing the frequency and amount of carbohydrate consumption, including avoiding between-meal snacks; and weaning infants from the bottle by approximately one year of age, if possible. Measures to help prevent baby bottle tooth decay include not allowing the baby to sleep with a bottle in the mouth, breast-feeding, or providing water bottles at night or at naptime.

National Associations & Support Groups

1419 American Dental Association
211 East Chicago Avenue
Chicago, IL 60611 312-440-2500
www.ada.org

Professional association of dentists to serving both the public and the profession of dentistry. Promotes the profession of dentistry by enhancing the integrity and ethics of the profession and strengthening the paatient/dentist relationship. Fulfills its mission by providing services and through its initiatives in education, research, advocacy and the development of standards.

1420 National Institute of Dental Research
31 Center Dr Msc 2290 Bldg 31
Bethesda, MD 20892 301-496-4261
Fax: 301-496-9988
www.nidr.nih.gov

Provides leadership for a national resarch program designed to understand, treat and prevent the infectious and inherited craniofacial-oral-dental diseases and disorders.

Web Sites

1421 Dental Consumer Advisory
www.toothinfo.com

1422 Dental Resources on the Web
dental-resources.com/

Books

1423 Understanding Dental Health
Francis G. Serio, D.M.D., M.S., author
University Press of Mississippi
3825 Ridgewood Road
Jackson, MS 39211 601-432-6205
800-737-7788
Fax: 601-432-6217
e-mail: press@ihl.state.ms.us
www.upress.ms.us

A user friendly manual on the basics of dental health.

128 pages
ISBN: 1-578060-09-5

DESCRIPTION

1424 DEPRESSION

Disorder Type: Mental, Emotional or Behavioral Disorder

Depression refers to an emotional state characterized by exaggerated feelings of sadness, discouragement, loneliness, low self-esteem, and despair. These feelings may follow a recent loss or other tragic event. However, if feelings of depression worsen and are prolonged, or occur for no apparent reason, this may indicate a chronic (endogenous or true) depressive disorder. Although endogenous depression occurs more commonly among the adult population, depression may be evident as early as infancy and is increasingly common among adolescents.

Symptoms and findings associated with depression are variable. Depression in infants may be precipitated by such events as sudden separation from the mother or caregiver after six months of age (anaclitic depression of infancy) and may be manifested by ceaseless crying, panic, apprehension, withdrawal, and eating and sleeping disturbances. Eventually, indifference and unresponsiveness may develop and result in deficiencies in intellectual, physical, and social development. Recovery may be possible if the mother or substitute caregiver is reintroduced to the child within a reasonably short period of time (i.e., one to three months). Symptoms associated with depression in school-age children include overwhelming feelings of sadness, crying, loss of interest in pleasurable activities, eating and sleeping irregularities, and, in some cases, suicidal thoughts. Some affected children may exhibit symptoms that belie a diagnosis of depression, such as overactivity and aggression. Adolescents with depression may have feelings of hopelessness and helplessness with no corresponding periods of happiness or well-being. However, inappropriate displays of euphoria together with such behavior as truancy, substance abuse, or other antisocial behaviors may also be symptomatic of depression. Other symptoms and findings associated with adolescent depression may include a decline in school grades, boredom, repetitive accidents, drug or alcohol abuse, absenteeism, feelings or delusions of guilt, and thoughts of suicide. Physical symptoms may sometimes include fatigue, headaches, and abdominal pain. Those who are psychotically depressed may experience delusions and hallucinations.

Endogenous depression may be caused by many different factors including genetic influences, hormonal disturbances, certain medications, infectious or neurologic disorders, physical conditions (i.e., stroke, etc.), tumorous growths, nutritional influences, and psychosocial factors. In addition, depression may occur in association with other psychological disorders such as bipolar or other mood disorders (e.g., schizoaffective disorder).

Treatment of depression may include the administration of certain antidepressant medications. In addition, children and adolescents with this disorder often require individual psychotherapy and, in many cases, group and family therapy. Children and adolescents with suicidal thoughts or tendencies require immediate intervention. Other treatment is supportive.

The following organizations in the General Resources Section can provide additional information: Federation of Families for Children's Mental Health, NIH/National Institute of Mental Health, Online Mendelian Inheritance in Man: www3.ncbi.nlm.nih.gov/Omim/searchomim.html

National Associations & Support Groups

1425 Anxiety Disorders Association of America
11900 Parklawn Drive Ste 100
Rockville, MD 20852   301-231-9350

Offers help, support and information for persons with anxiety disorders, manic and depressive disorders and mental illness.

1426 Depression & Related Affective Disorders Association
Meyer 3-181 600 North Wolfe Street
Baltimore, MD 21287   410-955-4647
                            Fax: 410-614-3241
                   e-mail: drada@jhmi.med.jhu.edu
                        www.med.jhu.edu/drada/

Organization that brings together people with affective disorders, their families and mental health professionals; and support research programs.

1427 National Alliance for Research on Schizophrenia and Affective Disorders
60 Cutter Mill Road Suite 404
Great Neck, NY 11021   516-829-0091
                            800-829-0091
                       Fax: 516-487-6930
                  e-mail: info@narsad.org
                        www.narsad.org

Raises and distributes funds for scientific research into the causes, cures, treatments, and prevention of severe mental illness, primarily schizophrenia and affective disorders.

William O'Reilly, Executive Director

1428 National Alliance for the Mentally Ill (NAMI)
Colonial Place Three, 2107 Wilson Blvd., Ste 300
Arlington, VA 22201   703-524-7600
                            800-950-6264
                       Fax: 703-524-9097
                       TDD: 703-516-7227
                            www.nami.org

Membership organization offering a mail order bookstore, many programs, conferences, symposia and group meetings for families and patients.

1429 National Anxiety Foundation
3135 Custer Drive
Lexington, KY 40517   606-272-7166
                   207.69.132.114/naf.htm

Offers information and help to persons with panic disorders, manic and depressive disorders and mental illness.

Stephen Cox, Medical Director

1430 National Depressive and Manic Depressive Association
730 N. Franklin Suite 501
Chicago, IL 60610   312-642-0049
                          800-826-3632

Offers information, research and support for persons suffering from manic and depressive disorders.

1431 National Foundation for Depression
2 Penn Plaza, Ste 1981
New York, NY 10121   212-268-4260

Amy Russell

1432 National Foundation for Depressive Illness
P.O. Box 2257
New York, NY 10116   212-268-4260
                            800-248-4344
                       Fax: 212-268-4434
                       www.depression.org

Corrects the myths and misconceptions surrounding the illness and helps to reverse the devastating effects of depression. Informs the public, health care providers, healthcare professionals and corporations about depression, manic depression and provides the information about correct diagnosis and treatment and the availability of qualified doctors and support groups. Psychiatric referral service and information packets on childhood, adolescent depression.

International

1433 Depression Alliance (UK)
35 Westminster Bridge Road
London Intl SE1 7JB,
United Kingdom
                        www.gn.apc.org/da/

1434 Mental Health Foundation (UK)
37 Mortimer St.
London Intl W1N 8J0,
United Kingdom
                   e-mail: mhf@mentalhealth.org.uk
                        www.mentalhealth.org.uk

Research Centers

1435 University of Pennsylvania, Depression Research Unit
School of Medicine, Dept. of Psychiatry
3600 Spruce Street
Philadelphia, PA 19104   215-662-3462
                            Fax: 215-662-6443

Focuses on mental health and depression.

Jay D. Amsterdam, MD, Director

1436 University of Texas, Mental Health Clinical Research Center
5323 Harry Hines Blvd.
Dallas, TX 75235   214-648-2951

Research activity of major and atypical depression.

Dr. A. John Rush, Director

1437 Yale University, Behavioral Medicine Clinic
Yale School of Medicine
333 Cedar Street
New Haven, CT 06510   203-785-4184

Focuses on mental disorders including schizophrenia and depression.

Hoyle Leigh, MD, Director

1438 Yale University, Ribicoff Research Facilities
CT Medical Health Center
34 Park Street
New Haven, CT 06511   203-789-7300
Fax: 203-562-7079

Clinical research in the areas of schizophrenia, depression and mental disorders.

George Heninger, MD, Director

Audio Video

1439 Depression and Manic Depression
Fanlight Productions
47 Halifax St
Boston, MA 02130   617-469-4999
Fax: 617-469-3379
e-mail: fanlight@tiac.net
www.fanlight.com

This video explores the realities of depression and manic depression, as well as providing an overview of available treatments, and a listing of other resources.

28 minutes

Web Sites

1440 AACAP
www.aacap.org/factsfam/index.htm

1441 Internet Mental Health
www.mentalhealth.com/

1442 Mental Health Net
www.cmhc.com

Books

1443 Anxiety & Depression In Adults & Children
Kenneth D. Craig, author
Sage Publications
2455 Teller Road
Newbury Park, CA 91320   805-499-0721

1994 304 pages Softcover
ISBN: 0-803970-21-8

1444 Ask the Doctor: Depression
Vincent Frieldewald, MD, author
Andrews McMeel Publishing
P.O. Box 419150
Kansas City, MO 64141   816-932-6700
800-826-4216
Fax: 660-859-6559

A look at depression, its symptoms, what causes it, and what you can do about it. Learn the difference between mood problems and genuine depression, and how to read warning signs such as sleep abnormalities, nervousness, and suicidal thoughts. Information on chemicals, genetics, and medical solutions.

128 pages Softcover
ISBN: 0-836227-11-5

1445 Coping with Depression
Lawrence Clayton, PhD, and Sharon Carter, author
Rosen Publishing Group
29 East 21st Street
New York, NY 10010   212-777-3017
800-237-9932
Fax: 212-436-4643
e-mail: rosenpub@tribeca.ios.com

With an emphasis on life's myriad difficulties, the authors help teens find practical ways to cope with depression.

ISBN: 0-823919-51-0

1446 Dealing with Depression: Five Ways to Help
Richard Dayringer, author
Haworth Press
10 Alice Street
Binghamton, NY 13904   607-722-8277
Fax: 607-722-1424

1995
ISBN: 1-560249-33-1

1447 Depression Sourcebook

Brian P. Quinn, CSW, PhD, author

Lowell House Press
2029 Century Park East
Los Angeles, CA 90067   310-556-2715
                              Fax: 310-552-7555

Everything anyone afflicted with a depressive disorder - or the people who care about them - need to know about unipolar and bipolar depression.

266 pages

1448 Depression and Its Treatment

Warner Books
1271 Avenue of the Americas
New York, NY 10020   212-522-7200

A layman's guide to help one understand and cope with America's #1 mental health problem.

157 pages

1449 Depression, the Mood Disease

Francis M. Mondimore, MD, author

Johns Hopkins University Press
2715 North Charles Street
Baltimore, MD 21218   410-516-6900
                             800-537-5487
                         Fax: 410-516-6998

This book explores the many faces of an illness that will affect as many as 36 million Americans at some point in their lives. Updated to reflect state-of-the-art treatment.

1993 240 pages
ISBN: 0-801851-84-X

1450 Depressive Illnesses: Treatments Bring New Hope

Superintendent of Documents
P.O. Box 371954
Pittsburgh, PA 15250   202-512-2250

Offers the general public an overview of the various depressive illnesses. Topics include causes, symptoms and types of depression, clinical evaluation and treatment, helpful suggestions for family and friends, and other sources of information.

28 pages

1451 Encyclopedia of Depression

Roberta Roesch, author

Facts on File
Department M274 11 Penn Plaza
New York, NY 10001   212-290-8090
                            800-322-8755
                        Fax: 212-678-3633

This volume defines and explains all terms and topics relating to depression.

170 pages Hardbound

1452 Essential Guide to Psychiatric Drugs

Jack M. Fgorman, MD, author

St. Martin's Press
175 Fifth Avenue
New York, NY 10010   212-674-5151
                            800-221-7945
                        Fax: 212-420-9314

Basic information on 123 drugs used for depression, anxiety and bipolar illness.

1453 Everything You Need To Know About Depression

Elanor H. Ayer, author

Rosen Publishing Group
29 East 21st Street
New York, NY 10010   212-777-3017
                            800-237-9932
                        Fax: 212-436-4643
                e-mail: rosenpub@tribeca.ios.com

An important resource for teens who are looking for help with depression.

Grades 7-12
ISBN: 0-823926-06-0

1454 Handbook of School-Based Interventions

Courage To Change
P.O. Box 1268
Newburgh, NY 12551
                            800-440-4003
                        Fax: 800-772-6499

Comprehensive volume that describes interventions for virtually every major problem behavior students may exhibit from K-12. All interventions are research-based and guidance is given for practical application of the techniques. Topics range from dishonesty, academic performance, procrastination and low self-esteem to obsessive-compulsive behavior, substance abuse, AIDS and depression.

512 pages Hardcover

1455 Help Me, I'M Sad

David G. Fassler, MD, author

Penguin Putnam
PO Box 999
Bergenfield, NJ 07621

800-526-0275
Fax: 800-227-9604

Helping and understanding a child with depression.

1456 Helping Your Child Cope with Depression and Suicidal Thoughts

Tonia K. Shamoo, Philip G. Patros, author

Jossey-Bass
350 Sansome Street
San Francisco, CA 94104

415-433-1740
800-956-7739
Fax: 800-605-2665
www.josseybass.com

Shows parents how to learn to talk, listen, and communicate effectively with a depressed child; signs to watch for and situations which may cause a wish to commit suicide.

192 pages
ISBN: 0-787908-44-4

1457 Helping Your Depressed Child

Lawrence L. Kerns, MD, author

Prima Publishing
PO Box 1260
Rocklin, CA 95677

916-624-5718

Reasurring guide to the causes and treatment of childhood and adolescent depression.

284 pages

1458 Mood Apart

Peter C. Whybrow, MD, author

Basic Books
10 East 53rd Street
New York, NY 10022

212-207-7057

An overview of the depression and manic depression and the available treatments for them.

363 pages

1459 Overcoming Depression

Demitri Papolos, MD, & Janice Papolos, author

Harper & Row
10 East 53rd Street
New York, NY 10022

212-207-7000

1987 318 pages Softcover

1460 Panic Disorder in the Medical Setting

Superintendent of Documents
P.O. Box 371954
Pittsburgh, PA 15250

202-512-2250

This book serves the primary care physicians as a helpful guide in recognizing and treating panic disorder in patients and in identifying those who need psychiatric consultation or rerferrals.

1993 135 pages

1461 Prozac Nation: Young & Depressed in America, A Memoir

Elizabeth Wurtzel, author

Houghton Mifflin Company
222 Berkeley St
Boston, MA 02116

617-351-3698
800-225-3362

Struck with depression at 11, now 27, Wurtzel chronicles her struggle with the illness. Witty, terrifying and sometimes funny, it tells the story of a young life almost destroyed by depression.

317 pages

1462 Psychotherapy of Severe and Mild Depression

Silvano Arieti and Jules Bemporad, author

Jason Aronson, Inc.
400 Keystone Industrial Park
Dunmore, PA 18521

800-782-0015
Fax: 201-840-7242
www.aronson.com

464 pages Softcover
ISBN: 1-568211-46-5

1463 Questions & Answers About Depression & Its Treatment

Ivan K. Goldberg, MD, author

Charles C. Thomas Publishing, Ltd.
2600 South First Street
Springfield, IL 62704

217-789-8980
800-258-8980
Fax: 217-789-9130

All the questions you'd like to ask, asked and answered.

136 pages

1464 Report of the Secretary's Task Force on Youth Suicide

Superintendent of Documents
P.O. Box 371954
Pittsburgh, PA 15250

202-512-2250

A comprehensive review of information about youth suicide. The task force recommendations are presented in Volume 1.

110 pages

1465 Suicide, Why?

Adina Wrobleski, author

National Alliance for the Mentally Ill
P.O. Box 753
Waldorf, MD 20604   703-524-7600
                          www.NAMI.org

An authoritative book, noting that suicide is usually caused by brain disorders.

1989

1466 Surprising Truth About Depression: Medical Breakthroughs That Can Work

Herbert Wagemaker, author

Zondervan
5300 Patterson SE
Grand Rapids, MI 49530   616-698-6900
                             Fax: 616-698-3439
                             www.zondervan.com

1994 224 pages Softcover
ISBN: 0-310401-01-1

1467 Treating Depressed Children

Charma D. Dudley, PH.D, author

New Harbinger Publications
5674 Shattuck Avenue
Oakland, CA 94609

                          800-748-6273
                       Fax: 510-652-5472
          e-mail: customerservice@newharbinger.com
                     www.newharbinger.com

This book explains a 12-session treatment program to help children change their negative thoughts, gain confidence and recognize their emotions. These actions are acheived with the help of cartoons and role-playing games.

160 pages Hardcover
ISBN: 1-572240-61-X

Laseu Pfaff, Publicist

1468 Treating Depression

Ira D. Glick, author

Jossey-Bass
350 Sansome Street
San Francisco, CA 94104   415-433-1740
                             800-956-7739
                          Fax: 800-605-2665
                          www.josseybass.com

This ket resource assists the clinician in deciding if it is appropriate to prescribe medication, if phychotherapy is the proper course of action, or if it is best to use a combination of medication and physcotherapy. Treating depression offers step-by-step guidelines and specific models for intervention in treating the numerous types and subtypes of depression.

1995
ISBN: 0-787901-44-0

1469 Understanding Depression

Patricia Ainsworth, M.D., author

University Press of Mississippi
3825 Ridgewood Road
Jackson, MS 39211   601-432-6205
                          800-737-7788
                       Fax: 601-432-6217
           e-mail: press@ihl.state.ms.us
                     www.upress.state.ms.us

A clear explanation for those who know the illness personally and for those who want to understand them.

120 pages
ISBN: 1-578061-68-7

1470 Understanding Your Teenager's Depression

Kathleen McCoy, author

Berkley Books
200 Madison Avenue
New York, NY 10016   212-951-8800

1994 352 pages Softcover
ISBN: 0-399518-56-8

1471 Working with Children and Adolescents in Groups
Courage*To*Change
P.O. Box 1268
Newburgh, NY 12551
                          800-440-4003
                       Fax: 800-772-6499

Step-by-step guide that discusses how to effectively treat problem behavior in children and adolescents using small groups. Based on empirical research and their own work with groups, the authors show how a variety of approaches can be effectively combined to help resolve such problem behaviors as fighting, low self-esteem.

384 pages Hard Cover

1472 Yesterday's Tomorrow

Barry L., author

Hazelden
15251 Pleasant Valley Road
Center City, MN 55012

612-257-4010
800-328-9000
Fax: 612-257-2195
www.hazelden.org

A meditation book that shows why and how recovery works, from the author's own experiences.

432 pages Softcover
ISBN: 1-568381-60-3

Children's Books

1473 Sad Days, Glad Days

Dewitt Hamilton, author

National Alliance for the Mentally Ill
P.O. Box 753
Waldorf, MD 20604

703-524-7600
www.NIMF.org

Introduces five to nine year olds to a parent's depression.

1995

Newsletters

1474 National Foundation for Depressive Illness
P.O. Box 2257
New York, NY 10116

212-268-4260
800-248-4344
Fax: 212-268-4434
www.depression.org

Information on the myths and misconceptions surrounding the illness, Informs the public, health care providers, healthcare professionals and corporations about depression, manic depression and provides the information about correct diagnosis and treatment and the availability of qualified doctors and support groups.

4 pages quarterly

Amy C. Russell, Editor

Pamphlets

1475 Depression Is a Treatable Illness: A Patients Guide
Department of Health & Human Services
2101 E. Jefferson St Ste 501
Rockville, MD 20852

301-217-1245

Tells about major depressive disorder, which is only one form of depressive illness. This booklet answers important questions regarding this disorder and gives information on where to go for more help.

1476 Let's Talk About Depression
Superintendent of Documents
P.O. Box 371954
Pittsburgh, PA 15250

202-512-2250

Targeted especially for inner-city youth. The colorful design will capture attention and focus on depression in a way that young people will understand and identify with.

1477 Let's Talk Facts About Childhood Disorders
American Psychiatric Association
1400 K Street NW
Washington, DC 20005

202-682-6220

Offers information on depression and depressive disorders including the causes, symptoms, treatments, anxiety, and various other phobias.

1478 Living Without Depression & Manic Depression: A Workbook

Mary Ellen Copeland, author

National Alliance for the Mentally Ill
P.O. Box 753
Waldorf, MD 20604

703-524-7600
www.NAMI.org

Workbook offering checklists and helpful advice targeted for individuals whose depressive illness is stabilized.

1994

1479 Now We Can Successfully Treat the Illness Called Depression
National Foundation for Depressive Illness (NAFDI)
P.O. Box 2257
New York, NY 10116

212-268-4260
800-248-4344
Fax: 212-268-4434
www.depression.org

Basic information on depression and manic depression, gives symptoms, encourages persons who have symptoms to seek medical treatment. Tips on managing depressive illness.

Amy C. Russell, Editor

1480 Panic Disorder
National Institutes of Health
5600 Fishers Lane Room 7C-02
Rockville, MD 20857

301-443-3706
Fax: 301-443-6349

Written for the lay public, this pamphlet contains a description of panic disorder, gives the symptoms, describes treatment methods, and encourages the person who has the symptoms to seek treatment.

1481 Plain Talk About Depression
Superintendent of Documents
P.O. Box 371954
Pittsburgh, PA 15250   202-512-2250

A flyer discussing types of depression, major depression, symptoms and causes.

1482 Understanding Panic Disorder
National Institutes of Health
5600 Fishers Lane Room 7C-02
Rockville, MD 20857   301-443-3706
                                       Fax: 301-443-6349

Offers information on what an panic disorder is, symptoms, causes, treatment, medications and therapy.

1483 Useful Information on Phobias and Panic
Superintendent of Documents
P.O. Box 371954
Pittsburgh, PA 15250   202-512-2250

This booklet provides information on both phobias and panic. Symptoms, causes and treatments of these disorders are referred to. If you know someone who is excessively fearful, this booklet will be of great help to them in understanding their problem.

40 pages 50 copies

1484 What to Do When a Friend Is Depressed: Guide for Students
Superintendent of Documents
P.O. Box 371954
Pittsburgh, PA 15250   202-512-2250

Offers information on depression and its symptoms and suggests things a young person can do to guide a depressed friend in finding help.

DESCRIPTION

1485 DEVELOPMENTAL DYSPLASIA OF THE HIP
Synonyms: CDH, Congenital dislocation of the hip, DDH, Developmental dysplasia of the hip
Disorder Type: Birth Defect
Covers these related disorders: Teratologic congenital dysplasia of the hip, Typical congenital dysplasia of the hip (Developmental dysplasia)
May involve these systems in the body (see Section III):
Prenatal & Postnatal Growth & Development, Skeletal System

Congenital dysplasia of the hip (CDH) refers to a condition present at birth or soon thereafter in which one or both hips are dislocated. This occurs when the ball-shaped head of the upper thigh bone (femur) does not fit appropriately into the hip socket of the pelvis. Congenital hip dysplasia may be classified as typical, which occurs shortly after birth in infants with no underlying neurologic irregularities, or teratologic, which develops before birth. The typical form of this condition is commonly referred to as developmental dysplasia of the hip.

The cause of developmental hip dysplasia is unknown, although it is more prevalent in newborns who were surrounded by an unusually small amount of amniotic fluid during the gestational period (oligohydramnios). Those infants who present in a breech position and those with other close family members with this condition may also be at increased risk for CDH. In addition, it is more predominant in girls than it is in boys by a ratio of nine to one. Teratologic dysplasia of the hip in the developing fetus may occur as part of a pattern of abnormalities associated with certain underlying disorders affecting the neuromuscular system such as arthrogryposis multiplex congenita and myelodysplasia.

Treatment during infancy may include manipulation of the hip joint into its proper position followed by immobilization and splinting of the thigh for a period of several months. Some infants may benefit from wearing two or three diapers at a time. In some patients, delayed detection of this birth defect may necessitate the use of traction; however, if the dislocation is not discovered until late childhood, surgery followed by fitting with a plaster cast may be necessary to correct this condition. Delayed treatment may result in chronic difficulties with walking. Untreated dysplasia of the hip may result in degenerative changes in the joint (osteoarthritis). Approximately 400 of every 100,000 infants are affected by congenital dysplasia of the hip; however, in approximately 70 percent of these children, the dislocation corrects itself.

The following organizations in the General Resources Section can provide additional information: Genetic Alliance, March of Dimes Birth Defects Foundation, NIH/National Institute of Child Health and Human Development

Web Sites

1486 Dr. Koop
www.drkoop.com/adam/mhc/top/000971.htm

DESCRIPTION

1487 DIGEORGE SYNDROME

Synonyms: DiGeorge sequence, Thymic agenesis immunodeficiency

Disorder Type: Birth Defect, Genetic Disorder

May involve these systems in the body (see Section III):

Immune System

DiGeorge syndrome is a disorder present at birth (congenital) that is characterized by absence (aplasia) or underdevelopment (hypoplasia) of the thymus and the parathyroid glands, malformations of the heart and its major blood vessels (cardiovascular abnormalities), and characteristic malformations of the head and facial (craniofacial) area. Due to absence or underdevelopment of the thymus, affected children may have abnormalities of the immune system, causing impaired resistance to certain infections. DiGeorge syndrome occurs as the result of abnormal development of certain embryonic structures (third and fourth pharyngeal pouches) that later develop into the thymus and parathyroid glands. In some cases, other embryonic structures that are forming during the same approximate period may also be affected, resulting in certain cardiovascular, craniofacial, or other malformations. The thymus, a lymphoid tissue organ located in the upper portion of the chest, plays an essential role in the immune system beginning at approximately the twelfth week of fetal development until puberty. It serves as a source of certain white blood cells (lymphocytes) before birth and then promotes the development of certain specialized lymphocytes, known as T lymphocytes, through secretion of particular hormones (e.g., thymosin). The actions of the T lymphocytes help to defend the body against certain microorganisms (i.e., cell-mediated immunity). The parathyroid glands, which are two pairs of small glands on the sides of the thyroid gland, produce parathyroid hormone, which helps to maintain normal levels of calcium in the blood.

DiGeorge syndrome usually occurs randomly (sporadically) and is caused by spontaneous, minute deletions of material from the long arm of chromosome 22 (22q11.2). DiGeorge syndrome may also occur in association with certain chromosomal abnormalities (e.g., chromosome 10, monosomy 10p; chromosome 22, monosomy 22q). There have also been some cases in which DiGeorge syndrome affected individuals within certain families (kindreds) yet did not appear to result from known chromosome syndromes. In some familial cases, DiGeorge syndrome may have autosomal dominant inheritance. The disorder is thought to affect approximately one in 20,000 newborns.

In infants and children with DiGeorge syndrome, associated sypmtoms and findings may be extremely variable. Patients who have absence or severe underdevelopment of the thymus are prone to frequent infections from fungi, viruses, and certain bacteria (such as Pneumocystis carinii). These patients often experience chronic inflammation of the mucous membranes of the nose (rhinitis), recurrent inflammation of the lungs (pneumonia), fungal infection of the mucous membranes of the mouth (oral candidiasis), recurrent diarrhea, or systemic infections in which invading microorganisms or their toxins are present in the blood circulation (septicemia). In some cases of serious infection, life-threatening complications may result. Infants and children with mild underdevelopment (hypoplasia) of the thymus are said to have partial DiGeorge syndrome and may have little difficulty with recurring infections. Because of absence or underdevelopment of the parathyroid glands (hypoparathyroidism), many affected infants experience certain symptoms and findings during the first days of life, including abnormally low calcium levels in the blood (hypocalcemia) and muscle twitching, tremors and cramps, (neonatal tetany) and even seizures. Such symptoms and findings can be treated with calcium infusion and are usually temporary but may recur later in life.

Some newborns with DiGeorge syndrome may also have defects of the heart and its great arteries such as interrupted aortic arch, tetralogy of Fallot, an abnormal opening in the fibrous partition that separates the upper chambers or the lower chambers of the heart (atrial or ventricular septal defects) infants with DiGeorge syndrome may have an unusually narrow or blind-ending esophagus (esophageal atresia) that does not form a passageway into the stomach. In addition, affected newborns may have characteristic malformations of the head and facial (craniofacial) area, such as widely spaced eyes (ocular hypertelorism); downwardly slanting eyelid folds (palpebral fissures); a small mouth; an unusually short, vertical groove in the center of the upper lip (philtrum); and low-set, notched ears. Some patients may also have mild to moderate mental retardation.

The treatment of infants and children with DiGeorge syndrome is symptomatic and supportive. Treatment measures may include the administration of calcium in those with hypoparathyroidism and hypocalcemia, therapies to help prevent and aggressively treat infections (e.g., antiviral, antifungal, and antibiotic agents) in patients with immunodeficiency, medical and surgical measures for cardiovascular malformations, or other measures as required. If patients with immunodeficiency require blood transfusions, donor blood must be exposed to high levels of radiation (irradiated) to kill the donor lymphocytes and thus prevent the occurrence of graft-versus-host disease, a serious disease caused by an immune response of donor cells against the recipient's tissues.

The following organizations in the General Resources Section can provide additional information: National Organization for Rare Disorders, Inc (NORD), NIH/Office of Rare Diseases, March of Dimes Birth Defects Foundation, Genetic Alliance, Online Mendelian Inheritance in Man:

www3.ncbi.nlm.nih.gov/Omim/searchomim.html

National Associations & Support Groups

1488 22Q and You Center
34th St and Civic Cntr Blvd
Philadelphia, PA 19104   215-590-2920
                                        Fax: 215-590-3298
                           e-mail: lunny@email.chop.edu
                                  cbil.humgen.upenn.edu

Services offered by the Department of Clinical Genetics in the Children's Hospital of Philadelphia, include literature, support groups and referrals.

1489 Chromosome 22 Central
232 Kent Ave
Timmins, Ontario,
Canada   705-268-3099
                                        Fax: 705-268-3099
                          e-mail: mum2_1@hotmail.com
                                              www.nt.net/

1490 Immune Deficiency Foundation
25 W. Chesapeake Ave, Ste 206
Townson, MD 21204   410-321-6647
                                              800-296-4433
                                        Fax: 410-321-9165
                                   e-mail: idf@clark.net
                                            www.clark.net

Offers every possible support avenue that people suffering from this defiency could turn to and use repeatedly.

Web Sites

1491 Congenital Heart Disease Resource Page
www.csun.edu/~hcmth011/heart/
                          e-mail: sheri.berger@csun.edu
                          www.csun.edu/~hcmth011/heart/

1492 International Patient Organization for Primary Immunodeficiencies
ipopi.org

1493 Jeffrey Modell Foundation
www.jmfworld.com/html/digeorge.html

1494 Kansas University Medical Center
www.kumc.edu/gec/support/velo.html

1495 Pedbase
www.icondata.com/health/pedbase/files/DI-GEORGE.HTM

DESCRIPTION

1496 DIPHTHERIA

Synonym: Bretonneau's disease
Disorder Type: Infectious Disease
Covers these related disorders: Cutaneous diphtheria, Respiratory tract diphtheria

Diphtheria is an acute, contagious bacterial disease caused by the bacterium Corynebacterium diphtheriae. The disease is characterized at its onset by sore throat and painful swallowing. Approximately one to four days after exposure, infected individuals may also develop a low-grade fever, headache, nausea and vomiting, chills, and a rapid heart rate (tachycardia). Other symptoms may include inflammation of the nasal membranes, nasal discharge, and other signs associated with upper respiratory tract infection. Within a few days, a grayish-brown pseudomembrane composed of bacteria, blood cells, and other substances may form over the tonsils, voice box (larynx), trachea (windpipe), and palate. The throat and underlying soft tissue may swell causing difficulties with breathing, eating, and drinking. In addition, the lymph nodes in the neck may become swollen and enlarged. Occasionally, the diphtheria bacterium causes infection in the mucous membranes of the eyes, ears, or genital tract. In some cases, this bacterium releases a toxin into the bloodstream, causing damage to the heart or central nervous system. The severity of heart damage may range from modest to potentially life-threatening. Central nervous system involvement occurs in progressive stages. Initially there may be paralysis of the soft palate of the throat, difficulty in swallowing, facial nerve weakness, and other symptoms that become apparent within the first to third week of onset of infection. Inflammation of the nerves of the eyes (optic neuritis) may occur in the fifth week and result in blurred vision and misalignment of the eye (strabismus). Weakness in the arms and legs due to nervous system inflammation usually occurs during the third to sixth week of infection.

Cutaneous diphtheria affects the skin and is characterized by the appearance of pus-filled ulcerations on the arms and legs. These lesions may also be covered with a grayish-brown membrane. Sometimes, cutaneous diphtheria affects the skin on the head or trunk. These nonprogressive lesions may be painful and tender. In some patients, cutaneous diphtheria may be limited to the appearance of a small number of yellow sores on the skin.

In the early part of the twentieth century, diphtheria was a major cause of disease and death in the United States; however, with the advent of immunization, there have been fewer than five recorded cases a year since 1980. Most cases of diphtheria are now restricted to developing countries, although there have been outbreaks in other areas. Because of the ease of travel and the immigration of people from developing countries into the U.S., national immunization programs remain important in preventing the spread of this disease. Diphtheria vaccine is usually combined with the vaccines for whopping cough (pertussis) and tetanus. This DPT combination is routinely given to children in a series, starting within the first few months of life. A booster dose of just diphtheria and a tetanus vaccines is also recommended between the ages of 11 and 16 years (if there has been a five-year lapse since the last vaccination). It is given every 10 years thereafter. In addition, individuals exposed to diphtheria or those who are carriers, but have no symptoms, are usually put on antibiotic therapy, given a diphtheria toxoid booster if they have not had one recently, and then monitored closely. Also, asymptomatic carriers may be put in isolation until cultures taken at prescribed intervals are negative.

In most cases, diphtheria is transmitted through droplets coughed or exhaled into the dry air by an infected individual; however, diphtheria bacteria may also spread through direct contact with secretions or discharge from the respiratory tract or infected skin lesions. Treatment for diphtheria is aimed toward elimination of the bacterial infection with antibiotic therapy as well as the removal of toxins from the body through the use of an antitoxin derived from immunized horses. In addition, if an individual is having difficulty in breathing due to an obstructed or swollen airway, a surgical procedure may be performed to create a temporary opening in the throat to assist breathing (tracheostomy). Individuals with diphtheria are usually isolated until there is no detectable infection. During the recovery period, fluids are administered, an appropriate diet is followed, and bedrest is maintained. Other treatment is symptomatic and supportive.

The following organizations in the General Resources Section can provide additional information: NIH/National Institute of Allergy and Infectious Diseases, World Health Organization, Centers for Disease Control (CDC), Child Health and Development (CHD) www.who.int/chd/

Web Sites

1497 CenterWatch/Drugs
www.centerwatch.com/drugs/DRU144.HTM

1498 Child Health Research Project
http://ih.njsph.edu/chr/chr.htm

DESCRIPTION

1499 DISCOLORATION OF THE TEETH

Disorder Type: Teeth
Covers these related disorders: Dental mottling, Permanent discoloration of the teeth, Temporary discoloration of the teeth

Permanent discoloration of the teeth is a dental abnormality caused by incorporation of particular substances into developing enamel, the hard, outermost covering of the teeth." Discoloration may result from"therapy with certain antibiotic medications (e.g., tetracyclines), excessive consumption of the mineral fluoride, particular pediatric conditions or disorders, or other factors.

Tetracycline medications are highly absorbed or incorporated into the teeth and bones. Therefore, such therapy during the development of enamel may result in thin, deficient tooth enamel (enamel hypoplasia) that is permanently stained an abnormal yellowish brown. The risk for such enamel hypoplasia and staining extends from about the fourth month of fetal development until about 10 months of age for the primary (deciduous) teeth and from approximately four months up to 16 years of age for the permanent (secondary) teeth. In addition, the potential risk is affected by the specific tetracycline medication prescribed, dosage level, and duration of therapy. Because enamel development is typically not complete in children until approximately eight years of age (with the exception of the third molars), tetracycline therapy is generally not recomme for children who are younger than eight years nor for women who are pregnant.

Excessive consumption of the mineral fluoride may also result in enamel hypoplasia and discoloration. This form of tooth discoloration, known as mottling, primarily affects infants and children who reside in areas where natural levels of fluoride in the water supply are much greater than recommended levels. Due to improper deposition of calcium salts in the teeth, tooth surfaces may wear down easily and tooth enamel is chalky white in color, gradually becoming a yellowish brown.

Permanent discoloration of the teeth may also result from certain vitamin deficiencies, particular infectious disorders, or certain pediatric conditions, such as excessive levels of the waste duct bilirubin in the blood after birth (neonatal hyperbilirubinemia). This condition may cause a bluish or blackish discoloration of the primary teeth and, in some cases, the tips of certain permanent teeth. In infants and children with permanent discoloration of the teeth, the use of certain specialized dental procedures and devices may help to minimize or cover such discoloration.

In some cases, infants and children may also experience temporary staining on the surfaces of the teeth due to abnormal accumulations of pigment-producing bacteria or certain dyes within foods. Because such stains affect only the surfaces rather than the substance of the teeth, they may be removed by tooth polishing during dental visits and may be prevented by regular, appropriate tooth cleaning and hygiene.

The following organizations in the General Resources Section can provide additional information: NIH/National Institute of Child Health and Human Development

National Associations & Support Groups

1500 American Dental Association
211 East Chicago Avenue
Chicago, IL 60611   312-440-2500
                                www.ada.org

Professional assocation of dentists dedicated to serving both the profession of dentistry. Promotes the profession of dentistry by enhancing the integrity and ethics of the profession and strengthening the patient/dentist relationship. Fulfills its mission by providing services and through its initiatives in education, research, advocacy and the development of standards.

1501 National Institute of Dental Research
31 Ctr Dr Msc 2290 Bldg 31 Rm 2c35
Bethesda, MD 20892   301-496-4261
                                Fax: 301-496-9988
                                www.nih.gov/nichd

Provides leadership for a national program designed to understand, treat and prevent the infectious and inherited craniofacial-oral-dental diseases and disorders.

Web Sites

1502 Dental Consumer Advisory
www.toothinfo.com

1503 Dental Resources on the Web
www.dental-resources.com

DESCRIPTION

1504 DOWN SYNDROME

Synonyms: Chromosome 21, trisomy 21, Trisomy 21 syndrome

Disorder Type: Birth Defect, Chromosomal Disorder, Developmental Milestones

Covers these related disorders: Trisomy 21 mosaicism, Trisomy 21 translocation

Down syndrome, also known as trisomy 21 syndrome, is a chromosomal disorder that affects approximately one in 660 newborns. The disorder is considered the most common chromosomal abnormality syndrome. Cells of the body (with the exception of reproductive cells) typically contain 23 pairs of chromosomes that are numbered from 1 to 22. The 23rd pair consists of one X chromosome from the mother and an X or Y chromosome from the father. However, in infants with Down syndrome, all or a portion of chromosome 21 is present three times rather than twice in cells of the body (trisomy). In rare cases, a certain percentage of cells contain the extra chromosome 21, whereas other cells have the normal two. This finding is known as chromosomal mosaicism.

The symptoms and physical findings associated with Down syndrome vary in range and severity and depend in part on the exact location and the percentage of body cells containing the extra chromosome 21. Many infants with Down syndrome have abnormally diminished muscle tone (hypotonia), a tendency to keep the mouth open, protrusion of the tongue, excessive mobility of the joints (hyperextensibility), absence of certain reflexes (i.e., Moro reflex), and excessive skin on the back of the neck. Other characteristic abnormalities may include a relatively small, short head (microbrachycephaly); flattened facial features; upwardly slanting eyelid folds (palpebral fissures) and vertical skin folds that may cover the eyes' inner corners (epicanthal folds); a highly arched roof of the mouth (palate); a small nose and depressed nasal bridge; and small, misshapen ears. Abnormalities of the limbs may also be present, including unusually short arms and legs; short, broad hands; improper positioning of the fifth fingers (clinodactyly); abnormal skin ridge patterns on the fingers, hands, toes, and feet (dermatoglyphics); and a wide gap between the first and second toes. Patients also tend to have relatively short stature, progressive delays in the acquisition of skills requiring the coordination of physical and mental activities (psychomotor delays), poor coordination, an awkward manner of walking (gait), and varying levels of mental retardation.

Approximately 40 percent of infants with Down syndrome may also have heart defects at birth (congenital heart defects). In some patients, such heart defects may require surgical repair. In addition, some individuals with Down syndrome are prone to recurrent respiratory infections and chronic inflammation of the membranes that line the eyes and eyelids (conjunctivitis) or the nasal cavity (rhinitis). Treatment of individuals with Down syndrome includes symptomatic and supportive measures, such as possible surgical correction of congenital heart defects, special education, and other appropriate measures.

Down syndrome is usually the result of errors during the division of a parent's reproductive cells (meiosis). Increased maternal age (over 35 years of age) is an additional risk factor. In other cases, the disorder may result due to a chromosome 21 translocation that is transmitted by a parent or occurs sporadically (de novo). Translocations are chromosomal abnormalities in which pieces of two or more chromosomes break off and are rearranged, resulting in an altered set of chromosomes.

The following organizations in the General Resources Section can provide additional information: Genetic Alliance, March of Dimes Birth Defects Foundation, NIH/National Institute of Child Health and Human Development, Online Mendelian Inheritance in Man: www3.ncbi.nlm.nih.gov/Omim/searchomim.html

National Associations & Support Groups

1505 ARC

500 East Border Street, Suite 300
Arlington, TX 76010

512-454-6694
800-433-5255
Fax: 817-277-3491
TDD: 817-277-0553
e-mail: thearc@metronet.com
thearc.org/welcome.html

The ARC of the United States works through education, research and advocacy to improve the quality of life for children and adults with mental retardation and their families and works to prevent both the causes and the effects of mental retardation.

1506 Aleh Foundation

Aleh Institustions U.S.A
5317 13th Avenue
Brooklyn, NY 11219

718-851-4596
www.aleh.org

Founded in 1983, the Aleh Rehabilitation Center in Bnei Break has served close to 200 children with multiple, physical and mental disabilities with our wide range of services in an atmosphere of warmth and love.

1507 Association for Children with Down Syndrome

4 Fern Place
Plainview, NY 11803

516-933-4700
Fax: 516-933-9524
e-mail: info@aods.org
www.aods.org

Combines national information and research dissemination with direct services at the local level from US national library and also provides direct services for children with Down syndrome from birth to 5.

Sam Nussbaum, Executive Director

1508 Down Syndrome Guild

P.O. Box 821174
Dallas, TX 75382

214-239-8771

Disabled Children's Computer Group, and a major corporation consisting of parents, consumers and professionals. It is one of the nation's largest resources to help children and adults who have disabilities gain access to the benefits of technology. Includes nationwide network of community-based assistive technology, resource centers, hands on consultants and product demonstrations.

1509 National Association for Down Syndrome

PO Box 4542
Oak Brook, IL 60522

www.nads.org

1510 National Down Syndrome Congress

7000 Peachtree-Dunwoody Rd
Atlanta, GA 30328

770-604-9500
800-232-6372
Fax: 770-604-9898
e-mail: ndsscenter@aol.com
www.carol-net/@ndsc/

Creates a national climate in which all persons will recognize and embrace the value and dignity of persons with Down syndrome. Promotes the availability of and accessibility to a full range of opportunities that meet family needs, builds a sense of community and fellowship for all persons concerned with Down syndrome, provides a network for linking over 500 parent groups and organizations which serve the needs of families, offers a journal, educational books and resources and a hotline.

Frank J. Murphy, Executive Director

1511 National Down Syndrome Society

666 Broadway, 8th Fl
New York, NY 10012

212-460-9330
800-221-4602
Fax: 212-979-2873
e-mail: info@ndss.org
www.ndss.org

Established in 1979 with the goals of promoting research, education and advocacy for individuals with Down syndrome and their families. NDSS works to obtain a better understanding of Down syndrome, the potential of people with Down syndrome, to support research about the condition, and to provide information and referral services for families and professionals.

Elizabeth F. Goodwin, President

1512 National Early Childhood Technical Assistance System

University of North Carolina, Chapel Hill
CB#8040, 500 NCNB Plaza
Chapel Hill, NC 27599

919-962-2001

Assists states and other entities in developing comprehensive services for children with special needs through the age of eight and their families.

1513 National Information Center for Children and Youth with Disabilities
P.O. Box 1492
Washington, DC 20013   202-884-8200
                            800-695-0285
mcrcr2.med.nyu.edu/murphp01/homenew.htm

Information clearinghouse that provides free information on disabilities and disability-related issues. Provides personal responses to questions on disability issues including early intervention, special education programs, and family, legal and adult transitional issues.

1514 Parents of Down Syndrome Children
11600 Nebel Street
Rockville, MD 20852   301-984-5792
                           Fax: 301-816-2429

Activities include formal and informal meetings, parent-to-parent counseling, contacting new parents of Down syndrome children to offer support and information on community resources, providing information on doctors, hospitals and professionals.

International

1515 National Center for Down Syndrome
9 Westbourne Rd
Edg Baston, Birmingham,
United Kingdom

State Agencies & Support Groups

Alabama

1516 Down Syndrome Clinic, Children's Hospital of Alabama
1600 7th Avenue South
Birmingham, AL 35233   205-939-9141
                           Fax: 205-975-6330

Dr. Diane K. Donley

Arizona

1517 Foundation for Children with Down Syndrome
17646 N Cave Creek Rd, Ste 152
Phoenix, AZ 85032   602-493-7688
                           Fax: 602-265-8216
                           www.ffcwds.org

California

1518 Children's Hospital Medical Center of Northern California
747 52nd Street
Oakland, CA 94609   510-428-3448

Dr. Richard Umansky

1519 Pediatric Disabilities Clinic, Down Syndrome Clinic
University of California Medical Center
400 Parnassus, Box 0374
San Francisco, CA 94143   415-476-2841

Dr. Lucy Crain

Illinois

1520 LaRabida Children's Hospital, Down Syndrome Clinic
65th & Lake Michigan
Chicago, IL 60649   773-363-6700
                           Fax: 773-363-7160

A clinic for children with Down syndrome where the medical problems and developmental status are reviewed.

Nancy Roizen, MD
Lynn Cunningham-Anderson

1521 Lutheran General Children's Medical Center
Nesset Center
1775 Ballard Road
Park Ridge, IL 60068   847-696-7344

Dr. Nancy Keck

Indiana

1522 Ann Whitehill Down Syndrome Program
James Whitcomb Riley Hospital for Children
702 Barnhill Drive, #1601
Indianapolis, IN 46202   317-631-5885
                           Fax: 317-274-4471

Dr. Marilyn Bell

Iowa

1523 Down Syndrome Clinic, Child & Young Adult Clinic
University Hospital School
100 Hawkins Drive
Iowa City, IA 52242   319-353-6900
                            Fax: 319-356-8284
                            www.uiowa.edu/uhs

Provides comprehensive health care and services
to people with disabilities of all ages and their
families through a combination of outpatient, inpatient, and community based programs. UHS
provides information, evaluation, treatment recommendations, and training related to aging
and disabilities. UHS provides both preservice
and inservice training programs for service
providers and others who provide services to individuals with disabilities.

Elayne Sexsmith, Assistant Administrator

Maryland

1524 Department of Pediatrics, University of Maryland
Down Syndrome Clinic
630 W. Fayette Street
Baltimore, MD 21201   410-328-2214
                            Fax: 410-328-3981

Dr. George Lentz, Jr.

1525 Kennedy Krieger Institute, Down Syndrome Clinic
707 N. Broadway
Baltimore, MD 21205   410-550-9000
                            Fax: 410-550-9292

Dr. George Capone

1526 Mt. Washington Pediatric Clinic
Down Syndrome Clinic
1708 W. Rogers Avenue
Baltimore, MD 21209   410-578-8600
                            Fax: 410-466-1715

Dr. Paul Rogers

1527 Parents of Children with Down Syndrome ARC of Montgomery County
11600 Nebel St
Rockville, MD 20852   301-984-5792

A support groups (PODS) for parents of children of all ages who have Down syndrome. They
train parents to provide individual support to
new parents. A new parent packet containing
helpful, relevant, accurate information is available.

Massachusetts

1528 Down Syndrome Program - Children's Hospital Boston
300 Longwood Avenue
Boston, MA 02115   617-735-6509
                          Fax: 617-735-7429

Dr. Allen Crocker

Minnesota

1529 Down Syndrome Clinic of Minneapolis Children's Medical Center
2525 Chicago Avenue South
Minneapolis, MN 55404   612-863-6957
                              Fax: 612-863-6953

Dr. Kim McConnell

Missouri

1530 Children's Mercy Hospital, Down Syndrome Clinic
2401 Gillham Road
Kansas City, MO 64108   816-234-3000
                              Fax: 816-842-6107

Dr. David Harris

1531 Down Syndrome Medical Clinic
Washington University Medical Center
400 S. Kingshighway Blvd.
St. Louis, MO 63110   314-454-6026

Dr. Arnold Strauss

New Hampshire

1532 Dartmouth Center for Genetics & Child Development
Down Syndrome Program
1 Medical Center Drive
Lebanon, NH 03756   603-650-7884
                          Fax: 603-650-8268

Dr. W. Carl Cooley

New Jersey

1533 Foundation for Children with Down Syndrome
355 Bennetts Mills Rd
Jackson, NJ 08527   732-833-1331
                                     www.ffcwds.org

New York

1534 Developmental Evaluation Clinic
Westchester Institute for Human Development
Westchester Medical Center
Valhalla, NY 10595   914-285-8178
                                     Fax: 914-285-1973

Dr. Taesun Chung

North Dakota

**1535 Children's Hospital Merit Care Down Syndrome
Service**
737 Broadway
Fargo, ND 58102   701-234-2568
                                     Fax: 701-234-6965

Dr. Guy Carter

Ohio

1536 Cincinnati Center for Developmental Disorders
Down Syndrome Clinic
Elland & Bethesda Avenues
Cincinnati, OH 45229   513-559-4691
                                     Fax: 513-559-9669

Dr. Bonnie Patterson

**1537 Clinical Genetics - Down Syndrome Children's
Hospital**
700 Children's Drive
Columbus, OH 43205   614-461-2663
                                     Fax: 614-460-7035

Dr. Anne Marie Sommer

1538 Down Syndrome Clinic, Department of Pediatrics
Medical College of Ohio, Health Center
Box 10008
Toledo, OH 43699   419-381-4000

Dr. Eileen Quinn

**1539 Down Syndrome Clinic, Rainbow Babies and
Children's Hospital**
2074 Abington Road
Cleveland, OH 44106   216-844-8260

Dr. Joanne Mortimer

Pennsylvania

1540 Children's Seashore House
Children's Hospital in Philadelphia
3405 Civic Center Blvd.
Philadelphia, PA 19104   215-590-1734

Dr. Ada Hayes

1541 Down Syndrome Center of Western Pennsylvania
3705 Fifth Avenue
Pittsburgh, PA 15213   412-692-7963
                                     Fax: 412-692-5723

Dr. William Cohen

1542 Down Syndrome Clinic
M.S. Hershey Medical Center, Division of Genetics
Box 850
Hershey, PA 17033   717-531-8414

Maria Mascari, PhD

Rhode Island

**1543 Child Development Center, Down Syndrome,
Inborn Errors of Metabolism Program**
Rhode Island Hospital
593 Eddy Street
Providence, RI 02903   401-444-8477
                                     Fax: 401-444-6115

Dr. Pueschel has been working in the fields of Down syndrome and Inborn Errors of Metabolism for more than thirty years. He has lectured on these subjects both in this country and abroad. Dr. Pueschel has published more than twenty five scientific papers and fifteen books.

S.M. Pueschel, MD, PhD, JD, MPH, Professor of Peds

Texas

1544 Down Syndrome Clinic - Texas
1935 Motor St., 4th Floor
Dallas, TX 75235   214-640-2357

Dr. Golder Wilson

Washington

1545 University of Washington - the Model Preschool Center for Children
Experimental Education Unit
CDMRC, WJ-10
Seattle, WA 98195   206-543-2100

Research Centers

1546 International Foundation for Genetic Research
500A Garden City Dr
Pittsburgh, PA 15146   412-823-6380
                        Fax: 412-373-7713
                        e-mail: tmf@pennet.com
                        www.pennet.com/chuckdet/index.html

Audio Video

1547 A Different Kind of Beginning
Association for Children with Down Syndrome
2616 Martin Avenue
Bellmore, Long Island, NY 11710   516-221-4700

Demonstrates the independence and capabilities of individuals with Down syndrome as seen in various settings from early intervention programs to adult employment.

1548 A New Set of Fears, a New Set of Hopes
Meyer Children's Rehabilitation Institute
Resource Center, 444 S. 44th St.
Omaha, NE 68131   402-559-7467
                        800-232-6372

Explores the way a family adjusts as they go through the life cycle with their child who has Down syndrome.

1549 A Special Love
Association for Children with Down Syndrome
2616 Martin Avenue
Bellmore, NY 11710   516-221-4700
                        Fax: 516-221-4311

A candid video of a 10 year old brother playing with his 6 year old sister with Down syndrome. The brother describes his perceptions of mental retardation and his feelings towards his sister.
4 minutes, b/w

D.B. Shalom, Editor

1550 Adaptation to the Initial Crisis
Lawren Productions
930 Pitner Avenue
Evanston, IL 60202   847-328-6700
                        800-421-2363

A family learns to adapt to the birth of a child with a handicap.

1551 Congratulations
New Challenges
96 Ogden Avenue
White Plains, NY 10605   914-287-0723

A film for parents which addresses some of the most commonly asked questions about raising a child with Down syndrome.

1552 Down Syndrome Preschool Program
Association for Children with Down Syndrome
2616 Martin Avenue
Long Island, NY 11710   516-221-4700

A look at preschool programs for children with Down syndrome birth to five years.

1553 Down Syndrome, See the Potential
Down Syndrome Association of Charlotte
7000 Peachtree Dunwood Road, Building 5 Suite 100
Atlanta, GA 30328   770-604-9500
                        Fax: 770-604-9898

Video highlighting the capability of children with Down syndrome.

1554 Gifts of Love
National Down Syndrome Society
666 Broadway Suite 800
New York, NY 10012   212-460-9330
     800-221-4602
     Fax: 212-979-2873
     e-mail: info@ndss.org
     www.ndss.org

Four families of children with Down syndrome talk about their feelings and experiences with their children, particularly during the first six years. All the children live at home and attend programs in their communities.

25 minutes

1555 Infant Motor Development: A Look At The Phases
Psychological Corporation, Order Service Center
P.O. Box 839954
San Antonio, TX 78283
     800-211-8378
     Fax: 800-232-1223

A video depicting development in and activities for infants birth through 12 months.

1556 New Expectations
Lawren Productions
930 Pitner Avenue
Evanston, IL 60202
     800-421-2363

Focuses on the emotional and technical aspects of Down syndrome. Highlights four persons at various life stages from infancy to adulthood in the areas of education and employment.

1557 Opportunities to Grow
National Down Syndrome Society
666 Broadway Suite 800
New York, NY 10012   212-460-9330
     800-221-4602
     Fax: 212-979-2873
     e-mail: info@ndss.org
     www.ndss.org

Sequel to Gifts of Love (separately listed) shows how people with Down syndrome, ages 6 to 26, participate equally in all phases of community life. Vignettes of 15 young men and women illustrate how inclusion, education, computer facilitation, socialization programs, and employment training help them to fulfill their potential.

25 minutes

1558 Stepping Stones
AIT
Box A
Bloomington, IN 47402
     800-457-4509

Series of video programs on teaching basic skills to at-risk, special needs and normally developed children.

Web Sites

1559 Pedbase
www.icondata.com/health/pedbase/files/DOWN-SYND.HTM

Books

1560 Adolescent with Down Syndrome
Down's Syndrome Association of Ontario
157 Hazlewood Drive
Whitby, Ontario, L1N 3L9, IT   905-619-0073

A book about teens and their families. Includes a study done of 90 families in England with a teenager with Down syndrome. Focuses on the range of skills, degree of independence, educational functions, friendships and more.

165 pages

Sue Buckley, Editor
Buckley Ben, Sacks

1561 Babies with Down Syndrome
Karen Stray-Gunderson, author

Woodbine House
6510 Bells Mill Road
Bethesda, MD 20817   301-468-8800
     800-843-7323
     Fax: 301-897-5838
     e-mail: info@woodbinehouse.com
     www.woodbinehouse.com

Praised as the finest book ever written for new parents, this book covers everything they need to know about rearing these beautiful and special children in a loving environment.

237 pages Softcover
ISBN: 0-933149-02-6

1562 Biomedical Concerns In Persons with Down Syndrome
Siegfried Pueschel, author

Paul H. Brookes Publishing Company
P.O. Box 10624
Baltimore, MD 21285   410-337-8539
     800-638-3775

Written by leading authorities and spanning many disciplines and specialties, this comprehensive resource provides vital information on biomedical issues concerning individuals with Down syndrome.

336 pages

1563 Communication Skills In Children with Down Syndrome

Libby Kumin, PhD, author

Woodbine House
6510 Bells Mill Road
Bethesda, MD 20817
301-468-8800
800-843-7323
Fax: 301-897-5838
e-mail: info@woodbinehouse.com
www.woodbinehouse.com

Offers parents a chance to learn what to expect as communication skills progress from infancy through early teenage years. Discussions are included on speech and language therapy, hearing problems, school performance and intelligibility issues.

150 pages Softcover
ISBN: 0-933149-53-0

1564 Count Us In: Growing Up with Down Syndrome

Mitchell Levitz, author

Harcourt Brace Jovanovich
6277 Sea Harbor Drive
Orlando, FL 32887
407-345-2000
Fax: 407-345-8388

1994 Softcover
ISBN: 0-156226-60-0

1565 Current Approaches to Down Syndrome

Greenwood Publishing Group, Inc.
88 Post Road West, P.O. Box 5007
Westport, CT 06880
203-226-3571
800-225-5800
Fax: 203-222-1502
e-mail: custserv@greenwood.com
www.greenwood.com

An exploration of current initiatives relating to Down syndrome in the medical, educational and social fields.

345 pages

David Lane, Editor
Lane Brian, Stratford

1566 Differences In Common: Straight Talk on Mental Retardation/Down Syndrome & Life

Marilyn Trainer, author

Woodbine House
6510 Bells Mill Road
Bethesda, MD 20817
301-468-8800
800-843-7323
Fax: 301-897-5838
e-mail: info@woodbinehouse.com
www.woodbinehouse.com

A collection of essays by the mother of an adult son who has Down syndrome. Focuses on mainstreaming, terminology, parent groups and advocacy.

M. Trainer, Editor

1567 Down Sydrome - Living and Learning in the Community

L. Nadel and D. Rosenthal, author

Books on Special Children
P.O. Box 305
Congers, NY 10920
914-638-1236
Fax: 914-638-0847

Four parents' personal observations, challenges of people with DS as they become integrated into community. Family role, cognitive development and acquisition of language, education, health care, idependent living arrangement.

1995 295 pages Hardcover
ISBN: 0-471034-13-4

1568 Down Syndrome - Advances in Medical Care

P.O.Box 305
Congers, NY 40920
606-638-1236
Fax: 606-638-0847
e-mail: bosc@j51.com
www.geocities.com/eureka/3830

Principles of development in Down syndrome. Clinical expression of the disorder, advances and update on endocrine disorders, advances and update on endocrine disorders and other specialties.

196 pages Hardcover
ISBN: 0-471561-81-9

1569 Down Syndrome - An Update and Review for Primary Care Physician's

Dartmouth-Hitchcock Medical Center
1 Medical Center Drive
Lebanon, NH 03756
603-650-5000

An excellent medical review of Down syndrome intended for physicians.

W.C. Cooley, Editor

1570 Down Syndrome: Advances In Medical Care
Books On Special Children
P.O. Box 305
Congers, NY 10920   914-638-1236
                           Fax: 914-638-0847

Discusses the principles of development in Down syndrome, clinical expressions of the disorder, advances and updates on endocrine disorders and other specialities.

196 pages Hardcover

I.T. Lott, Editor
Lott E., McCoy

1571 Down Syndrome: Birth to Adulthood
John Rynders & J. Margaret Horrobin, author

Love Publishing Company
9101 E. Kinyon Avenue
Denver, CO 80237   303-221-7333
                          Fax: 303-221-7444

Filled with photographs, this new book is an invaluable guide for parents of children with Down syndrome, as well as the professionals who help advance whole-family development. The authors, well known and respected leaders in the field, share case studies of families from the EDGE Project at the University of Minnesota, examining both large and small issues. Research findings from several sources are woven into pages in a clear, readable fashion, followed with numerous practical suggestions.

1995 356 pages Softcover
ISBN: 0-891082-36-0

1572 Down Syndrome: Living & Learning in the Community
Lynn Nadel & D Rosenthal, author

John Wiley & Sons
605 Third Avenue
New York, NY 10158   212-850-6000

1995 312 pages Softcover
ISBN: 0-471022-01-2

1573 Down Syndrome: The Facts
M. Selikowitz, author

Oxford University Press
2001 Evans Road
Cary, NC 27513   212-726-6000
                          800-451-7556
                          Fax: 212-726-6447
                          www.oup-usa.org

A book for parents who have a child with Down syndrome written by a pediatrician who works with Down syndrome children.

M. Selikowitz, Editor

1574 From 17 Months to 17 Years...A Look At Down Syndrome
Bonnie Lavender
RR-1, Box 102C
Richville, NY 13681   315-287-2973

Includes profiles of six families who have children with Down syndrome. Offers photographs and accompanying text that detail each family's experiences with Down syndrome.

B. Lavender, Editor
Lavender G.J., Lega

1575 Medical and Surgical Care for Children with Down Syndrome
D.C. Van Dyke, M.D., author

Woodbine House
6510 Bells Mill Road
Bethesda, MD 20817   301-468-8800
                          800-843-7323
                          Fax: 301-897-5838
                          e-mail: info@woodbinehouse.com
                          www.woodbinehouse.com

Provides detailed and easy-to-understand information for parents on a wide range of medical conditions and treatments including: heart disease, recurrent infections, thyroid problems, eye problems, skin conditions, ear, nose and throat problems, orthopedic conditions, leukemia, facial and dental concerns and neurological problems.

320 pages Softcover
ISBN: 0-933149-54-9

1576 Nursing Your Baby with Down Syndrome
Sarah Coulter Danner, author

Childbirth Graphics
P.O. Box 21207
Waco, TX 76702   254-755-6885

1577 Parent's Guide to Down Syndrome: Toward A Brighter Future

Siegfried M. Pueschel, author

Books on Special Children
P.O. Box 305
Congers, NY 10920   914-638-1236
                                     Fax: 914-638-0847

A comprehensive reference book especially for new parents but useful and informative to seasoned parents as well. Range of topics include a history of Down syndrome, physical characterisitcs, developmental expectations, early intervention, feeding the young child and the school years.

315 pages Softcover

1578 Parents of Down Syndrome Children
11600 Nebel Street
Rockville, MD 20852   301-984-5792

Activities include formal and informal meetings; parent-to-parent counseling; contacting new parents of Down syndrome children to offer support and information on community resources; providing information on doctors, hospitals and professionals.

1579 Screening for Down Syndrome

J.G. Grudzinskas, et al., author

Cambridge University Press
40 W. 20th Street
New York, NY 10011   212-924-3900
                                     Fax: 212-691-3239

*1995 286 pages
ISBN: 0-521452-71-6*

1580 Shattered Dreams - Lonely Choices: Birth Parents of Babies with Disabilities

Joanne Finnegan, author

Greenwood Publishing Group, Inc.
88 Post Road West, P.O. Box 5007
Westport, CT 06880   203-226-3571
                                     800-225-5800
                                     Fax: 203-222-1502
                                     e-mail: custserv@greenwood.com
                                     www.greenwood.com

Written by a mother who, without warning, gave birth to a boy with Down's Syndrome, this book is meant to help parents through the initial shock and the realization that they are not able to care for their child.

208 pages Hardcover

1581 Since Owen

Johns Hopkins University Press
701 West 40th Street
Baltimore, MD 21211   410-516-6960

A well written book displaying understanding from a veteran parent communicating with other parents of children with disabilities.

466 pages

Charles R. Callanan, Editor

1582 Teaching the Infant with Down Syndrome: A Guide for Parents and Professionals

Marci J. Hanson, author

8700 Shaol Creek Blvd.
Austin, TX 78757   512-451-3246
                                     800-897-3202
                                     Fax: 800-397-7633

A manual providing teaching ideas and activities that can be used to assist an infant's development.

*268 pages Large Format
ISBN: 0-890791-03-1*

1583 To Give An Edge: A Guide for New Parents of Children with Down Syndrome
Viking Press C/O Meg Colwell
7000 Washington Avenue South
Eden Prairie, MN 55435   612-941-8780

A guide for new parents designed to provide information about the disorder and how other parents of children with Down syndrome have coped.

J.E. Rynders, Editor
Rynders J.M., Horrobin

1584 Understanding Down Syndrome

Cliff Cunningham, author

Brookline Books/Lumen Editions
P.O. Box 1047
Cambridge, MA 02238   617-868-0360
                                     800-666-2665
                                     Fax: 617-868-1772
                                     e-mail: brooklinebks@delphi.com
                                     www.people.delphi.com/brooklinebks

The author provides answers and explanations to the countless questions directed to him during his twenty years' involvement with Down syndrome individuals and their families.

*Softcover
ISBN: 1-571290-09-5*

Children's Books

1585 Cara: Growing with a Retarded Child

M.M. Jablow, author

Temple University Press
USB Room 305, Broad & Oxford
Philadelphia, PA 19122   215-204-8787

The author offers information and experiences
on raising her daughter, Cara, who has Down
syndrome.

Newsletters

1586 Down Syndrome News

National Down Syndrome Congress
7000 Peachtree Dunwood Road, Building 5 Suite 100
Atlanta, GA 30328   770-604-9500
                           Fax: 770-604-9898

Contains book reviews, articles and items of interest to those touched by Down syndrome.

10x Annually

Frank J. Murphy, Executive Director

1587 Down Syndrome Today

Down Syndrome Today Publications
P.O. Box 212
Holtsville, NY 11742   516-654-3242

Offers information, articles, resources and materials for the parent and professional working
and nurturing patients and persons with Downs
syndrome.

Debra Hoeft, Publisher

1588 Exceptional Parent Magazine

209 Harvard Street
Brookline, MA 02146   617-730-5800
                             Fax: 617-730-8742

A publication dealing with many issues affecting
exceptional children and their families.

Monthly

1589 National Down Syndrome Society Update

666 Broadway
New York, NY 10012   212-460-9330
                            800-221-4602

Offers information on the activities of the society, new breakthroughs in medical technology,
articles offering state of the art information to
families and individuals with Down syndrome,
and answers to questions about the illness.

12 pages Quarterly

Fran Goldstein, Editor

Pamphlets

1590 Alzheimer's Disease and Down Syndrome

Ira T. Lott, MD, author

National Down Syndrome Society
666 Broadway
New York, NY 10012   212-460-9330
                            800-221-4602
                            e-mail: info@ndss.org
                            www.ndss.org

1995

1591 Down Syndrome

March of Dimes Resource Center
1275 Mamaroneck Avenue
White Plains, NY 10605   888-663-4637
                                Fax: 914-997-4763

1592 Life Planning and Down Syndrome

Janet S. Brown, MSW, ACSW, author

National Down Syndrome Society
666 Broadway
New York, NY 10012   212-460-9330
                            800-221-4602
                            Fax: 212-979-2873
                            e-mail: info@ndss.org
                            www.ndss.org

1593 New Parents

Association for Children with Down Syndrome
2616 Martin Avenue
Bellmore, Long Island, NY 11710   516-221-4700
                                         Fax: 516-221-4311

A bibliography compiled for parents who have
just given birth to a child with Down syndrome.

**1594 Speech and Language Skills in Children and Adults
with Down Syndrome**

Libby Kumin, MD, CCC-SLP, author

National Down Syndrome Society
666 Broadway
New York, NY 10012   212-460-9330
                             800-221-4602
                        Fax: 212-979-2873
                    e-mail: info@ndss.org
                         www.ndss.org

1995

DESCRIPTION

1595 DYSLEXIA

Disorder Type: Developmental Milestones

Dyslexia refers to a specific learning disability characterized by the impaired ability to process written symbols. Although individuals with dyslexia are able to see and recognize letters, this disorder impairs their ability to read, write, and spell. Affected individuals typically have no problems with the correct recognition of pictures and objects.

Young children with dyslexia may have difficulty remembering the correct names of letters and numbers. Articulating proper speech may be difficult. Some children of school age may reverse letters and words when writing. For example, affected children may substitute the letter p for q or the word was for saw, while transposing letters so that bets may become best. Children with dyslexia may also have difficulty reading due to an impaired ability to determine the sequence of letters within words and to distinguish right from left. The hallmark of this learning disability is the fact that, despite the difficulties associated with dyslexia, affected children are of average or above average intelligence as evidenced by I.Q. testing as well as their success in other scholastic achievements.

Early diagnosis of dyslexia is an important factor in treating this learning disability. Children nearing the end of first grade who exhibit difficulties with word skills or any children whose reading and writing ability is not commensurate with that of their other scholastic abilities may be tested for dyslexia. Although dyslexia is not related to eye defects, an ophthalmologic evaluation is beneficial in determining if ocular abnormalities may be eliminated as a cause of symptoms. Also, eye irregularities may be present in addition to dyslexia and, therefore, may be diagnosed and corrected at that time. Treatment for dyslexia is geared toward remedial teaching techniques specific to this disability.

Dyslexia is thought to be a familial disorder that may be inherited through an autosomal dominant trait. Boys are more frequently affected than girls.

The following organizations in the General Resources Section can provide additional information: NIH/National Institute of Child Health and Human Development, National Organization for Rare Disorders, Inc. (NORD), Genetic Alliance, March of Dimes Birth Defects Foundation

National Associations & Support Groups

1596 Association for Children and Adults with Learning Disabilities, Inc.
4156 Library Rd
Pittsburgh, PA 15234   412-341-1515

1597 Dyslexia Research Institute
4745 Centerville Rd
Tallahassee, FL 32308   850-893-2216
Fax: 850-893-2440
e-mail: pathard@aol.com
www.dyslexia-add.org

1598 National Network of Learning Disabled Adults
P.O. Box Z
Station Commerce, TX 75428   214-886-5937

1599 Orton Dyslexia Society
8600 La Salle Rd, Chester Bldg
Baltimore, MD 21286   301-296-0232
800-222-3123
Fax: 410-321-5069
e-mail: info@interdyx.org
www.pie.org/ods

Dyslexia is a neurological disorder that impairs reading. If undetected in children, it can create major learning problems.

Conferences

1600 International Dyslexia Association 50th Anniversary Conference
The Marriott
Chicago, IL
800-222-3123

Nov. 3-6, 2000

Dyslexia/Audio Video

Audio Video

1601 Dyslexia
Fanlight Productions
47 Halifax St
Boston, MA 02130   617-469-4999
Fax: 617-469-3379
e-mail: fanlight@fanlight.com
www.fanlight.com

Looks at the experiences of people with these
learning disabilities as well as the potential
value to society of their alternative ways of
learning. Dartmouth Hitchcock Medical Center
Series, The Doctor is In...

28 minutes

Web Sites

1602 British Dyslexia Association
www.inclusive.co.uk/support/bda.htm

1603 Davis Dyslexia Association
www.dyslexia.com

1604 International Dyslexia Association
http://interdys.org

1605 Mental Health Net
www.chmc.com/guide/dyslexia.htm

**1606 National Institute of Child Health and Human
Development**
www.cmhc.com/factsfam/dyslexia.htm

Books

**1607 How to Teach Your Dyslexic Child to Read: A
Proven Method for Parents and Teachers**
Bernice H. Baumer, author

Active Parenting Publishers
810 Franklin Court, Suite B
Marietta, GA 30067

800-825-0060
Fax: 770-429-0334
www.activeparenting.com

Easy-to-use instructional book with pictures,
charts and word lists for kindergarten through
grade three.

160 pages

**1608 Overcoming Dyslexia in Children, Adolescents, and
Adults**
8700 Shoal Creek Blvd.
Austin, TX 78757

800-897-3202
Fax: 800-397-7633

The second edition summarizes what science
knows today about what causes the forms of dyslexia that are related to left-brain language processing. This book also discusses in detail
nonverbal types of learning disabilities (LD) and
social and emotional types of LD. All forms of
dyslexia are described in detail with graphic illustrations of how dyslexia impacts classroom
learning, social behavior, emotional maturity
and development.

367 pages Softcover
ISBN: 0-890796-42-4

248

DESCRIPTION

1609 DYSTONIA

Disorder Type: Neuromuscular
Covers these related disorders: Dopa-responsive dystonia (DRD) or Segawa syndrome, Drug-induced dystonia, Dystonia musculorum deformans (DMD) or torsion, Fecal dystonia
May involve these systems in the body (see Section III):
 Nervous System

Dystonia is a neurologic movement disorder characterized by relatively slow, involuntary, writhing motions that may result in twisting or distorted posturing of affected muscles. The abnormal motions associated with dystonia result from unusually increased muscle rigidity due to simultaneous contractions of certain muscles termed agonists and antagonists. When voluntary movements occur, there are usually coordinated contractions and simultaneous relaxations of several muscles. Muscles known as agonists are primarily responsible for producing a particular movement, and other muscles, called synergists, contract to assist the agonist muscles. While these muscles contract, other muscles known as antagonists normally simultaneously relax, helping to ensure smooth rather than jerky, uncoordinated motions. However, in patients with dystonia, agonist and antagonist muscles simultaneously contract, resulting in abnormally distorted movements. Depending upon the form of dystonia present, abnormal motions may vary greatly in severity and may be limited to one muscle group or may affect many muscles of the body, causing severely distorted postures and significantly interfering with activities of daily living.

 Dystonias that are limited to certain specific muscle groups may be referred to as focal dystonias. Focal dystonias may be confined to muscles of the neck (cervical dystonia or spasmodic torticollis); the eyelids, causing near or complete closure of the eyelids (blepharosposm) and functional blindness;

the mouth and jaw (buccomandibular dystonia); the hand (writer's cramp); or certain other areas of the body. Although such conditions are considered the most prevalent forms of dystonia, they occur much more commonly in adults than children. The main causes of dystonia during childhood include certain genetic disorders, including dystonia musculorum deformans, dopa-responsive dystonia, Wilson disease, or Hallervorden-Spatz disease; lack of oxygen during labor, delivery, or immediately after birth (perinatal asphyxia), causing brain damage (hypoxicischemic encephalopathy); or exposure to particular medications.

The most pronounced form of dystonia is observed in a group of genetic disorders known as dystonia musculorum deformans (DMD) or torsion dystonia. One form of the disorder is thought to most commonly affect individuals of Eastern European Ashkenazi Jewish descent. Symptoms typically become apparent between the ages of six to 14 years and initially include involuntary movement or posturing of one area of the body, particularly the foot. Most patients first experience abnormal periodic bending of one foot with the toes downward (plantar flexion), potentially causing tip-toe walking. Such posturing of the foot gradually becomes constant, and muscles in other areas of the body, such as the shoulders, pelvis, and spine, begin to develop periodic, involuntary, spasmodic, twisting movements. With disease progression, spasms become frequent and, eventually, are ongoing, causing contortion and severely distorted posturing of affected muscles. Although dystonic movements may initially subside during sleep, they may eventually be present at all times, severely restricting activities of daily living and causing a high level of functional disability. Treatment may include administration of the drug trihexyphenidyl or certain other medications, such as carbamazepine, bromocriptine, levodopa, or diazepam.

 Dopa-responsive dystonia (DRD), also known as Segawa syndrome, is a genetic disorder that is thought to be transmitted as an autosomal dominant trait. The disorder more commonly affects females and usually becomes apparent between four to eight years of age. Initial symptoms often include periodic, involuntary stiffening and abnormal posturing of the foot. As the disease progresses, dystonia may also eventually affect muscles of the arms, torso, and, in some patients, the neck. Within about four to five years, all areas of the body are usually affected. Some patients may also have unusually slow movements (bradykinesia) and involuntary, rhythmic movements (tremors) of certain muscles while at rest. Symptoms usually subside with sleep and gradually worsen during the day. Administration of the medication levodopa, a biological forerunner or precursor of the neurotransmitter dopamine, typically causes a dramatic improvement of symptoms.

Wilson disease is an autosomal recessive disorder in which copper metabolism causes an abnormal accumulation of copper in the liver, brain, kidneys, corneas, and other tissues of the body. The disorder is often characterized by progressive liver disease, degenerative changes of the brain, kidney failure, and the presence of characteristic grayish-green or reddish-gold rings at the outer margins of the corneas (Kayser-Fleischer rings). Neurologic symptoms, which rarely become apparent before age 10, are thought to result from progressive involvement of a region of the brain that assists in regulating muscular movements (basal ganglia). Such symptoms usually initially include progressive dystonia that is characterized by abnormalities of muscle tone, muscle stiffness and rigidity, muscle spasms, and abnormal movement patterns and fixed postures, such as a fixed smile due to drawing back of the upper lip. Patients also experience involuntary, rhythmic, quivering movements of the extremities on one side of the body (unilateral) that eventually become generalized and disabling. The treatment of patients with Wilson disease often consists of administration of penicillamine, a medication that binds with copper and enables it to be excreted from the body; supplementation of vitamin B6; and a diet that is low in copper intake (less than one mg/day). Hallervorden-Spatz disease is a rare autosomal recessive disorder characterized by an abnormal accumulation of iron pigment in certain areas of the brain.

Symptoms usually develop during childhood and may include progressive dystonia characterized by muscle stiffness, rigidity, and relatively slow, involuntary, twisting and distorted posturing of affected muscles. By adolescence, patients may have restricted movements of certain muscles due to increased muscle rigidity (spasticity); an inability to coordinate voluntary movements (ataxia); difficulty speaking (dysarthria); and progressive confusion, disorientation, and deterioration of intellectual abilities (dementia). The treatment of patients with Hallervorden-Spatz disease is symptomatic and supportive.

In some children, the administration of certain drugs may cause a sudden (acute) development of dystonia, such as certain antiseizure (anticonvulsant) medications or antipsychotic drugs (phenothiazines). In addition, particular medications may cause acute or chronic progressive dystonia, such as the antiseizure medications phenytoin or carbamazepine, or the antipsychotic drug haloperidol. Treatment may include the withdrawal of the offending drug and intravenous administration of the medication diphenhydramine.

Depending upon its underlying cause or specific form, treatment measures for chronic dystonia may include the administration of certain medications (anticholinergic agents), such as trihexyphenidyl or ethopropazine. These drugs inhibit the transmission of particular nerve impulses to muscles. In addition, focal dystonias, such as dystonia limited to muscles of the neck (cervical dystoniodic torticollis), are often treated with periodic injections of botulin (botulinum toxin) into affected muscles. Botulin is a bacterial toxin that blocks the release of a particular neurotransmitter (acetylcholine), resulting in temporary paralysis and thus relief from discomfort and disability associated with muscle rigidity.

The following organizations in the General Resources Section can provide additional information: National Organization for Rare Disorders, Inc. (NORD), Genetic Alliance, March of Dimes Birth Defects Foundation, NIH/Office of Rare Diseases, NIH/National Institute of Neurological Disorders & Stroke, Online Mendelian Inheritance in Man:

www3.ncbi.nlm.nih.gov/Omim/searchomim.html

National Associations & Support Groups

1610 Dystonia Medical Research Foundation
One E Wacker Dr, Ste 2430
Chicago, IL 60601   312-755-0198
                    Fax: 312-803-0138
     e-mail: dystonia@dystonia-foundation.org/
              www.dystonia-foundation.org/

1611 Muscular Dystrophy Association
3300 E Sunrise Dr
Tuscon, AZ 85718   520-529-2000
          e-mail: mda@mdausa.org
              www.mdausa.org

Dedicated to supplying the general public with the knowledge to properly assess and choose their doctors and medical facilities.

1612 National Institute of Neurological Disorders & Stroke
31 Center Dr MSC 2540, Bldg 31, Rm 8806
Bethesda, MD 20892   301-496-5751
                          800-352-9424
                    Fax: 301-402-2186
                    www.ninds.nih.gov

Supports and conducts research and research training on the normal structure and function of the nervous system and on the causes, prevention, diagnosis and treatment of nervous system disorders including stroke, epilepsy, multiple sclerosis, Parkinson's disease, head and spinal cord injury, Alzheimer's disease and brain tumors.

1613 Society for Muscular Dystrophy Association
P.O. Box 479
Bridgewater, NS Canada, B4V   902-685-3961
                    Fax: 902-685-3962
          e-mail: smdi@auracom.com

1614 Worldwide Education and Advocacy for Movement Disorders
204 E 84th St
New York, NY 10024   212-241-8567
                          800-437-6682
          e-mail: wemove@wemove.org
                    www.wemove.org

Research Centers

1615 Dystonia Medical Research Foundation
One East Wacker Drive, Ste 2430
Chicago, IL 60601   312-755-0198
                    Fax: 312-803-0138
     e-mail: dystonia@dystonia-foundation.org
              www.dystonia-foundation.org/

It is dedicated to serving people with dystonia, a neurological disorder. The goals of the Foundation are to advance research into the causes of and treatments for dystonia; to build awareness of dystonia in both the medical and lay communities; and to sponsor patient and family support groups and programs.

Web Sites

1616 MHG Neurology Web Forums
http://neuro-www.mgh.harvard.edu/forum

Newsletters

1617 Dystonia Dialgoue
Dystonia Medical Research Foundation
One East Wacker Drive, Ste 2430
Chicago, IL 60601   312-755-0198
                    Fax: 312-803-0138
     e-mail: dystonia@dystonia-foundation.org
              www.dystonia-foundation.org/

Is the official publication of the Dystonia Medical Research Foundation. It is published quarterly to provide information to individuals with dystonia, their families, health care professionals, and supporters of the Foundation.

Quarterly

DESCRIPTION

1618 ECTODERMAL DYSPLASIAS

Disorder Type: Birth Defect, Genetic Disorder
May involve these systems in the body (see Section III):
Dermatologic System

Ectodermal dysplasias are a group of inherited disorders that are apparent at birth (congenital) and are characterized by abnormalities of the teeth, hair, nails, skin glands (i.e., eccrine and sebaceous glands), the skin, nervous system, ears and eyes, or the delicate mucous membranes that line the mouth and the anus. Ectodermal dyplasia is an integral part of several different syndromes that include anhidrotic ectodermal dysplasia, hidrotic ectodermal dysplasia, and EEC syndrome.

Anhidrotic ectodermal dysplasia, also known as hypohidrotic ectodermal dyplasia or Christ-Siemens-Touraine syndrome, is usually inherited as an X-linked recessive trait that is fully expressed in boys; however, some children may inherit this disorder as an autosomal recessive trait that affects boys and girls in equal numbers. Anhidrotic ectodermal dysplasia is characterized by absent (aplastic) or underdeveloped (hypoplastic) sweat glands, dental irregularities such as absent or widely-spaced, cone-shaped teeth, and sparse hair (hypotrichosis) that is light in color. Characteristic facial features may include a large chin; thick lips; bulging forehead (frontal bossing); flat nasal bridge; prominent, low-set ears; wrinkled, dark skin around the eyes; and other facial irregularities. Other findings may include light-colored, dry, and wrinkled skin that peels easily. Occasionally, children with anhidrotic ectodermal dysplasia have certain irregularities of the eyes such as cataracts, and abnormalities of the ears that can result in hearing loss. Affected children may be at increased risk for gastrointestinal infections as well as potentially life-threatening respiratory infections. Other life-threatening findings may include abnormally elevated body temperature coupled with an inability to sweat. Treatment for this disorder is preventive, cosmetic, symptomatic, and supportive. For example, parents and caregivers are counseled to protect children from high environmental temperatures. In addition, intervention for teeth and eye irregularities may include evaluation and treatment with dental appliances (e.g., bridgework, implants) and other dental and ocular corrective measures.

Hidrotic ectodermal dysplasia, also known as Clouston's syndrome, is inherited as an autosomal dominant trait. This form of the disorder is characterized by defective or absent nails, thickening of the skin on the palms of the hands and soles of the feet (palmar/plantar hyperkeratosis), and sparse hair. Other occasional findings may include abnormally increased coloration of the skin over major joints and the development of unusually small teeth that are prone to decay. Treatment is symptomatic and supportive.

EEC syndrome, also called ectrodactyly-ectodermal dysplasia-clefting syndrome, is inherited as an autosomal dominant trait. Symptoms and physical findings associated with this disorder are variable and may include lightly-pigmented skin, sparse hair and eyebrows, absent eyelashes, a split or opening (cleft) in the lip and palate, defective nails, tear duct irregularities, and absence of all or part of one or more fingers or toes (ectrodactyly). Other findings may include deafness and irregularities of the teeth, eyes, and urinary tract. Treatment is symptomatic and supportive.

The following organizations in the General Resources Section can provide additional information: Genetic Alliance, March of Dimes Birth Defects Foundation, NIH/National Institute of Arthritis and Musculoskeletal and Skin Diseases, Online Mendelian Inheritance in Man: www3.ncbi.nlm.nih.gov/Omim/searchomim.html

National Associations & Support Groups

1619 ARC
500 East Border Street, Suite 300
Arlington, TX 76010   817-261-6003
                             800-433-5255
                         Fax: 817-277-3491
                         TTY: 817-277-0553
               e-mail: thearc@metronet.com
                    thearc.org/welcome.html

The ARC of the United States works through
education, research and advocacy to improve
the quality of life for children and adults with
mental retardation and their families and works
to prevent both the causes and the effects of mental retardation.

1620 American Dental Association
211 East Chicago Avenue
Chicago, IL 60611   312-440-2500
                             www.ada.org

Professional association of dentists dedicating to
serving both the public and the professoin of
dentistry. Promotes the profession of dentistry
by enhancing the integrity and ethics of the profession and strengthening the patient/dentist relationship. Fulfills its mission by providing
services and through its initiatives in education,
research, advocacy and the development of
standards.

**1621 HED Hypohidrotic Ectodermal Dysplasia
Foundation & Related Disorders**
P.O. Box 9421
Hampton, VA 23670

1622 National Foundation for Ectomdermal Dysplasias
219 East Main Street PO Box 114
Mascoutah, IL 62258   618-566-2020
                         Fax: 618-566-4718
     e-mail: nfed1@aol.com and nfed2@aol.com
                             www.nfed.org

Disseminates information on this and related diseases for people of any age to access and use in
everyday life situations.

1623 National Institute of Dental Research
31 Ctr Dr Msc 2290 Bldg 31 Rm 2c35
Bethesda, MS 20892   301-496-4261
                         Fax: 301-496-9988
                         www.nidr.nih.gov/

Provides leadership for a national research program designed to understand, treat and prevent
the infectious and inherited craniofacial-oral-
dental diseases and disorders.

Web Sites

1624 American Dental Association
211 East Chicago Avenue
Chicago, IL 60611   312-440-2500
                             www.ada.org

Professional association of dentists dedicated to
serving both the public and the profession of
densitry. Promotes the profession of denstiry by
enhancing the integrity and ethics of the profession and strengthening the patient/dentist relationship. Fulfills its mission by providing
services and through its initiatives in education,
research, advocacy and the development of
standards.

1625 Dental Consumer Advisory
www.toothinfo.com

1626 Dental Resources on the Web
www.dental-resources.com

DESCRIPTION

1627 ECZEMA

Synonym: Eczematous dermatitis

Covers these related disorders: Allergic contact dermatitis, Atopic dermatitis, Dyshidrosis, Irritant contact dermatitis, Seborrheic dermatitis

May involve these systems in the body (see Section III):

Dermatologic System

Eczema is a common inflammatory condition of the skin (dermatitis) characterized by redness, itching, blistering, and oozing of affected areas. As the condition progresses, the skin often becomes abnormally dry and may scale, crust over, thicken, or develop increased or decreased areas of coloration. There are several different types of eczema that may be caused by various internal or external factors. Children are mostly affected by certain forms of the condition, including atopic dermatitis, irritant and allergic contact dermatitis, seborrheic dermatitis, or dyshidrosis.

Approximately two to eight percent of children develop atopic dermatitis, which is the most common form of childhood eczema. Also known as infantile eczema when it occurs during childhood, this form of eczema is characterized by an excessive immune response to particular substances that the body perceives as foreign (sensitizing antigen). Such responses, known as allergic or hypersensitive reactions, occur upon exposure to previously encountered, usually environmental substances (allergens). Patients with atopic dermatitis are thought to have an inherited tendency toward allergy. This may be supported by the fact that many affected infants and children later develop additional conditions due to exposure to certain allergens, particularly inflammation of the nose's mucous membranes (allergic rhinitis) and inflammation and narrowing of the airways (asthma).

Atopic dermatitis usually begins during the first year of life, and up to 90 percent of patients are affected by five years of age. The disorder often occurs with the introduction of particular foods into a child's diet, such as wheat, cow's milk, soy, eggs, or peanuts. Although atopic dermatitis tends to subside with advancing age, the condition may recur over many years before completely disappearing. Atopic dermatitis is characterized by the development of reddish, inflamed, intensely itchy (pruritic) patches that rapidly begin to ooze and crust over. During infancy, the condition usually initially affects the skin of the cheeks and gradually extends to involve the rest of the face; the neck, abdomen, wrists, and hands; the inside of the elbows; behind the knees; or other areas. Due to intense itching, infants may rub affected areas against their crib, their clothes, or other surfaces in an attempt to obtain relief. Secondary bacterial infections may occur as the result of the repeated rubbing or scratching. Over time, skin areas may become dry and scaly and develop changes in color. In addition, the skin may thicken, accentuating skin lines and causing an unusual, "bark-like" skin appearance (lichenification).

The treatment of atopic dermatitis may include measures to eliminate or avoid certain factors that may worsen the condition, such as certain foods, extremes of humidity and temperature, detergents or soaps, or potentially abrasive textures, such as wool. Affected children should be dressed in garments with smooth textures, such as cotton; their fingernails should be kept as short as possible to discourage scratching; and excessive bathing should be avoided. Adding bath oil to bath water and applying moisturizing lotions and creams to damp skin after bathing may help to alleviate some symptoms. In addition, when inflammation is severe, the application of wet dressings may reduce inflammation and associated itching. Treatment may also include the use of topical medicated skin creams and ointments, such as corticosteroid preparations, as well as certain medications such as oral antihistamines to help reduce itching. Secondary bacterial infections are treated with appropriate antibiotics.

Contact dermatitis, another common form of eczema, is a skin inflammation that is typically confined to a particular area and may have clearly defined boundaries. This disorder is often subdivided into irritant and allergic contact dermatitis. Irritant contact dermatitis is a skin inflammation caused by repetitive or prolonged exposure to certain substances that damage the skin. Allergic contact dermatitis is a hypersensitive, inflammatory response of the skin due to exposure to a previously encountered substance (allergen).

Irritant contact dermatitis may be caused by repetitive or prolonged exposure to certain soaps or detergents, citrus juices, saliva, bubble bath, or other substances. In many infants, saliva from drooling may cause inflammation of the skin of the face and neck folds. Diaper dermatitis is another common form of irritant contact dermatitis. Affected infants may develop reddish, scaling, blistering skin inflammation and secondary bacterial infections due to prolonged contact with waste materials, diaper soaps, and topical skin lotions. The treatment of irritant contact dermatitis includes removal or avoidance of the responsible irritants and administration of topical corticosteroid creams or ointments. In addition, affected areas should be carefully, regularly washed with warm water and a mild soap. To help prevent diaper dermatitis, physicians may recommend frequent changing of diapers; gentle, thorough cleansing of genitals with warm water and mild soaps and application of mild protective topical preparations during the diaper changes; or use of disposable diapers with absorbent materials.

Allergic contact dermatitis is characterized by a hypersensitive or allergic response to previously encountered allergens. Common causes include metal compounds in jewelry; particular plants, such as poison ivy, poison oak, or poison sumac; medications in skin creams, such as certain antibiotic- or antihistamine-containing creams; shoes; or clothing. Patients may develop intensely itchy, reddish, blistering skin inflammations that may later develop scaling, cracking, (fissuring), changes in color, or an abnormal thickened, bark-like appearance. Treatment includes removal or avoidance of the allergen and application of cool compresses, corticosteroid ointments or oral medications, antihistamine medications, and antibiotic therapy for secondary bacterial infections.

Seborrheic dermatitis is a chronic inflammatory disorder of unknown cause that may occur at any age and may appear to follow the distribution of sebaceous glands in skin tissue. These relatively small glands, which open into hair follicles, produce an oily secretion known as sebum that helps to lubricate the hair and skin and protect the skin from drying. In children, the condition most commonly occurs during infancy. Affected infants may initially develop localized or widespread crusting and scaling of the scalp, known as cradle cap. In some patients, this may be the only finding of the condition. Other infants may develop reddish, greasy, scaling patches that may be localized or may spread to affect most of the body. Affected areas often include the face, behind the ears, the neck, the diaper region, or under the arms. Patients may experience associated itching, hair loss, or changes in skin color. Treatment may include the use of special antiseborrheic shampoos or the application of wet compresses or topical corticosteroid creams or ointments.

Dyshidrosis, also known as pompholyx, is another form of eczema that may occur during childhood. This is a recurrent, potentially seasonal blistering condition that affects the palms of the hands and soles of the feet. The condition is initially characterized by recurrent crops of severely itchy blisters. Affected skin areas gradually become abnormally thickened and may have areas of cracking (fissuring). Many patients also experience excessive sweating (hyperhidrosis) in affected areas and may develop secondary bacterial infections due to scratching. Because this is typically a recurrent condition, patients should take appropriate measures to protect their hands and feet from harsh soaps, chemicals, the effects of excessive sweating or adverse weather, or other potential triggering factors. Treatment may include the application of wet dressings, topical corticosteroid ointments or creams, or mild topical preparations that promote skin softening and peeling (keratolytic agents) and the administration of antibiotics to treat secondary bacterial infections.

The following organizations in the General Resources Section can provide additional information: NIH/National Institute of Allergy and Infectious Diseases, NIH/National Institute of Arthritis and Musculoskeletal and Skin Diseases

National Associations & Support Groups

1628 Alergy Information Association
25 Poynter Drive Suite 7
Weston, Ontario, M9R
Canada

1629 Eczema Association for Science and Education
1211 SW Yanhill, Ste. 303
Portland, OR 97205   503-228-4430

Offers research and information to persons with eczema and other skin disorders.

1630 National Eczema Society
163 Eversholt Street
London,
United Kingdom

Pamphlets

1631 Eczema/Atopic Dermatitis
American Academy of Dermatology
930 N Meacham Road
Schaumberg, IL 60173   847-330-0230
                              Fax: 847-330-0050
                              www.aad.org

Explains how to recognize and treat dermatitis.
1995

1632 Hand Eczema
American Academy of Dermatology
930 N Meacham Road
Schaumberg, IL 60173   847-330-0230
                              Fax: 847-330-0050
                              www.aad.org

Shows examples of hand rashes, explains causes, lists protective measures and treatments.
1993

DESCRIPTION

1633 EHLERS-DANLOS SYNDROME

Disorder Type: Genetic Disorder
May involve these systems in the body (see Section III):
Connective Tissue

Ehlers-Danlos syndrome is a group of hereditary connective tissue disorders characterized by abnormalities of collagen, the major structural protein in the body. At least 10 forms of the disorder have been identified based upon underlying biochemical and genetic abnormalities and associated symptoms and findings. Although such subtypes were previously indentified by Roman numerals (e.g., I to X), different classification systems have since been proposed. Most forms of Ehlers-Danlos syndrome are thought to have autosomal dominant inheritance. However, other subtypes have been identified that may be inherited as an autosomal recessive or an X-linked recessive trait. Although certain symptoms and findings are commonly associated with Ehlers-Danlos syndrome, other abnormalities may be variable in range and severity, depending upon the form of the disorder present.

Although infants with Ehlers-Danlos syndrome often appear normal at birth, associated symptoms and findings soon become apparent. The main symptoms associated with the disorder may include abnormally thin, elastic skin that is excessively fragile and unusually loose, flexible (hyperextensible) joints that may be prone to recurrent dislocation. Due to abnormal fragility of the skin, blood vessels, and other tissues, patients may be prone to tearing or splitting of the skin, be susceptible to easy bruising and bleeding, and tend to heal slowly. Healing of skin wounds may leave distinctive, cigarette paper-like scars, such as over the knees, shins, elbows, and forehead. In addition, due to abnormal accumulations of scar tissue, patients may develop small, rounded skin growths that resemble tumors (molluscoid pseudotumors).

In some cases, small, round, hard lumps (calcified spheroids) may also develop under the skin.

Depending upon the form of the disorder present, affected children may have additional, variable symptoms, such as certain skeletal, blood vessel, or eye (ocular) abnormalities. Associated skeletal malformations may include front-to-back and sideways curvature of the spine (kyphoscoliosis); short, wide collarbones (clavicles); bowing of bones of the arms and legs; bone fragility; short stature; or other abnormalities. Fragility of certain blood vessels may lead to ballooning of the wall of the major artery in the body (aortic aneurysm) or spontaneous rupture of certain intermediate- or large-sized arteries, potentially causing life-threatening complications. In addition, in some patients, ocular abnormalities may include fragility of the front, transparent region of the eye (cornea); noninflammatory protrusion of the cornea (keratoconus); rupture of the cornea or the tough, fibrous, outer coating of the eye (sclera); or detachment of the nerve-rich membrane at the back of the eye (retina). Additional symptoms and findings may include diminished muscle tone (hypotonia); abnormal prominence of blood vessels under the skin; protrusion of one of the heart valves back into the left upper chamber (atrium) of the heart during contraction of the left lower heart chamber (mitral valve prolapse); severe inflammation of the tissues that surround and support the teeth (periodontitis), leading to premature tooth loss; rupture of the intestine; or other abnormalities.

The treatment of children with Ehlers-Danlos syndrome is symptomatic and supportive. Appropriate measures must be taken to avoid trauma and injuries, such as those that may occur in contact sports. Wearing protective clothing and padding may be beneficial. In addition, appropriate precautions must be taken during dental or surgical procedures.

The following organizations in the General Resources Section can provide additional information: National Organization for Rare Disorders, Inc (NORD), March of Dimes Birth Defects Foundation, NIH/Office of Rare Diseases, NIH/National Institute of Arthritis and Musculoskeletal and Skin Diseases, Genetic Alliance

National Associations & Support Groups

1634 Ehlers—Danlos National Foundation
6399 Willshire Blvd, Ste 510
Los Angeles, CA 90048   323-651-3038
e-mail: loosejoint@aol.com
www.ednf.org

Provides emotional support and updated information to the individual and their families who are affected by the disease. The foundation produces educational and support pamphlets, brochures, audiovisual aids, journal article reprints, newsletter, and a referral service.

International

1635 British Coalition of Heritable Disorders of Connective Tissue
Rochester House
5 Aldershot Road
Fleet, Hampshire,
United Kingdom
www.Business-Partners.co.uk/marfan

1636 Ehlers-Danlos Syndrome Support Group UK
1 Chandler Close
Richmond, N Yorkshire,
United Kingdom
e-mail: EDS_UK@compuserve.com

Web Sites

1637 Vanderbilt University
www.mc.vanderbilt.edu/peds/pidl/genetic/ehlers.htm

1638 Wheeless' Textbook of Orthopaedics
www.medmedia.com/o14/87.htm

Pamphlets

1639 Ehlers-Danlos Syndrome
Arthritis Foundation
P.O. Box 7669
Atlanta, GA 30357   404-872-7100
800-283-7800
Fax: 404-872-0457

DESCRIPTION

1640 ENCEPHALOCELE

Disorder Type: Birth Defect, Genetic Disorder
May involve these systems in the body (see Section III):
Central Nervous System, Prenatal & Postnatal Growth & Development

Encephalocele is an abnormality that is present at birth and belongs to a group of birth defects known as neural tube defects. These defects develop during the early stages of pregnancy at which time a specialized layer of tissue forms and extends along the back portion of the developing embryo. As the embryo grows, this tissue, known as the neural plate, forms a groove that is bordered by folds. This groove eventually deepens and closes to form the neural tube. Later in development, the neural tube gives rise to tissue that later forms the brain and spinal cord. The neural tube is surrounded and protected by the bones of the back (vertebrae). Failure in this sequence of developmental events results in a neural tube defect.

In newborns with encephalocele, a portion of the brain protrudes through a defect in the skull. This defect may be located at the back of the head (occipital region), the forehead (frontal region), or the area of the forehead and nose (nasofrontal region). Affected children may experience visual abnormalities, mental retardation, an abnormally small head (microcephaly), and seizures. Affected newborns may also have an increase in the volume of fluid surrounding the brain (hydrocephalus), possibly resulting in increased pressure within the skull, enlargement of the head, and convulsions.

Encephalocele may occur as the result of different genetic and environmental factors (multifactorial), alone or in combination. Such factors may include vitamin deficiencies or toxic factors. Genetic transmission in some children is supported by the fact that multiple cases of this neural tube defect have been reported in some families. In addition, encephalocele may sometimes be associated with other disorders. For example, physical characteristics of Meckel-Gruber syndrome, a rare, life-threatening disorder inherited as an autosomal recessive trait, include encephalocele in the back of the head; an abnormal ridge (cleft) or opening in the lip or palate; a sloping forehead, extra fingers or toes (polydactyly); and enlarged kidneys that contain multiple cysts (polycystic kidneys).

Treatment of encephalocele may often involve a team of medical specialists working together to determine the best course of treatment or management. Such treatment may include surgery, medication, or the insertion of a tube known as a shunt into the brain. This shunt diverts fluid away from the brain into the trunk of the body where it is harmlessly absorbed into the systemic circulation.

Researchers believe that folic acid supplementation, initiated before conception, may reduce the risk of neural tube defects. For this reason, women of child-bearing age, especially those at risk who may have previously delivered a child with a neural tube defect, are encouraged to take these supplements under the supervision of their physician.

The following organizations in the General Resources Section can provide additional information: March of Dimes Birth Defects Foundation, NIH/National Institute of Child Health and Human Development, NIH/National Institute of Neurological Disorders & Stroke

National Associations & Support Groups

1641 AboutFace USA
1407 N Wells
Chicago, IL 60610

800-665-3223
Fax: 815-444-1943
e-mail: aboutface2000@aol.com
www.aboutface2000.org

Provides information, services, emotional support and educational program for and on behalf of individuals with facial differences and their families. Working to increase understanding through public awareness and education.

3M members

Rickie Anderson, Executive Director

1642 Association of Birth Defect Children, Inc.
930 Woodcock Road, Suite 225
Orlando, FL 32803　　　　407-245-7035
　　　　　　　　　　　　800-313-2223
　　　　　　　　　　Fax: 407-895-0824
　　　　e-mail: abdc@birthdefects.org
　　　　　　　　www.birthdefects.org

Organization devoted to dissemination of data
pertaining to birth related malformations.

1643 Children's Craniofacial Association
P.O. Box 280297
Dallas, TX 75243　　　　972-994-9902
　　　　　　　　　　　　800-535-3643
　　　　　　　　　　Fax: 972-240-7607
　　　　e-mail: DNKM90A@prodigy.com
　　　　　　　　masterlink.com/children

Devoted to the dispersion of medical knowledge
of this and similar disorders, along with providing emotional support for the sufferers and their
families.

1644 Fighters of Encephaly Support Group
332 Brereton Street
Pittsburgh, PA 15219　　　　412-687-6437

1645 Forward Face, Inc
317 East 34th St, Room 901
New York, NY 10016　　　　212-684-5860

Provision of data and emotional assistance to
both sufferers and medical professionals.

1646 Guardians of Hydrocephalus Research Foundation
2618 Avenue Z
Brooklyn, NY 11235　　　　718-743-4473
　　　　　　　　　　　　800-458-8655

Provides people with the knowledge regarding
the facilities across the nation dedicated to this
disorder.

1647 Hydrocephalus Association
870 Market Street, Suite 705
San Francisco, CA 94102　　　415-732-7040
　　　　　　　　　　　　888-598-3789
　　　　　　　　　　Fax: 415-732-7044
　　　　e-mail: hydroassoc@aol.com
　　　　　　　　www.hydroassoc.org

A national nonprofit organization providing support, education, resource materials and advocacy to individuals, families and professionals.
Our resources include Prenatal Hydrocephalus-
A Book for Parents, About Hydrocephalus-A
Book for Families, About Normal Pressure Hy-
drocephalus- A Book for Adults and their Families. We publish a 12-page quarterly newsletter
and host a biannual national conference on hydrocephalus for families and professionals.

Emily. S. Fudge, Executive Director
Jennifer Henerlau, Assistant Director

1648 Hydrocephalus Support Group, Inc.
9245 Sky Park Court, Suite 130
San Diego, CA 92123　　　　619-268-8252

Provides education and support for hydrocephalus patients and their families. The HSG puts out
a quarterly newspaper, gives parent referrals
and has a library with articles and tapes about
hydrocephalus.

1649 National Craniofacial Foundation
3100 Carlisle Street, Suite 215
Dallas, TX 75204
　　　　　　　　　　　　800-535-1632

1650 National Hydrocephalus Foundation
22427 South River Road
Joliet, IL 60436　　　　815-467-6548
　　　　　　e-mail: hydrobrat@aol.com

Dedicated to supplying both audio and visual resources to victims of the disorder.

Debbie Fields, Executive Director

Web Sites

1651 Pediatric Database (PEDBASE)
www.icondata.com/health/ped-
base/files/ENCEPHAL.HTM

1652 Rare Genetic Diseases in Children (NYU)
http://mcrcr2.med.nyu.edu/murphp01/home-
new.htm

Newsletters

1653 AboutFace U.S.A.
AboutFace
1407 N Wells
Chicago, IL 60610

800-665-3223
Fax: 815-444-1943
e-mail: aboutface2000@aol.com
www.aboutface2000.org

8 pages

Rickie Anderson, Executive Director

DESCRIPTION

1654 ENCOPRESIS

Disorder Type: Mental, Emotional or Behavioral Disorder

Encopresis refers to the passage of feces in inappropriate or unacceptable places by children who have no detectable disorder or organic abnormality and who are past the age when toilet training is typically completed. This type of soiling may be considered primary encopresis, in which fecal incontinence persists from birth, or secondary encopresis, a regressive form of this disorder in which fecal incontinence occurs in children who were previously toilet trained. Children with this disorder may refuse to use a commode, may soil their clothing, or may defecate in secret places. Other associated findings may include chronic constipation leading to the presence of large, hardened fecal masses in the colon or rectum (fecal impaction) that, in turn, may result in an abnormally enlarged or dilated colon (megacolon). Encopresis occurs in approximately one percent of school children and is much more common in boys than it is in girls.

The causes of encopresis may sometimes be linked to anger, defiance, resistance, or fear of toilet training and, as such, may indicate the need for psychotherapeutic intervention that includes parents or caregivers, as well as the affected child. Treatment is often supportive. For example, a reward system may be established so that the child has an incentive to cooperate. In addition, the affected child may be encouraged to use the bathroom at specific times (e.g., after meals) and for specified periods of time. Parents are advised to remain nonjudgmental and nonretaliatory, so that consequences for noncompliance are minor. Additional treatment for primary encopresis may initially include the carefully monitored, short-term use of laxatives and enemas to relieve constipation and subsequent complications. Affected children may sometimes benefit from biofeedback, during which individuals learn how to control certain involuntary physiologic functions such as, in this case, the anal sphincter muscle. In addition, the careful administration of mineral oil, together with a high fiber diet, may be effective in relieving constipation and associated complications in children with secondary encopresis. Other treatment is symptomatic and supportive.

The following organizations in the General Resources Section can provide additional information: NIH/National Institute of Child Health and Human Development, March of Dimes Birth Defects Foundation, International Foundation for Functional Gastrointestinal Disorders: www.iffgd.org/

National Associations & Support Groups

1655 International Foundation for Functional Gastrointestinal Disorders
P.O. Box 17864
Milwaukee, WI 53217
414-964-1799
888-964-2001
Fax: 414-964-7176
e-mail: iffgd@execpc.com
www.execpc.com/iffgd

The organization offers responses to those commonly asked questions for families and individuals who's lives have been touched with the disorder.

Web Sites

1656 MentalHealth Net
http://suicide.cmhc.com/disorders/sx69.htm

DESCRIPTION

1657 EPIDERMOLYSIS BULLOSA

Disorder Type: Genetic Disorder
Covers these related disorders: Epidermolysis bullosa dystrophica, Epidermolysis bullosa simplex, Junctional epidermolysis bullosa
May involve these systems in the body (see Section III):
Dermatologic System

Epidermolysis bullosa is a group of inherited diseases that are often apparent at birth (congenital) and characterized by blistering of the skin after minor injury or trauma. In addition, blistering tends to worsen in warm temperatures. These disorders vary in severity, specific features, and mode of inheritance, and are classified under one of three groupings.

Epidermolysis bullosa simplex is a relatively mild, non-scarring form of this disorder that is inherited as an autosomal dominant trait. Epidermolysis bullosa simplex is further categorized as generalized or localized. The generalized type is usually apparent at birth or soon thereafter. The blisters, also known as bullae, are usually located on areas of the body that are prone to injury such as the hands, feet, elbows, knees, etc. Blistering tendencies usually lessen with advancing age with no long-term effects or scarring. The localized form of this disorder, known as Weber-Cockayne syndrome, affects the hands and feet and may not become apparent until walking commences or, in some cases, adolescence or adulthood. Blistering may be mild, but may severely worsen with such activities as extended walking. Treatment is symptomatic and supportive and may be directed toward prevention and treatment of secondary infections.

Junctional epidermolysis bullosa is inherited as an autosomal recessive trait and is apparent at birth or soon thereafter. Characteristic findings and symptoms associated with this potentially life-threatening form of the disorder may include severe blistering around the mouth and on the scalp, trunk, diaper area, and legs. In addition, slow-healing lesions may develop in the mucous membranes of the respiratory, gastrointestinal, and genitourinary tracts. Affected infants are also at increased risk for infections such as septicemia, a life-threatening condition in which harmful bacteria multiply in the bloodstream. In addition, the nails may appear defective and teeth may decay easily. Other findings may include growth retardation and abnormally low levels of circulating red blood cells (anemia). Treatment for junctional epidermolysis bullosa may include the administration of antibiotics to treat infections and blood transfusions to treat anemia. In addition, nutritional supplementation may be beneficial. Other treatment is symptomatic and supportive.

Epidermolysis bullosa dystrophica may be inherited as an autosomal dominant trait, an autosomal recessive trait, or it may appear sporadically. Findings associated with autosomal dominant inheritance are less severe than those of autosomal recessive transmission. This form of epidermolysis bullosa may be further categorized as the albopapuloid Pasini variant and the Cockayne-Touraine variant. The albopapuloid Pasini variant may first appear as early as infancy or as late as adolescence and is characterized by extensive, scarring-type blistering of the skin on the joints, arms, and legs; the appearance during adolescence of flesh-colored (albopapuloid) lesions on the trunk; and involvement of certain mucuous memberanes. The Cockayne-Touraine variant of this disorder develops during infancy or early childhood and is characterized by blisters that most commonly appear on the arms and legs. Epidermolysis bullosa dystrophica that is inherited as an autosomal recessive trait is a severe form of this disorder that may be characterized at birth by extensive blistering and erosions of the body surfaces and mucous membranes. As the lesions heal, scarring may result in deformity and limited mobility. In addition, healing of the mucous membranes of the esophagus may cause narrowing of this structure, leading to difficulties in feeding and eating. Treatment may include the implementation of a special diet or use of special feeding devices necessitated by scarring or narrowing of the esophagus. Additional treatment may be directed toward the prevention or care of associated secondary infections. Other treatment is symptomatic and supportive.

The following organizations in the General Resources Section can provide additional information: National Organization for Rare Disorders, Inc. (NORD), NIH/Office of Rare Diseases, Genetic Alliance, March of Dimes Birth Defects Foundation, NIH/National Institute of Arthritis and Musculoskeletal and Skin Diseases, Online Mendelian Inheritance in Man: www3.ncbi.nlm.nih.gov/Omim/searchomim.html

National Associations & Support Groups

1658 DEBRA: Dystrophic Epidermolysis Bullosa Research Foundation
40 Rector St
New York, NY 10006   212-513-4090
                           Fax: 212-513-4099
                           www.debra.org

Committed to providing referrals, patient advocacy and lobbying, offers networking services, and engages in patient and professional education.

1659 Dystrophic Epidermolysis Bullosa Research Association - United Kingdom DEBRA House
13 Wellington Business Park, Dukes Ride
Crowthorne, Berkshire,
United Kingdom
          e-mail: debra.uk@btinternet.com
                           www.debra.org.uk

Web Sites

1660 EB Medical Research Foundation
www-med.stanford.edu/school/dermatology/ebmrf/

1661 EB Web Ring
www.geocities.com/CollegePark/Lab/3326/ebring.htm

1662 Family Village
www.familyvillage.wisc.edu/lib_deb.htm

Books

1663 Epidermolysis Bullosa

Clinical, Epidemiologic, and Laboratory Advances and the Findings of the National Epidermolysis Bullosa Registry. The first comprehensive examination of EB employing a large, well-characterized research study population and using the latest epidemiological and biostatistical research principles. Includes the assessment of over 2,000 patients with EB. Topics discussed are molecular and cell biology, epidemiology, diagnosis, classification, medical and surgical treatments, and clinical outcomes.

510 pages
ISBN: 0-801860-24-5

Jo-David Fine, M.D., M.P.H., Editor
Eugene A. Bauer, M.D., Editor

DESCRIPTION

1664 ERB'S PALSY

Synonym: Erb-Duchenne paralysis

May involve these systems in the body (see Section III):

Neuromuscular

Erb's palsy is a form of paralysis in newborns resulting from injury to certain nerves (i.e., fifth and sixth cervical nerves of upper brachial plexus) that supply specific muscles of the shoulder and arm. Nerve injury may be the result of a difficult delivery (e.g., breech presentation, delivery of an unusually large newborn, etc.). During delivery, lateral traction of the head and neck may occur and lead to stretching of these nerves, potentially resulting in such injury.

Newborns with Erb's palsy typically experience swelling and inflammation of the affected nerves and paralysis of the affected shoulder and arm muscles (e.g., deltoid, biceps, brachialis). This causes the arm to hang loosely with the elbow extended and inwardly rotated. Newborns with the condition are unable to move the affected arm away from the shoulder or rotate the arm away from the body. In addition, although they may extend the forearm, affected newborns lack a startle reflex known as Moro's reflex on the affected side. Moro's reflex, which is usually present at birth, involves stretching of the arms and legs forward and out and extension of the fingers when startled. In some severe cases, paralysis and associated loss (atrophy) of the muscle mass in the shoulder area (deltoid muscle) may cause drop shoulder, which is characterized by depression of the affected shoulder below the level of the other. Some infants may experience impairment of sensation in affected areas. Movements of the hand are typically not affected.

The effectiveness of certain treatments for Erb's palsy may vary, depending upon whether affected nerves (i.e., fifth and sixth cervical nerves) were torn or injured in a manner that allows a return of function within a few months. Treatment meas-ures may include initial immobilization of the affected arm and shoulder with braces or splints and physical therapy including range of motion exercises, massage, and active and passive corrective exercises. Such therapy may help to improve muscle function and prevent permanent bending of affected joints in a fixed posture (flexion contractures). If paralysis continues at three to six months of age, surgical measures may be considered in some cases.

The following organizations in the General Resources Section can provide additional information: National Organization for Rare Disorders, Inc. (NORD), March of Dimes Birth Defects Foundation, NIH/National Arthritis and Musculoskeletal and Skin Diseases

National Associations & Support Groups

1665 Brachial Plexus Injury/Erb's Palsy Support & Information Network
P.O. Box 533
Manasha, WI 54952   441-836-3843

Furnishes a variety of support tools including reading and audio materials.

1666 Brachial Plexus/Erb's Palsy Support and Informational Network, Inc.
P.O. Box 23
Larsen, WI 54947   920-836-9955
Fax: 920-836-9587
e-mail: nationalbpi@powernetonline.com
www.customforum.com/nationalbpi

Furnishes a variety of support tools including reading and audio materials.

Web Sites

1667 Erb's Palsy Information & Resource Group
www.erbspalsy.org/chat.html

1668 Texas Children's Hospital
www.bcm.tmc.edu/pednsurg/disorder/brachial.htm

DESCRIPTION

1669 ERYTHEMA INFECTIOSUM

Synonyms: EI, Fifth disease, Sticker's disease

Disorder Type: Infectious Disease

May involve these systems in the body (see Section III):

Dermatologic System

Erythema infectiosum, or Fifth disease, is a mildly contagious infection caused by the human parvovirus B19. It is characterized by a three-stage rash. First there is the sudden appearance of a red rash on the face that may look as if the cheeks had been slapped. Then the rash progresses to a reddish, raised-spot, blotchy eruption that spreads to the trunk, buttocks, arms, and legs. When it begins to fade, the rash takes on a lacy-type appearance. The rash usually subsides within five to 10 days, but may reappear within a month's time, especially after exercise, stress, skin irritation, or exposure to sunlight. Transmission of this virus is through inhalation of droplets exhaled or coughed into the air by infected individuals.

Erythema infectiosum occurs most commonly in preschool and young school-age children. The first symptoms may be low-grade fever and headache. Once the rash appears or shortly thereafter, fever and other signs of illness may be absent. However, some older children and adults may develop mild itching (pruritus), joint pain (arthralgia), and inflammation of the joints (arthritis). In addition, under certain circumstances, exposure to human parvovirus B19 may result in more severe complications. For example, individuals with certain blood disorders such as thalessemia or sickle cell anemia may develop a temporary inability to produce red blood cells, resulting in a decrease in the body's capacity to supply oxygen to the tissues of the body (anemia). Symptoms associated with severe anemia may include fever, weakness, discomfort, pale skin (pallor), rapid breathing (tachypnea), and rapid heartbeat (tachycardia). In addition, those who have impaired immune function may experience severe consequences upon exposure to human parvovirus B19. For example, individuals undergoing certain types of chemotherapy, those with acquired immunodeficiency syndrome (AIDS), or those with certain types of primary, inherited immune defects may experience recurrent or prolonged infections, anemia, or other blood abnormalities.

Pregnant women infected with the EI virus may transmit it to their unborn children, resulting, in rare cases, in miscarriage or stillbirth; however, most of those exposed in utero are born with no apparent consequences. Other viral-exposed infants may have abnormal accumulations of fluid in the tissues or cavities of the body (hydrops). If this condition is diagnosed before birth, special blood transfusions delivered by way of the umbilical vein may be of benefit to the affected fetus. The incubation period for erythema infectiosum is approximately four to 14 days. Treatment for this viral infection is symptomatic.

The following organizations in the General Resources Section can provide additional information: National Organization for Rare Disorders, Inc. (NORD), March of Dimes Birth Defects Foundation, NIH/National Institute of Allergy and Infectious Disease, World Health Organization (WHO), Centers for Disease Control (CDC)

Web Sites

1670 Karolista Institute
www.mic.ki.se/Diseases/c2.html

1671 Kid's Health
kidshealth.org/parent/common/fifth.html

1672 New York State Department of Health
www.medhelp.org/lib/fifth.htm

1673 State of Hawaii
mano.icsd.hawaii.gov/health/cdd/cddfifth.htm

1674 State of Maryland
www.dhmh.state.md.us/cpha/edcp.html/fifth.html

1675 Virtual Hospital
www.medhelp.org/general2/ww000223.htm

DESCRIPTION

1676 ERYTHROPOIETIC PROTOPORPHYRIA

Synonyms: EPP, Erythrohepatic protoporphyria, Ferrochelatase deficiency, Protoporphyria

Disorder Type: Genetic Disorder, Metabolism

Erythropoietic protoporphyria is a hereditary metabolic disorder that belongs to a group of diseases known as the porphyrias. These disorders are characterized by enzyme deficiencies that result in the abnormal accumulation of chemicals known as porphyrins in certain tissues of the body. Porphyrins are formed during the manufacture of heme, the pigmented, iron-containing component of hemoglobin, which is the oxygen-carrying protein in red blood cells. The porphyrias may be classified as erythropoietic or hepatic porphyrias. The erythropoietic porphyrias are characterized by overproduction of porphyrins in the blood-forming tissue of the bone marrow. In individuals with hepatic porphyrias, there is abnormally increased production of porphyrins in the liver. The range and severity of associated symptoms and the age at onset are variable and depend on the underlying enzyme deficiency and the form of porphyria present. Erythropoietic protoporphyria is the most common form of erythropoietic porphyria and is thought to affect approximately one in 5,000 to 10,000 individuals.

In patients with erythropoietic protoporphyria, also known as EPP, deficiency of the enzyme ferrochelatase results in excessive accumulation of protoporphyrin in red blood cells and the fluid portion of the blood (plasma). Excessive protoporphyrin is also concentrated in a liquid secreted by the liver (bile) and is eliminated in the feces. In some patients, abnormal accumulations of protoporphyrin also become deposited within the liver itself.

Symptoms associated with EPP usually begin in childhood before age 10. The most common symptom is an abnormal sensitivity of the skin to sunlight and certain forms of artificial light (photosensitivity). Affected children typically ex-perience pain, burning, and itching of the skin within an hour of exposure to sunlight. Such symptoms are often followed hours later by redness and inflammation of the skin and abnormal accumulation of fluid (edema) beneath the skin in affected areas. However, abnormal burning sensations of the skin may occur in the absence of associated redness or fluid accumulation. Rarely, if sun exposure is prolonged, fluid-filled blisters (vesicles) may develop or there may be bleeding in the skin or mucous membranes, appearing as pinpoint purplish spots (petechiae) or small bluish-purple patches (purpura). Such blistering or bruising may persist for several days after exposure to the sun. In addition, prolonged, repeated sun exposure may cause mild scarring, abnormal thickening of the skin in certain areas, or an abnormality of the nails in which the nails become separated from the nail beds (onycholysis). Although symptoms associated with photosensitivity typically become apparent during infancy or early childhood, the condition sometimes does not occur until adolescence or adulthood.

Many patients with EPP may also develop lumps of solid matter in the gall bladder (gallstones or cholelithiasis) at an unusually early age. The gall bladder is a small, muscular sac under the liver that stores and concentrates bile from the liver. In addition, uncommonly, there may be mildly decreased levels of circulating red blood cells (anemia). Rarely, patients may develop progressive liver damage that may lead to liver failure.

EPP is caused by changes (mutations) in the gene that regulates the production of the enzyme ferrochelatase. This gene is located on the long arm of chromosome 18 (18q21.3). Several different mutations of the gene have been identified in individuals with the disorder. In most cases, EPP has autosomal dominant inheritance. However, there have been reports in which patients inherited two different mutations of the gene, one from each parent. In addition, some individuals who inherit one copy of the disease gene may have slightly elevated levels of protoporphyrin, yet do not experience symptoms associated with the disease.

Patients with EPP benefit from avoiding sunlight, using topical sunscreens, and wearing protective clothing, such as sunglasses, hats, long sleeves, and double layers. Administration of beta-carotene by mouth may help improve tolerance to sunlight. Therapy with cholestyramine, a medication that acts upon the liver's bile acids, may help to alleviate skin symptoms and liver disease. Additional treatment is symptomatic and supportive.

The following organizations in the General Resources Section can provide additional information: National Organization for Rare Disorders, Inc. (NORD), NIH/Office of Rare Diseases, March of Dimes Birth Defects Foundation, Genetic Alliance, NIH/National Institute of Child Health and Human Development, Research Trust for Metabolic Disaeases in Children, NIH/National Digestive Diseases Information Clearinghouse

National Associations & Support Groups

1677 American Porphyria Foundation
PObox 22712
Houston, TX 77227   713-266-9617
                           Fax: 713-871-1788
                           www.enterprise.net/apf/

1678 Canadian Porphyria Foundation, Inc.
PO Box 1206
Neepawa, Manitoba, R0J
Canada   204-476-2800

1679 Erythropoietic Protoporphyria Research and Education Fund
Channing Laboratory, Harvard Medical School
Bringham & Women's Hospital, 181 Longwood Avenue
Boston, MA 02115   617-525-2249
                           Fax: 617-731-1541
e-mail: mmmathroth@bics.bwh.harvard.edu

DESCRIPTION

1680 ESOPHAGEAL ATRESIA

Disorder Type: Birth Defect
May involve these systems in the body (see Section III):
Digestive System

Esophageal atresia is a defect that is present at birth (congenital). The esophagus, which is a muscular tube, is that portion of the digestive system that connects the throat and the stomach. In infants with esophageal atresia, the channel (lumen) within the tubular esophagus fails to develop properly, resulting in an esophagus that ends in a blind pouch, failing to provide a continuous passage to the stomach. In some infants, the upper section of the esophagus may be dramatically narrowed or it may be closed at its lower end. In others, the closed-end lower portion extends upward from the stomach and there is no through connection between the two. Most affected infants also have an abnormal tube-like connection or opening between the windpipe (trachea) and either the upper or lower portion of the esophagus. This is known as a tracheoesophageal fistula. In some children, there is a double connection in which there is an abnormal passage between the windpipe (trachea) and part of the esophagus as well as between the trachea and a lower region of the esophagus.

Infants with esophageal atresia cannot swallow at all and therefore salivate and regurgitate excessively. If a tracheoesophageal fistula exists between the windpipe and upper portion of the esophagus, fluid may enter the lungs, resulting in coughing, choking, a bluish discoloration of the nail beds, lips, and mucous membranes (cyanosis), and possibly pneumonia. The presence of an abnormal passage between the trachea and the lower section of the esophagus may allow air to enter the abdomen, resulting in excessive abdominal swelling (distension) that may interfere with normal breathing. In addition, contents of the abdomen may enter the lungs and severe inflammation may

occur. If esophageal atresia is present without a fistula, characteristic findings may include a boat-shaped abdomen that is devoid of air.

Treatment includes surgery to join or connect the two sections of the esophagus. This procedure is known as an esophageal anastomosis. Tracheoesophageal fistulas may be surgically corrected by ligation, a procedure in which the passageway is tied off. Before surgery, special care is taken to ensure the infants do not draw fluid (aspirate) into their lungs through the esophagus.

As many as 50 percent of infants with esophageal atresia have associated structural malformations of other organs. For example, if a tracheoesophageal fistula is present, other abnormalities of the trachea may also be apparent. In addition, approximately half of all affected infants have a complex of congenital anomalies (VATER syndrome) characterized by additional malformations involving the heart, skeleton, kidneys, and urinary and genital systems. Treatment for esophageal atresia includes management or correction of associated anomalies. Esophageal atresia occurs in approximately one in 3,500 births in the United States. About 33 percent of these infants are born prematurely.

The following organizations in the General Resources Section can provide additional information: National Organization for Rare Disorders, Inc. (NORD), Genetic Alliance, March of Dimes Birth Defects Foundation, NIH/Office of Rare Diseases, NIH/National Digestive Diseases Information Clearinghouse, Online Mendelian Inheritance in Man: www3.ncbi.nlm.nih.gov/Omim/searchomim.html

---

National Associations & Support Groups

1681 Digestive Disease National Coalition
507 Capital Courte, Suite 200
Washington, DC 20002   202-544-7497
                              Fax: 202-546-7105

Objective is to inform the public about technology improvements through several media forms.

Newsletters

1682 TEF/VATER

EA-TEF-VATER/VACTERL International
15301 Grey Fox Road
Upper Marlboro, MD 20772   301-952-6837
e-mail: tefvater@ix.netcom.com

Provides support to children and adults born
with esophageal atresia.

Newsletter

DESCRIPTION

1683 EWING'S SARCOMA

Synonym: Ewing's tumor

Disorder Type: Neoplasm: Benign or Malignant Tumor

Ewing's sarcoma is a malignant tumor that typically occurs in individuals under the age of 20 years. The tumor most often arises in the long bones of the shin (tibia), thigh (femur), or upper arm (humerus) or the flat bones of the pelvis, vertebrae, or chest wall. Ewing's sarcoma often invades surrounding soft tissues and tends to spread (metastasize) to other bones, the lungs, and, less frequently, the bone marrow or other organs. In some cases, the primary tumor may develop in soft tissue. Approximately 75 percent of these tumors occur in the legs or arms as well as the bones of the shoulders.

The most common symptoms of Ewing's sarcoma include fever, as well as pain, tenderness, and swelling in the area of the tumor. Some children may also experience weight loss, low levels of circulating red blood cells (anemia), and elevated levels of circulating white blood cells (leukocytosis). In addition, the tumor may weaken the surrounding bone and thus increase vulnerability to bone fracture. The diagnosis of Ewing's tumor is established through the use of x-rays along with examination of tissue samples obtained through biopsy. In addition, other procedures such as bone scanning, computed tomography (CT), and magnetic resonance imaging (MRI) may be used to confirm the presence of lung, bone, or other metastases.

Ewing's sarcoma develops most frequently between the ages of 10 and 20 years of age and affects boys more often than girls by a ratio of two to one. These tumors rarely occur in black children. Treatment of Ewing's sarcoma may include the use of chemotherapy and radiation. Patients are also evaluated for possible surgical removal of the tumor. Other treatment is symptomatic and supportive.

The following organizations in the General Resources Section can provide additional information: National Organization for Rare Disorders, Inc. (NORD), NIH/Office of Rare Diseases, American Cancer Society, Inc., Candlelighters Childhood Cancer Foundation, Candlelighters Childhood Cancer Foundation Canada, National Childhood Cancer Foundation, NIH/National Cancer Institute

Web Sites

1684 CancerCare:
www.cancercare.org/faq/cancer_faq.html

1685 CancerOnline:
www.stonecottage.com/canceronline/

1686 OncoLink: The University of Pennslyvania Cancer Center Resource
www.oncolink.upenn.edu

DESCRIPTION

1687 FAMILIAL DYSAUTONOMIA
   Synonyms: FD, HSAN-III, Riley-Day syndrome
   Disorder Type: Genetic Disorder, Neuromuscular

Familial dysautonomia (FD) is a rare inherited disorder of that part of the nervous system responsible for regulating various essential involuntary functions (autonomic nervous system). This disorder is characterized in infants by feeding difficulties, including excessive salivation and poor swallowing and sucking reflexes. The breathing in of liquid or other substances into the lungs (aspiration) may lead to repeated episodes of bronchial pneumonia. Other associated symptoms and findings include skin blotching, sweating, fluctuating extremes in body temperature, and defective tear secretion (lacrimation). Affected children develop an insensitivity and indifference to pain. This may lead to frequent injuries such as irritation of the corneas of the eyes. Corneal injury may also occur as the result of decreased tear production. In addition, slurred speech and drooling may become evident. Children with familial dysautonomia typically have weak reflex responses (hyporeflexia) and experience delays in walking accompanied by the inability to coordinate voluntary movements (motor incoordination). After three years of age, affected children often develop severe vomiting episodes (hyperemesis) that may occur three or four times an hour and, in some cases, may last for three days or more. These episodes may sometimes be accompanied by elevated blood pressure (hypertension), abdominal pain and swelling, increased irritability, or breathing difficulties. As children with this disorder reach adolescence, a sideward curvature of the spine (scoliosis) may become evident along with leg cramping and weakness. In addition, some children may experience a delay in the onset of puberty. Older children may develop emotional and behavioral changes, such as irritability and depression. Intolerance for anesthetics is a common finding among children with FD.

Treatment for familial dysautonomia is symptomatic and supportive. Artificial tears, drops, or ointments may be placed in the eyes to prevent injury to corneas. Certain medications known as antiemetics may be prescribed to help control episodes of vomiting. In addition, replacement fluids and electrolytes may be administered to prevent excessive fluid loss (dehydration) resulting from vomiting episodes. Other treatment may include surgery or the use of orthopedic aids to correct scoliosis.

Familial dysautonomia is inherited as an autosomal recessive trait and occurs most commonly among certain individuals of eastern European descent, particularly Ashkenazi Jews at a rate of one out of 10,000 to 20,000 births. The disease gene for this disorder is located on the long arm of chromosome 9 (9q31-33).

The following organizations in the General Resources Section can provide additional information: National Organization for Rare Disorders, Inc., (NORD), NIH/Office of Rare Diseases, Genetic Alliance, March of Dimes Birth Defects Foundation, NIH/National Institute of Neurological Disorders & Stroke, Online Mendelian Inheritance in Man: www3.ncbi.nlm.nih.gov/Omim/searchomim.html

---

National Associations & Support Groups

1688 Dysautonomia Foundation
20 E 46th St, 3rd Fl
New York, NY 10017
       212-949-6644
       Fax: 212-682-7325
       www.med.nyu.edu

Provides parents the knowledge regarding both national and international facilities that specialize in the treatment of the disorder.

1689 FD Familial Dysautonomia Foundation
343 Clark Ave
Thornhill Ontario, L4J
       905-764-5335
       Fax: 905-764-7752

Devoted to keeping families up-to-date on the medical knowledge surrounding the disorder and the facilities dealing with it.

1690 National Foundation for Jewish Genetic Diseases
  250 Park Ave Ste 1000
  New York, NY 10017   212-371-1030
                                         Fax: 212-319-5808

  Provides the information regarding this and related disorders for the people suffering from
  them.

Web Sites

1691 Family Village
  www.familyvillage.wisc.edu/lib_dysa.htm

1692 NYU
  www.med.nyu.edu/fd/fdcenter.html

DESCRIPTION

1693 FETAL ACQUIRED IMMUNE DEFICIENCY SYNDROME

Synonym: Fetal AIDS
Disorder Type: Infectious Disease

Fetal acquired immune deficiency syndrome (fetal AIDS) refers to the development of AIDS in children who acquire the HIV virus through transmission by an infected mother before or during birth. Acquired immune deficiency syndrome (AIDS) is an infectious disease characterized by acquired immunodeficiency and is caused by infection with the human immunodeficiency virus (HIV-1 or HIV-2). Most young children with AIDS contract the disease through in utero transmission; however, infants may occasionally acquire the infection through mother's milk. In addition, children with hemophilia and others who may have received transfusions of blood or blood products before HIV blood-screening became standard in 1985 may have become infected by contaminated blood. HIV may also be transmitted to young children and adolescents through sexual contact. Older children may acquire the infection through the sharing of infected needles used to inject drugs.

Some children with HIV infection develop symptoms in the first or second year of life, while the majority may not show signs of infection until several years have passed. AIDS is diagnosed in about 50 percent of HIV-infected children by three years of age. Early signs may include chronic or recurrent fevers and diarrhea, rashes, swollen lymph glands, enlarged liver and spleen (hepatosplenomegaly), and delays in growth and the development of the nervous system. Some infants and young children may have decreased levels of circulating red blood cells (anemia), weight loss, loss of appetite (anorexia), decreased energy, or progressive neurologic degeneration and irregularities of the heart and kidneys. In addition, some children may have an unusually small head (microcephaly) and other distinctive facial features. Early symptoms may include chronic or recurrent

bacterial infections and uncommon viral, fungal, and other types of opportunistic infections caused by microorganisms that do not ordinarily cause disease or infection except in those with impaired immune systems. As the immune system becomes increasingly weakened, children may develop lung inflammations such as lymphoid interstitial pneumonitis (LIP) and potentially life-threatening pneumocystis pneumonia. Children with AIDS are also at increased risk for certain types of malignant diseases such as non-Hodgkins lymphoma.

Most infants born to mothers with HIV show antibodies in their blood for approximately 12 to 14 months. In infants who are not infected with the virus, these passive antibodies disappear. For this reason, standardized HIV testing is not conclusive in children younger than 18 months. However, HIV infection in these children may often be detected through the use of virus cultures and a specialized DNA-copying technique called polymerase chain reaction or PCR.

Prevention of HIV and subsequent AIDS infection in infants may be directed toward counseling of at-risk women of child-bearing age who may be advised to avoid becoming pregnant. The strictly prescribed administration of the drug AZT during the last six months of pregnancy, as well as during labor and delivery, has been shown to greatly improve the chances of an HIV-infected mother delivering an infant who is not infected with HIV. Delivery by Cesarean section may also reduce risk of transmission to the newborn. In addition, mothers with HIV should refrain from breast-feeding their infants, as there is some evidence of HIV transmission from mother to child in women who may have contracted the virus after pregnancy.

Infants and children with HIV may be treated with antibiotics to prevent pneumocystis pneumonia. Intravenous gamma globulin therapy may be used to maintain or increase the ability of the immune system to fight the effects of secondary infections. In addition, certain steroidal drugs may be administered to treat lymphoid interstitial pneumonitis, while AZT, alone or in combination, is often used to treat children and has been found to be particularly effective against neurologic irregularities. Additional therapies are also being tested in children. Other treatment is symptomatic and supportive.

The following organizations in the General Resources Section can provide additional information: National Organization for Rare Disorders, Inc. (NORD), NIH/National Institute of Allergy and Infectious Disease, World Health Organization, Centers for Disease Control (CDC)

National Associations & Support Groups

1694 Family Empowerment Network: Supporting Families Affected by FAS/FAE
519 Lowell Hall, 610 Langdon St
Madison, WI 53703
608-262-6590
800-462-5254
Fax: 608-265-3352
e-mail: fen@mail.dcs.wisc.edu

Disabled Children's Computer Group, and a major corporation consisting of parents, consumers and professionals. It is one of the nations largest resources to help children and adults who have disabilities gain access to the benefits of technology. Includes nationwide network of community-based assistive technology, resource centers, hands on consultants and product demonstrations.

1695 Foundation for Children with AIDS
1800 Columbus Avenue
Roxbury, MA 02119
617-442-7442
Fax: 617-442-1705

A national, nonprofit organization founded to improve the quality of life for drug-effected and HIV-infected children and their families. The foundation raises funds for family and community-based services for children and their families affected by HIV infection and drug exposure. Offers Project STAR which is a child and family care program offering therapeutic child care, early intervention, transportation, counseling and case management services.

Geneva Woodruff, PhD, Executive Director

1696 Immune Deficiency Foundation
Immune Deficiency Foundation
25 West Chesapeake Avenue Suite 206
Towson, MD 21204
410-321-6647
800-296-4433
Fax: 410-321-9165
e-mail: IDF@primaryimmune.org
www.primaryimmune.org

The only national charitable organization aimed at fighting the primary immune deficiency diseases. The founders included parents of children with primary immune deficiency, immunologists who treat immune deficient patients and other individuals with an interest in helping others. The Foundation's main goal is to improve the care and treatment of adults and children with primary immune deficiency diseases and to promote public education and awareness about the diseases.

1697 National AIDS Hotline
c/o American Social Association
P.O. Box 13827
RTP, NC 27709
800-342-2437
Fax: 919-361-4855
TTY: 800-243-7889
www.sunsite.unc.edu/asha

Information and advocacy resources for families and professionals. Includes listings of organizations providing general information and organizations focusing on more specific areas of concern to families and young adults who have disabilities.

1698 National Abandoned Infants Assistance Resource Center
1950 Addison Street, Suite 104
Berkeley, CA 94704
510-643-8390
Fax: 510-643-7019
e-mail: ala@link4.berkeley.edu
www.socrates.berkeley.edu/~airc

The Centers vision is to enhance the quality of social and health services delivered to drug- and HIV-affected children and their families. Its strategy is to provide state-of-the-art training, technical assistance, research, and information to professionals who serve these families. Services include a national newsletter, telephone seminars, conferences, monographs, guides and reports.

Jeanne Pietrzak, Director

1699 National Association of People with AIDS
1413 K St, NW, 7th Fl, Ste 7
Washington, DC 20005
202-898-0414
Fax: 202-898-0435
e-mail: napwa@napwa.org
http://www.napwa.org

1700 Pediatric AIDS Foundation
2950 31st Street, Suite 125
Santa Monica, CA 90405   310-395-9051
                                800-499-4673
                                Fax: 310-314-1469

A national nonprofit organization dealing with
medical problems unique to children infected
with HIV/AIDS. The foundation is focused specifically on creating a future that will offer
hope, finding effective therapies and issues of
pregnancy and HIV. The foundation funds criti-
cally neS, encourages students to enter the
world of pediatric AIDS through a student in-
tern program and more.

1701 Support for Children with Aids Inc.
1222 T Street NW, Grandma's Hosue
Washington, DC 20009   202-462-8526

A support organization that provides service,
care, and preventive education for children and
adults with AIDS. It provides housing for children with AIDS (e.g. Grandma's House in Washington, DC).

Libraries & Resource Centers

**1702 Hawaii Department of Health - Communicable
Disease Division**
AIDS/Sexually Transmitted Diseases Control Branch
3627 Kilauea Avenue, Suite 305
Honolulu, HI 96816   808-735-5303
                            Fax: 808-735-5318

Offers research, education, surveillance and testing components. AIDS information and guidelines about the placement of infants, children
and adolescents who test positive for HIV in
nursery or school settings are also available.

Robert M. Worth, Chief

Research Centers

1703 Children's Clinical Research Center
New York Hospital, Cornell Medical Center
525 East 68th Street
New York, NY 10021   212-746-3484
                            Fax: 212-746-8821

Offers research into the study of pediatric AIDS
and other disorders.

Maria I.. New, Program Director

**1704 National Training Center for Professional AIDS
Education**
1800 Columbus Avenue
Roxbury, MA 02119   617-442-7442
                          Fax: 617-442-1705

Program training teachers, health care providers and other professionals who serve HIV-infected children and their families. Offers
education, site workshops, technical assistance,
regional conferences, printed materials and publication of articles in the media and professional
journals. Training is designed for providers
and administrators of early childhood/interven-
tion programs, public school, preschool and special education programs.

Geneva Woodruff, PhD, Executive Director

Massachusetts

1705 Developmental Evaluation Center
Children's Hospital
300 Longwood Avenue
Boston, MA 02115   617-355-6000
                          Fax: 617-735-7429

Studies developmental effects of infants at risk
and development effects of congenital HIV infection.

Allen C. Crocker, MD, Director

Audio Video

1706 Kid Called Troy
Terry Carlyon and Michael J. Rivette, author
Fanlight Productions
47 Halifax St
Boston, MA 02131   617-469-4999
                          Fax: 617-524-8838
                          e-mail: fanlight@tiac.net
                          www.fanlight.com

Troy, a seven-year-old from Australia, has lived
with the HIV virus his entire life. Narrated by
Troy's father, this film shows how Troy manages to remain happy and engaged and also offers a portrait of parental love and dedication.

54 minutes
ISBN: 1-572952-21-0

1707 Pediatric AIDS: A Time of Crisis
Association for the Care of Children's Health
8701 Hartsdale Avenue
Bethesda, MD 20817   301-493-5113

Families caring for children who are HIV positive speak about the kinds of services and programs they need to meet the needs of these children in the hospital, at home and in the community.

23 minutes

Web Sites

1708 AEGIS
www.aegis.com/

1709 AIDS Knowledge Base
http://hivinsite.ucsf.edu/akb/1994/3-4/ref50a.html

1710 Camp Heartland
www.campheartland.org/

1711 Children with AIDS Project
www.aidskids.org/

1712 Elizabeth Glazer Pediatric AIDS Foundation
www.pedaids.org/

1713 Food and Drug Administration
www.fda.gov/oashi/aids/hiv.html

1714 National Foundation for Children with AIDS
www.childrenwithaids.org/

1715 National Pediatric & Family HIV Resource Center
www.pedhivaids.org/

1716 National Pediatric AIDS Network
www.npan.org/

1717 Parents Helping Parents
http://php.com/

1718 Pediatric AIDS Clinical Trials Group
http://pactg.s-3/com/sites.htm

1719 Sunshine for HIV Kids
www.songshine.com/

1720 Wayne State University
http://cmmg.biosci.wayne.edu/asg/global-conf.html

Books

1721 AIDS and the Education of Our Children

US Department of Education, author

Consumer Information Center
Dept. ED
Pueblo, CO 81009   719-948-3334

A guide for parents and teachers offering helpful information on the topic of AIDS education.

1722 Community Service Delivery for Children with HIV Infection and Families

Geneva, Woodruff & Christopher Hanson, author

South Shore Mental Health Center
6 Fort Street
Quincy, MA 02169   617-847-1950

A manual providing guidelines for developing community-based, family-centered services for children with HIV infection and their families. Describes how services can be planned and delivered using guiding principles and practices of transagency case management.

1723 How Can I Tell You? Secrecy with Children When a Family Member Has AIDS

M. Tasker, author

Association for the Care of Children's Health
8701 Hartsdale Avenue
Bethesda, MD 20817   301-493-5113

Assists families and professionals as they explore issues surrounding the disclosure of an HIV diagnosis to children.

84 pages

Children's Books

1724 AIDS Awareness Library

Anna Forbes, MSS, author

Rosen Publishing Group
29 East 21st Street
New York, NY 10010   212-777-3017
                            800-237-9932
                            e-mail: rosenpub@ios.com

This series of eight 24 pg. books for grades K-4, speaks to children in nonthreatening langauge that provides vital information without graphic detail. This series is meant to be a gentle introduction to this frightening epidemic. Each book can also be purchased seperately for $13.95 (Set includes: Where did AIDS Come From; Myths and Facts; Living in a World with AIDS; What is AIDS; When Someone You Know Has AIDS; What You Can Do About AIDS; Heroes Against AIDS; Kids with AIDS.).

1996
ISBN: 0-823916-87-1

1725 Alex, the Kid with AIDS

Linda Wolvoord Girard, author

Albert Whitman & Company
6340 Oakton Street
Morton Grove, IL 60053   847-581-0033
                                800-225-7675
                          Fax: 847-584-0039
                          www.awhitmanco.com

This first person account presents a young peer's experience of going to school with a classmate who has AIDS. At first the class feels awkward around him, but then comes to accept him as any other boy. Also available in paperback.

32 pages Grades 2-5
ISBN: 0-807502-45-6

Joseph Boyd, President
Joe Campbell, Customer Service

1726 Be a Friend- Children Who Live with AIDS Speak

Weiner, Best, & Pizzo, et al, author

Compassion Books
477 Hannah Branch Road
Burnsville, NC 28714   704-675-9670
                        Fax: 704-675-9687

Through writings and drawings children living with HIV infection and AIDS candidly share their feelings, hopes, and fears.

Softcover

1727 You and HIV: A Day At a Time

L.S. Baker, author

Association for the Care of Children's Health
8701 Hartsdale Avenue
Bethesda, MD 20817   301-493-5113

Written for children and adolescents with HIV, this book guides patients and their families through the medical and psychological whats and whys of HIV.

258 pages

Newsletters

1728 Children with AIDS
Foundation for Children with AIDS
1800 Columbus Avenue
Roxbury, MA 02119   617-442-7442
                      Fax: 617-442-1705

Offers information on AIDS/HIV and hemophilia disorders affecting children. Gives housing information, medical research, projects, and publications for children and their families.

Bi-Monthly

1729 Just Kids
3 Corners, Inc.
5th Avenue
New York, NY 10014   212-634-4879

Covers medical and social issues faced by HIV-positive children, teens and their parents.

Annual

Pamphlets

1730 Children with AIDS: Guidelines for Parents and Caregivers
AIDS Task Force of Central New York
627 West Genesee Street
Syracuse, NY 13204   315-415-2430

Offers general information on AIDS, diet and feeding, household chores, and coping with the illness.

1731 Hope for Children with AIDS
Pediatric AIDS Foundation
2950 31st Street, Suite 125
Santa Monica, CA 90405   310-394-0661
                                888-499-4693
                          Fax: 310-314-1469
                          www.pedaids.org

A brochure offering information on the latest research and advances in the area of pediatric AIDS.

DESCRIPTION

1732 FETAL ALCOHOL SYNDROME

Synonym: FAS

Disorder Type: Teratogen

Fetal alcohol syndrome, or FAS, is a condition that is present at birth and the result of persistent maternal alcohol consumption during pregnancy. This condition is characterized by various birth defects such as low birth weight, short birth length, and an unusually small head (microcephaly) that may be associated with slowed development of the brain. Infants with FAS may also have several abnormalities of the face and skull including an unusually short opening between the margins of the upper and lower eyelids (palpebral fissures), vertical folds of skin that extend from the inner corners of the upper eyelids to the sides of the nose (epicanthal folds), an abnormally small lower jaw (micrognathia), or a poorly developed upper jaw (maxillary hypoplasia). Additional unusual features may include an abnormal opening in the roof of the mouth (cleft palate), a prominent forehead (frontal bossing), a flattened nasal bridge, and a thin upper lip. Other characteristic findings may include heart defects, abnormalities of the limbs and joints (e.g., dislocated hip, etc.), and irregular skin crease patterns on the palms of the hands. Within the first day of life, affected newborns may also exhibit characteristic symptoms of alcohol withdrawal such as tremor, increased irritability, muscle spasms, vomiting, or other problems. The development of the brain may also be impaired resulting in moderate to severe mental retardation. Approximately 20 percent of newborns with fetal alcohol syndrome risk life-threatening symptoms and complications within the first few weeks of life.

Alcohol consumption during pregnancy affects the growth and development of the fetus within the uterus and may result not only in birth defects but, in some cases, miscarriage or stillbirth. Although it is believed that fetal alcohol syndrome results from persistent moderate or heavy drinking, no safe levels of alcohol intake during pregnancy have been established; therefore, pregnant women are counseled to avoid alcohol consumption. It has, however, been determined that the more alcohol consumed, the greater the chances of giving birth to children with associated abnormalities. Therefore, treatment is directed toward identification, counseling, and education of women at risk. Other treatment is symptomatic and supportive.

The following organizations in the General Resources Section can provide additional information: March of Dimes Birth Defects Foundation, National Mental Health Association, National Mental Health Consumer Self-Help Clearinghouse, NIH/National Institute of Mental Health, NIH/National Institute of Child Health and Human Development

National Associations & Support Groups

1733 ARC
500 E. Border St, Ste 300
Arlington, TX 76010
817-261-6003
800-433-5255
Fax: 817-277-0553
TDD: 817-277-0553
e-mail: thearc@metronet.com
thearc.org/

1734 Family Empowerment Network: Supporting Families Affected by FAS/FAE
519 Lowell Hall
Madison, WI 53703
608-262-8971
800-462-5254
Fax: 608-265-3352
e-mail: fen@mail.dcs.wisc.edu

Disabled Children's Computer Group, and a major corporation consisting of parents, consumers, and professionals. It is one of the nations largest resources to help children and adults who have disabilities gain access to the benefits of technology. Includes nationwide network of community-based assistive technology, resource centers, hands on consultants and product demonstrations.

1735 Fetal Alcohol Education Program
7 Kent St
Brookline, MA 02146
617-739-1424
Fax: 617-566-4019

Works to educate the professional and community on the affects of alcohol consumption during pregnancy.

1736 Fetal Alcohol Syndrome Family Resource Institute
P.O. Box 2525
Lynwood, WA 98036   253-531-2878
800-999-3429
Fax: 253-531-2668
e-mail: vicfas@hotmail.com
www.accessone.com/~delindam/

1737 Institute on Alcohol Abuse and Alcoholism
6000 Executive Blvd Ste 400
Bethesda, MD 20892   301-443-3885
Fax: 301-443-7043

1738 NIH/Institute on Alcohol Abuse and Alcoholism
6000 Executive Blvd, Ste 400
Bethesda, MD 20892   301-443-3885
Fax: 301-443-7043

1739 National Organization on Fetal Alcohol Syndrome
216 G Street NE
Washington, DC 20002   202-785-4585
800-666-6327
Fax: 202-466-6456
e-mail: nofas@erols.com
www.nofas.org

Only national organization dedicated solely to raising public awareness about alcohol-related birth defects. Projects include national campaigns, conferences, and training for parents and professionals. Free informaction packet available.

1740 National Resource Center for Prevention of Perinatal Abuse of Alcohol
CSAP Division of Communications Programs
5600 Fishers Lane
Rockville, MD 20857   301-443-9936

Offers information and resources to pregnant women on substance abuse, alcoholism and drugs pertaining to their unborn child's health.

Books

1741 Alcohol, Tobacco and Other Drugs May Harm the Unborn
National Clearinghouse for Alcohol and Drug Info.
P.O. Box 2345
Rockville, MD 20847
800-729-6686

Presents the most recent findings of basic research and clinical studies conducted on the effects of alcohol, drugs and tobacco on the unborn.

1742 Drugs and Pregnancy: It's Not Worth The Risk
American Council On Drug Education
204 Monroe Street, Ste. 110
Rockville, MD 20850
800-488-3784

A scientific monograph for health care providers which teaches them to identify alcohol and drug problems in their patients.

48 pages

1743 Pregnancy and Exposure to Alcohol and Other Drug Use
National Clearinghouse for Alcohol and Drug Info.
P.O. Box 2345
Rockville, MD 20849
800-729-6686
www.health.org

This report is for health care professionals presenting the state-of-the-art information about preventing ATOD use among women of childbearing age.

1744 Prevention Resource Guide: Pregnant Postpartum Women and Their Infants
National Clearinghouse for Alcohol and Drug Info.
P.O. Box 2345
Rockville, MD 20849
800-729-6686
www.health.org

This resource guide targets health care providers, prevention program planners and counselors of pregnant and postpartum women between the ages of 15 and 44.

30 pages

Pamphlets

1745 Alcohol and Pregnancy, Make the Right Choice
March of Dimes Resource Center
1275 Mamaroneck Avenue
White Plains, NY 10605   888-663-4637
Fax: 914-997-4763

1746 Drinking During Pregnancy
March of Dimes Resource Center
1275 Mamaroneck Avenue
White Plains, NY 10605   888-663-4637
Fax: 914-997-4763

1747 Effects of Alcohol on Pregnancy National Clearinghouse for Alcohol Info
P.O. Box 2345
Rockville, MD 20847   301-468-2600

Free publications are available that discuss the effects of alcohol on pregnancy: Fetal Alcohol Syndrome; and The Fact Is Alcohol and Other Drugs Can Harm an Unborn Baby.

1748 Fetal Alcohol Syndrome
Brent Q. Hafen, author

Hazelden
15251 Pleasant Valley Road
Center City, MN 55012   612-257-4010
                                 800-328-9000
                          Fax: 612-257-1331
                          www.hazelden.org

A source of information about the effects of drinking while pregnant.

1749 Fight Drug Abuse at Home, Work, School and in the Community
American Council for Drug Education
204 Monroe Street, Ste. 110
Rockville, MD 20850
                                 800-488-3784

A catalog of print and video materials pertaining to substance abuse, alcoholism and drugs.

1750 How to Take Care of Your Baby Before Birth
National Clearinghouse for Alcohol and Drug Info.
P.O. Box 2345
Rockville, MD 20849
                                 800-729-6686
                          www.health.org

A low-literacy brochure aimed at pregnant women that describes what they should and should not do during pregnancy.

DESCRIPTION

1751 FETAL EFFECTS OF COCAINE
Synonyms: Cocaine embryopathy, Fetal effects of maternal cocaine
Disorder Type: Birth Defect, Teratogen

The use of any form of cocaine by a woman during pregnancy may result in characteristic birth defects and other findings in affected newborns. Cocaine is a drug that is obtained from coca leaves or produced artificially (synthetically). The drug, which is used as a local anesthetic, narrows blood vessels and stimulates brain activity, potentially causing feelings of exhilaration and other effects. Cocaine is a highly addictive substance that is categorized as a Schedule II drug under the United States' Controlled Substance Act of 1970. This federal law regulates the prescribing and dispensing of drugs that affect thinking processes, mood, and behavior (psychoactive drugs) according to five categories. Drugs are categorized based on their medical acceptance, their potential for abuse, and their ability to produce a state in which increasing quantities of the drug are required to prevent withdrawal symptoms (dependence).

The use of cocaine and cocaine addiction have significantly increased over the past several decades. Maternal use of cocaine in any form during pregnancy (including crack, a purified form of cocaine) may result in certain complications of pregnancy as well as characteristic birth defects and other findings. These abnormalities may depend upon the stage of fetal development during which cocaine exposure occurs; the dose and method of use, such as sniffing, smoking, or intravenous administration; and the regularity of maternal cocaine use. Other factors may include maternal nutritional habits, possible coexisting alcohol abuse, additional abuse of other drugs, or tobacco use. Complications of pregnancy associated with cocaine use may include early separation of the placenta from the mother's uterus (abruptio placentae), inadequate oxygen supply to fetal tissues (fetal hypoxia), and early (premature) labor.

In some severe cases, abruptio placentae may result in miscarriage and potentially life-threatening complications in the mother. In addition, affected newborns may have a low birth weight, localized loss of brain tissue resulting from interrupted blood supply, an unusually small head (microcephaly), and episodes of abnormally increased electrical activity in the brain (seizures). Additional birth defects may affect the digestive system, kidneys, genitals, heart, or skeleton. Patients also commonly experience delays in the acquisition of skills that require the coordination of physical and mental activities (psychomotor delays) and learning and behavioral problems.

Withdrawal symptoms are considered unusual in affected newborns. However, in rare cases, such symptoms may occur, including abnormally increased responses to environmental stimuli (hyperexcitability) and uncontrollable trembling. These symptoms may be more common when there was also maternal use of other drugs or alcohol.

The treatment of affected newborns is symptomatic and supportive. Such measures may include the use of certain medications to help prevent or control seizures (anticonvulsants), surgical correction of birth defects, and multidisciplinary measures, such as special education, for children affected with learning or behavioral problems. Women who experience premature separation of the placenta from the uterus may require an immediate emergency Cesarean section to prevent life-threatening complications. Counseling and education of women of child-bearing age concerning the fetal effects of maternal cocaine use play an essential role in helping to prevent pregnancy complications and birth defects associated with cocaine use.

The following organizations in the General Resources Section can provide additional information: March of Dimes Birth Defects Foundation, NIH/National Institute of Child Health and Human Development, National Organization for Rare Disorders, Inc., (NORD)

National Associations & Support Groups

1752 Center for Substance Abuse Prevention National Drug Hotline
Rockwall II
1515 Security Lane
Rockville, MD 20852   301-443-0373

1753 National Institute on Drug Abuse
5600 Fischer Lane
Rockville, MD 20857   301-443-1124
                            800-729-6686

Pamphlets

1754 Cocaine Use During Pregnancy
March of Dimes Resource Center
1275 Mamaroneck Avenue
White Plains, NY 10605   888-663-4637
                              Fax: 914-997-4763

1755 Making the Right Choices: The Facts About Drugs and Pregnancy
March of Dimes Resource Center
1275 Mamaroneck Avenue
White Plains, NY 10605   888-663-4637
                              Fax: 914-997-4763

DESCRIPTION

1756 FETAL RETINOID SYNDROME

Disorder Type: Birth Defect, Teratogen
Covers these related disorders: Etretinate embryopathy, Isotretinoin embryopathy, Retinol embryopathy

Fetal retinoid syndrome is a characteristic pattern of birth defects caused by exposure to vitamin A (retinol) or its derivatives during early pregnancy. The term retinoid refers to retinol or any natural or artificially created derivative of vitamin A. In newborns with fetal retinoid syndrome, characteristic symptoms and findings include small, low-set ears or complete absence of the outer ears and external ear canals (microtia); an abnormally small head (microcephaly); enlargement of the cavities within the brain (ventricles); and underdevelopment (hypoplasia) of the thymus, a small gland in the upper portion of the chest that functions as an essential part of the immune system during infancy and childhood.

Several studies have reported fetal retinoid syndrome in newborns as a result of maternal use of vitamin A derivatives such as isotretinoin during early pregnancy. In addition, an increasing number of studies reveal the occurrence of such birth defects due to maternal use of other vitamin A derivatives, particularly the medication etretinate, or large doses of vitamin A (e.g., greater than 15,000 units daily) during early embryonic development. Although the frequency of fetal retinoid syndrome is unknown, reported cases represent only a small percentage of actual occurrences of the syndrome. Moreover, there is ongoing concern that increasing use of high dose vitamin A preparations and of vitamin A derivatives to treat certain common skin conditions, such as cystic acne or psoriasis, may result in additional cases of fetal retinoid syndrome. Dosage levels and the stage of embryonic development during which retinoid exposure occurs are thought to be the major factors influencing the occurrence of fetal retinoid

syndrome. The period of greatest risk may occur between approximately two to five weeks after conception. The specific underlying abnormality that causes fetal retinoid syndrome is not known. Studies indicate that retinoid exposure may cause disrupted development in the embryonic region that later becomes the brain and spinal cord (neural crest). The role that genetic influences or other environmental factors may have in contributing to fetal retinoid syndrome is unknown.

Although the symptoms and findings associated with fetal retinoid syndrome vary somewhat from case to case, affected newborns typically have a characteristic pattern of malformations. Affected newborns may have abnormalities of the head and face, including premature closure of the fibrous joint between the bones forming the forehead (metopic craniosynostosis); downslanting eyelid folds (palpebral fissures); widely spaced eyes (ocular hypertelorism) that may be abnormally small (microphthalmia); a short or broad nose; a small jaw (micrognathia); or incomplete closure of the roof of the mouth (cleft palate) and a groove in the upper lip (cleft lip). Abnormalities of the brain and spinal cord (central nervous system) are also common and include obstruction of the flow of cerebrospinal fluid around the brain, causing the fluid to accumulate under increasing pressure within the cavities of the brain (hydrocephalus); loss of vision; or other abnormalities (e.g., holoprosencephaly, posterior fossa cyst). Additional neurologic problems may include paralysis of the nerves that supply muscles responsible for eye movements (oculomotor paralysis) or weakness or paralysis of the nerve that supplies the forehead, scalp, eyelids, cheeks, jaws, and muscles of facial expression (facial nerve palsy).

Newborns with fetal retinoid syndrome may also have clouding of the lenses of the eyes (congenital cataracts); malformations of the heart and its major blood vessels (e.g., ventricular septal defects, hypoplastic aortic arch, transposition of the great arteries); underdevelopment (hypoplasia) of the kidneys and tubes that carry urine from the kidneys into the bladder (ureters); and abnormalities of the liver. Many affected newborns may also have malformations of the arms, legs, hands, and feet, such as webbing or fusion of the fingers and toes (syndactyly); malformations of the bone on the thumb side of the forearm (radial defects); a defect in which the foot is twisted out of shape or position (clubfoot or talipes); or fusion of the lower legs and absence of the feet (sirenomelia). In some patients, life-threatening complications may occur soon after birth. Treatment of newborns with fetal retinoid syndrome includes symptomatic and supportive measures.

The following organizations in the General Resources Section can provide additional information: March of Dimes Birth Defects Foundation, National Organization for Rare Disorders, Inc., (NORD), NIH/Office of Rare Diseases, NIH/National Institute of Child Health and Human Development

National Associations & Support Groups

1757 Association of Children's Prosthetic/ Orthotic Clinics
6300 North River Road, Ste 727
Rosemont, IL 60018   847-698-1694
e-mail: hohimer@aaos.org
www.acpoc.org

Reassures sufferers through the support groups provided.

1758 National Rehabilitation Information Center
8455 Colesville Rd, Ste 935
Silver Springs, MD 20190   301-588-9284
e-mail: naric@capaccess.org
www.naric.com/naric

NARIC is a library and information center focusing in disability and rehabilitation research. Information specialists provide quick information and referrals free of charge. Other sevices include customized searches of REHABDATA, the priemer database of disability and rehabilitation literature.

International

1759 Reach: the Association for Children with Hand or Arm Deficiency
12 Wilson Way, Earls Barton
Northamptonshire,
United Kingdom
e-mail: reach@reach.org.uk
www.reach.org.uk

Newsletters

1760 Superkids, Inc.
60 Clyde St
Newton, MA 02430
www.super-kids.org

Newsletter for parents of children with limb reduction abnormalities

DESCRIPTION

1761 FETAL THALIDOMIDE SYNDROME
Synonym: Thalidomide embryopathy
Disorder Type: Birth Defect, Teratogen

Fetal thalidomide syndrome is a characteristic pattern of birth defects in a newborn caused by exposure to the drug thalidomide during early pregnancy. Maternal use of thalidomide during early embryonic growth may affect the normal development of almost any organ. However, in newborns with fetal thalidomide syndrome, the most common characteristic associated with the disorder is incomplete development of the arms, legs, hands, and feet (limb reduction deformities). Such deformities may range from underdevelopment (hypoplasia) of one or more fingers or toes to complete absence of the arms and legs (amelia). In many patients, one or both of the hands or feet may be attached to the trunk by short, irregularly shaped bones (phocomelia). Some newborns with fetal thalidomide syndrome may also have additional abnormalities, such as absence or underdevelopment of the anal canal (anal atresia), causing the rectum to end blindly. The rectum is the muscular tube that forms the lower region of the large intestine. Additional abnormalities may include narrowing of a portion of the small intestine (duodenal stenosis), absence of certain tissues of the eyes (coloboma), or a benign tumor in the mid-facial area composed of abnormal blood vessels (mid-facial hemangioma). Genital, kidney, and heart defects may also be present. Depending upon the range and severity of associated symptoms and findings, complications may include visual impairment or blindness, deafness, or potentially life-threatening symptoms soon after birth. The treatment of infants with fetal thalidomide syndrome is symptomatic and supportive, including appropriate medical and surgical measures to treat possible digestive, heart, kidney, bone, or other defects. Artificial limbs (prostheses), orthopedic appliances, mobility devices, and other measures may be used as required.

The stage of embryonic development during which thalidomide exposure occurs may be the major factor influencing the possible occurrence and severity of fetal thalidomide syndrome. According to researchers, the greatest period of risk may occur between four to six weeks after conception.

Thalidomide was widely used in Europe during the late 1950s and early 1960s as an anxiety-relieving medication. When it was discovered that the drug causes severe birth defects, the medication's use was discontinued in most countries. However, complete withdrawal, of thalidomide was delayed in some areas of the world. Between 1958 and 1963, approximately 8,000 to 10,000 newborns were affected by fetal thalidomide syndrome.

The following organizations in the General Resources Section can provide additional information: March of Dimes Birth Defects Foundation, National Organization for Rare Disorders, Inc., (NORD), NIH/Office of Rare Diseases, NIH/National Institute of Child Health and Human Development

National Associations & Support Groups

1762 Association of Children's Prosthetic/ Orthotic Clinics
6300 North River, Ste 727
Rosemont, IL 60018   847-698-1694
e-mail: hohimer@aaos.org
www.acpoc.org

Reassures sufferers through the support groups provided.

1763 National Rehabilitation Information Center
8455 Colesville Rd, Ste 935
Silver Springs, MD 20190   301-588-9284
e-mail: naric@capaccess.org
www.naric.com/naric

NARIC is a library and information center focusing in disability and rehabilitation research. Information specialists provide quick information and referrals free of charge. Other services include customized searches of REHABDATA, the premier database of disability and rehabilitation literature, and documents from NARIC's collection of more than 60,000 documents are available for nominal fee.

International

**1764 Reach: the Association for Children with Hand or
Arm Deficiency**
12 Wilson Way, Earls Barton
Northamptonshire,
United Kingdom

e-mail: reach@reach.org.uk
www.reach.org.uk

Newsletters

1765 Superkids, Inc.
60 Clyde St
Newton, MA 02460

www.super-kids.org

Newsletter for parents of children with limb reduction abnormalities.

DESCRIPTION

1766 FRAGILE X SYNDROME

Synonyms: Marker X Syndrome, Martin-Bell Syndrome

Disorder Type: Chromosomal Disorder, Developmental Milestones, Genetic Disorder, Mental, Emotional or Behavioral Disorder

Fragile X Syndrome, a disorder that results from an inherited defect of the X chromosome, is the most common cause of mental retardation in males. The disorder is thought to affect approximately one in 2,000 to 4,000 males and to be slightly less frequent in females. Although symptoms may be variable, the most common feature associated with fragile X syndrome is mental retardation.

Most males with fragile X syndrome have mild to profound mental retardation (e.g., an intelligence quotient or I.Q. ranging from approximately 30 to 55.) However, some may have an I.Q. that is considered borderline normal. Affected males with mild mental retardation may have a distinctive speech pattern characterized by rapid speech with a variable rhythm (cluttering). Those with more severe retardation typically communicate in bursts of repetitive speech. Affected males with severe or profound mental retardation may lack the ability to speak. In addition, most males with fragile X syndrome may have poor eye contact or experience emotional difficulties. Some may have poor concentration associated with hyperactivity or engage in autistic-like behaviors, such as hand biting or hand flapping.

In many cases, affected males may also have physical abnormalities. For example, many males with fragile X syndrome may have unusually large testes (macroorchidism), a finding that is most apparent after puberty; however, testicular function is normal. Affected males may also typically have characteristic facial features, such as a large head (macrocephaly) and forehead, a relatively long face and prominent jaw, thick lips, and prominent ears. Other findings may include crowding of the teeth, excessive flexibility of the finger joints, or flat feet (pes planus). In addition, approximately 50 percent of affected females have varying degrees of mental retardation or learning difficulties. In some cases, females with fragile X syndrome may also have physical abnormalities, such as irregular teeth or unusually flexible finger joints. The treatment of children with fragile X syndrome includes symptomatic and supportive measures, such as special education, speech therapy, and, in some cases, multidisciplinary techniques such as behavioral therapies to help manage hyperactivity or autistic-like behaviors.

Individuals with fragile X syndrome inherit a fragile area or site on the long arm (q) of the X chromosome (Xq27.3). Chromosomal analysis reveals that the genetic material on the end of this arm appears to be broken off. In reality, this genetic material is actually dangling from the end of the long arm. The disease gene within this area is known as the FRAXA gene. This region (locus) of the X chromosome contains abnormally long repeats (e.g., over 200 repeats) of coded DNA instructions (CGG trinucleotide repeat expansion). Males have only one X chromosome; therefore, if they inherit a fragile X locus containing more than 200 CGG repeats, they generally express the symptoms associated with this syndrome and are typically more severely affected than females. However, because females have two X chromosomes, certain disease traits may be masked by the presence of a normal gene on the other X chromosome, resulting in lower frequency and decreased severity of the disease among females.

The following organizations in the General Resources Section can provide additional information: National Organization for Rare Disorders, Inc. (NORD), Genetic Alliance, NIH/National Institute of Child Health and Human Development

National Associations & Support Groups

1767 ARC
500 East Border Street, Suite 300
Arlington, TX 76010   817-261-6003
                             800-433-5255
                        Fax: 817-277-3491
                        TTY: 817-277-0553
              e-mail: thearc@metronet.com
                    thearc.org/welcome.html

The ARC of the United States works through
education, research and advocacy to improve
the quality of life for children and adults with
mental retardation and their families and works
to prevent both the causes and the effects of mental retardation.

1768 FRAXA Research Foundation Newsletter
45 Pleasant Street
Newburyport, MA 01950   978-462-1866
                        Fax: 978-463-9985
                 e-mail: info@fraxa.org
                       www.fraxa.org

FRAXA supports research on fragile X syndrome, a genetic disorder which is the most common inherited cause of mental retardation.

2,500 members

Katherine Clapp, President

1769 National Fragile X Foundation
1441 York St Ste 303
Denver, CO 80206   303-333-6155
                             800-688-5765
                        Fax: 303-333-4369
              e-mail: natlfx@ix.netcom.com
                         www.infxf.org

Provides a wide variety data for people suffering
from the disorder to access at any time with ease.

Web Sites

1770 American College of Medical Genetics
www.faseb.org/genetics/acmg/pol-16.htm

1771 Pedbase
www.icondata.com/health/ped-
base/files/FRAGILEX.HTM

Newsletters

1772 FRAXA Research Foundation
FRAXA
45 Pleasant Street
Newburyport, MA 01950   978-462-1866
                        Fax: 978-463-9985
                 e-mail: info@fraxa.org
                       www.fraxa.org

FRAXA supports research on fragile X syndrome, a genetic disorder which is the most common inherited cause of mental retardation.

12 pages 4X

Katherine Clapp, Editor

DESCRIPTION

1773 GALACTOSEMIA

Disorder Type: Genetic Disorder, Metabolism
Covers these related disorders: Classic galactosemia, Galactokinase deficiency, Galactose epimerase deficiency (Deficiency of uridyl diphosphogal

Galactosemia is a genetic disorder transmitted as an autosomal recessive trait and characterized by the inability of the body to process or metabolize galactose, a simple sugar found in milk and milk products, certain fruits and vegetables, and seaweed. This inborn error of metabolism occurs as the result of a deficiency of one of three different enzymes and is thus divided into three distinct galactosemic disorders.

Classic galactosemia results from a deficiency of galactose-1-phosphate uridyl transferase, an enzyme that breaks down galactose-1-phosphate, a component of the milk sugar lactose. Galactose-1-phosphate begins to accumulate in the tissues of the body and may lead to damage of the functional tissues in the brain, liver, and kidneys. Symptoms may include a yellowish discoloration of the skin, eyes, and mucous membranes (jaundice); opacity of the lenses of the eyes (cataracts); vomiting; convulsions; increased irritability; sluggishness; difficulty in feeding; and failure to gain weight. Characteristic findings may include enlargement of the liver and spleen (hepatosplenomegaly), low blood sugar (hypoglycemia), the presence of amino acids in the urine (aminoaciduria), an abnormal accumulation of fluid in the abdomen (ascites), the formation of scar tissue in the liver (cirrhosis), and mental retardation. Treatment is directed toward the elimination of galactose from the diet to prevent the appearance of or progressive worsening of cirrhosis, mental retardation, cataracts, and other findings associated with galactosemia. In addition, a pregnant woman who has galactosemia or is aware that she carries the gene for this disorder should eliminate galactose-containing foods from her diet in order to prevent galactose from crossing the placental barrier, possibly resulting in injury to the fetus. Although strict dietary regulation may prevent many of the severe complications of classic galactosemia, some affected children and adults may experience delays in growth and development, speech irregularities, and difficulties with motor function. Approximately one of every 60,000 newborns is affected with classic galactosemia.

Galactokinase deficiency results from the absence of or decreased levels of galactokinase, an enzyme that is responsible for assisting in the first step of the chemical reaction that allows utilization of galactose. This deficiency results in findings associated with galactosemia, the presence of increased levels of galactose in the blood and urine, and the formation of cataracts. Treatment includes the institution of a galactose-free diet. Approximately one in 40,000 newborns is affected with galactosemia resulting from galactokinase deficiency.

Galactose epimerase deficiency, a very rare form of galactosemia, results from defective uridyl diphosphogalactose-4-epimerase (UDP glucose-4-epimerase), another enzyme that assists in the metabolism of galactose. This deficiency may be present in a benign form in which the deficiency is limited to the blood cells, usually resulting in no symptoms or long-term effects. However, in those with more widespread epimerase deficiency, symptoms, findings, and treatment may be similar to those of classic galactosemia.

The following organizations in the General Resources Section can provide additional information: National Organization for Rare Disorders, Inc., (NORD), Genetic Alliance, March of Dimes Birth Defects Foundation, NIH/Office of Rare Diseases, NIH/National Digestive Diseases Information Clearinghouse, Online Mendelian Inheritance in Man: www3.ncbi.nlm.nih.gov/Omim/searchomim.html

National Associations & Support Groups

1774 American Liver Foundation
75 Maiden Lane Suite 603
New York, NY 10038   212-668-1000
                                    800-465-4837
                                    Fax: 212-483-8179
                    e-mail: info@liverfoundation.org
                    www.liverfoundation.org

Organization provides several different medias
for answering questions and to help calrify any
uncertainties the individual may be experiencing.

1775 Parents of Galactosemic Children, Inc.
2148 Bryton Drive
Powell, OH 95252   614-840-0473
                    e-mail: gayled3@aol.com
                    www.galactosemia.org

Group provides support and educational information to affected families and professionals.
Also helps to facilitate communication between
the two groups.

International

1776 Research Trust for Metabolic Diseases in Children
Golden Gates Lodge
Weston Road
Crewe, Cheshire,
United Kingdom

Dedicated to providing the most up-to-date
knowledge for the families and friends of people
suffering from this and related diseases.

Web Sites

1777 American Liver Foundation
gi.ucsf.edu/alf/info/infogalactosemia.html

1778 Pedbase
www.icondata.com/health/pedbase/files/

1779 Rare Genetic Diseases in Children
mcrcr2.med.nyu.edu/murphp01/homenew.htm

1780 Tyler for Life Foundation
www.tylerforlife.com

1781 Women's and Children's Hospital
www.dircsa.org.au/pub/docs/galac.txt

DESCRIPTION

1782 GAUCHER'S DISEASE

Synonyms: Gaucher disease, Glucosylceramide lipidosis, Glucosyl cerebroside lipidosis

Disorder Type: Genetic Disorder, Metabolism

Covers these related disorders: Chronic Gaucher's disease (Adult or Classic Gaucher's disease), Infantile Gaucher's disease, Juvenile Gaucher's disease

Gaucher's disease is an inherited metabolic disorder characterized by a deficiency of the enzyme glucocerebrosidase (glucosylceramidase), which assists in the metabolism of certain fats. This deficiency results in the accumulation of certain fatty substances (glucocerebroside or glucosylceramide) throughout the body. Gaucher's disease is subdivided into three main types. The first, known as chronic, adult, or classic Gaucher's disease, may develop at any age from birth to 80 years old. This form of the disease is common among eastern European Jews, with an incidence rate of as many as one in 500 births. Findings associated with chronic Gaucher's disease include enlargement of the spleen (splenomegaly) or liver (hepatomegaly), or both (hepatosplenomegaly); a decrease in levels of hemoglobin in the blood (anemia); decreased numbers of circulating white blood cells (leukopenia); and abnormally low levels of circulating platelets (thrombocytopenia), which may lead to easy bruising or bleeding. Symptoms may include a brownish-pigmented skin; yellow spots in the eyes resulting from accumulation of fatty substances; and bone pain resulting from accumulations in the bone marrow. Treatment for chronic Gaucher's disease includes enzyme replacement therapy.

Infantile Gaucher's disease, a life-threatening form of this disorder, affects the central nervous system of the newborn. Symptoms and findings may include enlargement of the spleen, crossed eyes (strabismus); muscle spasms in the jaw (trismus or lockjaw); seizures; backward bending of the head; or a rigid, arched back. Additional abnormalities of the central nervous system may become apparent.

Juvenile Gaucher's disease may appear at any time during childhood. Characteristic findings may include enlargement of the liver and spleen (hepatosplenomegaly), bone abnormalities resulting in pain and swelling of the joints, anemia, and abnormally low levels of circulating white blood cells and platelets. Affected children may be pale, weak, and particularly susceptible to bleeding and recurring infection. Symptoms related to nervous system involvement include lack of motor coordination and loss of balance, inflammation of the nerves in the arms and legs accompanied by abnormal sensations and discomfort, muscle spasms, paralysis of the nerves of the eye (ophthalmoplegia), and impairment of mental function.

Enzyme replacement therapy is usually not effective in the treatment of the infantile and juvenile forms of Gaucher's disease. Alternative treatment may include removal of the spleen (splenectomy). Other treatment is symptomatic and supportive.

Gaucher's disease is inherited as an autosomal recessive trait. The gene responsible for the regulation of the enzyme glucocerebrosidase is located on the long arm of chromosome 1 (1q21-q31).

The following organizations in the General Resources Section can provide additional information: National Organization for Rare Disorders, Inc., (NORD), Genetic Alliance, March of Dimes Birth Defects Foundation, NIH/National Institute of Neurological Disorders & Stroke, Online Mendelian Inheritance in Man: www3.ncbi.nlm.nih.gov/Omim/searchomim.html

National Associations & Support Groups

1783 ARC
500 East Border Street, Suite 300
Arlington, TX 76010   817-261-6003
                             800-433-5255
                        TDD: 817-277-0553

Parent to Parent (P-P) programs provide informational and emotional support to parents who have a child, adolelscent, or adult family member with special needs. P-P programs offer an important connection for a parent who is seeking support for special disability issue, by matching him or her with a trained vetern parent who has already been there. Because the two parents share so many common concerns and interests, the support given and received is often uniquely meaningful.

1784 National Foundation for Jewish Genetic Diseases
250 Park Avenue, Suite 1000
New York, NY 10017   212-371-1030

Provides the information regarding this and related disorders for the people suffering from them.

1785 National Gaucher Foundation
11140 Rockville Pike, Ste. 350
Rockville, MD 20852   301-816-1515
                            800-428-2437
                      Fax: 301-816-1516
      e-mail: ngf@gaucherdisease.org
              www.gaucherdisease.org

A non-profit organization whose primary objective is to assist in perfecting a treatment program and discovering a cure for Gaucher disease. The Foundation supports medical research and clinical programs which enhance the current understanding of Gaucher disease.

1984 12-20 pages Quarterly

Rhonda P. Buyers, Executive Director
Robin Beima, Editor

1786 National Lipid Diseases Foundation
1201 Corbin Street
Elizabeth, NJ 07201   908-527-8000
                            800-527-8005
                      Fax: 908-527-8004

Focuses on the facilities that specialize on the disease and helping people choose the one that is right for them.

1787 Osteoporosis and Related Bone Diseases National Resource Center
1232 22nd Street NW
Washington, DC 20037   202-223-0344
                             800-624-2663
                       Fax: 202-293-2356
                       TTY: 301-565-2966
        e-mail: orbdnrc@nof.org
                www.osteo.org

The center seeks to educate patients, health professionals and the public on metabolic bone diseases, such as Paget's disease of the bone, osteoporosis, hyperparathyroidism and osteogenesis imoerfecta. It is opened under the NAtional Osteoporosis Foundation (NOF) and works in connection with the Paget Foundation and the Osteoporosis Imperfecta Foundation.

Jessica Branch, Health Information Specialist

1788 Tay-Sachs and Allied Diseases Association
2001 Beacon Street, Room 304
Brookline, MA 02164   617-277-4463

Dedicated to the treatment and preventy of Tay-Sachs and related diseases, and to provide information and support services to individuals and families affected by these diseases through education, research, genetic screening, family services and advocacy.

International

1789 Gauchers Association (UK)
25 West Cottages
London,
United Kingdom
        e-mail: gaucher@wisebuy.co.uk
        http://www.gaucher.org.uk

Firmly incorporated to provide the United Kingdom with a close and easy to access support foundation that they can turn to.

1790 Research Trust for Metabolic Diseases in Children
Golden Gates Lodge
Weston Road
Crewe, Cheshire,
United Kingdom

Dedicated to providing the most up-to-date medical knowledge for the families and friends of people suffering from this and related diseases.

1791 Vaincre Les Maladies Lysosomales
9 Place du Mars 1962 91035
Evry Cedex,
France

Faithful to disseminating the knowledge that is needed through several media outlets, including audio and visual.

Audio Video

1792 Pain & Hope

National Gaucher Foundation
11140 Rockville Pike, Ste. 350
Rockville, MD 20852   301-816-1515
                                         800-925-8885
                                 Fax: 301-816-1516
               e-mail: ngf@gaucherdisease.org
                        www.gaucherdisease.org

A patient and family perspective on Gaucher disease.

1984 free to members

Sharon Adams, Director of Membership

Web Sites

1793 Children's Gaucher Research Fund

www.childrensgaucher.com

1794 Gaucher Registry

www.gaucherregistry.com

1795 Pedbase

www.icondata.com/health/ped-base/files/GAUCHER.HTM

1796 Rare Genetic Diseases in Children

mcrcr2.med.nyu.edu/murphp01/homenew.htm

DESCRIPTION

1797 GERMAN MEASLES
  Synonyms: Rubella, Three-day measles
  Disorder Type: Infectious Disease

German measles, or rubella, is a contagious viral disease characterized by swollen lymph nodes and a fine, reddish-pink rash that persists for one to three days. Rubella is transmitted through inhalation of droplets that are coughed or exhaled into the air by an infected individual. Early symptoms and characteristic findings may include swollen lymph nodes, especially in the neck and back of the head; pain in the joints (arthralgia); low-grade fever; cold symptoms; and redness and discomfort of the throat. Within one or two days, a rash usually appears on the face and quickly spreads to the trunk, arms, and legs and is accompanied by a generalized, spreading red flush. This mildly itchy rash usually subsides after three days. In some cases, the spleen may become slightly enlarged (splenomegaly). Symptoms may be so slight in some children that they go unnoticed. In older children and adults, symptoms are typically more pronounced and may include fever, headache, and joint inflammation (arthritis) accompanied by pain and swelling. In addition, pregnant women with German measles are at risk of transmitting the infection to their unborn children, possibly resulting in miscarriage, stillbirth, or disease in the newborn (congenital rubella) characterized by developmental abnormalities.

Protection against German measles infection is provided through intramuscular rubella immunization, usually in combination with measles and mumps vaccine. Immunization is recommended to women of child-bearing age who have not had German measles or have not been previously vaccinated; however, in individuals with compromised immune systems or a sensitivity to live vaccine, this type of vaccination is usually not advised. The incubation period for this viral infection is anywhere from 12 to 23 days. Treatment for rubella is symptomatic.

The following organizations in the General Resources Section can provide additional information: Genetic Alliance, March of Dimes Birth Defects Foundation, National Organization for Rare Disorders, Inc. (NORD), National Institute of Child Health and Human Development, National Institute of Allergy and Infectious Disease, World Health Organization (WHO), Centers for Disease Control (CDC)

Web Sites

1798 Child Health Research Project
ih.jhsp.edu/chr/chr.htm

1799 Pathfinder
www.pathfinder.com/ParentTime/Health.germeas.html

1800 Slack
www.slackinc.com/child/idc.idchome.htm

DESCRIPTION

1801 GROWTH HORMONE DEFICIENCY
Synonym: GH deficiency
May involve these systems in the body (see Section III):
Endocrine System

Growth hormone deficiency is a condition characterized by deficient production or impaired response to growth hormone, resulting in growth impairment and short stature with normal proportions (pituitary dwarfism). Growth hormone, also known as GH, stimulates body growth and development by promoting the production of protein in cells, releasing energy from the breakdown of fats, and performing other vital functions. GH is secreted by the pituitary gland. Also known as the master gland, the pituitary gland is connected to a region of the brain known as the hypothalamus by a stalk of nerve fibers (pituitary stalk). The hypothalamus controls the functioning of the pituitary gland through direct nerve stimulation as well as through the actions of certain nerve cells that secrete hormones (hormone-releasing and hormone-inhibiting factors) into the bloodstream for transport directly to the pituitary gland. The region of the pituitary gland known as the anterior pituitary gland secretes GH in response to a particular hormone-releasing factor (growth hormone releasing factor) from the hypothalamus. Depending upon the underlying cause of GH deficiency, some patients may also have deficiencies of additional hormones that are produced by the anterior pituitary gland, such as thyroid-stimulating hormone (TSH), which stimulates the production of thyroid hormones, or adrenocorticotropic hormone (ACTH), which promotes the growth and production of hormones by cells in the outer region (adrenal cortex) of the adrenal gland. Inadequate functioning of the pituitary gland is known as hypopituitarism.

Growth hormone deficiency may be due to many different causes, including absence, underdevelopment, or malformation of the pituitary gland or hypothalamus at birth; tumors of the anterior pituitary gland, pituitary stalk, or hypothalamus, particularly pituitary tumors known as craniopharyngiomas; or radiation therapy for the treatment of certain malignancies in the brain or skull region. GH deficiency may also result from trauma affecting the pituitary gland or hypothalamus, such as injury during delivery or lack of oxygen to the brain (anoxia). In addition, the condition may occur in association with certain chromosomal or genetic syndromes or may appear to occur randomly for unknown reasons (idiopathic hypopituitarism). There are also genetic forms of hypopituitarism that may be limited to GH deficiency or may be characterized by additional anterior pituitary hormone deficiencies.

There are several genetic subtypes of isolated growth hormone deficiency (IGHD), including those that may be inherited as an autosomal recessive, autosomal dominant, or X-linked trait. Patients with autosomal recessive IGHD may have complete deletions of a particular gene, known as the GH1 gene, which is located on the long arm of chromosome 17 (17q22-24). This form of the disorder is typically characterized by marked growth delays after birth and severe short stature. Other patients with autosomal recessive IGHD have various abnormal changes (mutations) of the GH1 gene, causing variable degrees of growth failure and short stature. Some patients with autosomal dominant IGHD may also have mutations of the GH1 gene. The disease gene responsible for X-linked IGHD has not yet been located. Another genetic form of hypopituitarism, known as Laron syndrome, is thought to result from an impaired response to growth hormone and is characterized by abnormally increased levels of circulating GH.

Most children with GH deficiency appear to be of normal weight and length at birth. By the first year of life, children with severe GH deficiency or Laron syndrome may be significantly shorter than would be expected (e.g., more than four standard deviations below the mean) for their age and sex. Patients with less severe GH deficiency experience regular growth spurts that alternate with periods during which no growth occurs. Patients may continue to experience growth beyond the age when most individuals attain their adult height. This is due to abnormal delays in the fusion of the growing ends and the shafts of the long bones. If children with GH deficiency do not receive treatment, their adult height may range from four to 12 standard deviations below the mean.

Children with GH deficiency typically have normally proportioned arms and legs; however, they may have relatively small hands and feet. Many also have a characteristic facial appearance, including a short, broad face and relatively round head; and undeveloped upper and lower jaw; a small, saddle-shaped nose with a depressed nasal bridge; a small neck; delayed eruption and crowding of the teeth; and fine, sparse scalp hair. Due to abnormal smallness of the voice box (larynx), many patients have a high-pitched voice. Other findings may include underdeveloped genitals, delayed or absent sexual development, and abnormally low blood sugar (hypoglycemia).

Children with GH deficiency due to tumors of the pituitary gland or hypothalamus may develop additional symptoms, depending upon the location, nature, and growth of the tumor. In some patients, invasion and destruction of the pituitary gland cause degeneration (atrophy) of the thyroid gland, sex glands (gonads), and outer regions of the adrenal glands (adrenal cortex). Associated findings may include absence of sweating, weight loss, abnormal sensitivity to cold, delayed or absent sexual maturation, lack of response to certain stimuli (torpor), or other abnormalities. Tumor growth may also cause total growth failure, abnormally increased urination (polyuria), vomiting, headaches, visual disturbances, episodes of abnormally increased electrical activity in the brain (seizures), and other abnormalities.

The treatment of GH deficiency varies and depends on the underlying cause and nature of the condition. If the condition results due to tumor growth, treatment measures may include surgery, radiation therapy, or other appropriate measures to remove the tumor. Pituitary function should be carefully evaluated after such measures to determine any necessary therapies for pituitary abnormalities. The treatment of children with IGHD

includes early replacement therapy with synthetic growth hormone that is continued until there is no longer a response. The maximum response usually occurs during the first year of therapy with slower subsequent growth. Because such therapy may cause abnormally decreased activity of the thyroid gland (hypothyroidism), thyroid function should be regularly evaluated. Children who have deficiencies of other anterior pituitary hormones in association with GH deficiency may receive additional hormone replacement therapies as required. Additional treatment is symptomatic and supportive.

The following organizations in the General Resources Section can provide additional information: National Organization for Rare Disorders, Inc. (NORD), Genetic Alliance, March of Dimes Birth Defects Foundation, NIH/Office of Rare Diseases, Online Mendelian Inheritance in Man.: www3.ncbi.nlm.nih.gov/Omim/searchomim.hmtl

National Associations & Support Groups

1802 Human Growth Foundation
7777 Leesburg Pike, Suite 202 South
Falls Church, VA 22043   703-883-1773
                                     800-451-6434
                        e-mail: hgfound@erols.com
                                  www.genetic.org

Devoted to the dispersion of medical knowledge of this and similar disorders, along with providing support for the sufferers and their families.

1803 Little People of America, Inc.
P.O. Box 9897
Washington, DC 20016   301-589-0730
                                     800-243-9273

1804 MAGIC Foundation for Children's Growth
1327 N. Harlem Avenue
Oak Park, IL 60302   708-383-0808
                                     800-362-4423
                             Fax: 708-383-0899

Support and education provided to families of children with growth related disorders. Specialty divisions include: Growth Hormone Deficiency; Precocious Puberty; Congenital Adrenal Hyperplasia; McCune Albright Syndrome; Congenital Hypothyroidism; Down Syndrome with Growth Failure; Russell-Silver Syndrome; Tuners Syndrome.

Mary Andrews, Executive Director

1805 Short Stature Foundation
4521 Campus Dr. #130
Irvine, CA 92715 714-258-1833
800-243-9273

Improves everyday life through the dispersion of information for commonly asked questions and problems of these with growth-related disorders.

Research Centers

1806 Case Western Research University, Bolton Brush Growth Study Center
2123 Abington Road
Cleveland, OH 44106 216-368-3200

Investigations and research into the growth and development of the human body.

B. Holly Broadbent, Jr., DDS, Director

1807 International Center for Skeletal Dysplasia
St. Joseph Hospital 7620 York Road
Towson, MD 21204 301-337-1250

1808 Jackson Laboratory
600 Main Streeet
Bar Harbor, ME 04609 207-288-6000
Fax: 207-288-5079

Studies focusing on growth disorders and human genetics.

Kenneth Paigen, Director

1809 New Jersey Institute of Technology Center For Biomedical Engineering
323 Martin Luther King, Jr.
Newark, NJ 07102 973-596-3000
Fax: 973-596-8436

Offers research into facial and bone disorders.

David Kristol, Director

1810 R.F. Stolinsky Research Laboratories
University of Colorado
4200 E. 9th Street, Box C233
Denver, CO 80262 303-315-8017

Focuses on genetic disorders and growth diseases.

Stephen Goodman, MD, Director

1811 W.M. Krogman Center for Research In Child Growth and Development
4019 Erving Street
Philadelphia, PA 19104 215-898-1470

Focuses research and studies on growth disorders and birth defects.

Dr. Solomon Katz, Director

Web Sites

1812 Pediatric Database;
www.icondata.com/health/pedbase/files/GROW-THHO.HTM

1813 Society for Endocrinology
www.endocrinology.org

Books

1814 Growing Children: A Parent's Guide
Patricia Rieser, author

Human Growth Foundation
7777 Leesburg Pike Suite 202S
Falls Church, VA 22043 703-883-1773
800-451-6434

Offers parents information on the normal pattern of their child's growth, growth charts, recognition of growth problems, evaluation of growth problems and resources for more information.

1815 Short and OK
Human Growth Foundation
7777 Leesburg Pike Suite 202S
Falls Church, VA 22043 703-883-1773
800-451-6434

This is a guide for parents of short children offering information on behavior issues, medical issues and psychological warning signs.

54 pages

Pamphlets

1816 Dental Problems with Growth Hormone Deficiency
Human Growth Foundation
7777 Leesburg Pike Suite 202S
Falls Church, VA 22043   703-883-1773
                               800-451-6434

1817 Growth Hormone Deficiency
Human Growth Foundation
7777 Leesburg Pike Suite 202S
Falls Church, VA 22043   703-883-1773
                               800-451-6434

Causes and control of growth hormone deficiency.

1818 Most Frequently Asked Questions with Growth Hormone Deficiency
Human Growth Foundation
7777 Leesburg Pike Suite 202S
Falls Church, VA 22043   703-883-1773
                               800-451-6434

DESCRIPTION

1819 GUILLAIN-BARRE SYNDROME

Synonyms: Acute ascending polyneuritis, Acute febrile polyneuritis, Acute idiopathic polyneuritis, Acute postinfectious polyneuropathy, GBS, Landry's paralysis

Disorder Type: Autoimmune Disease

May involve these systems in the body (see Section III):

Nervous System

Guillain-Barre syndrome (GBS) is a progressive neurologic disorder that affects many nerves (polyneuropathy) and is characterized by unusual sensations (paresthesias) in the arms or legs, or both. GBS generally causes progressive muscle weakness over days and, in some cases, paralysis accompanied by lack of muscle tone. Guillain-Barre syndrome is thought to be an autoimmune disorder and may occur as a reaction to a previous viral infection, immunization, or bacterial infection (e.g., Lyme disease). The symptoms of GBS typically begin approximately one to three weeks following the triggering event. Autoimmune disorders involve the body's inappropriate immune response to its own healthy tissues.

Symptoms associated with Guillain-Barre syndrome range from mild to severe and may include numbness, tingling, muscle weakness, and sometimes paralysis that begins in the legs and then usually spreads upward toward the trunk, arms, muscles of the chest, and sometimes the face. Affected children may become irritable and unable or unwilling to walk. As weakness spreads to the chest and facial areas, muscles required for speech, breathing, and eating may become affected. In addition, if the nerves of the autonomic nervous system which control vital involuntary functions are affected, individuals with GBS may develop fluctuations in blood pressure and heart rate as well as other heart irregularities. A rare form of Guillain-Barre syndrome called the Miller-Fisher syndrome is characterized by paralysis of the nerves and muscles of the eyes (ophthalmoplegia), an absence of normal reflexes (areflexia), and an inability to coordinate voluntary movement (ataxia).

Most children with Guillain-Barre syndrome recover completely within two to three weeks. Some may experience ongoing muscular weakness. In addition, in rare cases, affected individuals may experience prolonged or recurring episodes of GBS that may last for months or years. These uncommon manifestations are referred to as chronic unremitting polyradiculoneuropathy and chronic relapsing polyradiculoneuropathy.

Guillain-Barre syndrome may be diagnosed through specialized tests of the fluid that surrounds the brain and spinal cord (cerebrospinal fluid) and other clinical findings. Early diagnosis and hospitalization allow for observation and monitoring of affected individuals. If the progression of muscle weakness or paralysis is very slow and limited, treatment may include observation and supportive care until recovery is complete. If, however, paralysis progresses to involve breathing and swallowing, appropriate support is necessary. Other treatment may include plasma exchange (plasmapheresis), a procedure during which blood is withdrawn and the liquid portion (plasma) removed in order to filter out harmful substances. A plasma substitute is then mixed with the blood, and the reconstituted blood is then returned to the body. Alternative treatment may include the intravenous administration of immunoglobulin (IVIG). Children with chronic disease may also benefit from the use of IVIG or ongoing plasmapheresis. In some cases, certain immunosuppressive drugs or corticosteroids may be effective. Physical therapy may aid in the maintenance of joint and muscle function. Other treatment is symptomatic and supportive.

The following organizations in the General Resources Section can provide additional information: National Organization for Rare Disorders, Inc., (NORD), NIH/Office of Rare Diseases, American Autoimmune Related Diseases Association, Inc., NIH/National Institute of Neurological Disorders & Stroke (NINDS)

National Associations & Support Groups

1820 Guillain Barre Syndrome Foundation International
P.O. Box 262
Wynnewood, PA 19096   610-667-0131
                                   Fax: 610-667-7036
                              e-mail: GBINTix.netcom.com
                                   www.webmast.com/gbs/

Provides emotional support and assistance to
people after this rare disease. Arranges personal visits to affected individuals in hospitals
and rehabilitation centers. Forstors research
into the cause, treatment, and other aspects of
the disorders; and directs affected individuals
with long-term disabilities to resources for vocational, financial, and other aspects of the disorder.

International

**1821 Guillan-Barre Syndrome Support Group of the
United Kingdom**
Lincolnshire Cnty Council Off.
Lincolnshire Intl
NG34 7EB,
United Kingdom

Web Sites

1822 GBS Support Group of the UK
www.gbs.org.uk/

DESCRIPTION

1823 HEAD INJURIES

May involve these systems in the body (see Section III):

Central Nervous System

Head injuries describe trauma to the head that results in damage to the scalp, skull, or brain and associated membranes, nerves, or blood vessels. Every year in the United States, approximately 100,000 children require hospitalization because of head injuries. Many of these injuries are the result of motor vehicle and bicycle accidents. The risk of sustaining head or brain injury during a vehicular or bicycle accident is reduced by the proper use of restraint systems such as approved car seats, seat belts, or helmets. There are different types of head injuries, some of which are minor and, after healing, often of no further significance; however, certain injuries that impact upon the brain may have severe complications and be potentially life-threatening. These include skull fractures, concussions, brain contusions and lacerations, and bleeding in the brain (e.g., subdural or epidural hematomas). Brain injury may result in mild, moderate, or severe functional disabilities, depending upon the particular area of brain tissue that is damaged or destroyed. Disabilities may affect physical, emotional, or intellectual development and include impairment in the comprehension or production of speech and language (aphasia); the inability to remember or perform certain familiar tasks requiring sequential movements (apraxia); the failure to remember past events or experiences (amnesia); the lack of ability to recognize familiar persons or objects (agnosia); and the development of episodes of uncontrolled electrical activity in the brain (post-traumatic epilepsy), usually within two years of the initial head injury.

In children with skull fractures, an open-head injury, there is an actual break in the skull bone (cranium). Many skull fractures do not interfere with normal brain function and will heal with no complications. However, in some patients, fractures may damage blood vessels or the membranes surrounding the brain (meninges), resulting in leakage of the fluid that surrounds the brain and spinal cord (cerebrospinal fluid). The break in the skull may also serve as an entry point for bacteria that may subsequently cause serious infection. A thorough evaluation is necessary to determine the extent of the injury. Surgical intervention may sometimes be necessary.

Concussions are closed-head injuries that occur as a result of a jarring of the brain within the skull. Symptoms and findings associated with this type of injury in children may include a temporary loss of consciousness, lack of muscle tone, poor or absent reflexes (areflexia), dilated pupils, blurred vision, irritability, or restlessness. These signs of concussion may be followed by rapid heartbeat (tachycardia), vomiting, listlessness, drowsiness, apathy, a pale skin color, or confusion. Treatment for concussion always involves observation. Although most children recover completely, hospitalization may be required for those whose level of consciousness continues to drop or those who appear listless, drowsy, or confused. Those who vomit excessively or experience seizures or other neurological symptoms may also require hospitalization.

Other closed-head injuries may include contusions, characterized by bruises on the brain; lacerations, characterized by tears in the brain tissue; subdural hematomas, characterized by accumulations of blood under the outermost membrane layer surrounding the brain (dura mater); and epidural hematomas, characterized by blood between the dura mater and the skull. Hematomas may result from ruptures or lacerations in certain blood vessels. Contusions and hematomas may cause the brain to swell with an accompanying buildup of fluid (edema). Increasing pressure within the skull may result in brain damage. Symptoms and findings may include headache; seizures; altered levels of consciousness sometimes leading to coma; loss of strength; numbness; paralysis; confusion; memory loss (amnesia); or life-threatening complications such as respiratory distress and heart irregularities. Treatment is aimed at the maintenance of respiratory and cardiovascular function in order to prevent further injury. If necessary, the upper spine (cervical spine) is stabilized. The monitoring and management of brain swelling and fluid accumulation may include the careful administration of intravenous fluids and medications, bed elevation, and the use of supplemental oxygen. In addition, surgical intervention may be required to relieve intracranial pressure, remove blood clots, or control bleeding around the brain. Further treatment may include medication for the control of seizures. Recovery from major head or brain trauma may be a very slow, progressive process and, as such, may require the assistance of a team of specialists who will work with the family or caregivers of the child to coordinate symptomatic and supportive care.

The following organizations in the General Resources Section can provide additional information: National Institute of Neurological Disorders and Stroke (NINDS)

National Associations & Support Groups

1824 American Brain Tumor Association Patient Line
2720 River Road
Des Plaines, IL 60018
800-886-2282

Offers emergency support, information and referrals for patients and their families.

1825 Brain Injury Association National Office
105 N. Alfred Street
Alexandria, VA 22314
703-236-6000
800-444-6443
Fax: 703-236-6001
e-mail: jnidhiry@biusa.org
www.biausa.org

A national non-profit that seeks to improve the quality of life for people with brain injuries and their families through information and resource referral, legislative advocacy, prevention awareness, and professional education.

Tara McDonough, Dir., Info./Resource

1826 Brain Injury Association Family Helpline
105 N Alfred Street
Alexandria, VA 22314
800-444-6443

1827 Coma Recovery Association, Inc.
100 E Old Country Rd, Ste 9
Mineola, NY 11501
516-746-7714
Fax: 516-749-7706
e-mail: office@comarecovery.org
http://comarecovery.org

1828 Head Injury Hotline
212 Pioneer Bldg.,PO Box 84151
Seattle, WA 98124
206-329-1371
Fax: 206-624-4961
e-mail: brain@headinjury.com
www.headinjury.com

Founded in 1989, sponsors public information seminars designed to bring together survivors of head injuries, their families and professionals for networking and information sharing, as well as operating a national helpline for people suffering from a head injury.

1829 Perspective Network
P.O. Box 1859
Cumming, GA 30128
770-844-6898
800-685-6302
Fax: 770-844-6898
www.tbi.org

State Agencies & Support Groups

1830 Brain Injury Association of Alabama
3600 8th Ave S
Birmingham, AL 35222
205-328-3505
800-433-8002
Fax: 205-328-2479

Kim Ferguson-Hooks, President
Ferguson-Hooks Charles, Priest

Alaska

1831 Brain Injury Association of Alaska
Richard Warrington
313 Cindy Circle
Kena, AK 99611
907-283-5711

Debbie Russell

Arizona

1832 Brain Injury Association of Arizona
4545 N 36th St Ste 125-A
Phoenix, AZ 85018   520-747-7140

Mary Jane Trunzo, President
Trunzo Ellen, Conroy

Arkansas

1833 Brain Injury Association of Arkansas
P.O. Box 26236
Little Rock, AR 72221   501-771-5011
800-235-2443
Fax: 501-227-8632

Tim S. Parker, President

California

1834 Brain Injury Association of California
P.O. Box 160786
Sacramento, CA 95816   916-442-1710
800-457-2443
Fax: 916-442-7305
freeyellow.com/members/BIAC/in

Claude Munday, President

Colorado

1835 Brain Injury Association of Colorado
6825 E. Tennessee Avenue Suite 405
Denver, CO 80224   303-355-9969
800-955-2443
Fax: 303-355-9968
e-mail: biacolo@aol.com

Provides information and resources, support
groups throughout the state, outdoor adventure
challenge - a week long outdoor recreation and
social experience for surviviors working one on
one with trained counselors.

Judy Dettmer, President
Helen O. Kellogg, Executive Director

Connecticut

1836 Brain Injury Association of Connecticut
1800 Silas Deane Highway Suite 224
Rocky Hill, CT 06067   860-721-8111
800-278-8242
Fax: 860-721-9008
www.connix.com/~dpyers/bia

Linda Detelich, President
Detelich Kathleen, Ryan

Delaware

1837 Brain Injury Association of Delaware
P.O. Box 9876
Newark, DE 19714   302-475-2286
800-411-0505

Sy Londoner, President

Florida

1838 Brain Injury Association of Florida
North Broward Medical Center
201 East Sample Road
Pompano Beach, FL 33064   954-941-8300
800-992-3442
Fax: 954-786-2437
e-mail: info@biaf.org
www.biaf.org

Robert A. Levitt, PhD, President
Levitt, PhD Elynor, Kazuk

Georgia

1839 Brain Injury Association of Georgia
1447 Peachtree Street NE, Ste. 810
Atlanta, GA 30309   404-817-7577
Fax: 404-817-7521

David Sotto, Chair
Sotto Gloria, Stahle

Hawaii

1840 Pacific Head Injury Association
1775 S. Beretania Rm 203
Honolulu, HI 96826   808-941-0372
www.waikiki-gallery.com/tbi.ht

Lyna Burnian

Idaho

1841 Brain Injury Association of Idaho
Marilyn Hern
1575 East Holly Street
Boise, ID 83712   208-336-7708
e-mail: melelina@aol.com

Contact either: Dennis S. Voorhees P.O. Box Z
Twin Falls, ID 83303-0090.

Illinois

1842 Brain Injury Association of Illinois
1127 S. Mannheim Road Suite 213
Westchester, IL 60154   708-344-4646
800-699-6443
Fax: 708-344-4680
e-mail: biail@yahoo.com
www.biausa.org/illinois/bia.htm

A nonprofit organization dedicated to providing
information, advocacy, education, and support
to people with brain injuries, their families, and
the professionals who serve them.

Cheryl Burda, President/ CEO
Julie Papieuis, Community Relations Coordinator

Indiana

1843 Brain Injury Association of Indiana
5506 East 16th Street Suite B-5
Indianapolis, IN 46218   317-356-7722
800-407-4246
Fax: 317-356-4241
140.254.20.2/ovchome/HIFIhome

Karen May, President
May Donna, Jackson

Iowa

1844 Brain Injury Association of Iowa
2101 Kimball Avenue LL7
Waterloo, IA 50702   319-272-2312
800-475-4442
Fax: 319-272-2109
e-mail: glauer@blue.weeg.uiowa.edu

Geof Lauer, President
Lauer Jean F., Kelley

Kentucky

1845 Brain Injury Association of Kentucky
113 South Hubbards Lane
Louisville, KY 40207   502-899-7141
800-592-1117
Fax: 502-899-7106
www.braincenter.org

Gwenevere Josey, President
Josey Robert E., Ayres

Louisiana

1846 Brain Injury Association of Louisiana
217 Buffwood Drive
Baker, LA 70714   504-775-2780
Fax: 504-387-6252

William Moak, President, Exec. Dir

Maine

1847 Brain Injury Association of Maine
211 Maine Avenue Suite 200
Farmingdale, ME 04344   207-582-4696
800-275-1233
Fax: 207-583-4803

Marcia Cooper, President
Cooper Patricia, Brinkman

Maryland

1848 Brain Injury Association of Maryland
c/o Kernan Hospital
2200 Kernan Drive Suite 810-E
Baltimore, MD 21207   410-448-2924
800-221-6443
Fax: 410-448-3541
www.neurolaw.com/biz/BIA_home

Frances Bateson, President
Bateson Patsy A., Kressig

Massachusetts

1849 Brain Injury Association of Massachusetts
Denholm Building
484 Main Street Suite 325
Worcester, MA 01608   508-753-5208
800-242-0030
Fax: 508-757-9109

Gayle Alfreds, President
Alfreds Arlene, Korab

Minnesota

1850 Brain Injury Association of Minnesota
43 Main Street S.E. Suite 135
Minneapolis, MN 55414   612-378-2742
                              800-669-6442
                        Fax: 612-378-2789
            e-mail: info@braininjurymn.org
                    www.braininjurymn.org

Solely commited to preventing brain injury and
enhancing the quality of life of all persons living
with brain injury and their families, through
support, education, and advocacy. Offers
classes, raises public awareness about brain injury through media relations, legislative advocacy, and education campaigns.

Tom Gode, Executive Director

Mississippi

1851 Brain Injury Association of Mississippi
P.O. Box 55912
Jackson, MS 39296   601-981-1021
                          800-641-6442
                    Fax: 601-981-1039
        e-mail: biaofms@aol.com
    members.aol.com/biaofms/index

Harriet Turner, President
Turner Gail, Rowland

Missouri

**1852 Brain Injury Association of Kansas & Greater
Kansas City**
1100 Pennsylvania Suite 4061
Kansas City, MO 64105   816-842-8607
                              800-783-1356
                        Fax: 816-842-1531

Suzanne Dotson, President
Dotson Elizabeth, Jenkins

**1853 Brain Injury Association of Kansas and Greater
Kansas City**
1100 Pennsylvania Avenue Suite 4061
Kansas City, MO 64105   816-842-8607
                              800-783-1356
                        Fax: 816-842-1531
                www.brain-injury-ks-gkc.org

Karen VanAsdale, President
VanAsdale Elizabeth, Jenkins

1854 Brain Injury Association of Missouri
10270 Page Suite 100
St. Louis, MO 63132   314-426-4024
                            800-377-6442
                      Fax: 314-426-3290
        e-mail: braininjury@aol.com
        www.biausa.org/missouri/bia

A glass roots organization of indivivuals with
brain injury, families and health service providers. Programs include I and R, support groups,
respite, camp, prevention/education and a men-
tor program.

500+ members

Lori Winter, Executive Director

Montana

1855 Brain Injury Association of Montana
MSU-B Montana Center Room 147
1500 North 30th Street
Billings, MT 59101   406-657-2907
                            800-241-6442
                      Fax: 406-657-2807

Karen Rimel, Co-President
Rimel Ann, Patrick

Nebraska

1856 Brain Injury Association of Nebraska
P.O. Box 124, 1108 Avenue H
Gothenburg, NE 69138   308-761-2781
                              800-743-4781
                        Fax: 308-761-2219

Tom Korn, PhD, President
Korn, PhD Jan, Kauffman

Nevada

1857 Brain Injury Association of Nevada
Dennis Luck
2820 W Charleston Blvd D37
Las Vegas, NV 89102   702-387-2318
                        Fax: 702-259-1907

An all volunteer non-profit organization of survivors, family, and care givers. Dedicated to support through social interaction, exchange of information, and prevention plus educational research.

200 members

Dennis Luck, Board of Directors

1858 Brain Injury Association of Northern Nevada
Carol Swan
P.O. Box 2789
Gardnerville, NV 89410   702-782-8336

New Hampshire

1859 Brain Injury Association of New Hampshire
2 1/2 Beacon Street Suite 171
Concord, NH 03301   603-225-8400
          800-773-8400
          Fax: 603-228-6749
          e-mail: nhbia@nh.ultranet.com
          www.bianh.org

Our mission is to promote awareness, understanding and prevention of brain injury through education, advocacy, research and community support services that lead toward reduced incidence and improved outcomes of children and adults with brain injuries.

Carolyn Ramsay, President
Steven Wade, Executive Director

New Jersey

1860 Brain Injury Association of New Jersey
1090 King George Post Rd. Suite 708
Edison, NJ 08837   732-738-1002
          800-669-4323
          Fax: 732-738-1132
          e-mail: info@bianj.org
          www.bianj.org

Dedicated to providing education, outreach, prevention, advocacy and support services to all persons affected by brain injury, their families and the general public.

Milton S. Hall, President
Hall Barbara, Geiger-Parker

New Mexico

1861 Brain Injury Association of New Mexico
2819 Richmond N.E.
Albuquerque, NM 87107   505-292-7414
          800-279-7480
          Fax: 505-883-1079

Charlotte Lough, President

New York

1862 Brain Injury Association of New York
10 Colvin Avenue
Albany, NY 12206   518-459-7911
          800-228-8201
          Fax: 518-482-5285
          e-mail: info@bianys.org
          www.bianys.org

A not-for-profit dedicated to improving the lives of persons, and their families, who have sustained traumatic brain injury. A clearinghouse providing information resources and referral, statewide support groups, and family support services coordinators, as well as educational programs to increase public and professional awarenesss.

Judith Avner, Executive Director

North Carolina

1863 Brain Injury Association of North Carolina
P.O. Box 748
133 Fayetteville St. Mall Suite 310
Raleigh, NC 27602   919-833-9634
          800-377-1464
          Fax: 919-833-5415
          e-mail: terry@bianc.org
          www.bianc.org

Betty Lilyquist, President
Lilyquist Cecil, Greene, Jr.

Ohio

1864 Ohio Brain Injury Association
1335 Dublin Road Suite 217D
Columbus, OH 43215   614-481-7100
          800-686-9563
          Fax: 614-481-7103
          e-mail: help@biaoh.org
          www.biaoh.org

State-wide advocacy and education organization affiliated with the National Brain Injury Association serving Ohioans with brain injury and their families through assistance in locating services, supports, educational materials, conferences, prevention initiatives and legislative advocacy. Membership fee is $50.00 for professionals

400 members

Suzanne Minnich, Executive Director/Helpline Staff

Oklahoma

1865 Brain Injury Association of Oklahoma
P.O. Box 88
Hillsdale, OK 73743   580-635-2237
800-765-6809
Fax: 580-635-2238
e-mail: rxot@ionet.net
www.ionet.net/~rxot/

Charles Bell, President
Charlotte Bell Bowen

Oregon

1866 Brain Injury Association of Oregon
1118 Lancaster Drive NE, Suite 345
Salem, OR 97301   503-585-0855
800-544-5243
Fax: 503-375-4918
e-mail: biaor@open.org
www.open.org/~/biaor

The mission of the Brain Injury Association of Oregon is to improve the quality of life for people with brain injury and their families. We serve as a clearing house of state wide community resources with new and enhanced information and referral services, participate in state legislative advocacy, support research, host educational programs, facilitate local support groups and encourage programs to prevent injuries.

250 members

Robyn Baim, Office Manager

Pennsylvania

1867 Brain Injury Association of Eastern Pennsylvania
Roger Schott
2006 Par Drive
Doylestown, PA 18901   215-491-9036
Fax: 215-491-1246

1868 Brain Injury Association of Western Pennsylvania
Charlotte Herbert c/o St. Andrews Church
304 Morewood Avenue
Pittsburgh, PA 15213   412-682-2520
e-mail: herbertc@mail.dec.com

Rhode Island

1869 Brain Injury Association of Rhode Island
Independence Square
500 Prospect Street
Pawtucket, RI 02860   401-722-9540
Fax: 401-727-2810

Frank Sparadeo, PhD, President
Sparadeo, PhD Sharon, Brinkworth

South Carolina

1870 South Carolina Brain Injury Task Force Affiliated with National Brain Injury
1030 Saint Andrews Road
Columbia, SC 29210   803-731-0588
800-290-6461
Fax: 803-731-0589
e-mail: scbraininjury@mindspring.com

Robert Bramble, MD, Executive Director

Tennessee

1871 Brain Injury Association of Tennessee
699 West Main Street Suite 208
Hendersonville, TN 37075   615-264-3052
800-480-6693
Fax: 615-264-3052
www.nashville.com/~colin.frahm

Joe Frahm, President
Frahm Gary, Driskill

Texas

1872 Brain Injury Association of Texas
6633 Highway 290 East Suite 306
Austin, TX 78723   512-326-1212
800-392-0040
Fax: 512-467-9035
e-mail: myoung@bcm.tmc.edu

Mary Ellen Young, PhD, President
Young, PhD Tad, Thayer

Utah

1873 Brain Injury Association of Utah
1800 S. West Temple
Suite 203 Box 22
Salt Lake City, UT 84115   801-484-2240
                                  800-281-8442
                            Fax: 801-484-5932
                       e-mail: biau@sisna.com
                    www.starpage.com/braininjury/

Barbara Hayward, President
Hayward Ron, Roskos

Vermont

1874 Brain Injury Association of Vermont
P.O. Box 1837 Station A
Rutland, VT 05701   802-446-3017

Richard Marceau, President
Marceau Emmie, Burke

Virginia

1875 Brain Injury Association of Virginia
3212 Cutshaw Avenue Suite 315
Richmond, VA 23230   804-355-5748
                            800-334-8443
                      Fax: 804-355-6381
                      www.bia.pmr.vcu.edu/

Non-profit organization offering information
and resources to individuals with brain injury,
their family members and professionals dealing
with brain injury. Lists of local support groups
available.

Ann Brown, President
Harry Weinstock, Executive Director

Washington

1876 Brain Injury Association of Washington
P.O. Box 52890
16315 N.E. 87th Street Suite B-4
Redmond, WA 98052   425-895-0047
                           800-523-5438
                           www.biawa.org

Ron Finlay, President
Finlay John W., Andrews

West Virginia

1877 Brain Injury Association of West Virginia
P.O. Box 574
Institute, WV 25112   304-766-4892
                             800-356-6443
                       Fax: 304-766-4940
                       e-mail: biawv@aol.com

Kenneth Wright, MD, President
Wright, MD Jennifer, Rhule

Wisconsin

1878 Brain Injury Association of Wisconsin
3505 North 124th Street, Suite 100
Brookfield, WI 53005   262-790-6901
                              800-882-9282
                        Fax: 262-790-6824

Gary L. Jackson, President
Jackson Patricia, David

Wyoming

1879 Brain Injury Association of Wyoming
246 South Center Suite 16
Casper, WY 82601   307-473-1767
                          800-643-6457
                    Fax: 307-237-5222

David Eudaley, President
Eudaley Lesley, Travers

Research Centers

**1880 Brain Research Institute - U.C.L.A. School of
Medicine**
University of California, Los Angeles
www.medsch.ucla.edu/som/bri   310-794-1195
                        www.medsch.ucla.edu/som/bri

Allan J. Tobin, PhD, Director
Arthur P. Arnold, PhD, Assoc. Dir. for Education

1881 Brain Trauma Foundation
523 E. 72nd St. 8th Floor
New York, NY 10021   212-772-0608
                           www.aitken.org

1882 Dana Alliance for Brain Initiatives
745 Fifth Ave. Suite 700
New York, NY 10151   202-737-9200
                           www.dana.org/brainweb

Dana Alliance is a non-profit organization made up of brain scientists working to advance brain research and educate the public.

1883 Rehabilitation, Research & Training Center For Persons with TBI
Mt. Sinai Med. Ctr., Dept. of Rehab. Med.
One Gustave L. Levy Place, Box 1240
New York, NY 10029   212-241-7917

Wayne A. Gordon, PhD, Director

1884 Rehabilitation, Research and Training Center in Traumatic Brain Injuries
Institute for Rehabilitation and Research
1333 Moursund Ave.
Houston, TX 77030   713-799-5000

L. Don Lehmkuhl, PhD, Director

California

1885 Southern California Neuropsychiatric Institute
6794 La Jolla Blvd.
La Jolla, CA 92037   619-454-2102
                           Fax: 619-454-2104

Sydney Walker, III, MD, Director

1886 University of California, Irvine Brain Imaging Center
146 Whitby Research Center
Irvine, CA 92717   949-856-4245

Offers PET scan analysis of brain functions focusing on brain damage, brain tumors and head injuries.

Monte S. Buchscaum, MD, Director

1887 University of California, San Francisco Laboratory for Neurotrauma
1001 Portero Road
San Francisco, CA 94110   415-206-8313

Research done into traumatic brain and head injuries.

Lawrence H. Pitts, MD

Massachusetts

1888 Boston University Aphasia Research Center
150 S. Huntington Avenue
Boston, MA 02130   617-739-3487

Research done into cognitive and language impairment following brain damage and closely related topics.

Dr. Harold Goodglass, Director

Michigan

1889 Brain Injury Association of Michigan
8619 W. Grand River Suite I
Brighton, MI 48116   810-229-5880
                           800-772-4323
                           Fax: 810-229-8947
                           e-mail: biaofmi@cac.net
                           www.biausa.org/michigan

A resource and information center addressing the needs of persons with brain injury, their families, and concerned professionals. Resources include written materials, videos, etc. on various topics regarding the understanding and rehabilitation of brain injury.

Michael Dabbs, President
Carolyn Laughton, Director of Administration

1890 Rehabilitation Institute of Michigan
261 Mack Blvd.
Detroit, MI 48201   313-745-1203
                           Fax: 313-745-9863

Physical medicine and rehabilitation medicine.

Marcel Sijkers, Dr., Dir. of Research

1891 Wayne State University, Guardjian-Lesser Biomechanics Laboratory
550 E. Canfield Ave.
Detroit, MI 48201   313-577-4603
                           Fax: 313-577-1342

Head and neck injury research.

Voigt R. Hodgson, Dr., Dir.

New York

1892 Brady Institute
Jamaica Hospital Medical Center
8900 Van Wyck Expressway
Jamaica, NY 11418   718-206-6000
                          e-mail: tbil@jh.org

The James and Sarah Brady Institute for Traumatic Brain Injury.

Pennsylvania

1893 Institutes for Achievement of Human Potential
Neil Harvey, Ph.D, IACBD, author

8801 Stenton Avenue
Wyndmoor, PA 19038   215-233-2050
                           800-344-8322
                           Fax: 215-233-3940
                     e-mail: institutes@iahp.org
                           www.iahp.org

A teaching institute that focuses on home-based neurological training for brain-injured children. Commited to the significant increases of the ability of all children to perform in the physical, intellectual and social realms. Our work has led to powerful insights about the brain and, especially, about its development in the neonate and very young children. We have developed exciting concepts and practices applied by parents at home, to mulitply the intelligence of tiny children.

500 members

Neil Harvey, Ph.D, Deans

1894 Thomas Jefferson University Infectious Disease Research Center
1020 Locust Street
Philadelphia, PA 19107   215-503-1272
                               Fax: 215-955-2073

Virginia

1895 Virginia Commonwealth University, Rehab Research and Training Center
Box 677, MCA Station
Richmond, VA 23298   804-828-0488
                           Fax: 804-371-6340

Focuses research on traumatic brain and head injuries.

Dr. Nathan Zasler, Diredctor

Web Sites

1896 Dana Alliance for Brain Initiatives
www.dana.org/brainweb

1897 Family Caregiver Alliance
www.caregiver.org

1898 National Institute of Neurological Disorders and Stroke
www.ninds.nih.gov

1899 Perspectives Network
www.tbi.org

1900 ReHab Net
www.rehabnet.com

1901 Traumatic Brain Injury Model Systems
www.tbims.org

1902 Web Site for the Neuroskills Program in California
www.neuroskills.com

Books

1903 Cognitive Effects of Early Brain Injury
Casey Dorman and Bilha Katzir, author

Johns Hopkins University Press
2715 North Charles Street
Baltimore, MD 21218   410-516-6900
                            800-537-5487
                            Fax: 410-516-6998

This book offers a detailed overview of the effects of genetic, prenatal, and perinatal brain disorders on cognitive development and learing in children. Summarizing the available data as well as presenting previously unpublished research, the book provides clinicians with practical information that will aid their disagnostic and therapeutic work with children who have sustained early brain injury.

1994 320 pages
ISBN: 0-801851-84-X

1904 Cognitive Rehabilitation for Persons with Traumatic Brain Injury
J.S. Kreutzer, P.H. Wehman, author

Books on Special Children
P.O. Box 305
Congers, NY 10920   914-638-1236
                          Fax: 914-638-0847

Virtually all persons with brain injury retain ability to learn. Cognitive rehab is a set of stategies to improve problems. Reports on theory, practices, research, consequences of brain trauma and assessment and intervention. Case studies.

1991 299 pages Hardbound

1905 Handbook of Head Truma: Acute Care to Recovery
Plenum Publishing Corporation
233 Spring Street
New York, NY 10013   212-620-8000
                            800-221-9369
                      Fax: 212-463-0742
              e-mail: books@plenum.com

1992 466 pages
ISBN: 0-306439-47-6

1906 Head Injury in Children and Adolescents: A Resource and Review

Vivian Begali, author

John Wiley & Sons, INC.
605 Third Avenue
New York, NY 10158   212-850-6000
                      Fax: 212-850-6088
                      www.wiley.com

This book examines the different implications of head injuries, as well as the recovery process in an educational setting. Also includes an appendix, glossary and references.

280 pages
ISBN: 0-471161-94-2

1907 Traumatic Brain Injury Survival Guide

Glen Johnson, author

The purpose of this book is to provide information about brain injury to family members and survivors in clear, easy to understand language. An overview of how the brain works, possible problems related to brain injury and suggestions on how to improve common problems are provided.

1908 What To Do About Your Brain Injured Child

Glenn Doman, author

8801 Stenton Avenue
Wyndmoor, PA 19038   215-233-2050
                            800-344-8322
                      Fax: 215-233-3940
                      www.iahp.org

ISBN: 0-944349-24-2

Journals

1909 Journal of Head Trauma Rehabilitation
Aspen Publishers, Inc.
1600 Research Blvd.
Rockville, MD 20850   301-251-8500
                            800-638-8437

Scholarly journal designed to provide information on clinical management and rehabilitation of the head-injured for the practicing professional.

Newsletters

1910 American Brain Tumor Association Message Line
2720 River Road
Des Plaines, IL 60018   847-827-9910
                              800-886-2282

Offers association news, events, fundraising and convention news, as well as medical and legislative updates for patients and their families.

Quarterly

1911 Brain Injury Association of Minnesota
43 Main Street S.E. Suite 135
Minneapolis, MN 55414   612-378-2742
                              800-669-6442
                        Fax: 612-378-2789
              e-mail: info@braininjurymn.org
                      www.braininjurymn.org

Published for the families and professionals who are involved with brain injuries. We also have an e-mail newsletter that reaches several hundred.

Quarterly

1912 Brain Injury Association of Oregon Newsletter
1118 Lancaster Drive NE, Suite 345
Salem, OR 97301   503-585-0855
                        800-544-5243
                  Fax: 503-375-4918
          e-mail: biaor@open.org
                  www.open.org/~/biaor

To provide information and resources to those with brain injuries, families and professionals.

Robyn Baim, Office Manager

1913 Brain Injury Association of Virginia Newsletter
3212 Cutshaw Avenue Suite 315
Richmond, VA 23230   804-355-5748
                           800-334-8443
                           Fax: 804-355-6381
                           www.bia.pmr.vcu.edu/

Information and resources for individuals with brain injury, their family members and professionals dealing with brain injury.

16 pages Quarterly

Stacy Lucas, Editor

1914 Ohio Brain Injury Association Newsletter
Ohio Brain Injury Association
1335 Dublin Road Suite 217D
Columbus, OH 43215   614-481-7100
                           800-686-9563
                           Fax: 614-481-7103
                           e-mail: help@biaoh.org
                           www.biaoh.org

The official newsletter of the Ohio Brain Injury Association to provide members with information on locating services, supports, educational materials, conferences, prevention initiatives and legislative advocacy. Membership fee is $50.00 for professionals.

16 pages quarterly

Suzanne Minnich, Editor

Michigan

1915 Brain Injury Association of Michigan
8619 W. Grand River Suite I
Brighton, MI 48116   810-229-5880
                           800-772-4323
                           Fax: 810-229-8947
                           e-mail: biaofmi@cac.net
                           www.biausa.org/michigan

Information center for persons with brain injury, their families, and concerned professionals.

Newsletter 3x

Michael Dabbs, President
Carolyn Laughton, Director of Administration

Camps

Michigan

1916 Brain Injury Association of Michigan
8619 W. Grand River Suite I
Brighton, MI 48116   810-229-5880
                           800-772-4323
                           Fax: 810-229-8947
                           e-mail: biaofmi@cac.net
                           www.biausa.org/michigan

Summer camp program during in May and August.

Michael Dabbs, President
Carolyn Laughton, Director of Administration

DESCRIPTION

1917 HEARING IMPAIRMENT/DEAFNESS

Covers these related disorders: Conductive deafness or hearing loss, Mixed hearing loss, Sensorineural deafness or hearing loss

Hearing impairment may be defined as a loss of the ability to hear that is sufficient enough to impede the ability to communicate. Deafness refers to severe or profound hearing loss. Hearing loss or deafness may occur as the result of hereditary factors or birth defects. Hearing loss may also be acquired and occur after birth (e.g., from disease or physical damage to the hearing mechanism); however, genetic factors are thought to be responsible for moderate to severe hearing loss in about half of affected children. Hearing loss may be further categorized into three types: conductive, sensorineural, or mixed.

Conductive hearing loss occurs as a result of the faulty transmission of sound through the external or middle ear to the inner ear. This transmission problem may be due to infections of the middle ear (otitis media), damage to the eardrum or bones of the middle ear, the absence or the narrowing of the ear canal, impacted earwax (cerumen), foreign bodies in the ear canal, or other physical causes. In addition, conductive hearing loss is sometimes inherited as a feature of certain syndromes such as Klippel-Feil syndrome, Crouzon syndrome, osteogenesis imperfecta, and others. In children with sensorineural hearing loss, sounds are conducted to the inner ear through the external and middle ear, but are not transmitted from there to the brain. This occurs as the result of a defect in the structure of the inner ear or problems with the nerve that conveys impulses from the inner ear to the brain (auditory nerve; acoustic nerve; eighth cranial nerve). Sensorineural hearing loss that results from defects of inner ear structures is considered sensory and include the absence or underdevelopment of the snail shell-type tubular structure of the inner ear (cochlea); damage to

hair cells or other inner ear structures from prolonged exposure to loud noise, certain drugs, viral infections or other diseases; and other irregularities. Sensorineural hearing loss that results from damage to the auditory nerve pathway is considered neural and may be due to brain lesions or tumors; childhood disorders such as German measles, mumps, inner ear infections, etc.; certain hereditary disorders (e.g., Waardenburg syndrome, Usher syndrome, etc.); diseases that affect the myelin sheath, which is the fatty, protective, insulating covering on certain nerve fibers (demyelinating diseases); or seizures. Mixed hearing loss refers to a combination of both conductive and sensorineural hearing loss.

Early screening for hearing loss is important in order to provide early intervention that will allow the best outcome for educational and social development. Treatment may require the cooperation of parents, caregivers, pediatricians, speech and language pathologists, and specialists in hearing loss (audiologists) who assess the extent of hearing loss through the use of specialized tests. Infant screening by specialists may include tests that gauge behavioral responses to noise through observation. Other tests may electronically assess hearing loss (audiometry); measure the head-turning response of an infant or toddler using animated aids in conjunction with sounds emitted through a loudspeaker (visual reinforcement audiometry or VRA); measure the lowest intensity at which certain words are heard or understood (speech recognition threshold or SRT); measure the ability of the middle ear to impede or resist sound energy (tympanometry); differentiate between sensory and neural hearing loss (auditory brain stem response); measure the integrity of the cochlea (otoacoustic emissions or OAEs); or other specialized tests. Treatment for conductive hearing loss may include the removal of fluid, earwax, or foreign bodies through drainage or other means. Surgical intervention may be indicated for the correction of structural abnormalities. Children as well as infants with hearing loss may benefit from the use of certain types of hearing aids; however, repeat testing is necessary to provide more exact hearing aid specification. In addition, cochlear implants are now available to children with severe or profound hearing loss. Other treatment is directed toward the teaching of communication skills such as lip-reading, sign language, and speech. Cooperation and support of family, medical specialists, and educators is important in determining the best approach for the education and social development of the individual child.

National Associations & Support Groups

1918 ADARA
P.O. Box 27
Roland, AR 72135   501-224-6678
                                Fax: 501-868-8812
                                TTY: 501-868-8850
                         e-mail: ADARAhuie@aol.com

Professional networking for excellence in service delivery with individuals who are deaf or hard of hearing. A partnership of national organizations, local affiliates, professional sections, and individual members working together to support social services and rehabilitation delivery for deaf and hard of hearing people.

Steve Larew, President
Larew Marie, Huite

1919 Academy of Rehabilitative Audiology
P.O. Box 26532
Minneapolis, MI 55426   612-920-0196
                                Fax: 612-920-6098
                           e-mail: ara@incnet.com
                                www.audrehab.org

Provides professional education, research, and interest in programs for hearing handicapped persons. Yearly journal avaialable.

350 members

Frances Laven, Assoc. Executive

1920 Advocates for Deaf & Hard of Hearing Youth, Inc.
P.O. Box 75949
Washington, DC 20013   202-651-5160

Information on deafness, hearing impairments, child welfare and advocacy.

Catherine Moses, President

1921 Alexander Graham Bell Association for the Deaf and Hearing Impaired
Alexander Graham Bell Association for the Deaf
3417 Volta Place N.W.
Washington, DC 20007   202-337-5220
                                   800-432-7543
                                Fax: 202-337-8314
                                TTY: 202-337-5220
                         e-mail: agbell2@aol.com
                                www.agbell.org

Gathers and disseminates information on hearing loss, promotes better public understanding of hearing loss in children and adults, provides scholarships and financial and parent-infant awards, and promotes early detection of hearing loss in infants. Advocates for appropriate technology and access for children and adults with hearing loss.

Donna L. Sorkin, MCP, Executive Director

1922 American Academy of Audiology
8201 Greensboro Drive-Suite 300
McLean, VA 22102   703-524-1923
                                   800-222-2336
                                Fax: 703-524-2303
                                TTY: 703-610-9022
                                www.audiology.org

A professional organization of individuals dedicated to providing high quality hearing care to the public. Provides professional development, education and research and provides increased public awareness of hearing disorders and audiologic services.

Barry Freeman, President
Freeman J.Bruce, Wardle

1923 American Association of the Deaf-Blind
814 Thayer Avenue, Room 302
Silver Spring, MD 20910
                                Fax: 301-588-8705
                                TTY: 301-588-6545
                         e-mail: aadb@erols.com

Promotes better opportunities and services for deaf-blind people. The mission of this organization is to assure that a comprehensive, coordinated system of services is accessible to all deaf-blind people, enabling them to achieve their maximum potential through increased independence.

Harry Anderson, President
Joy Larson, Program Manager

1924 American Auditory Society
512 East Canterbury Lane
Phoenix, AZ 85022   602-789-0755
                          Fax: 602-942-1486
           e-mail: aas@amauditorysoc.org
                www.amauditroysoc.org

Provides professional education and research
and publishes a journal.

Brenda Ryals, Ph.D, President
Wayne J. Staab, Ph.D, Secretary/Treasurer

1925 American Deafness and Rehabilitation Association
P.O. Box 251554
Little Rock, AK 72225   501-868-8850
                             Fax: 501-868-8812
                 e-mail: adarahuie@aol.com

1926 American Hearing Research Foundation
55 East Washington St., Ste. 2022
Chicago, IL 60602   312-726-9670
                          Fax: 312-726-9695

Supports medical research and education into
the causes, prevention, and cures of deafness,
hearing losses, and balance disorders. Also
keeps physicians and the public informed of the
latest developments in hearing research and education.

William L. Lederer, Executive Director

1927 American Society for Deaf Children
P O Box 3355
Gettysburg, PA 17325   717-334-7922
                              800-942-2732
                          Fax: 717-334-8808
                          TTY: 800-942-2732
                 e-mail: asdcl@aol.com
                  www.deafchildren.org

A nonprofit parent-helping-parent organization
promoting a positive attitude toward signing
and deaf culture. Also provides support, encouragement, and current information about deafness to families with deaf and hard of hearing
children.

Sandy Harvey, Executive Director

1928 American Speech, Language, Hearing Association
10801 Rockville Pike
Rockville, MD 20852   301-897-5700
                          Fax: 301-571-0457
                          TTY: 301-897-5700

The American Speech-Language-Hearing Foundation supports the advancement of knowledge
and improvement of practice in serving children
and adults with speech, language, and hearing
disorders.

Nancy Minghetti, Director

1929 Auditory-Verbal International, Inc.
2121 Eisenhower Avenue, Ste. 402
Alexandria, VA 22314   703-739-1049
                          Fax: 703-739-0395
                          TTY: 703-739-0874
           e-mail: audioverb@aol.com
                www.auditory-verbal.org

Dedicated to helping children who have hearing
losses learn to listen and speak. Promotes the
Auditory-Verbal Therapy approach, which is
based on the belief that the overwhelming majority of these children can hear and talk by using
their residual hearing and hearing aids. Membership dues for Canada is $55, International is
$60.

900 members

Sara Lake, Executive Director

1930 BEGINNINGS for Parents of Hearing Impaired Children
Ms. Lauren Edwards, Secretary
3900 Barrett Drive, Suite 100
Raleigh, NC 27609   919-571-4843
                          800-541-4327
                          Fax: 919-571-4846
                          TTY: 919-571-4843
           e-mail: jalberg@beginningssvcs.com
                www.beginningssvcs.com

BEGINNINGS provides: support to parents of
deaf and hard-of-hearing children in an unbiased, family-centered atmosphere; impartial information on communication options, placement
and educational programs; workshops for professional personnel who work with deaf and
hard-of-hearing children; advocacy and support
for young people from birth through age 21.

Joni Alberg, Executive Director
Lauren Edwareds, Administrative Assistant

1931 Better Hearing Institute
515 King Street Suite 420
Alexandria, VA 22314   703-684-3391
                          800-327-9355
                          Fax: 703-684-3394
                          TTY: 703-642-0580
           e-mail: mail@betterhearing.org
                www.betterhearing.org

A nonprofit educational organization that implements national public information programs on hearing loss and available medical, surgical, hearing aid, and rehabilitation assistance for millions with uncorrected hearing problems. Its award-winning series of television, radio, and print media public service messages include many celebrities who overcame hearing loss. BHI maintains a toll-free Hotline HelpLine telephone service that provides information on hearing loss and hearing help to callers.

1932 Center for the Advancement of Deaf Children
P.O. Box 1181
Los Alamitos, CA 90720   562-430-1467
                                     Fax: 562-430-1467
                                     TTY: 562-430-1467

1933 Center for the Education of the Infant Deaf
1810 Hopkins St
Berkeley, CA 94707   415-527-5544

Provides special education services for children between the ages of birth to 4 years old who have hearing losses or speech and language delays. Uses (Total Communication) approach that includes the simultaneous use of speech, hearing aids, and Signing Exact English (S.E.E.)

1934 Children's Rights Program
Alexander Graham Bell Association for the Deaf
3417 Volta Place N.W.
Washington, DC 20007   202-337-5220
                                          800-432-7543
                                     Fax: 202-337-8314
                                     TTY: 202-337-5220
                                     e-mail: agbell2@aol.com
                                          www.agbell.org

Actively advocates for the legal rights of children with hearing impairments and for legislation to upgrade the delivery of services to children and adults who are hearing impaired.

1935 Cochlear Implant Club International
5335 Wisconcin Ave NW
Washington, DC 20015   202-895-2781
                                     Fax: 202-895-2782
                                     e-mail: 6207.3114@compuserve.com

Dedicated to serving implant users, candidates, their families, and professional supporters. Promotes the opportunities afforded by the use of cochlear implants through mutual sharing of ideas and personal experiences; to function as a support group for cochlear implant candidates at both the pre- and postoperative stages; to enhance community awareness of hearing impairment and to promote a better understanding of cochlear implants.

1936 Council on Education of the Deaf
Deaf Studies Department, California State Univ.
18111 Nordhoff
Northridge, CA 91330   818-677-5116
                                     Fax: 818-677-5717
                                     TTY: 818-667-2335
                                     www.monster.educ.kent.edu/deaf

Offers information and referral services to the hearing impaired.

Lawrence R. Fleischer, Ed.D, President

1937 Deaf REACH
12th Street, N.E.
Washington, DC 20017   202-832-6681

1938 Deafness Research Foundation
575 5th Avenue, 11th Floor
New York, NY 10017   212-768-1181
                                     Fax: 212-599-0039
                                          www.drf.org

The nation's largest voluntary health organization entirely committed to public awareness and support for basic and clinical research into deafness and hearing disabilities. Sponsors a broad program of innovative research and education into causes, treatments and prevention of nerve deafness, supports the increasing the number of young scientists entering and engaged in otologics, and creates an understanding of serious hearing dysfunctions.

Jane Fortune, Chairman
Fortune Joanne, Abate

1939 Deafness and Communicative Disorders Branch
Department of Education
330 C Street SW, Room 3228
Washington, DC 20202   202-205-9152
                                     Fax: 202-205-9772
                                     TTY: 202-205-8352

Promotes improved and expanded rehabilitation services for deaf and hard of hearing people and individuals with speech or language impairments.

Victor Galloway, Ed.D., Branch Chief

1940 Dial-a-Hearing Screening Test
P.O. Box 1880
Media, PA 19063   610-544-7700
                                          800-222-3277
                                     Fax: 610-543-2802
                                     e-mail: dahst@aol.com
                                          www.dialatest.com

Hearing help information center. Provides local phone number for Dial-a-Hearing Screening Test and hearing information.

George Biddle, Executive Director

1941 EAR Foundation
2000 Church Street, Box 111
Nashville, TN 37236   615-329-7807
                            800-545-4327
                            Fax: 615-329-7935
                            TTY: 615-329-7849
                            www.theearfound.com

A national, non-profit organization committed to the goal of better hearing and balance through public and professional education programs including The Meniere's Network and the Young Ears program. The Meniere's Network is a national network of patient organized self-help groups which allow the exchange of experiences and coping strategies associated with Meniere's Disease.

R. Edward Thompson, Executive Director
Thompson Bridgette, Garza

1942 Gallaudet University: Laurent Clerk National Deaf Education Center
800 Florida Ave NE
Washington, DC 20002   202-651-5340
                            Fax: 202-651-5708
                            TTY: 202-651-5340
                            e-mail: Randall.Gentry@gallaudet.edu
                            www.gallaudet.edu;80/~precpweb

Serves deaf and hard of hearing children throughout the United States, as well as their families and professionals who serve them. Magazines, books, videos and curricula describe the work of the Clerc Center, as well as of collaborators across the country. Information and links are provided for deaf education, interpreting, speech and language development, pediatric audiology, and all other areas related to deaf education, deaf and hard of hearing children and their families.

Randall Gentry, Director

1943 Genetic Centers Center
800 Florida Ave NE, HMB
Washington, DC 20002   202-651-5258
                            800-451-8834
                            Fax: 202-651-5179
                            TDD: 202-651-5258
                            e-mail: kathleen.arnos@gallaudet.rda

Professional genetic services are available for: deaf and hard-of-hearing individuals and couples who wish to better understand the cause and future implications of their deafness; parents of deaf and hard-of-hearing children who want information about the cause of their children's hearing loss and the potential for having other chidren with hearing loss; and individuals with a history of hearing loss in their family who have questions about the effects on future generations

1944 Hands Organization
2501 West 103rd Street
Chicago, IL 60655   773-239-6632

Advocacy for the deaf and hard of hearing; information and referrals, educational events, sign language summer youth camps and newsletters.

1945 Hear Now
9745 E. Hampden Avenue, #300
Denver, CO 80231   303-695-7797
                          800-648-4327
                          Fax: 303-695-7789
                          TTY: 800-648-4327
                          e-mail: jostetter@aol.com
                          www.leisurelan.com/~hearnow

Committed to making technology accessible to deaf and hard of hearing individuals throughout the United States. Also raises funds to provide hearing aids, cochlear implants and related services to children and adults who have hearing losses but do not have financial resources to purchase their own devices.

Bernice Dinner, MA, CCC, President, Founder
Dinner, MA, CCC Elain, Hansen

1946 Hearing Aid Helpline
International Hearing Society
16880 Middlebelt Road, Suite 4
Livonia, MI 48154   734-522-7200
                          Fax: 734-522-0200
                          www.hearingihs.org

A hearing specialist is ready to answer questions of the consumer about hearing aids, hearing loss and treatments.

1947 Hearing Impairments Better Hearing Institute
P.O. Box 1840
Washington, DC 20013
                          800-327-9355
                          TTY: 800-EAR-WELL

1948 Hearing Impairments - A.D.A.R.E.
P.O. Box 251554
Little Rock, AR 72225   501-224-6678
                              TDD: 501-224-6678

1949 House Ear Institute
2100 West Third Street, 5th Floor
Los Angeles, CA 90057   213-483-4431
                          Fax: 213-483-8789
                          TTY: 213-484-2642
                              www.hei.org

A national non-profit otologic research and educational institute that provides information on hearing and balance disorders.

John W. House, M.D., President

1950 International Hearing Society
16880 Middlebelt Road, Suite 4
Livonia, MI 48152   734-522-7200
                               800-521-5247
                          Fax: 734-522-0200
                          www.hearingihs.org

A nonprofit professional association which represents Hearing Instrument Specialists world. The society is recognized for promoting and maintaining the highest possible standards for its members in the best interest of the consumer.

Robin L. Holm, Executive Director

1951 International Kaf/Tek,Inc.
P.O. Box 2431
Frmingham, MA 01703   617-620-1777
                          Fax: 617-626-0270
                          TTY: 508-620-1777
              e-mail: admin.deaftek@deaftek.sprint
                  www.dac.neu.edu/services/drc

International electronic mail service dedicated to communities that are deaf or hard of hearing; the service is used by individuals, organizations, agencies, schools, colleges and universities, service providers, and professionals in the field of deafness.

Brenda Monene, R.N., M.Ed., President

1952 International Organization for the Education of the Hearing Impaired
Alexander Graham Bell Association for the Deaf
3417 Volta Place N.W.
Washington, DC 20007   202-337-5220
                               800-432-7543
                          Fax: 202-337-8314
                          TTY: 202-337-5220
                  e-mail: agbell2@aol.com
                              www.agbell.org

IOEHI promotes excellence in education for children and adults who are deaf or hard of hearing, encourages scientific study of the educational and communicative processes and stimulates the exchange of information among educators through seminars.

Elizabeth Wilkes, Ph.D., Chairperson
Wilkes, Ph.D. Elizabeth, Quigley

1953 John Tracy Clinic
806 W. Adams Blvd.
Los Angeles, CA 90007   213-748-5481
                               800-522-4582
                          Fax: 213-749-1651
                          TTY: 213-747-2924
          e-mail: mmartindale@johntracyclinic.org
                      www.johntracyclinic.org

An educational facility for preschool age children who have hearing losses and their families. In addition to on-site services, worldwide correspondence courses in English and Spanish are offered to parents whose children are of preschool age and are hard of hearing, deaf, or deaf-blind.

Maura Martindale, Director of Education

1954 Junior National Association of the Deaf & Youth Leadership Camp
National Association of the Deaf
814 Thayer Avenue
Silver Spring, MD 20910   301-587-1788
                          Fax: 301-587-1791
                          TTY: 301-587-1789

Michele Listisard

1955 Lead Line
2100 W Third Ave, 5th Fl
Los Angeles, CA 90057
                               800-352-8888
                          TTY: 800-287-4763
                  e-mail: blincoln@hei.org
                              www.hei.org

1956 National Association for Hearing and Speech Action
10801 Rockville Pike
Rockville, MD 20852
301-571-0457
800-638-8255
Fax: 301-897-7348
TDD: 806-388-255

1957 National Association of the Deaf
814 Thayer Avenue, Suite 250
Silver Spring, MD 20910
301-587-1788
Fax: 301-587-1791
TTY: 301-587-1789
e-mail: nadhq@juno.com
www.nad.org

The nation's largest constituency organization safeguarding the accessibility and civil rights of 28 million deaf and hard of hearing Americans in education, employment, health care and tele-communications. NAD is a dynamic federation of 51 state association affiliates, organizational affiliates and direct members, focusing on advocacy, captioned media, deafness-related information/publications, legal assistance and more.

Nancy J. Bloch, Executive Director

1958 National Captioning Institute
1900 Gallows Rd, Ste 3000
Vienna, VA 22182
703-917-7600
TTY: 703-917-7600

Provides captioning for the hearing-impaired, deaf children and adults. With the help of a decoder, they can read the dialog of certain TV programs with home videocassettes, and cable. The captioning is also useful for chidlren with learning disabilities and learning English as a second language.

1959 National Center for Law and the Deaf
Gallaudet University, 800 Florida Ave NE
Washington, DC 20002
202-651-5373
Fax: 202-651-5887
TTY: 202-651-5373

1960 National Center for Voice and Speech
University of Iowa
330 WJSHC
Iowa City, IA 52242
319-335-6600
Fax: 319-335-8851
e-mail: titze@shc.uiowa.edu
www.shc.uiowa.edu/ncvs_home.

This is a consortium of the following institutions focusing on voice and speech disorders: University of Iowa, Denver Center for Performing Arts, University of Wisconsin-Madison, University of Utah. NCVS trains scientists interested in careers in voice and speech research, provides continuing education for professionals, and conducts research on voice and speech production.

Ingo Titze, Ph.D., Director
Titze, Ph.D. Cynthia, Kintigh, M.A.

1961 National Cued Speech Association
23970 Hermitage Rd.
Cleveland, OH 44122
216-292-6213
800-459-3529
TTY: 216-292-6213
e-mail: cuedspdisc@aol.com
www.cuedspeech.org

Provides instruction, support services and information pertaining to deafness and the application of Cued Speech. The center provides classes and workshops in Cued Speech, maintains a speakers bureau and provides counseling and support for hearing-impaired adults and their families.

Mary Elsie Daisey, Executive Director
Daisey

1962 National Family Association for Deaf-Blind
Paticia McCallum, Secretary
111 Middle Neck Roak
Sands Point, NY 11050
800-225-0411
Fax: 516-944-7302
TTY: 516-944-8637

NFADB advocates for all persons who are deaf-blind of any chronological age and cognitive ability, supports national policy to benefit people who are deaf-blind, encourages the founding and strengthening of family organizations in each state, shares information related to deaf-blindness, provides resources and referrals, collaborates with professionals, and assists in the development of materials and training seminars which benefit family members.

Ralph Warner, President

1963 National Information Center on Deafness
Gallaudet Univ. Press c/o Chicago Distrib. Center
11030 South Langley Avenue
Chicago, IL 60628   202-651-5000
                                     800-621-2736
                                Fax: 800-621-8476
                                TTY: 888-630-9347
        e-mail: david.gunton@gallaudet.edu
             www.gallaudet.edu/~gupress

Provides information or referrals on questions
about deafness, including general information,
education, research, legislation, assistive devices
and more. Offers a bibliography of readings
available on 30 topics relating to deafness.

Loraine DiPietro, Director

**1964 National Information Clearinghouse on Children
Who Are Deaf-Blind**
Teaching Research
345 N. Monmouth Avenue
Monmouth, OR 97361
                                     800-438-9376
                                Fax: 541-438-8150
                                TTY: 800-854-7013
                       e-mail: dblink@tr.wou.edu
                             www.tr.wou/dblink/

Collects, organizes and disseminates information
related to children and youth who are deaf-blind
and connects consumers of deaf-blind information to sources of information about deaf-blindness, assistive technology and deaf-blind people.

John Reiman, Ph.D., Director

**1965 National Organization for the Advancement of the
Deaf, Inc**
Lamar University Station
P.O. Box 10076
Beaumont, TX 77710   409-880-8921
                                Fax: 409-880-2265
                         e-mail: mbeany.aol.com

This organization is dedicated to facilitation
communication on issues related to the deaf and
providing technical assistance for professionals
and parents working with deaf and hard-of-hearing children, adolescents, and adults.

Michael Bienenstock, President

**1966 National Rehabilitation Information Center
(NARIC)**
10R Wayne Avenue, Suite 800
Silver Spring, MD 20910   301-562-2400
                                     800-346-2742
                                Fax: 301-562-2401
                       e-mail: naricinfo@kra.com
                                     www.naric.com

NARIC is a library and information center focusing on disability and rehabilitation research.
Information specialists provide quick information and referrals free of charge. Other services
include customized searches of REHABDATA,
the premier database of disability and rehabilitation literature, and document delivery from
NARIC's collection of more than 60,000 documents are available for nominal fees.

Mark Odum, Director

1967 National Technical Institute for the Deaf
Rochester Institute
Lyndon Baines Johnson Bldg,52 Lomb
Rochester, NY 14623   716-475-6400
                                TTY: 716-475-6400
                                     www.rit.edu

NTID is a College of the Rochester Institute of
Technology.

1968 Self Help for Hard of Hearing People
7910 Woodmont Avenue Suite 1200
Bethesda, MD 20814   301-657-2248
                                Fax: 301-913-9413
                                TTY: 301-657-2249
                       e-mail: national@shhh.org
                                     www.shhh.org

Dedicated to the well-being of people who do not
hear well, SHHH believes that such people can
help one another, be helped, and participate successfully in society. Their primary purpose is
education about the causes, nature, and complications of hearing loss, and what can be done
about it.

**1969 Signing Exact English Center Advancement of Deaf
Children**
P.O. Box 1181
Los Alamintos, CA 90720   562-430-1467
                                Fax: 562-795-6614
                        e-mail: seectr@aol.com
                                     seectr.com

Information and referral center for parents and educators of hearing impaired children. Conducts workshops on the use of Signing Exact English, educational interpreting, education-related communication topics. Sign skill evaluations for teachers/teachers aids, educational interpreters also available.

Esther Zawolkow, Director

1970 Telecommunications for the Deaf
8630 Fenton Street-Suite 604
Silver Spring, MD 20910   301-589-3786
                                 Fax: 301-589-3797
                                 TTY: 301-589-3006
                                 e-mail: tdiexdir@aol.com

A nonprofit consumer advocacy organization promoting full visual and other access to information and telecommunications for people who are deaf, hard of hearing, deaf-blind, and speech impaired.

Claude Stout, Executive Director

1971 Tripod
1727 W. Burbank Blvd.
Burbank, CA 91506
                                 800-352-8888
                                 Fax: 818-972-2090
                                 TTY: 818-972-2080
                                 e-mail: tripodschool@earthlink.net
                                 www.tripod.org

In partnership with the Burbank Unified School District, provides a co-enrollment educational program for deaf and hard of hearing children and support services for their families. The program begins with a parent-infant/toddler group and continues through the 12th grade. Additionally, TRIPOD Captioned Films, a public service of the TRIPOD Model School program, distributes first-run open feature films to deaf and hard of hearing movie-going audiences nationwide.

Debra Leavitt-Gilmore, Office Manager

1972 USA Deaf Sports Federation
3607 Washington Boulevard, Ste 4
Ogden, UT 84403   801-393-7916
                                 800-393-8710
                                 Fax: 801-393-2263
                                 TTY: 801-393-7916
                                 e-mail: deafsports@juno.com

Information on adaptive sports and recreation activities for people of many abilities. Including local chapters, referrals, fun and social interaction and support groups.

1973 VOICE for Hearing-Impaired Children
124 Englinton Avenue, W., Suite 420
Toronto, ON,
Canada   416-487-7719

Libraries & Resource Centers

Alabama

1974 University of Alabama Speech and Hearing Center
Box 870242
Tuscaloosa, AL 35487   205-348-7628

Dr. Eugene Cooper, Director

Arizona

1975 Arizona Hearing Resources
P.O. Box 27213
Tempe, AZ 85285   480-777-1145
                                 Fax: 480-777-0450
                                 TTY: 480-777-2307
                                 e-mail: listenhear@listenhear.org
                                 www.listenhear.org

Auditory oral habilitation program for individuals who are hearing impaired or deaf. Comprehensive audiology services including fitting of hearing aids for children and adults.

Linda Thompson, Executive Director

Arkansas

1976 Arkansas Rehabilitation Research and Training Center for Deaf Persons
University of Arkansas
4601 W. Markham Street
Little Rock, AR 72205   501-686-9691
                                 Fax: 501-686-9698

The center focuses on issues affecting the employability of deaf and hard-of-hearing rehabilitation clients.

Douglas Watson, Ph.D., Director

1977 Research and Training Center for Persons Who Are Deaf or Hard of Hearing
4601 W. Markham
Little Rock, AR 72205   501-686-9691

Rehabilitation of deaf and hearing impaired individuals.

Dr. Douglas Watson, Director

California

1978 Hear Center
301 E. Del Mar Blvd.
Pasadena, CA 91101   626-796-2016

Auditory and verbal program designed to help hearing impaired children, infants and adults lead normal and productive lives. Seeks to develop auditory techniques to aid people who have communication problems due to deafness.

Josephine Wilson, Executive Director

District of Columbia

1979 District of Columbia Public Library/ Librarian for the Deaf Community
901 G Street NW, Room 410
Washington, DC 20001   202-727-1186
          Fax: 202-727-1129

Offers reference services through TDD, portable TDD for public use at pay phone, signers for library programs, sign language classes, information about deafness, print and non-print materials for persons who are deaf.

1980 Gallaudet University, Center for Auditory and Speech Sciences
800 Florida Avenue NE
Washington, DC 20002   202-651-5000
          Fax: 202-651-5295

Develops new hearing tests that use speech sounds to measure hearing loss.

Sally G. Revoille, Director

1981 Volta Bureau Library
Alexander Graham Bell Association for the Deaf
3417 Volta Place N.W.
Washington, DC 20007   202-337-5220
          800-432-7543
          Fax: 202-337-8314
          TTY: 202-337-5220
          e-mail: agbell2@aol.com
          www.agbell.org

Contains one of the world's largest historical collections of publications, documents and information on deafness. In addition to the main collection, which includes books, periodicals and indexed clipping files dating from the turn of the century, the library also houses a significant archival collection dealing with the history of deafness since the 16th century. Membership dues for professionals is $50.

4500 members

Rebecca Parlakian, Director, Member Services

Illinois

1982 Loyola University of Children, Parmly Hearing Institute
6525 N. Sheridan Road
Chicago, IL 60626   773-274-3000
          Fax: 773-508-2719

Dr. William Yost, Director

Maine

1983 University of Maine, Conley Speech and Hearing Center
N. Stevans Hall
Orono, ME 04469   207-581-2006

Speech disorders of adults and children including hearing impairments and deafness.

Dr. John M. Petit, Coordinator

Maryland

1984 Captioned Films/Videos
National Association of the Deaf
814 Thayer Avenueet
Silver Spring, MD 20910   301-587-1788
          800-237-6213
          Fax: 301-587-1791
          TTY: 301-587-1789
          e-mail: info@cfv.org
          www.cfv.org

Free loans of educational and entertainment captioned films and videos for deaf and hard of hearing people.

Bill Stark, Project Director

Massachusetts

1985 Caption Center
WGBH Educational Foundation
125 Western Avenue
Boston, MA 02134   617-492-9225
Fax: 617-562-0590

A nonprofit service of the WGBH Educational Foundation with offices in Boston, New York and Los Angeles. Produces captions for every segment of the entertainment and advertising industries and offers clients off-line captions, real-time captions, and open captions.

Trisha O'Connell, Director

1986 Eaton-Peabody Laboratory of Auditory Physiology
Massachusetts Eye & Ear Institute
243 Charles Street
Boston, MA 02114   617-523-4545
Fax: 617-720-4408

Auditory system and auditory information processing, including ear-brain interactions in normal and pathologic hearing.

Nelson Y.S. Kiang, PhD, Director

Nebraska

1987 University of Nebraska, Lincoln Barkley Memorial Center
Barkley Center 301
Lincoln, NE 68583   402-472-2145
Fax: 402-472-7697

Focuses on hearing impairments and deaf research.

John Bernthal, Director

New Jersey

1988 Princeton University, Cutaneous Communication Laboratory
Psychology Department, Green Hall

Princeton, NJ 08544   609-258-5277
Fax: 609-258-1113

Dr. Roger Cholewiak

New York

1989 Wallace Memorial Library
Rochester Institute of Technology
1 Lomb Memorial Drive
Rochester, NY 14623   716-475-2505

Information on physical disabilities and deafness.

Melanie Norton, Reference Librarian

Oregon

1990 Regional Resource Center on Deafness
Western Oregon State College

Monmouth, OR 97361   503-838-8000

John Freeburg, Director

Virginia

1991 University of Virginia Communication Disorders Program
2205 Fontaine Avenue, Suite 202
Charlottesville, VA 22903   804-924-7107
Fax: 804-924-4621

Dr. Richard Talbott, Director

Research Centers

Alabama

1992 Civitan International Research Center
Circ 137 1530 3rd Ave., So.
Birmingham, AL 35294   205-934-8900
Fax: 205-975-6330
www.circ.uab.edu

Aims to improve the well-being and quality of life of individuals and families affected by mental retardation and developmental disabilities.

Dr. Craig Ramey, Co-Director
Dr. Sharon Ramey, Co-Director

Illinois

1993 University of Chicago, Temporal Bone Laboratory for Ear Research
5841 S. Maryland Avenue, Box 412
Chicago, IL 60637   773-702-6152
     Fax: 773-702-6809

Focuses on hearing impairments and deafness research.

Dr. Raul Hinojasa, Director

Michigan

1994 University of Michigan, Kresge Hearing Research Institute
1301 E. Ann Street, Rm. 5032
Ann Arbor, MI 48109   734-763-9600
     Fax: 734-764-0014

Focuses on hearing and auditory disorders.

Josef M. Miller, Director

Missouri

1995 Central Institute for the Deaf
818 South Euclid Avenue
St. Louis, MO 63110   314-977-0000
     Fax: 314-977-0025
     TTY: 314-997-0001
     e-mail: bf@cidmac.wustl.edu
     www.cidmac.wustl.edu/index.htm

Central Institute for the Deaf is a private, non-profit institute composed of research laboratories in which scientists study the normal aspects as well as the disorders of hearing, language, and speech; a school for children who have hearing impairments; speech, language, and hearing clinics; and professionals with hearing impairment, and communication sciences.

Nebraska

1996 Center for Hearing Loss in Children
555 North 30th Street
Omaha, NE 68131   402-498-6511
     800-282-6657
     Fax: 402-498-6638
     TTY: 402-498-6543
     e-mail: chilic@boystown.org
     www.boystown.org/chlc

The Center for Hearing Loss in Children unites professionals from a variety of disciplines to focus on research, research training, information dissemination, and continuing education in the area of childhood deafness.

New York

1997 New York Foundation for Otologic Research
920 Park Avenue
New York, NY 10021   212-980-3100

Unsolved hearing problems and deafness research.

Dr. Alan Austin Scheer, Director

1998 State University College at Plattsburgh Auditory Research Laboratory
107 Beaumont
Plattsburgh, NY 12901   518-564-7701

Dr. Roger Hamernik, Director

1999 Syracuse University, Institute for Sensory Research
Merrill Lane
Syracuse, NY 13244   315-443-4164
     Fax: 315-443-1184
     e-mail: robert-smith@isr5yr.edu
     www.isr.syr.edu/ben/

Sensory processing and hearing disorders.

Dr. Robert Smith, Director

2000 Yeshiva University, Institute of Communication Disorders
Montefiore Medical Center
111 East 210th Street
Bronx, NY 10467   718-920-4321
     Fax: 718-405-9014

Studies on communicative disorders including speech and hearing.

Robert Ruben, MD, Chairman

Oregon

2001 Oregon Health Sciences University Research Center
3181 SW Sam Jackson Park Road
Portland, OR 97201   503-494-7820
Fax: 503-494-5656

Hearing problems, including clinical and basic research into the field of hearing disorders.

Jack A. Vernon, PhD, Director

Pennsylvania

2002 Temple University, Section of Auditory Research
3440 Kruege, N. Broad Street
Philadelphia, PA 19140   215-221-3661

William Hal Martin, Director

Tennessee

2003 Bill Wilkerson Center
1114-19th Avenue South
Nashville, TN 37212   615-320-5353
Fax: 615-343-7705

Community-operated research and treatment center focusing studies on hearing sciences.

Dr. Fred H. Bess, Director

Texas

2004 Houston Ear Research Foundation
7737 SW Freeway, Ste. 630
Houston, TX 77074   713-771-9966
Fax: 713-771-0546
TTY: 713-771-9966
e-mail: jangil@hern.org

Aims to improve health care and education for deaf and hearing-impaired children; cochlear implant center.

Jan Gilden, Executive Director

Audio Video

2005 ABCs of AVT: Analyzing Auditory-Verbal Therapy
Alexander Graham Bell Association for the Deaf
3417 Volta Place N.W.
Washington, DC 20007   202-337-5220
800-432-7543
Fax: 202-337-8314
TTY: 202-337-5220
e-mail: agbell2@aol.com
www.agbell.org

This educational tool will enable therapists, teachers, speech-language pathologists, and audiologists to expand their professional auditory-verbal therapy skills by studying actual videotaped footage of therapy. They will learn how to identify a child's current development level and begin an auditory-verbal therapy program.

1995 98 pages 45 Minute video

Warren Estabrooks, Editor

2006 Basic Course in American Sign Language Videotape Package

Humphries, Padden, O'Rourke, author

T.J. Publishers, Inc.
817 Silver Spring Avenue, Suite 206
Silver Spring, MD 20910   301-585-4440
800-999-1168
Fax: 301-585-5930
TTY: 301-585-4440
TDD: 301-585-4441
e-mail: TJPubinc@aol.com

The first three tapes illustrate and demonstrate the exercises and dialogues presented in A Basic Course in American Sign Language. The fourth tape presents unrehearsed conversations among four deaf adults and offers excellent practice in reading signs. The fifth tape demonstrates each vocabulary word contained in all 22 lessons plus the alphabet and numbers. Includes the ABC text and Study Guide.

2007 Beginning Reading and Sign Language Video

Aylmer Press, author

T-J Publishers
817 Silver Spring Avenue, Suite 206
Silver Spring, MD 20910   301-585-4440
800-999-1186
Fax: 301-585-5930

Learning Sign improves reading, motor skills and visual perception and increases language acquisition abilities. For kids from 2 to 12, this video picture book features deaf actress Susan Bressler signing over a hundred words at the zoo, at home, and around the community.

Video

2008 Communication Rules for Hard of Hearing People

Samuel Trychin, PhD, author

Self Help for Hard of Hearing People, Inc.
7910 Woodmont Avenue Suite 1200
Bethesda, MD 20814   301-657-2248
                        Fax: 301-913-9413
                        TTY: 301-657-2249
                        e-mail: national@shhh.org
                            www.shhh.org

For use with manual (listed separately).

1987 Open-captioned

2009 Deaf Children Signers

Harris Communications
15159 Technology Drive
Eden Prairie, MN 55344   612-906-1180
                            800-825-6758
                        Fax: 612-902-1099
                        e-mail: mail@harriscomm.com
                            www.harriscomm.com

This 5-part collection of children signers is great for children, teachers, parents and interpreters.

2010 Getting In Touch

Elizabeth Cooley, author

Research Press
P.O. Box 9177
Champaign, IL 61826   217-352-3273
                            800-519-2707
                        Fax: 217-352-1221

Introduces teachers, staff and parents

Videocassette

2011 Getting Through Audiotape

Self Help for Hard of Hearing People, Inc.
7910 Woodmont Avenue Suite 1200
Bethesda, MD 20814   301-657-2248
                        Fax: 301-913-9413
                        TTY: 301-657-2249
                        e-mail: national@shhh.org
                            www.shhh.org

Simulates hearing loss for better understanding of communication difficulties. The tape features a hearing test.

Audiotape

2012 I Can Hear!

Alexander Graham Bell Association for the Deaf
3417 Volta Place N.W.
Washington, DC 20007   202-337-5220
                            800-432-7543
                        Fax: 202-337-8314
                        TTY: 202-337-5220
                        e-mail: agbell2@aol.com
                            www.agbell.org

This inspirational video describes the auditory-verbal approach for developing speech and language for hearing impaired children and adults.

1992 23 minutes

2013 I Can Hear-II

Alexander Graham Bell Association for the Deaf
3417 Volta Place N.W.
Washington, DC 20007   202-337-5220
                            800-432-7543
                        Fax: 202-337-8314
                        TTY: 202-337-5220
                        e-mail: agbell2@aol.com
                            www.agbell.org

An exciting videotape that gives more examples of auditory-verbal therapy and a variety of kids who have been taught to speak using this method.

1996 19 Minute video

2014 Joy of Signing

Lottie Riekehof, author

Gallaudet Univ. Press c/o Chicago Distrib. Center
11030 South Langley Avenue
Chicago, IL 60628   202-651-5000
                            800-621-2736
                        Fax: 800-621-8476
                        TTY: 888-630-9347
                        e-mail: david.gunton@gallaudet.edu
                            www.gallaudet.edu/~gupress

Three tapes full of useful information to help increase skill and comfort with sign.

1 Videotape

2015 Learning to Communicate: The First Three Years Videotape

Bill Wilkerson Center Press, author

Alexander Graham Bell Association for the Deaf
3417 Volta Place N.W.
Washington, DC 20007   202-337-5220
                            800-432-7543
                        Fax: 202-337-8314
                        TTY: 202-337-5220
                        e-mail: agbell2@aol.com
                            www.agbell.org

This video shows normal communication development in young children under three years of age. It discusses factors which can affect speech and language development, including anatomy and environment. Closed-captioned.

11 minutes

2016 Lipreading Made Easy

Audrey B. Greenwald, author

Alexander Graham Bell Association for the Deaf
3417 Volta Place N.W.
Washington, DC 20007   202-337-5220
                                                  800-432-7543
                                        Fax: 202-337-8314
                                        TTY: 202-337-5220
                                 e-mail: agbell2@aol.com
                                                  www.agbell.org

Uses actual photos of lips to teach the student to listen with their eyes.

Video & Book

2017 Teaching Strategies for the Development of Auditory Verbal Communication

Doreen Pollack, author

Alexander Graham Bell Association for the Deaf
3417 Volta Place N.W.
Washington, DC 20007   202-337-5220
                                                  800-432-7543
                                        Fax: 202-337-8314
                                        TTY: 202-337-5220
                                 e-mail: agbell2@aol.com
                                                  www.agbell.org

This educational series of five-hour videotapes demonstrates teaching strategies for developing auditory-verbal communication in young children with severe to profound hearing loss.

Set of 5

2018 Videos on Hearing-Impaired Children TRIPOD Grapevine

2901 N Keystone St
Burbank, CA 91504
                                                  800-352-8888
                                        TDD: 800-2TR-IPOD

TRIPOD Grapevine will loan to parents upon request two excellent videos (open captioned) for families with hearing-impaired children. 'Language Says It All' focuses on the importance of establishing clear communication in the home. Parents talk about concerns for their children. 'Once Upon a Time' reminds us how important story time is to parents and their hearing-impaired child. Parents describe the ways in which they learned to share a rich story heritage with their children

Computer Software

2019 Fingerspelling & Numbers Software

Sign Enhancers, Inc.
Dept. 98 P.O. Box 12687
Salem, OR 97309
                                        Fax: 503-304-1063
                                        TTY: 800-767-4461
                          e-mail: sign@signenhancers.com
                                        www.teleport.com/~sign

Fingerspelling practice partner that allows you to control the speed and vocabulary level. Requires Windows 3.1 or greater.

Software

2020 Foundation In Speech Perception Computer Program

Carolyn J. Brown, Ph.D., author

Alexander Graham Bell Association for the Deaf
3417 Volta Place N.W.
Washington, DC 20007   202-337-5220
                                                  800-432-7543
                                        Fax: 202-337-8314
                                        TTY: 202-337-5220
                                 e-mail: agbell2@aol.com
                                                  www.agbell.org

This computerized auditory training program for children, ages 3 and up, fosters learning and literacy by developing skills in speech perception, speech production, vocabulary, reading, writing, and computer skills in children with a variety of hearing impairments, this software progresses at the child's pace and allows unlimited exploration opportunities. Each module varies the amount of visual support that a child can use.

2021 SignFinder: A Software Program for Learning More Than 300 ASL Signs

James Nusbaum, author

Pro-Ed
8700 Shoal Creek Boulevard
Austin, TX 78757   512-451-3246
                                                  800-897-3202
                                        Fax: 512-451-8542
                                        www.proedinc.com

Easy-to-use, interactive program with animated and attractive illustrations which is also easy to install and takes up less than 2 megabytes of hard disk space. Macintosh or Windows.

2022 Software to Go

Ken Kurlychek, author

Gallaudet Univ. Press c/o Chicago Distrib. Center
11030 South Langley Avenue
Chicago, IL 60628
202-651-5000
800-621-2736
Fax: 800-621-8476
TTY: 888-630-9347
e-mail: david.gunton@gallaudet.edu
www.gallaudet.edu/~gupress

Lists and describes commercial software that may be borrowed by educators of hearing impaired students.

100 pages

Books

2023 A Basic Vocabulary: American Sign Language for Parents and Children

Terrence J. O'Rourke, author

T.J. Publishers, Inc.
817 Silver Spring Avenue, Suite 206
Silver Spring, MD 20910
301-585-4440
800-999-1168
Fax: 301-585-5930
TTY: 301-585-4440
TDD: 301-585-4441
e-mail: TJPubinc@aol.com

Carefully selected words and signs include those families use every day. Alphabetically organized vocabulary incorporates developmental lists helpful to both Deaf and hearing children and over 1,000 clear sign language illustrations.

240 pages Softcover
ISBN: 0-932666-00-0

2024 A Hug Just Isn't Enough

Caren Ferris, author

Gallaudet Univ. Press c/o Chicago Distrib. Center
11030 South Langley Avenue
Chicago, IL 60628
202-651-5000
800-621-2736
Fax: 800-621-8476
TTY: 888-630-9347
e-mail: david.gunton@gallaudet.edu
www.gallaudet.edu/~gupress

Photos of deaf children and excerpts from interviews with parents of deaf youngsters.

2025 A Journey Into the DEAF-WORLD

Harlan Lane, Robert Hoffmeister, and Ben Bahan, author

DawnSignPress
6130 Nancy Ridge Drive
San Diego, CA 92121
858-625-0600
800-549-5350
Fax: 858-625-2336
e-mail: dsp@dawnsign.com
www.dawnsign.com

Provides explanation about the nature and meaning of the DEAF-WORLD. Comprehensive work discusses latest findings and theories for Deaf Studies students and professionals working with deaf people.

528 pages Softcover
ISBN: 0-915035-63-4

Barry Howland, Marketing Director

2026 A Journey Into the Deaf World

Harlan Lane, author

DawnSignPress C/O T.J. Publishers
817 Silver Spring Avenue, Suite 206
Silver Spring, MD 20910
301-585-4440
800-999-168
Fax: 301-585-5930

Provides a clear explanation about the nature and meaning of the Deaf World. It combines thought-provoking intellectual perspectives with first-hand accounts of life in the Deaf World.

1996 513 pages Softcover
ISBN: 0-915035-63-4

2027 APT/HI: Auditory Perception Test for the Hearing Impaired

Susan G. Allen and Thomas S. Serwatka, author

Alexander Graham Bell Association for the Deaf
3417 Volta Place N.W.
Washington, DC 20007
202-337-5220
800-432-7543
Fax: 202-337-8314
TTY: 202-337-5220
e-mail: agbell2@aol.com
www.agbell.org

This test, modeled on children with hearing losses, allows speech therapists and audiologists to assess functional use of residual hearing. The test identifies auditory processing and auditory training, prioritizes speech targets and auditory functioning, and assesses amplification.

1994 25-Tests

2028 Academic Acceptance of ASL

Sherman Wilcox, author

Gallaudet Univ. Press c/o Chicago Distrib. Center
11030 South Langley Avenue
Chicago, IL 60628   202-651-5000
                                    800-621-2736
                              Fax: 800-621-8476
                              TTY: 888-630-9347
            e-mail: david.gunton@gallaudet.edu
                    www.gallaudet.edu/~gupress

This monograph presents a dozen articles that demonstrate clearly and convincingly that the study of ASL affords the same educational values and the same intellectual rewards as the study of any other foreign language.

196 pages

2029 Access for All: Integrating Deaf, Hard of Hearing and Hearing Preschoolers

Gail Solit, author

Gallaudet Univ. Press c/o Chicago Distrib. Center
11030 South Langley Avenue
Chicago, IL 60628   202-651-5000
                                    800-621-2736
                              Fax: 800-621-8476
                              TTY: 888-630-9347
            e-mail: david.gunton@gallaudet.edu
                    www.gallaudet.edu/~gupress

Describes a model program for integrating the deaf and hard of hearing in early education.

150 pages Book & Video

2030 Advanced Sign Language Vocabulary: A Resource Text

Janet R. Coleman, Elizabeth E. Wolf, author

Charles C. Thomas Publishing, Ltd.
2600 South First Street
Springfield, IL 62704   217-789-8980
                                    800-258-8980
                              Fax: 217-789-9130
                e-mail: books@ccthomas.com
                        www.ccthomas.com

This book is a collection of advanced sign language vocabulary intended for use by educators, interpreters, parents or anyone wishing to enlarge their sign vocabulary. Each sign is clearly illustrated and movement is both shown and described.

202 pages
ISBN: 0-398057-22-2

2031 Advocacy for Deaf Children

Hugh Prickett, author

Charles C. Thomas
2600 South First Street
Springfield, IL 62794   217-789-8980
                                    800-258-8980
                              Fax: 217-789-9130

Professional text on attitudes toward the deaf children in America.

114 pages

2032 American Deaf Culture

Sherman Wilcox, author

Gallaudet Univ. Press c/o Chicago Distrib. Center
11030 South Langley Avenue
Chicago, IL 60628   202-651-5000
                                    800-621-2736
                              Fax: 800-621-8476
                              TTY: 888-630-9347
            e-mail: david.gunton@gallaudet.edu
                    www.gallaudet.edu/~gupress

This book presents a collection of classic articles which have been selected to provide a variety of perspectives on language and culture of deaf people in America.

132 pages

2033 American Deaf Culture: An Anthology

Ed. Sherman Wilcox, author

Sign Media, Inc.
4020 Blackburn Lane
Burtonsville, MD 20866   301-421-0268
                                    800-475-4756
                              Fax: 301-421-0270
                              TTY: 301-421-4460
                        www.signmedia.com

Features deaf and hearing authors offering their experience and perspectives on cultural values, ASL, social interaction in the deaf community, education, folklore, and more.

1989
ISBN: 0-932130-09-7

Barbara Olmert, Director of Marketing

2034 American Sign Language: A Beginning Course - Teacher's Manual

Catherine Kettrick, author

National Association of the Deaf
814 Thayer Avenue
Silver Spring, MD 20910   301-587-1788
                              Fax: 301-587-1791
                              TTY: 301-587-1789

Provides a quick reference to the vocabulary and grammar in the student text, with lists of props and pictures needed for each lesson, and stories and dialogues for classroom instruction.

2035 American Sign Language: A Beginning Course

Catherine Kettrick, author

National Association of the Deaf
814 Thayer Avenue
Silver Spring, MD 20910   301-587-1788
                                 Fax: 301-587-1791
                                 TTY: 301-587-1789

An interactive approach to teaching and learning American Sign Language, with 700 sign illustrations, each accompanied by an object drawing.

2036 Amplification for Children with Auditory Deficits

Fred H. Bess, author

Alexander Graham Bell Association for the Deaf
3417 Volta Place N.W.
Washington, DC 20007   202-337-5220
                              800-432-7543
                              Fax: 202-337-8314
                              TTY: 202-337-5220
                              e-mail: agbell2@aol.com
                              www.agbell.org

This text offers an overview of the field of pediatric amplification and is a valuable addition to any audiologist's reference collection. Based on papers presented at the International Symposium on Amplification for children with Auditory Defects, this volume of work represents years of study related to amplification devices and the various issues facing the children who wear them.

1996 578 pages

2037 Approaching Equality

Frank Bowe, author

T.J. Publishers, Inc.
817 Silver Spring Avenue, Suite 206
Silver Spring, MD 20910   301-585-4440
                                 800-999-1168
                                 Fax: 301-585-5930
                                 TTY: 301-585-4440
                                 TDD: 301-585-4441
                                 e-mail: TJPubinc@aol.com

Written by the former chair of the Commission on the Education of the Deaf, this book reviews the dramatic developments in the education of Deaf children.

1991 112 pages Softcover
ISBN: 0-932666-39-6

2038 Assessment and Management of Mainstreamed Hearing-Impaired Children

Ross, Brackett, Maxon, author

Pro-Ed
8700 Shoal Creek Boulevard
Austin, TX 78757   512-451-3246
                          800-897-3202
                          Fax: 512-451-8542
                          www.proedinc.com

Covers the development of appropriate programming for children with hearing impairments (primarily oral/aural).

415 pages Hardcover
ISBN: 0-890794-58-8

2039 Assessment of Hearing Impaired People

Frank R. Zieziula, author

Gallaudet Univ. Press c/o Chicago Distrib. Center
11030 South Langley Avenue
Chicago, IL 60628   202-651-5000
                           800-621-2736
                           Fax: 800-621-8476
                           TTY: 888-630-9347
                           e-mail: david.gunton@gallaudet.edu
                           www.gallaudet.edu/~gupress

This is a comprehensive review of 62 tests used by educational institutions, rehabilitation agencies, and mental health centers.

128 pages Softcover

2040 Auditory Enhancement Guide

B. David Shea, author

Alexander Graham Bell Association for the Deaf
3417 Volta Place N.W.
Washington, DC 20007   202-337-5220
                              800-432-7543
                              Fax: 202-337-8314
                              TTY: 202-337-5220
                              e-mail: agbell2@aol.com
                              www.agbell.org

For the teacher and professional, this handbook presents strategies which emphasize the student's total auditory development and shows how to assess the appropriate auditory learning approach and how to plan classroom placement.

1992 222 pages

2041 Auditory Training

Norman P. Erber, Ph.D., author

Alexander Graham Bell Association for the Deaf
3417 Volta Place N.W.
Washington, DC 20007   202-337-5220
                              800-432-7543
                              Fax: 202-337-8314
                              TTY: 202-337-5220
                              e-mail: agbell2@aol.com
                              www.agbell.org

Experience with hearing-impaired children to develop a practical hearing guide for teachers and parents of hearing-impaired children.

1982 197 pages

2042 Auditory-Verbal Therapy for Parents and Professionals

Warren Estabrooks, M.Ed., author

Alexander Graham Bell Association for the Deaf
3417 Volta Place N.W.
Washington, DC 20007   202-337-5220
                              800-432-7543
                         Fax: 202-337-8314
                         TTY: 202-337-5220
                  e-mail: agbell2@aol.com
                              www.agbell.org

A comprehensive book introducing auditory-verbal therapy and its impact on children with hearing impairments and their families.

1994 300 pages

2043 Aural Habilitation

Daniel Ling, Ph.D. and Agnes Ling Phillips, Ph.D., author

Alexander Graham Bell Association for the Deaf
3417 Volta Place N.W.
Washington, DC 20007   202-337-5220
                              800-432-7543
                         Fax: 202-337-8314
                         TTY: 202-337-5220
                  e-mail: agbell2@aol.com
                              www.agbell.org

This classic text for professionals, educators and parents teaches how to assess and plan individualized educational programs for young children with hearing impairments.

1978 324 pages

2044 Basic Course in Manual Communication

Terrence J. O'Rourke, author

National Association of the Deaf
814 Thayer Avenue
Silver Spring, MD 20910   301-587-1788
                            Fax: 301-587-1791
                            TTY: 301-587-1789

Over 700 signs are grouped according to shape, location, and movement. Also includes dialogues for practice.

2045 Basic Sign Communication: Student Materials

William Newell, author

National Association of the Deaf
814 Thayer Avenue
Silver Spring, MD 20910   301-587-1788
                            Fax: 301-587-1791
                            TTY: 301-587-1789

Includes study and reference materials for all three levels of Basic Sign Communication.

2046 Basic Sign Communication: Vocabulary

William Newell, author

National Association of the Deaf
814 Thayer Avenue
Silver Spring, MD 20910   301-587-1788
                            Fax: 301-587-1791
                            TTY: 301-587-1789

Features sections on Sign Vocabulary, Numbers, and Classifiers. Contains 1000 illustrated signs, organized alphabetically by gloss for quick reference.

2047 Basic Vocabulary and Language Thesaurus for Hearing-Impaired Children

Daniel Ling, Ph.D. and Agnes Ling Phillips, Ph.D., author

Alexander Graham Bell Association for the Deaf
3417 Volta Place N.W.
Washington, DC 20007   202-337-5220
                              800-432-7543
                         Fax: 202-337-8314
                         TTY: 202-337-5220
                  e-mail: agbell2@aol.com
                              www.agbell.org

This simple thesaurus lists spontaneous vocabulary used by normally hearing children and lets patients and teachers check so that children with hearing losses have mastered these words.

1977 76 pages

2048 Being In Touch

Gallaudet Univ. Press c/o Chicago Distrib. Center
11030 South Langley Avenue
Chicago, IL 60628   202-651-5000
                              800-621-2736
                         Fax: 800-621-8476
                         TTY: 888-630-9347
            e-mail: david.gunton@gallaudet.edu
                  www.gallaudet.edu/~gupress

Provides information on hearing and vision loss.

80 pages

2049 Ben's Story: A Deaf Child's Right to Sign

Lorraine Fletcher, author

T.J. Publishers, Inc.
817 Silver Spring Avenue, Suite 206
Silver Spring, MD 20910   301-585-4440
                                 800-999-1168
                            Fax: 301-585-5930
                            TTY: 301-585-4440
                            TDD: 301-585-4441
                       e-mail: TJPubinc@aol.com

This is a mother's story of how she responded to the diagnosis of her son's deafness, and how she struggled to have her son educated using sign language.

267 pages Softcover
ISBN: 0-930323-47-5

2050 Blueprint for Conversational Competence

Patrick Stone, Ed.D., author

Alexander Graham Bell Association for the Deaf
3417 Volta Place N.W.
Washington, DC 20007   202-337-5220
                              800-432-7543
                         Fax: 202-337-8314
                         TTY: 202-337-5220
                    e-mail: agbell2@aol.com
                         www.agbell.org

A book that develops conversational skills in children with hearing impairments.

1988 175 pages

2051 Book of Name Signs

Samuel Supalla, author

Gallaudet Univ. Press c/o Chicago Distrib. Center
11030 South Langley Avenue
Chicago, IL 60628   202-651-5000
                           800-621-2736
                      Fax: 800-621-8476
                      TTY: 888-630-9347
          e-mail: david.gunton@gallaudet.edu
               www.gallaudet.edu/~gupress

This text discusses the rules for ASL name sign formulation and their appropriate uses and presents a list of over 400 name signs.

112 pages

2052 CHATS: The Miami Cochlear Implant, Auditory & Tactile Skills Curriculum

Kathleen Vergara & Lynn Weissler Miskiel, author

Alexander Graham Bell Association for the Deaf
3417 Volta Place N.W.
Washington, DC 20007   202-337-5220
                              800-432-7543
                         Fax: 202-337-8314
                         TTY: 202-337-5220
                    e-mail: agbell2@aol.com
                         www.agbell.org

A comprehensive curriculum for educators and clinicians providing educational tools and techniques to maximize the potential of children with hearing impairments who wear sensory aids.

1994 327 pages

2053 CUED Speech Resource Guide for Parents of Deaf Children

R. Orin Cornett, Ph.D. and Mary Elsie Daisey, author

Alexander Graham Bell Association for the Deaf
3417 Volta Place N.W.
Washington, DC 20007   202-337-5220
                              800-432-7543
                         Fax: 202-337-8314
                         TTY: 202-337-5220
                    e-mail: agbell2@aol.com
                         www.agbell.org

A comprehensive book describing Cued Speech, getting started, your child's rights in and out of school, and families expectations with special attention on siblings and peer relationships.

1992 832 pages Hardcover

2054 Can't Your Child Hear?

Roger D. Freeman, author

Gallaudet Univ. Press c/o Chicago Distrib. Center
11030 South Langley Avenue
Chicago, IL 60628   202-651-5000
                           800-621-2736
                      Fax: 800-621-8476
                      TTY: 888-630-9347
          e-mail: david.gunton@gallaudet.edu
               www.gallaudet.edu/~gupress

Is deafness a difference to be accepted or a defect to be corrected? This comprehensive reference will help parents, as well as educators and other professionals, recognize their options in understanding and handling a child who is deaf.

340 pages Softcover

2055 Can't Your Child Hear? A Guide for Those Who Care About Deaf Children

Clifton F Carbin, Robert J Boese, & Roger Freeman, author

Pro-Ed
8700 Shoal Creek Boulevard
Austin, TX 78757

512-451-3246
800-897-3202
Fax: 512-451-8542
www.proedinc.com

The first complete and compassionate book for parents of children who are deaf. Answers the questions parents most often ask about deafness.

368 pages Illustrated
ISBN: 0-936104-40-6

2056 Carolina Picture Vocabulary Test For Deaf and Hearing Impaired Children

Thomas L. Layton, & David W. Holmes, author

Pro-Ed
8700 Shoal Creek Boulevard
Austin, TX 78757

512-451-3246
800-897-3202
Fax: 512-451-8542
www.proedinc.com

The CPVT is a norm-referenced, validated, individually administered, receptive sign vocabulary test for children between the ages of 4 and 11 1/2 who are deaf or hearing impaired.

4-11 1/2

2057 Challenge of Educating Together

Paul C. Higgins, author

Charles C. Thomas Publishing, Ltd.
2600 South First Street
Springfield, IL 62704

217-789-8980
800-258-8980
Fax: 217-789-9130
e-mail: books@ccthomas.com
www.ccthomas.com

This book is for those who have this challenge of education; the author believes that deaf and hearing youth can be educated together and without outrageously expensive devices and programs.

198 pages $28.95 paper
ISBN: 0-398056-65-X

2058 Children with Hearing Difficulties

Alec Webster, author

Paul H. Brookes Publishing Co.
P.O. Box 10624
Baltimore, MD 21285

800-638-3775

Based on 10 years of research into hearing and hearing-impaired children, this book looks at the impact of deafness on all aspects of the development and education of young children.

192 pages Softcover
ISBN: 0-304317-24-1

2059 Choices In Deafness

Sue Schwartz Ph.D, author

Woodbine House
6510 Bells Mill Road
Bethesda, MD 20817

301-468-8800
800-843-7323
Fax: 301-897-5838
e-mail: info@woodbinehouse.com
www.woodbinehouse.com

Offers clear, objective descriptions of five communication methods for children with hearing impairments or deafness.

212 pages Softcover
ISBN: 0-933149-09-3

2060 Choices In Deafness: A Parent's Guide to Communication Options

Sue Schwartz Ph.D., author

Alexander Graham Bell Association for the Deaf
3417 Volta Place N.W.
Washington, DC 20007

202-337-5220
800-432-7543
Fax: 202-337-8314
TTY: 202-337-5220
e-mail: agbell2@aol.com
www.agbell.org

Serving as an invaluable guide to the world of deaf education, this expanded edition covers a wide variety of communication options for children with hearing impairments. Provides medical, audiological, and educational information and numerous case studies.

1996 304 pages

2061 Cochlear Implant Auditory Training Guidebook

Dave Sindrey, Cert.AVT, author

Alexander Graham Bell Association for the Deaf
3417 Volta Place N.W.
Washington, DC 20007

202-337-5220
800-432-7543
Fax: 202-337-8314
TTY: 202-337-5220
e-mail: agbell2@aol.com
www.agbell.org

Designed for parents and professionals working with children ages 4 and up who have cochlear implants. It includes an easy to follow hierarchy for listening goals and a quick placement test to help you find where to start.

236 pages

2062 Cochlear Implant Rehabilitation in Children and Adults

Rlexander Graham Bell Association for the Deaf
3417 Volta Place N.W.
Washington, DC 20007   202-337-5220
                              800-432-7543
                         Fax: 202-337-8314
                         TTY: 202-337-5220
                    e-mail: agbell2@aol.com
                              www.agbell.org

This text focuses on the rehabilitation of cochlear implant users as a process rather than a series of training tasks. Each chapter reveals unique aspects of this process. A variety of exercises are dispersed throughout the text and most of these can be adapted to a variety of languages.

1996 325 pages

Dianne J. Allum, Editor

2063 Cochlear Implantation for Infants and Children

Grame M. Clark and Robert S. Cowan, author

Alexander Graham Bell Association for the Deaf
3417 Volta Place N.W.
Washington, DC 20007   202-337-5220
                              800-432-7543
                         Fax: 202-337-8314
                         TTY: 202-337-5220
                    e-mail: agbell2@aol.com
                              www.agbell.org

This comprehensive text presents the surgical, medical, audiological speech and language, and habilitation aspects of cochlear implants in infants and children.

1997 263 pages

2064 Cochlear Implants and Children

Nancy Tye-Murray, PhD, author

Alexander Graham Bell Association for the Deaf
3417 Volta Place N.W.
Washington, DC 20007   202-337-5220
                              800-432-7543
                         Fax: 202-337-8314
                         TTY: 202-337-5220
                    e-mail: agbell2@aol.com
                              www.agbell.org

Designed to educate readers about cochlear implants, including surgery, the importance of rehabilitation, and the significance of parents' and professionals' roles.

189 pages Softcover

2065 Cognition, Education, and Deafness

David S. Martin, author

Gallaudet Univ. Press c/o Chicago Distrib. Center
11030 South Langley Avenue
Chicago, IL 60628   202-651-5000
                           800-621-2736
                      Fax: 800-621-8476
                      TTY: 888-630-9347
            e-mail: david.gunton@gallaudet.edu
                 www.gallaudet.edu/~gupress

The work of 54 authors is gathered in this definitive collection of current research on deafness and cognition. The articles are grouped into seven sections: cognition, problem solving, thinking processes, language development, reading methodologies, measurement of potential and intervention programs.

260 pages Hardcover

David S. Martin, Editor

2066 Come Sign with Us: Sign Language Activities for Children

Jan Hafer and Robert Wilson, author

T.J. Publishers, Inc.
817 Silver Spring Avenue, Suite 206
Silver Spring, MD 20910   301-585-4440
                                 800-999-1168
                            Fax: 301-585-5930
                            TTY: 301-585-4440
                            TDD: 301-585-4441
                     e-mail: TJPubinc@aol.com

Illustrated activities manual contains more than 300 line drawings of adults and children signing familiar words, phrases, and sentences using ASL in English word order.

144 pages Softcover
ISBN: 0-930321-56-3

2067 Communication Access for Persons with Hearing Loss

Alexander Graham Bell Association for the Deaf
3417 Volta Place N.W.
Washington, DC 20007   202-337-5220
                              800-432-7543
                         Fax: 202-337-8314
                         TTY: 202-337-5220
                    e-mail: agbell2@aol.com
                              www.agbell.org

Filled with information about available technologies, this book explores equipment and options available uner the ADA. The book stresses that technology is a tool, not a solution, for combination hearing loss and for improving communication.

1994 306 pages

2068 Communication Issues Among Deaf People

Mervin Garretson, author

Gallaudet Univ. Press c/o Chicago Distrib. Center
11030 South Langley Avenue
Chicago, IL 60628   202-651-5000
                                 800-621-2736
                          Fax: 800-621-8476
                          TTY: 888-630-9347
        e-mail: david.gunton@gallaudet.edu
               www.gallaudet.edu/~gupress

Monograph discussing important aspects of communication including total communication and the value of ASL.

138 pages

2069 Communication Issues Among Deaf People - Eyes, Hands, and Voices

Mervin D. Garretson, author

National Association of the Deaf
814 Thayer Avenue
Silver Spring, MD 20910   301-587-1788
                          Fax: 301-587-1791
                          TTY: 301-587-1789

Includes over thirty relevant articles reflecting a wide range of perceptions and attitutes on communication among deaf people.

2070 Communication Issues Related to Hearing Loss

Samuel Trychin, PhD, author

Self Help for Hard of Hearing People, Inc.
7910 Woodmont Avenue Suite 1200
Bethesda, MD 20814   301-657-2248
                          Fax: 301-913-9413
                          TTY: 301-657-2249
           e-mail: national@shhh.org
                    www.shhh.org

An overview of causes and effects of hearing loss on those who experience it - both people with hearing loss and their families. Helpful also to professionals who provide services to people with hearing loss.

1993

2071 Communication Rules for Hard of Hearing People

Samuel Trychin, PhD, author

Self Help for Hard of Hearing People, Inc.
7910 Woodmont Avenue Suite 1200
Bethesda, MD 20814   301-657-2248
                          Fax: 301-913-9413
                          TTY: 301-657-2249
           e-mail: national@shhh.org
                    www.shhh.org

Presents scenarios with discussions to solve communication problems. Manual for accompanying video (listed separately).

1987

2072 Communication Training for Hearing- Impaired Children and Teenagers

Nancy Tye-Murray, author

Pro-Ed
8700 Shoal Creek Boulevard
Austin, TX 78757   512-451-3246
                                 800-897-3202
                          Fax: 512-451-8542
                    www.proedinc.com

Program combines speechreading, listening, and repair strategy training using speech materials that are meaningful to children and teenagers. The training activities are simple to present and do not require advance preparation.

2073 Comprehensive Signed English Dictionary

Harris Communications
15159 Technology Drive
Eden Prairie, MN 55344   612-906-1180
                                 800-825-6758
                          Fax: 612-902-1099
        e-mail: mail@harriscomm.com
               www.harriscomm.com

Complete dictionary offers 3100 signs, including signs reflecting contemporary vocabulary.

457 pages

2074 Conversational Sign Language II An Intermediate Advanced Manual

Harris Communications
15159 Technology Drive
Eden Prairie, MN 55344   612-906-1180
                                 800-825-6758
                          Fax: 612-902-1099
        e-mail: mail@harriscomm.com
               www.harriscomm.com

This book presents English words and their American Sign Language equivalents.

218 pages

2075 Cued Speech Curriculum: Acquiring Receptive & Expressive Cued Speech

Karen Koehler-Cesa, author

Alexander Graham Bell Association for the Deaf
3417 Volta Place N.W.
Washington, DC 20007   202-337-5220
                             800-432-7543
                        Fax: 202-337-8314
                        TTY: 202-337-5220
                   e-mail: agbell2@aol.com
                             www.agbell.org

This is a curriculum to teach receptive and expressive cueing skills to students with hearing losses ranging in age from 8 years old to adult. These nine-week lessons teach proper hand and mouth shapes for vowel and consonant sets, word and sentence lists, hand and mouth shape diagrams, classroom worksheets, and homework sheets. The student's workbook contains worksheets, tests, and simple charts.

1990 315 pages

2076 Curriculum Guide: Hearing-Impaired Children, Birth to Three Years

Winifred H. Northcott, Ph.D., author

Alexander Graham Bell Association for the Deaf
3417 Volta Place N.W.
Washington, DC 20007   202-337-5220
                             800-432-7543
                        Fax: 202-337-8314
                        TTY: 202-337-5220
                   e-mail: agbell2@aol.com
                             www.agbell.org

An invaluable book providing guidelines for professionals in the organization and administration of an auditory-oral infant/preschool program for children with hearing impairments stressing an equal partnership between parents and the team of teachers.

1977 291 pages

2077 Deaf Children in Public Schools Placement, Context, and Consequences

Claire L. Ramsey, author

Gallaudet Univ. Press c/o Chicago Distrib. Center
11030 South Langley Avenue
Chicago, IL 60628   202-651-5000
                          800-621-2736
                     Fax: 800-621-8476
                     TTY: 888-630-9347
          e-mail: david.gunton@gallaudet.edu
                www.gallaudet.edu/~gupress

Assesses the progress of three second-grade deaf students to demonstrate the importance of placement, context, and language in their development.

August 1997 250 pages
ISBN: 1-563680-62-9

2078 Deaf Children, Their Families, and Professionals: Dismantling Barriers

Sarah Beazley and Michele Moore, author

David Fulton Publishers
2 Barbon Close, Great Ormond Street
London, WCIN   171-405-5606
                 Fax: 171-831-4840

Concerns the growing need among parents of deaf children and professionals (including student practitioners) who work with them for clear illustrations of what deaf children and their families have to say for themselves about their experiences.

1995 176 pages Softcover
ISBN: 1-853463-29-9

2079 Deaf Heritage: Student Text and Workbook

Felicia Mode Alexandria and Jack R. Gannon, author

National Association of the Deaf
814 Thayer Avenue
Silver Spring, MD 20910   301-587-1788
                            Fax: 301-587-1791
                            TTY: 301-587-1789

Each chapter is followed by a vocabulary section and workbook activities including questions and follow-up activities for students.

2080 Deafness - 1993-2013

Mervin D. Garretson, author

National Association of the Deaf
814 Thayer Avenue
Silver Spring, MD 20910   301-587-1788
                            Fax: 301-587-1791
                            TTY: 301-587-1789

Over 30 articles cover such topics as magnet schools, deaf identity, technology, multicultural education, communication, leadership, and sign language research.

2081 Deafness and Child Development

Kathryn Meadow, author

Gallaudet Univ. Press c/o Chicago Distrib. Center
11030 South Langley Avenue
Chicago, IL 60628   202-651-5000
        800-621-2736
        Fax: 800-621-8476
        TTY: 888-630-9347
        e-mail: david.gunton@gallaudet.edu
        www.gallaudet.edu/~gupress

Provides rational, informed and balanced approaches to the effects of deafness in child development.

236 pages

2082 Directory of Auditory-Oral Programs

Alexander Graham Bell Association for the Deaf
3417 Volta Place N.W.
Washington, DC 20007   202-337-5220
        800-432-7543
        Fax: 202-337-8314
        TTY: 202-337-5220
        e-mail: agbell2@aol.com
        www.agbell.org

This directory lists auditory-oral programs in public and private schools, auditory-oral programs in speech and hearing centers, and therapists who offer private tutoring and auditory-oral therapy.

1995 204 pages

2083 Discovering Sign Language

Eva Barsh Dicker and Laura Greene, author

Gallaudet Univ. Press c/o Chicago Distrib. Center
11030 South Langley Avenue
Chicago, IL 60628   202-651-5000
        800-621-2736
        Fax: 800-621-8476
        TTY: 888-630-9347
        e-mail: david.gunton@gallaudet.edu
        www.gallaudet.edu/~gupress

Fascinating book explaining different kinds of hearing losses and the significance of when the loss occurred.

104 pages Softcover

2084 Ear Book

David Marty, author

Gallaudet Univ. Press c/o Chicago Distrib. Center
11030 South Langley Avenue
Chicago, IL 60628   202-651-5000
        800-621-2736
        Fax: 800-621-8476
        TTY: 888-630-9347
        e-mail: david.gunton@gallaudet.edu
        www.gallaudet.edu/~gupress

A how-to book on obtaining and using an otoscope, recognizing and managing common ear disorders, when to call the doctor and when your child needs ear tubes.

136 pages Softcover

2085 Ear Gear: A Student Workbook on Hearing and Hearing Aids

Carole Bugosh Sinko, author

Gallaudet Univ. Press c/o Chicago Distrib. Center
11030 South Langley Avenue
Chicago, IL 60628   202-651-5000
        800-621-2736
        Fax: 800-621-8476
        TTY: 888-630-9347
        e-mail: david.gunton@gallaudet.edu
        www.gallaudet.edu/~gupress

Attractive workbook designed to teach elementary-age children about hearing loss and the use of hearing aids.

75 pages

2086 Educating Deaf Children Bilingually

Shawn Mahshie, author

Gallaudet Univ. Press c/o Chicago Distrib. Center
11030 South Langley Avenue
Chicago, IL 60628   202-651-5000
        800-621-2736
        Fax: 800-621-8476
        TTY: 888-630-9347
        e-mail: david.gunton@gallaudet.edu
        www.gallaudet.edu/~gupress

Discusses perspectives and practices of educating deaf children with goals of age-level achievement.

120 pages

2087 Education of the Hearing Impaired Child

F. Powell, author

A book of information about educational programs and devices used in teaching the hearing impaired child.

180 pages Softcover

2088 Educational Audiology for the Limited- Hearing Infant and Preschooler

D. Pollack, D. Goldberg, N. Coleffe-Schenck, author

Charles C. Thomas Publishing, Ltd.
2600 South First Street
Springfield, IL 62704   217-789-8980
        800-258-8980
        Fax: 217-789-9130
        e-mail: books@ccthomas.com
        www.ccthomas.com

The third edition of this popular book focuses on current concepts and practices in audio-logic screening, evaluation and the role of parents.

410 pages $66.95 paper
ISBN: 0-398067-50-3

2089 Educational and Development Aspects of Deafness

Donald F. Moores and Kathryn P. Meadow-Orlans, author

Gallaudet Univ. Press c/o Chicago Distrib. Center
11030 South Langley Avenue
Chicago, IL 60628   202-651-5000
                                      800-621-2736
                                  Fax: 800-621-8476
                                  TTY: 888-630-9347
              e-mail: david.gunton@gallaudet.edu
                      www.gallaudet.edu/~gupress

Book detailing the ongoing revolution in the education of deaf children.

415 pages

Donald F. Moores, Editor
Kathryn P. Meadow-Orlans, Editor

2090 Effectiveness of Cochlear Implants and Tactile Aids for Deaf Children

Ann E. Geers, Ph.d., author

Alexander Graham Bell Association for the Deaf
3417 Volta Place N.W.
Washington, DC 20007   202-337-5220
                                      800-432-7543
                                  Fax: 202-337-8314
                                  TTY: 202-337-5220
                      e-mail: agbell2@aol.com
                              www.agbell.org

This monograph presents a fascinating study to evaluate differences in the rate of change in speech perception, speech production and spoken language skills among children using the Nucleus 22-channel cochlear implant, tactile aids and conventional hearing aids. This monograph also offers teaching strategies in perception, lipreading, and spoken language.

232 pages Softcover

2091 Encyclopedia of Deafness and Hearing Disorders

Facts on File
Department M274, 11 Penn Plaza
New York, NY 10001
                                      800-322-8755
                                  Fax: 800-678-3633

A comprehensive guide to all aspects of hearing impairments.

2092 FM Trainers: A Winning Choice for Students, Teachers and Parents

Linda Brewer Hammond, author

Alexander Graham Bell Association for the Deaf
3417 Volta Place N.W.
Washington, DC 20007   202-337-5220
                                      800-432-7543
                                  Fax: 202-337-8314
                                  TTY: 202-337-5220
                      e-mail: agbell2@aol.com
                              www.agbell.org

A practical guide to the selection and use of FM trainers in class or at home.

1991 67 pages

2093 Facilitating Hearing and Listening in Young Children

Howard E. "Rocky" Stone, author

SHHH Publications
7800 Wisconsin Avenue
Bethesda, MD 20814   301-657-2248

Emphasizes the need to create an auditory world. Up-to-date information on many faces of hearing loss, amplification technology, cohlear implants, federal laws and listening strategies.

2094 Facilitating Hearing and Listening in Young Children

Carol Flexer, Ph.D., author

Alexander Graham Bell Association for the Deaf
3417 Volta Place N.W.
Washington, DC 20007   202-337-5220
                                      800-432-7543
                                  Fax: 202-337-8314
                                  TTY: 202-337-5220
                      e-mail: agbell2@aol.com
                              www.agbell.org

A straightforward book maximizing hearing and listening through practical recommendations about maintaining optimal listening and learning environments for young children with hearing impairments.

1994 257 pages

2095 Families and Their Hearing-Impaired Children

Dale Atkins, author

Alexander Graham Bell Association for the Deaf
3417 Volta Place N.W.
Washington, DC 20007   202-337-5220
                                      800-432-7543
                                  Fax: 202-337-8314
                                  TTY: 202-337-5220
                      e-mail: agbell2@aol.com
                              www.agbell.org

Looks at specific family issues that have not had much play in the literature to date. Discussions include a range of family members, problems, solutions and more.

150 pages

2096 Foundations of Spoken Language For Hearing Impaired Children

Daniel Ling, Ph.D., author

Alexander Graham Bell Association for the Deaf
3417 Volta Place N.W.
Washington, DC 20007   202-337-5220
800-432-7543
Fax: 202-337-8314
TTY: 202-337-5220
e-mail: agbell2@aol.com
www.agbell.org

This guide traces the individual progress of a child's speech development.

1978 87 pages

2097 Free Hand: Education of the Deaf

Margaret Walworth, author

T-J Publishers
817 Silver Spring Avenue, Suite 206
Silver Spring, MD 20910   301-585-4440
800-999-1186
Fax: 301-585-5930

Based on the proceedings of a 1990 symposium on the educational uses of ASL, A Free Hand presents papers by prominent educators, researchers and linguists in the changing role of American Sign Language in the classroom.

1992 204 pages Softcover
ISBN: 0-932666-40-X

2098 Functional Signs: A New Approach from Simple to Complex

Harry Bornstein, I. King Jordan, author

Pro-Ed
8700 Shoal Creek Boulevard
Austin, TX 78757   512-451-3246
800-897-3202
Fax: 512-451-8542
www.proedinc.com

A unique dictionary of 330 American Sign Language signs for persons with disabilities. Each of the signs has been analyzed for a percentage of understandability.

2099 Gallaudet Encyclopedia of Deaf People and Deafness

John Van Cleve, author

Gallaudet Univ. Press c/o Chicago Distrib. Center
11030 South Langley Avenue
Chicago, IL 60628   202-651-5000
800-621-2736
Fax: 800-621-8476
TTY: 888-630-9347
e-mail: david.gunton@gallaudet.edu
www.gallaudet.edu/~gupress

Three-volume set of research and information on deaf people and deafness.

1400 pages

2100 Growing Together: Information for Parents of Deaf & Hard of Hearing Children

National Information Center On Deafness, author

Gallaudet Univ. Press c/o Chicago Distrib. Center
11030 South Langley Avenue
Chicago, IL 60628   202-651-5000
800-621-2736
Fax: 800-621-8476
TTY: 888-630-9347
e-mail: david.gunton@gallaudet.edu
www.gallaudet.edu/~gupress

This publication answers questions often asked by parents of children with a hearing loss.

92 pages

2101 Guidelines for Evaluating Auditory-Oral Programs for Children

Alexander Graham Bell Association for the Deaf
3417 Volta Place N.W.
Washington, DC 20007   202-337-5220
800-432-7543
Fax: 202-337-8314
TTY: 202-337-5220
e-mail: agbell2@aol.com
www.agbell.org

Use these guidelines to evaluate quality auditory-oral educational programs.

1993 5 pages

2102 Hear: Solutions, Skills and Sources for People with Hearing Loss

Anne Pope, author

Alexander Graham Bell Association for the Deaf
3417 Volta Place N.W.
Washington, DC 20007   202-337-5220
800-432-7543
Fax: 202-337-8314
TTY: 202-337-5220
e-mail: agbell2@aol.com
www.agbell.org

Hearing Impairment/Deafness/Books

This practical, well-designed self-help guide is a
valuable resource for people who are hard of
hearing and their families and friends. HEAR
features real-life case studies and interviews
with people who have become hard of hearing.
The reader will learn about sound and how we
hear; tips for making changes, finding self-help
groups, and knowing your rights; about types of
hearing loss and hearing tests; about different
devices that manage hearing loss, from hearing
aids to cochlear implant.

1997 128 pages Hardcover

**2103 Hear: Solutions, Skills, and Sources for
Hard-of-Hearing People**

Anne Pope, author

Self Help for Hard of Hearing People, Inc.
7910 Woodmont Avenue Suite 1200
Bethesda, MD 20814   301-657-2248
                            Fax: 301-913-9413
                            TTY: 301-657-2249
                            e-mail: national@shhh.org
                            www.shhh.org

Offers practical communication strategies that
will enable people with hearing loss to make the
most of the hearing they have. Also explains
how the ear works and what can go wrong.

1997 Hardcover

2104 Hearing Aid Handbook: User's Guide for Children

Donna S. Wayner, Ph.D., author

Alexander Graham Bell Association for the Deaf
3417 Volta Place N.W.
Washington, DC 20007   202-337-5220
                              800-432-7543
                              Fax: 202-337-8314
                              TTY: 202-337-5220
                              e-mail: agbell2@aol.com
                              www.agbell.org

1990

2105 Hearing Care for Children

Frederick N. Martin and John Greer Clark, author

Alexander Graham Bell Association for the Deaf
3417 Volta Place N.W.
Washington, DC 20007   202-337-5220
                              800-432-7543
                              Fax: 202-337-8314
                              TTY: 202-337-5220
                              e-mail: agbell2@aol.com
                              www.agbell.org

This professional text for audiologists provides a
comprehensive overview of childhood hearing
loss and rehabilitation options. Among the topics covered are the causes and effects of childhood hearing loss, the identification and
evaluation of such hearing loss, counseling options for affected children and their families, amplification and auditory stimulation, and
intervention and education options for children
with hearing losses.

1996 372 pages Hardcover

Mark Ross, Editor

2106 Hearing Impaired Children and Youth

Eveyln Cherow, author

Gallaudet Univ. Press c/o Chicago Distrib. Center
11030 South Langley Avenue
Chicago, IL 60628   202-651-5000
                           800-621-2736
                           Fax: 800-621-8476
                           TTY: 888-630-9347
                           e-mail: david.gunton@gallaudet.edu
                           www.gallaudet.edu/~gupress

Offers insights from 24 experts to help clarify relationships between hearing impairments and developmental difficulties.

416 pages

2107 Hearing Impairments in Young Children

Arthur Boothroyd, Ph.D., author

Alexander Graham Bell Association for the Deaf
3417 Volta Place N.W.
Washington, DC 20007   202-337-5220
                              800-432-7543
                              Fax: 202-337-8314
                              TTY: 202-337-5220
                              e-mail: agbell2@aol.com
                              www.agbell.org

A useful text that helps educators and professionals effectively manage early intervention programs for children with hearing impairments
from birth to five years of age and their families.

1988 239 pages

2108 Hearing Loss Help

Alec Combs, author

National Association of the Deaf
814 Thayer Avenue
Silver Spring, MD 20910   301-587-1788
                                 Fax: 301-587-1791
                                 TTY: 301-587-1789

Self-help guide provides factual information on how we hear, and on the causes and symptoms of hearing loss. Gives practical information on ways to improve everyday communication and create better listening conditions, including assistive listening devices.

2109 Hearing-Impaired Child

Antonia Maxon, author

Alexander Graham Bell Association for the Deaf
3417 Volta Place N.W.
Washington, DC 20007   202-337-5220
                                          800-432-7543
                                          Fax: 202-337-8314
                                          TTY: 202-337-5220
                                          e-mail: agbell2@aol.com
                                          www.agbell.org

This indispensable book provides speech-language pathologists and audiologists with essential information to help diagnose and treat children with all degrees of hearing loss.

183 pages

2110 Hearing-Impaired Children and Youth with Developmental Disabilities

Evelyn Cherow, author

Gallaudet Univ. Press c/o Chicago Distrib. Center
11030 South Langley Avenue
Chicago, IL 60628   202-651-5000
                                    800-621-2736
                                    Fax: 800-621-8476
                                    TTY: 888-630-9347
                                    e-mail: david.gunton@gallaudet.edu
                                    www.gallaudet.edu/~gupress

The insights of 24 experts help clarify relationships between hearing impairment and developmental difficulties and propose interdisciplinary cooperation as an approach to the problems created.

416 pages

2111 Hearing-Impaired Children in the Mainstream

Alexander Graham Bell Association for the Deaf
3417 Volta Place N.W.
Washington, DC 20007   202-337-5220
                                          800-432-7543
                                          Fax: 202-337-8314
                                          TTY: 202-337-5220
                                          e-mail: agbell2@aol.com
                                          www.agbell.org

This comprehensive book advises educators to integrate students with hearing impairments into regular classrooms and covers many areas that will help students to become appropriately mainstreamed from elementary school to the college level.

1990 336 pages

Mark Ross, Editor

2112 How to Survive a Hearing Loss

Charlotte Himber, author

Gallaudet Univ. Press c/o Chicago Distrib. Center
11030 South Langley Avenue
Chicago, IL 60628   202-651-5000
                                    800-621-2736
                                    Fax: 800-621-8476
                                    TTY: 888-630-9347
                                    e-mail: david.gunton@gallaudet.edu
                                    www.gallaudet.edu/~gupress

This book presents the results of the author's intensive research about hearing and the ear.

241 pages

2113 I Heard That! A Developmental Sequence of Listening Activities for the Young Child

Winifred H. Northcott, Ph.D, Editor, author

Alexander Graham Bell Association for the Deaf
3417 Volta Place N.W.
Washington, DC 20007   202-337-5220
                                          800-432-7543
                                          Fax: 202-337-8314
                                          TTY: 202-337-5220
                                          e-mail: agbell2@aol.com
                                          www.agbell.org

This handbook provides a practical framework for teachers, clinicians, and parents by setting objectives and designing activities to develop listening skills in children with hearing losses. Includes auditory communication, listening skill development, auditory learning objectives, and experience charts.

1978 360 pages

2114 I.D.E.A. Advocacy for Children Who Are Deaf or Hard of Hearing

Bonnie P. Tucker, Esq, author

Alexander Graham Bell Association for the Deaf
3417 Volta Place N.W.
Washington, DC 20007   202-337-5220
                                          800-432-7543
                                          Fax: 202-337-8314
                                          TTY: 202-337-5220
                                          e-mail: agbell2@aol.com
                                          www.agbell.org

This book offers up to date information about the 1997 Individuals with Disabilities Education Act which affects children who are deaf or hard of hearing.

1997 96 pages

2115 Inclusion?

Gallaudet Univ. Press c/o Chicago Distrib. Center
11030 South Langley Avenue
Chicago, IL 60628   202-651-5000
                                   800-621-2736
                              Fax: 800-621-8476
                              TTY: 888-630-9347
          e-mail: david.gunton@gallaudet.edu
                  www.gallaudet.edu/~gupress

This book defines quality education for deaf and hard of hearing students.

213 pages

2116 Infants and Toddlers with Hearing Loss: Family Centered Assessment/Intervention

Jackson Roush & Noel D. Matkin, author

Alexander Graham Bell Association for the Deaf
3417 Volta Place N.W.
Washington, DC 20007   202-337-5220
                                   800-432-7543
                              Fax: 202-337-8314
                              TTY: 202-337-5220
                 e-mail: agbell2@aol.com
                         www.agbell.org

A scholarly title for early intervention professionals examining clinical, legislative, and philosophical issues affecting the delivery of early intervention services to hearing impaired and hard of hearing children.

1994 360 pages

2117 International Directory of Periodicals Related to Deafness

Steven Frank, author

Gallaudet Univ. Press c/o Chicago Distrib. Center
11030 South Langley Avenue
Chicago, IL 60628   202-651-5000
                                   800-621-2736
                              Fax: 800-621-8476
                              TTY: 888-630-9347
          e-mail: david.gunton@gallaudet.edu
                  www.gallaudet.edu/~gupress

Offers information on more than 500 magazines and journals related to deafness.

150 pages

2118 Introduction to Communication

Gallaudet Univ. Press c/o Chicago Distrib. Center
11030 South Langley Avenue
Chicago, IL 60628   202-651-5000
                                   800-621-2736
                              Fax: 800-621-8476
                              TTY: 888-630-9347
          e-mail: david.gunton@gallaudet.edu
                  www.gallaudet.edu/~gupress

Curriculum materials exploring the areas of sound, hearing and interpersonal communication.

100 pages

2119 Journey Into the World of the Deaf

Oliver Sacks, author

T-J Publishers
817 Silver Spring Avenue, Suite 206
Silver Spring, MD 20910   301-585-4440
                                   800-999-1186
                              Fax: 301-585-5930

Well known for his exploration of how people respond to neurological impairments, Dr. Sacks explores the world of the deaf and discovers how deaf people respond to their loss of hearing and how they develop language. A highly readable introduction to deaf people, deaf culture and American Sign Language.

180 pages Softcover
ISBN: 0-913580-99-6

2120 Joy of Listening: An Auditory Training Program

Janice Baliker Light, author

Alexander Graham Bell Association for the Deaf
3417 Volta Place N.W.
Washington, DC 20007   202-337-5220
                                   800-432-7543
                              Fax: 202-337-8314
                              TTY: 202-337-5220
                 e-mail: agbell2@aol.com
                         www.agbell.org

This manual contains lessons to improve listening skills, auditory discrimination, attention span, memory, and sequencing in children with hearing losses. The lessons can be used when working with children alone, or in small groups.

1978 160 pages

2121 Joy of Signing

Lottie Riekehof, author

National Association of the Deaf
814 Thayer Avenue
Silver Spring, MD 20910   301-587-1788
                              Fax: 301-587-1791
                              TTY: 301-587-1789

Illustrated sign language text with descriptions of the origin of selected signs and examples of how each is used. Second edition.

2122 Kaleidoscope of Deaf America

Frank Turk, author

Harris Communications
15159 Technology Drive
Eden Prairie, MN 55344   612-906-1180
                               800-825-6758
                          Fax: 612-902-1099
             e-mail: mail@harriscomm.com
                     www.harriscomm.com

Puts you in touch with trends, events and thinking that is shaping the future of deaf Americans.

79 pages

2123 Kendall Demonstration Elementary School Curriculum Guides

Gallaudet Univ. Press c/o Chicago Distrib. Center
11030 South Langley Avenue
Chicago, IL 60628   202-651-5000
                          800-621-2736
                     Fax: 800-621-8476
                     TTY: 888-630-9347
        e-mail: david.gunton@gallaudet.edu
              www.gallaudet.edu/~gupress

These guides provide detailed information to help teachers organize curriculum, structure classes and develop individualized education programs.

18 months+

2124 Keys to Living with Hearing Loss

Marcia B. Dugan, author

Self Help for Hard of Hearing People, Inc.
7910 Woodmont Avenue Suite 1200
Bethesda, MD 20814   301-657-2248
                       Fax: 301-913-9413
                       TTY: 301-657-2249
               e-mail: national@shhh.org
                         www.shhh.org

Guidebook that provides helpful advice on a wide range of topics, from living alone with a hearing loss, to going to the hospital, to legal rights.

1997 Softcover

2125 Keys to Raising a Deaf Child

Virginia Frazier-Maiwald and Lenore M. Williams, author

Barron's Education Series, Inc.
250 Wireless Blvd
Hauppauge, NY 11788   516-434-3311
                            800-645-3476
                       Fax: 516-434-3723
             e-mail: info@barronsedu.com
                     www.barronseduc.com

Two educators offer positive advice and encouragement on helping children adapt to deafness. They show how problems related to deafness can be overcome so that the child interacts as a social and intellectual equal with children who can hear. The authors recommend bimodal communication - having the child, parents, and other non-deaf family members combine sign language and speech as a first step in normal communication.

208 pages Softcover
ISBN: 0-764107-23-2

2126 Kid-Friendly Parenting with Deaf and Hard of Hearing Children

Denise Chapman Weston & Daria Medwid, author

Gallaudet Univ. Press c/o Chicago Distrib. Center
11030 South Langley Avenue
Chicago, IL 60628   202-651-5000
                          800-621-2736
                     Fax: 800-621-8476
                     TTY: 888-630-9347
        e-mail: david.gunton@gallaudet.edu
              www.gallaudet.edu/~gupress

A step-by-step guide offering parents hundreds of ideas and play activities for children ages 3 to 12.

336 pages

2127 Language - Children Living with Deafness

Thomas Bergman, author

Gareth Stevens
1555 North River Center Drive
Milwaukee, WI 53212   414-225-0333
                            800-341-3569
                       Fax: 414-225-0377

Did you know you can't whisper in sign language? To share a secret, you have to be sure that no one else can see what you're signing. Linda is nearly deaf, and some of her friends at school can't hear at all. Read about how they speak to each other with their hands, in sign language. Learn what special dangers deaf children face. Find out how you can play and talk with children who are deaf.

ISBN: 1-555329-16-0

2128 Language Learning Practices with Deaf Children

McAnally, Rose, Quigley, author

Pro-Ed
8700 Shoal Creek Boulevard
Austin, TX 78757   512-451-3246
                         800-897-3202
                    Fax: 512-451-8542
                    www.proedinc.com

Describes the variety of language development theories and practices used with children who are deaf without advocating any one group.

321 pages
ISBN: 0-890793-25-5

2129 Language in Motion Exploring the Nature of Sign

Jerome D. Schein and David A. Stewart, author

National Association of the Deaf
814 Thayer Avenue
Silver Spring, MD 20910   301-587-1788
                           Fax: 301-587-1791
                           TTY: 301-587-1789

Introduces sign language and communication, follows with a history of sign languages in general, and then tells about the structure of American Sign Language.

2130 Learning to See: American Sign Language as a Second Language

Sherman Wilcox, author

Gallaudet Univ. Press c/o Chicago Distrib. Center
11030 South Langley Avenue
Chicago, IL 60628   202-651-5000
                         800-621-2736
                    Fax: 800-621-8476
                    TTY: 888-630-9347
          e-mail: david.gunton@gallaudet.edu
              www.gallaudet.edu/~gupress

Provides a comprehensive introduction to the history and structure of ASL to the deaf community.

134 pages

2131 Learning to Sign Special Needs Project

3463 State St, Ste 282
Santa Barbara, CA 93105   805-683-9633
                            800-333-6867

An illustrated guide for mastering the current basic signs used to communicate with deaf or hearing-impaired people in either the word order of the English language or in the American Sign Language pattern.

2132 Least Restrictive Environment

Lawrence M. Siegel, author

Gallaudet Univ. Press c/o Chicago Distrib. Center
11030 South Langley Avenue
Chicago, IL 60628   202-651-5000
                         800-621-2736
                    Fax: 800-621-8476
                    TTY: 888-630-9347
          e-mail: david.gunton@gallaudet.edu
              www.gallaudet.edu/~gupress

Presents compelling legal and emotional arguments for educating children with disabilities outside the regular school environment.

290 pages

2133 Least Restrictive Environment: The Paradox of Inclusion

Lawrence M. Siegel, author

National Association of the Deaf
814 Thayer Avenue
Silver Spring, MD 20910   301-587-1788
                           Fax: 301-587-1791
                           TTY: 301-587-1789

Analyzes relevant federal law and the inclusion reform movement, and discusses the premise that forcing one generic placement on all children will be more problematic.

2134 Legal Rights of Hearing-Impaired People

National Association of the Deaf, author

Gallaudet Univ. Press c/o Chicago Distrib. Center
11030 South Langley Avenue
Chicago, IL 60628   202-651-5000
                         800-621-2736
                    Fax: 800-621-8476
                    TTY: 888-630-9347
          e-mail: david.gunton@gallaudet.edu
              www.gallaudet.edu/~gupress

Includes updated interpretations of legislation affecting hearing-impaired people, including chapters dealing with the ADA.

297 pages

2135 Let's Converse

Nancy Tye-Murray, Ph.D., author

Alexander Graham Bell Association for the Deaf
3417 Volta Place N.W.
Washington, DC 20007   202-337-5220
                              800-432-7543
                        Fax: 202-337-8314
                        TTY: 202-337-5220
                     e-mail: agbell2@aol.com
                              www.agbell.org

Written for parents, teachers and professionals, this guide introduces techniques and exercises for facilitating conversation between children and adults.

1994 229 pages

2136 Let's Learn About Deafness

Rachael Harris, author

Gallaudet Univ. Press c/o Chicago Distrib. Center
11030 South Langley Avenue
Chicago, IL 60628   202-651-5000
                             800-621-2736
                       Fax: 800-621-8476
                       TTY: 888-630-9347
            e-mail: david.gunton@gallaudet.edu
                    www.gallaudet.edu/~gupress

Hands-on school classroom activities for the deaf student.

82 pages

2137 Listening and Talking

Elizabeth Cole, Ed.D., author

Alexander Graham Bell Association for the Deaf
3417 Volta Place N.W.
Washington, DC 20007   202-337-5220
                              800-432-7543
                        Fax: 202-337-8314
                        TTY: 202-337-5220
                     e-mail: agbell2@aol.com
                              www.agbell.org

This research-based text for professionals promotes communication by developing language, audition, and speech in early intervention programs for young children with hearing loss.

191 pages Softcover

2138 Listening to Learn: A Handbook for Parents with Hearing-Impaired Children

Arlie Adam, Pam Fortier, Gail Schiel, et al., author

Alexander Graham Bell Association for the Deaf
3417 Volta Place N.W.
Washington, DC 20007   202-337-5220
                              800-432-7543
                        Fax: 202-337-8314
                        TTY: 202-337-5220
                     e-mail: agbell2@aol.com
                              www.agbell.org

Developed by teachers, this handbook provides parents with the essential steps necessary to develop effective spoken communication with their children.

1990 98 pages

2139 Look Now, Hear This: Combined Auditory Training and Speechreading Instruction

Janet Jeffers and Margaret Barley, author

Charles C. Thomas Publishing, Ltd.
2600 South First Street
Springfield, IL 62704   217-789-8980
                               800-258-8980
                         Fax: 217-789-9130
                  e-mail: books@ccthomas.com
                          www.ccthomas.com

1979 230 pages Softcover
ISBN: 0-398061-81-5

2140 Looking Back: A Reader on the History of Deaf Communities & Sign Language

Renate Fischer and Harlan Lane, author

Gallaudet Univ. Press c/o Chicago Distrib. Center
11030 South Langley Avenue
Chicago, IL 60628   202-651-5000
                             800-621-2736
                       Fax: 800-621-8476
                       TTY: 888-630-9347
            e-mail: david.gunton@gallaudet.edu
                    www.gallaudet.edu/~gupress

Renowned researchers from around the world present provocative findings in six areas relating to the deaf culture.

558 pages

2141 Mainstreaming Deaf and Hard of Hearing Students

National Information Center on Deafness, author

Gallaudet Univ. Press c/o Chicago Distrib. Center
11030 South Langley Avenue
Chicago, IL 60628   202-651-5000
                             800-621-2736
                       Fax: 800-621-8476
                       TTY: 888-630-9347
            e-mail: david.gunton@gallaudet.edu
                    www.gallaudet.edu/~gupress

Booklet presenting mainstreaming as one educational option.

40 pages

2142 Manual Communication: A Basic Text and Workbook With Practical Exercises

Dean A. Christopher, author

Pro-Ed
8700 Shoal Creek Boulevard
Austin, TX 78757
512-451-3246
800-897-3202
Fax: 512-451-8542
www.proedinc.com

An excellent textbook with practical exercises for students in training as audiologists, speech pathologists, psychologists, and educator of persons who are deaf.

illustrated

2143 Mental Health Services for Deaf People

Barbara A. Willigan, author

Gallaudet Univ. Press c/o Chicago Distrib. Center
11030 South Langley Avenue
Chicago, IL 60628
202-651-5000
800-621-2736
Fax: 800-621-8476
TTY: 888-630-9347
e-mail: david.gunton@gallaudet.edu
www.gallaudet.edu/~gupress

Contains information on over 350 mental health programs and services for deaf people across the United States.

210 pages

2144 My First Book of Sign

Pamela J. Baker, author

T.J. Publishers, Inc.
817 Silver Spring Avenue, Suite 206
Silver Spring, MD 20910
301-585-4440
800-999-1168
Fax: 301-585-5930
TTY: 301-585-4440
TDD: 301-585-4441
e-mail: TJPubinc@aol.com

Full-color book gives alphabetically grouped signss for 150 words most frequently used by young children.

76 pages Hardcover

2145 Negotiating the Special Education Maze

Winifred Anderson and Stephen Chitwood, author

Alexander Graham Bell Association for the Deaf
3417 Volta Place N.W.
Washington, DC 20007
202-337-5220
800-432-7543
Fax: 202-337-8314
TTY: 202-337-5220
e-mail: agbell2@aol.com
www.agbell.org

This guidebook, written primarily for parents, teachers, and school administrators, provides easy to understand information about developing and effective educational program for children with special needs.

1996 296 pages

2146 Operation SHHH

Self Help for Hard of Hearing People, Inc.
7910 Woodmont Avenue Suite 1200
Bethesda, MD 20814
301-657-2248
Fax: 301-913-9413
TTY: 301-657-2249
e-mail: national@shhh.org
www.shhh.org

Features SHHHerman, the lion who does not roar. This program is designed for elementary school children. Includes video, posters, brochures, and more.

2147 Our Forgotten Children

Julia Davis, author

Alexander Graham Bell Association for the Deaf
3417 Volta Place N.W.
Washington, DC 20007
202-337-5220
800-432-7543
Fax: 202-337-8314
TTY: 202-337-5220
e-mail: agbell2@aol.com
www.agbell.org

This simple book describes characteristics of hard-of-hearing children in the school and discusses their educational requirements, psychological and social needs and amplification options.

1990 68 pages

2148 Our Forgotten Children: Hard of Hearing Pupils in the Schools

Julia Davis, PhD, author

Self Help for Hard of Hearing People, Inc.
7910 Woodmont Avenue Suite 1200
Bethesda, MD 20814
301-657-2248
Fax: 301-913-9413
TTY: 301-657-2249
e-mail: national@shhh.org
www.shhh.org

Important resource about the educational environment.

1990

2149 Parents Guide to Middle Ear Infections

Dorinne S. Davis, MA, CCC-A, author

Alexander Graham Bell Association for the Deaf
3417 Volta Place N.W.
Washington, DC 20007   202-337-5220
                             800-432-7543
                             Fax: 202-337-8314
                             TTY: 202-337-5220
                             e-mail: agbell2@aol.com
                             www.agbell.org

Written for parents and educators, this book discusses middle ear infections in young children
and suggests ways to enhance communication.

1994 138 pages

**2150 Parents and Teachers: Partners in Language
Development**

Audrey Simmons-Martin, Ph.D., author

Alexander Graham Bell Association for the Deaf
3417 Volta Place N.W.
Washington, DC 20007   202-337-5220
                             800-432-7543
                             Fax: 202-337-8314
                             TTY: 202-337-5220
                             e-mail: agbell2@aol.com
                             www.agbell.org

Outlines the essential role of the teacher and parent in the development of language in the school-
aged child with hearing impairment.

1990 386 pages

2151 Parents' Guide to Speech and Deafness

Donald R. Calvert, author

Alexander Graham Bell Association for the Deaf
3417 Volta Place N.W.
Washington, DC 20007   202-337-5220
                             800-432-7543
                             Fax: 202-337-8314
                             TTY: 202-337-5220
                             e-mail: agbell2@aol.com
                             www.agbell.org

A guide to help parents play an active role in the
speech development of children with hearing impairment.

2152 Patrick Gets Hearing Aids

Maureen Cassidy Riski and Nikolas Klakow, author

Alexander Graham Bell Association for the Deaf
3417 Volta Place N.W.
Washington, DC 20007   202-337-5220
                             800-432-7543
                             Fax: 202-337-8314
                             TTY: 202-337-5220
                             e-mail: agbell2@aol.com
                             www.agbell.org

A children's book where Patrick the rabbit
finds himself out of touch because he has a hearing loss.

1994 spanish avail.

2153 Pediatric Audiology 0 to 5 Years, 2nd Ed.

Barry McCormick, author

Alexander Graham Bell Association for the Deaf
3417 Volta Place N.W.
Washington, DC 20007   202-337-5220
                             800-432-7543
                             Fax: 202-337-8314
                             TTY: 202-337-5220
                             e-mail: agbell2@aol.com
                             www.agbell.org

A professional title that examines childhood
hearing impairments and the impact of hearing
loss on speech and language.

1993 446 pages

2154 Pediatric Cochlear Implants

Judith Barnes, Darla Franz and Wallace Bruce, author

Alexander Graham Bell Association for the Deaf
3417 Volta Place N.W.
Washington, DC 20007   202-337-5220
                             800-432-7543
                             Fax: 202-337-8314
                             TTY: 202-337-5220
                             e-mail: agbell2@aol.com
                             www.agbell.org

Created for educators, parents, implant teams,
and rehabilitation specialists, this resource book
investigates the education and rehabilitation of
successful children with cochlear implants.

1994 250 pages

**2155 Psychoeducational Assessment of Hearing-Impaired
Students**

Sharon Bradley-Johnson, Larry D. Evans, author

Pro-Ed
8700 Shoal Creek Boulevard
Austin, TX 78757   512-451-3246
                             800-897-3202
                             Fax: 512-451-8542
                             www.proedinc.com

Issues and procedures related to the assessment
of students with hearing impairments. Summarizes the strengths and limitations of all tests
and subtests.

251 pages
ISBN: 0-890794-55-3

2156 Psychoeducational Assessment of Hearing- Impaired Students

Sharon Bradley, author

Pro-Ed
8700 Shoal Creek Boulevard
Austin, TX 78758   512-451-3246
                         Fax: 512-451-8542

This book includes a comprehensive presentation of issues and procedures related to the assessment of hearing-impaired students.

251 pages Softcover
ISBN: 0-890794-55-3

2157 Raising Your Hearing-Impaired Child

Shirley MacArthur, author

Alexander Graham Bell Association for the Deaf
3417 Volta Place N.W.
Washington, DC 20007   202-337-5220
                            800-432-7543
                       Fax: 202-337-8314
                       TTY: 202-337-5220
                  e-mail: agbell2@aol.com
                          www.agbell.org

This practical book is written by the mother of two children with hearing impairments offering support, information, and practical suggestions for parents who discover their child has a hearing problem.

1982 238 pages

2158 Reading and Deafness

Cynthia M. King and Stephen P. Quigley, author

Pro-Ed
8700 Shoal Creek Boulevard
Austin, TX 78758   512-451-3246
                         Fax: 512-451-8542

Three areas are covered: deaf children's pre-reading development of real-world knowledge; cognitive abilities; and linguistic skills.

422 pages Hardcover
ISBN: 0-887441-07-6

2159 Rhode Island Test of Language Structure RITLS
8700 Shoal Creed Blvd
Austin, TX 78757
                            800-897-3202
                       Fax: 800-397-7633

The Rhode Island Test of Language Structure (RITLS) provides a measure of English language development and assessment data. It is designed primarily for use with children who are hearing impaired, but also useful in other areas where level of language development is of concern, including mental retardation, learning disability, and bilingual programs. The RITLS focuses on syntax, unlike other tests compared with other reading, language, intelligence, and achievement tests frequently used.

2160 Rural Habilitation

Daniel Ling, author

Alexander Graham Bell Association for the Deaf
3417 Volta Place N.W.
Washington, DC 20007   202-337-5220
                            800-432-7543
                       Fax: 202-337-8314
                       TTY: 202-337-5220
                  e-mail: agbell2@aol.com
                          www.agbell.org

Provides essential information to the planning of individual educational programs for hearing-impaired children from early infancy to emphasize the optimal use of residual hearing, the assessment of each child for placement in the least restrictive educational setting and more.

336 pages

2161 Say it in Sign: A Workbook of Sign Language Exercises

Carol B. Carpenter, Sue F.V. Rakow, author

Charles C. Thomas Publishing, Ltd.
2600 South First Street
Springfield, IL 62704   217-789-8980
                            800-258-8980
                       Fax: 217-789-9130
              e-mail: books@ccthomas.com
                          www.ccthomas.com

Emphasis is placed on practice in language and on increasing receptive and expressive skills in sign language, not on the formation of signs or the various sign systems used. The materials presented in this book are adaptable for use with individuals or small groups, and they are designed to save the instructor hours of preparation time.

266 pages
ISBN: 0-398047-79-0

2162 Schedules of Development for Hearing Impaired Infants and Their Parents

Agnes Ling Phillips, Ph.D., author

Alexander Graham Bell Association for the Deaf
3417 Volta Place N.W.
Washington, DC 20007   202-337-5220
                              800-432-7543
                         Fax: 202-337-8314
                         TTY: 202-337-5220
                       e-mail: agbell2@aol.com
                              www.agbell.org

Written for parents and teachers, this assessment record of verbal learning will help to evaluate each child's language development.

1977 14 pages

2163 Science Curriculum: Clarke Curriculum Series

Clarke School for the Deaf, author

Alexander Graham Bell Association for the Deaf
3417 Volta Place N.W.
Washington, DC 20007   202-337-5220
                              800-432-7543
                         Fax: 202-337-8314
                         TTY: 202-337-5220
                       e-mail: agbell2@aol.com
                              www.agbell.org

This comprehensive science curriculum for young students with hearing losses teaches classroom units about the process of science, technology, and society. Teaches science through language activities, central science concepts, scientific processes, objectives, resources, and related children's literature.

1994 455 pages

2164 Science of Sound

Norman Lederman, author

Gallaudet Univ. Press c/o Chicago Distrib. Center
11030 South Langley Avenue
Chicago, IL 60628   202-651-5000
                              800-621-2736
                         Fax: 800-621-8476
                         TTY: 888-630-9347
                 e-mail: david.gunton@gallaudet.edu
                         www.gallaudet.edu/~gupress

This exciting book is carefully designed to help hearing-impaired students understand, use and enjoy the principles of sound.

32 pages

2165 Screening Children for Auditory Function

Fred H. Bess, author

Alexander Graham Bell Association for the Deaf
3417 Volta Place N.W.
Washington, DC 20007   202-337-5220
                              800-432-7543
                         Fax: 202-337-8314
                         TTY: 202-337-5220
                       e-mail: agbell2@aol.com
                              www.agbell.org

This current source of information on early recognition of children with hearing impairments from infancy to school-age is based on papers by 58 distinguished authors.

1992 560 pages Hardcover

2166 Self-Advocacy for Students Who Are Deaf or Hard of Hearing

Kristina M. English, author

Pro-Ed
8700 Shoal Creek Boulevard
Austin, TX 78757   512-451-3246
                              800-897-3202
                         Fax: 512-451-8542
                              www.proedinc.com

Explores the safety net of special education. Helps to prepare for and evaluate one's participation in the development of the Individualized Transition Plan (ITP).

125 pages spiral bound

2167 Sign Communication: A Family Affair

Mark Goldfarb, author

Gallaudet Univ. Press c/o Chicago Distrib. Center
11030 South Langley Avenue
Chicago, IL 60628   202-651-5000
                              800-621-2736
                         Fax: 800-621-8476
                         TTY: 888-630-9347
                 e-mail: david.gunton@gallaudet.edu
                         www.gallaudet.edu/~gupress

Book designed to help hearing parents communicate effectively with their deaf children on issues of good health and personal growth.

132 pages

2168 Sign Language Coloring Books

Ralph Miller, author

Gallaudet Univ. Press c/o Chicago Distrib. Center
11030 South Langley Avenue
Chicago, IL 60628   202-651-5000
                              800-621-2736
                         Fax: 800-621-8476
                         TTY: 888-630-9347
                 e-mail: david.gunton@gallaudet.edu
                         www.gallaudet.edu/~gupress

A mischievous mouse and a spinning top, a doll on the sofa, a hobo clown with his friend the elephant: these coloring books are a FUNtastic way for children to learn to sign, fingerspell, read and write.

2169 Sign Language Talk

Laura Greene, author

Franklin Watts c/o Grolier
90 Old Sherman Tpke
Danbury, CT 06816
203-797-3500
800-621-1115
Fax: 203-797-3197
www.grolier.com

Using 300 easy-to-follow illustrations, this book introduces the structure of sign language, shows how sentences are formed and how signed conversations differ from spoken ones.

96 pages
ISBN: 0-531105-97-0

2170 Sign with Me Books

Susan P. Shroyer, author

Gallaudet Univ. Press c/o Chicago Distrib. Center
11030 South Langley Avenue
Chicago, IL 60628
202-651-5000
800-621-2736
Fax: 800-621-8476
TTY: 888-630-9347
e-mail: david.gunton@gallaudet.edu
www.gallaudet.edu/~gupress

Bold, colorful pictures and accurate diagrams make it fun to learn everyday signs. Titles in this series include ABC Sign With Me; Colors Sign With Me; and 1,2,3 Sign With Me.

2171 Signed English Starter

Harry Bornstein, author

Harris Communications
15159 Technology Drive
Eden Prairie, MN 55344
612-906-1180
800-825-6758
Fax: 612-902-1099
e-mail: mail@harriscomm.com
www.harriscomm.com

The first book to use when learning Signed English.

208 pages

2172 Signing Illustrated

Mickey Flodin, author

Gallaudet Univ. Press c/o Chicago Distrib. Center
11030 South Langley Avenue
Chicago, IL 60628
202-651-5000
800-621-2736
Fax: 800-621-8476
TTY: 888-630-9347
e-mail: david.gunton@gallaudet.edu
www.gallaudet.edu/~gupress

A guide presenting illustrations of over 1,350 signs.

85 pages

2173 Signs of Sharing: An Elementary Sign Language and Deaf Awareness Curriculum

Sue F.V. Rakow, Carol B. Carpenter, author

Charles C. Thomas Publishing, Ltd.
2600 South First Street
Springfield, IL 62704
217-789-8980
800-258-8980
Fax: 217-789-9130
e-mail: books@ccthomas.com
www.ccthomas.com

A unique set of materials that provides educators whose responsibilities include the integration of hearing-impaired children, with a multifaceted tool to teach sign language and deaf awareness.

380 pages
ISBN: 0-398058-51-2

2174 Silent Garden Raising Your Deaf Child

Paul W. Ogden, author

Gallaudet Univ. Press c/o Chicago Distrib. Center
11030 South Langley Avenue
Chicago, IL 60628
202-651-5000
800-621-2736
Fax: 800-621-8476
TTY: 888-630-9347
e-mail: david.gunton@gallaudet.edu
www.gallaudet.edu/~gupress

Provides parents with a firm foundation for making the difficult decisions necessary for their deaf child's future. Includes information on critical concerns, communication, technological alternative, and reassurance through case studies and interviews.

304 pages Softcover
ISBN: 1-563680-58-0

2175 Sociolinguistics in Deaf Communities

Ceil Lucas, author

Gallaudet Univ. Press c/o Chicago Distrib. Center
11030 South Langley Avenue
Chicago, IL 60628   202-651-5000
                          800-621-2736
                     Fax: 800-621-8476
                     TTY: 888-630-9347
          e-mail: david.gunton@gallaudet.edu
               www.gallaudet.edu/~gupress

The first volume in a series offering assessments
and up-to-date information on sign language lin-
guistics.

280 pages

Ceil Lucas, Editor

**2176 Sound and Sign, Childhood Deafness and Mental
Health**

Hilde Schlesinger, author

Gallaudet Univ. Press c/o Chicago Distrib. Center
11030 South Langley Avenue
Chicago, IL 60628   202-651-5000
                          800-621-2736
                     Fax: 800-621-8476
                     TTY: 888-630-9347
          e-mail: david.gunton@gallaudet.edu
               www.gallaudet.edu/~gupress

Presents research to support beliefs that deaf
children should be educated using a combination manual and oral communication in residual
hearing and speech.

265 pages

2177 Speech and Deafness

Donald R. Calvert, author

Alexander Graham Bell Association for the Deaf
3417 Volta Place N.W.
Washington, DC 20007   202-337-5220
                             800-432-7543
                        Fax: 202-337-8314
                        TTY: 202-337-5220
               e-mail: agbell2@aol.com
                       www.agbell.org

Practical examination of the major current methodologies of teaching of the deaf. There are
more down-to-earth recommendations for selecting and assessing the appropriate approach for
each child.

304 pages

2178 Speech and the Hearing-Impaired Child

Daniel Ling, author

Alexander Graham Bell Association for the Deaf
3417 Volta Place N.W.
Washington, DC 20007   202-337-5220
                             800-432-7543
                        Fax: 202-337-8314
                        TTY: 202-337-5220
               e-mail: agbell2@aol.com
                       www.agbell.org

Provides a systematic approach to the teaching
of speech and a challenge to all involved in the
development of spoken language skills in hearing-impaired children.

402 pages

2179 Speechreading: A Way to Improve Understanding

Harriet Kaplan, Scott J. Balk and Carol Garretson,
author

Gallaudet Univ. Press c/o Chicago Distrib. Center
11030 South Langley Avenue
Chicago, IL 60628   202-651-5000
                          800-621-2736
                     Fax: 800-621-8476
                     TTY: 888-630-9347
          e-mail: david.gunton@gallaudet.edu
               www.gallaudet.edu/~gupress

This useful guide for teachers and therapists approaches speechreading instruction with the
help of context cues.

32 pages

2180 Sport Signs

Harley Hamilton, author

Modern Signs Press, Inc.
P.O. Box 1181
Los Alamitos, CA 90720   562-596-8548
                               800-572-7332
                          Fax: 562-795-6614
                          TTY: 310-493-4168

Objects and actions are depicted with illustrations, and manual signs are shown with the
printed words.

1985 Six Book Series

2181 Standards of Care

Randall R. Myers, LCSW-C, author

National Association of the Deaf
814 Thayer Avenue
Silver Spring, MD 20910   301-587-1788
                            Fax: 301-587-1791
                            TTY: 301-587-1789

Contains a wide range of resources designed to assist consumers, parents, professionals, and administrators identify and access quality mental health services for deaf and hard of hearing persons and their families.

3-ring binder

2182 Substance Abuse and Recovery: Empowerment of Deaf Persons

Gallaudet Univ. Press c/o Chicago Distrib. Center
11030 South Langley Avenue
Chicago, IL 60628   202-651-5000
800-621-2736
Fax: 800-621-8476
TTY: 888-630-9347
e-mail: david.gunton@gallaudet.edu
www.gallaudet.edu/~gupress

Professionals in the field of substance abuse and deafness present their views on abuse.

217 pages

2183 Supporting Young Adults Who Are Deaf-Blind in Their Communities

Jane M. Everson, PhD, author

National Association of the Deaf
814 Thayer Avenue
Silver Spring, MD 20910   301-587-1788
Fax: 301-587-1791
TTY: 301-587-1789

Provides specific strategies to help individuals who are deaf-blind to achieve greater integration into the community.

2184 Talk with Me

Ellyn Altman, Ph.D., author

Alexander Graham Bell Association for the Deaf
3417 Volta Place N.W.
Washington, DC 20007   202-337-5220
800-432-7543
Fax: 202-337-8314
TTY: 202-337-5220
e-mail: agbell2@aol.com
www.agbell.org

Written by a clinical psychologist and mother, this book educates parents and professionals about crucial early decisions that affect the speech, language, auditory, social and emotional development of children with hearing impairments.

1988 222 pages

2185 Teaching English to the Deaf as a Second Language
Depart. of English, Gallaudet University

Washington, DC 20002   202-651-5580

Publishes articles of practical interest to classroom teachers of hearing impaired and second language students.

Kendall Green

2186 Teaching Reading to Deaf Children

Beatrice Ostern Hart, author

Alexander Graham Bell Association for the Deaf
3417 Volta Place N.W.
Washington, DC 20007   202-337-5220
800-432-7543
Fax: 202-337-8314
TTY: 202-337-5220
e-mail: agbell2@aol.com
www.agbell.org

Developed by Lexington School for the deaf, this practical hand book for educators and parents presents a step by step program to guide children's reading growth.

1978 221 pages

2187 Teaching and Talking with Deaf Children

David Wood; Heather Wood; Amanda Griffiths, author

John Wiley & Sons, Inc.
605 Third Avenue
New York, NY 10158   212-806-6000
Fax: 212-850-6088
www.wiley.com

214 pages
ISBN: 0-471933-27-9

2188 Test of Early Reading Ability- Deaf or Hard of Hearing

Reid, Hresko, Hammill, author

Pro-Ed
8700 Shoal Creek Boulevard
Austin, TX 78757   512-451-3246
800-897-3202
Fax: 512-451-8542
www.proedinc.com

This is the only individually administered test of reading designed for children with moderate to profound sensory hearing loss (i.e. ranging from 41 to beyond 91 decibels, corrected).

Hearing Impairment/Deafness/Books

2189 There's a Hearing Impaired Child in my Class

Debra Nussbaum, author

Gallaudet Univ. Press c/o Chicago Distrib. Center
11030 South Langley Avenue
Chicago, IL 60628   202-651-5000
800-621-2736
Fax: 800-621-8476
TTY: 888-630-9347
e-mail: david.gunton@gallaudet.edu
www.gallaudet.edu/~gupress

This complete package provides basic facts about deafness, practical strategies for teaching hearing impaired children, and the question-and-answer information for all students.

44 pages

2190 They Grow in Silence

Eugene D. Mindel, author

Taylor & Francis, Inc.
47 Runaway Dr. # G
Levittown, PA 19057   215-269-0400
800-821-8312
Fax: 201-785-5515
www.taylorandfrancis.com

Gives a comprehensive picture of the deaf child in society, not looking at the individual but also, at the related problems for the family, community and the professional. Only by the examination of such a broad perspective can questions on the position and circumstances of the deaf child be fully considered.

223 pages Softcover

2191 They Grow in Silence: Understanding Deaf Children and Adults

Pro-Ed
8700 Shoal Creek Boulevard
Austin, TX 78757   512-451-3246
800-897-3202
Fax: 512-451-8542
www.proedinc.com

Data about psychological and educational processes important for the families and professionals working with children who are deaf with an examination of the whole of these children's life circumstances as an integrated process.

204 pages
ISBN: 0-890793-25-5

Eugene D. Mindel, Editor
McCay Vernon, Editor

2192 Today's Hearing Impaired Child: Into The Mainstream of Education

Vira Froehlinger, author

Alexander Graham Bell Association for the Deaf
3417 Volta Place N.W.
Washington, DC 20007   202-337-5220
800-432-7543
Fax: 202-337-8314
TTY: 202-337-5220
e-mail: agbell2@aol.com
www.agbell.org

A practical guide to the educational rights of hearing-impaired children under the law, guidelines for mainstreaming, educational assessment, special instructions for the regular classroom teacher, suggestions for developing and enhancing reading skills necessary for successful mainstreaming and an overview of hearing impairment for the regular classroom teacher.

240 pages

2193 Toward Effective Public School Programs for Deaf Students

Thomas N. Kluwin, Donald F. Moores, author

Baker & Taylor, Int'l
1200 US Highway 22 East
Bridgewater, NJ 08807   908-429-4074
Fax: 908-429-4037
e-mail: intsale@bakertaylor.com

Examining various options for providing effective education-including the highly controversial practice of mainstreaming. The editors base their study on one of the largest and longest-running studies ever of public school programs for the deaf.

1992 272 pages
ISBN: 0-807733-56-3

Martha Gonter Gaustad, Editors

2194 Understanding Ear Infections

Peter Allen, M.D., author

Alexander Graham Bell Association for the Deaf
3417 Volta Place N.W.
Washington, DC 20007   202-337-5220
800-432-7543
Fax: 202-337-8314
TTY: 202-337-5220
e-mail: agbell2@aol.com
www.agbell.org

355

Based on medical research, this clinical aid for medical and hearing professionals explains ear infections and their complications to patients and their families. Sturdily designed of cardboard, each page has photos and diagrams that explain each topic and answer commonly-asked questions about ear infections.

1993 27 pages

2195 We CAN Hear and Speak

Parents of Natural Communication, Inc., author

Alexander Graham Bell Association for the Deaf
3417 Volta Place N.W.
Washington, DC 20007　　　　　202-337-5220
　　　　　　　　　　　　　　　800-432-7543
　　　　　　　　　　　Fax: 202-337-8314
　　　　　　　　　　　TTY: 202-337-5220
　　　　　　　　e-mail: agbell2@aol.com
　　　　　　　　　　　　www.agbell.org

Written by parents for families of children who are deaf or hard of hearing, this work describes auditory-verbal terminology and approaches and contains personal narratives written by parents and their children who are deaf or hard of hearing.

171 pages Softcover

2196 We Can!

Robin Star, author

Alexander Graham Bell Association for the Deaf
3417 Volta Place N.W.
Washington, DC 20007　　　　　202-337-5220
　　　　　　　　　　　　　　　800-432-7543
　　　　　　　　　　　Fax: 202-337-8314
　　　　　　　　　　　TTY: 202-337-5220
　　　　　　　　e-mail: agbell2@aol.com
　　　　　　　　　　　　www.agbell.org

Hearing-impaired children need hearing-impaired role models. Written at a 4th-grade level, the books can also be used in the classroom for career education, as well as for reading and language instruction.

96 pages

2197 When Your Child is Deaf: A Guide for Parents

David M. Luterman with Mark Ross, Ph.D., author

Alexander Graham Bell Association for the Deaf
3417 Volta Place N.W.
Washington, DC 20007　　　　　202-337-5220
　　　　　　　　　　　　　　　800-432-7543
　　　　　　　　　　　Fax: 202-337-8314
　　　　　　　　　　　TTY: 202-337-5220
　　　　　　　　e-mail: agbell2@aol.com
　　　　　　　　　　　　www.agbell.org

This book gives encouragement and advice to parents on their essential roles in teaching speech to their child.

1991 182 pages

2198 When a Hug Won't Fix the Hurt

Karen Dockery, author

Alexander Graham Bell Association for the Deaf
3417 Volta Place N.W.
Washington, DC 20007　　　　　202-337-5220
　　　　　　　　　　　　　　　800-432-7543
　　　　　　　　　　　Fax: 202-337-8314
　　　　　　　　　　　TTY: 202-337-5220
　　　　　　　　e-mail: agbell2@aol.com
　　　　　　　　　　　　www.agbell.org

This compassionate book provides support to and suggests methods for parents whose child is in crisis, due to emotional problems, illness or disability.

1993 175 pages

2199 Writer's Workshop

Sandy Fischer, author

Gallaudet Univ. Press c/o Chicago Distrib. Center
11030 South Langley Avenue
Chicago, IL 60628　　　　　　202-651-5000
　　　　　　　　　　　　　　800-621-2736
　　　　　　　　　　　Fax: 800-621-8476
　　　　　　　　　　　TTY: 888-630-9347
　　　　　e-mail: david.gunton@gallaudet.edu
　　　　　　　www.gallaudet.edu/~gupress

Offers suggestions to teachers who are interested in turning the classroom into an environment where students learn to express themselves in writing.

95 pages

2200 Written-Language Assessment and intervention: Links To Literacy

Alexander Graham Bell Association for the Deaf
3417 Volta Place N.W.
Washington, DC 20007　　　　　202-337-5220
　　　　　　　　　　　　　　　800-432-7543
　　　　　　　　　　　Fax: 202-337-8314
　　　　　　　　　　　TTY: 202-337-5220
　　　　　　　　e-mail: agbell2@aol.com
　　　　　　　　　　　　www.agbell.org

Assessment is an important part of a written-language program because it helps to identify students' strengths and weaknesses, determine instructional objectives, monitor students' progress, and provide feedback to students on their performance.

1996 215 pages

2201 You and Your Deaf Child

John W. Adams, author

Gallaudet Univ. Press c/o Chicago Distrib. Center
11030 South Langley Avenue
Chicago, IL 60628   202-651-5000
                                 800-621-2736
                           Fax: 800-621-8476
                           TTY: 888-630-9347
            e-mail: david.gunton@gallaudet.edu
                    www.gallaudet.edu/~gupress

This guide for parents explores how families interact to deal with the special impact of a child who is hearing impaired.

1997 224 pages 2nd edition

**2202 You and Your Hearing Impaired Child: A
Self-Instructional Parents Guide**

John W. Adams, author

T.J. Publishers, Inc.
817 Silver Spring Avenue, Suite 206
Silver Spring, MD 20910   301-585-4440
                                 800-999-1168
                           Fax: 301-585-5930
                           TTY: 301-585-4440
                           TDD: 301-585-4441
                e-mail: TJPubinc@aol.com

Designed specifically for parents who have children newly diagnosed as hearing impaired. Provides vital information on hearing impairment, setting limits, behavior management, nonverbal behavior and much more.

142 pages Softcover

2203 Young Deaf Child

Ellen Kurtzer-White and Richard C. Seewald, author

Alexander Graham Bell Association for the Deaf
3417 Volta Place N.W.
Washington, DC 20007   202-337-5220
                                 800-432-7543
                           Fax: 202-337-8314
                           TTY: 202-337-5220
                e-mail: agbell2@aol.com
                        www.agbell.org

With a foreward by Mark Ross, Ph.D., this book is based on experience by the three authors and outlines the best approach for the child, early intervention, maximization of technology and strong family involvment.

1999

Children's Books

2204 ABC's of Finger Spelling

Michael Geiger, author

Modern Signs Press, Inc.
P.O. Box 1181
Los Alamitos, CA 90720   562-596-8548
                                 800-572-7332
                           Fax: 562-795-6614
                           TTY: 310-493-4168

Helps teach upper and lower case letters of the alphabet. Includes printed letters and easy-to-follow drawings of the hand shapes.

60 pages

2205 Advocacy Handbook

Alexander Graham Bell Association for the Deaf
3417 Volta Place N.W.
Washington, DC 20007   202-337-5220
                                 800-432-7543
                           Fax: 202-337-8314
                           TTY: 202-337-5220
                e-mail: agbell2@aol.com
                        www.agbell.org

A comprehensive guide including sections on effective advocacy, parent concerns, special education and IEPs, adolescence, the Americans with Disabilities Act, inclusion, technology, and taxes.

1995 150 pages

2206 Be Happy Not Sad

Kristen Gough, author

Modern Signs Press, Inc.
P.O. Box 1181
Los Alamitos, CA 90720   562-596-8548
                                 800-572-7332
                           Fax: 562-795-6614
                           TTY: 310-493-4168

These books help children understand hard to explain emotions through signing. Includes Be Happy Not Sad coloring workbook.

1988 2 Book Set

2207 Chris Gets Ear Tubes

Betty Pace, and Kathryn Hutton, author

Gallaudet Univ. Press c/o Chicago Distrib. Center
11030 South Langley Avenue
Chicago, IL 60628   202-651-5000
                                 800-621-2736
                           Fax: 800-621-8476
                           TTY: 888-630-9347
            e-mail: david.gunton@gallaudet.edu
                    www.gallaudet.edu/~gupress

A helpful book for parents and children to share concerning ear tubes and hospitals.

44 pages

2208 Come Sign with Us Sign Language Activities for Children

Jan C. Hafer and Robert M. Wilson, author

Gallaudet Univ. Press c/o Chicago Distrib. Center
11030 South Langley Avenue
Chicago, IL 60628   202-651-5000
                                      800-621-2736
                          Fax: 800-621-8476
                          TTY: 888-630-9347
          e-mail: david.gunton@gallaudet.edu
                 www.gallaudet.edu/~gupress

Revised version, offering more follow-up activities, including many in context, to teach children sign language. Features more than 300 line drawings of both adults and children signing familiar words, phrases, and sentences using ASL. Shows how to form each sign exactly and also presents the origins of ASL, facts about deafness, and the Deaf community.

160 pages Softcover
ISBN: 1-563680-51-3

2209 Discovering Sign Language

Laura Greene & Eva Barash Dicker, author

Gallaudet Univ. Press c/o Chicago Distrib. Center
11030 South Langley Avenue
Chicago, IL 60628   202-651-5000
                                      800-621-2736
                          Fax: 800-621-8476
                          TTY: 888-630-9347
          e-mail: david.gunton@gallaudet.edu
                 www.gallaudet.edu/~gupress

Fascinating book explaining different kinds of hearing losses and the significance of when the loss occurred.

104 pages

2210 Finger Alphabet

S. Harold Collins, author

Gallaudet Univ. Press c/o Chicago Distrib. Center
11030 South Langley Avenue
Chicago, IL 60628   202-651-5000
                                      800-621-2736
                          Fax: 800-621-8476
                          TTY: 888-630-9347
          e-mail: david.gunton@gallaudet.edu
                 www.gallaudet.edu/~gupress

Includes activities for improving fingerspelling.

30 pages

2211 Hearing Loss

Karin N. Mango, author

Franklin Watts c/o Grolier
90 Old Sherman Tpke
Danbury, CT 06816   203-797-3500
                                      800-621-1115
                          Fax: 203-797-3197
                          www.grolier.com

Offers a concise explanation of how and why hearing losses occur, how the ear works and how to protect your hearing.

144 pages Grades 7-12
ISBN: 0-531125-19-0

2212 Living with Deafness

Barbara Taylor, author

Franklin Watts c/o Grolier
90 Old Sherman Tpke
Danbury, CT 06816   203-797-3500
                                      800-621-1115
                          Fax: 203-797-3197
                          www.grolier.com

Shows how deaf persons can overcome their disability and live happy, productive lives.

32 pages Grades 5-7
ISBN: 0-531108-42-2

2213 None So Deaf - Student Text

Sarah Val, author

National Association of the Deaf
814 Thayer Avenue
Silver Spring, MD 20910   301-587-1788
                          Fax: 301-587-1791
                          TTY: 301-587-1789

A student history of the education of deaf people and the development of sign language. Stories about deaf children illustrate the struggle toward equal recognition and the right to education, and modern systems of communication.

2214 Reading Between the Lips

Lew Golan, author

Alexander Graham Bell Association for the Deaf
3417 Volta Place N.W.
Washington, DC 20007   202-337-5220
                                      800-432-7543
                          Fax: 202-337-8314
                          TTY: 202-337-5220
          e-mail: agbell2@aol.com
                 www.agbell.org

In a frank and witty celebration of the advantages and pitfalls of speaking and lipreading, the author shows that total deafness is not an impenetrable barrier but one to get over or around.

1995 363 pages

2215 Secret Signing: A Sign Language Activity Book

Susan P. Shroyer, author

Gallaudet Univ. Press c/o Chicago Distrib. Center
11030 South Langley Avenue
Chicago, IL 60628   202-651-5000
800-621-2736
Fax: 800-621-8476
TTY: 888-630-9347
e-mail: david.gunton@gallaudet.edu
www.gallaudet.edu/~gupress

Children will enjoy this activity book with signs.
64 pages Level K-1

2216 Sign-Me-Fine

Laura Greene and Eva Barash Dicker, author

Gallaudet Univ. Press c/o Chicago Distrib. Center
11030 South Langley Avenue
Chicago, IL 60628   202-651-5000
800-621-2736
Fax: 800-621-8476
TTY: 888-630-9347
e-mail: david.gunton@gallaudet.edu
www.gallaudet.edu/~gupress

Written for young adults, this book introduces American Sign Language and how it differs from English.
120 pages

2217 Signing for Kids

Mickey Flodin, author

Gallaudet Univ. Press c/o Chicago Distrib. Center
11030 South Langley Avenue
Chicago, IL 60628   202-651-5000
800-621-2736
Fax: 800-621-8476
TTY: 888-630-9347
e-mail: david.gunton@gallaudet.edu
www.gallaudet.edu/~gupress

Contains 17 chapters dealing with special areas of interest to children like pets, family, friends and people.
142 pages

2218 Signs for Me: Basic Sign Vocabulary for Children, Parents, & Teachers

Ben Bahan and Joe Dannis, author

DawnSignPress
6130 Nancy Ridge Drive
San Diego, CA 92121   858-625-0600
800-549-5350
Fax: 858-625-2336
e-mail: dsp@dawnsign.com
www.dawnsign.com

ASL/English vocabulary primer filled with all the basics for preschoolers. The focus is on learning ASL signs and English words for better language development. Illustrates the meaning of the sign, the sign itself, and the English word in bold print.
128 pages
ISBN: 0-915035-27-8

Barry Howland, Marketing Director

2219 Silent Garden: Raising Your Deaf Child

Paul W. Ogden, author

Alexander Graham Bell Association for the Deaf
3417 Volta Place N.W.
Washington, DC 20007   202-337-5220
800-432-7543
Fax: 202-337-8314
TTY: 202-337-5220
e-mail: agbell2@aol.com
www.agbell.org

This book provides parents of deaf children with crucial information on the possibilities afforded their children. Ogden, deaf since birth and a professor of deaf studies offers parents the foundation for making the difficult decisions necessary to start their children on the road to realizing their full potential.
1996 313 pages

2220 Very Special Friend

Dorothy Levin, author

Gallaudet Univ. Press c/o Chicago Distrib. Center
11030 South Langley Avenue
Chicago, IL 60628   202-651-5000
800-621-2736
Fax: 800-621-8476
TTY: 888-630-9347
e-mail: david.gunton@gallaudet.edu
www.gallaudet.edu/~gupress

Six-year-old Frannie finds a very special friend who talks in sign language. She learns to sign and the two become best friends.
32 pages Hardcover
ISBN: 0-930323-55-6

2221 You Make the Difference In Helping Your Child Learn

Ayala Monolson, author

Alexander Graham Bell Association for the Deaf
3417 Volta Place N.W.
Washington, DC 20007   202-337-5220
800-432-7543
Fax: 202-337-8314
TTY: 202-337-5220
e-mail: agbell2@aol.com
www.agbell.org

This simple, attractive book will help parents and children connect in ways that foster children's self-esteem and language learning. Full of clear cartoons, these easily understood messages are uncomplicated and perfect for parents of all children, especially those whose language and social skills are delayed or at risk.

1994 30 pages

Magazines

2222 American Association of the Deaf-Blind
814 Thayer Avenue, Room 302
Silver Spring, MD 20910
Fax: 301-588-8705
TTY: 301-588-6545
e-mail: aadb@erols.com

Information on better opportunities and services for deaf-blind people, to assure that a comprehensive, coordinated system of services is accessible to all deaf-blind people, enabling them to achieve their maximum potential through increased independence.

50 pages Quarterly

Jamie McNamara, Editor

2223 American Auditory Society
Lippincort Williams and Wilkins
512 East Canterbury Lane
Phoenix, AZ 85022
602-789-0755
Fax: 602-942-1486
e-mail: aas@amauditorysoc.org
www.amauditroysoc.org

Information on the American Auditory Society.

540 pages 6x/Year
ISSN: 01960202

Susan Jergen, Ph.D, Editor

2224 Deaf Life
C/O MSM Productions, Ltd.
P.O. Box 23380
Rochester, NY 14692
716-442-6370
Fax: 716-442-6371
TTY: 716-442-6370
e-mail: deaflife@deaflife.com
www.deaflife.com

This magazine focuses on profiles, news, controversial issues, cultural topics and more relating to the Deaf community, first published in 1988.

64 pages Monthly
ISSN: 0898-719x

Matthew Moore, Publisher

2225 Deaf USA
Eye Festival Communications, Inc.
6917-B Woodley Avenue
Van Nuys, CA 91406
Fax: 818-902-9840

Provides news coverage on all activities and issues of interest to deaf and hard of hearing readers as well as professionals and associates within this specialized market.

Monthly

David Rosenbaum, Editor

2226 Hearing Health
P.O. Box 2663
Corpus Christi, TX 78403
512-884-8388
Fax: 512-884-3314

A publication for deaf and hard-of-hearing people, as well as hearing health care professionals, libraries, agencies, schools and organizations.

BiMonthly

Paula Bartone-Bonillas, Editor

2227 Language, Speech and Hearing Services in the Schools
American Speech-Language-Hearing Association
10801 Rockville Pike
Rockville, MD 20852
301-897-5700
800-638-8255

Professional journal for clinicians, audiologists and speech-language pathologists.

Russell L. Malone, Ph.D., Editor

2228 Perspectives in Education and Deafness
Gallaudet Univ. Press c/o Chicago Distrib. Center
11030 South Langley Avenue
Chicago, IL 60628
202-651-5000
800-621-2736
Fax: 800-621-8476
TTY: 888-630-9347
e-mail: david.gunton@gallaudet.edu
www.gallaudet.edu/~gupress

A practical, reader-friendly magazine, offering help and advice in and beyond the classroom, tuned to the needs of today's students, teachers, and families.

5x Annually

Mary Abrams Perica, Editor

2229 Volta Voices
Alexander Graham Bell Association for the Deaf
3417 Volta Place N.W.
Washington, DC 20007   202-337-5220
                              800-432-7543
                              Fax: 202-337-8314
                              TTY: 202-337-5220
                              e-mail: agbell2@aol.com
                              www.agbell.org

A magazine highlighting inspirational stories
from parents of children who are deaf, legislative news, technology update, and stories pertaining to speech, speech-reading, and the use of
residual hearing.

BiMonthly

Brooke Rigler, Editor

Journals

2230 American Annals of the Deaf
Convention of American Instructors of the Deaf
Fowler Hall 409, 800 Florida Avenue NE
Washington, DC 20002   202-651-5340
                              Fax: 202-651-5708
        www.gallaudet.edu:80/~penmpaad/index.htm

Scholarly journal at the forefront of research related to the education of deaf people. Annual reference Issue identifies programs and services for
deaf people nationwide.

5x Annually

Donald F. Moores, Editor
Mary Ellen Carew, Managing Editor

2231 Journal of Speech-Language-Hearing Research
American Speech-Language-Hearing Association
10801 Rockville Pike
Rockville, MD 20852   301-897-5700
                             800-638-8255

Russell L. Malone, Ph.D., Editor

2232 SHHH Journal
Self Help for Hard of Hearing People, Inc.
7910 Woodmont Avenue, Ste. 1200
Bethesda, MD 20814   301-657-2248
                            Fax: 301-913-9413
                            TTY: 301-657-2249

An educational journal about hearing loss for
hard-of-hearing people.

BiMonthly

Barbara G. Harris, Editor

Newsletters

2233 ADARA Updated
ADARA
P.O. Box 251554
Little Rock, AR 72225   501-224-6678
                               Fax: 501-868-8812

Updates readers on events, resources, legislation, information of national interest, conferences, workshops and employment
opportunities. Information from and about local chapters, special interest sections, and national organizations is included in this
publication.

Quarterly

Nanncy Long, Ph.D., Editor

2234 Deaf American Monograph Series
National Association of the deaf
814 Thayer Avenue
Silver Spring, MD 20910   301-587-1788
                                 Fax: 301-587-1791
                                 TTY: 301-587-1789

Each monograph in the series contains more
than 30 articles on a single theme. Past themes
have included communication issues, perspectives on deafness, viewpoints on deafness, and
deafness — the next twenty years.

Annual

Mervin D. Garretson, Editor

2235 Endeavor
American Society for Deaf Children
P O Box 3355
Gettysburg, PA 17325   717-334-7922
                              800-942-2732
                              Fax: 717-334-8808

Newsletter for parents of deaf children.

Quarterly

Barbara Aschembrenner, Editor

2236 Gallaudet Today

Vickie Walter, Editor, author

Gallaudet Univ. Press c/o Chicago Distrib. Center
11030 South Langley Avenue
Chicago, IL 60628   202-651-5000
                          800-621-2736
                          Fax: 800-621-8476
                          TTY: 888-630-9347
                          e-mail: david.gunton@gallaudet.edu
                          www.gallaudet.edu/~gupress

A university alumni publication with both general and special issues on deafness-related topics. A suscription to the magazine also includes the Gallaudet Today - newsletter which is sent out three times a year.

44 pages Quarterly

Roz Prickett, Publications Manager

2237 Hear

Deafness Research Foundation
15 West 39th Street
New York, NY 10018   212-768-1181

Offers information on the Foundation's activities and events, technical updates on assistive devices, legislative and medical information on the latest breakthroughs and laws for the hearing impaired, book reviews and resources.

Monte H. Jacoby, Executive Director

2238 National Association of the Deaf

814 Thayer Avenue, Suite 250
Silver Spring, MD 20910   301-587-1788
                                Fax: 301-587-1791
                                TTY: 301-587-1789
                                e-mail: NADinfo@nad.org
                                www.nad.org

Information on the nation's largest constituency organization safeguarding the accessibility and civil rights of 28 million deaf and hard of hearing Americans in education, employment, health care and telecommunications. Focus on advocacy, captioned media, deafness-related information/publications, legal assistance and more.

32-40 pages 11x/Year

Dawn Bradley, Editor

2239 Newsletter of American Hearing Research

American Hearing Research Foundation
55 E Washington St, 2022
Chicago, IL 60602   312-726-9670

Concerned with hearing research and education.

William Lederer, Editor

2240 Newsline

Sertoma Foundation
1912 East Meyer Blvd.
Kansas City, MO 64132   816-333-8300

Reports on activities of the Sertoma Foundation in the field of speech and hearing impairments.

2241 Signs for Me: Basic Sign Vocabulary for Children, Parents, and Teachers

Ben Bahan and Joe Dannis, author

T.J. Publishers, Inc.
817 Silver Spring Avenue, Suite 206
Silver Spring, MD 20910   301-585-4440
                                800-999-1168
                                Fax: 301-585-5930
                                TTY: 301-585-4440
                                TDD: 301-585-4441
                                e-mail: TJPubinc@aol.com

Sign language vocabulary for preschool and elementary school children introduces household items, animals, family members, actions, emotions, safety concerns and other concepts.

112 pages Softcover

2242 Speech and Deafness Newsletter

Hearing, Speech
1620 18th Avenue
Seattle, WA 98122   206-323-5770

Agency newsletter for membership and community.

8 pages

Patty Tumberg, Editor

2243 Volta Review

Alexander Graham Bell Association for the Deaf
3417 Volta Place N.W.
Washington, DC 20007   202-337-5220
                            800-432-7543
                            Fax: 202-337-8314
                            TTY: 202-337-5220
                            e-mail: agbell2@aol.com
                            www.agbell.org

Offers the latest theory, research, current perspectives and practical guidance from noted specialists in education, audiology, speech and language sciences and psychology. Each issue contains a Special Focus - a group of chapters exploring a specific topic in detail.

Quarterly

2244 World Federation of the Deaf News
Ilkantie 4, P.O. Box 65
SF-00401 Helsinki Finland,   358-580-831
                               Fax: 358-580-770

The official magazine of the World Federation of the Deaf, features information on the work of the EFD, the latest news and interviews with people active in the deaf communities throughout the world.

Quarterly

Antti Makipaa, Editor

Pamphlets

2245 25 Ways to Promote Spoken Language in Your Child with a Hearing Loss

Amanda Mangiardi, author

Alexander Graham Bell Association for the Deaf
3417 Volta Place N.W.
Washington, DC 20007   202-337-5220
                               800-432-7543
                          Fax: 202-337-8314
                          TTY: 202-337-5220
                   e-mail: agbell2@aol.com
                          www.agbell.org

This pamphlet teaches twenty-five golden rules about preparing your child to listen and to speak.

1995 62 pages

2246 Between Two Worlds of Hearing and Not Hearing
Self Help for Hard of Hearing People, Inc.
7910 Woodmont Avenue Suite 1200
Bethesda, MD 20814   301-657-2248
                          Fax: 301-913-9413
                          TTY: 301-657-2249
                   e-mail: national@shhh.org
                          www.shhh.org

2247 Books for Parents of Deaf and Hard of Hearing Children
National Information Center on Deafness
800 Florida Ave. NE
Washington, DC 20002   202-651-5051
                          Fax: 202-651-5054
                          TTY: 202-651-5052

Identifies books written for parents and everday experiences of deaf and hard of hearing children.

2248 Can Your Baby Hear?
Alexander Graham Bell Association for the Deaf
3417 Volta Place N.W.
Washington, DC 20007   202-337-5220
                               800-432-7543
                          Fax: 202-337-8314
                          TTY: 202-337-5220
                   e-mail: agbell2@aol.com
                          www.agbell.org

This simple card for parents lists risk indicators and warning signs of hearing loss in babies.

2249 Care of the Ears and Hearing for Health
American Hearing Research Foundation
55 East Washington Street
Chicago, IL 60602   312-726-9670

Offers information on ear infections relating to chronic progressive deafness.

2250 Child's Perspective
Self Help for Hard of Hearing People, Inc.
7910 Woodmont Avenue Suite 1200
Bethesda, MD 20814   301-657-2248
                          Fax: 301-913-9413
                          TTY: 301-657-2249
                   e-mail: national@shhh.org
                          www.shhh.org

2251 Commonly-Asked Questions About Children with Minimal Hearing Loss in the Class
Self Help for Hard of Hearing People, Inc.
7910 Woodmont Avenue Suite 1200
Bethesda, MD 20814   301-657-2248
                          Fax: 301-913-9413
                          TTY: 301-657-2249
                   e-mail: national@shhh.org
                          www.shhh.org

2252 Communicating with People who Have a Hearing Loss

Carol L. Williams, author

Alexander Graham Bell Association for the Deaf
3417 Volta Place N.W.
Washington, DC 20007   202-337-5220
                               800-432-7543
                          Fax: 202-337-8314
                          TTY: 202-337-5220
                   e-mail: agbell2@aol.com
                          www.agbell.org

This brochure describes ways to communicate more effectively with people who have hearing losses.

1994

2253 Deafness: A Fact Sheet
National Information Center On Deafness
800 Florida Ave. NE
Washington, DC 20002   202-651-5051
                         Fax: 202-651-5054
                         TTY: 202-651-5052

2254 Developing Cognition in Young Children Who are Deaf

Susan Watkins, author

Hope, Inc.
55 East 100 North
Logan, UT 84321   435-752-9533
                    Fax: 435-752-9533

Presents interesting, updated information on the importance of early cognition development in young children who are deaf. Contains many ideas for ways to promote early thinking skills, especially those that promote and enhance early communication and language development.

2255 Educating Deaf Children: An Introduction
National Information Center on Deafness
800 Florida Ave. NE
Washington, DC 20002   202-651-5051
                         Fax: 202-651-5054
                         TTY: 202-651-5052

Describes the different settings in which deaf children are currently educated.

2256 Educational Perspective
Self Help for Hard of Hearing People, Inc.
7910 Woodmont Avenue Suite 1200
Bethesda, MD 20814   301-657-2248
                       Fax: 301-913-9413
                       TTY: 301-657-2249
                       e-mail: national@shhh.org
                       www.shhh.org

2257 Getting Beyond Hearing Loss: A Guide for Families
Self Help for Hard of Hearing People, Inc.
7910 Woodmont Avenue Suite 1200
Bethesda, MD 20814   301-657-2248
                       Fax: 301-913-9413
                       TTY: 301-657-2249
                       e-mail: national@shhh.org
                       www.shhh.org

2258 Hearing Alert! Informational Brochures
Alexander Graham Bell Association for the Deaf
3417 Volta Place N.W.
Washington, DC 20007   202-337-5220
                         800-432-7543
                         Fax: 202-337-8314
                         TTY: 202-337-5220
                         e-mail: agbell2@aol.com
                         www.agbell.org

These brochures encourage early detection of hearing loss in young children; for medical facilities, speech and hearing clinics, and schools.

2259 Helping Your Hard-of-Hearing Child Succeed
Susan Coffman, Stephen Epstein, M.D. & Carol Fisch, author

Alexander Graham Bell Association for the Deaf
3417 Volta Place N.W.
Washington, DC 20007   202-337-5220
                         800-432-7543
                         Fax: 202-337-8314
                         TTY: 202-337-5220
                         e-mail: agbell2@aol.com
                         www.agbell.org

Offers information on how to help children succeed in school with speech and language development.

2260 How Does Your Child Hear and Talk?
American Speech-Language-Hearing Association
10801 Rockville Pike
Rockville, MD 20852   301-897-8682
                        800-638-8255

Offers a chart to parents on children's growth pertaining to their hearing and speech.

2261 Leading National Publications of and for Deaf People
National Information Center On Deafness
800 Florida Ave. NE
Washington, DC 20002   202-651-5051
                         Fax: 202-651-5054
                         TTY: 202-651-5052

Identifies publications with national circulations to deaf audiences.

2262 Listen! Hear! for Parents of Hearing Impaired Children
Alexander Graham Bell Association for the Deaf
3417 Volta Place N.W.
Washington, DC 20007   202-337-5220
                         800-432-7543
                         Fax: 202-337-8314
                         TTY: 202-337-5220
                         e-mail: agbell2@aol.com
                         www.agbell.org

Offers information that parents of deaf and hard of hearing children need to be aware of. Also includes information on hearing aids, hearing loss and the association in general.

2263 National Information Center on Deafness Brochure
National Information Center On Deafness
800 Florida Ave. NE
Washington, DC 20002   202-651-5051
                             Fax: 202-651-5054
                             TTY: 202-651-5052

A description of services offered by NICD.

2264 Parent Packets
Alexander Graham Bell Association for the Deaf
3417 Volta Place N.W.
Washington, DC 20007   202-337-5220
                             800-432-7543
                             Fax: 202-337-8314
                             TTY: 202-337-5220
                             e-mail: agbell2@aol.com
                             www.agbell.org

These educational packets for parents are specifically designed to address important age-related topics about your child with a hearing impairment.

Packet

2265 Parents' Perspective
Self Help for Hard of Hearing People, Inc.
7910 Woodmont Avenue Suite 1200
Bethesda, MD 20814   301-657-2248
                           Fax: 301-913-9413
                           TTY: 301-657-2249
                           e-mail: national@shhh.org
                           www.shhh.org

2266 Personal Quest for Educational Excellence for a Hard of Hearing Child
Self Help for Hard of Hearing People, Inc.
7910 Woodmont Avenue Suite 1200
Bethesda, MD 20814   301-657-2248
                           Fax: 301-913-9413
                           TTY: 301-657-2249
                           e-mail: national@shhh.org
                           www.shhh.org

2267 Perspectives Folio: Parent-Child

Pre-College Outreach, author

Gallaudet Univ. Press c/o Chicago Distrib. Center
11030 South Langley Avenue
Chicago, IL 60628   202-651-5000
                          800-621-2736
                          Fax: 800-621-8476
                          TTY: 888-630-9347
                          e-mail: david.gunton@gallaudet.edu
                          www.gallaudet.edu/~gupress

Seven articles emphasizing family communication while providing important information for parents about deafness and the deaf culture.

29 pages

2268 Publications From the National Information Center on Deafness
National Information Center on Deafness
800 Florida Ave. NE
Washington, DC 20002   202-651-5051
                             Fax: 202-651-5054
                             TTY: 202-651-5052

Order form and explanations of NICD publications.

2269 Questions and Answers on Hearing Loss
Self Help for Hard of Hearing People, Inc.
7910 Woodmont Avenue Suite 1200
Bethesda, MD 20814   301-657-2248
                           Fax: 301-913-9413
                           TTY: 301-657-2249
                           e-mail: national@shhh.org
                           www.shhh.org

2270 Situation is Serious But Not Hopeless: The Psychological Benefits of Hearing Loss
Self Help for Hard of Hearing People, Inc.
7910 Woodmont Avenue Suite 1200
Bethesda, MD 20814   301-657-2248
                           Fax: 301-913-9413
                           TTY: 301-657-2249
                           e-mail: national@shhh.org
                           www.shhh.org

2271 So You Have Had An Ear Operation...What Next?
American Hearing Research Foundation
55 East Washington Street
Chicago, IL 60602   312-726-9670

Offers information on ear infections and surgery.

2272 Speechreading: Methods and Materials
Self Help for Hard of Hearing People, Inc.
7910 Woodmont Avenue Suite 1200
Bethesda, MD 20814   301-657-2248
                           Fax: 301-913-9413
                           TTY: 301-657-2249
                           e-mail: national@shhh.org
                           www.shhh.org

2273 Statewide Services for Deaf and Hard of Hearing People
National Information Center on Deafness
800 Florida Ave. NE
Washington, DC 20002   202-651-5051
                              Fax: 202-651-5054
                              TTY: 202-651-5052

A resource list of states that have established commissions and other offices to serve deaf people.

2274 World of Sound
International Hearing Society
16880 Middlebelt Road, Suite 4
Livonia, MI 48154   734-522-7200
                           Fax: 734-522-0200
                           www.hearingihs.org

The purpose of this booklet is to provide basic information for those with questions about hearing loss, hearing aids and Hearing Instrument Specialists.

DESCRIPTION

2275 HEMANGIOMAS AND LYMPHANGIOMAS

Disorder Type: Neoplasm: Benign or Malignant Tumor

Covers these related disorders: Capillary hemangiomas, Cavernous hemangiomas, Cystic hygromas, Disseminated hemangiomatosis, Mixed hemangiomas, Port-wine stains, Salmon stains

Hemangiomas are the most common benign tumors in infants. In addition, during childhood, lymphangiomas, also known as lymphatic malformations, are the second most common benign tumors affecting vessels of the body. Hemangiomas consist of an abnormal distribution of relatively small blood vessels (e.g., capillaries) due to malformation of developing fetal tissue from which the vessels arise. Lymphangiomas consist of masses of abnormally enlarged (dilated), newly formed lymph vessels, which are the channels that transport lymphatic fluid throughout the body. Lymph, a thin bodily fluid that consists of proteins, fats, and certain white blood cells (lymphocytes), accumulates in spaces between tissue cells and flows back into the bloodstream via lymph vessels.

Hemangiomas usually affect blood vessels of the skin (cutaneous hemangiomas). They most commonly develop in the head and neck regions and are rarely fully formed at birth. These tumors, which occur more frequently in females than males, are usually single growths that occur randomly for unknown reasons (sporadically). However, some multigenerational families (kindreds) have been reported in which several individuals developed isolated hemangiomas. In such cases, the condition may be transmitted as an autosomal dominant trait. In addition, in rare cases, certain forms of hemangiomas may occur in association with particular underlying syndromes.

Hemangiomas that affect blood vessels of the skin (cutaneous hemangiomas) may be superficial (capillary hemangiomas), deep (cavernous he-

mangiomas), or both (mixed hemangiomas). Capillary hemangiomas are considered the most common type of hemangioma, affecting approximately 60 percent of patients. These hemangiomas include port-wine stains (a form of nevus flammeus) and strawberry hemangiomas (strawberry nevi). Port-wine stains are present at birth (congenital) and are typically permanent defects. These lesions consist of mature, abnormally widened capillaries; are flat (macular) with sharply defined borders; and are usually reddish purple in color. They may vary greatly in size and typically develop on the head, face, and neck areas. As patients reach adulthood, port-wine stains may darken and form elevated (papular) areas that may occasionally bleed. Port-wine stains must be differentiated from salmon patches, which are flat, salmon-colored lesions that are typically present during infancy on certain facial areas, such as over the eyelids, on the middle of the forehead, or between the eyes. Salmon patches typically fade completely over time. Port-wine stains may be an isolated condition or may occur in association with several rare underlying syndromes (e.g., Klippel-Trenaunay-Weber syndrome, Sturge-Weber syndrome, etc.). Treatment may include a variety of measures, such as laser therapy, destruction of affected tissue through the use of extreme cold (cryosurgery), surgical removal (excision), transplantation of skin tissues (grafting), or masking with cosmetics.

Strawberry hemangiomas are dull or bright red and elevated, have clearly defined borders, and consist of immature capillaries. The lesions, which may develop as single or multiple growths, may affect any area of the body; however, they are most common on the scalp, face, chest, or back. Strawberry hemangiomas usually appear within approximately two months after birth. In most patients, the hemangiomas initially grow rapidly, cease such growth (stationary phase), and then gradually begin to regress in size (involution). After the lesions have reduced in size, approximately 10 percent of patients have residual discoloration or puckering of affected skin. In rare cases, complications associated with strawberry hemangiomas may include infection; destruction of the skin's surface, resulting in open sores and inflammation (ulceration); bleeding (hemorrhaging); or extensive growth that interferes with necessary functions, such as breathing difficulties due to tumor growth affecting the airways. Because most strawberry hemangiomas spontaneously regress, treatment typically consists of careful, ongoing observation. However, if hemangiomas rapidly grow, potentially causing tissue destruction of associated removal, use of elastic bandages, or other measuers in selected patients. If there is rapid growth that may ultimately cause life-threatening complications, treatment may include the administration of corticosteroids by injection or mouth; therapy with an artificial (synthetic) form of interferon (interferon alpha-2a); or, in potentially life-threatening cases, radiation therapy. Interferons are natural proteins that are produced by the body's immune system in response to certain invading viruses or other stimuli. Other treatment is symptomatic and supportive.

Cavernous hemangiomas are deep hemangiomas that may be firm or form cysts. The skin overlying such hemangiomas is often bluish in color. Mixed hemangiomas include a deep or cavernous area with an overlying, thin capillary hemangioma. Cavernous hemangiomas initially grow rapidly, cease such growth (stationary phase), and then gradually begin to regress in size (involution). In most patients, treatment includes careful, ongoing observation. However, if physicians suspect that underlying structures may be affected, specialized imaging techniques, such as CT scanning or ultrasonography, are conducted to detect and characterize such involvement. When treatment other than observation is required such measures may include the administration of corticosteroids by mouth or injection or therapy with a synthetic form of interferon (interferon alpha-2a). Rarely, some patients develop multiple hemangiomas. In such cases, affected children may have numerous small, red or purplish, raised (papular) hemangiomas on the skin. In addition, internal hemangiomas may be present involving certain organs, particularly the liver, lungs, brain and spinal cord, and organs of the gastrointestinal tract. In such cases, affected children are said to

have disseminated hemangiomatosis. Life-threatening complications may potentially arise due to bleeding (hemorrhage), tissue compression (e.g., neural tissue compression), obstruction of the airways, or an inability of the heart to effectively pump blood to the lungs and throughout the body (heart failure). Treatment may include corticosteroid therapy, potentially with interferon therapy; radiation therapy; surgical measures; and symptomatic and supportive measures. In some cases, multiple internal and cutaneous hemangiomas occur in association with certain rare, underlying syndromes (e.g., macrocephaly with pseudopapilledema). In other patients, multiple cutaneous hemangiomas may be present in the absence of internal hemangiomas.

Lymphangiomas may be localized or widely distributed growths that, in some cases, may have hemangioma-like components. In almost all affected children, lymphangiomas are apparent by approximately age three. Lymphangiomas most commonly develop in the neck and facial regions, in the chest area (thorax), or under the arms (axillae). For example, some affected children may have an abnormal cystic growth consisting of dilated lymph vessels beneath the skin in the neck area (cystic hygroma). Lymphangiomas, such as cystic hygroma, may occur as isolated findings or in association with certain underlying syndromes (e.g., Noonan syndrome). Unlike hemangiomas, lymphangiomas rarely spontaneously regress. In some patients, they may expand in size and may obstruct the gastrointestinal tract or the airways, potentially causing life-threatening complications without appropriate treatment. Because most lymphangiomas are relatively widely distributed (diffuse), treatment often includes removal of the growths in several stages (staged surgical resection). Additional treatment includes symptomatic and supportive measures.

The following organizations in the General Resources Section can provide additional information: NIH/National Institute of Arthritis and Musculoskeletal and Skin Diseases

National Associations & Support Groups

2276 American Academy of Dermatology
930 North Meacham Road, P.O.Box 4014
Schaumburg, IL 60168   708-330-0230
                              www.aad.org

Largest and most representative of all dermatologic associations. Committed to the highest quality standards in continuing medical education. Developed a platform in which to promote and advance the science and art of medicine and surgery related to the skin; promotes the highest possible standards in clinical practice, education and research in dermatology and related disciplines; and supports and enhances patient care.

2277 American Skin Association
150 East 58th Street, 33rd Floor
New York, NY 10155   212-753-8260
                            800-499-7546
                            Fax: 212-688-6547
          e-mail: AmericanSkin@compuserve.com

2278 Hemangioma Support System
Cynthia Schumerth
1215 Monterey Terrace
Depere, WI 54115   920-336-9399

Provides moral support to families affected by hemangiomas. Offers inforamtion on Capilary and Cavernous Hemangiomas and networking services to affected families, enabling them to exchange information, support, and resources.

2279 Hemangioma and Vascular Birthmarks Foundation
P.O. Box 106
Latham, NY 12110   518-782-9637
                 e-mail: HVBF@aol.com
                 www.birthmark.org

2280 Sturge-Weber Foundation
P.O. Box 418
Mt. Freedom, NJ 07970   973-895-4114
                            800-627-5482
                 Fax: 973-895-4846
                 e-mail: SWF@pobox.com
                 www.pobox.com/~swf

Dedicated to acting as a clearinghouse of information on all aspects of Sturge-Weber syndrome and offering support to all interested parties. Provides appropriate referrals and offers a variety of educational and support materials.

Web Sites

2281 Arkansas Children's Program
www.hemangioma.org/

2282 Cystic Hygroma and Hemangioma Online Support Group
http://members.tripod.com/~chsupport/

DESCRIPTION

2283 HEMOLYTIC DISEASE OF THE NEWBORN

Synonyms: Erythroblastosis fetalis, Erythroblastosis neonatorum

May involve these systems in the body (see Section III):

Blood (Hematologic)

Hemolytic disease of the newborn, also known as erythroblastosis neonatorum, is characterized by destruction of a newborn's red blood cells by antibodies that crossed the placenta from the mother's bloodstream during pregnancy. Antibodies are produced by certain white blood cells in response to foreign proteins (antigens), such as those present in foreign cells and invading microorganisms. Because the condition begins during fetal development, it may also be referred to as erythroblastosis fetalis. In most cases, the condition occurs when a developing fetus has Rh-positive blood (i.e., inherited from the father), but the mother has Rh-negative blood.

In approximately 85 percent of individuals, red blood cells contain an antigen called the Rh factor. Those with this antigen are said to have Rh-positive blood, whereas those without the antigen have Rh-negative blood. The blood plasma does not naturally contain antibodies to inactivate or destroy the Rh antigen (anti-Rh antibodies). However, if a fetus has Rh-positive blood and the mother is Rh negative, the presence of the Rh factor in the fetus' red blood cells causes the mother's body to produce anti-Rh antibodies. If the woman becomes pregnant again and the developing fetus has Rh-positive blood, the mother's antibodies may react with the fetus' Rh-positive cells, resulting in erythroblastosis fetalis. In many cases, mothers who are known to have Rh-negative blood may be treated with a protein to help prevent them from producing anti-Rh antibodies (e.g., injection of human anti-D globulin), thereby lowering the risk of erythroblastosis fetalis during future pregnancies.

In infants affected by hemolytic disease of the newborn, associated symptoms and findings may vary. These may range from a mild breakdown of red blood cells (mild hemolysis) to severely low levels of circulating red blood cells (severe anemia); paleness of the skin (pallor); tiny reddish, purplish spots on the skin (petechiae) due to abnormal bleeding under the skin's surface; enlargement of the liver and spleen (hepatosplenomegaly); or development of abnormal yellowish coloring of the mucous membranes, whites of the eyes; and skin (jaundice). In extremely severe cases, affected newborns may experience low levels of oxygen supply (hypoxia), difficulties breathing (respiratory distress), heart (cardiac) failure, severe abnormal accumulations of fluid in body tissues and cavities (hydrops), and potentially life-threatening complications. Depending upon the severity of the condition, treatment may include transfusions (e.g., partial or full exchange transfusions with Rh-negative blood cross-matched against the mother's serum; compatible packed red blood cells in cases of severe hemolytic anemia) and supportive measures, such as ventilation assistance.

In some cases, hemolytic disease of the newborn may also result due to other blood type incompatibilities, primarily if a mother is type O and the developing fetus is type A or B. However, the condition develops in only about 10 percent of such cases of ABO incompatibility. In addition, the condition is typically less severe than that associated with Rh incompatibility. In cases of ABO blood type incompatibility, the development of jaundice approximately a day after birth may be the only associated symptom.

The following organizations in the General Resources Section can provide additional information: NIH/National Institute of Child Health and Human Development, NIH/National Heart, Lung and Blood Institute, National Organization for Rare Disorders, Inc. (NORD), Online Mendelian Inheritance in Man: www3.ncbi.nlm.nih.gov/Omim/searchomim.html

National Associations & Support Groups

2284 American Autoimmune Related Diseases Association, Inc.
15475 Gratiot Avenue
Detroit, MI 48205   313-371-8600
                                e-mail: aarda@aol.com
                                www.aarda.org

Focused on the dissemination of information to a wide public base of similar diseases.

2285 National Hemophilia Foundation
110 Greene Street, Ste 303
New York, NY 10012   212-328-3700

Jody Corngold

Web Sites

2286 Cliniweb
www.ohsu.edu/cliniweb/C15/C15.378.71.htm

2287 National Institutes of Health/Office of Rare Diseases
http://rarediseases.info.nih.gov/ord/

DESCRIPTION

2288 HEMOPHILIA

Synonyms: AHF, Antihemophilic factor deficiency, Classic hemophilia, Factor VIII deficiency, Hemophilia A

Covers these related disorders: Hemophilia A, Hemophilia B (Christmas disease; Factor IX deficiency), Von Willebrand's disease (Factor VIIIR deficiency; Vascular hemop

May involve these systems in the body (see Section III):

Blood (Hematologic), Genetic Disorder

The term hemophilia refers to a group of bleeding disorders including hemophilia A, hemophilia B, and von Willebrand's disease. Each of these diseases is characterized by the deficiency of a specific blood-clotting protein (factor). Hemophilia A, the most common form of the disease, affects approximately 80 percent of people with hemophilia and is caused by a deficiency of factor VIII. Hemophilia B, accounting for approximately 12 to 15 percent of all cases, results from a deficiency in clotting factor IX. In both forms of hemophilia, the severity of the disease and associated symptoms depend upon the level of coagulating activity of the individual clotting factors; the lower the activity of these factors, the more severe the disease. The most common symptoms, usually appearing at about 18 months when the child becomes more physically active, include easy bruising and bleeding into the joints (hemanthrosis) and muscles. Pain and swelling in the ankles, knees, and elbows may follow and eventually lead to degenerative changes and limited range of motion. Bleeding episodes may occur after injury, trauma, minor surgery, and, in some cases, for no apparent reason (spontaneously). Von Willebrand's disease involves a deficiency of factor VIIIR and is characterized by easy bruising, nose bleeds into the gastrointestinal tract. In affected females, excessive uterine bleeding may occur during menstruation or childbirth. In some patients, blood may be present in the urine (hematuria). Unlike hemophilia A or B, bleeding into the joints is rare and the disorder seems to improve with advancing age.

Treatment of hemophilia A and B includes transfusions of appropriate clotting factor when a bleeding episode occurs. These concentrates may also be regularly self-administered to prevent bleeds. Other preventive measures may include the administration of certain clot-aiding drugs before surgery, the avoidance of certain drugs that may exacerbate bleeding problems, and avoidance of participation in contact sports or other similar activities that could provoke a bleeding episode. The treatment of von Willebrand's disease may include the infusion of DDAVP or VW protein prior to surgery or childbirth.

Hemophilia A and hemophilia B are transmitted as x-linked recessive traits and affect males almost exclusively. Approximately 10 males out of every 100,000 are born with hemophilia A, while the rate of occurrence of hemophilia B is about two males out of every 100,000. For the most part, von Willebrand's disease is inherited as an autosomal dominant disorder. In rare instances, the disease may be inherited as a recessive gene.

The following organizations in the General Resources Section can provide additional information: Online Mendelian Inheritance in Man - www3.ncbi.nlm.nih.gov/Omim/searchomim.html

National Associations & Support Groups

2289 American Red Cross Blood Services
1616 N. Fort Myer Drive 17th Floor
Arlington, VA 22209
703-312-8724
Fax: 703-312-8738
www.crossnet.org

Distributes a wide variety of plasma therapeutics to benefit people with hemophilia A and B, immune disorders and hypoalbuminemia.

Sandra L. Mertz, Product Manager

2290 Canadian Hemophilia Society
625 President Kennedy, Suite 1210
Montreal, Quebec H3A1K2,
Canada
514-848-0503
800-668-2686
Fax: 514-848-9661
e-mail: chs@odyssee.net

2291 Children's Blood Foundation
333 East 38th Street, Room 830
New York, NY 10016   212-297-4336
                            Fax: 212-297-4340
                            e-mail: cbf@nyh.med.cornell.edu

Devoted to supplying families and friends of children diagnosed, with the knowledge and facts they require.

2292 Hemophilia Health Services
6820 Charlotte Pike
Nashville, TN 37209   615-320-0400
                            Fax: 615-352-2588

Craig Alsup, Chief Officer
Alsup Louise, Hardaway

2293 National Hemophilia Foundation
116 West 23rd Street, 11th Floor
New York, NY 10001   212-328-3700
                            800-424-2634
                            Fax: 212-328-3777
                            e-mail: handi@hemophilia.org
                            www.hemophilia.org

Dedicated to the treatment and the cure of hemophilia, related bleeding disorders and complications of those disorders or their treatment, including HIV infection, as well as improving the quality of life of all those affected through the promotion and support of research, education and other services.

Jodie L. Corngold, Director of Communications

2294 National Hemophilia Foundation - Info Center
116 West 23rd Street, 11th Floor
New York, NY 10001   212-328-3700
                            800-424-2634
                            Fax: 212-328-3777
                            e-mail: info@hemophilia.org
                            www.hemophilia.org

Offers various information, articles, resources, books and more for the hemophilia and HIV/AIDS community.

2295 World Federation of Hemophilia
1310 Greene Avenue, Suite 500
Montreal, Quebec H3Z2B2,
Canada   514-933-7944
                            Fax: 514-933-8916
                            e-mail: wfh@wfh.org

State Agencies & Support Groups

Alabama

2296 Alabama Chapter of the National Hemophilia Foundation
802 Midland Avenue
Muscle Shoals, AL 35661   205-381-5925

California

2297 Central California Chapter of the National Hemophilia Foundation
2804 Tioga Way
Sacramento, CA 95821   916-489-0276
                             Fax: 916-489-1569

A very small and family-oriented chapter. Offers an active youth group, an annual summer camp, a men's and women's group and various family activities for persons living in the central California valley from its center in Sacramento to the borders of Nevada and Oregon.

Carola Russell

2298 Hemophilia Association of San Diego County
P.O. Box 23099
San Diego, CA 92193   858-560-8373
                            Fax: 858-467-4788
                            e-mail: hemoofsd@aol.com
                            www.hemophilia.org

Provides summer camp programs for young persons with hemophilia, sponsors educational programs for the general public, sponsors support groups for parents to help them deal with hemophilia, monitors legislation pertaining to hemophilia and HIV and provides representation on the San Diego County Task Force on AIDS.

Jessica E. Swann, Executive Director

2299 Northern California Chapter of the National Hemophilia Foundation
7700 Edgewater Drive, Ste. 710
Oakland, CA 94621   510-568-6243
                          Fax: 510-568-2048

A volunteer, nonprofit organization serving the needs of people with hemophilia and other related bleeding disorders in 35 counties in Northern California. Provides hemophilia literature, scholarships, youth programs, annual summer camps, blood credits, medical alert tags, AIDS education committee and an emergency assistance fund for hemophiliacs and persons with HIV/AIDS.

Colorado

2300 Hemophilia Society of Colorado
10020 E. Girrard Ave,. Suite 100
Denver, CO 80231   303-750-6990
                          800-687-2568
                     Fax: 303-750-7035
              e-mail: HSC@ohisp.org
                     www.cottemo.org

The society exist to asvocate for assist and educate persons and families with hemophilia, Von Willebrand's disease, coagulation and other blood disorders. The society also distributes information to educate the general public.

96 members

Florida

2301 Florida Chapter of the National Hemophilia Foundation
17810 Litlewood Drive
Sprinhill, FL 34610   727-856-7057
                             888-880-8330
                        Fax: 727-856-2257
           e-mail: hemophsoll@aol.com
           www.gcocities.com/hotsprings/1809

1,000 members

Natalie Philips, Executive Director

Georgia

2302 Hemophilia Foundation of Georgia
8800 Rosweel Road, Suite 170
Atlanta, GA 30350   770-518-8272
                      Fax: 770-518-3310
                           www.hot.org

Established to help Georgia residents with hemophilia lead normal and productive lives. Comprised of patients, their friends and families, it provides the best in personalized and comprehensive services. Support services include home care programs, medical services, education and information on hemophilia and support groups and counseling to patients and families.

Elene Scaglotti, Director

Hawaii

2303 Hemophilia Foundation of Hawaii
Kapiolani Medical Center
1164 Bishop Street, Suite 1501
Honolulu, HI 96813   808-521-5483
                       Fax: 808-528-7430

Illinois

2304 Hemophilia Foundation of Illinois
332 S. Michigan Ave., Ste. 812
Chicago, IL 60604   312-427-1495
                      Fax: 312-427-1602

Serves as an information source, referral service and advocate for persons with hemophilia and their families. The mission of this chapter is to provide counseling, educational information and support services to persons affected by hemophilia and related blood disorders. Services provided include an annual summer camp for boys, family counseling, support groups, crisis intervention, financial counseling, video and reading library and health education.

Gary Steagall, ACSW, Social Worker

Indiana

2305 Hemophilia Foundation of Indiana
2216 East 44th Street
Indianapolis, IN 46205   317-543-1299
                                800-241-2873
                           Fax: 317-543-1291

Kentucky

2306 Kentuckian Hemophilia Foundation
Kosair Charities Center
982 Eastern Parkway
Louisville, KY 40217   502-637-7696
                            800-532-2873
                         Fax: 502-634-9995

Cynthia S. Hall, Executive Director

Louisiana

2307 Louisiana Chapter of the National Hemophilia Foundation
3636 S. Sherwood Forest Blvd.
Baton Rouge, LA 70816   504-293-4693
                            Fax: 504-291-1679

Maryland

2308 National Hemophilia Foundation, Maryland Chapter
8043 Kimberly Road
Baltimore, MD 21222   410-288-3955
                            800-424-2634
                         Fax: 410-285-3271
                         www.hemophilia.org

Massachusetts

2309 Massachusetts, New England Hemophilia Association
180 Rustcraft Road, Suite 101
Dedham, MA 02026   781-326-7645
                        800-228-6342
                     Fax: 781-329-5122

This chapter serves persons with hemophilia and other bleeding disorders in Massachusetts, Maine, New Hampshire and Vermont. Services include hemophilia and HIV/AIDS education, information and referrals, insurance and legislative updates, lending library, support group meetings and a resource referral network.

Jan Wilson, Executive Director

Michigan

2310 Hemophilia Foundation of Michigan
117 N. First St.,Suite 40
Ann Arbor, MI 48104   734-761-2535
                          800-482-3041
                       Fax: 734-761-3267

2311 Michigan Hemophilia Foundation
117 N. First St., Ste. 40
Ann Arbor, MI 48104   734-761-2535
                          800-482-3041
                       Fax: 734-761-3267

Educational materials on hemophilia, von Willebrand and other hereditary, bleeding disorders and complications (i.e. HIV and hepatitis). HFM provides direct services, and serves as a referral source for genetic information treatment and resources.

Lisa Teton, Outreach Specialist
Teton Isabel, Lin

Minnesota

2312 Hemophilia Foundation of Minnesota and the Dakotas
2066 First Ave. North, Suite 204
Anoka, MN 55303   612-232-7406
                       Fax: 612-323-7564

A nonprofit organization established to lead the community and inspire members to impact their own lives, with the ultimate aim of cures for both hemophilia and HIV/AIDS. The mission of the foundation is to meet the needs of persons who live with hemophilia and related inherited bleeding disorders, and complications including HIV/AIDS.

Mississippi

2313 Mississippi Hemophilia Foundation
309 Peach Street, Box 224
Flora, MS 39071   601-856-6157

Missouri

2314 National Hemophilia Foundation, Heart of America Chapter
Route 1, Box 98
Leasburg, MO 65535   573-245-6851
                          800-424-2634

Nebraska

2315 Nebraska Chapter of the National Hemophilia Foundation
3610 Dodge Street #110-W
Omaha, NE 68131
402-342-3329
Fax: 402-342-4326

The mission of this chapter is to provide support, education, communication and advocacy for all who are challenged by hemophilia. Services provided include a toll free telephone hotline for persons seeking information on HIV and hemophilia, comprehensive library services, outreach services providing HIV education, financial assistance, crisis intervention and a free speakers bureau.

Julie Sutcliffe

New York

2316 Hemophilia Center of Western New York
426 Gider Street
Buffalo, NY 14215
716-896-2470
Fax: 716-896-3119

2317 Mary M. Gooley Hemophilia Center of the National Hemophilia Foundation
1415 Portland Avenue, Ste. 425
Rochester, NY 14621
716-544-3630
Fax: 716-266-0772

Carol Orto, RN BS, Program Director

2318 Upper Hudson Valley Chapter of National Hemophilia Foundation
P.O. Box 3707
Albany, NY 12203
518-272-5082

North Carolina

2319 Hemophilia Foundation of North Carolina
2 Centerview Drive, Ste. 51
Greensboro, NC 27407
336-852-4788

A nonprofit organization that serves as an information source for the hemophilia community of North Carolina. Supplies up-to-date information concerning hemophilia and hemophilia related HIV/AIDS through newsletters, brochures and other patient services.

Wallace Revels, Administrative Mgr.

Ohio

2320 Central Ohio Chapter of the National Hemophilia Foundation
1312 Smallwood Drive
Columbus, OH 43235
614-457-0027

2321 Northern Ohio Chapter of the National Hemophilia Foundation
5755 Granger Rd, Ste 790
Cleveland, OH 44131
216-739-1755
800-554-4366
Fax: 216-739-1758

2322 Northwest Ohio Hemophilia Association
Davis Building
1 Stranahan Square, Suite 540
Toledo, OH 43604
419-241-9587
Fax: 419-242-6316

2323 Southwestern Ohio Chapter of the National Hemophilia Foundation
184 Salem Avenue
Dayton, OH 45406
937-220-6633
Fax: 937-220-6609

Serves persons with hemophilia and blood clotting disorders in an 11 county area. Offers educational opportunities about the physical, psychological and social aspects of these disorders, workshops, seminars, support groups, volunteer services, telephone and walk-in education, information, counseling and referrals.

Oklahoma

2324 Oklahoma Chapter of the National Hemophilia Foundation
525 N. W. 13th Street
Oklahoma City, OK 73103
405-236-1414
800-735-3855
Fax: 405-272-0436

Oregon

2325 Hemophilia Foundation of Oregon
5319 S.W. Westgate Drive, Suite 126
Portland, OR 97221
503-297-7207
Fax: 503-297-0127

Michial Fillman, Executive Director

Pennsylvania

2326 Delaware Valley Chapter of the National Hemophilia Foundation
222 S. Easton Road, Suite 119
Glenside, PA 19038   215-885-6500

2327 Western Pennsylvania Chapter of the National Hemophilia Foundation
580 South Aiken Avenue, Suite 220
Pittsburgh, PA 15232   412-685-2231
                              Fax: 412-683-2568

Brings together medical and social service providers, people with hemophilia and their families, educators and the general public. This chapter combines service, education and advocacy programs.

Rhode Island

2328 Rhode Island Hemophilia Foundation
160 Plainfield Street
Providence, RI 02909   401-944-6950
                              Fax: 401-944-4161

South Carolina

2329 Hemophilia Association of South Carolina
375 Sweetgum
Fort Mill, SC 29715   864-225-2139

Tennessee

2330 TN Hemo & Bleeding Disorders Foundation
7003 Chadwick Drive, Suite 269
Brentwood, TN 37027   615-373-0351
                             Fax: 615-373-4394
                             e-mail: thbdf@worldnet.att.net
                             http://home.att.net/-thbdf

Education and advocacy agency for TN Hemophiliac and public communities. Literature, referrals, summer camp, ages 7-15; scholarships; group events; limited emergency financial assistance; medically related transportation assistance; HIV/AIDS services.

Tina Majors, Executive Director

Texas

2331 Lone Star Chapter of the National Hemophilia Foundation
1407 North Durham
Houston, TX 77008   281-862-7707
                           Fax: 281-864-5538

Utah

2332 National Hemophilia Foundation, Utah Chapter
5635 South Waterbury Way Suite C-102
Salt Lake City, UT 84121   801-273-7471
                                  800-424-2634
                                  Fax: 801-273-7488
                                  www.hemophiliautah.org

Virginia

2333 Hemophilia Association of the Capital Area
3251 Old Lee Highway, Ste. 3
Fairfax, VA 22030   703-352-7641
                           Fax: 703-352-2145

A nonprofit organization serving persons with bleeding disorders and their families in northern Virginia, Washington, DC and Montgomery and Prince George's Counties in Maryland. This chapter's mission is to improve the quality of life for persons with hemophilia and Von Willebrand's disease and their families, to educate, act as an advocate, and provide member services.

Washington

2334 Hemophilia Foundation of Washington
Ryther Child Center
2400 N.E. 95th Street
Seattle, WA 98115   253-373-9094
                           Fax: 252-373-8280

West Virginia

2335 West Virginia Chapter
Route 2, Box 231
Milton, WV 25541   304-743-3966

Wisconsin

2336 Great Lakes Hemophilia Foundation
P.O. Box 13127, 8739 Watertown Road
Wauwatosa, WI 53213   414-257-0200
                             Fax: 414-257-1225

The only Wisconsin organization that addresses the physical, emotional, social and financial needs of individuals affected by hemophilia. This chapter supports high-quality, cost-effective programs for patient care, education, research and public awareness.

Libraries & Resource Centers

Alabama

2337 Hemophilia Clinic - Childrens' Rehabilitation Service
1616 Sixth Avenue South
Birmingham, AL 35233   205-939-5900

Nancy Woodall, RN

2338 Mobile Hemophilia Clinic
Children's Rehabilitation Service
1870 Pleasant Avenue
Mobile, AL 36617   334-479-8617

Arizona

2339 Mountain States Regional Hemophilia Center
University of Arizona Health Sciences Center
1501 North Campbell, Box 245073
Tucson, AZ 85724   520-626-6527
                             Fax: 520-626-4220

Comprehensive diagnosis and management of children and adults with congenital bleeding or clotting disorders.

John J. Hutter, Jr. MD, Director

2340 St. Joseph's Hemophilia Center
2927 North Seventh Avenue
Phoenix, AZ 85013   602-406-3770

Rachel Stuart, RN

Arkansas

2341 Hemophilia Center of Arkansas
Arkansas Children's Hospital
800 Marshall Street
Little Rock, AR 72202   501-320-1018

Nikki Shock

California

2342 Hemophilia Comprehensive Care Center at The Children's Hospital of L.A.
4650 Sunset Blvd.
Los Angeles, CA 92354   909-669-2339

Elaine Deavenport, PNP

2343 Orthopaedic Hospital's Hemophilia Treatment Center
2400 South Flower Street
Los Angeles, CA 90007   213-742-1000

Carol K. Kasper, MD

2344 UCD Northern Central California Hemophilia Program
2516 Stockton Blvd.
Sacramento, CA 95817   916-734-3461

Charles F. Abildgaard, MD

2345 UCSD Comprehensive Hemophilia Treatment Center
225 Dixsonson Street
San Diego, CA 92103   619-543-6737

George Davignon, MD

Connecticut

2346 Yale Hemophilia Center
Yale University School of Medicine

New Haven, CT 06510   203-785-4672

Diana S. Beardsley, MD, PhD

District of Columbia

2347 Hemophilia Treatment Center at Children's National Medical Center
Department of Hematology/Oncology

Washington, DC 20010   202-745-2140

Gordon L. Bray, MD

Florida

2348 Comprehensive Pediatric Hemophilia Center
University of South Florida
12901 Bruce B. Downs Blvd.
Tampa, FL 33612   813-974-2201

Sara Griggs, RN

2349 University of Florida Hemophilia Treatment Center
University of Florida

Gainesville, FL 32610   352-392-4061

Paulette Mehta, MD

Hawaii

2350 Hemophilia Foundation of Hawaii/ Kapiolani Medical Center
Comprehensive Hemophilia Treatment Center
1100 Ward Avenue, Ste. 1010
Honolulu, HI 96814   808-521-5483

Robert Wilkinson, MD

Illinois

2351 Regional Comprehensive Hemophilia Center of Central and Northern Illinois
530 N. East Glen Oak
Peoria, IL 61637   309-665-3889

Emily Czapek, MD

Indiana

2352 Riley Hemophilia and Thrombophilia Center
Riley Hospital for Children
702 Barnhill Drive, Room 2720
Indianapolis, IN 46202   317-274-5000
800-769-2848
Fax: 317-278-0816
e-mail: sslinbac@iupui.edu
pediatrics.iupui.edu

Sherry Linback, RN, PNP, Nurse Coordinator

Iowa

2353 Great Plains Regional Hemophilia Center
University of Iowa Hospitals

Iowa City, IA 52242   319-353-7877

Julie Mckillip, RN, BSN

Louisiana

2354 Louisiana Comprehensive Hemophilia Care Center
1430 Tulane Avenue
New Orleans, LA 70112   504-588-5433

W. Abe Andes, MD

Massachusetts

2355 Boston Hemophilia Center
Fegan 5 Children's Hospital

Boston, MA 02115   617-735-6369

Jocelyn Bessette, PNP

2356 Hemophilia Center of the New England Medical Center
750 Washington Street
Boston, MA 02111   617-956-6227

Bruce Furie, MD

Michigan

2357 Eastern Michigan Hemophilia Center
St. Joseph Hospital
302 Kensington
Flint, MI 48116   810-762-8656

Leslie Kirschke

2358 Greater Grand Rapids Pediatric Hemophilia Program
Butterworth Hospital
225 Wildwood Avenue
Woburn, MI 01801   781-928-2500
800-366-2665
Fax: 781-446-6520

James B. Fahner, MD

2359 Hemophilia Treatment Center at Munson Medical Center
1105 Sixth Street
Traverse City, MI 49684   616-922-7227

Jane Wares

2360 Michigan State University Hemophilia Comprehensive Care Clinic
1800 E. Grand River
Lansing, MI 48909   517-353-9385

Kathy Bosma, RN

2361 Regional Hemophilia Treatment Center
Children's Hospital of Michigan
3901 Beaubien Blvd.
Detroit, MI 48201   313-745-5437

Jeanne M. Lusher, MD

2362 University of Michigan Hemophilia Center
1500 E. Medical Center Dr.
Ann Arbor, MI 48109   734-936-3236

Raymond Hutchinson, MD

2363 West Michigan Regional Hemophilia Center
252 East Lowell Street
Kalamazoo, MI 49007   616-341-7966

Brian Eddy, MD

Minnesota

2364 Mayo Comprehensive Hemophilia Center
200 1st Street SW
Rochester, MN 55905   507-284-2021
800-344-7726
Fax: 507-284-8286

A World Federation of Hemophilia-Training Center, providing multidisciplinary assessment and care of persons with bleeding disorders. Offers consultation with hemotologists specializing in the care of pediatric and adult patients, a special consultation laboratory testing center and more.

2365 University of Minnesota Comprehensive Hemophilia Center
Harvard St. At E. River Road
Minneapolis, MN 55455   612-626-6455
800-688-5252
Fax: 612-625-4955

Serves over 700 adults and children with inherited bleeding disorders. Offers access to current technologies and treatments, including HIV and hemophilia research opportunities.

Missouri

2366 Missouri Illinois Regional Hemophilia Comprehensive Treatment Center
1465 S. Grand Blvd.
St. Louis, MO 63104   314-577-5332

Kathleen P. Gioia, RN

Nebraska

2367 Nebraska Regional Hemophilia Center
University of Nebraska Medical Center

Omaha, NE 68198   402-559-4227

Frances Tennant, RN, MA

Nevada

2368 University Medical Center Hemophilia Program
1800 W. Charleston Blvd.
Las Vegas, NV 89102   702-383-2000

Jack Lazerson, MD

New Hampshire

2369 Dartmouth Hitchcock Hemophilia Center
Medical Center - Section of Hematology
2 Maynard Street
Hanover, NH 03756   603-646-5486

Laurel J. McKernan, RN

New Jersey

2370 Nadeene Brunini Comprehensive Hemophilia Care Center
St. Michael's Medical Center
268 Dr Martin Luther King Jr
Newark, NJ 07102   973-877-5000

Yale S. Arkel, MD

New Mexico

2371 Ted R. Montoya Hemophilia Program
University of New Mexico, Ambulatory Care Center
3rd Floor
Albuquerque, NM 87131   505-272-5551

T. John Gribble, MD

New York

2372 Adult & Pediatric Hemophilia Clinics SUNY Health Sciences Center
750 East Adams Street
Stony Brook, NY 11794   516-689-8333

Mae B. Hultin, MD

2373 Albany New York Regional Comprehensive Hemophilia Center
Albany Medical College, MSX 12 Hematology
New Scotland Avenue
Albany, NY 12208   518-445-5827

Linda Whipple, RN

2374 Hemophilia Center of Western New York
Adult Unit - Erie County Medical Center
462 Grider Street, 5th Floor
Buffalo, NY 14215   716-896-2470

The center provides a variety of services to the hemophilia and HIV/AIDS community. Included among these services are diagnostics, registration, outpatient treatment, home care programs, home visits, school visits, dental services and counseling services. Offers an adult unit and a pediatric unit.

2375 Southern Tier Hemophilia Center
United Health Services - Wilson Hospital
Harrison Street
Johnson City, NY 13790   607-763-6130

Doris Michalovic, RN

North Carolina

2376 Bowman Grey School of Medicine - Hemophilia Diagnostic Center
Wake Forest University
Department of Pediatrics
Winston-Salem, NC 27157   919-716-2235

Christine A. Johnson, MD

2377 Comprehensive Hemophilia Diagnostic and Treatment Center
University of North Carolina - Chapel Hill
Box 7015
Chapel Hill, NC 27599   919-966-4736
                Fax: 919-962-8224

Haley Hall

North Dakota

2378 North Dakota Comprehensive Hemophilia Center
Roger Maris Cancer Center
820 4th Street North
Fargo, ND 58122   701-234-7544
                800-437-4010
                Fax: 701-234-7592

A treatment center for diseases of hemotosis and thrombosis which includes a clinical research program in bleeding disorders. Hemotologists are available for consultation 24 hours a day.

Ohio

2379 Children's Hospital Hemophilia Treatment Center
Elland & Bethesda Avenue
Cincinnati, OH 45229   513-559-4269

Ralph Gruppo, MD

2380 Northwest Ohio Hemophilia Treatment Center
2142 N. Cove Blvd.
Toledo, OH 43606   419-471-4225

Sue Ohler, RN

2381 University Treatment Center of University Hospitals of Cleveland
2074 Abingdon Road, Room 787
Cleveland, OH 44106   216-844-3376

Susan B. Shurin, MD

2382 West Central Ohio Hemophilia Center
One Children's Plaza
Dayton, OH 45404   937-226-8472

Complete care for individuals and families with hemophilia and related bleeding disorders. Some of the services offered include a comprehensive clinic, emergency treatment network, consultations, diagnostic coagulation laboratory, home infusion programs, HIV/AIDS education and counseling and more.

Leticia Valdez, M.D., Co-Director
Valdez, M.D. Robert, Stout, M.D.

2383 Youngstown Hemophilia Center
Western Reserve Care System South Medical Center
345 Oak Hill Avenue
Youngstown, OH 44501   330-747-0777

Lawrence M. Pass, MD

Oklahoma

2384 Oklahoma Comprehensive Hemophilia Diagnostic Treatment Center
P.O. Box 26307
Oklahoma City, OK 73126   405-271-3661

Beverly Stevens, RN

Pennsylvania

2385 Albert Einstein Medical Center Hemophilia Program
York And Tabor Roads
Philadelphia, PA 19141   215-456-7890

Mehdi K. Kajani, MD

2386 Children's Hospital of Philadelphia Hemophilia Program
Division of Hematology
34th St. & Civic Center Blvd.
Philadelphia, PA 19104   215-590-3438

Alan R. Cohen, MD

2387 Hemophilia Center of Central Pennsylvania
M.S. Hershey Medical Center
Pennsylvania State University
Hershey, PA 17033   717-531-7468

M. Elaine Eyster, MD

2388 Hemophilia Center of Western Pennsylvania
3636 Blvd. of the Allies
Pittsburgh, PA 15219   412-622-7280

Margaret V. Ragni, MD

2389 Thomas Jefferson University, Cardenza Foundation for Hematologic Research
1015 Walnut Street
Philadelphia, PA 19107   215-955-8875

Sandor Shapiro, MD, Director

Rhode Island

2390 Hemophilia Center of Rhode Island
Rhode Island Hospital
Aldrich House #258
Providence, RI 02903   401-444-3563

Peter Smith, MD

South Carolina

2391 Richland Memorial Comprehensive Pediatric Hemophilia Center
Children's Hospital for Cancer & Blood Disorders
5 Richland Medical Park
Columbia, SC 29203   803-765-7000

Robert S. Etinger, MD

South Dakota

2392 Sioux Falls Hemophilia Treatment Center
1000 E. 21st Street, Ste. 3100
Sioux Falls, SD 57105   605-339-7595
800-658-3030
Fax: 605-333-8460

Provides comprehensive care based on family
centered/community based health care. Hemophilia specialists are available 24 hours a day.

Tennessee

2393 East Tennessee Comprehensive Hemophilia Center
1924 Alcoa Highway
Knoxville, TN 37920   423-544-9625

Cheryl Zimmerman, RN

2394 First Regional Hemophilia Center
James H. Quillen College of Medicine
P.O. Box 21, 160A, ETSU
Johnson City, TN 37614   423-929-6362

Sheri Miller, RN

2395 University of Tennessee Hemophilia Clinic
3 North Dunlap, 3rd Floor
Memphis, TN 38163   901-528-6454

Marion Dugdale, MD

2396 Vanderbilt Comprehensive Hemophilia Center
2901 TVC
Nashville, TN 37232   615-322-3891

Robert L. Janco, MD

Texas

2397 Gulf States Hemophilia Diagnostic and Treatment Center
University of Texas Health Science Center Houston
6410 Fanin Street, Ste. 416
Houston, TX 77030   713-704-6025

Christopher Wicker

2398 North Texas Comprehensive Pediatric Hemophilia Center
1935 Motor Street
Dallas, TX 75235   214-920-2382

Andrea Johnson, RN, PNP

2399 South Texas Comprehensive Hemophilia Center - Santa Rosa Health Corp.
Children's Hospital
519 W Houston Street, 8th Fl
San Antonio, TX 78207   210-704-2201

John Drake, RN

Vermont

2400 Vermont Regional Hemophilia Center
1193 North Avenue
Burlington, VT 05402   802-863-7292

Miriam Husted, RN

Virginia

2401 Hemophilia Treatment Center of Tidewater Virginia
Division of Pediatric Hematology
800 West Olney Road
Norfolk, VA 23507   757-628-7000

Eric J. Werner, MD

2402 University of Virginia Hemophilia Treatment Center
Kluge Children's Rehabilitation Center
2270 Ivy Road
Charlottesville, VA 22901   804-924-5161

Julie A. Kopco, RN

Washington

2403 Puget Sound Blood Center
921 Terry Avenue
Seattle, WA 98104   206-292-6500

Arthur R. Thompson, MD, PhD

West Virginia

2404 Hemophilia Center of West Virginia
University Health Sciences Center

Morgantown, WV 26506   304-293-4639

John S. Rogers II, MD

2405 Huntington Area Hemophilia Association
Marshall University of School of Medicine
1600 Medical Center Drive Ste 3500
Huntington, WV 25701   304-691-1386
                              Fax: 304-691-1333

Andrew L. Perdleton MD

Wisconsin

2406 American Red Cross Hemophilia Center
Box 5905
Madison, WI 53705   608-233-9300

Diane Nugent, MD

2407 Eau Claire Hemophilia Center
Sacred Heart Hospital

Eau Claire, WI 54701   715-839-4121

Vicky Anderson, RN

2408 Gundersen Clinic Comprehensive Hemophilia Treatment Center
Gundersen Clinic

LaCrosse, WI 54601   608-782-7300

Susan Bock, RN

2409 Hematology Treatment Center of the Great Lakes Hemophilia Foundation
8739 Watertown Plank Road
Wauwatosa, WI 53213   414-257-2424

Joan Gill, MD

2410 Northeastern Wisconsin Hemophilia Center
St. Vincent Hospital

Green Bay, WI 54307   920-433-0111

S.E. Adair, MD

Audio Video

2411 Song of Superman
National Hemophilia Foundation
116 West 32nd Street 11th Floor
New York, NY 10001

                    800-424-2634
                    Fax: 212-328-3799
                    e-mail: info@hemophilia.org
                    www.hemophilia.org

Designed to help young people with bleeding disorders come to terms with their HIV status, sexuality, and living with HIV. The video explores issues of disclosure in relationships and safer sex through dramatic scenes and testimonials by young people living with hemophilia and/or HIV. The companion workbook contains group exercises that follow the main topics of the video and encourage discussion.

1993 49 pages

Web Sites

2412 Hemophilia Newsgroup
tile.net/news/altsupporthemophilia.html

2413 Pedbase
www.icondata.com/health/pedbase/files/HEMOPHIL.HTM

2414 Usenet: alt.support.hemophilia
www.kelleycom.com/infohtc.html

Books

2415 Avoiding Indecision and Hesitation With Hemophilia-Related Emergencies
Michael A. Coyne, MD, author

American Health Consultants
3525 Piedmont Road NE, #400
Atlanta, GA 30305

                    800-688-2421

Provides detailed information necessary for physicians, and ED staff to deal effectively and expeditiously with hemophilia emergencies.

12 pages

2416 Hemophilia Handbook
Hemophilia of Georgia, Inc
8800 Roswell Road, Suite 170
Atlanta, GA 30350
770-518-8272
800-866-4366
Fax: 770-518-3310
www.hog.org

Offers information on what hemophilia is, common factors in hemophilia, the cost and treatments offered to hemophiliacs and more.

2417 Procedure Coding for Hemophilia Treatment
Armour Pharmaceutical Company
500 Arcola Road
Collegeville, PA 19426
215-454-3720

Educational guide designed to facilitate the appropriate use of CPT codes for the hemophilia community.

Children's Books

2418 Adventures of Maxx
Nova Factor
1620 Century Centery Pky, Suite 109
Memphis, TN 38137
901-348-8129
800-424-2634
Fax: 901-385-3778

An activity book for children with hemophilia, this publication is intended to be both educational and entertaining.

1991 15 pages

2419 Harold Talks About How He Inherited Hemophilia
Hemophilia Foundation
982 Eastern Parkway
Louisville, KY 40217
502-634-8161

Children's brochure explaining hemophilia causes, symptoms and living a regular life.

2420 Understanding Hemophilia: A Young Person's Guide
Armour Pharmaceuticals Company
500 Arcola Road
Collegeville, PA 19426
800-424-2634

This publication is designed for young persons with hemophilia. Presented in very basic and accessible language, this text with colored illustrations points out what hemophilia is, how to cope and more.

1988 91 pages

Magazines

2421 HEMALOG
208 51st Street, Box No. 234
New York, NY 10022
212-725-5151
Fax: 212-725-2794
e-mail: mmca@earthlink.net

The purpose of Hemalog is to serve as a national forum for the hemophilia community, providing current news, information, opinion, and contact with others in the community. The material contained in this journal reflects the experience and opinion of a wide range of people connected with hemophilia, and encourages story and art contributions.

Quarterly

Barbara Robin Slonevsky, Publisher
Robin Slonevsky Janet, Spencer-King

2422 HemAware
National Hemophilia Foundation
116 West 32nd Street 11th Floor
New York, NY 10001
800-424-2634
Fax: 212-328-3799
e-mail: info@hemophilia.org
www.hemophilia.org

NHF magazine that offers treatment news about bleeding disorders and provides comprehensive articles on the latest developments in treatment and research as well as highlighting new programs and new resources in the field.

Bi-Monthly

2423 Human Factor
Hemophilia Health Services, Inc.
6820 Charlotte Pike
Nashville, TN 37209
800-800-6606

This journal is provided as a free service for the purpose of informing, educating and empowering the hemophilia community.

Quarterly

Newsletters

2424 Affirmations
Hemophilia Foundation of Greater Florida
4210 NW 37th Place, Suite 200
Gainesville, FL 32606
352-384-0899
800-293-6527
Fax: 352-384-0890

State association news and information.

Quarterly

Wanda Bedell, Executive Director

2425 Artery
Hemophilia Foundation of Michigan
117 N 1st Street, Suite 40
Ann Arbor, MI 48104   734-761-2535
                                   800-482-3041
                                   Fax: 734-761-3267
                                   e-mail: hfm@ic.net
                                   www.ic.net/~hfm

Offers information on the chapter's activities
and events, support groups and hotlines, technical and medical updates pertaining to the hemophilia and HIV/AIDS community.

Quarterly

Susan Lerch, Editor

2426 Big Red Factor
Nebraska Chapter - National Hemophilia Foundation
3610 Dodge Street, Suite 110-W
Omaha, NE 68105   402-342-3329
                                   Fax: 402-342-4329

Chapter newsletter offering legislative and medical updates, technology, resources, assistive devices and more for persons affected by
hemophilia and other blood disorders.

2427 Bloodlines
Hemophilia Association of San Diego County
3636 4th Avenue, Ste. 305
San Diego, CA 92103   619-560-8373

Updates membership on the newest techniques
and technologies on the treatment of hemophilia.

Quarterly

2428 Community Alert
National Hemophilia Foundation
116 West 32nd Street 11th Floor
New York, NY 10001   888-463-6643
                                  800-424-2634
                                  Fax: 212-966-9247
                                  www.infonhf.org

Features advocacy updates and medical news for
the entire bleeding disorders community.

8 pages Bi-Monthly

Christopher Rael, Editor

2429 Concentrate
Hemophilia of North Carolina
2 Centerview Drive, Ste. 51
Greensboro, NC 27407   919-852-4788

Offers information on summer camps, resources, book reviews, parent information and
articles pertaining to hemophilia.

Monthly

2430 Factor Nine News
Coalition for Hemophilia B
712 Fifth Avenue 43rd Floor
New York, NY 10019   212-554-6823
                                  Fax: 212-554-6900
                                  e-mail: cfb@web-depot.com
                                  www.web-depot.com/users/cfb

Offers information on FDA approvals, annual
meetings and the latest in technology and information regarding hemophilia.

Four/year

Kimberly Phelan, Vice President

2431 Hemophilia Headlines
Oregon Chapter - National Hemophilia Foundation
320 SW Stark St., Room 404
Portland, OR 97204   503-227-2901

Offers information on summer camps, programs
and activities of the chapter, member updates
and educational articles pertaining to hemophilia and HIV.

Quarterly

Michial Fillman, Executive Director

2432 Hemophilia Newsbriefs
Great Lakes Hemophilia Foundation
8739 Watertown Plank Road
Wauwatosa, WI 52313   414-257-0200

2433 Infusion
Kentuckian Hemophilia Foundation
982 Eastern Parkway
Louisville, KY 40217   502-634-8161
                                  800-582-2873

Offers information on summer camps, association activities and events, national projects
touching on hemophilia and HIV related disorders and articles on the newest breakthroughs
and technology for fighting bleeding disorders.

Quarterly

2434 Infusions
Northern California Chapter of the NHF
7700 Edgewater Dr, Ste 710
Oakland, CA 94621   650-568-NCHF

Informs members of medical, dental and orthopedic treatment advances and the latest research
in the field. Helps to keep people with hemophilia and their families aware of relevant local
and national meetings and includes important
updates regarding research and treatment.

Bi-Monthly

2435 Linking Factor
National Hemophilia Foundation, Utah Chapter
5635 South Waterbury Way Suite C-102
Salt Lake City, UT 84121   801-273-7471
                                  800-424-2634
                             Fax: 801-273-7488
                        www.hemophiliautah.org

A newsletter offering chapter association news
and information.

Bi-Monthly

Charles Hand, Executive Director
Hand Linda, Aagard

2436 New England Hemophilia Association Newsletter
180 Rustercraft Road
Dedham, MA 02026   781-326-7645
                          800-228-6342

Offers information on the activities and events
of the chapter, support groups, hotlines, book reviews and more pertaining to the world of the hemophiliac and their families.

Quarterly

Kevin Kelley, Editor

Pamphlets

2437 Anyone Can Have a Bleeding Problem
Hemophilia Foundation of Michigan
117 North 1st Street, Suite 40
Ann Arbor, MI 48104   734-761-2535
                             800-482-3041
                        Fax: 734-761-3267
                        e-mail: hfm@ic.net
                        www.ic.net/~hfm

Offers information on hemophilia and Von
Willebrand's Disease. How persons can get it,
prevention and causes of the illnesses.

2438 Article Reprint Exchange
HANDI - The National Hemophilia Foundation
116 West 32nd Street, 11th Floor
New York, NY 10001   212-328-3700
                            800-424-2634
                       Fax: 212-328-3777
                       e-mail: info@hemophilia.org
                       www.hemophilia.org

Offers various reprinted articles concerning hemophilia and the newest medical technology.

2439 Clotting Agents Are Lifesavers
Hemophilia Foundation of Michigan
117 N 1st Street, Suite 40
Ann Arbor, MI 48104   734-761-2535
                        Fax: 734-761-3261
                        e-mail: hfm@ic.net
                        www.ic.net/~hfm

Offers information on what hemophilia is, treatments, occurances, heredity, Von Willebrand's
Disease, patient services and direct services for
hemophiliacs and HIV/AIDS patients.

**2440 Comprehensive Services for Persons With
Hemophilia**
Hemophilia Foundation of Minnesota/Dakotas
2304 Park Avenue
Minneapolis, MN 55404   612-871-3340
                          Fax: 612-871-1359

Offers information on what hemophilia is and information and resources for persons with hemophilia and other bleeding disorders.

2441 Countdown to a Cure
Louisiana Chapter - National Hemophilia Foundation
3636 S Sherwood Forest, 390
Baton Rouge, LA 70816   504-291-1675

Offers information on chapter resources and
services for hemophiliacs and their families.

2442 Fight Hemophilia with Facts Not Fiction
Great Lakes Hemophilia Foundation
8739 Watertown Plank Road
Wauwatosa, WI 53213   414-257-0200
                          Fax: 414-257-1225

Offers information on what hemophilia is, research information and treatments.

2443 Guidelines for Finding Childcare

Elizabeth H. Fung, MSW, author

National Hemophilia Foundation
116 West 32nd Street 11th Floor
New York, NY 10001

800-424-2634
Fax: 212-328-3799
e-mail: info@hemophilia.org
www.hemopilia.org

Information for parents on how to hire a good
babysitter, information on daycare centers, how
to tell daycare staff about hemophilia, cooperative childcare and suggested reading for parents.

1987 10 pages

2444 Hemophilia, Sports, and Exercise

Marvin S. Gilbert, MD, et al, author

National Hemophilia Foundation
116 West 32nd Street 11th Floor
New York, NY 10001

800-424-2634
Fax: 212-328-3799
e-mail: info@hemophilia.org
www.hemophilia.org

Presents information for the person with a bleeding disorder or his/her parents considering participation in sports activities. Topics include
conditioning, stretching and flexibility, strength,
weight training, prophylaxis, and physical activities for children of all ages. A safety rating for
many sports activities is provided.

1996 30 pages

2445 Hemophilia: Current Medical Management

Dr. Jonathan Goldsmith, author

National Hemophilia Foundation
116 West 32nd Street 11th Floor
New York, NY 10001

800-424-2634
Fax: 212-328-3799
e-mail: info@hemophilia.org
www.hemophilia.org

Provides an overview of all aspects of hemophilia treatment, including prophylaxis, home
therapy, inhibitors, orthopedic solutions, surgery, and dental care.

1994 30 pages

**2446 How to Control Bleeds: Inspired by Vince, an
8-year-old Boy with Hemophilia**

Nora Schwetz, author

Bayer
400 Morgan Lane
West Haven, CT 06516   203-937-2765

An educational comic book story about hemophilia and treatment for bleeds.

26 pages

2447 Living with HIV: For Adolescents with Hemophilia

Bobbie Steinhart, LCSW, author

National Hemophilia Foundation
116 West 32nd Street 11th Floor
New York, NY 10001

800-424-2634
Fax: 212-328-3799
e-mail: info@hemophilia.org
www.hemophilia.org

A publication with information on living with
HIV and for adolescents with hemophilia who
are HIV-infected.

1990 8 pages

**2448 Student with Hemophilia: A Resource for the
Educator**

William A. Beiersdorfer, Maribel J. Clements, author

National Hemophilia Foundation
116 West 32nd Street 11th Floor
New York, NY 10001

800-424-2634
Fax: 212-328-3799
e-mail: info@hemophilia.org
www.hemophilia.org

Written for teachers, nurses, and other school
personnel, this booklet aims to dispel the myths
and fears surrounding hemophilia.

1995 16 pages

Carol Weisman, MSW and ACSW

2449 What Is Hemophilia?

Hemophilia of Georgia, Inc
8800 Roswell Road, Suite 170
Atlanta, GA 30350   770-518-8272
800-866-4366
Fax: 770-518-3310
www.hog.org

Offers information on what hemophilia is, common factors in hemophilia, the cost and treatments offered to hemophiliacs and more.

2450 What You Should Know About Bleeding Disorders

National Hemophilia Foundation
116 West 32nd Street 11th Floor
New York, NY 10001

800-424-2634
Fax: 212-328-3799
e-mail: info@hemophilia.org
www.hemophilia.org

Defines hemophilia, explains its effects, and provides a historical overview of treatment and treatment complications.

1991 13 pages

Camps

2451 NHF Camp Directory
National Hemophilia Foundation
116 West 32nd Street 11th Floor
New York, NY 10001

800-424-2634
Fax: 212-328-3799
e-mail: info@hemophilia.org
www.hempohilia.org

Lists camps in the United States for children with hemophilia and other coagulation disorders. Now available on web site.

16 pages

DESCRIPTION

2452 HEREDITARY FRUCTOSE INTOLERANCE
Synonym: Deficiency of phosphofructaldolase
Disorder Type: Genetic Disorder, Metabolism

Hereditary fructose intolerance is a metabolic disorder characterized by a deficiency of the enzyme phosphofructaldolase (fructose-1,6-bisphosphate aldolase), resulting in the body's inability to process or metabolize fructose, a simple carbohydrate. Fructose, found in honey, certain sweet fruits, baby food and baby formula sweeteners, and in combination with more complex sugars (disaccharides and polysaccharides), is converted in the liver into glucose that in turn is either distributed immediately for use as energy or converted into glycogen and stored in the liver, muscle, or fat for later energy use. The deficiency of the enzyme phosphofructaldolase results in the accumulation in the body of fructose-1-phosphate, a compound in the chain of fructose metabolism. This accumulation inhibits glucose production as well as the glycogen processing into energy-producing glucose.

Ingestion of fructose by affected infants may result in extremely low blood sugar (hypoglycemia), yellowing of the skin, eyes, and mucous membranes (jaundice), enlargement of the liver (hepatomegaly), bleeding from within the digestive tract, kidney involvement (i.e., proximal tubular dysfunction), vomiting, sluggishness, sweating, tremors, irritability, and seizures. Affected children have an aversion to sweets and fruits and typically do not have dental cavities (caries). However, physical findings and symptoms may be variable in their severity and manifestation.

Treatment for hereditary fructose intolerance includes total elimination of fructose from the diet. Vigilance is extremely important in that fructose is present in many foods and medicines as an additive. Other treatment may include administration of supplemental glucose to counteract the effects of hypoglycemia.

Hereditary fructose intolerance is transmitted as an autosomal recessive trait. The defective gene for this disorder is located on the long arm of chromosome 9 (9q22). Approximately one of every 40,000 is affected with this disorder.

The following organizations in the General Resources Section can provide additional information: National Organization for Rare Disorders, Inc., (NORD), Genetic Alliance, March of Dimes Birth Defects Foundation, NIH/Office of Rare Diseases, NIH/National Digestive Diseases Information Clearinghouse, Online Mendelian Inheritance in Man: www3.ncbi.nlm.nih.gov/Omim/searchomim.html

National Associations & Support Groups

2453 Research Trust for Metabolic Diseases in Children
Golden Gates Lodge
Weston Road, Crewe, Cheshire CW1
1XN United Kingdom,

Web Sites

2454 Boston University
http://bio.bu.edu/~vfunari/

2455 Oxford University
oxmedinfo.jr2.ox.ac.uk/Pathway/Disease/36355.htm

2456 Rare Genetic Diseases in Children
http://mcrcr2.med.nyu.edu/murphp01/home-new.htm

DESCRIPTION

2457 HERPES SIMPLEX

Disorder Type: Infectious Disease
Covers these related disorders: Herpes simplex virus type 1 (HSV-1), Herpes simplex virus type 2 (HSV-2)

Herpes simplex refers to a contagious infection caused by the herpes simplex virus. This infection is characterized by the formation of small, sometimes painful, fluid-filled, blister-like lesions on the skin and various mucous membranes. There are two strains of herpes simplex virus: type 1 (HSV-1) and type 2 (HSV-2). Although there is some overlapping, HSV-1 is usually responsible for lesions of the lips such as cold sores (herpes labialis), the mouth (herpetic gingivostomatitis), and the eyes (e.g., corneal lesions, conjunctivitis, etc.). HSV-2 usually produces genital herpes and herpes associated with infections of the newborn that occur before or during birth (congenital herpes). HSV-1 is transmitted by direct contact, while HSV-2 is generally transmitted through direct sexual contact. In addition, HSV-2 may be acquired by the fetus of an infected mother through the placenta or by direct contact during the birthing process.

Symptoms and findings associated with an initial or primary infection with herpes simplex virus usually appear in one to two weeks after contact and may range from no significant illness to the appearance of flu-like symptoms, sometimes in conjunction with blister-like lesions that usually scab and heal in a week to 10 days. However, newborns, malnourished infants, and individuals with compromised immune function may develop severe infection involving the entire body (systemic infection). After the primary infection, HSV becomes inactive but remains in nerve cells near the primary infection site. Recurrent episodes may be triggered by such factors as sun exposure, fever, physical and emotional stress, suppression of the immune system, the ingestion of certain medications or specific foods, and other factors. Such episodes may begin with mild irritation, itching, burning, tingling, or sometimes severe pain in the affected area followed a few hours or days later by the formation of small, fluid-filled blisters that often merge to form one large lesion. Associated symptoms and findings may include itching or discomfort in the affected area, fever, and swollen lymph nodes in the neck. The lesions sometimes become infected, especially in children. Typically, however, the lesions ulcerate and form a yellowish crust within a few days, with healing complete in about three weeks.

Symptoms associated with primary oral herpes infection (herpetic gingivostomatitis) usually appear suddenly and include pain, fever, excessive salivation, bad breath, and difficulty eating. Lesions may appear anywhere in the mouth, although the tongue and the cheeks are most frequently involved. In addition, the gums are usually inflamed and nearby lymph nodes may become enlarged. Primary episodes typically persist for about five to nine days. Lesions associated with recurrent oral herpes infection are often accompanied by itching, pain, or tingling that usually subsides within a week. Recurrent cold sore lesions sometimes precede oral herpes infections. Eye lesions may result from both primary and recurrent infections and include inflammation of the delicate mucous membranes that line the inside of the eyelids and the whites of the eyes (conjunctivitis) or inflammation and dryness involving the corneas as well as the conjunctiva.

Genital herpes most often affects adolescents and adults and is usually caused by HSV-2; however, approximately 10 to 25 percent of primary genital herpes infection results from HSV-1 through such factors as oral-genital transmission. This type of infection may be characterized by fever, painful urination, and swollen glands in the genital area. Females may develop herpetic lesions on the cervix and, less commonly, in the vagina and on the external genitalia while males typically develop lesions on the penis. Many patients exhibit few symptoms during an episode; however, the virus may be transmitted during this time through sexual activity or from a mother to her newborn.

Additional findings and complications associated with herpes simplex include a condition called herpetic whitlow, which is an infection of the finger resulting from transmission of HSV through a skin break. Whitlow is characterized by painful blistering and swelling at the fingertip. Eczema herpeticum is a severe condition in which patients with certain preexisting inflammatory skin conditions are infected with HSV and develop widespread blistering. Potentially life-threatening associated findings include high fever; excessive fluid loss (dehydration); decreases in the levels of essential elements known as electrolytes in the fluid portion of the blood (e.g., calcium, potassium, and sodium); spread of HSV to the brain and other organs; and bacterial infection. In addition, patients with suppressed immune systems are at risk for potentially life-threatening complications resulting from spread of disease to the liver, lungs, central nervous system, and other organs.

Treatment for herpes simplex is dependent upon the site affected as well as the severity and type of infection. For example, keeping affected areas dry is an important aspect of treatment as moisture tends to promote bacterial infection. Therefore, mild infections such as those associated with herpes of the lip may be treated by cleansing of the affected area with soap and water followed by careful drying of the lesion. Secondary bacterial infections may be treated with antibiotics. In addition, antiviral drugs such as acyclovir are often effective in treating various types of infection as well as preventing recurrences if administered during high-risk periods. Adolescents and young adults may require counseling or training in order to reduce the risk of transmission. Other treatment is symptomatic and supportive.

The following organizations in the General Resources Section can provide additional information: National Organization for Rare Disorders, Inc. (NORD), March of Dimes Birth Defects Foundation, NIH/National Institute of Allergy and Infectious Disease, World Health Organization (WHO), Centers for Disease Control (CDC)

Web Sites

2458 American Social Health Association
www.bcpl.lib.md.us/~psmith/ashahelp.html

2459 Child Health Research Project
ih.jshph.edu/chr/chr.htm

2460 HerpeSite
members.aol.com/herpesite/index.html

2461 Herpes.com
www.herpes.com/

2462 International Herpes Management Forum
www.ihmf.org/

2463 NOAH
www.noah.cuny.edu/aids/gmhc/herpes.html

2464 Slack
www.slackinc.com/child/idc/idchome.htm

2465 Vanderbilt University
www.mc.vanderbilt.edu/peds/pidl.infect/herpes.htm

2466 Virtual Hospital
www.vh.org/Providers/Teachingfiles/CNSin

Books

2467 Understanding Herpes

Lawrence R. Stanberry, M.D., Ph.D., author

University Press of Mississippi
3825 Ridgewood Road
Jackson, MS 39211
601-432-6205
800-737-7788
Fax: 601-432-6217
e-mail: press@ihl.state.ms.us
www.upress.ms.us

A most informative overview of herpes written for the general reader.

120 pages
ISBN: 1-578060-40-0

DESCRIPTION

2468 HIRSCHSPRUNG DISEASE

Synonyms: Aganglionic megacolon, Congenital aganglionic megacolon

Disorder Type: Birth Defect, Genetic Disorder

May involve these systems in the body (see Section III):

Digestive System

Hirschsprung disease is a gastrointestinal disorder that is usually apparent within the first few days after birth. However, in some affected infants, symptoms may not become apparent until the first weeks of life. Hirschsprung disease is characterized by absence of groups of certain nerve cell bodies (ganglia) in the smooth muscle wall of the large intestine. In most affected infants, the affected segment begins at the ring-shaped involuntary muscle of the anus (internal anal sphincter) and extends to the lowest region of the colon (sigmoid colon). However, in some cases, this segment may extend to involve the entire colon.

In infants with Hirschsprung disease, absence of these nerve groups results in impairment or absence of rhythmic contractions that propel food through the digestive system (peristalsis). Due to impaired peristalsis, most affected newborns have inadequate or delayed passage of meconium, the thick, sticky, darkish green material that accumulates in the fetal intestines and forms a newborn's first stools. Although some affected newborns may pass meconium normally, they may subsequently experience chronic constipation. In infants with Hirschsprung disease, failure to properly pass stools results in widening of the colon (megacolon) above the affected segment and severe abdominal bloating (abdominal distension). Additional symptoms and findings may include episodes of diarrhea, nausea and vomiting, dehydration, loss of appetite (anorexia) and malnutrition, failure to grow and gain weight at the expected rate (failure to thrive), listlessness (lethargy), and other abnormalities. In addition, widening of the colon may result in deterioration of the colon's mucous membranes (mucosal barrier), potentially allowing increased reproduction of certain bacteria and associated inflammation of the colon (i.e., enterocolitis). In severe cases, severe diarrhea and potentially life-threatening complications may result.

In infants with Hirschsprung disease, treatment includes surgical removal of the affected area of the colon and rejoining of healthy areas of the colon and rectum. In some patients, before surgical correction, a temporary colostomy may be required. Colostomy is a procedure in which the lower end of the healthy region of the colon is connected to a surgically created opening in the abdominal wall.

Hirschsprung disease affects approximately one in 5,000 newborns and is considered the most common cause of lower intestinal obstruction in infants during the first month of life. The condition is about four times as common in males as females. Hirschsprung disease may occur in association with other disorders or conditions that are apparent at birth (congenital disorders) or as an isolated finding for unknown reasons (sporadic occurrence). In addition, there have been many reports of Hirschsprung disease in infants within certain families (kindreds). Researchers suggest that sporadic and familial cases may result from abnormal changes or mutations of one of several different genes expressed either alone or together (polygenic). Depending upon the specific disease gene or genes, the condition may have autosomal dominant, autosomal recessive, or polygenic inheritance.

The following organizations in the General Resources Section can provide additional information: National Organization for Rare Disorders, Inc., (NORD), Genetic Alliance, March of Dimes Birth Defects Foundation, NIH/Office of Rare Diseases, Online Mendelian Inheritance in Man: www3.ncbi.nlm.nih.gov/Omim/searchomim.html, NIH/National Digestive Diseases Information Clearinghouse

National Associations & Support Groups

2469 American Hirschprung Disease Association
22 1/2 Spruce Street
Brattleboro, VT 05301   802-257-0603

2470 American Pseudo-Obstruction and Hirschsprung's Disease Society
158 Pleasant Street
North Andover, MA 01845   978-685-4477
Fax: 978-685-4488
e-mail: aphs@tiac.net
www.tiac.net/users/aphs

Promotes public awareness of gastrointestinal motility disorders, in particular intestinal pseudo-obstruction and Hirschsprung's disease; provides education and support to individuals and families of children who have been diagnosed with these disorders through parent-to-parent contact, publications, and educational symposia; and encourages and supports medical research in the area of gastrointestinal motility disorders.

2471 Hirschsprung Disease-American Pseudo Obstruction/Hirschsprung Disease Society
P.O. Box 772
Medford, MA 02155   617-395-4225

2472 Intestinal Pseudoobstruction (IP) Support Network
34929 Elm
Wayne, MI 48184   313-729-7912

2473 Pull-Through Network
1126 Grant Street
Wheaton, IL 60187   312-665-1268

2474 Support for Parents of Ostomy Children
Division of United Ostomy Association
11385 Cedarbrook Road
Roscoe, IL 61073   815-623-8034

2475 United Ostomy Association
36 Executive Park, Suite 120
Irvine, CA 92714   714-660-8624
800-826-0826

Web Sites

2476 NIH News Advisory
www.nih.gov/news/pr/jan98/nhgri-0.9.htm

2477 Online Pediatric Surgery
home.coqui.net/titolugo/handbook.htm#IIIF

2478 PedBase
www.icondata.com/health/ped-base/files/HIRSCHSP.HTM

2479 Vanderbilt University
www.mc.vanderbilt.edu/peds/pidl/gi/agang-meg.htm

Newsletters

2480 Pull-thru Network News
4 Woody Lane
Westport, CT 06880   203-221-7530
e-mail: pullthru@aol.com
www.members.aol.com/

Provides emotional support and information to patients and families of children who have had or will have pull-through surgery to correct an imperforate anus or associated malformation, Hirschsprung's disease, or other fecal incontinence problems; sponsors online discussion groups.

Pamphlets

2481 Hirschsprung's Disease
Nat'l Digestive Diseases Information Clearinghouse
2 Information Way
Bethesda, MD 20892   301-654-3810
Fax: 301-907-8906
e-mail: nddic@info.niddk.nih.gov
www.niddk.nih.gov

DESCRIPTION

2482 HISTIOCYTOSIS

Synonyms: Class I histiocytoses, Langerhans cell histiocytosis, LCH

Disorder Type: Neoplasm: Benign or Malignant Tumor

Histiocytosis X, also known as Langerhans cell histiocytosis, LCH, or Class I histiocytoses, refers to a group of three similar disorders called eosinophilic granuloma, Hand-Schuller-Christian disease, and Letterer-Siwe disease. These disorders are all characterized by the excessive production and accumulation of certain types of tissue cells known as histiocytes, resulting in benign growth or scar formation. Characteristic findings and symptoms are variable and depend upon the organ or organ system affected; however, approximately 80 percent of individuals with LCH have skeletal involvement. Associated bone lesions may appear in isolation or in many parts of the body. These lesions occur most often in the skull, although their appearance in other areas of the skeleton is not uncommon. Some individuals may also experience complications resulting from bone involvement. For example, involvement of certain bone (i.e., mastoid) near the ear may result in chronic ear infections and persistent drainage. Involvement of certain weight-bearing bones may result in fractures.

Letterer-Siwe disease occurs during early childhood, usually before three years of age. This disease is characterized by skin eruptions, enlargement of the liver and spleen (hepatosplenomegaly) and certain lymph nodes, and abnormally low levels of circulating red blood cells resulting in anemia. In addition, some children may experience involvement of the lungs, sometimes resulting in lung collapse (pneumothorax). Hand-Schuller-Christian disease often appears during early childhood and is characterized by bulging of the eyeballs (exophthalmos); excessive urinary excretion (polyuria), a decrease in body fluid volume (dehydration), and excessive thirst; elevated cholesterol levels; and involvement of soft tissues and bone. Eosinophilic granulomas most often occur during the second to fourth decade of life; however, they develop during childhood, especially between the ages of five to 10 years. Benign growths may develop in the skull, jaw, and the long bones of the arms and legs, sometimes resulting in pain and fractures. In addition, lung involvement may result in respiratory symptoms such as coughing and shortness of breath, fever, and lung collapse.

Other findings and symptoms sometimes associated with Class I histiocytoses may include growth retardation, thyroid deficiency, and other abnormalities resulting from disruption in pituitary gland function or involvement of another gland in the brain known as the hypothalamus; difficulty walking and other neurologic symptoms resulting from involvement of the central nervous system; and additional irregularities of the blood resulting from involvement of the bone marrow.

Although the exact cause of each of the disorders that comprise Class I histiocytoses is unknown, it is believed that Letterer-Siwe disease may be inherited as an autosomal recessive trait and that the diseases develop as a result of disturbances within the immune system. Treatment for LCH depends upon the extent and severity of involvement. For example, if only one organ or organ system (e.g., skeletal or skin, etc.) is affected, the disease is often self-limited; therefore, treatment may be directed toward control and resolution of specific lesions through low-dose radiation therapy or removal by means of a scraping procedure (curettage). If more than one system of the body is affected, treatment may involve a chemotherapy regimen that includes the use of one or two specific drugs (i.e., etoposide and vinblastine). More resistant disease may necessitate the use of other immunosuppressive drugs, bone marrow transplantation, or other experimental treatments. Other treatment is symptomatic and supportive.

The following organizations in the General Resources Section can provide additional information: National Organization for Rare Disorders, Inc., (NORD), NIH/Office of Rare Diseases, March of Dimes Birth Defects Foundation, Genetic Alliance, Online Mendelian Inheritance in Man: www3.ncbi.nlm.nih.gov/Omim/searchomim.html, NIH/National Cancer Institute

National Associations & Support Groups

2483 Histiocytosis Association of America
302 N Broadway
Pitman, NJ 08071　　　　　609-589-6606
　　　　　　　　　　　　800-548-2758
　　　　　　　　　　　Fax: 609-589-6614
　　　　　　　　e-mail: hisiocyte@aol.com
　　　　　　　　　　　　www.histio.org

Committed to the promotion of scientific research into the Histiocytosis and the development of improved control and management of these diseases. Promotes public education and produces educational materials.

2484 Histiocytosis Support Group UK
23 Maple Grove, Woburn, Sands, Milton Keynes Intl
MK17 8ON,
United Kingdom
　　　　　　e-mail: hsguk@mcmail.com
　　　　http://www.histiocytosis.mcmail.com

2485 Histiocytosis-X Association of America
609 New York Road
Glassboro, NJ 08208　　　　609-881-4911
　　　　　　　　　　　　800-548-2758
　　　　　　　　　　　Fax: 609-589-6614

Web Sites

2486 National Histicytosis Organizations
www.histio.rog/

2487 Texas Children's Cancer Center
www.tccc.tch.tmc.edu

DESCRIPTION

2488 HODGKIN'S DISEASE

Synonym: Hodgkin's lymphoma

Disorder Type: Neoplasm: Benign or Malignant Tumor

Covers these related disorders: Hodgkin's disease, lymphocyte depletion type, Hodgkin's disease, lymphocyte predominance type, Hodgkin's disease, mixed cellularity type, Hodgkin's disease, nodular sclerosing type

May involve these systems in the body (see Section III):

Lymphatic System

Hodgkin's disease is a malignant disorder (cancer) characterized by painless, progressive enlargement of the lymph nodes, spleen, and other lymphoid tissues (lymphoma). The lymphatic system includes a network of vessels that collect a fluid known as lymph from different areas of the body and drain this fluid into the bloodstream. As lymph moves through the lymphatic system, it is filtered by a network of lymph nodes, which are small structures located along the course of the lymphatic vessels. Most lymph nodes that can be felt (palpable) are located in the neck, mouth, and groin and under the arms (axillae). Lymph nodes store certain white blood cells and are thought to play a role in producing antibodies, thus functioning as part of the body's immune system.

Malignancies of lymph tissue, known as lymphomas, are the third most common form of cancer affecting children in the United States. Approximately 13 per one million children are affected by lymphoma in the U.S. each year. There are two main categories of lymphoma, including Hodgkin's disease and non-Hodgkin's lymphoma. Although Hodgkin's disease may affect individuals of any age, it usually occurs between the ages of 15 and 35 or after age 50. In children, the disease is most common during late childhood or early adolescence and rarely affects those younger than five years of age. About 6,000 to 7,000 cases of the disease occur in the U.S. annually. Hodgkin's dis-ease most commonly affects males, Caucasians stein-Barr virus (EBV) plays some role. In addition, some familial cases have been reported, suggesting potential genetic mechanisms.

Hodgkin's disease is characterized by the presence of relatively large, abnormal white blood cells that have more than one nucleus and a distinctive appearance under a microscope. These cancerous cells, known as Reed-Sternberg cells, may be seen during the microscopic examination of small tissue samples removed from affected lymph nodes or other lymphoid tissues. Hodgkin's disease is categorized into four main subtypes based upon the number and relative proportion of such cells as well as the proportions of certain other white blood cells (e.g., plasma cells, eosinophils, macrophages, etc.). The frequency of the different subtypes varies with age. For example, nodular sclerosing type is the most common form of the disease and affects approximately 50 percent of children and up to 70 percent of adolescents with Hodgkin's disease. Another subtype, known as the mixed cellularity type, affects about 40 to 50 percent of patients, and the lymphocyte predominance type of the disease primarily occurs in males and younger patients. The fourth subtype, called lymphocyte depletion type, is the rarest and most aggressive form of the disorder and occurs in fewer than 10 percent of patients.

Hodgkin's disease usurse of the lymphatic vessels. As the disease progresses, the malignancy may spread from lymph nodes and infiltrate certain organs, particularly the spleen, lungs, liver, and bone marrow. Most patients initially experience painless swelling of lymph nodes in the neck or, in some cases, under the arm or in the groin area. Some may gradually develop generalized symptoms including fever, night sweats, fatigue, listlessness (lethargy), generalized itching (pruritus), loss of appetite (anorexia), and weight loss. Involvement of other organs or tissues may cause varying symptoms. For example, if the lungs are affected, patients may experience coughing and breathlessness. Advanced involvement of the bone marrow may result in abnormally low levels of circulating red blood cells (anemia), platelets (thrombocytopenia), or certain white blood cells (neutropenia). Advancing disease may cause progressive impairment of the body's immune system, resulting in an increased susceptibility to certain infections. In patients with severe disease progression, infection with certain microorganisms that typically cause no or only minor symptoms in healthy individuals may result in severe or potentially life-threatening complications.

Hodgkin's disease is classified into four major stages based upon the groups of lymph nodes affected, any other involved organs, and certain associated findings. Treatment of patients with the disease varies, depending on the stage of the disease and other factors. For patients in early stages who have localized disease and have obtained full growth, radiation therapy alone may be effective. However, up to 15 percent of such patients may experience recurrences, requiring therapy with certain anticancer drugs (combination chemotherapy). In patients with advanced disease, combination chemotherapy may include the drugs doxorubicin (Adriamycin), bleomycin, vinblastine, and dacarbazine (known as ABVD) or mechlorethamine, vincristine (Oncovin), procarbazine, and prednisone (called MOPP). Physicians who specialize in the treatment of childhood cancers (pediatric oncologists) often select alternating therapy with MOPP and ABVD in combination with low-dose radiation therapy due to its high success and a reduction in certain long-term effects potentially associated with treatment for Hodgkin's disease. For example, such combination chemotherapy/radiation therapy may help reduce the risk of potential growth defects in affected children, damage to heart and lung tissue, infertility, or the development of certain secondary malignancies later in life, such as acute myeloid leukemia (AML) or certain solid tumors. Patients should receive ongoing monitoring throughout life to ensure prompt detection and treatment of possible recurrences or secondary malignancies.

The following organizations in the General Resources Section can provide additional information: Candlelighters Childhood Cancer Foundation, Candlelighters Childhood Cancer Foundation Canada, National Childhood Cancer Foundation, National Cancer Foundation, NIH/National Cancer Institute

National Associations & Support Groups

2489 Cure for Lymphoma Foundation
215 Lexington Avenue
New York, NY 10016
212-213-9595
Fax: 212-213-1987
e-mail: infocfl@aol.com
www.cfl.org

2490 Leukemia Society of America, Inc.
600 Third Avenue, 4th Floor
New York, NY 10016
212-573-8484
800-955-4572
Fax: 212-856-9686
e-mail: infocenter@leukemia.org
www.leukemia.org

The Leukemia Society will give the caller the address and phone number for the nearest local chapter. Application for financial aid is made to the local chapter. It is important to apply as soon as possible after diagnosis.

2491 Lymphoma Association (UK)
P.O. Box 275, Haddenham, Aylesbury
Bucks Intl HP17 8JJ UK,
England
www.lymphoma.org.uk

2492 Lymphoma Research Foundation Canada
2100-1075 West Georgia St
Vancouver, BC, Canada, V6E
Canada
Fax: 604-631-3232
e-mail: pmanson@lymphoma.ca
www.lymphoma.ca

2493 Lymphoma Research Foundation of America
8800 Venice Boulevard, Suite 207
Los Angeles, CA 90034
310-204-7040
800-500-9976
Fax: 310-204-7043
e-mail: LRFA@aol.com
www.lymphoma.org

Pamphlets

2494 Hodgkin's Disease and Non-Hodgkin's Lymphomas
Leukemia and Lymphoma Society

800-955-4572

Explanation of the disease, its symptoms, diagnosis, prognosis and treatment, psychological responses to a confirmed diagnosis and current research.

36 pages

DESCRIPTION

2495 HOMOCYSTINURIA

Disorder Type: Genetic Disorder, Metabolism
Covers these related disorders: Homocystinuria Type I (Classic homocystinuria), Homocystinuria Type II, Homocystinuria Type III

Homocystinuria is a metabolic disorder characterized by an inborn error in the metabolism of the amino acid methionine. There are three types of homocystinuria, each resulting from a deficiency or defect of a specific enzyme or compound that is essential in the processing of methionine.

Homocystinuria Type I (Classic homocystinuria) is caused by a deficiency of the enzyme cystathionine synthase. Although symptoms and physical findings are not apparent at birth, early symptoms may include delays in development and failure to thrive. Characteristic findings, which are often not apparent until after the age of three years, may include eye abnormalities such as dislocation of the lens of the eyes (ectopia lentis), followed by nearsightedness (myopia) and tremors of the iris (iridodonesis). Other physical findings may include skeletal abnormalities such as osteoporosis, sideways curvature of the spine (scoliosis), either a sunken or prominent chest, and a condition known as genu valgum in which the legs curve inward causing the knees to touch (knock-knee) and the space between the feet to increase. Affected children often have a fair complexion, blue eyes, sparse blonde hair, and a characteristic flushed face (malar flush). In addition, blood clots (thromboemboli), particularly in the brain, may occur at any time, possibly resulting in paralysis, seizures, heart problems, and high blood pressure. Laboratory findings may include elevated levels of both methionine and the sulfur compound homocystine in body fluids. Mental retardation is apparent in approximately 65 percent of affected people. It is estimated that about 50 percent of patients experience some form of psychiatric disorder.

Treatment for classic homocystinuria includes aggressive vitamin B6 supplementation. In addition, restriction of foods that contain methionine is recommended in conjunction with supplementation of cysteine, also a sulfur-containing amino acid. In some affected individuals who do not respond to vitamin B6 treatment, administration of betaine may be effective. Classic homocystinuria is inherited as an autosomal recessive trait and occurs in approximately one in 200,000 live births. The gene for cystathionine synthase is located on the long arm of chromosome 21 (21q22.3).

Homocystinuria Type II is transmitted as an autosomal recessive trait and results from a defect in the formation of methylcobalamin. Characteristic symptoms and findings depend on the particular underlying defect. Some children with homocystinuria type II may also have a condition called methylmalonic aciduria characterized by excessive methylmalonic acid in the urine. Symptoms usually develop in the early months of life and may include difficulty in feeding, listlessness, vomiting, diminished muscle tone (hypotonia), and delays in development. Treatment for this form of homocystinuria includes vitamin B12 supplementation.

Homocystinuria Type III, a very rare form of this disorder, results from a deficiency of the enzyme methylenetetrahydrofolate reductase, also essential to the maintenance of methionine. Symptoms and physical findings are extremely variable and depend upon the extent of the deficiency. Complete absence of this enzyme may result in life-threatening episodes of respiratory distress as well as seizure-like muscle contractions (myoclonus). A partial enzyme deficiency may cause convulsions, an abnormally small head (microcephaly), mental retardation, and muscular irregularities. Occasional findings may include psychiatric disturbances, abnormalities of certain blood vessels, and inflammation or degenerative changes of specific nerves. In addition, blood clot activity may be apparent in some affected individuals.

Treatment for homocystinuria type III may include supplementation with folic acid, vitamin B6, vitamin B12, methionine, and betaine. Early intervention with betaine has a particularly effective outcome. Homocystinuria Type III is transmitted as an autosomal recessive trait. The gene for methylenetetrahydrofolate reductase is located on the short arm of chromosome 1 (1p36.3).

The following organizations in the General Resources Section can provide additional information: Genetic Alliance, National Organization of Rare Disorders, Inc., (NORD), March of Dimes Birth Defects Foundation, Online Mendelian Inheritance in Man: www3.ncbi.nlm.nih.gov/Omim/searchomim.html, NIH/National Digestive Diseases Information Clearinghouse

National Associations & Support Groups

2496 ARC
500 East Border Street, Suite 300
Arlington, TX 76010   817-261-6003
                             800-433-5255
                    TDD: 817-277-0553

Parent to Parent (P-P) programs provide informational and emotional support to parents who have a child, adolescent, or adult family member with special needs. P-P programs offer an important connection for a parent who is seeking support for special disability issue, by matching him or her with a trained vetern parent who has already been there.

2497 National Digestive Diseases Information Clearinghouse
9000 Rockville Pike
Bethesda, MD 20892   301-654-3810
                           800-891-5389
                    Fax: 301-907-8906

Conducts and supports research and provides leadership for a national program on diabetes, endocrinology and metabolic diseases; digestive diseases and nutrition; and kidney, urologic and hematologic diseases.

2498 Research Trust for Metabolic Diseases in Children
Golden Gates Lodge Weston Rd
Crewe, Cheshire, UK, CW1   127-025-0021

Dedicated to providing the most up-to-date medical knowledge for the families and friends of people suffering from this and related diseases.

Web Sites

2499 Maryland Department of Health
www.dhmh.state.md.us/cpha/ohd/html/homocys.htm

2500 Oxford University
oxmedinfo.jr2.ox.ac.uk/Pathway/Disease/23584.htm

2501 Pedbase
www.icondata.com/health/pedbase/files/HOMOCYST.HTM

2502 Rare Genetic Diseases in Children (NYU)
http://mcrcr2.med.nyu.edu/murphp01/homosup.htm

2503 Tyler for Life Foundation
www.tylerforlife.com

DESCRIPTION

2504 HYDROCEPHALUS

Synonym: Hydrocephaly

Covers these related disorders: Acute hydrocephalus, Occult tension hydrocephalus, Overt tension hydrocephalus

May involve these systems in the body (see Section III):

Nervous System

Hydrocephalus is a general term used to describe a group of conditions characterized by the accumulation of cerebrospinal fluid (CSF) around the brain. This fluid, which acts as a protective shock absorber for the brain and spinal cord, flows through the four cavities in the brain (ventricles); through the cavity containing the spinal fluid (spinal canal); and between layers of the membrane that surrounds the brain and spinal cord (subarachnoid space). Obstructed flow or impaired absorption of the CSF results in increasing fluid pressure within the brain, which may lead to abnormal enlargement of the cavities in the brain. Hydrocephalus is thought to affect approximately one in 500 to 1,500 births. The condition may occur as a result of certain malformations that are present at birth, such as Arnold-Chiari malformation or Dandy-Walker syndrome, certain infectious diseases, head injuries, bleeding within the brain, or certain tumors.

Symptoms associated with hydrocephalus may vary, depending upon the nature of the underlying abnormality, the age of onset, and the rate and duration of increasing pressure within the brain. Hydrocephalus may be apparent at birth (congenital) or develop during the first few months or years of life. Because the fibrous joints of the skull have not fused or completely closed, rapid enlargement of the head may occur. The forehead appears abnormally prominent; the skin over the skull is thin with obvious scalp veins; and the face may appear relatively small. Additional symptoms and findings may include difficulties feeding, irritability, sluggishness, lack of interest in surroundings,

lack of normal reflex responses, and downward turning of the eyes. Progression of the condition without treatment may result in extreme drowsiness, episodes of uncontrolled electrical disturbances in the brain (seizures), and potentially life-threatening complications.

In other children, hydrocephalus becomes apparent after the bones of the skull are fused (i.e., after two years of age). Some children may have no apparent symptoms, whereas others may have mild, intermittent, or progressive symptoms. These symptoms may include headaches, easy distractibility, poor memory, and progressively impaired walking and balance. Others may experience an acute form of hydrocephalus in which there is rapidly increasing intracranial pressure, causing severe headache, vomiting, visual disturbances, increasing drowsiness over the period of minutes or hours, potential coma, and possibly life-threatening complications.

Treatment of infants and children with hydrocephalus depends upon the underlying cause of the condition. Therapeutic measures may include use of certain medications, such as acetazolamide and furosemide, that help to reduce the rate of cerebrospinal fluid production. Other treatment options may include surgical removal of any obstruction or surgical implantation of a specialized device known as a shunt. Shunts allow excess fluid to drain away from the brain to another part of the body for absorption into the bloodstream. After treatment, many affected children may continue to have associated impairment, such as intellectual deficits, impaired memory, and visual abnormalities. Physicians may regularly monitor affected children and suggest a variety of multidisciplinary measures.

The following organizations in the General Resources Section can provide additional information: Genetic Alliance, March of Dimes Birth Defects Foundation, NIH/National Institute of Neurological Disorders and Stroke, Online Mendelian Inheritance in Man: www3.ncbi.nlm.nih.gov/Omim/searchomim.html

National Associations & Support Groups

2505 Association for Spina Bifida and Hydrocephalus
ASBAH House, 42 Park Road
Peterborough, PE1-2UQ UK,
England

www.asbah.demon.co.uk/

Organization that provides services to those
with spina bifida or hydrocephalus and the people that care for them. Also provides advocacy
and education.

2506 Association of Birth Defect Children, Inc.
930 Woodcock Road, Suite 225
Orlando, FL 32803   407-245-7035
                                    800-313-2223
                            Fax: 407-895-0824
            e-mail: abdc@birthdefects.org
                       www.birthdefects.org

Organization devoted to dissemination of data
pertaining to birth related malformations.

**2507 Association of Hydrocephalus Education Advocacy
& Discussion (AHEAD)**
1730 Autumn Leaf Lane
Huntington Valley, PA 19006   215-355-4728

Organized by young adults with hydrocephalus
for the purpose of providing telephone support
nationwide.

Lane Borden, NE Regional Contact

2508 Guardians of Hydrocephalus Research Foundation
National Headquarters
2618 Avenue Z
Brooklyn, NY 11235   718-743-4473
                                    800-458-8655
                            Fax: 718-743-1171
            e-mail: ghrf2618@aol.com

The Foundation offers an information and referral service to the afflicted hydrocephalic, nationwide. Our goal is to wipe out hydrocephalus.
Includes referral to doctors, video, newsletter
and satellite information center and parenting
network.

10,500 members

Michael Fischetti, Founder
Soriano Katherine, National Vice President

2509 Hydrocephalus Association
870 Market Street Suite 955
San Francisco, CA 94102   415-732-7040
                            Fax: 415-732-7044
            e-mail: hydroassoc@aol.com
        www.heurosurgery.mgh.harvard.edu/ha/

The Association provides support, education
and advocacy for families and professionals.
The goal is to insure that families and individuals dealing with the complexities of hydrocephalus receive: personal support, comprehensive
educational materials, and on-going medical
care.

Emily S. Fudge, Executive Director
Fudge Jennifer, Henerlau

2510 Hydrocephalus Foundation Inc.
910 Rear Broadway
Saugus, MA 01906   617-942-1161
            www.neurosurgery.mgh.harvard.edu

Foundation established to assist patients and
their families in the transition from diagnosis to
the return to a normal life. Also offers emotional support and assistance in research for
treatment.

2511 Hydrocephalus Parent Support Group
9425 Sky Park Court, Ste 130
San Diego, CA 92123   619-268-8252

2512 Hydrocephalus Support Group, Inc.
P.O. Box 4236
Chesterfield, MO 63006   314-532-8228
                            Fax: 314-995-4108
            e-mail: hydro@inlink.com

Provides education and support for hydrocephalus patients and their families. The HSG puts out
a quarterly newspaper, gives parent referrals
and has a library with articles and tapes about
hydrocephalus.

2513 National Hydrocephalus Foundation
12413 Centralia Road
Lakewood, CA 90715   562-402-3523
                                    888-260-1789
                            Fax: 562-924-6666
            e-mail: hydrobrat@earthlink.net
        www.geocities.com/HotSprings/Villa/2300

Dedicated to supplying both audio and visual resources to victims of the disorder.

Debbie Fields, Executive Director

**2514 Society for the Rehabilitation of the Facially
Disfigured, Inc.**
550 First Avenue
New York, NY 10016   212-340-5400

2515 Spina Bifida and Hydrocephalus Association of Canada
220-388 Donald Street
Winnipeg, Canada, MA R3B   204-925-3650
                                  800-565-9488
                             Fax: 204-925-3654
                        e-mail: spinab@mts.net
                                  www.sbhac.ca

Dedicated to improving the quality of life of individuals with spina bifida and/or hydrocephalus and their families through awareness, education, and research. Offers a variety of educational guides and materials for schools, professionals, parents, and the general public.

International

2516 International Federation for Hydrocephalus and Spina Bifida
Attn. David Bagares
c/o RBU Gata 3
Stockholm,
Sweden

                        www.asbah.demon.co.uk

Provides information, assistance, and support to inidviduals affected by hydrocephalus and their family members. Offers patient referrals, engages inpatient advocacy, offers networking serices and promotes research.

State Agencies & Support Groups

California

2517 Hydrocephalus Parent Support Group
9245 Sky Park Court, Suite 130
San Diego, CA 92123   619-268-8252

Determined to provide support to the parent and relatives of the children stricken with the disorder.

2518 Hydrocephalus Support Group of Southern California
412 North Coast Highway, #131
Laguna Beach, CA 92651   949-551-6865
                           Fax: 949-497-5518

Founded in 1976, this group was formed as a group of concerned families and patients with hydrocephalus to share information and experiences in dealing with this disease, locally and nationwide.

Fay Lavoy, President
Lavoy Marilee, Stockman

2519 Sacramento Area Hydrocephalus Group
7588 Sylvan Creek Court
Citrus Heights, CA 95610   916-721-9986

Founded in 1992, the group is divided into age groups for support.

Janet Kirkman

Massachusetts

2520 Hydrocephalus Support Group
55 Lake Avenue North
Wooster, MA 01655   617-856-3403

Recently founded, the group provides support and education to families in central Massachusetts and southern New Hampshire.

Dorothy Hutchins, Co-Facilitator
Hutchins Kathleen, Davidson

Michigan

2521 Hydrocephalus Support Group - Michigan
Children's Hospital of Michigan
3901 Beaubien
Detroit, MI 48201   313-745-5437
                      Fax: 313-993-8744

Founded in 1992, this group provides information to families and gives them support.

Mary Smellie-Decker, RN/MSN, Clinical Nurse Spec.

New Jersey

2522 Hydrocephalus Parents Support Group
329 West Frech Avenue
Manville, NJ 08835   908-722-4691

Founded in 1993, the group provides support for parents of children with hydrocephalus.

Andrea Liptak, Founder

New York

2523 New York University Medical Center Auxillary of Tisch Hospital
560 - 1st Avenue
New York, NY 10016   212-263-5040

Conducts national symposiums on hydrocephalus.

Doris Farrelly, Contact

Pennsylvania

2524 Hydrocephalus Association of Philadelphia
P.O. Box 2099
Boothwyn, PA 19061

Founded in 1992, the Association provides support, information, advocacy and telephone support to families in Pennsylvania, New Jersey, and Delaware.

Rita McAdams, Contact

Rhode Island

2525 Hydrocephalus Association of Rhode Island
P.O. Box 343
Valley Falls, RI 02864   401-723-6065
                               Fax: 401-722-1166

Founded in 1993, the mission of this Association is to provide information, support and advocacy for individuals with hydrocephalus and for friends and family members.

Gabriella Halmi, Director

Texas

2526 Hydrocephalus Association of North Texas
P.O. Box 670552
Dallas, TX 75637   903-528-2877
                         Fax: 903-528-8097

Founded in 1987, the mission is to provide information and support to parents of children with hydrocephalus in Texas and neighboring states.

Jana Dransfield, Director

Washington

2527 Hydrocephalus Support Group of Seattle
2001 Eastlake Avenue E, #1
Seattle, WA 98102   206-324-4084

Founded in 1993, the group of Seattle provides support to individuals with hydrocephalus.

Kim Anderson, Director

Wisconsin

2528 Fox Valley Hydrocephalus Support Group
W5929 Highway KK
Appleton, WI 54915   920-739-1751

Founded in 1990, the group provides referrals for parents and information to the community and throughout Wisconsin.

Donna Uitenbroek, Director

Research Centers

2529 Hydrocephalus Research Foundation, Inc.
1670 Green Oak Circle
Lawrenceville, GA 30243   770-995-9570
                           Fax: 770-995-8982
                  e-mail: ann_liakos@atlmug.org

Provides information, assistance, and support to individuals affected by hydrocephalus and their family members. Offers patient referrals, engages inpatient advocacy, offers networking services, and promotes research.

2530 Seeking Techniques Advancing Research in Shunts (STARS)
1289 North Glenhurst
Birmingham, MI 48009   248-644-7827
                         Fax: 248-647-5711

Audio Video

2531 Hydrocephalus, a Neglected Disease
Guardians of Hydrocephalus Research Foundation
2618 Avenue Z
Brooklyn, NY 11235   718-748-4473
                            800-458-8658
                       Fax: 718-743-1171

Web Sites

2532 Beth Israel Medical Center-Hydrocephalus
www.bimc.edu

2533 HYCEPH-L
www.geocities.com/HotSprings/Villa/2020/

2534 Hudrocephalus Brochure
www.aans.org/pubpages/patres/hydrobroch

2535 Hydrocephalus Fact Sheet (Harvard)
neurosurgery.mgh.harvard.edu/ha/fact-sht.htm

2536 Hydrocephalus Facts & Links
members.nova.org/~twinkee/HydroLinks

2537 Hydrocephalus Index
www.bgsm.edu/bgsm/surg-sci/ns/hyceph

2538 Hydrocephalus Links
www.ufbi.ufl.edu/~joneslab/hclinks.htm
e-mail: hjones@college.med.ufl.edu.
www.ufbi.ufl.edu/~joneslab/hclinks.htm

2539 Hydrocephalus Project at the Cleveland Clinic Foundation
www.neus.ccf.org:80/Hydroceph

2540 Hydrohaven Chat Room
www.geocities.com/Heartland/6950/HydroHa

2541 Pediatric Neurosurgery-Hydrocephalus
cpmcnet.columbia.edu/dept/nsg/PNS/Hydroc

2542 Rare Genetic Diseases in Children (NYU)
mcrcr2.med.nyu.edu/murphp01/homenew.htm

2543 University of Adelaide Hydrocephalus Department
www.health.adelaide.eduau/paed-neuro/

2544 Usenet
alt.support.spina-bifida

Books

2545 A Guide to Hydrocephalus
Spina Bifida Association of America
4590 MacArthur Blvd. N.W. Suite 250
Washington, DC 20007   202-944-3285
800-621-3141
Fax: 202-944-3295
e-mail: spinabifida@aol.com
www.infohiway.com/spinabifida

2546 Hydrocephalus: A Guide for Patients, Families, and Friends
Chuck Toporek, Kellie Robinson, author

O'Reilly & Associates, Inc.
101 Morris Street
Sebastopol, CA 95472

800-998-9938
Fax: 707-829-0104
e-mail: patientguides@oreilly.com
www.patientcenters.com

This book educates families so they can select a skilled neurosurgeon, understand treatments, participate in care and know what symptoms need attention, keep records needed for follow-up treatments and make wise lifestyle choices.

379 pages Softcover
ISBN: I-565924-10-X

Newsletters

2547 Hydrocephalus Association Newsletter
Hydrocephalus Association
870 Market Street, Ste. 955
San Francisco, CA 94102   415-776-4713

Offers information on association news, conference articles, meetings, support and educational groups.

12 pages Quarterly

Emily S. Fudge, Executive Director

2548 Hydrocephalus News & Notes
National Hydrocephalus Foundation
1670 Green Oak Circle
Lawrenceville, GA 30243   770-995-9570
800-831-8093
Fax: 770-995-8982

Membership news.
Quarterly

Ann Marie Lakos, Editor

Pamphlets

2549 About Hydrocephalus - A Book for Parents
Hydrocephalus Association
870 Market Street Suite 955
San Francisco, CA 94102   415-732-7040
Fax: 415-732-7044
e-mail: hydroassoc@aol.com

A booklet in either English or Spanish, detailing all aspects of hydrocephalus from diagnosis and treatment to complications and follow-up care.

36 pages Softcover

2550 Directory of Pediatric Neurosurgeons
Hydrocephalus Association
870 Market Street Suite 955
San Francisco, CA 94102   415-732-7040
Fax: 415-732-7044
e-mail: hydroassoc@aol.com

162 neurosurgeons are listed with addresses, both alphabetically and geographically.

Emily S. Fudge, Executive Director

2551 Eye Problems Associated with Hydrocephalus in Children
Hydrocephalus Association
870 Market Street Suite 955
San Francisco, CA 94102   415-732-7040
Fax: 415-732-7044
e-mail: hydroassoc@aol.com

2552 Fact Sheet: Hydrocephalus
Hydrocephalus Association
870 Market Street Suite 955
San Francisco, CA 94102   415-732-7040
Fax: 415-732-7044
e-mail: hydroassoc@aol.com

Available in Spanish.

2553 Headaches and Hydrocephalus
Hydrocephalus Association
870 Market Street Suite 955
San Francisco, CA 94102   415-732-7040
Fax: 415-732-7044
e-mail: hydroassoc@aol.com

2554 Hospitalization Tips
Hydrocephalus Association
870 Market Street Suite 955
San Francisco, CA 94102   415-732-7040
Fax: 415-732-7044
e-mail: hydroassoc@aol.com

2555 How to be an Assertive Parent on the Treatment Team
Hydrocephalus Association
870 Market Street Suite 955
San Francisco, CA 94102   415-732-7040
Fax: 415-732-7044
e-mail: hydroassoc@aol.com

2556 Individualized Education Program (IEP) - Communication Skills for Parents
Hydrocephalus Association
870 Market Street Suite 955
San Francisco, CA 94102   415-732-7040
Fax: 415-732-7044
e-mail: hydroassoc@aol.com

2557 LINK Directory Information
Hydrocephalus Association
870 Market Street Suite 955
San Francisco, CA 94102   415-732-7040
Fax: 415-732-7044
e-mail: hydroassoc@aol.com

A nationwide network of individuals listed in directory format giving members direct access to others in similar circumstances.

Emily S. Fudge, Executive Director

2558 Learning Disabilities in Children with Hydrocephalus
Hydrocephalus Association
870 Market Street Suite 955
San Francisco, CA 94102   415-732-7040
Fax: 415-732-7044
e-mail: hydroassoc@aol.com

Available in Spanish.

2559 National Directory of Hydrocephalus Support Groups
Hydrocephalus Association
870 Market Street Suite 705
San Francisco, CA 94102   415-732-7040
888-598-3789
Fax: 415-732-7044
e-mail: hydroassoc@aol.com
www.hydroassoc.org

Published in 1994, the Directory lists information on sixteen hydrocephalus groups nationwide.

2560 Preparing Your Child for Surgery
Hydrocephalus Association
870 Market Street Suite 705
San Francisco, CA 94102   415-732-7040
                                 888-598-3789
                            Fax: 415-732-7044
                     e-mail: hydroassoc@aol.com
                          www.hydroassoc.org

2561 Resource Guide
Hydrocephalus Association
870 Market Street Suite 705
San Francisco, CA 94102   415-732-7040
                                 888-598-3789
                            Fax: 415-732-7044
                     e-mail: hydroassoc@aol.com
                          www.hydroassoc.org

A comprehensive listing of 380 articles on all aspects of hydrocephalus. Articles may be ordered for a small fee.

Emily S. Fudge, Executive Director

2562 Social Skills Development in Children with
    Hydrocephalus
Hydrocephalus Association
870 Market Street Suite 705
San Francisco, CA 94102   415-732-7040
                                 888-598-3789
                            Fax: 415-732-7044
                     e-mail: hydroassoc@aol.com
                          www.hydroassoc.org

2563 Survival Skills for the Family Unit
Hydrocephalus Association
870 Market Street Suite 705
San Francisco, CA 94102   415-732-7040
                                 888-598-3789
                            Fax: 415-732-7044
                     e-mail: hydroassoc@aol.com
                          www.hydroassoc.org

DESCRIPTION

2564 HYPOSPADIAS

Disorder Type: Birth Defect
May involve these systems in the body (see Section III):
Reproductive Systems

Hypospadias is a developmental abnormality that affects approximately one in 500 newborn males. In most males, the opening of the urethra, the tube that carries urine from the bladder to the exterior of the body, is located at the tip of the glans penis, the conical expansion at the end of the penis. However, in male newborns with hypospadias, the opening of the urethra is located on the underside of the penis or near or at the junction between the penis and the pouch that contains the testes (scrotum). In severe cases, the urethral opening may be located in the region behind the scrotum and in front of the anus (perineum). Hypospadias may have varying degrees of severity, depending upon the location of the urethral opening and possible associated abnormalities. For example, with increasing degrees of severity, there may be abnormal downward curvature of the penis (chordee) and progressive shortening of the urethra. In the most severe cases, the urethra may open into the perineum and affected males may have severe curvature of the penis and associated malformation of the scrotum (e.g., bifid scrotum, scrotal transposition). In addition, in approximately 10 percent of males with hypospadias, the testes may fail to descend into the scrotum and portions of the intestines may abnormally protrude into the canal that passes through lower muscular layers of the abdominal wall (inguinal canal). In affected male newborns, routine removal of the foreskin (circumcision) should be avoided since the foreskin is often essential in the surgical repair of hypospadias later during childhood. In most patients, hypospadias is surgically corrected before the age of 18 months. In mild cases, surgical repair may be undertaken for cosmetic purposes. In more severe cases, surgical repair may be necessary to enable normal passage of urine, prevent potential psychologic consequences, and enable proper sexual functioning.

Although the exact underlying causes of hypospadias are unknown, the condition is thought to result from failed fusion of a shallow groove (urethral groove) that becomes the penile urethra during fetal development. Hypospadias may occur in association with other congenital abnormalities or syndromes or may occur as an isolated finding. In some cases of isolated hypospadias, the condition may result from genetic changes (mutations) that occur spontaneously for unknown reasons (sporadically). There have been reports of multiple cases of isolated hypospadias within certain families (kindreds). Researchers suggest that sporadic and familial cases may result from mutations of one of several different genes expressed either alone or together (polygenic). Depending upon the specific disease gene or genes, the condition may have autosomal dominant, autosomal recessive, or polygenic inheritance.

The following organizations in the General Resources Section can provide additional information: March of Dimes Birth Defects Foundation, Genetic Alliance, NIH/National Institute of Child Health and Human Development, Online Mendelian Inheritance in Man: www3.ncbi.nlm.nih.gov/Omim/searchomim.html

Web Sites

2565 Children's Hospital Boston
www.duj.com/hypospadias.html

2566 European Society for Paediatric Urology
www.espu.org/

2567 University of Michigan
www.um-urology.com/clinic/pediatric/hypospadias.html

DESCRIPTION

2568 HYPOTHYROIDISM

Covers these related disorders: Acquired
hypothyroidism, Congenital hypothyroidism
**May involve these systems in the body (see Section
III):**
Endocrine System

Hypothyroidism is a condition characterized by
decreased activity of the thyroid gland, an endocrine gland that consists of two lobes on either side
of the windpipe. Certain specialized cells within
the thyroid gland secrete the thyroid hormones
thyroxine (T-4) and triiodothyronine (T-3), which
assist in regulating the rate of metabolism. Metabolism refers to the chemical activities within cells
that release energy from nutrients or consume
energy to create certain substances. The thyroid
hormones also play a vital role in the normal mental and physical development and growth of infants and children. Other specialized cells in the
thyroid gland secrete the hormone calcitonin,
which helps to regulate concentrations of calcium
in the body by inhibiting the loss of bone.

Hypothyroidism may result from an underlying
defect that is present at birth (congenital). In
children with congenital hypothyroidism, associated symptoms may begin at birth or be delayed
until later during childhood, depending upon the
nature of the underlying abnormality. Congenital
hypothyroidism may result from several underlying causes, such as abnormal development (dysplasia) or absence (aplasia) of the thyroid gland;
abnormalities in the production of certain hormones due to particular biochemical defects; or
fetal exposure to particular medications or therapies (e.g., radioiodine therapy) during pregnancy.
In children with malformation of the thyroid
gland or abnormalities in hormonal production,
the condition may appear to occur randomly for
unknown reasons (sporadically) or may be familial. Congenital hypothyroidism affects approximately one in 4,000 infants worldwide and is about
twice as common in females as in males.

Hypothyroidism may also occur later during
childhood (acquired hypothyroidism) due to an
autoimmune disorder in which the immune system
develops antibodies against cells of the thyroid
gland (Hashimoto's disease) or in association with
other underlying disorders (e.g., nephropathic
cystinosis, histiocytosis). Acquired hypothyroidism may also develop due to the use of particular
medications or surgical removal of all or a portion
of the thyroid gland as a treatment for certain
diseases or conditions (e.g., thyroid cancer, thyro-
toxicosis).

In newborns and infants with congenital hypothyroidism, associated symptoms may vary in
range, severity, and rate of progression, depending upon the degree of thyroid hormone deficiency. Some patients may have an abnormally
enlarged thyroid gland (goiter), causing swelling
in front of the neck. In addition, early symptoms
may include yellowish discoloration of the skin,
mucous membranes, and whites of the eyes (jaundice); sluggishness; and feeding difficulties, including choking episodes during nursing. Many
patients also have a large abdomen; a weakening
of the abdominal wall muscles (umbilical hernia);
constipation; widely open soft spots (fontanels)
under the front and back of the scalp; and respiratory difficulties, including episodes in which
there is a temporary cessation of spontaneous
breathing (apnea). Some patients may have progressive retardation of mental and physical development that becomes increasingly severe without
early diagnosis and prompt treatment. Patients
may experience delays in obtaining certain developmental milestones, such as sitting up and standing; may not learn to speak; and may be
increasingly lethargic. Additional physical findings associated with severe hypothyroidism include delayed skeletal maturation; a short, thick
neck; short fingers and broad hands; a thick, protruding tongue; delayed eruption of the teeth (den-
tition); dry, scaly skin; coarse, scanty hair; and an
abnormal, progressive accumulation of fluid
within body tissues and associated swelling, par-

ticularly in the genital area, eyelids, and backs of the hands (myxedema).

The symptoms and findings associated with acquired hypothyroidism may also vary, depending upon the underlying cause, the age at onset, and the degree of thyroid hormone deficiency. Children with acquired hypothyroidism may experience an abnormally decreased rate of growth, decreased energy, puffiness of the skin (myxedematous changes), constipation, cold intolerance, headaches, visual problems, or other abnormalities.

In the United States, thyroid hormone levels in the blood are routinely tested in all newborns shortly after birth. Early diagnosis and prompt treatment of congenital hypothyroidism are essential for normal brain development during infancy. Such treatment includes thyroid hormone replacement therapy (e.g., sodium-L-thyroxine by mouth). The treatment of children with acquired hypothyroidism also includes thyroid hormone replacement therapy. Additional treatment is symptomatic and supportive.

The following organizations in the General Resources Section can provide additional information: NIH/National Digestive Diseases Information Clearinghouse, Genetic Alliance, March of Dimes Birth Defects Foundation, Online Mendelian Inheritance in Man: www3.ncbi.nlm.nih.gov/Omim/searchomim.html, MedHelp International: www.medhelp.org/

Web Sites

2569 American Association of Clinical Endocrinologists
www.aace.com/

2570 Elibrary.com
www.elibrary.com/id/238/222/search.cgi

2571 Online Mendelian Inheritance in Man
www3.ncbi.nlm.nih.gov

2572 Thyroid Federation International
www.thyroid-fed.org/

Pamphlets

2573 Congenital & Acquired Hypothyroidism
Human Growth Foundation
7777 Leesburg Pike Suite 202S
Falls Church, VA 22043   703-883-1773
                               800-451-6434

DESCRIPTION

2574 ICHTHYOSIS

Covers these related disorders: Collodion baby, Congenital ichthyosiform erythroderma, Epidermolytic hyperkeratosis, Harlequin fetus, Ichthyosis vulgaris, X-linked ichthyosis
May involve these systems in the body (see Section III):
Dermatologic System

Ichthyosis is a group of disorders characterized by abnormal thickening, dryness, and scaling of the skin due to abnormalities in the production of keratin, a protein that is the primary component of the skin, hair, and nails. Most forms of ichthyosis are genetic disorders that are usually apparent at birth (congenital) or during the first months of life. The disease genes that cause some genetic forms of ichthyosis have been mapped to particular chromosomes. Ichthyosis may also be due to other underlying genetic syndromes or may be an acquired condition due to certain nutritional deficiencies, the administration of particular drugs, or certain conditions, such as abnormally decreased activity of the thyroid gland (hypothyroidism) or Hodgkin's disease, a malignancy of the lymphatic system.

One form of ichthyosis that is present at birth (congenital) is known as harlequin fetus. This form of the disease may result from several different genetic abnormalities, most of which are thought to be transmitted as an autosomal recessive trait. Affected newborns may be covered with thickened, ridged, armor-like plates that confine the fingers and toes, restrict movements of the joints, and flatten the nose and ears. Additional features may include eyelids that are turned outward (ectropion), causing eyes to be indistinct; gaping lips; and absent hair and nails. Newborns with the condition may experience difficulties breathing, be susceptible to repeated skin infections, and develop life-threatening complications during the first days or weeks of life.

Another congenital form of ichthyosis, known as collodion baby, may also result from many different genetic abnormalities. Affected newborns are covered by a thick membrane that resembles an oiled parchment (collodion membrane), causing flattening of the nose and ears, abnormalities of the eyelids (ectropion), gaping of the lips, or other abnormalities. The membrane begins to crack as patients begin to breathe and is gradually shed in large sheets. This condition is usually an early manifestation of certain genetic forms of ichthyosis (e.g., lamellar ichthyosis or congenital ichthyosiform erythroderma). Patients may develop potentially life-threatening symptoms due to skin infection, inflammation of the lungs (pneumonia), excessive loss of bodily fluids (dehydration), or other abnormalities.

Congenital ichthyosiform erythroderma is an autosomal recessive disorder that typically becomes apparent shortly after birth and may often present as collodion baby. This form of ichthyosis is characterized by abnormal redness of the skin (erythroderma); generalized, fine, white scaling of the skin; and potentially severe itching (pruritus). Many children also have abnormally thickened skin (hyperkeratosis) on the palms of the hands and soles of the feet as well as around the knees, ankles, and elbows. Additional findings may include unusually sparse hair and abnormalities of the nails. Another form of the disorder, known as lamellar ichthyosis or nonbullous congenital ichthyosiform erythroderma, is usually inherited as an autosomal recessive trait. This form of ichthyosis becomes apparent shortly after birth and may also present as collodion baby. After the collodion membrane is shed, the skin becomes covered with relatively large, coarse scales. Scaling often affects all surfaces of the body and may be associated with severe itching. Patients may also have thickened skin on the palms and soles, usually small ears, outward turning of the eyelids (ectropion), and abnormally sparse, fine hair.

Another form of the disorder, known as X-linked ichthyosis, is often apparent at birth or during early infancy. Although males are primarily affected, some females who carry a single copy of the disease gene may also experience some symptoms.

Patients develop prominent darkened scales on the scalp, ears, neck, arms and legs, torso, or other areas. Scaling may gradually worsen in severity and progress to affect other areas of the skin. By late childhood or adolescence, many patients develop clouding of the corneas (corneal opacities) that does not interfere with vision.

The most common form of the disorder is ichthyosis vulgaris, also known as ichthyosis simplex, an autosomal dominant disorder that affects about one in 250 to 300 children. Symptoms, which typically become apparent by the age of six months, may include slight roughness and scaling of the skin, particularly of the back and the legs. Scaling may worsen upon exposure to cold temperatures and may subside during warm months of the year. There may also be overgrowth of hair follicles (keratosis pilaris), particularly those of the thighs and upper arms, as well as abnormal thickening of the skin of the palms and soles. The condition may gradually improve or subside with age.

Another form of ichthyosis, known as epidermolytic hyperkeratosis or bullous congenital ichthyosiform erythroderma, may occur randomly for unknown reasons (sporadic) or be inherited as an autosomal dominant trait. This form of ichthyosis typically becomes apparent shortly after birth and is characterized by generalized reddening of the skin (erythroderma), severe skin thickening (hyperkeratosis) in certain areas, and small, rough, wart-like scales over body surfaces. Skin overgrowth may be most apparent on the neck and hips, under the arms, or at the elbows or knees and may affect the skin of the palms and soles. Recurrent blistering (bullae) may also develop, particularly on the lower legs, knees, or elbows.

There are also additional genetic forms of ichthyosis that have similar symptoms and findings. However, the specific range, severity, and extent of associated abnormalities and the age of onset may vary, depending upon the form of the disorder present.

The methods used to treat ichthyosis may depend upon the specific disorder type as well as the severity and extent of associated symptoms. In severe neonatal forms, such as collodion baby and harlequin fetus, supportive measures may include administration of fluids to prevent dehydration; use of specialized support equipment such as an incubator that provides a heated, appropriately moisturized (humidified) environment; and use of measures to help prevent or aggressively treat infections. Treatment may also include the administration of certain vitamin A derivatives (retinoids) or emulsifying ointments or lubricants. Bathing with oils may help to moisten the skin, and the application of certain emulsifying ointments and lubricants that soften the skin may alleviate dryness and scaling. In addition, applying topical agents that promote skin softening and peeling (keratolytic agents) may facilitate the removal of scales. In some patients, the use of air conditioning in warmer months and exposure to a high-humidity environment during the colder months may also be beneficial. Additional treatment is symptomatic and supportive.

The following organizations in the General Resources Section can provide additional information: National Organization for Rare Disorders, Inc. (NORD), NIH/Office of Rare Diseases, March of Dimes Birth Defects Foundation, NIH/National Institute of Arthritis and Musculoskeletal and Skin Diseases, NIH/National Institute of Allergy and Infectious Diseases, NIH/National Institute of Child Health and Human Development, Genetic Alliance

National Associations & Support Groups

2575 FIRST: Foundation for Ichthyosis and Related Skin Types
650 N. Cannon Ave. Suite 17
Lansdale, PA 19446   215-631-1411
800-545-3286
Fax: 215-631-1413
e-mail: ichthyosis@aol.com

Dedicated to helping individuals and families affected by the inherited skin diseases collectively called the Ichthyoses. Provides support, information, education, and advocacy for individuals and families affected by ichthyosis.

2576 National Registry for Ichtyosis and Related Disorders
University of Washington, Dermatology Department
Box 356524, 1959 NE Pacific
Seattle, WA 98195   206-616-3179
                                     800-595-1265
                              Fax: 206-616-4302
                   e-mail: fleck@u.washington.edu
     weber.u.washington.edu/~geoff/ichthyosis.registry/

Web Sites

2577 Family Village
laran.waisman.wisc.edu/fv/www/lib_icht.htm

2578 Ichthyosis Information
www.ichthyosis.com/

DESCRIPTION

2579 INFECTIOUS GASTROENTERITIS

Disorder Type: Infectious Disease

Infectious gastroenteritis refers to an infection of the gastrointestinal tract caused by various microorganisms such as certain bacteria, viruses, and parasites and is usually characterized by diarrhea and vomiting. Such microorganisms may be transmitted through fecal-oral contamination or contamination of food or water. Bacterial infection may result from the release of toxins or by bacterial growths inside or outside the walls of the intestines. Viral infection by gastroenteritis viruses, especially the rotavirus, is a major source of diarrhea-causing infection in the United States. However, parasitic gastroenteritis is more common outside of the U.S. Although infectious gastroenteritis often resolves on its own (spontaneously), some patients experience acute or prolonged symptoms that may require treatment as well as identification of the causative agent.

Symptoms and findings associated with infectious gastroenteritis depend upon the cause of the infection and the age and general health of the patient. Although some children and adults exhibit no symptoms, the most common manifestation of infection is watery or bloody diarrhea that usually appears suddenly and lasts from a few days to two weeks or longer. Other symptoms may include nausea, vomiting, loss of appetite, and abdominal cramping or distress. Infants, the elderly, and those with compromised immune systems are at risk for potentially severe illness. For example, within one day of onset, diarrhea and vomiting in infants younger than six months, or in older children if severe, may result in a potentially life-threatening and excessive fluid loss (dehydration) as well as the loss of essential substances, known as electrolytes, in the fluid portion of the blood (e.g., sodium, potassium, and calcium). Symptoms associated with dehydration may include fever, thirst, less-than-average urinary output, dry mouth, and poor feeding. In addition, severely dehydrated infants and older children may become weak, listless, or sleepy and their eyes may have a sunken, dry appearance. Bacteria associated with gastroenteritis sometimes cause infection outside the gastrointestinal tract and may involve the urinary tract, the eyes, the vulva and vaginal areas in females, as well as inflammation of the membranes surrounding the brain and spinal cord (meningitis), the liver (hepatitis), the lungs (pneumonia), the bone and bone marrow (osteomyelitis), and other tissues. In addition, certain foodborne or waterborne infections caused by bacterial or other toxins may produce severe, sudden, and potentially life-threatening symptoms including neurologic involvement such as numbness and paralysis.

Prevention of some types of infectious gastroenteritis may include vaccination against certain infectious diseases when traveling to countries in which these illnesses are widespread. In addition, care in handling and preparing foods may help to alleviate certain types of foodborne illnesss. Treatment is first directed toward the replacement of body fluids and electrolytes through oral preparations or, in the case of more severe dehydration, through intravenous administration. If indicated, identification of the cause may then be established through evaluation of family history including recent travels, foods eaten, other similar family illness as well as physical examination and testing of stool specimens. Bacterial infections may be treated with appropriate antibiotics. Additional treatment may include measures to prevent the spread of infection to other family members or associates. Such precautions may include good hygienics such as frequent hand washing, etc. Other treatment is symptomatic and supportive.

The following organizations in the General Resources Section can provide additional information: NIH/National Institute of Allergy and Infectious Diseases, NIH/National Digestive Diseases Information Clearinghouse, Centers for Disease Control (CDC), World Health Organization

National Associations & Support Groups

2580 Digestive Disease National Coalition
507 Capital Court, Suite 200
Washington, DC 20002   202-544-7497
                             Fax: 202-546-7105

Objective is to inform the public about technical improvements through several media.

2581 International Foundation for Functional Gastrointestinal Disorders
P.O. Box 17864
Milwaukee, WI 53217   414-964-1799
                             888-964-2001
                        Fax: 414-964-7176
                 e-mail: iffgd@execpc.com
                    www.execpc.com/iffgd

The organization offers responses to those commonly asked questions for families and individuals who are affected with these disorders.

2582 Intestinal Disease Foundation
1323 Forbes Avenue, Suite 200
Pittsburgh, PA 15219   412-261-5888
                             Fax: 412-471-2722

Encourages the individuals who have been diagnosed to have a positive outlook through support groups and reading materials.

Web Sites

2583 American Gastroenterological Association
www.gastro.org/brochure.html

Books

2584 Digestive Diseases Dictionary
Nat'l Digestive Diseases Information Clearinghouse
2 Information Way
Bethesda, MD 20892   301-654-3810
                           Fax: 301-907-8906
              e-mail: nddic@info.niddk.nih.gov
                          www.niddk.nih.gov

2585 Digestive Diseases in the United States: Epidemiology and Impact
Nat'l Digestive Diseases Information Clearinghouse
2 Information Way
Bethesda, MD 20892   301-654-3810
                           Fax: 301-907-8906
              e-mail: nddic@info.niddk.nih.gov
                          www.niddk.nih.gov

800 pages

2586 Directory of Digestive Diseases Organizations for Patients
Nat'l Digestive Diseases Information Clearinghouse
2 Information Way
Bethesda, MD 20892   301-654-3810
                           Fax: 301-907-8906
              e-mail: nddic@info.niddk.nih.gov
                          www.niddk.nih.gov

2587 Directory of Digestive Diseases Organizations for Professionals
Nat'l Digestive Diseases Information Clearinghouse
2 Information Way
Bethesda, MD 20892   301-654-3810
                           Fax: 301-907-8906
              e-mail: nddic@info.niddk.nih.gov
                          www.niddk.nih.gov

2588 Research Opportunities & Programs in the Digestive Diseases & Nutrition
Nat'l Digestive Diseases Information Clearinghouse
2 Information Way
Bethesda, MD 20892   301-654-3810
                           Fax: 301-907-8906
              e-mail: nddic@info.niddk.nih.gov
                          www.niddk.nih.gov

2589 What I Need To Know About Hepatitis A
Nat'l Digestive Diseases Information Clearinghouse
2 Information Way
Bethesda, MD 20892   301-654-3810
                           Fax: 301-907-8906
              e-mail: nddic@info.niddk.nih.gov
                          www.niddk.nih.gov

2590 What I Need To Know About Hepatitis B
Nat'l Digestive Diseases Information Clearinghouse
2 Information Way
Bethesda, MD 20892   301-654-3810
                           Fax: 301-907-8906
              e-mail: nddic@info.niddk.nih.gov
                          www.niddk.nih.gov

2591 What I Need To Know About Hepatitis C
Nat'l Digestive Diseases Information Clearinghouse
2 Information Way
Bethesda, MD 20892   301-654-3810
                           Fax: 301-907-8906
              e-mail: nddic@info.niddk.nih.gov
                          www.niddk.nih.gov

2592 Why Am I Constipated?
Nat'l Digestive Diseases Information Clearinghouse
2 Information Way
Bethesda, MD 20892   301-654-3810
                           Fax: 301-907-8906
              e-mail: nddic@info.niddk.nih.gov
                          www.niddk.nih.gov

2593 Why Do I Have Gas?
Nat'l Digestive Diseases Information Clearinghouse
2 Information Way
Bethesda, MD 20892   301-654-3810
                                    Fax: 301-907-8906
        e-mail: nddic@info.niddk.nih.gov
                        www.niddk.nih.gov

2594 Why Does Milk Bother Me?
Nat'l Digestive Diseases Information Clearinghouse
2 Information Way
Bethesda, MD 20892   301-654-3810
                                    Fax: 301-907-8906
        e-mail: nddic@info.niddk.nih.gov
                        www.niddk.nih.gov

Pamphlets

2595 Anal Fissure
Nat'l Digestive Diseases Information Clearinghouse
2 Information Way
Bethesda, MD 20892   301-654-3810
                                    Fax: 301-907-8906
        e-mail: nddic@info.niddk.nih.gov
                        www.niddk.nih.gov

2596 Appendicitis
Nat'l Digestive Diseases Information Clearinghouse
2 Information Way
Bethesda, MD 20892   301-654-3810
                                    Fax: 301-907-8906
        e-mail: nddic@info.niddk.nih.gov
                        www.niddk.nih.gov

2597 Autoimmune Hepatitis
Nat'l Digestive Diseases Information Clearinghouse
2 Information Way
Bethesda, MD 20892   301-654-3810
                                    Fax: 301-907-8906
        e-mail: nddic@info.niddk.nih.gov
                        www.niddk.nih.gov

2598 Bleeding in the Digestive Tract
Nat'l Digestive Diseases Information Clearinghouse
2 Information Way
Bethesda, MD 20892   301-654-3810
                                    Fax: 301-907-8906
        e-mail: nddic@info.niddk.nih.gov
                        www.niddk.nih.gov

2599 Celiac Disease
Nat'l Digestive Diseases Information Clearinghouse
2 Information Way
Bethesda, MD 20892   301-654-3810
                                    Fax: 301-907-8906
        e-mail: nddic@info.niddk.nih.gov
                        www.niddk.nih.gov

2600 Chronic Hepatitis C: Current Disease Management
Nat'l Digestive Diseases Information Clearinghouse
2 Information Way
Bethesda, MD 20892   301-654-3810
                                    Fax: 301-907-8906
        e-mail: nddic@info.niddk.nih.gov
                        www.niddk.nih.gov

2601 Cirrhosis of the Liver
Nat'l Digestive Diseases Information Clearinghouse
2 Information Way
Bethesda, MD 20892   301-654-3810
                                    Fax: 301-907-8906
        e-mail: nddic@info.niddk.nih.gov
                        www.niddk.nih.gov

2602 Constipation
Nat'l Digestive Diseases Information Clearinghouse
2 Information Way
Bethesda, MD 20892   301-654-3810
                                    Fax: 301-907-8906
        e-mail: nddic@info.niddk.nih.gov
                        www.niddk.nih.gov

2603 Constipation in Children
Nat'l Digestive Diseases Information Clearinghouse
2 Information Way
Bethesda, MD 20892   301-654-3810
                                    Fax: 301-907-8906
        e-mail: nddic@info.niddk.nih.gov
                        www.niddk.nih.gov

2604 Crohn's Disease
Nat'l Digestive Diseases Information Clearinghouse
2 Information Way
Bethesda, MD 20892   301-654-3810
                                    Fax: 301-907-8906
        e-mail: nddic@info.niddk.nih.gov
                        www.niddk.nih.gov

2605 Cyclic Vomiting Syndrome
Nat'l Digestive Diseases Information Clearinghouse
2 Information Way
Bethesda, MD 20892   301-654-3810
                                    Fax: 301-907-8906
        e-mail: nddic@info.niddk.nih.gov
                        www.niddk.nih.gov

2606 Diagnostic Tests
Nat'l Digestive Diseases Information Clearinghouse
2 Information Way
Bethesda, MD 20892   301-654-3810
                                    Fax: 301-907-8906
        e-mail: nddic@info.niddk.nih.gov
                        www.niddk.nih.gov

2607 Diagnostic Tests for Liver Disease
Nat'l Digestive Diseases Information Clearinghouse
2 Information Way
Bethesda, MD 20892   301-654-3810
                                  Fax: 301-907-8906
                    e-mail: nddic@info.niddk.nih.gov
                                   www.niddk.nih.gov

2608 Diarrhea
Nat'l Digestive Diseases Information Clearinghouse
2 Information Way
Bethesda, MD 20892   301-654-3810
                                  Fax: 301-907-8906
                    e-mail: nddic@info.niddk.nih.gov
                                   www.niddk.nih.gov

2609 Diverticulosis & Diverticulitis
Nat'l Digestive Diseases Information Clearinghouse
2 Information Way
Bethesda, MD 20892   301-654-3810
                                  Fax: 301-907-8906
                    e-mail: nddic@info.niddk.nih.gov
                                   www.niddk.nih.gov

2610 Facts & Fallacies About Digestive Diseases
Nat'l Digestive Diseases Information Clearinghouse
2 Information Way
Bethesda, MD 20892   301-654-3810
                                  Fax: 301-907-8906
                    e-mail: nddic@info.niddk.nih.gov
                                   www.niddk.nih.gov

2611 Fecal Incontinence
Nat'l Digestive Diseases Information Clearinghouse
2 Information Way
Bethesda, MD 20892   301-654-3810
                                  Fax: 301-907-8906
                    e-mail: nddic@info.niddk.nih.gov
                                   www.niddk.nih.gov

2612 Gallbladder and Biliary Tract Diseases
Nat'l Digestive Diseases Information Clearinghouse
2 Information Way
Bethesda, MD 20892   301-654-3810
                                  Fax: 301-907-8906
                    e-mail: nddic@info.niddk.nih.gov
                                   www.niddk.nih.gov

2613 Gallstones
Nat'l Digestive Diseases Information Clearinghouse
2 Information Way
Bethesda, MD 20892   301-654-3810
                                  Fax: 301-907-8906
                    e-mail: nddic@info.niddk.nih.gov
                                   www.niddk.nih.gov

2614 Gas in the Digestive Tract
Nat'l Digestive Diseases Information Clearinghouse
2 Information Way
Bethesda, MD 20892   301-654-3810
                                  Fax: 301-907-8906
                    e-mail: nddic@info.niddk.nih.gov
                                   www.niddk.nih.gov

2615 Gastritis
Nat'l Digestive Diseases Information Clearinghouse
2 Information Way
Bethesda, MD 20892   301-654-3810
                                  Fax: 301-907-8906
                    e-mail: nddic@info.niddk.nih.gov
                                   www.niddk.nih.gov

2616 Gastroesophageal Reflux Disease (Hiatal Hernia and Heartburn)
Nat'l Digestive Diseases Information Clearinghouse
2 Information Way
Bethesda, MD 20892   301-654-3810
                                  Fax: 301-907-8906
                    e-mail: nddic@info.niddk.nih.gov
                                   www.niddk.nih.gov

2617 Gastroesophageal Reflux Disease in Children
Nat'l Digestive Diseases Information Clearinghouse
2 Information Way
Bethesda, MD 20892   301-654-3810
                                  Fax: 301-907-8906
                    e-mail: nddic@info.niddk.nih.gov
                                   www.niddk.nih.gov

2618 Gastroparesis in Diabetes
Nat'l Digestive Diseases Information Clearinghouse
2 Information Way
Bethesda, MD 20892   301-654-3810
                                  Fax: 301-907-8906
                    e-mail: nddic@info.niddk.nih.gov
                                   www.niddk.nih.gov

2619 Helicobacter Pylori and Peptic Ulcer
Nat'l Digestive Diseases Information Clearinghouse
2 Information Way
Bethesda, MD 20892   301-654-3810
                                  Fax: 301-907-8906
                    e-mail: nddic@info.niddk.nih.gov
                                   www.niddk.nih.gov

2620 Hemochromatosis
Nat'l Digestive Diseases Information Clearinghouse
2 Information Way
Bethesda, MD 20892   301-654-3810
                                  Fax: 301-907-8906
                    e-mail: nddic@info.niddk.nih.gov
                                   www.niddk.nih.gov

2621 Ileostomy, Colostomy, & Ileoanal Reservoir Surgery
Nat'l Digestive Diseases Information Clearinghouse
2 Information Way
Bethesda, MD 20892 301-654-3810
Fax: 301-907-8906
e-mail: nddic@info.niddk.nih.gov
www.niddk.nih.gov

2622 Indigestion (Dyspepsia)
Nat'l Digestive Diseases Information Clearinghouse
2 Information Way
Bethesda, MD 20892 301-654-3810
Fax: 301-907-8906
e-mail: nddic@info.niddk.nih.gov
www.niddk.nih.gov

2623 Inguinal Hernia
Nat'l Digestive Diseases Information Clearinghouse
2 Information Way
Bethesda, MD 20892 301-654-3810
Fax: 301-907-8906
e-mail: nddic@info.niddk.nih.gov
www.niddk.nih.gov

2624 Irritable Bowel Syndrome
Nat'l Digestive Diseases Information Clearinghouse
2 Information Way
Bethesda, MD 20892 301-654-3810
Fax: 301-907-8906
e-mail: nddic@info.niddk.nih.gov
www.niddk.nih.gov

2625 Irritable Bowel Syndrome (IBS) in Children
Nat'l Digestive Diseases Information Clearinghouse
2 Information Way
Bethesda, MD 20892 301-654-3810
Fax: 301-907-8906
e-mail: nddic@info.niddk.nih.gov
www.niddk.nih.gov

2626 Lactose Intolerance
Nat'l Digestive Diseases Information Clearinghouse
2 Information Way
Bethesda, MD 20892 301-654-3810
Fax: 301-907-8906
e-mail: nddic@info.niddk.nih.gov
www.niddk.nih.gov

2627 Liver Transplantation
Nat'l Digestive Diseases Information Clearinghouse
2 Information Way
Bethesda, MD 20892 301-654-3810
Fax: 301-907-8906
e-mail: nddic@info.niddk.nih.gov
www.niddk.nih.gov

2628 Menetrier's Disease
Nat'l Digestive Diseases Information Clearinghouse
2 Information Way
Bethesda, MD 20892 301-654-3810
Fax: 301-907-8906
e-mail: nddic@info.niddk.nih.gov
www.niddk.nih.gov

2629 NDDIC Brochure
Nat'l Digestive Diseases Information Clearinghouse
2 Information Way
Bethesda, MD 20892 301-654-3810
Fax: 301-907-8906
e-mail: nddic@info.niddk.nih.gov
www.niddk.nih.gov

2630 NDDIC News
Nat'l Digestive Diseases Information Clearinghouse
2 Information Way
Bethesda, MD 20892 301-654-3810
Fax: 301-907-8906
e-mail: nddic@info.niddk.nih.gov
www.niddk.nih.gov

2631 NSAIDs and Peptic Ulcer
Nat'l Digestive Diseases Information Clearinghouse
2 Information Way
Bethesda, MD 20892 301-654-3810
Fax: 301-907-8906
e-mail: nddic@info.niddk.nih.gov
www.niddk.nih.gov

2632 Ostomy and Surgical Alternatives
Nat'l Digestive Diseases Information Clearinghouse
2 Information Way
Bethesda, MD 20892 301-654-3810
Fax: 301-907-8906
e-mail: nddic@info.niddk.nih.gov
www.niddk.nih.gov

2633 Overview of Digestive Diseases
Nat'l Digestive Diseases Information Clearinghouse
2 Information Way
Bethesda, MD 20892 301-654-3810
Fax: 301-907-8906
e-mail: nddic@info.niddk.nih.gov
www.niddk.nih.gov

2634 Polyps
Nat'l Digestive Diseases Information Clearinghouse
2 Information Way
Bethesda, MD 20892 301-654-3810
Fax: 301-907-8906
e-mail: nddic@info.niddk.nih.gov
www.niddk.nih.gov

2635 Porphyria
Nat'l Digestive Diseases Information Clearinghouse
2 Information Way
Bethesda, MD 20892   301-654-3810
Fax: 301-907-8906
e-mail: nddic@info.niddk.nih.gov
www.niddk.nih.gov

2636 Primary Biliary Cirrhosis
Nat'l Digestive Diseases Information Clearinghouse
2 Information Way
Bethesda, MD 20892   301-654-3810
Fax: 301-907-8906
e-mail: nddic@info.niddk.nih.gov
www.niddk.nih.gov

2637 Primary Sclerosing Cholangitis
Nat'l Digestive Diseases Information Clearinghouse
2 Information Way
Bethesda, MD 20892   301-654-3810
Fax: 301-907-8906
e-mail: nddic@info.niddk.nih.gov
www.niddk.nih.gov

2638 Proctitis
Nat'l Digestive Diseases Information Clearinghouse
2 Information Way
Bethesda, MD 20892   301-654-3810
Fax: 301-907-8906
e-mail: nddic@info.niddk.nih.gov
www.niddk.nih.gov

2639 Rapid Gastric Emptying (Dumping Syndrome)
Nat'l Digestive Diseases Information Clearinghouse
2 Information Way
Bethesda, MD 20892   301-654-3810
Fax: 301-907-8906
e-mail: nddic@info.niddk.nih.gov
www.niddk.nih.gov

2640 Short Bowel Syndrome
Nat'l Digestive Diseases Information Clearinghouse
2 Information Way
Bethesda, MD 20892   301-654-3810
Fax: 301-907-8906
e-mail: nddic@info.niddk.nih.gov
www.niddk.nih.gov

2641 Travelers' Diarrhea
Nat'l Digestive Diseases Information Clearinghouse
2 Information Way
Bethesda, MD 20892   301-654-3810
Fax: 301-907-8906
e-mail: nddic@info.niddk.nih.gov
www.niddk.nih.gov

2642 Ulcerative Colitis
Nat'l Digestive Diseases Information Clearinghouse
2 Information Way
Bethesda, MD 20892   301-654-3810
Fax: 301-907-8906
e-mail: nddic@info.niddk.nih.gov
www.niddk.nih.gov

2643 Vaccination for Hepatitis A and B
Nat'l Digestive Diseases Information Clearinghouse
2 Information Way
Bethesda, MD 20892   301-654-3810
Fax: 301-907-8906
e-mail: nddic@info.niddk.nih.gov
www.niddk.nih.gov

2644 Whipple's Disease
Nat'l Digestive Diseases Information Clearinghouse
2 Information Way
Bethesda, MD 20892   301-654-3810
Fax: 301-907-8906
e-mail: nddic@info.niddk.nih.gov
www.niddk.nih.gov

2645 Your Digestive System & How it Works
Nat'l Digestive Diseases Information Clearinghouse
2 Information Way
Bethesda, MD 20892   301-654-3810
Fax: 301-907-8906
e-mail: nddic@info.niddk.nih.gov
www.niddk.nih.gov

2646 Zollonger-Ellison Syndrome
Nat'l Digestive Diseases Information Clearinghouse
2 Information Way
Bethesda, MD 20892   301-654-3810
Fax: 301-907-8906
e-mail: nddic@info.niddk.nih.gov
www.niddk.nih.gov

DESCRIPTION

2647 INSULIN-DEPENDENT DIABETES MELLITUS

Insulin-dependent diabetes mellitus (IDDM) is a disorder in whch insufficient production of insulin by the pancreas results in abnormally high levels of the sugar glucose in the blood. Insulin is a hormone that regulates and stabilizes blood glucose levels by promoting the movement of energy-rich glucose into body cells for energy production or into the liver and fat cells for storage. IDDM may also cause impaired fat metabolism and long-term complications affecting certain large and small blood vessels (angiopathy), the nerve-rich membranes at the back of the eyes (retinas), skin, kidneys, nerves, or other tissues of the body. The exact cause of IDDM is unknown. However, researchers speculate that certain environmental factors, such as a viral infection, may inappropriately trigger the immune system to destroy insulin-producing cells within the pancreas (beta cells), resulting in severe insulin deficiency. Genetic factors are also thought to play some role in causing a predisposition for the disorder.

IDDM is the major form of diabetes affecting children. Another form of diabetes, known as non-insulin-dependent diabetes mellitus, may be characterized by a resistance to the effects of insulin. Although this type of diabetes may occur at any age, it most commonly becomes apparent after age 40, is rare during childhood or adolescence, and is most common in obese patients. In some children, various forms of diabetes may occur secondary to certain genetic multisystemic disorders that affect the pancreas, such as cystic fibrosis; other endocrine disorders, such as Cushing's syndrome; the administration of particular drugs; or exposure to certain poisons.

Insulin-dependent diabetes mellitus typically becomes apparent before the age of 30, and most patients affected between the ages of five and seven or by early adolescence. By age 16, approximately one in 360 children in the United States is affected by the disorder. In most children with IDDM, associated symptoms and findings may appear to occur suddenly and may include excessive urine production by the kidneys, causing increased urination (polyuria) and excessive thirst (polydipsia); weight loss; and abnormally increased hunger (polyphagia). Additional abnormalities may include exhaustion, blurred vision, abnormal sensations (paresthesias) in the hands and feet, and increased irritability. Without prompt diagnosis and treatment, symptoms may rapidly progress to a metabolic condition known as ketoacidosis. Because of deficient insulin prodcution, the body's cells begin to rely on sources of energy other than glucose, causing an excessive breakdown of fats and an abnormal accumulation of certain chemical compounds (ketones) in bodily tissues and fluids. Early symptoms associated with ketoacidosis may be relatively mild, including increased urination, vomiting, and excessively low levels of bodily fluids (dehydration). In more severe cases, patients may have an abnormal acetone-like odor on the breath and develop unusually deep, rapid breathing; abdominal pain; confusion; and, without appropriate treatment, coma and potentially life-threatening complications. The treatment of ketoacidosis may include the immediate administration of intravenous fluids; replacement of electrolytes, such as sodium and potassium; initation of intravenous insulin therapy; measures to prevent or appropriately treat increased fluid pressure within the brain; and other therapies as required.

Patients with IDDM may eventually develop certain long-term complications associated with the disease. However, careful control of blood sugar levels may help to prevent, delay, or slow the progression of such complications. Complications associated with IDDM may include thickening and leaking of the walls of certain small blood vessels, narrowing of medium and large-size arteries due to plaque development (atherosclerosis), abnormally high blood pressure (hypertension), poor blood circulation, and problems affecting the eyes, kidneys, nerves, and skin. For example, kidney damage may result in impaired kidney function and kidney failure; damage to blood vessels within the nerve-rich membranes at the back of the eyes (diabetic retinopathy) may lead to visual impairment; and nerve damage may cause weakness or the loss of certain sensations, such as changes in temperature or pressure, increasing the risk of injury. In addition, impaired blood supply to certain skin areas may increase the risk of developing skin sores (ulcers). Poor wound healing and susceptibility to infected foot ulcers may lead to localized loss of tissue (necrosis), potentially requiring amputation.

National Associations & Support Groups

2648 American Association of Diabetes Educators
100 W Monroe Street, Fl 4
Chicago, IL 60603

312-424-2427
800-832-6874
www.aabenet.org

An independent, multidisciplinary organization of health professionals involved in teaching persons with diabetes. The mission is to enhance the competence of health professionals who teach persons with diabetes education and care for all those affected by diabetes.

Cheryl Hunt, RN, MSED, CDE, President

2649 American Diabetes Association
N. Beauregard Street
Alexandria, VA 22311

703-549-1500
800-342-2383
Fax: 703-549-6995
www.diabetes.org

The nation's leading voluntary organization concerned with diabetes and its complications. The mission of the organization is to prevent and cure diabetes and to improve the lives of persons with diabetes. Offers a network of 52 affiliates with over 55,000 volunteers, including a professional membership of more than 10,000 physicians, social workers, nutritionists, educators and nurses.

Bruce R. Zimmerman, MD

2650 Juvenile Diabetes Foundation International
120 Wall Street
New York, NY 10005

212-785-9500
800-533-2873
Fax: 212-785-9595
e-mail: info@jdfcure.com

Focuses energies on fund-raising, referrals, educational materials and information pertaining to juvenile diabetes.

Stephen H. Leeper, DDS, President

2651 National Diabetes Action Network for the Blind
National Federation of the Blind
1800 Johnson Street Suite 2
Baltimore, MD 21230

410-659-9314
Fax: 410-685-5653

Leading support and information organization of persons losing vision due to diabetes. Provides personal contact and resource information with other blind diabetics about non-visual techniques of independently managing diabetes, monitoring glucose levels, measuring insulin and other matters concerning diabetes. Publishes Voice of the Diabetic, the leading publication about diabetes and blindness.

2652 National Diabetes Information Clearinghouse
One Information Way
Bethesda, MD 20205

301-468-2162
301-907-8906
e-mail: ndic@aerie.com
www.kiddk.nih.gov

Offers various materials, resources, books, pamphlets and more for persons and families in the area of diabetes.

Audio Video

2653 Diabetes: Not No Sweet
Fanlight Productions
47 Halifax St
Boston, MA 02130

617-469-4999
Fax: 617-469-3379
e-mail: fanlight@fanlight.com
www.fanlight.com

Exciting new approaches to the prevention and control of diabetes, and a look at its prevalence in Native American communities in particular.
47 minutes

2654 Juvenile Diabetes
Fanlight Productions
47 Halifax St
Boston, MA 02130

617-469-4999
Fax: 617-469-3379
e-mail: fanlight@fanlight.com
www.fanlight.com

Features a number of youngsters with diabetes, and stresses the importance of young people managing as much of their own care as possible.
28 minutes

Web Sites

2655 Mediconsult

www.mediconsult.com

Provides links to information on disease, illness and disorders, including such content areas as conference highlights, educational material, journal articles, research, news, and support.

2656 National Diabetes Information Clearinghouse

www.kiddk.nih.gov

Offers various materials, resources, books, pamphlets and more for persons and families in the area of diabetes.

Books

2657 Diabetes

Barbara Goodheart, author

Looks at the differences between juvenile and adult-onset diabetes, discusses the history of the disease, causes, complications and treatments.

2658 Diabetes 101

Betty Page Brackenridge, author

Chronimed Publishing
PO Box 59032
Minneapolis, MN 55459   612-513-6475
                               800-848-2793
                               Fax: 612-443-2806

Revised and expanded second edition. A layman's guide to everything you need to know to live healthfully with diabetes.

175 pages
ISBN: 1-565610-24-5

2659 Diabetes Dictionary

National Diabetes Information Clearinghouse
2 Information Way
Bethesda, MD 20892   301-654-3810
                          Fax: 301-907-8906
          e-mail: nddic@info.niddk.nih.gov
                     www.niddk.nih.gov

illustrated glossary of more than 300 diabetes-related terms.

2660 Diabetes Medical Nutrition Therapy

American Diabetes Association
1660 Duke Street Suite 100
Alexandria, VA 22314
                              800-232-3472
                         Fax: 703-549-6995
                         www.diabetes.org

A professional guide to management and nutrition education resources. provides in-depth coverage of nutrition assessment, goal setting, intervention, and outcome evaluation. Information is provided on specific resources and case studies are cited for practical examples.

2661 Diabetes Teaching Guide for People Who Use Insulin

Joslin Diabetes Center
1 Joslin Pl
Boston, MA 02215   617-732-2400

Discusses the causes of diabetes, the role of diet and exercise, meal planning and complications. Also provide information on drawing blood, mixing and injecting insulin.

2662 If Your Child Has Diabetes: An Answer Book for Parents

Putnam Publishing Group
200 Madison Ave
New York, NY 10016   212-951-8400

Provides information and recommendations for parents of children with diabetes on subjects such as school, recreation, medical and life insurance and employment as well as general information about diabetes.

2663 Life with Diabetes: A Series of Teaching Outlines

American Diabetes Association
1660 Duke Street Suite 100
Alexandria, VA 22314
                              800-232-3472
                         Fax: 703-549-6995
                         www.diabetes.org

Presents a comprehensive curriculum for diabetes education. Each outline includes a statement of purpose, preequisites for attending the session, materials needed for teaching the session, recommended teaching method, a content outline, instructor notes, and evaluation and documentation plan, and suggested readings relatede to each topic.

2664 Raising a Child with Diabetes a Guide for Parents

American Diabetes Association
1660 Duke Street Suite 100
Alexandria, VA 22314
                              800-232-3472
                         Fax: 703-549-6995
                         www.diabetes.org

You'll learn how to help your child adjust to insulin to allow for favorite foods, have a busy schedule and still feel healthy and strong, negotiate the twists and turns of being different, and much more.

2665 Resource and Activities Guide

Patricia Moynihan, author

Chronimed Publishing
PO Box 59032
Minneapolis, MN 55459

612-513-6475
800-848-2793
Fax: 612-443-2806

For use with the Diabetes Youth Curriculum. Contains 300 educational activities that correspond with the text in the Curriculum and can easily be removed for photocopying.

ISBN: 0-937721-50-6

Children's Books

2666 Dinosaur Tamer

25 fictional stories that will entertain, enlighten, and ease your child's frustrations about having diabetes. Each tale evaporates the fear of insulin shots,k blood test, going to diabetes camp, and more.

2667 Even Little Kids Get Diabetes

Connie Pirner, author

Albert Whitman & Company
6340 Oakton Street
Morton Grove, IL 60053

847-531-0033
800-255-7675
Fax: 847-531-0039
www.awhitmanco.com

A preschooler tells how it was discovered when she was only two, that she has this common disease and describes her daily treatment and the precautions her family must ovserve.

ISBN: 0-807521-58-2

Joseph Boyd, President
Joe Campbell, Customer Service

2668 Everyone Likes to Eat

Hugo J. Hollerorth, author

Chronimed Publishing
PO Box 59032
Minneapolis, MN 55459

612-513-6475
800-848-2793
Fax: 612-443-2806

Revised and up-to-date second edition. How children can eat most of the foods they enjoy and still take care of their diabetes. Intended for elementary-school-age children, this guide is filled with activities, puzzles, and problem-soloving exercieses.

ISBN: 1-565610-26-1

2669 Grilled Cheese

American Diabetes Association
1660 Duke Street Suite 100
Alexandria, VA 22314

800-232-3472
Fax: 703-549-6995
www.diabetes.org

story designed to ease children's fears and frustrations of having diabetes.

2670 In Control: A Guide for Teens with Diabetes

Chronimed Publishing
PO Box 59032
Minneapolis, MN 55459

612-513-6475
800-848-2793
Fax: 612-443-2806

dispels myths and tackles the real issues that teens with diabetes face. Teaches how to care for their diabetes without letting it get in the way of their lives.

ISBN: 1-565610-61-X

2671 It's Time to Learn About Diabetes: A Workbook on Diabetes for Children

Jean Betschart, author

Chronimed Publishing
PO Box 59032
Minneapolis, MN 55459

612-513-6475
800-848-2793
Fax: 612-443-2806

Contains everything school-age kids need to know about diabetes, from fun exercises to family vacations. Addresses fears concerning insulin shots and blood tests. A 24-minute companion video is also available (see separate lishting).

ISBN: 1-565610-80-6

2672 Kiss the Candy Days Good-Bye

Vincent T. Dacquino, author

Delacorte Press
1540 Broadway
New York, NY 10036

212-354-6500

This book focuses on Jimmy who is surprised to learn he has diabetes after seeming so healthy and fit. The story contains information on symptoms and the dangers of untreated diabetes.

Magazines

2673 Countdown
Juvenile Diabetes Foundation International
432 Park Ave S
New York, NY 10016   212-889-7575
                          Fax: 212-725-7259

Offers the latest news and information in diabetes research and treatment to everyone from an international arena of diabetes investigators to parents of small children with diabetes, from physicians to school teachers, from pharmacists to corporate executives.

Sandy Dylak, Editor

2674 Diabetes
American Diabetes Association
1660 Duke Street Suite 100
Alexandria, VA 22314
                          800-232-3472
                          Fax: 703-549-6995
                          www.diabetes.org

A peer-reviewed journal focusing on laboratory research.

2675 Diabetes Care
American Diabetes Association
166 Duke Street Suite 100
Alexandria, VA 22314
                          800-232-3472
                          Fax: 703-549-6995
                          www.diabetes.org

A peer-reviewed journal emphasizing reviews, cdomentaries and original research on topics of interest to clinicians.

2676 Diabetes Forecast
American Diabetes Association
166 Duke Street Suite 100
Alexandria, VA 22314
                          800-232-3472
                          Fax: 703-549-6995
                          www.diabetes.org

The monthly lifestyle magazine for people with diabetes, featuring complete, in-depth coverage of all aspects of living with diabetes.

2677 Diabetes Spectrum: From Research to Practice
American Diabetes Association
166 Duke Street Suite 100
Alexandria, VA 22314
                          800-232-3472
                          Fax: 703-549-6995
                          www.diabetes.org

A journal translating research into practice and focusing on diabetes education and counseling.

2678 Understanding Gestational Diabetes
2 Information Way
Bethesda, MD 20892   301-654-3810
                          Fax: 301-907-8906
                          e-mail: nddic@info.niddk.nih.gov
                          www.niddk.nih.gov

2679 Voice of the Diabetic
National Federation of the Blind
1800 Johnson Street Suite 2
Baltimore, MD 21230   410-659-9314
                          Fax: 410-685-5653

The leading publication in the diabetes field. Each issue addresses the probhlems and concerns of diabetes, with a special emphasis for those who have lost vision due to diabetes. Available in print and on cassette.

Newsletters

2680 Clinical Diabetes
American Diabetes Association
166 Duke Street Suite 100
Alexandria, VA 22314
                          800-232-3472
                          Fax: 703-549-6995
                          www.diabetes.org

A bi-monthly newsletter providing practical treatment information for primary care physicians.

2681 Diabetes Advisor
American Diabetes Association
166 Duke Street Suite 100
Alexandria, VA 22314
                          800-232-3472
                          Fax: 703-549-6995
                          www.diabetes.org

Offers informative articles and research in the area of diabetes for professionals and patients. Offers facts and research on diagnosis, symptoms, technology and the newest devices for persons with diabetes, as well as referral and hotline numbers.

2682 Diabetes Dateline
National Diabetes Information Clearinghouse
2 Information Way
Bethesda, MD 20892   301-654-3810
                              Fax: 301-907-8906
              e-mail: nddic@info.niddk.nih.gov
                          www.niddk.nih.gov

2683 Diabetes Educator
American Association of Diabetes Educators
444 N Michigan Ave Suite 1240
Chicago, IL 60611   312-644-2233
                              Fax: 312-644-4411

Offers information to health professionals working with persons with diabetes.

James J. Balija, Executive Director

2684 Kid's Corner
American Diabetes Association
166 Duke Street Suite 100
Alexandria, VA 22314

                              800-232-3472
                              Fax: 703-549-6995
                              www.diabetes.org

A mini-magazine for kids that offers word
searches, puzzles and jokes - plus an encouraging story in each issue about kids with diabetes.

Pamphlets

2685 Children with Diabetes
2 Information Way
Bethesda, MD 20892   301-654-3810
                              Fax: 301-907-8906
              e-mail: nddic@info.niddk.nih.gov
                          www.niddk.nih.gov

**2686 Complementary and Alternative Therapies for
Diabetes Treatment**
2 Information Way
Bethesda, MD 20892   301-654-3810
                              Fax: 301-907-8906
              e-mail: nddic@info.niddk.nih.gov
                          www.niddk.nih.gov

2687 Diabetes Insipidus
2 Information Way
Bethesda, MD 20892   301-654-3810
                              Fax: 301-907-8906
              e-mail: nddic@info.niddk.nih.gov
                          www.niddk.nih.gov

2688 Diabetes Overview
2 Information Way
Bethesda, MD 20892   301-654-3810
                              Fax: 301-907-8906
              e-mail: nddic@info.niddk.nih.gov
                          www.niddk.nih.gov

2689 Diabetes in African Americans
2 Information Way
Bethesda, MD 20892   301-654-3810
                              Fax: 301-907-8906
              e-mail: nddic@info.niddk.nih.gov
                          www.niddk.nih.gov

2690 Diabetes in Hispanic Americans
2 Information Way
Bethesda, MD 20892   301-654-3810
                              Fax: 301-907-8906
              e-mail: nddic@info.niddk.nih.gov
                          www.niddk.nih.gov

2691 Diabetic Neuropathy: the Nerve Damage of Diabetes
2 Information Way
Bethesda, MD 20892   301-654-3810
                              Fax: 301-907-8906
              e-mail: nddic@info.niddk.nih.gov
                          www.niddk.nih.gov

2692 Diabetics Control and Complications Trial
2 Information Way
Bethesda, MD 20892   301-654-3810
                              Fax: 301-907-8906
              e-mail: nddic@info.niddk.nih.gov
                          www.niddk.nih.gov

2693 I Have Diabetes: How Much Should I Eat?
2 Information Way
Bethesda, MD 20892   301-654-3810
                              Fax: 301-907-8906
              e-mail: nddic@info.niddk.nih.gov
                          www.niddk.nih.gov

2694 I Have Diabetes: What Should I Eat?
2 Information Way
Bethesda, MD 20892   301-654-3810
                              Fax: 301-907-8906
              e-mail: nddic@info.niddk.nih.gov
                          www.niddk.nih.gov

2695 I Have Diabetes: When Should I Eat?
2 Information Way
Bethesda, MD 20892   301-654-3810
                              Fax: 301-907-8906
              e-mail: nddic@info.niddk.nih.gov
                          www.niddk.nih.gov

DESCRIPTION

2696 JUVENILE RHEUMATOID ARTHRITIS

Synonym: JRA

Disorder Type: Autoimmune Disease

Covers these related disorders: Pauciarticular juvenile arthritis, Systemic-onset juvenile arthritis (Still's disease), Type I polyarticular juvenile arthritis, Type II polyarticular juvenile arthritis

May involve these systems in the body (see Section III):

Muscular System, Skeletal System

Juvenile rheumatoid arthritis (JRA) is a group of disorders of childhood characterized by inflammation (arthritis), tenderness, pain, and swelling of one or more joints, potentially causing impaired development, limited movements, and permanent bending or extension of affected joints in various fixed postures (contractures). The symptoms and findings associated with JRA occur as the result of inflammation of the synovial membrane of affected joints (synovitis). Synovial membranes are connective tissue membranes that line the spaces between joints and bones and secrete a thick fluid to lubricate the joints. Although the cause of JRA is unknown, researchers speculate that the disorder may be the result of infection by an unidentified microorganism, an excessive immune response to a substance that the body perceives as foreign (hypersensitivity response), or abnormal immune responses against the body's own cells or tissues (autoimmune response). Certain antibodies often present in the blood of adults with rheumatoid arthritis (e.g., rheumatoid factors) are only rarely present in children with JRA. In such cases, researchers indicate that affected children may have some genetic predisposition for certain forms of JRA. Approximately 250,000 children are thought to be affected by JRA in the United States. Females are more commonly affected than males.

There are three major categories of JRA: polyarticular, pauciarticular, and systemic-onset juvenile arthritis. Polyarticular juvenile arthritis, which affects approximately 35 percent of children with JRA, typically involves several joints. Associated symptoms and findings include inflammation, swelling, abnormal warmth, tenderness, and pain of affected joints. This form of JRA often affects joints of the elbows, wrists, fingers, knees, feet, and ankles. In addition, patients may have involvement of joints of the jaw (temporomandibular joints), causing limited opening of the mouth; the neck (cervical spine), resulting in neck pain and stiffness; and the hips, causing pain, stiffness, and limited movements. Normal growth may be delayed during periods of active disease, causing such abnormalities as unusually short fingers, small feet, or underdevelopment of the jaw (micrognathia). Some children with polyarticular juvenile arthritis may also experience more generalized symptoms, such as low fever, lack of appetite (anorexia), increased irritability, a mild decrease in the level of circulating blood cells (anemia), swelling of certain lymph nodes (lymphadenopathy), or mild enlargement of the liver and spleen (hepatosplenomegaly).

In pauciarticular juvenile arthritis, four or fewer joints are affected during the first six months after the onset of the disease. Type I pauciarticular juvenile arthritis primarily affects females, has an early onset, and affects approximately 30 to 40 percent of children with JRA. Affected joints typically include the elbows, knees, and ankles. In addition, other joints may sometimes be affected, such as those of a single finger or toe, the wrists, the neck, or the jaw. Patients are also at risk for chronic inflammation of the colored region of the eye (iris) and its muscle (iridocyclitis). One or both eyes may be affected. Some patients may experience associated redness, sensitivity to light (photophobia), pain, or decreased clearness of vision (visual acuity). Without appropriate treatment, visual impairment or, in severe cases, blindness may result. Generalized symptoms may include a general feeling of ill health (malaise), low fever, mild enlargement of the liver and spleen (hepatosplenomegaly), and mild anemia. Type II pauciarticular juvenile arthritis, which affects about 10 to 15 percent of children with JRA, is most common in males older than age eight. Affected joints usually include those of the hips, knees, toes, and heels. In some patients, joints of the elbows, fingers, wrists, or jaw may also be affected. In patients with this form of JRA, associated foot and hip pain may sometimes be disabling. In addition, chronic, progressive, inflammatory disease of joints of the spine (spondyloarthropathy) may develop. Symptoms may include pain, stiffness, and loss of mobility of joints of the upper and lower back (ankylosing spondylitis). In addition, some affected children may experience sudden (acute) episodes of iridocyclitis.

Systemic-onset juvenile arthritis occurs in about 10 to 20 percent of patients with JRA and appears to affect females and males equally. This form of JRA usually begins with generalized symptoms, such as a high, intermittent fever that rapidly returns to normal; a characteristic rash; anemia; enlargement of the liver and spleen (hepatosplenomegaly); enlargement of the lymph nodes (lymphadenopathy); mild liver dysfunction; and, in about one third of patients, inflammation of the membranous sac surrounding the heart (pericarditis) or the membrane lining the lungs and chest cavity (pleuritis). The fever associated with systemic JRA tends to rise in the evenings, although it may also be elevated in the mornings, and is often associated with shaking chills. During fever episodes, a temporary, salmon-colored rash often appears on the trunk or arms or legs (extremities), although it may appear anywhere on the body. Such a rash may also temporarily appear in association with heat exposure or stress. In patients with systemic disease, joint inflammation, swelling, stiffness, and pain may occur at disease onset or months later. Joint involvement is usually similar to that seen in patients with polyarticular juvenile arthritis. Systemic symptoms and findings typically have a self-limited course that lasts for several months. However, such findings may recur in some patients.

In approximately 75 percent of affected children, symptoms associated with JRA completely disappear with little loss of function or deformity. However, other patients, particularly those with multiple joint involvement or rheumatoid factor,

may experience repeated or chronic joint inflammation and permanent stiffness, limited movement, and deformity of certain affected joints. In addition, some patients with pauciarticular juvenile arthritis may experience additional later joint involvement (polyarthritis) or ongoing symptoms due to progressive, inflammatory disease of joints of the spine (spondyloarthropathy).

Children with JRA should receive regular eye (e.g., slit-lamp) examinations to ensure early detection and treatment of iridocyclitis. Treatment of iridocyclitis includes the use of corticosteroid eyedrops and drugs that widen (dilate) the pupil. Joint inflammation, pain, and stiffness may be alleviated with aspirin, nonsteroidal anti-inflammatory drugs (NSAIDS), medications such as methotrexate, or, in extremely severe cases, corticosteroids administered by mouth (orally). Due to the potential association of aspirin and the occurrence of Reye's syndrome, NSAIDS (e.g., tolmetin, naproxen, etc.) are currently being prescribed more frequently than aspirin as a treatment for JRA. Children with JRA who do not respond to NSAIDS therapy may be treated with low-dose methotrexate. If JRA is severe and systemic or, in patients in whom iridocyclitis is uncontrolled by corticosteroid eyedrops, oral corticosteroid therapy may be prescribed. However, oral corticosteroid therapy is usually avoided in children, if possible, since such therapy may slow the growth rate. In addition, splints may be used during the day to help rest inflamed joints and at night to minimize the risk of contracture development and associated deformity. Special exercises may also be recommended to help reduce possible muscle wasting and contractures. In some patients, surgery may be required to help correct contractures.

The following organizations in the General Resources Section can provide additional information: National Organization for Rare Disorders, Inc. (NORD), NIH/Office of Rare Diseases, Genetic Alliance, Online Mendelian Inheritance in Man.: www3.ncbi.nlm.nih.gov/Omim/searchomim.html, NIH/National Institute of Arthritis and Musculoskeletal and Skin Diseases

National Associations & Support Groups

2697 American Juvenile Arthritis Organization (AJAO)
Arthritis Foundation
P.O. Box 7669
Atlanta, GA 30357
404-872-7100
800-283-7800
Fax: 404-872-9559
e-mail: jaustin@arthritis.org
www.arthritis.com

A council established by the Arthritis Foundation which serves the special needs of young people with arthritis and their families. Provides information, inspiration and advocacy by identifying the needs of children with arthritis, and speaks out on their behalf.

2698 Arthritis Foundation
1330 West Peachtree Street
Atlanta, GA 30309
703-236-6000
800-283-7800
www.arthritis.org

The Arthritis Foundation was the genesis of today's arthritis research programs and has nurtured its growth in both the private and public sectors. The Foundation has spent more than $200 million to support more than 1,700 scientists and physicians in arthritis research.

2699 Arthritis Society
393 University Avenue Suite 1700
Toronto, Ontario, M4G
Canada
416-967-1414
Fax: 416-967-7171
e-mail: jkonecny@arthritis.ca
www.arthritis.ca

2700 Kids on the Block Arthritis Programs
Arthritis Foundation
1330 West Peachtree Street
Atlanta, GA 30329
404-872-7100
800-283-7800
Fax: 404-872-0457
e-mail: help@arthritis.org
www.arthritis.org

State and local programs that use puppetry to help children understand what it is like for children and adults who have arthritis.

Research Centers

2701 Affiliated Children's Arthritis Centers of New England
New England Medical Center
750 Washington Street, Box 286
Boston, MA 02111
617-636-5528
Fax: 617-350-8388

Research organization comprised of a network of 15 pediatric centers throughout New England and based at the Floating Hospital of New England Medical Center.

Jane G. Schaller, M.D., Coordinator

2702 Pediatric Rheumatoid Clinic
Duke Medical Center
Box 3212
Durham, NC 27710
919-684-6575

Clinical and laboratory pediatric rheumatoid studies.

Dr. Deborah Kredich, Chairman

Web Sites

2703 CUNY-NOAH
www.noah.cuny.edu/arthritis/arthritis.html

2704 Duquesne University
www.duq.edu/PT/RA/TableOfContents.html

Books

2705 Educational Rights for Children With Arthritis: A Parents Manual
AJAO
P.O. Box 7669
Atlanta, GA 30357
404-872-7100
Fax: 404-872-9559
e-mail: help@arthritis.org
www.arthritis.org

A self-instructional manual helping parents to identify and obtain school services needed by their child with arthritis. Covers laws and special services, explores strategies for working with school personnel and stresses good communication and advocacy techniques.

2706 Understanding Juvenile Rheumatoid Arthritis
American Juvenile Arthritis Organization
P.O. Box 19000
Atlanta, GA 30326
800-283-7800

A manual for health professionals to use in teaching children with JRA and their families about disease management and self-care.

372 pages

2707 We Can: A Guide for Parents of Children With Arthritis
AJAO
P.O.Box 7669
Atlanta, GA 30357
404-872-7100
Fax: 404-872-9559
e-mail: help@arthritis.org
www.arthritis.org

Offers parents tips for daily living and practical points for helping their child toward independent adulthood.

Children's Books

2708 Arthritis

Madelyn Klein Anderson, author

Franklin Watts c/o Grolier
90 Old Sherman Tpke
Danbury, CT 06816
203-797-3500
800-621-1115
Fax: 203-797-3197
www.grolier.com

This book offers a clear explanation of the various forms and effects of the disease of arthritis and what treatments are available.

96 pages Grades 7-12
ISBN: 0-531108-01-5

2709 JRA and Me
American Juvenile Arthritis Organization
P.O. Box 19000
Atlanta, GA 30326
800-283-7800

A workbook for school-aged children who have juvenile arthritis. This book offers a variety of educational games, puzzles and worksheets to teach children about their illness and how to take care of themselves.

57 pages

2710 Living with Arthritis

Dr. John Shenkman, author

Franklin Watts c/o Grolier
90 Old Sherman Tpke
Danbury, CT 06816
203-797-3500
800-621-1115
Fax: 203-797-3197
www.grolier.com

Shows how people with arthritis can overcome their pain and lead productive, full lives.

32 pages Grades 5-7

2711 Yard Sale Coloring Book
American Juvenile Arthritis Organization
P.O. Box 19000
Atlanta, GA 30326
800-283-7800

A coloring/activity book based on a Kids on the Block script, written for third and fourth grade students. It can be used with Kids on the Block performances, as a stand-alone piece or with a free lesson plan packet.

Newsletters

2712 AJAO Newsletter
American Juvenile Arthritis Organization
1330 West Peachtree Street
Atlanta, GA 30309
404-872-7100
Fax: 404-872-9559
e-mail: kgatmail@arthritis.org

This reliable and comprehensive newsletter for families coping with childhood arthritis and related conditions contains the latest research findings, responsible advice from pediatric specialists, practical methods to help improve quality of life, and informative updates about medications and how they affect children. Articles are written in clear understandable language. Timely medical insights and life enhancing information that provides solutions to everyday problems.

Quarterly

Beth Blaney, Editor

Pamphlets

2713 Arthritis Information: Children
Arthritis Foundation
P.O. Box 7669
Atlanta, GA 30357
404-872-7100
800-283-7800
Fax: 404-872-0457

List of materials for children with arthritis, their families and the health professionals who care for them.

2714 Arthritis in Children
NAMSIC, National Institutes of Health
1 AMS Circle
Bethesda, MD 20892
301-495-4484
Fax: 301-587-4352
TTY: 301-565-2966
www.nih.gov/niams/

2715 Arthritis in Children and La Artritis Infantojuvenil
American Juvenile Arthritis Organization
P.O. Box 19000
Atlanta, GA 30326

800-283-7800

A medical information booklet about juvenile
rheumatoid arthritis. This booklet is written for
parents or other adults and includes details
about different forms of JRA, medications,
therapies and coping issues.

**2716 Arthritis in Children: Resources for Children,
Parents and Teachers**
National Arthritis and Skin Diseases Clearinghouse
9000 Rockville Pike
Bethesda, MD 20892   301-495-4484

A resource offering information on juvenile arthritis, causes, treatments and prevention.

38 pages

2717 Rheumatoid Arthritis
NAMSIC, National Institutes of Health
1 AMS Circle
Bethesda, MD 20892   301-495-4484
Fax: 301-587-4352
TTY: 301-565-2966
www.nih.gov/niams/

Offers an introduction and definition of rheumatoid arthritis, treatments, causes, objectives,
daily living, resources and medical information.

**2718 When Your Student Has Arthritis: A Guide for
Teachers**
Arthritis Foundation
P.O. Box 7669
Atlanta, GA 30357   404-872-7100
800-283-7800
Fax: 404-872-0457

A medical information booklet written for teachers or other adults who have arthritis. The booklet describes different forms of juvenile
arthritis, how arthritis might affect the child at
school, and how to help the child work around
these problems.

DESCRIPTION

2719 KAWASAKI DISEASE

Synonyms: MLNS, Mucocutaneous lymph node syndrome

May involve these systems in the body (see Section III):

Cardiovascular System

Kawasaki disease is a syndrome of unknown origin that primarily affects infants and young children. The disease was initially observed in Japanese children after World War II. Kawasaki disease is becoming increasingly frequent in the United States, has been reported worldwide, and is currently considered the leading cause of acquired heart disease in children in the U.S. Although Kawasaki disease has been reported in people in all racial groups, individuals of Japanese descent appear to be most commonly affected. The disease may occur commonly in a random or an isolated manner (sporadic form) or, rarely, may suddenly affect large numbers of individuals (epidemic form). Although the cause of Kawasaki disease is unknown, researchers suspect that toxic substances produced by certain bacteria (e.g., staphylococcal toxins) may play some role. There is no evidence of transmission of the disease from one affected individual to another (person-to-person transmission).

Kawasaki disease most commonly affects children who are five years of age or younger. Affected children typically develop a sudden, sustained, high fever that is often greater than 104 degrees and unresponsive to therapy with fever-reducing (antipyretic) medications. Most patients also have inflammation of the whites of both eyes and the lining inside the eyelids (bilateral conjunctivitis), causing redness but no associated discharge; dry, red (erythematous), cracked (fissured) lips; a strawberry-red tongue; and swelling of one or several lymph nodes, particularly those of the neck (cervical lymphadenopathy). Patients also typically develop a reddish skin rash that may consist of flat, discolored spots and small, raised areas (maculopapular) or appear similar to that seen in measles (morbilliform). The trunk, the hands and feet, and the face may be affected. Patients usually experience subsequent swelling and associated pain of the hands and feet. By approximately the second to third week, affected skin may begin to peel (desquamation) from the palms of the hands, the soles of the feet, and the tips of the fingers and toes. Such peeling may also involve other affected areas, such as the trunk. In addition, children with Kawasaki disease are usually irritable and may develop joint swelling and pain (arthritis), abdominal pain, diarrhea, vomiting, coughing, inflammation of the gall bladder, or enlargement of the liver and spleen (hepatosplenomegaly). Additional symptoms and findings may include inflammation of certain muscles (myositis), discharge of a thin nasal fluid (rhinorrhea), episodes of increased electrical activity in the brain (seizures), mild inflammation of the protective membrane surrounding the brain (aseptic meningitis), or other abnormalities.

The most serious complication potentially associated with Kawasaki disease is involvement of the heart. Within the first few weeks after disease onset, approximately 25 percent of untreated patients develop inflammation of arteries that carry blood to the heart muscle (coronary arteritis) and associated widening or bulging (aneurysms) of the walls of these arteries. In rare cases, affected children, particularly those under the age of one year, may experience few early symptoms associated with the disease, yet later develop coronary arteritis. Patients with cardiac involvement may develop inflammation of heart muscle (myocarditis); deficient blood supply to heart muscle (myocardial ischemia), resulting in localized loss of tissue (infarction); and inflammation of the membranous sac surrounding the heart (pericarditis). Additional findings may include inflammation of the membrane lining the internal surfaces of the cavities of the heart (endocarditis), an inability of the heart to sufficiently pump blood to the lungs and the rest of the body (heart failure), or abnormalities of the rhythm or rate of the heartbeat (arrythmias). In some cases, without appropriate treatment, patients with severe cardiac involvement may experience potentially life-threatening complications.

All patients with diagnosed or suspected Kawasaki disease should undergo specialized diagnostic tests, such as chest x-rays, electrocardiograms, and echocardiograms. Additional testing (e.g., two-dimensional echocardiogram) may also be conducted during the first two weeks of disease. The treatment of children with Kawasaki disease should include intravenous (IV) infusion with a preparation of antibodies (immunoglobulins) obtained from plasma, the liquid portion of the blood (intravenous gammaglobulin), and therapy with aspirin (salicylate therapy). Early (within 10 days of fever onset) intravenous gammaglobulin therapy helps to alleviate fever and other associated symptoms; in addition, controlled studies have demonstrated that such therapy decreases heart involvement to 25% of patients. Once the fever has subsided, patients may receive therapy with lower doses of aspirin. Such therapy typically continues until coronary arteritis resolves. In the rare patient with large or multiple coronary aneurysms, treatment may include therapy with anticlotting medications, such as warfarin or heparin. Other treatment is symptomatic and supportive. All children diagnosed with Kawasaki disease receive outpatient follow-up with a pediatric cardiologist.

The following organizations in the General Resources Section can provide additional information: NIH/National Heart, Lung and Blood Institute, NIH/National Institute of Child Health and Human Development, NIH/National Institute of Allergy and Infectious Diseases, National Organization for Rare Disorders, Inc. (NORD), NIH/Office of Rare Diseases, Center for Disease Control (CDC)

National Associations & Support Groups

2720 Kawasaki Families' Network
46-111 Nahewai Place
Kaneohe, HI 96744   808-525-8053
                         Fax: 808-525-8055
                 e-mail: kawasaki@compuserve.com
         ourworld.compuserve.com/homepage/kawasaki

Web Sites

2721 Vanderbilt University
www.mc.vanderbilt.edu/peds/pidl/infect/kawasak2.htm

DESCRIPTION

2722 KELOIDS

Synonym: Cheloids

May involve these systems in the body (see Section III):

Dermatologic System

Keloids are firm, nodule-like overgrowths of scar tissue that occur at the sites of surgery, injury, or trauma to the skin. These overgrowths result from the formation, during the healing process, of excessive amounts of the fibrous protein collagen, which is a major structural component of connective tissue. These elevated scars may be itchy and are usually pink in color, shiny, smooth, irregularly shaped, firm, and rubbery. Some keloids may be tender or painful. Although keloids may appear on the face, neck, earlobes, legs, or other areas, they most often occur over the breastbone (sternum) and the shoulders.

Keloid development may sometimes result following surgery, body piercing, and other types of trauma to the skin such as burns or scalds. In addition, keloids may develop in association with severe acne and occasionally with certain connective tissue disorders such as Ehlers-Danlos syndrome or skin disorders such as Touraine-Solente-Gole syndrome. In some cases, keloid development may be inherited as an autosomal recessive or autosomal dominant trait. In addition, keloids are more common in black individuals.

Without treatment, keloids tend to flatten out and become less obvious within a period of months or years. However, monthly injections of certain corticosteroid drugs directly into the lesions may successfully decrease their size and reduce itching, but treatment should be initiated early in their development. Treatment of large keloids may include surgical removal followed by corticosteroid injections into the lesions. Surgery alone most often results in a recurrence of the keloid. Other treatment may include the direct application of silicone patches or sheeting to promote shrinkage.

The following organizations in the General Resources Section can provide additional information: NIH/National Institute of Arthritis and Musculoskeletal, and Skin Disorders

---

National Associations & Support Groups

2723 American Academy of Dermatology
930 North Meacham Road, P.O.Box4014
Schaumburg, IL 60168   708-330-0230
                              www.aad.org

Largest, most representative of all dermatologic associations. Committed to the highest quality standards in continuing medical education. Developed a platform in which to promote and advance the science and art of medicine and surgery related to the skin; promotes the highest possible standards in clinical practice, education and research in dermatology and related disciplines; and supports and enhances patient care.

2724 American Skin Association
150 East 58th Street, 33rd Floor
New York, NY 10155   212-753-8260
                            800-499-7546
                      Fax: 212-688-6547
e-mail: AmericanSkin@compuserve.com

Web Sites

2725 Project Image
http://projectimagine.org/

DESCRIPTION

2726 KERATOSIS PILARIS

May involve these systems in the body (see Section III):

Dermatologic System

Keratosis pilaris is a relatively common condition of the skin that is characterized by the appearance of small, scaly pimples or papules that form at the site of hair follicles. Although pimple formation may involve most of the body surface, it most commonly appears on the skin of the upper arms, buttocks, and thighs. In affected children, the face is usually involved. Keratosis pilaris often is referred to as having a gooseflesh appearance.

Keratosis pilaris occurs when the openings of the hair follicles become clogged with plugs composed of dead cells that are naturally shed from the skin's upper layer. Although the pimples are not inflamed, they may become irritated, resulting in inflammation of the hair follicles themselves (folliculitis). Because dry skin appears to be more prone to the formation of the characteristic papules associated with keratosis pilaris, this condition is much more prevalent in the winter than it is in the summer. Keratosis pilaris most often occurs during early childhood, adolescence, and young adulthood. In addition, this condition tends to develop more commonly in obese individuals as well as those with a chronic inflammatory skin disorder called atopic dermatitis.

Treatment of keratosis pilaris is dependent upon the extent of the pimple formation. Mild eruptions may be treated by the application of a petroleum jelly and cold cream mixture, petroleum jelly and water preparation, or other mild, soothing, lubricating agents. More generalized or severe eruptions may be treated with regular applications of a salicylic acid and paraffin mixture, retinoic acid (tretinoin) preparation, alpha hydroxy acid agents, or other similar preparations. Keratosis pilaris often recedes or resolves when affected individuals reach their 20s or 30s.

The following organizations in the General Resources Section can provide additional information: National Institute of Arthritis and Musculoskeletal and Skin Diseases

National Associations & Support Groups

2727 American Academy of Dermatology
930 North Meacham Road, P.O.Box4014
Schaumburg, IL 60168   708-330-0230
                              www.aad.org

Largest, most influential and most representative of all dermatologic associations. Committed to the highest quality standards in continuing medical education. Developed a platform in which to promote and advance the science and art of medicine and surgery related to the skin; promote the highest possible standards in clinical practice, education and research in dermatology and related disciples; and support and enhance patient care and promote the public interest relating to dermatology.

2728 American Skin Association
150 East 58th Street, 33rd Floor
New York, NY 10155   212-753-8260
                              800-499-7546
                         Fax: 212-688-6547
           e-mail: AmericanSkin@compuserve.com

DESCRIPTION

2729 KERNICTERUS

Synonym: Bilirubin encephalopathy

Disorder Type: Metabolism

May involve these systems in the body (see Section III):

Central Nervous System

Kernicterus refers to a neurologic condition in which excessive amounts of bilirubin accumulate in the brain of affected newborns, resulting in damage to the central nervous system. Bilirubin, a reddish-yellow pigment present in bile, is derived from the breakdown of the red protein in red blood cells (hemoglobin). Premature infants and newborns with certain congenital disorders (e.g., erythroblastosis fetalis and Criglar-Najjar syndrome) are at risk for this life-threatening condition. In premature infants, the processes needed for bilirubin excretion may not be fully developed. Factors that put extra strain on this immature metabolic process may result in increased levels of bilirubin in the blood (hyperbilirubinemia). If these levels become excessive and are left untreated, bilirubin may be deposited in the brain. For example, in infants with erythroblastosis fetalis, antibodies from the mother's blood cross the placental barrier and destroy red blood cells of the fetus, resulting in release of excessive amounts of bilirubin. In some cases, bilirubin builds up faster than the liver is able to eliminate it, resulting in hyperbilirubinemia. Signs of this condition include a yellowing of the eyes, skin, and mucous membranes (jaundice).

Criglar-Najjar syndrome results from the deficiency of an enzyme that is required to convert bilirubin to a form that may be excreted from the body, thus causing hyperbilirubinemia. Other conditions or disorders that cause hyperbilirubinemia place the newborn, especially those who are born prematurely, at risk for kernicterus.

Symptoms of kernicterus usually become apparent within the first week of life. However, hyperbilirubinemia that occurs anytime within the first month of life may result in kernicterus. Symptoms and characteristic findings may include difficulty in feeding; vomiting; lethargy; and lack of a normal response to sudden, loud noises (Moro or startle reflex). Further signs of this condition may include breathing difficulties; severe muscle spasms resulting in a backward arching of the back and neck (opisthotonos); twitching of the arms, legs, and face; a high-pitched cry; and convulsions. In some affected infants, severe involvement of the central nervous system may cause life-threatening complications. In others, findings associated with permanent disability may be observed periodically until the third year of life when the complete neurologic picture emerges. Symptoms may include involuntary spasms of the muscles, hearing loss, eye movement irregularities, deficiencies in motor development, difficulties in speech, seizures, and mental retardation. Some infants who experience only slight kernicterus may experience mild irregularities in neuromuscular coordination, moderate deafness, and slight retardation.

Treatment of kernicterus is directed toward prevention involving the correction of hyperbilirubinemia and jaundice before kernicterus can develop. Treatment may include phototherapy in which, under careful monitoring, the infant's bare skin is exposed to high-intensity fluorescent light. Although phototherapy is often effective in reducing levels of bilirubin, the underlying cause of hyperbilirubinemia and jaundice must be identified and treated as well. Some infants, especially those in whom early signs of kernicterus are evident, may be effectively treated with exchange blood transfusions in which small amounts of the infant's circulating blood are repeatedly withdrawn and replaced with equal amounts of whole blood from a donor until about 80 percent of the newborn's blood has been replaced. Other treatment is symptomatic and supportive.

The following organizations in the General Resources Section can provide additional information: Genetic Alliance, National Organization for Rare Disorders, Inc., (NORD), March of Dimes Birth Defects Foundation, Online Mendelian Inhertiance in Man: www3.ncbi.nlm.nih.gov/Omim/searchomim.html, NIH/National Digestive Diseases Information Clearinghouse, NIH/National Institute of Child Health and Human Development

National Associations & Support Groups

2730 American Liver Foundation
75 Maiden Lane Suite 603
New York, NY 10038

212-668-1000
800-465-4837
Fax: 212-483-8179
e-mail: info@liverfoundation.org
www.liverfoundation.org

Organization provides several different medias for answering questions and to clarify any uncertainties the individual may be experiencing.

2731 Research Trust for Metabolic Diseases in Children
Golden Gates Lodge
Weston Road, Crewe, Cheshire CW1
1XN United Kingdom,

2732 United Liver Foundation
11646 West Pico Boulevard
Los Angeles, CA 90064

213-445-4204

Web Sites

2733 About.com
babyparenting.miningco.com/library/blillness5.htm

2734 Rare Genetic Diseases in Children (NYU)
http://mcrcr2.med.nyu.edu/murphp01/home-new.htm

2735 Tyler for Life Foundation
www.tylerforlife.com

DESCRIPTION

2736 KLINEFELTER SYNDROME

Synonyms: Chromosome XXY, XXY syndrome

Disorder Type: Chromosomal Disorder,
Developmental Milestones

Covers these related disorders:
45,X/46,XY/47,XXY mosaicism, 46,XY/47,XXY
mosaicism, 46,XY/48,XXYY mosaicism,
46,XX/47,XXY mosaicism, 48,XXXY, 49,XXXYY

May involve these systems in the body (see Section III):
Endocrine System

Klinefelter syndrome is a chromosomal disorder that appears to affect approximately one in 1,000 males. Males usually have one X and one Y chromosome; however, those with Klinefelter syndrome have an extra X chromosome in cells of the body. In some patients, only a certain percentage of cells contain the XXY chromosomal abnormality. This finding is known as chromosomal mosaicism. Other cells may have the normal XY chromosomal pair or other sex chromosome abnormalities (e.g., XX, XXYY, etc.). Some males may have Klinefelter variants in which some or all cells contain more than two X chromosomes.

Because only a few or subtle symptoms may be associated with Klinefelter syndrome, the disorder is rarely diagnosed before puberty. Males with the disorder may have extremely variable I.Q.s (intelligence quotients), ranging from well above to far below average; however, most affected males have an I.Q. within average limits (mean of 85 to 90). Some children with Klinefelter syndrome may have learning problems, such as difficulties with verbal expression, reading, and spelling, potentially requiring special assistance or full-time special education classes. Children with the disorder also tend to have behavioral problems, such as immaturity, excessive shyness, anxiety, poor judgment, aggressive activity, and poor social skills. Such behavioral difficulties tend to begin when affected children begin school.

Many children with Klinefelter syndrome have slim, tall stature; long legs; and small testes and a relatively small penis (hypogenitalism). As affected males enter puberty, they may experience partial, inadequate development of secondary sexual characteristics (impaired virilization). For example, facial hair tends to be unusually sparse, the testes remain unusually small, and, in many cases, there is abnormal enlargement of the breasts (gynecomastia). In addition, many affected males experience inadequate production of the male hormone testosterone and deficient production of male reproductive cells (azoospermia), resulting in infertility. In males with deficient testosterone production, treatment may include testosterone replacement therapy beginning at approximately 11 to 12 years of age. In most cases, Klinefelter syndrome results from errors during the division of a parent's reproductive cells (meiosis). In rare cases, the disorder may result from errors during cellular division after fertilization (mitosis).

In males with XY/XXY mosaicism (i.e., a percentage of cells containing the normal XY chromosomal pair), the range and severity of associated symptoms and findings may be less severe, and there may be an increased likelihood of fertility and improved psychosocial adjustment. Affected males with Klinefelter variants (i.e., in which cells contain more than two X chromosomes) may have more severe symptoms and findings, such as a greater risk of mental retardation and impaired virilization and fertility as well as additional physical abnormalities, including malformations of the head and facial (craniofacial) areas and other skeletal abnormalities.

The following organizations in the General Resources Section can provide additional information: National Organization for Rare Disorders, Inc., (NORD), Genetic Alliance, NIH/National Institute of Child Health and Human Development

National Associations & Support Groups

2737 49 XXY Syndrome Association
10001 NE 74th St
Vancouver, WA 98662   360-892-7547
e-mail: kimbj@juno.com

2738 Klinefelter Syndrome and Associates
P.O. Box 119
Roseville, CA 95678   916-773-2999
888-999-9428
Fax: 916-773-1449
e-mail: ksinfo@genetic.org
www.genetic.org/ks/index/shtml

Klinefelter Syndrome and Associates is a non-
profit education and support organization for
the genetic condition Klinefelter Syndrome
(XXY) and its variants. This organization provides a wealth of information on this underdiagnosed condition.

2739 Klinefelter's Syndrome Association, Inc.
Route 1, Box 93
Pine River, WI 54965   414-987-5782

**2740 Support and Educational Exchange for Klinefelter
Syndrome**
1417 25th Avenue, Drive West
Bradenton, FL 34205   813-750-8044

Web Sites

2741 CORN Council
www.cc.emory.edu/PEDIATRICS/corn/corn.htm

2742 Klinefelter Syndrome Support Group
www.klinefeltersyndrome.org/

Sue Cook, National Contacts Co-ordinator

2743 National Institute of Mental Health (NIMH)
http://klinefeltersyndrome.org/nimh.htm

Newsletters

2744 Klinefelter Syndrome Newsletter
P.O. Box 119
Roseville, CA 95678   916-773-2999
888-999-9428
Fax: 916-773-1449
e-mail: ksinfo@genetic.org
www.genetic.org/ks/index/shtml

News on Klinefelter Syndrome, education and
support. You'll find a wealth of information on
this very common, but underdiagnosed condition.

DESCRIPTION

2745 KLIPPEL-FEIL SYNDROME

Synonym: KFS

Disorder Type: Birth Defect

Covers these related disorders: Klippel-Feil syndrome Type I, Klippel-Feil syndrome Type II, Klippel-Feil syndrome Type III

May involve these systems in the body (see Section III):

Skeletal System

Klippel-Feil syndrome (KFS) is a congenital malformation characterized by the fusion of two or more vertebrae, especially in the neck or cervical region (congenital synostosis) or by the absence of one or more cervical vertebrae. Klippel-Feil syndrome Type I involves extensive fusion of several cervical vertebrae and thoracic vertebrae located in the upper back. Type II involves fusion of a limited number of incompletely developed vertebrae (hemivertebrae) and vertebrae, fusion of the uppermost cervical vertebra with the bone at the back of the skull (occipital bone), and other irregularities. Klippel-Feil syndrome Type III is characterized by fusion of the cervical, lower thoracic, or lumbar vertebrae. Physical findings associated with Klippel-Feil syndrome may include a short neck with limited range of motion, a low hairline, and irregularities of the urinary tract and reproductive, cardiovascular, pulmonary, and nervous systems. Additional abnormalities may include curvatures of the spine (scoliosis or kyphosis), an inclination of the neck to one side (torticollis), webbing of the neck (pterygium colli) and fingers (syndactyly), and other irregularities of the bones and muscles.

Treatment of Klippel-Feil syndrome may be directed toward the particular physical findings and symptoms associated with this disorder. Such treatment may include measures to correct or halt the progression of various spinal irregularities and to correct other abnormalities as warranted. Other treatment is supportive.

In some children, Klippel-Feil syndrome is transmitted as an autosomal dominant trait, while transmission by autosomal recessive inheritance is possible in others. In addition, some affected children have no recognizable pattern of genetic transmission.

The following organizations in the General Resources Section can provide additional information: March of Dimes Birth Defects Foundation, Online Mendelian Inheritance in Man: www3.ncbi.nlm.nih.gov/Omim/searchomim.html, NIH/National Institute of Arthritis and Musculoskeletal and Skin Diseases, NIH/National Institute of Child Health and Human Development, National Organization for Rare Disorders, Inc., (NORD)

National Associations & Support Groups

2746 Klippel-Feil Syndrome Support Group
311 Bracken Avenue
Pittsburgh, PA 15227   412-884-2969
          www.members.aol.com/kfsconxpgs/index/htm

Klippel-Feil Syndrome describes congenital fusion of at least two of the seven vertebrae in the cervical-spine. In addition there may be fusion or anomalies of vertebrae in the thoracic or lumbar-spine.

2747 Osteoporosis and Related Bone Diseases National Resource Center
1232 22nd Street NW
Washington, DC 20037   202-223-0344
          800-624-2663
          Fax: 202-293-2356
          TTY: 301-565-2966
          e-mail: orbdnrc@nof.org
          www.osteo.org

Distributes information to health professionals, and the public on osteoporosis, Paget's disease of bone, osteogenesis imperfecta, and other metabolic bone diseases. Includes prevention, early detection, and treatment of these diseases.

Web Sites

2748 Rare Genetic Diseases in Children (NYU)
http://mcrcr2.med.nyu.edu/murphp01/home-new.htm

2749 Wheeless' Textbook of Orthopaedics
www.medmedia.com/o11/52.htm

DESCRIPTION

2750 KYPHOSIS

Disorder Type: Birth Defect, Genetic Disorder
Covers these related disorders: Congenital
kyphosis, Idiopathic kyphosis (Scheuermann's
disease), Postural kyphosis
**May involve these systems in the body (see Section
III):**
 Prenatal & Postnatal Growth & Development,
Skeletal System

The term kyphosis refers to a condition characterized by an exaggerated backward curvature of
the spine in the thoracic vertebral area. Children
with poor posture resulting in mild kyphosis who
have no associated spinal irregularities may be
treated by maintaining good posture habits. Congenital kyphosis, however, results from various
malformations in the spinal column and may
range from mild to severe deformity. As affected
children grow, progression of the spinal abnormality may continue until growth is complete, possibly resulting in partial paralysis. Idiopathic
kyphosis or Scheuermann's disease is a form of
kyphosis that is common to both adolescent boys
and girls. Although selected family histories suggest that this may be an inherited form of the
disease, no defined pattern has been established
and the cause remains unknown. Examination
and x-ray screening may determine whether
kyphosis is postural or a result of a spinal malformation. Symptoms of Scheuermann's disease may
include mild but chronic back pain and a round-
shouldered appearance.

Treatment options are dependent upon severity
of symptoms, age of the patient, and degree of
discomfort. Children with mild disease may be
advised to refrain from strenuous activities and
exercise, while those with more severe symptoms
may benefit from sleeping on a very firm mattress
or, perhaps, application of a spinal brace or corrective plaster cast. Although surgery is rarely
needed, it may be indicated for those who, once

their growth pattern is complete, experience persistent pain and severe deformity.

Kyphosis may also result from other underlying
disorders or abnormalities. Among these are reduction of bone mass (osteoporosis) and tumors or
fractures of the vertebrae. Treatment is directed
toward the underlying cause.

**The following organizations in the General
Resources Section can provide additional
information:** NIH/National Institute of Child Health
and Human Development, March of Dimes Birth
Defects Foundation, NIH/National Institute of
Arthritis and Musculoskeletal and Skin Diseases

Web Sites

2751 Wheeless' Textbook of Orthopaedics
www.medmedia.com/o11/47.htm

DESCRIPTION

2752 LEGG-CALVE-PERTHES DISEASE

Synonyms: LCPD, Perthes disease

Disorder Type: Genetic Disorder

May involve these systems in the body (see Section III):

Muscular System, Skeletal System

Legg-Calve-Perthes disease (LCPD) belongs to a group of disorders in which abnormalities of the growth centers of certain bones result in degeneration and gradual regeneration of the affected bone. This group of disorders is known as the osteochondroses. LCPD affects the growing end of the head of the thigh bone (femoral capital epiphysis). In most affected children, the thigh bone (femur) on one side of the body is affected (unilateral); however, in approximately 20 percent of patients, the disorder may eventually involve the other femur (bilateral). The age of onset and the severity and duration of the disease are variable. Legg-Calve-Perthes disease typically becomes apparent between the ages of two to 12 years, with the average age of onset approximately seven years of age. Males are affected four to five times as often as females; however, females may tend to have more severe symptoms. LCPD is thought to affect approximately one in 1,000 to 5,000 children.

Degeneration of the head of the femur is thought to occur due to insufficient blood supply (ischemia) to this area of bone, resulting in the localized loss of bone and cartilage as well as the loss of bone mass. The onset of symptoms associated with LCPD is typically slow and progressive. Many affected children initially experience muscle spasms, a limp, or mild or periodic pain that may affect the thigh, hip, knee, or groin area. As the disorder progresses, additional symptoms and findings often include delayed maturation of the thigh bone (delayed bone age); mild restriction of movements of the affected hip; potential degeneration of the front thigh muscles; abnormal positioning of the hip and thigh toward the body (internal rotation); and, in some patients, mild short stature. LCPD is considered a self-limiting disorder because, even without medical intervention, new blood supplies are eventually spontaneously reestablished (revascularization) to the femoral head, causing the formation of new bone tissue in the affected area. This may occur approximately two to four years after the onset of symptoms. In some affected children, new bony growth may be misshapen, potentially causing the affected leg to be relatively shorter than the unaffected leg, an associated limp, and an increased risk for degenerative changes of the hips, resulting in swelling, pain or tenderness, and stiffness (osteoarthritis).

Because Legg-Calve-Perthes disease is a self-limiting disorder, treatment usually is directed toward preventing deformity of the femoral head and secondary osteoarthritis. Such measures may include ongoing clinical assessment and specialized x-ray tests to monitor the progress of the disease; bed rest or special stretching exercises; the use of braces or casts; or surgery.

In most cases, Legg-Calve-Perthes disease is thought to occur randomly for unknown reasons (sporadically). There have also been reports of several affected individuals within certain families (kindreds) that suggest autosomal dominant inheritance. Some researchers suspect that LCPD may be caused by the interaction of several different genes, possibly in association with the involvement of certain environmental factors (multifactorial disorder).

The following organizations in the General Resources Section can provide additional information: National Organization for Rare Disorders, Inc. (NORD), NIH/National Institute of Arthritis and Musculoskeletal and Skin Diseases, March of Dimes Defects Foundation, NIH/National Information Center for Children & Youth with Disabilities, NIH/National Institute of Child Health and Human Development

Web Sites

2753 Pedbase
www.icondata.com/health/pedbase/files/LEGG-CAL.HTM

2754 Wheeless' Textbook of Orthopaedics
www.medmedia.com/orthoo/242.htm

DESCRIPTION

2755 LEUKODYSTROPHIES

Disorder Type: Genetic Disorder, Metabolism
May involve these systems in the body (see Section III):
Central Nervous System

The leukodystrophies are a group of inherited neurodegenerative diseases that affect the white matter of the brain and are characterized by the destruction of the fatty, protective covering around the nerve fibers (myelin sheaths). The symptoms of some forms of these diseases become obvious during childhood. These diseases include adrenoleukodystrophy (ALD), adrenomyeloneuropathy, Krabbe disease, metachromatic leukodystrophy, and Pelizaeus-Merzbacher disease.

Classic adrenoleukodystrophy, or ALD, is a metabolic disorder transmitted as an X-linked recessive trait that is fully expressed in boys. This type of adrenoleukodystrophy becomes apparent between the ages of five and 15 years and is characterized by behavioral disturbances, mental deterioration, seizures, lack of coordination, and motor weakness or partial paralysis with increased muscle tone in the arms and legs accompanied by exaggerated reflex responses (spasticity). In addition, boys with ALD may have difficulty with swallowing, language development, and speech. Vision may be impaired. Other findings include insufficient adrenal gland function characterized by a darkening or tanning of the skin. Experimental treatments include bone marrow transplantation and dietary considerations. Other treatment is symptomatic and supportive. The gene for classic ALD is located on the long arm of the X chromosome (Xq28). Adrenomyeloneuropathy is considered a milder, adult form of adrenoleukodystrophy, although its onset may occur as early as late adolescence.

Neonatal adrenoleukodystrophy is inherited as an autosomal recessive trait and is characterized by seizures, severe delays in skills that involve the coordination of mental and muscular activities (psychomotor coordination), and insufficiency of the adrenal glands. Treatment is symptomatic and supportive.

Krabbe disease, sometimes called globoid cell leukodystrophy, is a rare neurodegenerative disorder that is inherited as an autosomal recessive trait. This life-threatening, progressive disease results from a deficiency of the enzyme galactocerebrosidase and is characterized during early infancy by irritability, vomiting, extremely high fevers, difficulty feeding, and failure to thrive. Seizures may develop followed by muscular rigidity, convulsions, paralysis, seizures, loss of vision and hearing, mental deterioration, or other irregularities. Krabbe disease may sometimes have a later onset with symptoms and findings developing during childhood or adolescence. Treatment is symptomatic and supportive. The gene for Krabbe disease is located on the long arm of chromosome 14 (14q21-q31).

Metachromatic leukodystrophy (MLD) is inherited in an autosomal recessive pattern and occurs as the result of a deficiency of the enzyme sulfatase A. Late infantile MLD usually occurs in the first or second year of life and is characterized by progressive irregularities in the manner of walking (gait), frequent falling, developmental delays, seizures, diminished muscle tone in the arms and legs, and weak deep tendon reflexes. As the disease progresses, children may be unable to stand and signs of intellectual degeneration become apparent. Additional findings include impaired speech and deteriorating visual activity or blindness. Approximately one year after symptom onset, most children are unable to sit without support and may experience swallowing and eating difficulties. Life-threatening complications such as pneumonia may develop. Juvenile MLD occurs from the ages of four to 12 years and is characterized by behavioral and intellectual deterioration followed by walking and speech difficulties, urinary incontinence, lack of coordination, impaired muscle tone, and convulsions. This form of MLD has a slower progression than that of late infantile MLD. One variant of juvenile MLD results from a deficiency of a protein that aids in the activation of cerebroside sulfatase. Adult MLD usually begins anywhere from the sixteenth year of life to the sixth decade and is characterized initially by behavioral disturbances and deterioration of intellectual functions followed by slowly progressive neurologic involvement. The gene for metachromatic leukodystrophy is located on the long arm of chromosome 22 (22q13.31-qter).

Pelizaeus-Merzbacher disease is inherited as an X-linked recessive trait. This disorder occurs during infancy or early childhood and progresses slowly into adolescence or adulthood. This life-threatening form of leukodystrophy is characterized in infancy by head-nodding and eye irregularities such as involuntary, rhythmic movement of the eyes (nystagmus). Boys with this disorder experience developmental delays followed by tremors; well-coordinated but involuntary jerky, writhing movements; a mask-like, frozen expression (parkinsonian facies); difficulty with speech; and deterioration of mental function. Treatment is symptomatic and supportive. The gene for Pelizaeus-Merzbacher disease is located on the long arm of the X chromosome (Xq22).

The following organizations in the General Resources Section can provide additional information: National Organization for Rare Diseases, Inc. (NORD), NIH/Office of Rare Diseases, Genetic Alliance, March of Dimes Birth Defects Foundation, Online Mendelian Inheritance in Man.: www3.ncbi.nlm.nih.gov/Omim/searchomim.html, NIH/National Institute of Neurological Disorders & Stroke

National Associations & Support Groups

2756 Association for Neuro-Metabolic Disorders
5223 Brookfield Lane
Sylvania, OH 43506   419-885-1497

Organization that is comprised of families of children with disorders that affect the nervous system and the brain. It provides assistance and information through conferences, meetings and phone calls.

2757 National Tay-Sachs and Allied Diseases Association, Inc.
2001 Beacon St, Ste 204
Brighton, MA 02135   617-277-4463
800-906-8723
Fax: 617-277-0134
e-mail: NTSAD-Boston@worldnet.att.net
www.ntsad.org

Dedicated to the treatment and prevention of Tay-Sachs and related diseases, and to provide information and support services to individuals and families affected by these diseases through public and professional education, research, genetic screening, family services and advocacy.

2758 United Leukodystrophy Foundation
2304 Highland Drive
Sycamore, IL 60178   815-895-2432
800-728-5483
Fax: 812-895-2432
e-mail: ulf@ceet.niu.edu
www.ulf.org/

Organization that aids those with leukodystrophy and those who care for them.

Research Centers

2759 Research Trust for Metabolic Diseases in Children
Goldengates Lodge Weston Rd., Crewe
Cheshire,
United Kingdom

Dedicated to providing the most up-to-date medical knowledge for the families and friends of people suffering from this and related diseases.

Web Sites

2760 AMD/ALD Chat and Bullitin Board
www.amn.ald.ourfamily.com/

2761 Doctor.net Links
www.comedserv.com/ald.htm

2762 Medical College of Wisconsin
chorus.rad.mcw.edu/doc/00231.html

2763 NYU
www.med.nyu.edu/Research/E.Kolodny-res.html

2764 Neuropathy Association
www.neuropathy.org/

2765 Pedbase
www.icondata.com/health/pedbase/files/ADRENOLE.HTM

2766 Virtual Hospital
www.vh.org/Providers/Teaching-
Files/RCW/012696.html

DESCRIPTION

2767 LIMB REDUCTION DEFECTS

Disorder Type: Birth Defect
Covers these related disorders: Amelia, Central ray defects, Hemimelia, Limb hypoplasia, Meromeliaplasia, Micromelia, Phocomelia, Radial reduction defects
May involve these systems in the body (see Section III):
  Skeletal System

Limb reduction defects are the incomplete or disrupted development of the arms, legs, hands, or feet (limbs) during fetal growth. This results in absence of all or a portion of a limb or limbs at birth. Such defects may range from abnormal smallness or underdevelopment (hypoplasia) of one or more fingers or toes to complete absence (aplasia) of the arms and legs. Limb reduction defects may occur as isolated findings, in association with other birth defects, or due to several underlying malformation syndromes. In other patients, such malformations may result from exposure to certain medications, such as thalidomide, or other environmental factors (teratogens) during fetal development. According to some studies, limb reduction defects are thought to affect approximately six in 10,000 newborns.

Several classification systems have been proposed to categorize limb reduction defects. However, in general, such malformations may be classified as meromelia, meaning congenital absence of any region of a limb, or amelia, indicating complete absence of a limb or limbs. Many newborns with limb reduction defects have incomplete development or absence of the first bone in the body of the hand (first metacarpal), the thumb, and, in some patients, the bone of the thumb side of the forearm (radius). Such malformations, known as hemimelia or radical reduction defects, may also be associated with absence or incomplete development of the bone of the pinky side of the forearm (ulnar) and an abnormally small or absent bone in the upper arm (humerus). Some patients may have abnormalities affecting bones of the second, third, or fourth fingers (phalanges), known as central ray defects. Less commonly, newborns may have complete absence of the arms and legs (amelia) or a malformation in which one or both of the hands or feet are attached to the trunk by short, irregularly shaped bones (phocomelia). Such malformations are a primary feature associated with fetal thalidomide syndrome, a characteristic pattern of birth defects in newborns caused by maternal use of the drug thalidomide during early pregnancy.

Approximately 75 percent of limb reduction defects affect the hands or arms, whereas 25 percent involve the lower limbs. About half of newborns with such malformations also have associated birth defects, particularly additional musculoskeletal abnormalities or defects of the heart and its major blood vessels, the digestive system, or the genital and urinary tracts.

The treatment of infants and children with limb reduction defects is symptomatic and supportive. Such measures may include the use of artificial limbs (prostheses), orthopedic appliances, and mobility devices; surgery; physical and rehabilitative therapy; or other measures as required. In patients with additional birth defects, treatment may include medical and surgical measures to treat associated bone, digestive, genital, urinary, or other defects.

The following organizations in the General Resources Section can provide additional information: National Organization for Rare Disorders, Inc., (NORD), Genetic Alliance, March of Dimes Birth Defects Foundation, NIH/National Institute of Child Health and Human Development, NIH/National Institute of Arthritis and Musculoskeletal and Skin Disorders

National Associations & Support Groups

2768 CHERUB—Association of Families and Friends of Children with Limb Disorders
936 Delaware Avenue
Buffalo, NY 14209

Answers the questions and problems that families of juveniles diagnosed with a disorder may be experiencing.

Web Sites

2769 Association for Children with Hand or Arm Deficiency (REACH)
www.reach.org.uk/

2770 ICAN (International Child Amputee Network)
www.amp-info.net/childamp.htm

Newsletters

2771 Superkids, Inc.
60 Clyde Street
Newton, MA 02160

Newsletter for families and friends of children with limb differences.

DESCRIPTION

2772 LISSENCEPHALY

Synonym: Agyria

Disorder Type: Birth Defect, Genetic Disorder

Covers these related disorders: Isolated lissencephaly sequence, Miller-Dieker lissencephaly syndrome, Norman-Roberts lissencephaly syndrome, Walker-Warburg syndrome, X-linked lissencephaly

May involve these systems in the body (see Section III):

Central Nervous System

Lissencephaly is a developmental abnormality in which the brain has a relatively smooth surface due to incomplete formation of the folds or convolutions (gyri) of the surface of the brain (cerebral cortex). In most patients, the folds are not fully developed or are absent. Although lissencephaly was once thought to be a rare malformation, this developmental abnormality is now considered more common. This is largely due to an increase in the number of diagnosed cases resulting from the use of advanced imaging techniques.

Lissencephaly has multiple causes and may occur as an isolated finding or in association with several underlying syndromes. Affected newborns typically have a small head (microcephaly), episodes of uncontrolled electrical disturbances within the brain (seizures), and mental retardation. When an underlying syndrome is present, patients may have additional physical abnormalities. In some patients, life-threatening complications may develop during infancy or childhood. Isolated lissencephaly, which is an autosomal dominant trait, results due to changes (mutations) of a gene known as the LIS 1 gene. The gene is located on the short arm (p) of chromosome 17 (17p13.3). In addition, there are reports of numerous cases of lissencephaly in a multigenerational family due to mutations of a gene on the long arm (q) of chromosome X (Xq22.3-q23). In affected males, associated findings may include seizures that are resistant to treatment (intractable), growth failure, mental retardation, absence of the thick band

of nerve fibers that connect the two cerebral hemispheres (agenesis of the corpus callosum), an abnormally small penis (microphallus), and life-threatening complications shortly after birth. In affected females who inherit a single copy of the disease gene (heterozygotes), associated abnormalities, which are milder than those in affected males, include an unusual band of brain tissue under the cerebral cortex (subcortical heterotopia) and mild mental retardation and seizures.

Lissencephaly may also occur in association with several syndromes. For example, Miller-Dieker lissencephaly syndrome is thought to result from deletions of several genes located on the short arm (p) of chromosome 17. This syndrome, which is an autosomal dominant trait, is associated with lissencephaly, profound mental retardation, seizures, agenesis of the corpus callosum, poor feeding, and failure to grow and gain weight at the expected rate (failure to thrive). Malformations of the head and face may include a small head, a prominent forehead and back portion of the head, a short nose with upturned nostrils (anteverted nares), a small jaw, and a prominent upper lip. In Norman-Roberts lissencephaly syndrome, an autosomal recessive trait, affected infants have profound mental retardation and seizures, severe growth deficiency after birth, abnormally increased muscle tone (hypertonia), and exaggerated reflexes (hyperreflexia). Abnormalities of the head and face may include a low, sloping forehead and prominent back portion of the head, widely set eyes (ocular hypertelorism), and a broad nasal bridge. In Walker-Warburg syndrome, also an autosomal recessive disorder, affected infants have lissencephaly associated with seizures and an abnormally small head. Malformations of the eyes may include atypical development of the nerve-rich membrane at the back of the eyes (retinal dysplasia), abnormally small eyes (microphthalmia), and clouding of the lenses (cataracts) and corneas (corneal opacities). In addition, some affected infants may experience restriction of the flow of fluid surrounding the brain and spinal cord (hydrocephalus) and abnormal widening of the cavities of the brain. The treatment of lissencephaly includes symptomatic and supportive measures.

The following organizations in the General Resources Section can provide additional information: March of Dimes Birth Defects Foundation, NIH/National Institute of Child Health and Human Development, NIH/National Institute of Neurological Disorders and Stroke, NIH/National Information Center for Children & Youth with Disabilities, Online Mendelian Inheritance in Man.: www3.ncbi.nlm.nih.gov/Omim/searchomim.html

National Associations & Support Groups

2773 AboutFace U.S.A.
1407 N Wells
Chicago, IL 60610

800-665-3223
Fax: 815-444-1943
e-mail: aboutface2000@aol.com
www.aboutface2000.org

To provide information, services, emotional support and educational programs for and on behalf of individuals with facial difference and their families. Working to increase understanding through public awareness and education.

Rickie Anderson, Executive Director

2774 Association of Birth Defect Children
930 Woodcock Road, Suite 225
Orlando, FL 32803

407-245-7035
800-313-2223
Fax: 407-895-0824
e-mail: abdc@birthdefects.org
www.birthdefects.org

Organization devoted to dissemination of data pertaining to birth related malformations.

2775 Children's Craniofacial Association
P.O. Box 280297
Dallas, TX 75243

972-994-9902
800-535-3643
Fax: 972-240-7607
e-mail: DNKM90A@prodigy.com
masterlink.com/children

Devoted to the dispersion of medical knowledge of this and similar disorders, along with providing emotional support for the sufferers and their families.

2776 FACES: The National Craniofacial Association
P.O. Box 11082
Chattanooga, TN 37401

423-266-1632
e-mail: faces@faces-cranio.org
www.faces-cranio.org

Disperses information to the public on the medical professionals specializing in this field.

2777 Fighters for Encephaly Support Group
332 Brereton Street
Pittsburgh, PA 15219

412-687-6437

2778 Forward Face, Inc.
317 East 34th Street, Room 901
New York, NY 10016

212-684-5860

Provision of data and emotional assistance to both sufferers and medical professionals.

2779 Lissencephaly Contact Group
12 Didsbury Park, Didsbury
Manchester, M20 5LJ,
United Kingdom

Organization that networks families affected by lissencephaly. It promotes awareness of the disorder and related brain conditions.

2780 Lissencephaly Network, Inc.
716 Autumn Ridge Lane
Fort Wayne, IN 46804

219-432-4310
Fax: 219-432-4310
e-mail: lta1@is2.nyu.edu
www.lissenphaly.org

Lissencephaly is a genetic disorder that can be inherited from the parents or can occur during cell division. This web site is provided for the parentes, siblings, physicians and therapists of children born with lissencephaly (smooth brain), and other neuronal migration disorders.

2781 National Craniofacial Foundation
3100 Carlisle Street, Suite 215
Dallas, TX 75204

2782 National Hydrocephalus Foundation
22427 S River Rd
Joliet, IL 60436

815-467-6548
e-mail: hydrobrat@aol.com

2783 National Information Center for Children & Youth with Disabilities
P.O. Box 1492
Washington, DC 20013   202-884-8200
                                              800-695-0285
mcrcr2.med.nyu.edu/murphp01/homenew.htm

A clearinghouse that provides free information on disabilities and disability-related issues.

2784 Society for the Rehabilitation of the Facially Disfigured, Inc.
550 First Avenue
New York, NY 10016   212-340-5400

2785 Support Network for Pachygyria, Agyria, Lissencephaly
2410 South 24th Street, #9102
Kansas City, KS 66106
                          Fax: 913-432-7453

2786 World Craniofacial Foundation
P.O. Box 515838
Dallas, TX 75251   972-566-6669
                              800-533-3315

Not-for-profit foundation for persons with facial deformities.

Web Sites

2787 Independent Holoprosencephaly Support Site
www.team17.com/~tsmith/HPE/
          e-mail: Tim.Smith@gashead.demon.co.uk
                  www.team17.com/~tsmith/HPE/

This site contains information, advice and expertise from parents of HPE-affected children in their roles as carers.

2788 Pedbase
www.icondata.com/health/pedbase/files/LIS-SENCE.HTM

2789 Rare Genetic Diseases in Children (NYU)
mcrcr2.med.nyu.edu/murphp01/homenew.htm

DESCRIPTION

2790 LISTERIOSIS
  Synonym: Circling disease
  Disorder Type: Infectious Disease

Listeriosis, an infectious disease caused by the bacterium Listeria monocytogenes, may be present in birds, poultry, shellfish, spiders, and mammals. This disease is spread through direct contact with infected animals and, in some cases, through person-to-person contact; ingestion of contaminated raw and precooked meat or dairy products; contact with contaminated soil, livestock feed, and sewage; or mother-to-fetus transmission through the placenta. Newborns, the elderly, and individuals with compromised immune systems are especially vulnerable to this infection. Listeriosis may affect most parts of the body with symptoms varying according to the infection site and the age and overall health of the person affected. Many otherwise healthy children and adults develop only mild aches and pains; however, symptoms and findings may include the appearance of a dark, reddish rash on the trunk and legs, fever, lethargy, weakness, and generalized discomfort. In addition, listeriosis may cause inflammation of the membranes that surround the brain and spinal cord (meningitis) accompanied by a high fever, stiff neck, and severe headache. Enlargement of the lymph nodes as well as the spleen (splenomegaly) and liver (hepatomegaly) may also occur. In some cases, infection may develop in the heart valves, resulting in circulatory irregularities or heart failure. Most cases of listeriosis in newborns are transmitted from infected mother to child during the birthing process; however, some cases occur as a result of fetal infection transmitted via the placenta. Listeria infection transmitted through the placenta from mother to the developing fetus may result in miscarriage or premature labor and stillbirth; however, infected pregnant women do not always transmit the disease to their unborn children. Symptoms and findings associated with listeriosis in the newborn may be obvious immediately after birth or within several weeks. These may include meningitis, inflammation of the brain (encephalitis), or cardiorespiratory distress. Widespread bacterial contamination of the bloodstream (septicemia) may cause diarrhea, nausea, or vomiting.

Prevention of listeriosis may include precautions such as avoidance of uncooked meats or improperly stored precooked meats. Proper hygiene, including thorough and frequent hand washing, is advised in neonatal units and other hospital and institutional settings. Treatment of listeriosis includes the use of one or more antibiotics. Other treatment is symptomatic and supportive.

The following organizations in the General Resources Section can provide additional information: National Organization for Rare Disorders, Inc. (NORD), NIH/National Institutes of Allergy and Infectious Diseases, World Health Organization, Centers for Disease Control (CDC)

National Associations & Support Groups

2791 Food & Drug Administration (FDA) Office of Consumer Affairs
5600 Fishers Lane (HFE-88)
Rockville, MD 20857

www.fda.gov

Web Sites

2792 International Symposium on Problems of Listeriosis
www.isopol.com/

2793 Listeria: The Organism and the Disease
http://disabilities.miningco.com/msub111.htm

2794 Pedbase
www.icondata.com/health/pedbase/files/LISTE-RIO.HTM

DESCRIPTION

2795 MACROCEPHALY

Synonyms: Macrocephalia, Megalocephaly

Covers these related disorders: Benign familial macrocephaly

May involve these systems in the body (see Section III):

Nervous System

Macrocephaly is a term that is often used to describe an isolated or primary condition in which an infant's or a child's head circumference is more than two standard deviations above the mean for age and sex. Patients with overgrowth of the brain (megalencephaly) have normally sized or slightly enlarged cavities of the brain (ventricles) and no evidence of underlying conditions, such as certain metabolic disorders (metabolic megalencephaly).

Primary macrocephaly may be apparent at birth or during early infancy. In some affected infants and children, overgrowth of the brain results in varying degrees of mental retardation. Associated symptoms and findings may include episodes of uncontrolled electrical disturbances in the brain (seizures); unusually large or small stature; and motor abnormalities ranging from diminished muscle tone (hypotonia) to muscle rigidity and associated restrictions of movement (spasticity). Although affected infants and children may have abnormal delays in the acquisition of skills requiring the coordination of physical and mental activities (psychomotor delays), they do not experience regression of such skills, a finding that is typically associated with infantile metabolic megalencephaly or certain other underlying conditions.

Some infants and children with primary macrocephaly experience no associated mental retardation or other neurologic deficits. Several such cases have been reported in individuals within certain multigenerational families (kindreds). This form of benign or nonsyndromic macrocephaly, known as benign familial macrocephaly, is thought to have autosomal dominant inheritance.

Although infants with primary macrocephaly experience increasing head size, they typically do not have symptoms and findings associated with increased cerebrospinal fluid (CSF) pressure within the brain (intracranial pressure). This is in contrast to hydrocephalus, a condition in which the brain swells due to an abnormal accumulation of CSF under increasing pressure within the brain's ventricles. However, some infants with primary macrocephaly may have a slight separation of the fibrous joints (cranial sutures) between certain bones in the skull.

Although the specific underlying cause of primary macrocephaly is not understood, overgrowth of the brain is due to the presence of abnormally large or an unusually increased number of brain cells. The outer region of the brain (cerebral cortex) appears normal in some cases; however, others have structural abnormalities.

As mentioned above, overgrowth of the brain may occur as a secondary finding associated with certain progressive infantile metabolic diseases, such as Tay-Sachs disease, or other underlying genetic disorders, such as neurofibromatosis. The condition may also occur as a result of certain structural abnormalities of the brain, such as absence of the band of nerve fibers that joins the two cerebral hemispheres (agenesis of corpus callosum), or due to a localized accumulation of blood between the outer and middle layers of the membrane that surrounds and protects the brain and spinal cord (subdural hematoma). Infants and children with macrocephaly who experience psychomotor regression should receive thorough clinical, neurologic, metabolic, and other appropriate evaluations to rule out or confirm the presence of certain underlying disorders or conditions.

The treatment of infants and children with isolated or primary macrocephaly includes symptomatic and supportive measures. These may include the prescription of certain medications to help treat or control seizures (e.g., anticonvulsants) and physical therapy, special education, and other multidisciplinary measures to ensure that patients with motor impairments and mental retardation reach their potential. In infants and children with secondary macrocephaly, treatment includes appropriate therapies for any diagnosed, underlying causes of the condition.

The following organizations in the General Resources Section can provide additional information: Genetic Alliance, NIH/National Institute of Child Health and Human Development, NIH/National Institute of Neurological Disorders and Stroke, National Organization for Rare Disorders, inc. (NORD), Online Mendelian Inheritance in Man.: www3.ncbi.nlm.nih.gov/Omim/searchomim.html

National Associations & Support Groups

2796 ARC
500 East Border Street, Suite 300
Arlington, TX 76010   817-261-6003
                                 800-433-5255
                          TDD: 817-277-0553

Parent to Parent (P-P) programs provide informational and emotional support to parents who have a child, adolescent, or adult family member with special needs. P-P programs offer an important connection for a parent who is seeking support for special disability issue, by matching him or her with a trained vetern parent who has already been there. Because the two parents share so many concerns and interests, the support given and received is often uniquely meaningful.

2797 Association of Birth Defect Children
930 Woodcock Road, Suite 225
Orlando, FL 32803   407-245-7035
                                 800-313-2223
                           Fax: 407-895-0824
             e-mail: abdc@birthdefects.org
                        www.birthdefects.org

National clearinghouse that provides services to parents and professionals caring for children with disabilities. Services include data on over 300 categories of birth defects and developmental disabilities, search for links between birth defects and the mother's/father's exposure to drugs or environmental agents. Matching families of children with similar birth defects for mutual sharing and support, diagnosis and treatment. Support group information. Newsletter on Internet.

Betty Mekdeci, Executive Director

2798 National Information Center for Children & Youth with Disabilities
P.O. Box 1492
Washington, DC 20013   202-884-8200
                                     800-695-0285
     mcrcr2.med.nyu.edu/murphp01/homenew.htm

A clearinghouse that provides free information on disabilities and disability-related issues.

DESCRIPTION

2799 MALOCCLUSION

Disorder Type: Teeth
Covers these related disorders: Class I malocclusion, Class II malocclusion (retrognathis), Class III malocclusion (prognathism)

Malocclusion is a dental condition in which there is improper positioning of the teeth of the upper jaw (maxilla) in relation to those of the lower jaw (mandible). The different types of malocclusion were originally classified in a system established by an American orthodontist, Edward Hartley Angle. The classification system, known as Angle's Classification of Malocclusion, has been modified and is currently used to categorize three main classes of malocclusion.

In proper contact (occlusion) of the teeth, the front teeth (i.e., the incisors and canines) of the upper jaw slightly overlap the front teeth of the lower jaw. In addition, the ridges (cusps) of the back teeth (i.e., premolars and molars) in the lower jaw interlock slightly ahead and inside the cusps of the corresponding teeth in the upper jaw. Such occlusion results in a normal facial profile and provides for efficient chewing, tearing, and grinding of food (mastication).

In class I malocclusion, there is proper positioning of the upper jaw in relation to the lower jaw and appropriate contact of the upper and lower molars; however, other upper and lower teeth do not have appropriate contact due to abnormal rotation or spacing (e.g., crowding). In individuals with class II malocclusion, which is considered the most common occlusive abnormality, the cusps of the back teeth in the lower jaw are positioned behind and inside the cusps of the corresponding teeth in the upper jaw. Class II malocclusion (also known as retrognathism) is associated with a receding chin. In class III malocclusion, the cusps of the back teeth in the lower jaw are abnormally positioned in front of corresponding maxillary teeth and the front teeth of the lower jaw meet or

protrude beyond the upper front teeth. This least common form of malocclusion (also known as prognathism) is associated with a protruding chin.

Malocclusion usually occurs during childhood as the bones of the jaws grow and the teeth develop. In most cases, the different forms of malocclusion are genetic. In addition, in some cases, malocclusion may result due to other dental abnormalities, such as improper development or crowding of teeth. It may also be due to almost constant thumbsucking. Preventive measures are ideally performed during childhood and adolescence and are directed toward establishing proper relationships between the teeth of the upper and lower jaws. Preventive techniques or corrective measures to treat malocclusion may avoid strain, stiffness, or pain that may result from an abnormal bite; improve facial appearance; and prevent tooth decay and loss. During adulthood, malocclusion is a primary cause of tooth loss. Treatment may include a variety of measures, such as tooth extraction in cases of dental crowding; the use of orthodontic appliances such as braces to correct the positioning of teeth; or, in some severe cases, surgical correction of abnormal protrusion or recession of the lower jaw (orthognathic surgery).

The following organizations in the General Resources Section can provide additional information: National Institute of Dental Research, National Institute of Child Health and Human Development

National Associations & Support Groups

2800 American Dental Association
211 East Chicago Avenue
Chicago, IL 60611   312-440-2500
                                       www.ada.org

Professional association of dentists dedicated to serving both the public and the profession of dentistry. Promotes the profession of dentistry by enhancing the integrity and ethics of the profession and strengthening the patient/dentist relationship. Fulfills its mission by providing services and through its initiatives in education, research, advocacy and the development of standards.

2801 National Institute of Child Health and Human Development
9000 Rockville Pike, Bldg 31
Bethesda, MD 20892   301-496-5133
Fax: 301-496-7101
www.nih.gov/nichd

Research on fertility, pregnancy, growth, development, and medical rehabilitation strives to ensure that every child is born healthy and wanted and grows up free from disease and disability.

Research Centers

2802 National Institute of Dental Research
31 Cntr Dr.,Msc 2290,Bldg31,Rm2c35
Bethesda, MD 20892   301-496-4261
Fax: 301-496-9988
nidr.nih.gov/

Provides leadership for a national research program designed to understand, treat and prevent the infectious and inherited craniofacial-oral-dental diseases and disorders.

Web Sites

2803 American Academy of Pediatric Dentistry
aapd.org/

2804 American Association of Orthodontics
www.aaortho.org/

2805 Dental Resources on the Web
dental-resources.com/

2806 Straight Talk about Orthodontics
oao.on.ca/faq.htm

DESCRIPTION

2807 MAPLE SYRUP URINE DISEASE
Synonyms: Branched chain ketoaciduria, MSUD
Disorder Type: Genetic Disorder, Metabolism
Covers these related disorders: Classic MSUD, Mild (intermediate) MSUD, Intermittent MSUD, Thiamine-responsive MSUD

Maple syrup urine disease (MSUD) is a metabolic disorder characterized by the deficiency of certain enzymes of the branched-chain alpha-ketoacid dehydrogenase complex that break down (catabolize) three essential organic compounds. These compounds are known as amino acids and are the building blocks of protein. These amino acids include leucine, isoleucine, and valine. A deficiency of any enzyme within this complex results in the symptoms of MSUD. There are four basic types of maple syrup urine disease.

Classic MSUD, the most severe form of this disorder, becomes apparent within the first week of life and is recognizable by a characteristic maple syrup odor of the urine and on the body. Symptoms and physical findings associated with this life-threatening form of MSUD include listlessness, drowsiness, exaggerated muscular tension (hypertonicity) and rigidity with periods of loss of muscle tone (flaccidity), severe muscle spasms resulting in a backward arching of the back and neck (opisthotonus), convulsions, and coma. Additional findings include low blood sugar (hypoglycemia) and higher-than-normal acidic levels in the blood as well as abnormally low bicarbonate levels (metabolic acidosis). In addition, severe life-threatening complications may occur following infection, surgery, or other stressful events. Such complications include an excessive accumulation of fluid around the brain (cerebral edema) and acidosis accompanied by excessive levels of certain organic compounds in the tissues and body fluids (ketosis). Many affected children experience neurologic and mental deficiencies.

Treatment for classic MSUD includes the removal of leucine, isoleucine, valine, and certain other related elements from the blood by a procedure known as peritoneal dialysis. Subsequent therapy includes a diet low in leucine, isoleucine, and valine.

Intermittent MSUD develops suddenly in children who had previously exhibited no signs of the disease. Though this form of the disease is intermittent, the characteristic findings, symptoms, severity of complications, and treatment are similar to those of classic MSUD. In addition, children with this form of the disorder may exhibit more activity of certain enzymes than those with the classic form.

Mild or intermediate MSUD is a less severe form of this disorder that usually affects children after the first month of life. Affected infants may be mildly retarded and usually emit the characteristic maple syrup odor in their urine, sweat, and earwax (cerumen).

Characteristic findings and symptoms associated with thiamine-responsive MSUD are similar to those of intermittent or intermediate disease. The distinguishing feature is that treatment with high doses of vitamin B1 (thiamine) often results in a favorable response.

Maple syrup urine disease is inherited as an autosomal recessive trait. Approximately one in 200,000 people in the United States is affected by this disorder.

The following organizations in the General Resources Section can provide additional information: Genetic Alliance, March of Dimes Birth Defects Foundation, National Organization for Rare Disorders, Inc., (NORD), NIH/Office of Rare Diseases, NIH/National Digestive Diseases Information Clearinghouse (NDDIC)

National Associations & Support Groups

2808 ARC
500 East Border Street, Suite 300
Arlington, TX 76010   817-261-6003
                             800-433-5255
                        TDD: 817-277-0553

457

Parent to Parent (P-P) programs provide informational and emotional support to parents who have a child, adolescent, or adult family member with special needs. P-P programs offer an important connection for a parent who is seeking support for disability issue, by matching him or her with a trained vetern parent who has already been there. Because the two parents share so many common concerns and interests, the suppor given and received is often uniquely meaningful.

2809 Association for Neuro-Metabolic Disorders
5223 Brookfield Lane
Sylvania, OH 43506   419-885-1497

Organization that is comprised of families of children with disorders that affect the nervous system and the brain. It provides assistance and information through conferences, meetings and phone calls.

2810 Families with Maple Syrup Urine Disease
Route 2, Box 24-19
Flemingsburg, KY 41041   606-849-4679

2811 Maple Syrup Urine Disease Organic Acidemia Association
14600 41st Ave N
Plymouth, MN 55446   612-694-1797
Fax: 612-564-0017
e-mail: oaanews@aol.com
www.oaanews.com

Organization that provides support opportunities for those with the disease and their families through eudcational conferences, brochures and a symposium.

International

2812 Research Trust for Metabolic Diseases in Children
Golden Gates Lodge Weston Road, Crewe
Cheshire,
United Kingdom

Dedicated to providing the most up-to-date medical knowledge for the families and friends of people suffering from this and related diseases.

Web Sites

2813 Family Village
www.familyvillage.wisc.edu/lib_msud.htm

2814 Pedbase
www.icondata.com/health/pedbase/files/MAPLESYR.HTM

DESCRIPTION

2815 MARFAN SYNDROME
Synonym: MFS
Disorder Type: Genetic Disorder
Covers these related disorders: Neonatal or
infantile Marfan syndrome
May involve these systems in the body (see Section III):
Connective Tissue

Marfan syndrome is a connective tissue disorder that may result in heart (cardiac), blood vessel, skeletal, and eye (ocular) abnormalities. Children with Marfan syndrome tend to be unusually tall and slim; in some cases, this may be apparent at birth. Many affected infants also have deficiency of the layer of fat under the skin and abnormally diminished muscle tone (hypotonia) that may contribute to motor delays. In addition, in some infants with Marfan syndrome, several additional characteristic symptoms and findings may be apparent during later childhood. Neonatal or infantile Marfan syndrome is characterized by abnormal flexions (contractures), dislocations, and limited ranges of movement; an abnormally long head and face (dolichocephaly); a highly arched roof of the mouth (palate); unusually large corneas of the eyes (megalocornea); abnormal quivering movements of the colored portions of the eyes (irides); and heart defects (e.g., aortic root dilatation, mitral valve prolapse).

Older children with Marfan syndrome also tend to have an unusually long, narrow face as well as a narrow, highly arched palate and abnormal crowding of the teeth. Affected children and adults also have unusually long, thin arms and legs; a wide arm span; and long, thin fingers (arachnodactyly) with abnormally increased extension (hyperflexibility). Additional skeletal abnormalities are often present, such as unusually thin, fragile ribs; abnormal protrusion or depression of the breastbone (pectus carinatum or excavatum); and, in older children and adolescents, progressive abnormal sideways curvature (scoliosis) or front-to-back curvature (kyphosis) of the spine.

In many cases, affected children also have additional ocular abnormalities, such as dislocation (subluxation) of the lenses of the eyes (ectopia lentis); abnormal bluish coloration of the tough, outer membrane of the eyes; and severe nearsightedness (myopia). In addition, in some cases, the nerve-rich membrane at the back of the eyes (retinas) may become detached.

Most individuals with Marfan syndrome also experience abnormalities of the heart and certain blood vessels (cardiovascular defects) that may be life-threatening. These may include progressive widening of the major artery of the body (aorta), causing leakage of blood through the valve between the left ventricle and the aorta (aortic regurgitation). In addition, the valve between the left ventricle and the left upper chamber (atrium) of the heart may bulge backward (prolapse) into the atrium, causing leakage of blood into the atrium.

The treatment of Marfan syndrome is directed toward preventing potential complications associated with progression of the disease. Affected children should receive regular evaluations to detect ocular defects, abnormal spinal curvatures, or cardiovascular defects. Treatment includes symptomatic and supportive measures, such as orthopedic techniques to help prevent or treat scoliosis or kyphosis; therapy with certain medications (beta-adrenergic blocking agents, e.g., propranolol) that may help to prevent or reduce the progression of certain cardiovascular abnormalities (e.g., aortic dilatation and associated complications); or surgical correction of cardiovascular defects as required. In addition, affected individuals should be provided with antibiotic medications (antibiotic prophylaxis) before dental visits and surgical procedures.

Marfan syndrome results from abnormal changes (mutations) in a gene (fibrillin gene) located on the long arm of chromosome 15 (15q21.1). Such mutations may occur spontaneously (sporadically) for unknown reasons or may be inherited as an autosomal dominant trait. In individuals with the disease gene, the range and severity of associated symptoms and findings may vary from case to case (variable expressivity). Marfan syndrome is thought to affect about one in 10,000 individuals.

The following organizations in the General Resources Section can provide additional information: National Organization for Rare Disorders, Inc., (NORD), Genetic Alliance, March of Dimes Birth Defects Foundation, NIH/Office of Rare Diseases, NIH/National Institute of Arthritis and Musculoskelatal and Skin Diseases

National Associations & Support Groups

2816 National Marfan Foundation
382 Main St
Port Washington, NY 11050   516-883-8712
                                   800-862-7326
                                   Fax: 516-883-8040
                                   e-mail: staff@marfan.org
                                   www.marfan.org

The National Marfan Foudation was founded in 1981 to distribute information about the disorder to patients, families and healthcare providers, offer support for patients and families, and support and fostor research.

Carolyn Levering, Executive Director

International

2817 British Coalition of Heritable Disorders of Connective Tissue
Rochester House, 5 Aldershot Road, Fleet
Hampshire,
United Kingdom
          www.business-partners.co.uk/marfan

Association that unites member organizations that provide information, assistance and support to those affected by connective tissue disorders and their families.

2818 European Marfan Support Network
70 Greenways, Courtmoor Fleet
Hampshire,
United Kingdom
          e-mail: marfan@thenet.co.uk
          www.thenet.co.uk/~marfan

Network that acts as liaison with Marfan Syndrome Parent Organizations throughout Europe by advocacy and support groups.

Web Sites

2819 Marfan Matters Newsletter
home.talkcity.com/LOLWay/uncle_dan/marfan/index.htm

2820 Usenet Newsgroup
Alt.Support.Marfan

2821 Wheeless' Textbook of Orthopaedics
www.medmedia.com/o14/83.htm

Pamphlets

2822 Marfan Syndrome
March of Dimes Resource Center
1275 Mamaroneck Avenue
White Plains, NY 10605   888-663-4637
                               Fax: 914-997-4763

DESCRIPTION

2823 MCCUNE-ALBRIGHT SYNDROME

Synonyms: Albright syndrome, MAS, PFD, POFD,
Polyostotic fibrous dysplasia, Precocious puberty
with polyostotic

Disorder Type: Genetic Disorder

May involve these systems in the body (see Section III):

Skeletal System

McCune-Albright syndrome is a genetic disorder characterized by multiple areas of abnormal, fiber-like tissue growths (bone lesions) that replace normal bone tissue (polyostotic fibrous dysplasia); irregular, patchy areas of light brown pigmentation on the skin (cafe-au-lait spots); and abnormalities of certain hormone-producing glands that assist in regulating the body's growth, controlling the rate of metabolism, and promoting the development of secondary sexual characteristics. Although bone lesions are most common in the pelvis and the long bones of the arms and legs, other bones may be affected, including the ribs, skull and facial bones, and bones of the spinal column (vertebrae). These bone lesions may cause abnormal thickness and deformity of affected bones, susceptibility to fractures, and bone pain. In addition, lesions may cause corresponding bones to develop unevenly. For example, one leg may appear unusually short, or one side of the face may appear different from the other (facial asymmetry). Bone lesions of the skull and face may eventually result in hearing loss and visual impairment.

Many girls with McCune-Albright syndrome undergo early development of secondary sexual characteristics (precocious puberty), including early breast development and onset of menstrual cycles (menstruation). Some boys with the disorder may also experience precocious puberty, including genital development and unusually accelerated growth. In many patients, additional endocrine abnormalities may be present. For example, some affected children may produce excessive amounts of the hormone cortisol, resulting in Cushing's syndrome. This disorder is characterized by excessive weight gain in the chest and abdominal area; a moon-shaped, rounded face; abnormal pads of fat in certain areas of the body; high blood pressure (hypertension); weakening of bones, causing increased susceptibility to fractures; thin, fragile skin; or other symptoms and findings.

Some children with McCune-Albright syndrome may also produce excessive amounts of thyroid hormones (hyperthyroidism), potentially leading to heart palpitations, anxiety, heat intolerance, excessive sweating, muscle weakness, or weight loss. In addition, some affected children may be prone to developing tumors of the pituitary gland, resulting in increased secretion of growth hormone, which stimulates body growth and development. Affected children may experience enlargement of bones and soft tissues of the hands, feet, and face (acromegaly); lengthening and coarsening of the face; and enlargement of certain organs (e.g., heart). In some patients, excessive growth during childhood (gigantism) and tall stature may occur.

McCune-Albright syndrome may be obvious at birth because of unusual skin pigmentation. Alternatively, it may not be apparent until late infancy or early childhood due to precocious puberty or bone lesions. The disorder is caused by spontaneous (sporadic) changes (mutations) of a gene known as the GNAS1 gene. The disease gene is located on the long arm (q) of chromosome 20 (20q13.2). Because the gene mutation is present in only some cells of the body (mosaicism), symptoms and findings may vary among affected individuals, depending upon the specific body cells affected. Treatment of McCune-Albright syndrome includes symptomatic and supportive measures. These may include drug therapy to help prevent or treat precocious puberty, surgical removal of pituitary tumors or the thyroid gland, and appropriate treatment of bone lesions and associated abnormalities.

The following organizations in the General Resources Section can provide additional information: National Organization for Rare Disorders, Inc., (NORD), March of Dimes Birth Defects Foundation, Genetic Alliance, NIH/National Institute of Arthritis and Musculskeletal and Skin Diseases, NIH/National Institute of Child Health and Human Development

National Associations & Support Groups

2824 International Center for Skeletal Dysplasia
Saint Joseph's Hospital
7620 York Road
Towson, MD 21204

2825 MAGIC Foundation for Children's Growth
1327 North Harlem Avenue
Oak Park, IL 60302   708-383-0808
                           800-362-4423
                           Fax: 708-383-0899
            e-mail: mary@magicfoundation.org
                 www.magicfoundation.org

Support and education provided to families of children with growth related disorders. Specialty divisions include Growth Hormone Deficiency; Precocious Puberty; Congenital Adrenal Hyperplasia; McCune Albright Syndrome; Congenital Hypothyroidism; Russell-Silver Syndrome; Tuners Syndrome; Sepo Optic Dysplasia.

10,000 members

Mary Andrews, Executive Director

Web Sites

2826 Pediatric Database (PEDBASE)
www.icondata.com/health/ped-base/files/MCCUNE-A.HTM

2827 University Alabama Birmingham
www.uab.edu/pedradpath/albright.html

Pamphlets

2828 McCune-Albright Syndrome
Human Growth Foundation
7777 Leesburg Pike Suite 202S
Falls Church, VA 22043   703-883-1773
                                800-451-6434

DESCRIPTION

2829 MEASLES
Synonyms: Morbilli, Nine-day measles, Rubeola
Disorder Type: Infectious Disease

Measles is a highly contagious infection caused by the measles virus, a member of the Paramyxovirus family. This infection is characterized by a typical, spreading rash and other symptoms. Infected individuals may be contagious from as early as the seventh day after exposure to until five days after the appearance of the rash. Measles is typically a disease of the young, but may develop at any age and is spread mainly through airborne droplets of throat, mouth, or nasal secretions from an infected individual. One measles infection usually imparts lifetime immunity to those previously infected.

The early symptoms of measles develop anywhere from seven days to two weeks after exposure and usually include low-grade fever; inflammation of the nasal mucous membranes (rhinitis); runny nose; hacking cough; inflammation of the membranes that line the eyelids and whites of the eyes (conjunctivitis); and increased sensitivity to light (photophobia). These symptoms may last approximately four days, followed two or three days later by the development of tiny, grayish-white specks, each surrounded by an irregular red ring (Koplik's spots), that appear on the inside of the cheeks, usually near the back teeth. Koplik's spots usually disappear within 18 hours. A rash, accompanied by a high fever, may develop within three to five days after the onset of symptoms, characterized by faint, reddish flat spots that first appear behind the ears, at the hairline, and on the neck. The rash may become increasingly raised in character as it rapidly spreads to cover the entire body within the next two or three days. The rash fades in the same order in which it appears and its severity is directly proportionate to the severity of the infection. Other findings associated with measles may include enlargement of certain lymph nodes and the spleen (splenomegaly). Complications sometimes associated with measles may include bacte-

rial infection of the middle ear (otitis media) or of the lungs (pneumonia). In rare cases, inflammation of the brain (encephalitis) may develop, accompanied by headache, vomiting, fatigue, and high fever. In addition, encephalitis may sometimes result in mental retardation or life-threatening seizures and coma. In extremely rare cases, a complication of measles called subacute sclerosing panencephalitis may appear months or years after the original infection. This progressive, life-threatening disease is characterized by fever, blindness, behavioral and personality changes, seizures, uncontrollable muscular jerks, and mental deterioration.

In the United States, protection against measles is routinely provided by immunization, usually in combination with mumps and German measles (rubella) vaccines. Newborns acquire an immunity to measles from maternal antibodies transmitted through the placenta from immunized mothers or those who have had measles. This immunity offers protection for a good part of the first year of life; therefore, vaccination is typically administered at 12 to 15 months of age. Because the vaccine may not provide 100 percent immunity, a second immunization is usually administered upon entering school. Live vaccine is not recommended for children with leukemia or those receiving drugs that suppress the immune system, due to increased risk of certain types of infection (e.g., giant cell pneumonia). After exposure to measles, protection may be provided to infants, children with leukemia or on immunosuppressive drugs, and chronically ill children by passive immunization with certain types of immune gamma globulin.

Treatment of measles may include the use of medication to reduce fever, antibiotics to combat secondary bacterial infections, and increased fluid intake. In addition, bed rest in a warm, humidified room is often recommended. Sensitivity to light may necessitate protection from bright or strong light. Other treatment is symptomatic and supportive.

The following organizations in the General Resources Section can provide additional information: National Organization for Rare Disorders, Inc., (NORD), March of Dimes Birth Defects Foundation, NIH/National Institute of Allergy and Infectious Diseases, World Health Organization (WHO), Centers for Disease Control (CDC)

Web Sites

2830 Child Health Research Project
www.ih.jhsph.edu/chr/chr.htm

2831 Kid's Health
kidshealth.org/parent/common/measles.htm

2832 Medical Sciences Bulletin
www.pharminfo.com/pubs/msbped_dis.html

2833 Slack
www.slackinc.com/child/idc/idchome.htm

DESCRIPTION

2834 MECONIUM ASPIRATION SYNDROME

May involve these systems in the body (see Section III):
Respiratory System

Meconium aspiration syndrome is a respiratory condition that affects newborns. It is characterized by blockage and irritation of the airways of the lungs (bronchial airways) due to passage of meconium before birth and inhalation (aspiration) of meconium before or during delivery. Meconium, which primarily consists of secretions of the fetal intestinal glands and the liver, is the thick, sticky, darkish green material that accumulates in the fetal intestines and forms a newborn's first stools. Newborns typically pass meconium during the first 24 to 48 hours after birth. However, in some cases, a fetus may pass meconium into the amniotic fluid before birth and then inhale meconium-contaminated fluid into the lungs either in the uterus or with the first few breaths after birth. Amniotic fluid surrounds and protects the developing embryo and fetus during pregnancy. An increased risk for meconium aspiration syndrome is present if an infant is born postmaturely (post-term, i.e., after 40 weeks' gestation) or a fetus receives insufficient levels of oxygen (hypoxia) via the placenta. The condition may be most severe in post-term infants who were surrounded by decreased levels of amniotic fluid and typically have abnormally thick meconium, increasing the risk of severe airway obstruction. Meconium-stained fluid is present in approximately five to 15 percent of term or post-term infants.

The skin of newborns with meconium aspiration syndrome is usually stained with meconium. In severe cases, additional findings may include diminished muscle tone (hypotonia), an abnormally slow heartbeat (bradycardia), or absence of spontaneous respiration at birth (i.e., fetal distress), requiring emergency resuscitation measures, such as artificial ventilation, cardiac techniques, or correction of acid-base imbalance. In addition, due to blockage of the airways and associated collapse of the bronchial air sacs (alveoli), some newborns with meconium aspiration syndrome may have increasing difficulties breathing (respiratory distress) within the first hours after birth. In severe cases of respiratory distress, affected newborns may experience abnormally rapid breathing (tachypnea), grunting upon exhaling, drawing in of the chest wall while inhaling, and bluish discoloration of the skin and mucous membranes (cyanosis) due to increased levels of oxygen-poor hemoglobin in the blood. Hemoglobin is the oxygen-carrying protein in red blood cells. In some affected newborns, air may abnormally collect in the chest cavity surrounding the lung(s) (pneumthorax), causing the lung(s) to collapse.

In newborns with meconium aspiration syndrome, prompt treatment measures may help to delay the onset or decrease the severity of respiratory distress and potentially associated symptoms or complications. Treatment may include immediate suctioning of an affected newborn's mouth, throat, and nose and placement of a tube into the windpipe (endotracheal intubation) to remove meconium from the airways as well as measures to help prevent or treat respiratory distress (e.g., use of an oxygen hood or a ventilator, surfactant drug therapy, etc.). In most affected newborns, improvement usually occurs in approximately three days, although abnormally rapid breathing (tachypnea) may continue for several days or weeks. In some severe cases, life-threatening complications may occur shortly after birth.

The following organizations in the General Resources Section can provide additional information: Genetic Alliance, March of Dimes Birth Defects Foundation, NIH/National Institute of Child Health and Human Development

DESCRIPTION

2835 MENINGITIS

Covers these related disorders: Bacterial
meningitis, Chronic meningitis, Neonatal meningitis,
Viral meningitis
**May involve these systems in the body (see Section
III):**
 Central Nervous System

Meningitis is characterized by inflammation of the
protective membranes that surround the brain
and spinal cord (meninges). The condition is usually caused by infection with microorganisms,
such as certain bacteria (bacterial meningitis) or
viruses (viral meningitis). Meningitis primarily affects infants and young children.

 Meningitis that occurs within the first month of
life, known as neonatal meningitis, may cause a
different pattern of symptoms than that seen in
older infants and children. The condition affects
approximately 0.2 to 0.4 in every 1,000 newborns,
and the frequency increases among infants who
are born before 37 weeks of pregnancy (premature
infants). In newborns, meningitis may be caused
by infection with certain bacteria, viruses, protozoa, or fungi. These invading microorganisms usually reach the protective membranes of the brain
and spinal cord by circulating through the bloodstream (sepsis). Rarely, neonatal meningitis may
be due to local infection. Affected newborns may
initially experience generalized symptoms, including fever, abnormal yellowish discoloration of the
skin and mucous membranes (jaundice), and
breathing difficulties. Neurologic symptoms may
or may not occur. When present, such symptoms
typically include listlessness (lethargy), drowsiness, and episodes of abnormally increased electrical activity in the brain (seizures). In addition,
pus-filled pockets of infection (abscesses) may develop in the brain, causing increased fluid pressure in the brain, bulging of the soft spots where
bones of the skull have not fully fused (fontanels),

enlargement of the head, and vomiting. In some
cases, life-threatening complications may result.

 The treatment of newborns with neonatal meningitis includes the immediate administration of appropriate intravenous medications. Because
certain bacteria are the most common causes of
meningitis, such therapy may initially include a
number of different antibiotics. Once the specific
bacterium or other microorganism is identified,
different drugs may be substituted to most effectively treat the infection. Additional treatment is
symptomatic and supportive.

 Bacterial meningitis is a serious condition that
most commonly affects children between the ages
of one month to five years. Although older children and adults are rarely affected, small epidemics may periodically occur in environments where
many people have close contact, such as in certain
school settings, dormitories, or military camps. In
children aged approximately two months to 12
years, bacterial meningitis is most commonly
caused by three types of bacteria: i.e., Neisseria
meningitidis, Haemophilus influenzae type b, or
Streptococcus pneumoniae. These microorganisms are spread by the inhalation of airborne
droplets that contain the bacteria or through contact with infected respiratory secretions. Meningitis that results from the bacterium Neisseria
meningitidis in the bloodstream (meningococcal
sepsis with meningitis) may cause a sudden onset
of rapidly progressive symptoms that may lead to
life-threatening complications within 24 hours.
The bacteria Haemophilus influenzae type b or
Streptococcus pneumoniae less commonly cause
rapidly progressive illness; instead, such bacteria
usually initially cause several days of upper respiratory or digestive symptoms. General symptoms
associated with bacterial meningitis may include
fever, lack of appetite (anorexia), joint and muscle
aches, or small areas of abnormal bleeding within
skin layers, causing the appearance of small purplish spots on the skin (petechia). Inflammation of
the meninges may cause stiffness of the neck and
back pain; however, such symptoms are less common in children younger than 18 months of age.
Patients may also experience increased fluid pressure in the brain, vomiting, severe headache, pa-

ralysis of nerves controlling certain eye and facial movements, and, in young children, abnormal bulging of the soft spots and widening of the fibrous joints between bones of the skull. Additional symptoms may include breathing difficulties, episodes of abnormally increased electrical activity in the brain (seizures), and abnormal sensitivity to light (photophobia). Without prompt treatment, patients may become irritable, confused, and increasingly drowsy; become unaware of their surroundings (stupor); progress to a coma; and develop potentially life-threatening complications.

Prompt diagnosis and immediate treatment of bacterial meningitis is essential to help prevent brain damage and potentially life-threatening complications. Treatment requires immediate therapy with intravenous antibiotics and appropriate measures to treat increased fluid pressure in the brain. A number of different antibiotics may initially be administered, based on the different bacteria that are most likely responsible for the condition. Once the specific bacterium is identified, different drugs may be substituted as required to most effectively treat the infection. Additional treatment of children with bacterial meningitis is symptomatic and supportive. Preventive antibiotic therapy may be recommended for individuals who have had close contact with patients diagnosed with bacterial meningitis. In addition, routine childhood immunization with the Haemophilus influenzae type b vaccine now plays an essential role in preventing one of the most common causes of childhood bacterial meningitis.

Viral meningitis is a more common condition that occurs as the result of infection with a virus. This condition typically causes milder symptoms than those associated with bacterial meningitis. Patients often develop mild flu-like symptoms, including fever, headache, a general feeling of ill health (malaise), abdominal pain, nausea, and stiffness of the neck and back. Symptoms generally subside within one to two weeks. Treatment is usually symptomatic and supportive. However, in some more severe cases, antiviral medications may be prescribed.

Some patients may develop inflammation of the protective membranes of the brain and spinal cord that lasts for a month or longer. This condition, known as chronic meningitis, may occur secondary to certain infections. In addition, chronic meningitis may be due to noninfectious causes, such as certain disorders that may affect the brain, such as sarcoidosis or multiple sclerosis; administration of particular medications, such as certain anticancer drugs; or other factors. Individuals with impaired immune systems may be more susceptible to chronic meningitis. Patients generally develop associated symptoms over a few weeks. Such symptoms may include fever, headache, a stiff neck, back pain, confusion, nausea, and vomiting. The treatment of chronic meningitis is based on the underlying cause of the condition.

The following organizations in the General Resources Section can provide additional information: National Organization for Rare Disorders, Inc., (NORD), March of Dimes Birth Defects Foundation, NIH/National Institute of Allergy and Infectious Disease, Centers for Disease Control (CDC)

Web Sites

2836 MHG Neurology Web Forum
neuro-www.mgh.harvard.edu/forum/

2837 Maryland Department of Public Health
edcp.org/html/vir_men.html

2838 Meningitis Foundation of America
www.musa.org

2839 Meningitis Foundation of Texas
www.mft.org

2840 World Health Organization
www.who.org/inf-fs.en/fact105.html

DESCRIPTION

2841 MENTAL RETARDATION
Synonym: Mental deficiency
Disorder Type: Developmental Milestones

Mental retardation is characterized by impaired or below average intellectual functioning that results in deficits in learning ability and adaptive behaviors. The disorder is thought to affect approximately three percent of the general population. About 80 to 90 percent of patients have mild mental retardation, whereas 10 to 20 percent are affected by moderate to profound degrees of impairment.

The causes of mental retardation may be biological as well as psychosocial or sociocultural in nature. In other words, the disorder may be due to a combination of several factors and influenced both by biological abnormalities of the brain as well as the nature of a child's life experiences, such as those resulting from parent-child interactions and overall family dynamics. Biological causes of mental retardation may include fetal exposure to certain drugs, maternal infections, or radiation therapy; premature birth; or certain underlying disorders, such as inborn errors of metabolism, chromosomal abnormalities including Down syndrome and fragile X syndrome, or other genetic disorders. Mental retardation may also result from head injuries or low levels of oxygen to the brain during delivery, childhood exposure to lead, or certain infections during infancy or early childhood, such as inflammation of the protective membranes surrounding the brain and spinal cord (meningitis). Some underlying causes may be correctable before mental retardation occurs, such as phenylketonuria (PKU), which is a metabolic disorder, or hypothyroidism, a condition characterized by decreased activity of the thyroid gland. Additional contributing factors may include malnutrition; dysfunctional interactions between caregivers and infants; or other psychosocial or sociocultural factors. In many children with mental retardation, the specific causes remain unknown. The condition may occur as the result of the interactions of several genes (polygenic inheritance), possibly in association with certain environmental influences (multifactorial).

During normal development, infants and children acquire mental, physical, and behavioral skills in certain stages known as developmental milestones. Although the particular rate of development is variable, most children acquire such skills at certain ages. However, infants and children with mental retardation typically experience delays in achieving certain developmental milestones. For example, with severe levels of mental retardation, patients may initially have delays in the acquisition of certain motor skills. With more moderate levels of retardation, children may achieve early motor milestones yet be delayed in acquiring certain skills that require the coordination of physical and mental abilities (psychomotor delays), such as delayed speech and language skills. In children with mild or borderline impairment, below average intellectual functioning may not be suspected until the early school years. Varying degrees of mental retardation are based upon the different levels of support that may be required for daily functioning as well as intelligence quotient (I.Q.), which is a standardized, age-related measure of intelligence. Mental retardation may be defined as having an I.Q. below 70 and is often subdivided into mild, moderate, severe, and profound mental retardation. Most individuals in the general population have an I.Q. between 80 and 120.

Children with what is known as borderline intellectual functioning have very mild intellectual deficits (e.g., I.Q. between 70 to 85) and minor impairments in adaptive behaviors. These behaviors include certain adaptive skills, such as social, self-care, communication, and vocational skills. Patients with mild retardation (I.Q. between 50 and 70) may develop academic skills up to the sixth grade level. In addition, with appropriate support, they may achieve social skills that enable them to function relatively independently during adulthood. Patients with moderate impairment (I.Q. between 35 and 50) may learn to communicate and tend to have only fair motor development.

Although these patients rarely develop academic skills up to the second grade level, they may benefit from vocational training and achieve limited independence with appropriate supervision. Children with severe mental retardation (I.Q. between 20 and 35) typically have poor motor development and little speech or communication skills. With appropriate education and support, they may develop speech by late adolescence. In addition, with close supervision, they may learn basic hygienic skills and simple tasks by adulthood. Although children with profound impairment (I.Q. under 20) may learn some basic hygienic skills, they typically have limited psychomotor development and require close, ongoing supervision.

In infants with suspected mental retardation, a number of specialized laboratory tests may be conducted to rule out certain underlying disorders, such as fragile X syndrome or other chromosomal or genetic syndromes. The management of mental retardation is individualized for each child and may include therapeutic and special educational services as well as special social support and counseling services. Early diagnosis and the prompt development of an individualized, comprehensive intervention program may be essential in helping affected children reach their potential. Primary care pediatricians may play an important role in consulting with specialists and other health care providers as required and developing an appropriate intervention program. As patients with mild to moderate impairment reach adolescence, specialized services may include a focus on vocational training and community living.

National Associations & Support Groups

2842 ARC
500 E Border St, Ste 300
Arlington, TX 76010   817-261-6003
800-433-5255
Fax: 817-277-3491
TTY: 817-277-0553
e-mail: thearc@metronet.com
www.thearc.org/welcome.html

Parent to Parent (P-P) programs provide informational and emotional support to parents who have a child, adolescent, or adult family member with special needs. P-P programs offer an important connection for a parent who is seeking support for special disability issue, by matching him or her with a trained vetern parent who has already been there. Because the two parents share so many common concerns and interests, the support given and received is often uniquely meaningful.

2843 Bethpage
2245 Midway Rd
Carrolton, TX 75006   972-866-9989
Fax: 972-991-0834
e-mail: psanchez@bethpage.org

2844 Bethpage Mission, Inc.
4980 2 118th St, Ste A
Omaha, NE 68137   402-896-3884
Fax: 402-896-1511
e-mail: psanchez@bethpage.org
www.bethpage.org

2845 People First International
P.O. Box 12642
Salem, OR 97309   503-362-0336
Fax: 503-585-0287
e-mail: heathd@open.org
www.open.org/people1/people1/:htm

Developmentally disabled people joining together to learn how to speak for themselves. Offers support, information, assistance and advocacy.

2846 Voice of the Retarded
5005 Newport Dr, Ste 108
Rolling Meadows, IL 60008   847-253-6020
Fax: 847-253-6054
e-mail: vor@compuserve.com

National organization that offers information, support and advocacy for those affected by mental retardation with its educational materials.

Web Sites

2847 American Association on Mental Retardation
www.aamr.org

Books

2848 Art Projects for the Mentally Retarded Child

Ellen J. Sussman, author

Charles C. Thomas Publishing, Ltd.
2600 South First Street
Springfield, IL 62704   217-789-8980
                              800-258-8980
                         Fax: 217-789-9130
            e-mail: books@ccthomas.com
                      www.ccthomas.com

108 pages Softcover
ISBN: 0-398057-93-1

2849 Children with Mental Retardation

Romayne Smith, M.A., CCC-SLP, author

Woodbine House
6510 Bells Mill Road
Bethesda, MD 20817   301-468-8800
                              800-843-7323
                         Fax: 301-897-5838
       e-mail: info@woodbinehouse.com
                  www.woodbinehouse.com

A book for parents of children with mild to moderate mental retardation, whether or not they have a diagnosed syndrome or condition. It provides a complete and compassionate introduction to their child's medical, therapeutic, and edaucational needs, and discusses the emotional impact on the family. New parents can rely on Children with Mental Retardation to provide that solid foundation and confidence they need to help their child reach his or her highest potential.

437 pages Softcover

2850 Music Curriculum Guidelines for Moderately Retarded Adolescents

Mary R. Beal, Janet P. Gilbert, author

Charles C. Thomas Publishing, Ltd.
2600 South First Street
Springfield, IL 62704   217-789-8980
                              800-258-8980
                         Fax: 217-789-9130
            e-mail: books@ccthomas.com
                      www.ccthomas.com

122 pages
ISBN: 0-398047-57-X

2851 Retarded Isn't Stupid, Mom!

Sandra Z. Kaufman, author

Brookes Publishing
P.O. Box 10624
Baltimore, MD 21285   410-337-9580
                              800-638-3775
                         Fax: 410-337-8539
         e-mail: custserv@pbrookes.com
                www.brookespublishing.com

This book goes through the triumphs and sorrows of one young woman and her family; the emotions and events encountered as her daughter moves toward adulthood.

256 pages Softcover

Magazines

2852 Mental Retardation

American Association on Mental Retardation
444 North Capitol St. NW Suite 846
Washington, DC 20001   202-387-1968
                              800-424-3688
                         Fax: 202-387-2193
         e-mail: AAMR@access.digex.net
                          www.aamr.org

Provides information on the latest program advances, current research, and information on products and services in the developmental disabilities field.

Bi-monthly

DESCRIPTION

2853 MICROCEPHALY

Synonyms: Microcephalia, Microcephalism

May involve these systems in the body (see Section III):

Nervous System

Microcephaly is a developmental abnormality in which an infant's or child's head circumference is smaller than would be expected for his or her age and sex (i.e., two or three standard deviations below the mean). In most affected infants and children, underdevelopment of the brain (microencephaly) may result in varying degrees of mental retardation. Microcephaly is considered a relatively common condition, particularly among individuals affected by mental retardation.

In some affected infants and children, microcephaly occurs as an isolated genetic condition. Familial cases of isolated microcephaly have been reported that appear to have autosomal recessive or dominant inheritance. Autosomal recessive microcephaly is characterized by a narrow, sloping forehead; a flat back portion of the head (occiput); varying levels of mental retardation (although severe retardation is most common); and, in some cases, episodes of uncontrolled electrical disturbances in the brain (seizures). Autosomal dominant microcephaly may be characterized by mild slanting of the forehead, upslanting eyelid folds (palpebral fissures), prominent ears, short stature, and borderline or mild mental retardation. In others, the condition occurs in association with certain underlying genetic disorders, such as Cornelia de Lange syndrome. It may also be part of chromosomal malformation syndromes, such as trisomy 13 and trisomy 18 syndromes.

Microcephaly may also occur secondary to particular environmental factors, such as exposure before birth to radiation, certain chemical agents (e.g., alcohol), or certain maternal infections (e.g., rubella). In addition, the condition may result from particular conditions (e.g., meningitis, hyperthermia, etc.) during periods of rapid brain development after birth, particularly during the first two years of life.

When infants and children have a very small head circumference, the underlying abnormality may have begun during early embryonic or fetal development. Although the exact cause is not understood, the condition is thought to result from abnormal development of the outer region of the brain (cerebral cortex).

When infants or children are diagnosed with microcephaly, physicians typically take thorough family histories to determine whether other family members are affected or other disorders or syndromes may be present that are associated with microcephaly. The head circumference is measured periodically for a direct comparison to measurements at birth. Head circumference measurements may also be taken of both parents and any siblings. Additional testing may be undertaken to rule out potential underlying disorders or associated conditions. These tests may include advanced imaging techniques (e.g., CT scanning, MRI) of the brain, chromosomal testing (karyotyping), or certain laboratory tests to detect antibodies against certain infectious agents (e.g., rubella titers) in the child's and mother's bloodstream. Treatment of infants and children with microcephaly includes symptomatic and supportive measures, such as the prescription of certain medications to help treat or control seizures (e.g., anticonvulsants) and special education and other multidisciplinary measures to help ensure that affected children with mental retardation reach their potential.

The following organizations in the General Resources Section can provide additional information: Genetic Alliance, NIH/National Institute of Neurological Disorders and Stroke, Online Mendelian Inheritance in Man: www3.ncbi.nlm.nih.gov/Omim/searchomin.html, NIH/Office of Rare Diseases: rarediseases.info.nih.gov/ord/

National Associations & Support Groups

2854 ARC
500 E. Border Street, Suite 300
Arlington, TX 76010   817-261-6003
                            800-433-5255
                        TDD: 817-277-0553

The ARC of the United States works through
education, research and advocacy to improve
the quality of life for children and adults with
mental retardation and their families and work
to prevent both the causes and the effects of mental retardation.

2855 Association of Birth Defect Children
930 Woodcock Road, Suite 225
Orlando, FL 32803   407-245-7035
                            800-313-2223
                        Fax: 407-895-0824
              e-mail: abdc@birthdefects.org
                        www.birthdefects.org

Organization devoted to dissemination of data
pertaining to birth related malformations.

**2856 National Information Center for Children & Youth
with Disabilities**
P.O. Box 1492
Washington, DC 20013   202-884-8200
                            800-695-0285
        mcrcr2.med.nyu.edu/murphp01/homenew.htm

A clearinghouse that provides free information
on disabilities and disability-related issues.

Web Sites

2857 Pediatric Database
www.icondata.com/health/pedbase/files/MICRO-
CEP.HTM

DESCRIPTION

2858 MICRODONTIA

Synonym: Microdontism

Disorder Type: Birth Defect, Genetic Disorder, Teeth

May involve these systems in the body (see Section III):

Prenatal & Postnatal Growth & Development

Microdontia is a term that refers to a developmental dental irregularity in which one or more teeth are abnormally small. This tooth abnormality often occurs in association with certain disorders, conditions, and syndromes and usually affects a single tooth or specific groups of teeth, namely the second or lateral incisors and the molars of the upper jaw. However, in rare instances, microdontia occurs in association with certain other disorders and may affect all or most of the teeth. These other disorders may include pituitary dwarfism, Down's syndrome, and certain forms of congenital heart disease.

Children with certain abnormalities of the face or skull (craniofacial defects) may often exhibit some form of microdontia. These disorders include Turner syndrome, a chromosomal disorder affecting females and characterized by various symptoms including a narrow palate and a small jaw (micrognathia); Crouzon's disease, an autosomal dominant disorder characterized by underdevelopment of the upper jaw and protrusion of the lower jaw (prognathism), a beaked nose, and other symptoms; and cleft lip, a congenital defect in which there is a split or fissure (cleft) in the upper lip. Microdontia is also manifested in several other disorders (e.g., focal dermal hypoplasia, progeria, oculomandibulodyscephaly, oculo-auriculo-vertebral anomaly, and others). Small teeth with a characteristic cone shape are often present in conjunction with missing teeth (anodontia) in certain syndromes known as ectodermal dysplasias, in which there is abnormal development of embryonic tissues that give rise to tooth enamel, hair, nails, skin glands, the outermost

layer of the skin (epidermis), the nervous system, the ears and eyes, and mucous membranes of the anus and mouth. Other syndromes that involve microdontia include Williams syndrome, in which the second primary molar of the upper jaw is abnormally small. Aglossia-adactylia syndrome is characterized by partial or total absence of the tongue and missing or abnormally small incisors in the lower jaw.

Microdontia is thought to be genetically transmitted and results from an unknown factor or factors that affect the normal development of the main component of teeth (dentin) and their outermost covering (enamel). This condition is slightly more prevalent in females than males. Treatment may include oral surgery, orthodontic procedures, tooth restoration, and the use of implants or other dental appliances.

The following organizations in the General Resources Section can provide additional information: NIH/National Institute of Child Health and Human Development

National Associations & Support Groups

2859 American Dental Association

211 East Chicago Avenue
Chicago, IL 60611   312-440-2500
www.ada.org

Professional assocation of dentists dedicated to serving both the public and the profession of dentistry. Promotes the profession of dentistry by enhancing the integrity and ethics of the professions and strengthening the patient/dentist relationship. Fulfills its mission by providing services and through its initiatives in education, research, advocacy and the development of standards.

2860 National Institute of Dental Research

31 Cntr Dr,Msc 2290,Bld 31,Rm2c35
Bethesda, MD 20892   301-496-4261
Fax: 301-496-9988
nidr.nih.gov/

Provides leadership for a national research program designed to understand, treat and prevent the infectious and inherited craniofacial-oral-dental diseases and disorders.

Web Sites

2861 Dental Consumer Advisory
toothinfo.com/

2862 Dental Resources on the Web
dental-resources.com/

DESCRIPTION

2863 MIGRAINE HEADACHES

Covers these related disorders: Common migraine (Migraine without aura), Classic migraine (Migraine with aura)
May involve these systems in the body (see Section III):
Central Nervous System, Cardiovascular System

The term migraine refers to a headache that is recurring and accompanied by three or more symptoms or findings that include the presence of certain visual, motor, or other sensations (aura or prodrome) preceding onset; head throbbing; pain on one side of the head; nausea; vomiting; and abdominal pain. Additional associated findings include cessation of pain following sleep and a history of migraines in other family members. Migraines are the most common type of recurrent headaches that occur among children. In children younger than 10 years of age, boys are slightly more apt to develop migraines, while adolescent girls and adult females are more prone to migraines than are adolescent boys or adult men. Migraines may be caused by several different factors, alone or in combination. Such factors include genetic influences; stress-related factors; certain foods such as chocolate, citrus fruit, cheese, etc.; red wine; stimuli such as bright lights, loud noises, etc.; medications such as birth control pills; menstruation; and other factors. Pain associated with migraines results from the narrowing and subsequent widening of the arteries that lead to the brain. This action triggers the pain receptors in that region, thus producing the characteristic pain of migraine headaches.

Common migraine, or migraine without aura, is the type of migraine most likely to occur in children. Common migraine is characterized by a pounding or throbbing pain in the front or side(s) of the head. This headache may or may not be one-sided, may persist from one to 24 hours, and is usually accompanied by nausea, vomiting, and abdominal pain. Other associated symptoms may include fever, an unusual sensitivity to light (photophobia), numbness or tingling of the hands and feet, and dizziness or lightheadedness.

Classic migraine, or migraine with aura, is characterized by similar symptoms and findings to those associated with common migraine; however, classic migraine is always preceded by an aura that occurs from 10 to 30 minutes before onset of the headache. This phenomenon may be characterized by visual, motor, or other sensations such as the appearance of shimmering or flashing lights (photopsia) as well as distorted images, loss of vision in part of the visual field (blind spot or scotoma), dizziness, tingling or weakness in an arm or leg, prickling or burning sensation around the mouth, and other irregularities.

In addition to the two primary types of migraine headaches, some children may develop unusual migraine headaches, called migraine variants, that may be characterized by vomiting that recurs at irregular intervals, sudden attacks of dizziness, and confusion. Children with this type of migraine, especially infants, may experience monthly episodes of severe vomiting resulting in excessive fluid loss (dehydration); the loss of essential compounds, known as electrolytes, in the fluid portion of the blood (i.e., sodium, calcium, and potassium); and associated fever, abdominal pain, and diarrhea. Children with migraine variants may at times appear disoriented, hyperactive, and nonresponsive. Other types of migraine include complicated migraine and cluster headaches. Complicated migraines refer to migraine headaches accompanied by neurologic findings that persist beyond the headache and may be further categorized as basilar migraine, ophthalmoplegic migraine, and hemiplegic migraine. These types of headaches may sometimes indicate the presence of an underlying lesion. Basilar migraine is characterized by problems with equilibrium, double or blurred vision, loss of vision in part of the visual field, lack of muscular coordination (ataxia), seizures, or other irregularities. Ophthalmoplegic migraine, which is characterized by paralysis of the eye muscles on the same side as the migraine, does not commonly occur in children. Amaurosis fugax, a variant of complicated migraine, is characterized by reversible blindness or partial blindness in one eye. Hemiplegic migraine is characterized by numbness and muscular weakness or paralysis affecting only one side of the body. It is rare for children to experience more than one hemiplegic migraine episode. Cluster headaches do not commonly occur in children.

Treatment for migraine headaches may first be directed toward prevention by identifying and removing or avoiding stimulating influences such as certain foods, medications, or underlying stress factors. Many children may benefit from simply resting in a quiet, darkened room. Treatment for pain and vomiting associated with migraine headaches may include administration of pain relievers such as acetominophen or ibuprofen along with drugs to reduce vomiting (antiemetics). These drugs are often administered rectally in suppository form. In more severe episodes, older children and adolescents may require the administration of a preparation called ergotamine, which is most effective if taken during the early stages of the migraine episode. Ergotamine should not be administered to children with hemiplegic migraines. Some children and adolescents may benefit from behavior management therapy. Other treatment is symptomatic and supportive.

The following organizations in the General Resources Section can provide additional information: NIH/National Institute of Neurological Disorders & Stroke, NIH/National Eye Institute

National Associations & Support Groups

2864 American Academy of Neurology
1080 Montreal Avenue
St. Paul, MN 55116　　　　　651-695-1940
　　　　　　　　　　　　　　www.aan.com/

A professional organization representing neurologists worldwide.

2865 American Council for Headache Education (ACHE)
19 Mantua Rd
Mt. Royal, NJ 08061　　　　　856-423-0258
　　　　　　　　　　　　　　800-255-2243
　　　　　　　　　　　　　　Fax: 856-423-0082

Organization that promotes the treatment and management of headache through its support group network, referrals, advocacy and printed materials.

2866 Migraine Association of Canada
356 Bloor Street East Suite 1912
Toronto, Ontario,
Canada　　　　　　　　　　　416-920-4916
　　　　　　　　　　　　　　800-663-3557
　　　　　　　　　　　　　　Fax: 416-920-3677
　　　　　　　　　　　　　　www.migraine.ca

Supports migraine sufferers, provides educational materials, and increases knowledge and awareness of general public and supports research into a cure. Activities include the development of educational materials and information on the latest treatments available, programs for child migraine sufferers, workplace seminars; also supports 24-hour information hotline (416-920-4917).

7,000 members

Frances McKenzie, Office Manager

2867 Migraine Awareness Group: A National Understanding for Migraineurs
113 South Saint Asaph Suite 300
Alexandria, VA 22314　　　　　703-739-9384
　　　　　　　　　　　　　　Fax: 703-739-2432
　　　　　　　　　　　　　　www.migraines.org/

Works to raise public awareness, utilizing the electronic, print, and artistic mediums, of the fact that migraine is a true organic neurological disease.

2868 National Headache Foundation
428 West Street James Place 2nd Flr
Chicago, IL 60614　　　　　773-388-6399
　　　　　　　　　　　　　　888-643-5552
　　　　　　　　　　　　　　Fax: 773-525-7357
　　　　　　　　　　　　　　www.headaches.org

A non-profit organization established in 1970 dedicated to serve as an information resource to headache sufferers, their families, and the physicians who treat them; to promote research into potential headache causes and treatments; and to educate the public to the fact that headaches are serious disorders and sufferers need understanding and continuity of care.

Suzanne E. Simons, Executive Director

Research Centers

2869 Baltimore Headache Institute
2330 West Joppa Road
Lutherville, MD 21093   410-583-7171
                              Fax: 410-583-7173

Brian E. Mondell, M.D., Medical Director

Books

2870 Conquering Headache: An Illustrated Guide to Understanding & Control of Headaches
Alan Rapoport & Fred Sheftell, author

Login Publishers Consortium
1436 W. Randolph Street
Chicago, IL 60607   312-733-8228
                              Fax: 312-666-2680

1994 154 pages Softcover
ISBN: 0-969778-16-3

2871 Freedom From Headaches
Seper & Magee, author

Simon & Schuster Order Department
200 Old Tappan Road
Old Tappan, NJ 07675

                              800-999-5479

ISBN: 0-671254-04-9

2872 Handbook of Headache Disorders
Arthur H. Elkind, author

EMIS, Inc.
Box 1607
Durant, OK 74702   580-924-0643
                              800-225-0694
                              Fax: 580-924-9414
                              www.emispub.com

This book is intended as a quick reference for use by practitioners in the treatment of their headache patients. Includes information on mechanisms of head pain, and pharmacologic and prophylatic therapies.

1993 Softcover
ISBN: 0-929240-62-6

Arthur H. Elkind, Author

2873 Handbook of Headache Management: A Practical Guide to Diagnosis & Treatment
Joel R. Saper, author

Williams & Wilkins
351 West Camden Street
Baltimore, MD 21201   301-528-4000
                            800-638-0672

1993 224 pages
ISBN: 0-683058-01-0

2874 Headache Book: Prevention & Treatment For All Types of Headaches
Frank Mimirth, author

Nelson Publications
One Gateway Plaza
Port Chester, NY 10573   914-937-8400

1994
ISBN: 0-785282-56-4

2875 Management of Headache & Headache Medications
Lawrence D. Robbins, author

Spring-Verlag
175 5th fifth Ave., 19th Fl.
New York, NY 10010   212-460-1500
                            800-777-6497

1994 217 pages
ISBN: 0-387940-40-5

2876 Migraine and Other Headaches: Vascular Mechanisms
Raven Press
1185 Avenue of the Americas
New York, NY 10036   212-930-9500
                            800-777-2295

Leading international experts present new concepts on the mechanisms of migraine and other vascular headaches and detail the latest strategies for diagnosis and treatment of migraine with and without aura, tension-type headaches, cluster headaches and other vascular disorders.

368 pages
ISBN: 0-881677-95-7

2877 Treating the Headache Patient
Roger K. Cady & Anothny W. Fox, author

John H. Dekker & Sons
2941 Clydon Street SW
Grand Rapids, MI 49509   616-538-5160
                            Fax: 616-538-0720

1994 384 pages
ISBN: 0-824791-09-6

2878 Wolff's Headaches & Other Head Pain

Donald J. Dalessio, author

Oxford University Press
2001 Evans Road
Cary, NC 27513   212-726-6000
                                  800-451-7556
                                  Fax: 212-726-6447
                                  www.oup-usa.org

1993
ISBN: 0-195082-50-8

Newsletters

2879 NHF Head Lines

National Headache Foundation
428 W. St. James Place, 2nd Floor
Chicago, IL 60614

                                  888-643-5552
                                  Fax: 773-525-7357
                                  www.headches.org

Offers the latest information on headaches,
causes and treatments. Contains news on drugs
and medical forums, in-depth discussions of
headaches and preventions and a question and
answer section in which physicians respond to
reader inquiries and support group information.

1970 16 pages Bimonthly

International

2880 Migraine Association of Canada Newsletter

356 Bloor Street East Suite 1912
Toronto, Ontario, M4W   416-920-4916
                                  800-663-3557
                                  Fax: 416-920-3677
                                  www.migraine.ca

A newsletter providing information to migraine
sufferers. The cost is free to those who donate
$35 or more per year to the Migraine Associa-
tion of Canada.

Quarterly

Pamphlets

2881 52 Proven Stress Reducers

National Headache Foundation
428 W. St. James Place, 2nd Floor
Chicago, IL 60614

                                  888-643-5552
                                  Fax: 773-525-7357
                                  www.headaches.org

1970

2882 About Headaches

National Headache Foundation
428 W. St. James Place, 2nd Floor
Chicago, IL 60614

                                  888-643-5552
                                  Fax: 773-525-7357
                                  www.headches.org

Contains an in-depth look at headaches, tips on
when to seek medical advice, methods of treatment and more.

1970 16 pages

2883 Analgesic Rebound Headaches - Fact Sheet

National Headache Foundation
428 W. St. James Place, 2nd Floor
Chicago, IL 60614

                                  888-643-5552
                                  Fax: 773-525-7357
                                  www.headches.org

Offers information on analgesic agents or drugs
used to control pain including migraine and
other types of headaches.

1970

2884 Cluster Headache - Fact Sheet

National Headache Foundation
428 W. St. James Place, 2nd Floor
Chicago, IL 60614

                                  888-643-5552
                                  Fax: 773-525-7357
                                  www.headaches.org

Offers information on cluster headaches and the
treatment available for them.

1970

2885 Diet and Headache - Fact Sheet

National Headache Foundation
428 W. St. James Place, 2nd Floor
Chicago, IL 60614

                                  888-643-5552
                                  Fax: 773-525-7357
                                  www.headaches.org

Offers information on what foods should be
avoided, and what foods trigger headaches in all
migraine sufferers.

1970

2886 Headache Handbook

National Headache Foundation
428 W. St. James Place, 2nd Floor
Chicago, IL 60614

                                  888-643-5552
                                  Fax: 773-525-7357
                                  www.headaches.org

Gives information on causes and types of headaches as well as treatments available.

1970 8 pages

2887 Headache Q & A
National Headache Foundation
428 W. St. James Place, 2nd Floor
Chicago, IL 60614

888-643-5552
Fax: 773-525-7357
www.headaches.org

Handy, fact-filled card contains the most frequently asked questions and answers concerning headache triggers and treatments.

1970

2888 Headache in Children - Fact Sheet
National Headache Foundation
428 W. St. James Place, 2nd Floor
Chicago, IL 60614

888-643-5552
Fax: 773-525-7357
www.headaches.org

Offers information on vascular headaches, tension-type headaches, traction and inflammatory headaches and treatment.

1970

2889 How to Talk to Your Doctor About Headaches
National Headache Foundation
428 W. St. James Place, 2nd Floor
Chicago, IL 60614

888-643-5552
Fax: 773-525-7357
www.headaches.org

Learn how to keep a headache diary to pinpoint symptoms and effective diagnosis.

1970

2890 Migraine - Fact Sheet
National Headache Foundation
428 W. St. James Place, 2nd Floor
Chicago, IL 60614

888-643-5552
Fax: 773-525-7357
www.headaches.org

Offers information on migraines and treatments.

1970

2891 Tap the Best Resource
National Headache Foundation
428 W. St. James Place, 2nd Floor
Chicago, IL 60614

888-643-5552
Fax: 773-525-7357
www.headaches.org

Informational brochure offering facts and statistics on headaches. Everything from muscle contraction, vascular headaches, sinus headaches, TMJ, and much more.

1970

DESCRIPTION

2892 MUCOLIPIDOSES
Synonym: ML
Disorder Type: Genetic Disorder, Metabolism

The mucolipidoses are inborn errors of metabolism that belong to a group of diseases known as lysosomal storage disorders. Lysosomes are the major digestive structures within cells. Certain proteins known as enzymes break down or digest nutrients, such as particular fats or carbohydrates. The mucolipidoses are characterized by a deficiency or the abnormal functioning of certain lysosomal enzymes, causing the abnormal accumulation of complex carbohydrates (glycosaminoglycans) and fats (lipids) in cells within particular tissues. Such tissues may include those of the brain and spinal cord (central nervous system), skeleton, joints, heart, liver, spleen, or eyes. The different forms of mucolipidosis (ML) are caused by deficiency of different lysosomal enzymes. The mucolipidoses are thought to be inherited as an autosomal recessive trait.

Specific names as well as Roman numerals are used to classify the different forms of ML. Different types of mucolipidosis include I-Cell disease (ML II), pseudo-Hurler polydystrophy (ML III), and Berman syndrome (ML IV). Some forms of ML are further divided into different subtypes, such as sialidosis (ML I) types I and II, based on age of onset, associated symptoms, or other factors.

In children with mucolipidosis, associated symptoms and findings may be variable, depending upon the specific form of ML that is present. However, certain abnormalities occur in association with most forms of ML. Such findings include mild to severe coarsening of facial features, characteristic skeletal abnormalities (known as dysostosis multiplex), changes of the joints, and varying levels of mental retardation. In children with ML, skeletal malformations may include short stature; abnormal front-to-back or sideways curvature of the spine (kyphosis or scoliosis) or both; improper development of the hips (hip dysplasia); abnormally short neck; or premature fusion of the fibrous joints (sutures) between certain bones of the skull. Many affected children may develop joint stiffness and abnormal bending of certain joints in a fixed position (contractures). In addition, in some patients, neuromuscular abnormalities may be present, such as unusually decreased muscle tone (hypotonia) followed by abnormally exaggerated reflexes (hyperreflexia); shock-like contractions of certain muscles or muscle groups (myoclonus); or involuntary, rapid or writhing movements of the arms and legs (choreoathetoid movements).

Some forms of ML may also be associated with distinctive eye abnormalities, such as clouding of the corneas (corneal opacities), the development of abnormal red circular areas of the middle layer of the eyes (cherry-red spots), or other defects, causing visual impairment. Additional physical abnormalities associated with ML may include bulging of part of the intestine through a weak area in the abdominal wall (hernias), enlargement of the liver or spleen, enlargement of the heart or other heart defects, or increased susceptibility to repeated respiratory infections. Some children with these disorders may also experience delays in the acquisition of skills that require the coordination of physical and mental activities (psychomotor retardation) and may develop progressively severe mental retardation. Other patients may experience mild, nonprogressive mental retardation. Some of the mucolipidoses may result in potentially life-threatening complications during childhood, adolescence, or young adulthood.

The treatment of children with mucolipidosis is symptomatic and supportive. Such measures may include therapies to help prevent or aggressively treat respiratory infections; surgical correction of joint contractures, heart abnormalities, hernias, or other defects; physical therapy; special education; or other measures as required.

The following organizations in the General
Resources Section can provide additional
information: NIH/Office of Rare Diseases, National
Organization for Rare Disorders, Inc. (NORD),
March of Dimes Birth Defects Foundation,
Healthfinder: www.healthfinder.net/, Online
Mendelian Inheritance in Man:
www3.ncbi.nlm.nih.gov/Omim/searchomim.html

National Associations & Support Groups

2893 Research Trust for Metabolic Diseases in Children
Golden Gates Lodge Weston Rd
Crewe, Cheshire, UK, CW1   127-025-0021

Dedicated to providing the most up-to-date medical knowledge for the families and friends of people suffering from this and related diseases.

Web Sites

2894 Mucolipidosis IV Foundation
www.ml4.org

DESCRIPTION

2895 MUCOPOLYSACCHARIDOSES

Synonym: MPS
Disorder Type: Genetic Disorder, Metabolism

The mucopolysaccharidoses are hereditary metabolic disorders that belong to a group of diseases known as lysosomal storage disorders. Lysosomes are the major digestive units within cells. Enzymes within lysosomes break down nutrients, such as certain fats and carbohydrates. The mucopolysaccharidoses are characterized by deficiency of certain lysosomal enzymes, causing the abnormal accumulation of complex carbohydrates in cells within particular tissues of the body. Affected tissues and organs typically include the skeleton, joints, brain and spinal cord (central nervous system), heart, liver, spleen, and eyes. The different forms of mucopolysaccharidosis (MPS) result from deficiency of different lysosomal enzymes. The genes that encode most of these enzymes have been mapped to particular chromosomes. All of the mucopolysaccharidoses are inherited as an autosomal recessive trait, with the exception of Hunter syndrome, which has X-linked recessive inheritance. Collectively, these disorders are thought to affect approximately one in 10,000 newborns.

The various forms of MPS are typically designated by a Roman numeral and a specific name, such as Hunter syndrome (MPS II) or Sanfilippo syndrome (MPS III). In addition, some forms of MPS are divided into different subtypes, such as Hurler syndrome (MPS I H) and Hurler-Scheie syndrome (MPS I H/S), based on different changes (mutations) of the disease gene, age of onset, clinical course, or other factors. The range and severity of associated symptoms and findings may vary, depending upon the specific form of MPS that is present. However, certain findings are common to most forms of MPS, such as characteristic skeletal abnormalities (known as dysostosis multiplex), changes of the joints, growth delays, a characteristic facial appearance, and progressive mental retardation. For example, beginning in the first year of life or during later childhood, many patients develop progressively coarse facial features. Many children with MPS also experience delays in the acquisition of skills requiring the coordination of physical and mental activities (psychomotor retardation), a gradual loss of previously acquired skills (developmental regression), and progressively severe mental retardation. However, in a few forms of MPS, children may have average intelligence.

Many children with MPS also have short stature; sideways or front-to-back curvature of the spine (scoliosis or kyphosis) or both; other bone abnormalities; joint stiffness; and abnormal bending of certain joints in a fixed position (contractures). Other common findings include clouding of the corneas of the eyes and associated visual impairment, abnormal bulging of part of the intestine through a weak area in the abdominal wall (hernias), and enlargement of the liver and spleen (hepatosplenomegaly). Some patients also have associated abnormalities of the heart and its major blood vessels (cardiovascular defects), such as narrowing of the arteries supplying the heart; improper closure of one of the heart valves, allowing blood to leak back into the left upper chamber of the heart (mitral insufficiency); or other cardiac defects. Many of these disorders may result in potentially life-threatening complications during childhood or adolescence.

The treatment of children with MPS includes symptomatic and supportive measures, such as surgical correction of hernias, cardiovascular defects, joint contractures, or other abnormalities as required; physical therapy; or special education. In patients with some forms of MPS, enzyme replacement therapy has been shown to provide some temporary benefit. In addition, bone marrow transplantation may be effective in some patients with certain forms of mucopolysaccharidosis (e.g., Hurler syndrome).

Mucopolysaccharidoses/National Associations & Support Groups

The following organizations in the General Resources Section can provide additional information: NIH/Office of Rare Diseases, National Organization for Rare Disorders, Inc., (NORD), March of Dimes Birth Defects Foundation, Healthfinder: www.healthfinder.net/, Online Mendelian Inheritance in Man: www3.ncbi.nlm.nih.gov/Omim/searchomim.html

National Associations & Support Groups

2896 Association for Neuro-Metabolic Disorders
5223 Brookfield Ln
Sylvania, OH 43506   419-885-1497

Organization that is comprised of families of children with disorders that affect the nervous system and the brain. It provides assistance and information through conferences, meetings and phone calls.

2897 National Mucopolysaccharidosis Society
17 Kraemer St
Hicksville, NY 11801   516-931-6338
Fax: 516-822-2041
e-mail: cohenzec@aol.com
www.members.aol.com/mpssociety/index.htm

Organization that serves as a support group for those affected by mucopolysaccharidoses. Raises funds to promote research and increases awareness of the disorder.

Research Centers

International

2898 Research Trust for Metabolic Diseases in Children
Goldengates Lodge Weston Rd., Crewe
Cheshire,
United Kingdom

Dedicated to providing the most up-to-date medical knowledge for the families and friends of people suffering from this and related diseases.

Web Sites

2899 Canadian Society for Mucopolysaccharide & Related Disease, Inc.
neuro-www2.mgh.harvard.edu/MPS/mpsmain.html

2900 CliniWeb
www.ohsu.edu/cliniweb/C17/C17.300.550.htm

2901 Dysmorphic Syndromes
www.hgmp.mrc.ac.uk/dhmhd-bin/hum-look-up

2902 Mucopolysaccharidses & Related Diseases
www.neuro-www2.mgh.harvard.edu/MPS/

2903 National MPS Society
www.mpssociety.org/

2904 PedBase
www.icondata.com/health/pedbse/files/MUCOPOLY.HTM

2905 Society for Mucopolysaccharide Disease
www.home.btconnect.com/mps/

DESCRIPTION

2906 MUMPS
Synonyms: Epidemic parotitis, Infectious parotitis
Disorder Type: Infectious Disease

Mumps is an acute, infectious viral disease caused by a paramyxovirus and is characterized by swelling or enlargement of the salivary glands, particularly those that lie below and in front of the ears (parotid glands). This disease usually affects children from the ages of five through 15 years, but may develop at any age. Mumps is spread through airborne droplets or direct contact with saliva, or possibly urine, from an infected individual. Although mumps may occur during any season, outbreaks most often occur in late winter or early spring. The mumps virus may be present in the saliva as early as six days before parotid gland swelling and as late as nine days after symptoms begin; however, affected individuals appear to be contagious within one or two days preceding the swelling through three days after the swelling has resolved. Infection usually, but not always, results in lifelong immunity.

Symptoms of mumps may appear within two weeks to 24 days after exposure. Early symptoms may include fever, neck pain, weakness, discomfort, and headache. In addition to or following these symptoms, one or both of the parotid glands may become enlarged and tender to the touch. Chewing and swallowing (especially of citrus fruit juices) may become increasingly painful. If only one parotid gland is swollen, the other may swell as the first returns to normal size. Other findings may include a fever of 101 to 104 degrees, swelling of other salivary glands (i.e., sublingual and submandibular glands), and swelling of the throat. The swelling of the parotid glands usually resolves in a week to 10 days.

Several complications are associated with mumps infection. Among these are inflammation of the membranes surrounding the brain and spinal cord (meningitis), characterized by sensitivity to light (photophobia), severe headache, stiff neck, fever, and profound drowsiness. Other complications may include swelling and inflammation of the joints (arthritis), the pancreas (pancreatitis), the heart muscle (myocarditis), the kidneys (nephritis), and the thyroid gland (thyroiditis). Inflammation may also occur in the eyes. Affected girls who have already reached puberty may develop inflammation of the ovaries (oophoritis), characterized by pain and tenderness in the pelvic region. In affected adolescent boys and adult men, one or both of the testes may become inflamed (orchitis), accompanied by tenderness, swelling, fever, chills, headache, nausea, and lower abdominal pain. In some cases, after the swelling subsides, the affected testis may decrease in size (atrophy).

Newborns acquire a six to eight month immunity to mumps from maternal antibodies transmitted through the placenta. Protection against mumps is typically administered in a combination measles, mumps, German measles (rubella) vaccine form 12 to 15 months of age and once again before entering school. Treatment for mumps is symptomatic and supportive.

The following organizations in the General Resources Section can provide additional information: NIH/National Institute of Allergy and Infectious Disease, World Health Organization (WHO)

Web Sites

2907 About.com
babyparenting.miningco.com

2908 Centers for Disease Control
www.cdc.gov/epo/mmwr/other/case_def/mumps.html

2909 Duke University
www.botany.duke.edu/microbe/mumps.htm

2910 Encarta
www.encarta.msn.com

2911 Kid's Health
kidshealth.org/parent/common/mumps/html

2912 Virtual Hospital
www.vh.org

DESCRIPTION

2913 MUSCULAR DYSTROPHIES

Disorder Type: Genetic Disorder, Neuromuscular

Muscular dystrophies are a group of inherited neuromuscular disorders characterized by the progressive weakness and degeneration of muscles without accompanying nerve tissue involvement. Each of these disorders is different from the others with respect to its age of onset, clinical manifestations, severity, course, and underlying genetic defect.

Duchenne muscular dystrophy, the most common of these disorders, is transmitted as an X-linked recessive trait and, as such, is fully expressed in boys; however, on rare occasions, girls who are carriers of the disease gene may exhibit mild symptoms. The incidence rate for this disorder is about one out of every 3,600 newborn boys. Although some affected infants may exhibit signs of diminished muscle tone such as poor head control, most boys do not develop symptoms until three to seven years of age. Early symptoms may include weakness in the pelvic or girdle area that may be manifested by an unusual method of moving from the supine position to the standing position (Gowers' sign). In addition, boys with this disorder may develop a waddling manner of walking (Trendelenburg gait), be prone to stumbling and falling, or having difficulty climbing stairs and standing up from a sitting position. As the disease progresses, muscles around the joints may contract resulting in the inability to fully extend the knees and elbows. In addition, the spine may develop a side-to-side curve (scoliosis) and muscles, especially of the calves, become bulky due to the enlargement (hypertrophy) of the muscle fibers, the infiltration of fat into the muscles, and the increase of connective tissue protein (collagen) in the muscles. Other findings include involvement of the heart muscle (cardiomyopathy) and intellectual impairment ranging from learning disabilities to mental retardation. Most boys with Duchenne muscular dystrophy are able to walk until the age of 10 or 12 years, at which time they may be confined to a wheelchair. Life-threatening complications such as pneumonia, respiratory failure, and congestive heart failure often occur during late adolescence or early adulthood. This disorder is believed to result from the deficiency of the essential muscle protein dystrophin. The gene for Duchenne muscular dystrophy is located on the short arm of the X chromosome (Xp21).

Duchenne muscular dystrophy is initially diagnosed through evaluation of physical findings and through tests that show increased blood levels of the enzyme creatinine kinase. Additional diagnostic screening may include the use of an electrical muscle function test called electromyography or EMG. Confirmation, however, must be determined through microscopic examination of a muscle tissue sample (biopsy). Treatment is symptomatic and supportive. For example, nutritional vigilance and immunizations against flu and other childhood diseases may help to avoid complications. The administration of digitalis medications may help to alleviate certain heart-related complications. Some children may benefit from physical therapy, exercise, or surgical intervention to aid in walking.

Becker muscular dystrophy results in symptoms similar to those of Duchenne muscular dystrophy; however, these symptoms are usually less severe, do not appear until about the age of 10 years, and follow a long course. The gene for Becker muscular dystrophy is also located on the short arm of the X chromosome (Xp21); however, the essential muscle protein dystrophin is defective and dysfunctional rather than deficient.

Less common forms of muscular dystrophy include facioscapulohumeral muscular dystrophy (Landouzy-Dejerine disease), limb-girdle muscular dystrophy, and others. Facioscapulohumeral muscular dystrophy, which is an autosomal dominant disorder occurring in both males and females, is characterized by facial and shoulder muscle weakness and sometimes weakness in the lower legs. This is a relatively mild disease that usually occurs between seven years of age and early or mid-adulthood. The gene for this disorder is located on the long arm of chromosome 4 (4q35). Limb-girdle muscular dystrophy is usually transmitted as an autosomal recessive trait, although autosomal dominant inheritance has also been documented. This disorder usually occurs in late childhood or early adulthood and is characterized by the progressive weakness and degeneration of the muscles of the hips and shoulders. Treatment for these types of muscular dystrophy is symptomatic and supportive.

National Associations & Support Groups

2914 Duchenne Parent Project
125 Marymouth Court
Middletown, OH 45042

513-424-7452
800-714-5491
Fax: 513-425-9907
e-mail: patfurlong@aol.com
www.parentdmd.org

2915 Muscular Dystrophy Association
3300 E Sunrise Dr
Tucson, AZ 85718

520-529-2000
800-572-1717
Fax: 520-529-5300
e-mail: mda@mdausa.org
www.mdausa.org

A primary objective of MDA is the support of scientific investigators seeking the causes of and effective treatments for muscular dystrophy and related neuromuscular disorders. The worldwide research program supports over 400 scientific investigations annually and represents the largest single effort to advance knowledge of neuromuscular diseases. In addition, MDA offers a comprehensive program of patient and community services, with access to over 230 MDA-supported clinics nationwide.

Robert Ross, Executive Director
Bob Mackle, Director of Publications

2916 Parent to Parent Support for Muscular Dystrophy
Haiser Permanente Hospital/Conference Room 3
2025 Morse Avenue
Sacremento, CA 95825

916-863-8936
e-mail: darkrose@2xtreme.net

A nonprofit organization whose goal is to provide compassionate support for families living with Muscular Dystrophy. This group meets every second Saturday of the month from 11:00 am to 1:00 pm.

Craig Strunk, Contact
Strunk Marilyn, Strunk

International

2917 Muscular Dystrophy Association of Canada
2345 Yonge Street Suite 900
Toronto, Ontario, M4P
Canada

416-488-0030
800-567-2873
Fax: 416-488-7523
e-mail: motter@mdac.ca
www.mdac.ca

A national volunteer agency commited to funding, leading research to find the causes, treatments, prevention and cures for each of over 40 neuromuscular diorders. Provides funding assistance to registered clients for mobility items. It provides community referral and recycled equipment as well as disorder related information and newsletters.

1000+ members

Margaret Otter, RN, Director of Client Services
Yurs Savoie, National Executive Director

Research Centers

Minnesota

2918 Mayo Clinic and Foundation

Rochester, MN 55902   507-284-3250

Neuromuscular clinical research center with a primary research interest in neuropathies.

Peter J. Dyck, MD

New York

2919 Columbia Presbyterian Medical Center
710 West 168th Street
New York, NY 10032   212-305-3880

Neuromuscular clinical research center.

Lewis P. Rowland, MD

2920 Columbia University Clinical Research Center for Muscular Dystrophy
College of Physicians & Surgeons
630 W. 168th Street
New York, NY 10032   212-305-5131
Fax: 212-305-3986

Salvatore DiMauro, Codirector

2921 New York University
Jerry Lewis Neuromuscular Disease Center
Dept. of Rehab. Medicine, 400 E. 34th St, Rm: RG-2
New York, NY 10016   212-263-6350
Fax: 212-263-5499

Focuses on Muscular Dystrophy and related bone disorders.

Matthew Lee, MD, Professor

Ohio

2922 Parent Project for Muscular Dystrophy Research, Inc
125 Maymont Court
Middletown, OH 45042

800-714-5437
Fax: 513-425-9907
www.parentdmd.org

This organization of families around the world who have children diagnosed with DMD/BMD. Our goal is to invest significant amounts of money raised into medical research with clinical application.

Pennsylvania

2923 Hospital of the University of Pennsylvania
3400 Spruce Street
Philadelphia, PA 19104   215-662-3263

Research program centering its efforts on finding better ways to prevent and treat neuromuscular disorders.

David Pleasure, MD

Texas

2924 Baylor College of Medicine
Jerry Lewis Neuromuscular Disease Research
6501 Fannin
Houston, TX 77030   713-798-3200

Offers research into biochemistry, molecular genetics and neuromuscular disorders.

Stanley H. Appel, MD, Co-Director

Utah

2925 University of Utah
Laboratory for the Study of Hereditary Disorders
15 North 2030 East, Room 2100
Salt Lake City, UT 84112   801-581-6461
www.genetics.utah.edu

Focuses research on human muscular dystrophies.

Books

2926 Clinician's View of Neuromuscular Diseases
Michael H. Brooke, MD, author

Williams & Wilkins
351 West Camden Street
Baltimore, MD 21201   301-528-4000
800-638-0672

2927 Muscular Dystrophy
James A. Corrick, author

Franklin Watts c/o Grolier
90 Old Sherman Tpke
Danbury, CT 06816   203-797-3500
800-621-1115
Fax: 203-797-3197
www.grolier.com

2928 Muscular Dystrophy and Other Neuromuscular Diseases
Haworth Press
10 Alice Street
Binghamton, NY 13904

800-429-6784
Fax: 607-722-1424

A thoughtful new book from professionals who assist persons afflicted with neuromuscular disorders to help them and their families adapt to lifestyle changes accompanying the onset of these disorders.

2929 Physical Medicine and Rehab Advances in Neuromuscular Diseases

William M. Fowler, Jr., M.D., author

Hanley & Belfus, Inc.
210 South 13th Street
Philadelphia, PA 19107   212-546-4995

Vol. 2, #4

2930 Psychosocial Aspects of Muscular Dystrophy and Allied Diseases - Coping
Foundation of Thanatology
161 Fort Washington Ave.
New York, NY 10032   212-928-2066

1984

2931 Realities in Coping with Progressive Neuromuscular Diseases

Charash, Lovelace, Wolf, Kitscher, Roye and Leach, author

Charles C. Thomas Publishing, Ltd.
2600 South First Street
Springfield, IL 62704   217-789-8980
                                800-258-8980
                          Fax: 217-789-9130

1987

Children's Books

2932 Muscular Dystrophy

James A. Corrick, author

Franklin Watts c/o Grolier
90 Old Sherman Tpke
Danbury, CT 06816   203-797-3500
                            800-621-1115
                      Fax: 203-797-3197
                      www.grolier.com

Discusses the nature of muscular dystrophy, causes, treatments and the latest research into treatments and cures.

112 pages Grades 7-12
ISBN: 0-531125-40-8

2933 My Life - Melinda's Story
Children's Hospice International
901 N. Washington Street Suite 700
Alexandria, VA 22314

                              800-242-4453

Written by Melinda, a child with muscular dystrophy. This heartwarming story teaches children and their families how to cope with the illness.

2934 Precious Time: Children Living with Muscular Dystrophy

Thomas Bergman, author

Gareth Stevens, Inc.
1555 North River Center Drive
Milwaukee, WI 53212   414-225-0333
                        Fax: 414-225-0377
                          www.gsinc.com

ISBN: 0-836815-97-1

Magazines

2935 Quest Magazine
Muscular Dystrophy Association
3300 E. Sunrise Drive
Tucson, AZ 85718   520-529-2000

Presents news related to muscular dystrophy and other neuromuscular diseases including research, personal profiles, fund raising activities, and patient services.

Bimonthly

Pamphlets

2936 A Teacher's Guide to Duchenne Muscular Dystrophy
Muscular Dystrophy Association
3300 E. Sunrise Drive
Tucson, AZ 85718   520-529-2000
                      Fax: 520-529-5300

A source of guidance and information to educators detailing Duchenne muscular dystrophy, how it affects school participation, and ways that teachers can help meet the needs of students affected by the disorder.

18 pages

2937 Everybody's Different, Nobody's Perfect

Irwin Siegel, MD, author

Muscular Dystrophy Association
3300 E. Sunrise Drive
Tucson, AZ 85718   520-529-2000
                      Fax: 520-529-5300

Explains how muscular dystrophy affects children and describes how people are different from each other in many ways. Emphasizing fun, friendship, and caring, this booklet is ideal for heightening awareness and encouraging understanding of persons with disabilities.

11 pages

2938 Facts About Metabolic Diseases of Muscle
Muscular Dystrophy Association
3300 E. Sunrise Drive
Tucson, AZ 85718   520-529-2000
                                     Fax: 520-529-5300

Provides an overview of the 11 heritable metabolic diseases of muscle encompassed by MDA's program. Addresses commonly asked questions and highlights MDA's research efforts aimed at finding the causes of and effective treatments for these disorders.

2939 Facts About Muscular Dystrophy
Muscular Dystrophy Association
3300 E. Sunrise Drive
Tucson, AZ 85718   520-529-2000
                                     Fax: 520-529-5300

Answers many questions commonly asked about the nine forms of the disease encompassed by MDA's program.

2940 Facts About Myopathies
Muscular Dystrophy Association
3300 E. Sunrise Drive
Tucson, AZ 85718   520-529-2000
                                     Fax: 520-529-5300

Describes the eight inheritable myopathies encompassed by MDA's program, as well as current methods for diagnosing and managing these disorders.

2941 Hey! I'm Here, Too!

Irwin M. Siegel, MD, author

Muscular Dystrophy Association
3300 East Sunrise Drive
Tucson, AZ 85718   520-529-2000
                                     Fax: 520-529-5300
                                     www.mdausa.org

Help for siblings of boys with Duchenne muscular dystrophy. Explores how they feel about themselves, their brothers, and their families. Also provides specific answers to some questions that siblings may wonder about.

2942 Learning to Live with Neuromuscular Disease: A Message To Parents

Sylvia E. McGriff, author

Muscular Dystrophy Association
3300 E. Sunrise Drive
Tucson, AZ 85718   520-529-2000
                                     Fax: 520-529-5300

Intended to help parents and families cope with the knowledge that their child has a neuromuscular disease and with the impact the disease will have on everyday life.

2943 MDA Camp - A Special Place
Muscular Dystrophy Association
3300 E. Sunrise Drive
Tucson, AZ 85718   520-529-2000
                                     Fax: 520-529-5300

Highlights the activities of MDA summer camps for youngsters diagnosed with one of the 40 diseases in MDA's program. Shares camper and volunteer reactions.

2944 MDA Fact Sheet
Muscular Dystrophy Association
3300 E. Sunrise Drive
Tucson, AZ 85718   520-529-2000
                                     Fax: 520-529-5300

Outlines the history of MDA, the diseases included in MDA's program, and the services available through the Association.

2945 MDA Services for the Individual, Family and Community
Muscular Dystrophy Association
3300 E. Sunrise Drive
Tucson, AZ 85718   520-529-2000
                                     Fax: 520-529-5300

Contains a list of the diseases covered by MDA as well as eligibility criteria for MDA's services program, a list of MDA-sponsored clinics nationwide, and the services available through these clinics.

DESCRIPTION

2946 NARCOLEPSY

Synonyms: Gelineau's syndrome, Hypnolepsy, Paroxysmal sleep

Disorder Type: Mental, Emotional or Behavioral Disorder

Narcolepsy refers to a sleep disorder characterized by profound drowsiness during the day and sudden daytime attacks of sleep that may last from a few seconds to one or more hours. These episodes are sometimes accompanied by a condition characterized by sudden attacks of muscular weakness and diminished muscle tone (hypotonia) in response to emotional stimuli such as anger, fear, joy, or surprise (cataplexy). During a cataplectic episode, the patient remains conscious but is not able to speak or move. Some patients experience sleep paralysis and are unable to move at the onset of sleep or immediately upon waking. Hypnagogic hallucinations are disquieting occurrences that take place at onset of sleep or, less commonly, upon awakening. During these hallucinations, patients may see or hear things that are not grounded in reality. In most cases, narcolepsy begins during adolescence or early adulthood and persists throughout the life of the affected individual. Sleep attacks associated with narcolepsy may occur at any time and may take place many times during the day; however, most individuals may be easily awakened.

Very few people with narcolepsy exhibit all the symptoms associated with this disorder and, occasionally, children and adults who do not have this disorder may experience the signs and symptoms of cataplexy, sleep paralysis, or hypnagogic hallucinations. For this reason, diagnosis of narcolepsy may necessitate confirmation by a sleep study which uses a procedure called electroencephalography (EEG), during which electrical brainwave activity is recorded. An EEG may demonstrate an abnormal sleep pattern in which rapid eye movement or REM-type sleep occurs at the onset of sleep. In individuals who do not have narcolepsy, REM sleep or periods of deep sleep normally follow nonrapid eye movement sleep (NREM). The cause of narcolepsy is unknown, but researchers think that, in some cases, it may be related to genetic influences as evidenced by the tendency of this disorder to occur within families. Approximately 200,000 people in the United States are affected by narcolepsy.

Treatment for narcolepsy may include regular napping and the administration of stimulant medications to control attacks of drowsiness and sleep, while antidepressant medications may help control episodes of cataplexy. Because this disorder may increase the risk of accidents, appropriate care and caution is advised in the performance of certain tasks or jobs. Other treatment is symptomatic and supportive.

The following organizations in the General Resources Section can provide additional information: National Organization for Rare Disorders, Inc., (NORD), NIH/Office of Rare Diseases, Genetic Alliance, NIH/National Institute of Neurological Disorders and Stroke, Online Mendelian Inheritance in Man: www3.ncbi.him.nlm.gov/Omim/searchomim.html

National Associations & Support Groups

2947 American Sleep Disorders Association
6301 Bandel Rd NW
Rochester, MN 55901
507-287-6006
Fax: 507-287-6008
www.asda.org

Provides full diagnostic and treatment services to improve the quality of care for patients with all types of sleep disorders.

James Barrett, Executive Director

2948 Association of Professional Sleep Societies
6301 Bandel Rd
Rochester, MN 55901
507-287-6006

Works to facilitate the research and development of sleep disorders medically by encouraging exchange of information among members.

Carol C. Westbrook, Executive Director

2949 Narcolepsy Association
1255 Post Sreet, E F Towers, Ste 404
San Francisco, CA 94109   415-788-4793

2950 Narcolepsy Institute
Montefiore Medical Center
111 East 210th Street
Bronx, NY 10467   718-920-6799
                             Fax: 718-654-9580

Offers services such as screening, information
on narcolepsy, counseling and referrals for individuals and their families with problems arising
as a consequence of narcolepsy, adult and teenage support groups to help individuals develop
positive self-image and self-confidence at an annual conferences for patients and professionals.
Newsletter and video on narcolepsy available.
$10 for two issues of newsletter per year. Non-
pharmacological approaches to the management
of narcolepsy are stressed.

Dr. Meeta Goswami, Director

2951 Narcolepsy Network, Inc.
10921 Reed Hartman Highway, Suite 119
Cincinnati, OH 45242   513-891-3522
                             Fax: 513-891-3836
                         e-mail: narnet@aol.com

Non-profit organization consisting of member-
ships by people who have narcolepsy (or related
sleep disorders), their families and friends, and
professionals involved in treatment, research,
and public education. Participate also in support and protection of rights.

2952 Narcolepsy and Cataplexy Foundation of America
445 East 68th Street
New York, NY 10021   212-570-5506

Organization that provides information on narcolepsy and cataplexy. Also provides referrals,
research and educational materials.

2953 National Institute of Neurological Disorders and Stroke
31 Center Dr MSC 2540, Bldg 31, Rm 8806
Bethesda, MD 20892   301-496-5751
                                 800-352-9424
                             Fax: 301-402-2186
                            www.ninds.nih.gov

Information and advocacy resources for families
and professionals. Includes listings of organizations providing general tips and organizations focusing on more specific areas of concern to
families and young adults who have disabilities.

2954 National Narcolepsy Registry
729 15th Street NW 4th Floor
Washington, DC 20005   202-347-3471
                             Fax: 202-347-3472
                        e-mail: natsleep@erols.com
                          www.sleepfoundation.org

Organization that provides information to researchers that will further research, diagnosis
and treatment of the disorder.

2955 National Sleep Foundation
729 15th Street NW 4th Floor
Washington, DC 20005   202-347-3471
                             Fax: 202-347-3472
                        e-mail: natsleep@erols.com
                          www.sleepfoundation.org

Works to improve the quality of life for millions
of Americans who suffer from sleep disorders,
and to prevent the catastrophic accidents that
are related to poor or disordered sleep through
research, education and the dissemination of information towards the cause of Narcolepsy Project. Seeks patients to aid new research project
targeting the cause of the disorder.

Allan I. Pack, M.D., Ph.D., Medical Director

2956 Sleep/Wake Disorders Canada
3080 Yonge Street Suite 5055
Toronto, Ontario, M4N
Canada   416-483-9654
                                 800-387-9253
                             Fax: 416-483-7081
                       e-mail: swdc@globalserve.net
                       www.geocities.com/~sleepwake/

2957 Young Adults with Narcolepsy
1451 West 31st Street Third Floor
Minneapolis, MN 55408   612-824-1355
                           e-mail: yawn@yawn.org
                                 www.yawn.org

State Agencies & Support Groups

Alabama

2958 Knollwoodpark Hospital Sleep Disorders Center
5600 Girby Road
Mobile, AL 39993   334-660-5757
                             Fax: 334-660-5254
                   e-mail: 71054.2530@compuserve.com

Arizona

2959 Arizona Sleep Disorders Center
College of Medicine Room 7303
Tucson, AZ 85724   520-626-6112
                         Fax: 520-626-4884

Stuart F. Quan, Director

2960 Loma Linda University Sleep Disorders Clinic
VA Hospital, Medical Services Center
11201 Benton Street
Loma Linda, CA 92357   909-422-3063

Dr. Ralph Downey, III, Director

California

2961 Scripps Clinic Sleep Disorders Center
Sleep Disorders Center, Scripps Clinic
10666 North Torrey Pines Road
La Jolla, CA 92037   619-554-8087
                         Fax: 619-554-2502

Milton K. Erman, MD, Medical Director
Merrill M. Erman MD

2962 Sleep Disorders Center at California Pacific Medical Center
2340 Clay Street Suite 237
San Francisco, CA 94115   415-923-3336
                              Fax: 415-923-3584
              e-mail: 76307.2221@compuserve.com

2963 Stanford University Center for Narcolepsy
1201 Welch Road Room P-112
Stanford, CA 94305   650-723-7863
                         Fax: 650-498-7761
              e-mail: mignot@leland.standford.edu

Dr. William Dement, Director

Connecticut

2964 Gaylord Rehab and Sleep Center
1 Longwharf Drive
New Haven, CT 06511   203-624-3140
                          Fax: 203-495-8569
                          www.gaylord.org

Robert K. Watson, PhD, Director

District of Columbia

2965 Georgetown University Sleep Disorders Center
3307 M Street NW
Washington, DC 20007   202-687-8635
                           Fax: 202-687-8899

Dr. Samuel Potolicchio, Jr., Director

Indiana

2966 Methodist Hospital Sleep Center
Rehab Centers
303 East 89th Avenue
Merrillville, IN 46410   219-736-4074
                             Fax: 219-738-6624

2967 MidWest Medical Center - Sleep Disorders Center
3232 North Meridian Street
Indianapolis, IN 46208   317-927-2100

Kenneth Wiesert, MD

2968 Sleep Alertness Center, Lafayette Home Hospital
2400 South Street
Lafayette, IN 47903   765-447-6811

Frederick Robinson, MD

2969 Sleep Disorders Center, Good Samaritan Hospital
520 South 7th Street
Vincenne, IN 47591   812-885-3877

Henry S. Matick, DO

2970 Sleep/Wake Disorders Center, Community Hospitals of Indianapolis
1500 N. Ritter Avenue
Indianapolis, IN 46219   317-355-4275

Marvin E. Vollmer, MD

Maryland

2971 Johns Hopkins University Sleep Disorders Center
Francis Scott Key Medical Center
301 Bayview Boulevard
Baltimore, MD 21224   410-550-0545

Phillip L. Smith, Director

Massachusetts

2972 Center for Sleep Diagnostics
1400 Centre Street #101
Newton Centre, MA 02159   617-735-1850
Fax: 617-630-0142

Michael Biber, MD, Director

2973 Sleep Disorders Unit, Beth Israel Hospital
330 Brookline Avenue, KS430
Boston, MA 02215   617-735-3237

Jean K. Matheson, MD

Michigan

2974 Sleep Disorders Center of Henry Ford Hospital
2799 W. Grand Blvd CFP3
Detroit, MI 48202   313-916-4417
Fax: 313-916-5150

Thomas Roth, Director

Missouri

2975 Midwest Sleep Diagnostics
13975 Manchester Road Suite #9
Manchester, MO 63011   314-227-8787
Fax: 314-227-8610

Anthony Masi, MD, Director

New Hampshire

**2976 Dartmouth-Hitchcock Sleep Disorders Center
Dartmouth Medical Center**
One Medical Center Drive
Lebanon, NH 03756   603-650-5000

Michael Sateia, MD

2977 Sleep/Wake Disorders Center, Hampstead Hospital
East Road
Hampstead, NH 03841   603-329-5311

Deborah Sewitch, PhD

New Jersey

2978 Sleep Disorders Center, Newark Beth Israel Medical Center
201 Lyons Avenue
Newark, NJ 07112   973-926-7163

Monroe S. Karetzky, MD

New York

2979 Capital Regional Sleep-Wake Disorders Center
St. Peter's Hospital & Albany Medical Center
25 Hackett Boulevard
Albany, NY 12208   518-525-1550

Cheryl Carlucci, MD

2980 Center for Sleep Medicine of the Mount Sinai Medical Center
Box 1232, One Gustave L. Levy Place
New York, NY 10029   212-241-5098
Fax: 212-987-5584

Gabriele Barthlen, MD
Carol Rosenbaum, MD

2981 Columbia Presbyterian Medical Center Sleep Disorders Center
161 Fort Washington Avenue
New York, NY 10032   212-305-3953

Neil B. Kavey, MD

2982 Sleep Center, Community General Hospital
Broad Road
Syracuse, NY 13215   315-492-5795

Robert Westlake, MD

2983 Sleep Disorders Center of Rochester, St. Mary's Hospital
2110 Clinton Avenue South
Rochester, NY 14618   716-442-4141

Donald Greenblat, MD

2984 Sleep Disorders Center of Western New York
Millard Fillmore Hospital
3 Gates Circle
Buffalo, NY 14209　　　　　　　716-884-9253

Edwin J. Manning, MD

2985 Sleep Disorders Center, University Hospital
MR 120A
Stony Brook, NY 11794　　　　　516-444-2916

Wallace Mendelson, MD

2986 Sleep-Wake Disorders Center, Montefiore Sleep
Disorders Center
111 East 210th Street
Bronx, NY 10467　　　　　　　718-920-4841
　　　　　　　　　　　　　　Fax: 718-798-4352

Center that provides diagnostic and treatment
services for children with sleep disorders, such
as sleep apnea, narcolepsy, insomnia, daytime
sleepiness, sleepwalking, or night terrors.

Michael J. Thorpy, MD
Karen Balaban-Gil, MD

2987 Sleep-Wake Disorders Center, New York
Presbyterian Hospital
Cornell Medical Center
21 Bloomingdale Road
White Plains, NY 10605　　　　914-997-5751
　　　　　　　　　　　　　　800-694-7533
　　　　　　　　　　　　Fax: 914-682-6911
　　　　　　　e-mail: mmoline@med.cornell.edu

Provides outpatient diagnostic evaluation and
treatment for adults and children with problems
associated with sleeping and waking. More common pediatric sleep problems include complaints of: difficulty falling asleep and staying
asleep, snoring, sleep apnea, sleepwalking, sleep
terrors, nightmares, excessive diffculty waking
up, bedweting, and narcolepsy. Many can be successfully treated in one or several visits although
some may require an overnight or daytime sleep
study.

Margaret Moline, PHD, Director

2988 St. Joseph's Hospital Health Center Sleep
Laboratory
301 Prospect Avenue
Syracuse, NY 13203　　　　　315-448-5870

Edward T. Downing, MD, Director

2989 Winthrop-University Hospital Sleep Disorders
Center
222 Station Plaza North
Mineola, NY 11501　　　　　516-663-2169

Steven H. Feinsilver, MD

Ohio

2990 Bethesda Oak Hospital, Sleep Disorders Center
619 Oak Street
Cincinnati, OH 45206　　　　513-569-6111

Milton Kramer, MD

2991 Center for Sleep & Wake Disorders, Miami Valley
Hospital
One Wyoming Street Suite G200
Dayton, OH 45409　　　　　937-220-2515

James P. Graham, MD, Director

2992 Cleveland Clinic Foundation, Sleep Disorders Center
9500 Euclid Avenue S53
Cleveland, OH 44195　　　　216-444-2200

Dudley S. Dinner, MD

2993 Kettering Medical Center, Sleep Disorders Center
3535 Southern Boulevard
Kettering, OH 45429　　　　937-298-4331

Donna Arand, PhD, Director

2994 Northwest Ohio Sleep Disorders Center
Toledo Hospital
2142 North Cove Boulevard
Toledo, OH 43606　　　　　419-471-4000

Frank O. Horton, III, MD, Director

2995 Ohio Sleep Medicine Institute
4975 Bradenton Avenue
Dublin, OH 43017　　　　　614-766-0773

Betty Palmer, Director

2996 Ohio State University Hospitals, Sleep Disorders Center
410 West 10th Avenue
Columbus, OH 43210   614-293-8333

Gregory Landholt, Director

2997 St. Vincent Medical Center, Sleep Disorders Center
2213 Cherry Street
Toledo, OH 43608   419-251-3232

Joseph Schaffer, PhD, Director

Pennsylvania

2998 Community Medical Center, Sleep Disorders Clinic
1822 Mulberry Street
Scranton, PA 18510   717-969-8000

John Goodnow, Director

2999 Crozer-Chester Medical Center
Sleep Disorders Center
Department of Neurology
Upland-Chester, PA 19013   610-447-2689

Calvin Stafford, MD, Director

3000 Geisinger Wyoming Valley Medical Center, Sleep Disorders Center
100 E. Mountain Drive
Wilkes-Barre, PA 18711   717-826-7809

John Della Rosa, Jr., Director

3001 Lankenau Hospital, Sleep Disorders Center
100 Lancaster Avenue
Wynnewood, PA 19096   610-645-2000

Mark R. Pressman, PhD, Director

3002 Medical College of Pennsylvania, Sleep Disorders Center
3200 Henry Avenue
Philadelphia, PA 19129   215-842-6990

June M. Fry, MD, PhD, Director

3003 Mercy Hospital of Johnstown, Sleep Disorders Center
1020 Franklin Street
Johnstown, PA 15905   814-533-1661

Richard Parcinski, Director

3004 Penn Center for Sleep Disorders, Hospital of the University of Pennsylvania
3400 Spruce Street, 11 Gates
Philadelphia, PA 19104   215-898-5268

Joanne Getsy, MD, Director

3005 Presbyterian-University Hospital, Pulmonary Sleep Evaluation Center
DeSoto At O'Hara Street
Pittsburgh, PA 15213   412-647-3475

Mark Sanders, MD, Director

3006 Thomas Jefferson University Sleep Disorders Center
Jefferson Medical College
1025 Walnut Street
Philadelphia, PA 19107   215-955-6980
                                Fax: 215-923-8219

Karl Doghramji, M.D., Director

3007 Western Psychiatric Institute & Clinic, Sleep Evaluation Center
3811 O'Hara Street
Pittsburgh, PA 15213   412-624-2100

Charles F. Reynolds, III, MD, Director

Rhode Island

3008 Sleep Apnea Laboratory, Rhode Island Hospital
593 Eddy Street, APC 479-A
Providence, RI 02903   401-444-4269

Richard Millman, MD, Director

Texas

3009 Sleep Disorders Center for Children
Children's Medical Center of Dallas
1935 Motor Street
Dallas, TX 75235   214-640-2000

Dr. John Herman, Director

3010 Sleep Medicine Associates of Texas
8140 Walnut Hill Lane Suite 100
Dallas, TX 75231   214-750-7776
                                   Fax: 214-750-4621
                                   e-mail: smat@sleepmed.com

3011 University of Texas Sleep/Wake Disorders Center
Southwestern Medical Center
5323 Harry Hines Boulevard
Dallas, TX 75235   214-648-4283

Studies sleep/wake disorders including insomnia, apnea and narcolepsy.

Howard Roffwrag, MD, Director

International

3012 Sleep Disorders Centre of Metropolitan Toronto
2888 Bathurst Street
Toronto, Ontario, M6B
Canada   416-785-1128
                                   Fax: 416-782-2740
                                   e-mail: 75567.3155@compuserve.com

Jeffrey Lipsitz, MD, Director

Research Centers

California

3013 Mercy Sleep Laboratory
6601 Coyle Avenue
Carmicheal, CA 95606   530-966-5552
                                   Fax: 530-966-2426

Richard Stack, MD, Director

Illinois

3014 Center for Narcolepsy Research at the University of Illinois at Chicago
(M/C 802) College of Nursing
845 So. Damen Avenue Room 538
Chicago, IL 60612   312-996-5176
                                   Fax: 312-996-7008
                                   e-mail: narcolep@listserv.uic.edu

Maine

3015 Sleep Laboratory, Maine Medical Center
22 Bramhall Street
Portland, ME 04102   207-871-2279

George E. Bokinsky, Jr.

Ohio

3016 Center for Research in Sleep Disorders
1275 E. Kemper Road
Cincinnati, OH 45246   513-671-3101
                                   e-mail: sleepsat1@aol.com

Martin Scharf, PhD

Texas

3017 Baylor College of Medicine, Sleep Disorder and Research Center
1 Baylor Plaza
Houston, TX 77030   713-798-4945
                                   Fax: 713-796-9718

Internal unit of the College that focuses on research into sleep and sexual dysfunction in males.

Ismet Karacan, MD, Director

3018 University of Texas Medical Branch at Galveston, Clinical Research Center

Galveston, TX 77550   409-761-1950

Research focusing on sleep disorders including apnea and narcolepsy.

Charles A. Stuart, Program Director

Audio Video

3019 Narcolepsy
M. Mahowald, author

American Sleep Disorders Association
6301 Bandel Road NW, Suite 101
Rochester, MN 55901   507-287-6006
                                   Fax: 507-287-6008
                                   www.aasmnet.org

Addresses the etiology, pathophysiology, diagnosis and management of narcolepsy.

58 slides

Web Sites

3020 Sleep Home Page
bisleep.medsch.ucla.edu

Books

3021 Narcolepsy Primer

Meeta Goswami, MPD, PhD, author

Montefiore Medical Center
111 East 210th Street
Bronx, NY 10467   212-920-6799

A guide for physicians, patients and their families on the affects, causes and prevention of narcolepsy.

3022 Psychological Aspects of Narcolepsy
Haworth Press
10 Alice Street
Binghamton, NY 13904

800-342-9678
Fax: 607-722-6362

Addresses the diagnosis, treatment and management of narcolepsy with particular emphasis on psychological and social aspects of care.

Hardcover

Newsletters

3023 Eye Opener
American Narcolepsy Association
425 California St, Ste. 201
San Francisco, CA 94104   415-788-4793

Offers information on sleep disorders including a question and answer column for persons suffering from disorders.

Pamphlets

3024 Narcolepsy
American Sleep Disorders Association
1610 14th Street NW Suite 300
Rochester, MN 55901   507-287-6006
Fax: 507-287-6008
www.asda.org

Describes the causes, symptoms and treatments of a disorder characterized by excessive sleepiness.

Lot of 50

3025 Understanding Narcolepsy
National Sleep Foundation
1367 Conn. Ave NW, #200
Washington, DC 20036   202-785-2300

Offers an introduction to narcolepsy, symptoms, causes, treatments and daily living.

3026 When You Can't Sleep
Narcolepsy Network, Inc.
P.O. Box 42460
Cincinnati, OH 45242   513-891-3522
Fax: 513-891-9936
e-mail: narnet@aol.com

A primer on sleep basics, including getting enough sleep, why sleep is important, and sleep stealers. Plus a sleep quotient quiz.

DESCRIPTION

3027 NEONATAL HERPES SIMPLEX
Synonym: Congenital herpes
Disorder Type: Birth Defect, Infectious Disease

Neonatal herpes simplex refers to an infection of the newborn caused by the herpes simplex virus that is transmitted before birth from mother to fetus through the placenta, or more commonly, during birth as the baby passes through the birth canal. There are two strains of herpes simplex virus known as HSV-1 and HSV-2. Herpes simplex virus type 1 commonly causes infections of the skin and mucous membranes of the lips, mouth, and eyes, while type 2 typically causes genital herpes as well as approximately 75 percent of all neonatal herpes simplex infections.

Herpes simplex may be categorized as an initial (primary) infection or a recurrent infection. After an initial infection, the virus becomes inactive or latent; however, the virus may be reactivated by many different factors including stress, sun exposure, suppression of the immune system, and certain foods or drugs. Mothers with a primary genital herpes simplex virus infection have an approximately 45 percent chance of transmitting HSV-2 to their infants, while risk of transmission from a recurrent infection is less than five percent. In addition, newborns are at risk for HSV-1 transmission through such direct contact as kissing near the eyes or mouth by someone with a cold sore.

Symptoms of HSV infection transmitted through contact with infectious secretions during the birthing process may occur anywhere from one to four weeks after birth and may sometimes commence with the appearance of small, fluid-filled blisters on the skin or inflammation of the front part of the eyeball (cornea) and the delicate mucous membranes (conjunctiva) that line the inside of the eyelids and the whites of the eyes (keratoconjunctivitis). Other findings may include fever, drowsiness, loss of muscle tone, irritability, seizures, and inflammation of the liver (hepatitis) and brain (encephalitis), as well as other severe irregularities. If left untreated, HSV infection may cause potentially life-threatening complications. Some infants may have no skin involvement but manifest such symptoms as fluctuating temperature, listlessness, poor sucking, chills, shaking, nausea, vomiting, and diarrhea.

Transmission of the herpes simplex virus through the placenta is a rare but potentially life-threatening occurrence. This type of infection usually affects the skin, eyes, and central nervous system and is characterized by blister-type rashes and scarring, abnormally small eyes (microphthalmia) and other eye abnormalities, an abnormally small head (microcephaly), and brain and spinal cord irregularities. Some infants may also have an inflammation of the liver (hepatitis) or lung involvement.

Prevention of neonatal herpes simplex infection may include delivery by Cesarean section, especially if the mother has a primary genital herpes infection. Treatment is directed toward early diagnosis and intervention. Such therapy may include the intravenous administration of antiviral drugs such as acyclovir in conjunction with regular testing to preclude possible associated toxic side effects related to kidney dysfunction. Eye involvement may indicate the application of antiviral ointments or drops directly into the eyes. Other treatment is symptomatic and supportive.

The following organizations in the General Resources Section can provide additional information: National Health Information Center, National Institute of Allergy and Infectious Diseases

---

Web Sites

3028 American Social Health Association
www.bcpl.lib.md.us/~psmith/ashahelp.html

3029 Child Health Research Project
ih.jshph.edu/chr/chr.htm

3030 HerpeSite
members.aol.com/herpesite/index.html

3031 Herpes.com
www.herpes.com/

3032 International Herpes Management Forum
www.ihmf.org/

3033 NOAH
www.noah.cuny.edu/aids/gmhc/herpes.html

3034 Slack
www.slackinc.com/child/idc/idchome.htm

3035 Virtual Hospital
www.vh.org/Providers/Teachingfiles/CNSin

Books

3036 Understanding Herpes

Lawrence R. Stanberry, M.D., Ph.D., author

University Press of Mississippi
3825 Ridgewood Road
Jackson, MS 39211   601-432-6205
                          800-737-7788
                     Fax: 601-432-6217
          e-mail: press@ihl.state.ms.us
                     www.upress.ms.us

A most informative overview of herpes written
for the general reader.

120 pages
ISBN: 1-578060-40-0

DESCRIPTION

3037 NEONATAL JAUNDICE

Synonym: Icterus neonatorum
Disorder Type: Metabolism
May involve these systems in the body (see Section III):
Digestive System

Neonatal jaundice refers to a condition of the newborn in which high blood levels of the reddish-orange bile pigment bilirubin cause a yellowing of the skin, eyes, and mucous membranes. Bilirubin is derived from the breakdown of protein hemoglobin in red blood cells. Neonatal jaundice may be the result of many different factors including metabolic disturbances or deficiencies; certain genetic disorders; conditions associated with an increased rate of red blood cell destruction (hemolysis); conditions that affect liver function; and certain types of infections.

Blood levels of bilirubin may be somewhat elevated after the first day of life, usually peak by the fourth day, and fall to normal levels by the end of the first week. This temporary rise, frequently accompanied by jaundice, results from the increased destruction of fetal red blood cells and the inability of a still-developing metabolic mechanism to efficiently eliminate bile from the body. In addition, an enzyme present in the intestines of newborns may convert bilirubin to a form that allows it to be reabsorbed into the blood, resulting in even higher bilirubin blood levels. Premature infants are particularly at risk for jaundice. If no other underlying cause is responsible, jaundice typically resolves spontaneously along with bilirubin level stabilization.

The appearance of jaundice in a newborn is carefully evaluated for underlying causes. Factors that may indicate the presence of an underlying disorder may include jaundice within the first 24 hours of life; a higher and faster-than-expected rise in bilirubin levels; birth defects, especially those that affect the liver such as biliary atresia; a family history of diseases that cause the early destruction of red blood cells such as hemolytic disease of the newborn; or rare disorders associated with hyperbilirubinemia (e.g., Crigler-Najjar syndrome, transient familial neonatal hyperbilirubinemia, etc.). Other suspect findings may include an enlarged liver (hepatomegaly), enlarged spleen (splenomegaly), lethargy, unusual paleness, difficulty in feeding, vomiting, or excessive weight loss.

Treatment of neonatal jaundice depends upon the underlying cause. Some infants with jaundice associated with breast-feeding may benefit from phototherapy. During this treatment, which is carefully monitored, the infant's bare skin is exposed to high intensity fluorescent lights that speed up the excretion and elimination of bilirubin in the skin. Other treatment is symptomatic and supportive.

The following organizations in the General Resources Section can provide additional information: NIH/Office of Rare Diseases, National Organization for Rare Disorders, Inc., (NORD), March of Dimes Birth Defects Foundation, NIH/National Digestive Diseases Information Clearinghouse, NIH/National Institute of Child Health and Human Development (NICHD), Online Mendelian Inheritance in Man: www3.ncbi.nlm.nih.gov/Omim/searchomim.html

National Associations & Support Groups

3038 American Liver Foundation
75 Maiden Lane Suite 603
New York, NY 10038

212-668-1000
800-465-4837
Fax: 212-483-8179
e-mail: info@liverfoundation.org
www.liverfoundation.org

Organization provides several different medias for answering questions and to clarify any uncertainties the individual may be experiencing.

3039 Digestive Disease National Coalition
507 Capital Courte, Suite 200
Washington, DC 20002

202-544-7497
Fax: 202-546-7105

Promotes federal investment in biomedical research. Serves as a resouce for consumer-directed educational information, and has local support groups. Offers a toll-free hotline, patient networking services.

3040 United Liver Foundation
11646 West Pico Boulevard
Los Angeles, CA 90064   213-445-4204

Web Sites

3041 Cliniweb
www.ohsu.edu/cliniweb/C23/C23.888.html#C23.888.498

3042 Pedbase
www.icondata.com/health/pedbase/files/JAUNDICE.HTM

3043 University of Iowa
www.vh.org/Providers/ClinRef/FPHandbook/Chapter10/03

DESCRIPTION

3044 NEUROFIBROMATOSIS

Synonym: NF

Disorder Type: Genetic Disorder, Neoplasm:
Benign or Malignant Tumor

Covers these related disorders: Neurofibromatosis
type I (von Recklinghausen disease) (NF1),
Neurofibromatosis type II (NF2)

May involve these systems in the body (see Section III):

Dermatologic System, Nervous System

The term neurofibromatosis is often used to refer to neurofibromatosis type I (NF1), an autosomal dominant disorder that affects approximately one in 3,500 to 4,000 individuals. Neurofibromatosis type I, also known as von Recklinghausen disease, is characterized by the appearance of pale tan or light brown discolorations (macules) on the skin (cafe-au-lait spots) and multiple benign, fibrous tumors of nerves and skin (neurofibromas). A second, distinctive form of neurofibromatosis (NF), known as neurofibromatosis type II (NF2), accounts for about 10 percent of all cases of NF. Neurofibromatosis type II, also an autosomal dominant disorder, is characterized by the development of benign tumors on both acoustic nerves (bilateral acoustic neuromas), resulting in progressive hearing impairment.

In most children with neurofibromatosis type I, skin discoloration may develop by the age of one year. Such skin lesions typically increase in number and size over time, and most affected individuals have six or more spots measuring 1.5 centimeters or more in diameter after the onset of puberty. Although these cafe-au-lait spots are often distributed in various areas of the body, they are most commonly present on the trunk. In addition, after three years of age, areas of freckling, particularly under the arms (axillary) and in the groin (inguinal) area, may also be present.

In approximately 95 percent of children with NF1 over six years of age, two or more benign, tumor-like nodules, known as Lisch nodules, are present

on the pigmented areas of the eyes. Benign, fibrous tumors of the skin (cutaneous neurofibromas) tend to develop during the second decade of life, typically appearing as small, soft, raised, and slightly purplish discolorations of the overlying skin. These tumors, which rarely develop before six years of age, may increase in number and size during puberty. In addition, large benign tumors composed of bundles of nerves (plexiform neurofibromas) may be apparent at birth or during early childhood. Approximately two to four percent of individuals with NF1 may develop malignant tumors (e.g., neurofibrosarcomas). Physical findings that may be associated with malignant transformation include increasing tumor size, associated pain, or various neurologic symptoms due to tumor growth. Approximately 15 percent of affected individuals may also develop tumors of the optic nerve (optic glioma), which is the cranial nerve that carries visual impulses from the back of the eye (retina) to the brain. These tumors are usually considered relatively benign and may cause no associated symptoms (asymptomatic). However, in some cases, depending upon their specific location, growth, and nature, such tumors may affect vision. In these patients, associated findings may include visual impairment; degeneration (atrophy) of the optic nerve; abnormal deviation of the eye (strabismus); or involuntary, rhythmic eye movements (nystagmus). In addition, some affected individuals may have an increased risk of developing tumors of the brain and spinal cord (e.g., astrocytomas, meningiomas, neurilemmomas, etc.).

Some individuals with NF1 may also experience associated skeletal abnormalities, such as bowing of the lower legs; improper development of a bone at the base of the skull (sphenoid wing dysplasia), potentially causing pronounced bulging of the eyes (exophthalmos); and progressive sideways curvature of the spine (scoliosis). Additional abnormalities may be present, such as mild short stature, abnormal largeness of the head (macrocephaly), and episodes of uncontrolled electrical activity in the brain (seizures). In addition, many affected children may have learning disabilities and speech abnormalities. Neurofibromatosis type I is caused by abnormal changes (mutations) of a gene located on the long arm of chromosome 17 (17q11.2). In approximately 50 percent of patients, the disease gene is inherited an an autosomal dominant trait; the remaining cases result from new (sporadic) mutations of the gene that occur for unknown reasons.

Neurofibromatosis type II (NF2) is characterized by benign tumors of certain cranial nerves (bilateral acoustic neuromas) that are responsible for carrying sound impulses from the inner ear to the brain. Symptoms may become apparent during childhood or the second or third decades of life. These may include a facial numbness or weakness, headache, dizziness, unsteadiness, and progressive hearing loss. Individuals with NF2 may also develop clouding of the lenses of the eyes (i.e., posterior subcapsular opacities), have an increased risk of developing tumors of the brain and spinal cord (e.g., gliomas, meningiomas, schwannomas, etc.), or experience progressive visual impairment. NF2 is caused by a disease gene located on the long arm of chromosome 22 (22q12.2). This gene may be inherited as an autosomal dominant trait. Other cases may be caused by new (sporadic) mutations of the gene that occur for unknown reasons.

The treatment of neurofibromatosis is directed toward ensuring early detection and prompt, appropriate treatment of potentially associated findings or complications. Affected individuals are typically regularly monitored with complete neurologic evaluations (e.g., including visual and auditory screening) and thorough examinations to detect potential complications associated with NF. In some cases, tumors may be surgically removed or treated using other appropriate methods (e.g., radiation or chemotherapy for certain malignancies). Other treatment is symptomatic and supportive.

The following organizations in the General Resources Section can provide additional information: National Organization for Rare Disorders, Inc., (NORD), NIH/Office of Rare Diseases, Genetic Alliance, March of Dimes Birth Defects Foundation, Online Mendelian Inheritance in Man: www3.ncbi.nlm.nih.gov/Omim/searchomim.html, NIH/National Institute of Neurological Disorders & Stroke

National Associations & Support Groups

3045 National Brain Tumor Foundation
414 - 13th Street, Suite 700
Oakland, CA 94612
510-839-9777
800-934-2873
Fax: 510-839-9779
e-mail: nbtf@braintumor.org
www.braintumor.org

Provides data and technology updates regarding neurological disorders and ways to assist people diagnosed with them.

3046 National Coalition for Research in Neurological Disorders
1250 24th NW Suite 300
Washington, DC 20037
202-293-5453
Fax: 202-466-0585

Represents voluntary health agencies and professional societies concerned with obtaining funds for neurology.

L.S. Hoffheimer, Executive Director

3047 National Neurofibromatosis Foundation
95 Pine Street, 16th Floor
New York, NY 10005
212-344-6633
Fax: 212-747-0004
TTY: 800-323-7938
e-mail: nnff@aol.com
www.nf.org

To improve the well-being of patients and families affected by NF1 and NF2. The Foundation sponsors scientific research aimed at finding the causes and cures for people who have neurofibramatosis. It also promotes the development of cess and provides patient support services.

Peter Bellermann, President

3048 Neurofibromatosis, Inc.
8855 Annapolis Road Suite 110
Lanham, MD 20706   301-577-8984
800-942-6825
Fax: 301-577-0016
e-mail: nfinc1@aol.com
www.nfinc.org/

An organization of independent state and regional chapters that provides support and services to NF families. Works closely with clinical and research professionals who specialize in the treatment of NF. Has a newsletter and other printed materials.

State Agencies & Support Groups

Colorado

3049 NNFF of Colorado
11776 Glencoe Street
Thornton, CO 80233   303-452-1334
e-mail: kent.1.draper@saic.com

Kent Draper, Chapter President

Connecticut

3050 NNFF of Connecticut
206 Lucille Street
Fairfield, CT 06430   203-374-6664

Steve Sandler, Chapter President

Florida

3051 NNFF of Florida
31 Oakleigh Lane
Maitland, FL 32751

800-540-5721
e-mail: PBI.com@juno.com

Joe Polich, Jr., Chapter President

Georgia

3052 NNFF of Georgia
P.O. Box 1948
Hiram, GA 30141   770-445-4224
e-mail: bridges3@bellsouth.net

Rhonda Bridges, Chapter President

Hawaii

3053 NNFF of Hawaii
852 Kaahue Street
Honolulu, HI 96825   808-395-4505

Ruth Watanabe, Chapter President

Idaho

3054 NNFF of Idaho
4419 East Linden
Caldwell, ID 83605   208-459-6022
e-mail: bcrisci@micron.net

Suzy Crici, Chapter President

Illinois

3055 NNFF of Illinois
26 W 351 Madarin Lane
Bartlett, IL 60103   630-307-8497
e-mail: Melanie_B_ferengul@notes.ntrs.com

Neurofibromatosis information and support, raises funds for NF resesarch and programs through annual walk, run and NF Daisy Days.
2500 members

Melanie Ferengul, Co-President

Indiana

3056 NNFF of Indiana
5125 Maple Lane
Indianapolis, IN 46219   317-356-2580
e-mail: dcwhitehurst@earthlink.net

Dottie Whitehurst, Chapter President

Iowa

3057 NNFF of Iowa
429 56 Street
Des Moines, IA 50312   515-277-8494
e-mail: Drev@aol.com

Sheila Drevyanko, Chapter President

Kentucky

3058 NNFF of Kentucky
5482 B. Jamison Street
Fort Knox, KY 40121   502-943-0861
                e-mail: rrogers@bbtel.com

Lisa Rogers, Chapter President

Maryland

3059 NNFF of Maryland - Mid-Atlantic Region
3357 Garrison Circle
Abingdon, MD 21009   410-887-5576

Chapter of the National Neurofibromatosis
Foundation.

Mike Daughaday, Chapter President

Massachusetts

3060 NNFF of Massachusetts
347 Washington Street
Dedham, MA 02026   781-326-4775
                e-mail: nnffma@aol.com

Vincent Eagles, Executive Director

Michigan

3061 NNFF of Michigan
6069 Brynthrop
Shelby Township, MI 48316   810-731-7811

Peter Dingeman, Chapter President

Missouri

3062 NNFF of Missouri
200 North Broadway Suite 1495
St. Louis, MO 63102   314-436-6877
                888-848-6633
                Fax: 314-436-0524
                e-mail: nfmissouri@aol.com

Deborah Medbury, Executive Director

Nevada

3063 NNFF of Nevada
Prudential SW Realty
2950 South Rancho Drive Suite 200
Las Vegas, NV 89102

David Scherer, Chapter President

New Hampshire

3064 NNFF of Northern New England
3 Friar Tuck
Nashua, NH 03062   603-882-5405

Jeff Brown

New Jersey

3065 NNFF of New Jersey
P.O. Box 417
New Milford, NJ 07646   201-265-3296
                Fax: 201-871-8389
                e-mail: DonnaNF@aol.com

Donna Oettinger, Vice President

New York

3066 NNFF of New York/New Jersey
95 Pine Street 16th Floor
New York, NY 10005   212-344-6633
                Fax: 212-747-0004

Thomas Livingston, Chapter President

Ohio

3067 NNFF of Ohio
1377 Collinsdale
Cincinnati, OH 45230   513-231-2240

Jenny Ely, Chapter President

Oklahoma

3068 NNFF of Oklahoma
16 7th NW
Ardmore, OK 73401   580-223-3513
                e-mail: rhedr35594@aol.com

Richard Hedrick, President

Gino Bulso, Chapter President

Oregon

3069 NNFF of Oregon - Patient Information and Support Only
3845 SE 42nd St
Portland, OR 97206   503-775-5852

Terri Wardell

Rhode Island

3070 NNFF of Rhode Island - Coventry
52 Stone Street
Coventry, RI 02816   401-823-4421

Diane Sisson, Chapter Co-President

3071 NNFF of Rhode Island - Warwick
43 Ithaca Street
Warwick, RI 02886   401-732-6094

Deb Thornlimb, Chapter Co-President

South Carolina

3072 NNFF of South Carolina
P.O. Box 358
Cordova, SC 29039   803-534-0962

Stu Wright, Chapter President

South Dakota

3073 NNFF of South Dakota - Northern Plains
6008 Tecumseh Court
Sioux Falls, SD 57106   605-362-7279
          e-mail: dakotanf@aol.com

Bobbie Milton, Chapter President

Tennessee

3074 NNFF of Tennessee
9025 Old Smyrna Road
Brentwood, TN 37027   615-252-2360
          e-mail: gbulso@bccb.com

Utah

3075 NNFF of Utah
6179 South Impressions Drive
Kearns, UT 84118   801-968-3664
          Fax: 801-968-0981

Jennifer Newman, Chapter President

Washington

3076 NNFF of Washington
6628 212th Street SW
Lynnwood, WA 98036   425-672-9610
          Fax: 425-774-5870
          e-mail: NNFFWA@aol.com
          www.nf.org

Provides information, support services and referrals for patients and families afffected by neurfibromatosis, while supporting medical research toward effective treatments and a cure.

Susan Blalock, Executive Director

Wisconsin

3077 NNFF of Wisconsin

Milwaukee, WI   414-438-0985
          800-323-7938
          e-mail: NNFF@nf.org
          www.nf.org

Elaine Pankow, President

Wyoming

3078 NNFF of Wyoming
307 South 5th Avenue
Casper, WY 82604   307-473-7723
          e-mail: ngood13@juno.com

Norma Good, Chapter President

Web Sites

3079 Harvard
neurosurgery.mgh.harvard.edu/NFR/

3080 NF, Inc.
www.nfinc.org/

3081 Pedbase
www.icondata.com/health/ped-
base/files/NEUROFIB.HTM

Pamphlets

3082 Achieving in Spite of
National Neurofibromatosis Foundation, Inc.
95 Pine Street, 16th Floor
New York, NY 10005   212-344-6633
                            800-323-7938
                       Fax: 212-747-0004
                   e-mail: nnff@nf.org
                            www.nf.org

A booklet on learning disabilities. 50% of children with neurofibromatosis will experience
some form of learning disabilities.

3083 Child with Neurofibromatosis 1
National Neurofibromatosis Foundation, Inc.
95 Pine Street, 16th Floor
New York, NY 10005   212-344-6633
                            800-323-7938
                       Fax: 212-747-0004
                   e-mail: nnff@nt.org
                            www.nf.org

Offers information on the prognosis, management, complications, genetic implications, and
sources of support for children with neurofibromatosis 1.

3084 Guide for Teens
National Neurofibromatosis Foundation, Inc.
95 Pine Street, 16th Floor
New York, NY 10005   212-344-6633
                            800-323-7933
                       Fax: 212-747-0004
                   e-mail: nnfa@nf.org
                            www.nf.org

Offers information for teenagers on how to face
neurofibromatosis on a daily basis.

3085 Neuro*fibroma*tosis
National Neurofibromatosis Foundation, Inc.
95 Pine Street, 16th Floor
New York, NY 10005   212-344-6633
                            800-323-7938

A pamphlet offering information for patients
and families.

3086 Neurofibramatosis
March of Dimes Resource Center
1275 Mamaroneck Avenue
White Plains, NY 10605   888-663-4637
                           Fax: 914-997-4763

**3087 Neurofibromatosis Type 2: Information for Patients
and Families**
National Neurofibromatosis Foundation, Inc.
95 Pine Street, 16th Floor
New York, NY 10005   212-344-6633
                            800-323-7938

Offers extensive information on what NF2 is and
answers the most asked about questions regarding the illness.

3088 Neurofibromatosis: Questions and Answers
National Neurofibromatosis Foundation, Inc.
95 Pine Street, 16th Floor
New York, NY 10005   212-344-6633
                            800-323-7938
                       Fax: 212-747-0004
                   e-mail: nnff@nf.org
                            www.nf.org

Offers information on the disease.

DESCRIPTION

3089 NEUROBLASTOMA
Synonym: NB
Disorder Type: Neoplasm: Benign or Malignant Tumor

Neuroblastomas are malignant tumors that account for approximately eight to 10 percent of childhood cancers. They are the most common solid tumors that develop outside the skull in children. About 500 to 600 new cases are reported each year in the United States, with males affected slightly more frequently than females. In approximately 90 percent of affected infants and children, neuroblastoma is diagnosed before age five. Neuroblastoma sometimes occurs in members of certain families (kindreds), although the specific underlying cause is unknown.

Neuroblastomas may originate in any part of the sympathetic nervous system but most commonly develop in the inner region of the adrenal gland (adrenal medulla). In other patients, neuroblastomas may arise in the chest. The sympathetic nervous system controls certain involuntary activities during times of stress, such as raising blood pressure and increasing the heart rate. The adrenal glands, two relatively small organs that curve over the top of each kidney, secrete certain hormones directly into the bloodstream.

A neuroblastoma often invades surrounding tissues and spreads to small, node-like structures located along the course of the lymphatic vessels (lymph nodes). The tumor may then spread to other parts of the body (metastasize), particularly the liver, skeleton, and bone marrow. Rarely, neuroblastomas spread to the lungs or the brain. Associated symptoms and findings are highly variable and depend upon the specific location of the tumor and the extent to which it may have spread. Many infants and children may have a hard, solid, painless lump or mass in the neck or a large mass that may be felt in the abdomen or on the back. Patients often have a general feeling of ill health (malaise) and appear pale (pallor). Those with

skeletal involvement typically experience tumor-associated bone pain. In addition, because the bone marrow is a blood-producing tissue, tumor infiltration of the bone marrow may result in abnormally decreased levels of the different blood cells, including circulating red blood cells (anemia), platelets (thrombocytopenia), and certain white blood cells, including circulating red blood cells (anemia), platelets (thrombocytopenia), and certain white blood cells (neutropenia). Due to low levels of platelets, patients may experience abnormal bleeding and easy bruising. Decreased levels of white blood cells may cause an increased susceptibility to certain infections.

Depending upon the location and potential spread of the tumor, additional symptoms and findings may occur. If a neuroblastoma spreads to the bony cavities surrounding the eyes, associated symptoms may include abnormal protrusion of the eyes (proptosis) and the appearance of bluish-purple patches (ecchymosis) around the eyes. Tumor development near the spinal cord may result in weakness or paralysis of the legs (paresis). In addition, involvement of the liver typically causes abnormal liver enlargement (hepatomegaly). Tumor growth within the adrenal glands may cause excessive secretion of the hormones epinephrine and norepinephrine, resulting in increased irritability, high blood pressure (hypertension), increased heart rate (tachycardia), flushing of the skin, severe diarrhea, and other symptoms.

Some patients may also develop Horner's syndrome, which is characterized by drooping of the upper eyelid (ptosis), absence of sweating (anhidrosis), and narrowing of the pupil of the eye (miosis). Skin abnormalities may also be present, including firm, bluish nodules under the skin or skin lesions on the scalp. Approximately four percent of patients experience a sudden onset of neuromuscular symptoms due to abnormal functioning of the cerebellum (acute cerebellar encephalopathy). The cerebellum is a region of the brain that plays an essential role in maintaining normal postures, sustaining balance, and producing coordinated movements. These symptoms may include an impaired ability to coordinate voluntary movements (cerebellar ataxia); random, rapid, uncontrolled eye movements (opsoclonus); and shock-like contractions of certain muscles or muscle groups (myoclonic jerks).

In infants and children with neuroblastoma, treatment may depend upon the location of the tumor, whether it has spread, the patient's age, or other factors. If the tumor is contained and has not spread, treatment may consist of surgical removal of the tumor. When the tumor may not be removed surgically or has spread to other parts of the body, treatment measures may include the use of certain drugs (chemotherapy) or radiation therapy. Additional treatments for advanced disease may be considered.

The following organizations in the General Resources Section can provide additional information: National Organization for Rare Disorders, Inc. (NORD), NIH/National Cancer Institute, NIH/Office of Rare Diseases, Candlelighters Childhood Cancer Foundation, NIH/National Insitute of Neurological Disorders & Stroke, Genetic Alliance, Candlelighters Childhood Cancer Foundation Canada, Online Mendelian Inheritance in Man.: www3.ncbi.nlm.nih.gov/Omim/searchomim.html

National Associations & Support Groups

3090 Neuroblastoma Children's Cancer Society
P.O. Box 957672
Hoffman Estates, IL 60195   847-490-4240
800-532-5162
Fax: 847-490-0705
www.granitewebworks.com/nccs.htm

Web Sites

3091 CancerCare
www.cancercare.org/faq/cancer_faq.html

3092 Children's Cancer Web
www.ncl.ac.uk/~nchwww/guides/guide2n.htm

DESCRIPTION

3093 NEUTROPENIA

Covers these related disorders: Chronic
neutropenia, Transient neutropenia
May involve these systems in the body (see Section III):
Blood (Hematologic)

Neutropenia is a blood condition characterized by decreased numbers of circulating white blood cells known as neutrophils. These white blood cells play an essential role in fighting bacterial infections by detecting, engulfing, and digesting invading bacteria (phagocytosis). Neutrophils mature in the bone marrow and are then released into the bloodstream, where they may circulate for approximately six to eight hours. When responding to invading microorganisms or inflammation, neutrophils may leave the blood circulation, move into affected tissues, and digest microbes or other invaders as required.

Neutropenia is specifically defined as the presence of fewer than 1,500 neutrophils per microliter of blood. The condition may result from deficient production of neutrophils by the bone marrow or abnormally increased loss of neutrophils from the blood circulation. Depending upon the nature of the condition, its underlying cause, and other factors, neutropenia may occur for only days or weeks (transient neutropenia) or be present for months or a patient's lifetime (chronic neutropenia). In addition, the findings potentially associated with neutropenia are extremely variable and may include no apparent symptoms (asymptomatic), mild infections of the mucous membranes and the skin, or, in severe cases, potentially life-threatening complications.

In children, transient neutropenia may be caused by certain viral or bacterial infections; a deficiency of folic acid or vitamin B12; or the administration of certain medications, such as particular antipsychotic drugs (phenothiazines), penicillin preparations, nonsteroidal anti-inflammatory

agents, or anticancer drugs that may suppress bone marrow production. Chronic neutropenia also has several different causes and occurs in many different forms. Benign chronic neutropenia is a condition of childhood in which patients have chronically low levels of circulating neutrophils in the blood. This may result in increased susceptibility to recurrent infections of the skin, the mouth, or other areas. The condition typically resolves on its own by age four. Patients with immune deficiency disorders that are present at birth (primary inherited immunodeficiencies) or acquired (such as acquired immune deficiency syndrome) often develop chronic neutropenia during infancy or early childhood. These children often fail to grow and gain weight at the expected rate (failure to thrive) and may experience recurrent bacterial infections, enlargement of the liver and spleen (hepatosplenomegaly), and potentially life-threatening complications.

Other uncommon forms of childhood neutropenia include cyclic neutropenia and Kostmann's disease. In patients with cyclic neutropenia, neutropenia recurs in regular cycles (e.g., every 18 to 21 days). When circulating neutrophils are abnormally decreased, these patients may experience fever, a general feeling of ill health (malaise), and susceptibility to mouth ulcers and infections of the skin, mucous membranes, and tissues that surround and support the teeth. Cyclic neutropenia typically becomes apparent during childhood and often runs in certain families. Kostmann's disease, also known as genetic infantile agranulocytosis, is a rare, autosomal recessive disorder characterized by persistent, extremely low levels of circulating neutrophils (fewer than 200 per microliter), frequent bacterial infections, and potentially life-threatening complications by approximately age three.

Neutropenia may also occur as a component of certain genetic, multisystemic diseases, such as Shwachman syndrome and metaphyseal chondrodysplasia, or in association with certain cancers, including leukemia and lymphoma.

The treatment of children with neutropenia depends upon the condition's severity and its underlying cause. In those with mild neutropenia, treatment may not be required. If a particular medication is responsible for the condition, such drug therapy is discontinued if possible. In patients with chronic neutropenia, physicians may recommend steps to help prevent bacterial infection and institute immediate antibiotic therapy should infections occur. In severe cases of bacterial infection, hospitalization may be required. In addition, in some patients with severe neutropenia, therapies may be administered to help stimulate the bone marrow's production of neutrophils (granulocyte colony-stimulating factor [G-CSF]).

The following organizations in the General Resources Section can provide additional information: Online Mendelian Inheritance in Man: www3.ncbi.nlm.nih.gov/Omim/searchomim.html, Genetic Alliance, March of Dimes Birth Defects Foundation, NIH/National Heart, Lung and Blood Institute, NIH/National Institute of Child Health and Human Development

National Associations & Support Groups

3094 American Autoimmune Related Diseases Assocation, Inc.
22100 Gratiot Ave
Detroit, MI 48021   810-776-3900
                                     800-598-4668
                              Fax: 810-776-3903
                        e-mail: aarda@aol.com
                             www.aarda.org/

The American Autoimmune Related Disease Association is dedicated to the eradication of autoimmune diseases and the alleviation of suffering and the socioeconomic impact of autoimmunity through fostering and facilitating collaboration in the areas of education, public awareness, research, and patient services in an effective, ethical and efficient manner. AARDA is the only national nonprofit health agency dedicated to bringing a national focus to the major cause of serious chronic diseases.

Patricia Barber, Education Program Specialist

3095 National Neutropenia Network
P.O. Box 205,6348 N Milwaukee Ave
Chicago, IL 60646
                                     800-638-8768
                        e-mail: Bolyard@U.Washington.EDU

Supports general and clinical research and provides information to the families, the medical community, and the general public. Also committed to helping affected families and individuals work with hospitals, physicians, nurses, and other health care professionals.

3096 Neutropenia SCN International Registry
1325 4th Avenue Suite 620
Seattle, WA 98101   206-543-9749
                                     800-726-4463
                              Fax: 206-543-3668
                   e-mail: registry@u.washington.edu
                     www.scnir.medicine.washington.edu

3097 Neutropenia Support Association, Inc
P.O. Box 243, 905 Corydon Avenue
Winnepeg, Canada, MA R3M   204-489-8454
                                     800-663-8876
                       e-mail: stevensl@neutropenia.ca
                             www.neutropenia.ca

Services are geared for affected indivduals, families, and include genetic counseling from medical advisors, support groups, public and profesional education, an international disease registry, networking opportunities, and advocating for patient/family rights and more legislation. Offers a toll-free hotline and several published materials are available.

3098 Severe Chronic Neutropenia International Registry
Puget Sound Plz,1325 4th Ave,St#620
Seattle, WA 98101   206-543-9749
                                     800-726-4463
                              Fax: 206-543-3668
                   e-mail: registry@u.washington.edu
                    weber.u.washington.edu/~registry/

The SCNIR is a disease registry which was established in Australia, Canada, the European Community, and the United States in March, 1994, and is directed by a advisory board of physicians from around the world who care for SCN patients. The mission of the Registry is to establish a worldwide database of treatment and disease-related outcomes for persons diagnosed with SCN.

Web Sites

3099 Severe Chronic Neutropenia International Registry Australia
2nd Floor Marian House
St. John of God Hospital, 1002 Mair Street
Ballarat, 3350,
Australia
                   e-mail: scnirau@ballarat.edu.au
                    freyja.ballarat.edu.au:8080~scnirau/

The SCNIR is a disease registry which was established in Austria, Canada, the European Community, and the United States in March, 1994, and is directed by an advisory board of physicians from around the world who care for SCN patients. The mission of the Registry is to establish a worldwide database of treatment and disease-related outcomes for persons diagnosed with SCN.

DESCRIPTION

3100 NIGHTMARES

Disorder Type: Mental, Emotional or Behavioral Disorder

Nightmares are a type of sleep disturbance that occurs during the rapid eye movement (REM) phase of sleep, or deep sleep stage. Vivid, disturbing dreams often evoke feelings of extreme and inescapable fear, terror, anxiety, and distress. Nightmares are often so intense that they awaken the sleeping individual, who is then usually able to recall all or most details of the dream.

Nightmares are quite common in children, particularly in the eight to 10 year old age group. Girls are more prone to this type of sleep disturbance than boys. Precipitating factors vary and may include breathing irregularities caused by the common cold or other illnesses; violent movies or television programs, especially in younger children; separation anxiety; and other traumatic experiences or events. In addition, children with certain types of psychological disturbances (e.g., affective, mood, or anxiety disorders) may experience repeated episodes of nightmares.

It is common for most children to experience occasional nightmares and, until the anxiety or fear of the experience passes, understanding and comfort by parents or caregivers is usually helpful. However, children who experience frequent nightmares may require a careful evaluation to determine if these episodes are a manifestation of an underlying psychologic disorder or other irregularity. If this is the case, treatment may be directed toward the underlying condition. Other treatment is supportive. For example, parents and caregivers are encouraged to be reassuring, understanding, and firm but nonthreatening. Reading or other quiet or soothing activities or rituals before bedtime may also be beneficial. In addition, night lights or other reasonable accommodations may be provided to reassure or comfort affected children.

The following organizations in the General Resources Section can provide additional information: Federation of Families for Children's Mental Health, National Sleep Foundation, National Mental Health Association, National Mental Health Consumer Self-Help Clearinghouse, NIH/National Institute of Mental Health

National Associations & Support Groups

3101 American Mental Health Foundation (AMNF)
1049 5th Avenue
New York, NY 10028
USA
212-639-1561
Fax: 212-737-9027

Dedicated to the extensive and intensive research in the theories and techniques of treatment of emotional illness and to the implementation of reforms in the mental health system. Efforts have resulted in development of better and less expensive treatment methods. Findings are disseminated in English and other major languages.

Monroe W. Spero, MD

3102 Association for Persons with Mental and Developmental Disabilities
132 Fair Street
Kingston, NY 12401
USA
914-334-4336
800-331-5362
Fax: 914-331-4569
e-mail: nadd@mhv.net

Non-profit organization designed to promote interest of professional and parent development with resources for individuals who have the co-existence of mental illness and mental retardation. Provides conference, educational services and training materials to professionals, parents, concerned citizens and service organizations. Formerly known as the National Association for the Dually Diagnosed.

Robert Fletcher, Executive Director

3103 Center for Family Support
333 7th Ave.
New York, NY 10001
212-629-7939
Fax: 212-239-2211
www.cfsny.org

Provides comprehensive answers to the most commonly asked questions and situations.

Steven Vernickofs, Executive Director

3104 Center for Mental Health Services Knowledge Exchange Program
U.S. Department of Health and Human Services
P.O. Box 42490
Washington, DC 20015

800-789-2647
Fax: 301-984-8796
e-mail: ken@mentalhealth.org
www.mentalhealth.org

Supplies the public with responses to their commonly asked questions.

3105 Center for Self-Help Research
1918 University Ave, Ste 3D
Berkeley, CA 94704

510-849-0731
Fax: 510-849-3402

Unites various groups to examine the different features of the public health care systems.

Steven P. Segal, Director
Carol J. Silverman, Program Director

3106 Christian Horizons, Inc.
P.O. Box 334
Williamstown, MI 48895

517-655-3463

Devoted to assisting individuals, with mental disabilities, on a day-to-day basis.

Adonna Jory, Executive Secretary
Noel Churchman, Board President

3107 Mental Illness Foundation
772 W 168th Street
New York, NY 10032

212-682-4699
Fax: 212-682-4896

Supports community housing, treatment, research, outreach and public-awareness efforts for people with mental illness. Publications: Mental Illness Foundation, quarterly newsletter. Directory that lists mental illnesses and provides information on how to contact related associations. Annual meeting.

3108 National Alliance for the Mentally Ill
200 North Glebe Road #1015
Arlington, VA 22203

703-524-7600
800-950-6264
TDD: 703-516-7991
e-mail: membership@nami.org
www.nami.org

Aids families and individuals find the emotional and physical answers to the habitual forming disorders through several media resources.

Web Sites

3109 Cyber Psych
www.cyberpsych.org/

3110 Planetpsych
www.planetpsych.com

3111 Psych Central
www.psychcentral.com

3112 Sleep Home Page
bisleep.medsch.ucla.edu

Books

3113 American Academy of Somnology-Membership Directory
David L. Hopper, PhD, author
P.O. Box 29124
Las Vegas, NV 89126

702-450-5353
800-513-5833
Fax: 702-450-5833
e-mail: drdavelv@aol.com

Covers about 75 physcians, dentists, nurses, psychologists, technicians, and students and sponsoring organizations, including associations, institutions, and corporations, with a special interest in sleep.

3114 Concise Guide to Evaluation and Management of Sleep Disorders
American Psychiatric Press, Inc.
1400 K St., NW
Washington, DC 20005

202-682-6262
800-368-5777
Fax: 202-789-2648
e-mail: order@appi.org
www.appi.org

Over view of sleep disorders medicine, sleep
physiology and pathology, insomnia complaints,
excessive sleepiness disorders, parasomnias,
medical and psychiatric disorders and sleep,
medications with sedative-hypnotic properties,
special problems and populations.

1997 304 pages Softcover

3115 Depression and Sleep
American Psychiatric Press, Inc.
1400 K St., NW
Washington, DC 20005   202-682-6262
                             800-368-5777
                        Fax: 202-789-2648
                  e-mail: order@appi.com
                        www.appi.com

Contents include normal sleep, neurochemistry
of sleep, sleep in depression, neurochemistry of
depression, antidepressent drugs and sleep, and
clinical management of sleep disorders in depression.

1996 64 pages

**3116 Sleep Disorders Diagnosis and Treatment: Current
Clinical Practice Series**
American Psyciatric Publishing Group
1400 K St., NW
Washington, DC 20005   202-682-6262
                             800-368-5777
                        Fax: 202-789-2648
                  e-mail: order@appi.com
                        www.appi.com

1998 250 pages

3117 Snoring From A to Zzzz
Spencer Press
2525 NW Lovejoy St, Ste 402
Portland, OR 97210   503-223-4959
                        Fax: 503-223-1608
                  e-mail: reallip@aol.com
            www.foxcontent.com/snoring/htm

Covers organizations, associations, support
groups, and manufactorers of sleep-related medical products relevant to sleep disorders. Discussess every aspect of snoring abd sleep apnea
from causes to cures.

1999 248 pages

DESCRIPTION

3118 NIGHT TERRORS

Synonyms: Pavor nocturnus, Sleep-terror disorder
Disorder Type: Mental, Emotional or Behavioral Disorder

Night terrors is a sleep disorder characterized by episodes of sudden awakening from sleep in an extremely anxious or terrified state. This sleep disturbance occurs in from two to five children out of every hundred, and, in most cases, begins during the fourth to seventh year of life. Sleep-terror disorder more commonly affects boys than girls and often disappears before the onset of adolescence.

Episodes of night terrors usually take place during the third or fourth stage of the nonrapid eye movement or NREM phase of sleep. Each stage of NREM sleep is a successively deeper sleep leading up to rapid eye movement sleep or a deep REM during which dreams may occur. Typically, affected children awaken abruptly and may be screaming and extremely frightened. They may be in a semiconscious state and unaware of or unable to recognize people or surroundings. These children are generally inconsolable and may exhibit such physical symptoms as sweating; widening (dilation) of the pupils; elevated heart rate (tachycardia); abnormally deep, rapid breathing (hyperventilation); and violent thrashing. In about 33 percent of patients, sleepwalking (somnambulism) may also occur. Children are usually able to fall back to sleep within minutes of these short-lived episodes and have no memory of the event when they awaken.

Sleep disorders such as night terrors often result from childhood fears or anxieties. For example, some young children may be apprehensive about going to bed because this actually represents a temporary separation from their parents (separation anxiety). In addition, any issues affecting the family or child (e.g., separation, divorce, death, school performance, social interactions, etc.) may translate into disturbances in normal sleep patterns. Other contributing factors may include the presence of an elevated temperature, a state of depression, or other emotional disorders.

Although the administration of certain antianxiety and antidepressant drugs may, in some cases, be of benefit, treatment of night terrors is mainly supportive. If the precipitating cause can be determined, steps may then be taken to alleviate the fear or anxiety. In any case, parents or caregivers are encouraged to be supportive and firm, but nonjudgmental. Excitement before bedtime is discouraged; however, reading or other quiet, pleasurable activities may be beneficial.

The following organizations in the General Resources Section can provide additional information: Federation of Families for Children's Mental Health, National Sleep Foundation, National Mental Health Association, National Mental Health Consumer Self-Help Clearinghouse, NIH/National Institute of Mental Health

National Associations & Support Groups

3119 American Mental Health Foundation (AMNF)
1049 5th Avenue
New York, NY 10028
USA   212-639-1561
                                  Fax: 212-737-9027

Dedicated to the extensive and intensive research in the theories and techniques of treatment of emotional illness and to the implementation of reforms in the mental health system. Efforts have resulted in development of better and less expensive treatment methods. Findings are disseminated in English and other major languages.

Monroe W. Spero, MD

3120 An Association for Persons with Mental and Developmental Disabilities
132 Fair Street
Kingston, NY 12401
USA   914-334-4336
                                       800-331-5362
                                  Fax: 914-331-4569
                              e-mail: nadd@mhv.net

Non-profit organization designed to promote interest of professional and parent development with resources for individuals who have the co-existence of mental illness and mental retardation. Provides conference, educational services and training materials to professionals, parents, concerned citizens and service organizations. Formerly known as the National Association for the Dually Diagnosed.

Robert Fletcher, Executive Director

3121 Center for Family Support
333 7th Ave.
New York, NY 10001   212-629-7939
                                   Fax: 212-239-2211
                                   www.cfsny.org

Provides comprehensive answers to the most commonly asked questions and situations.

Steven Vernickofs, Executive Director

3122 Center for Mental Health Services Knowledge Exchange Program
U.S. Department of Health and Human Services
P.O. Box 42490
Washington, DC 20015
                                   800-789-2647
                                   Fax: 301-984-8796
                                   e-mail: ken@mentalhealth.org
                                   www.mentalhealth.org

Supplies the public with responses to their commonly asked questions.

3123 Center for Self-Help Research
1918 University Ave, Ste 3D
Berkeley, CA 94704   510-849-0731
                                   Fax: 510-849-3402

Unites various groups to examine the different features of the public health care systems.

Steven P. Segal, Director
Carol J. Silverman, Program Director

3124 Christian Horizons, Inc.
P.O. Box 334
Williamstown, MI 48895   517-655-3463

Devoted to assisting individuals, with mental disabilities, on a day-to-day basis.

Adonna Jory, Executive Secretary
Noel Churchman, Board President

3125 Mental Illness Foundation
772 W 168th Street
New York, NY 10032   212-682-4699
                                   Fax: 212-682-4896

Supports community housing, treatment, research, outreach and public-awareness efforts for people with mental illness. Publications: Mental Illness Foundation, quarterly newsletter. Directory that lists mental illnesses and provides information on how to contact related associations. Annual meeting.

3126 National Alliance for the Mentally Ill
200 North Glebe Road #1015
Arlington, VA 22203   703-524-7600
                                  800-950-6264
                                  TDD: 703-516-7991
                                  e-mail: membership@nami.org
                                  www.nami.org

Aids families and individuals find the emotional and physical answers to the habitual forming disorders through several media resources.

Web Sites

3127 Cyber Psych
www.cyberpsych.org/

3128 Planetpsych
www.planetpsych.com

3129 Psych Central
www.psychcentral.com

3130 Sleep Home Page
bisleep.medsch.ucla.edu

Books

3131 American Academy of Somnology-Membership Directory
David L. Hopper, PhD, author
P.O. Box 29124
Las Vegas, NV 89126   702-450-5353
                                  800-513-5833
                                  Fax: 702-450-5833
                                  e-mail: drdavelv@aol.com

Covers about 75 physcians, dentists, nurses, psychologists, technicians, and students and sponsoring organizations, including associations, institutions, and corporations, with a special interest in sleep.

3132 Concise Guide to Evaluation and Management of Sleep Disorders
American Psychiatric Press, Inc.
1400 K St., NW
Washington, DC 20005   202-682-6262
                              800-368-5777
                         Fax: 202-789-2648
                    e-mail: order@appi.org
                              www.appi.org

Over view of sleep disorders medicine, sleep physiology and pathology, insomnia complaints, excessive sleepiness disorders, parasomnias, medical and psychiatric disorders and sleep, medications with sedative-hypnotic properties, special problems and populations.

1997 304 pages Softcover

3133 Depression and Sleep
American Psychiatric Press, Inc.
1400 K St., NW
Washington, DC 20005   202-682-6262
                              800-368-5777
                         Fax: 202-789-2648
                    e-mail: order@appi.com
                              www.appi.com

Contents include normal sleep, neurochemistry of sleep, sleep in depression, neurochemistry of depression, antidepressent drugs and sleep, and clinical management of sleep disorders in depression.

1996 64 pages

3134 Sleep Disorders Diagnosis and Treatment: Current Clinical Practice Series
American Psyciatric Publishing Group
1400 K St., NW
Washington, DC 20005   202-682-6262
                              800-368-5777
                         Fax: 202-789-2648
                    e-mail: order@appi.com
                              www.appi.com

1998 250 pages

3135 Snoring From A to Zzzz
Spencer Press
2525 NW Lovejoy St, Ste 402
Portland, OR 97210   503-223-4959
                         Fax: 503-223-1608
                    e-mail: reallip@aol.com
              www.foxcontent.com/snoring/htm

Covers organizations, associations, support groups, and manufactorers of sleep-related medical products relevant to sleep disorders. Discussess every aspect of snoring abd sleep apnea from causes to cures.

1999 248 pages

DESCRIPTION

3136 NOCTURNAL ENURESIS

Synonym: Bed-wetting

Disorder Type: Mental, Emotional or Behavioral Disorder

May involve these systems in the body (see Section III):

Nervous System, Urinary System

Nocturnal enuresis or bed-wetting refers to the discharge of urine during the night by children who have achieved urinary control during other periods of the day. This type of bed-wetting is considered primary enuresis if nightly urinary incontinence has persisted since birth. Nocturnal enuresis that occurs in children who were previously continent during the night for a period of one year or more is considered secondary enuresis, a regressive form of this abnormality. Bed-wetting is a very common problem that occurs more often in boys than in girls and tends to run in families. In most cases, enuresis resolves spontaneously. The causes of nocturnal enuresis are varied and may include delayed maturation of certain functions of the nervous system that regulate bladder control, psychological influences, spinal abnormalities (e.g., spina bifida), structural abnormalities or defects, underlying disease (e.g., diabetes mellitus), urinary tract infection, or other physical causes. Secondary enuresis may be precipitated by stressful or traumatic events such as the birth of another child, death, divorce, or other situations that impact on the normal day-to-day routine.

Children with enuresis may undergo evaluation in order to determine if the condition is caused by neurological or physical problems. If this is the case, treatment is geared toward the underlying problem. Other treatment may include such supportive measures as establishing a reward system to give the child incentive to cooperate, charting the child's progress in order to offer positive reinforcement, limiting liquid intake before bedtime, having the child urinate directly before going to bed, and having affected older children take part in laundering soiled clothing and remaking the bed. Parents and caregivers are typically counseled to remain supportive and nonjudgmental. Additional treatment may include behavioral therapy and other counseling that involves both the parents or caregivers and the affected child. Bed-wetting alarms that detect small amounts of urine and certain types of medication (e.g., imipramine and desmopressin acetate nasal spray) may also be used to control enuresis. Imipramine is an antidepressant drug that is usually effective within two weeks; however, relapses are common after the drug is gradually stopped and, therefore, a longer course of administration may become necessary. Desmopressin acetate nasal spray reduces urine output in approximately 70 percent of affected children; however, its beneficial effect is temporary. Other treatment is supportive.

The following organizations in the General Resources Section can provide additional information: National Sleep Foundation, Federation of Families for Children's Mental Health, National Mental Health Association, National Mental Health Consumer Self-Help Clearinghouse, NIH/National Institute of Mental Health

National Associations & Support Groups

3137 American Foundation for Urologic Diseases
1128 North Charles St
Baltimore, MD 21201   410-468-1808
                                     800-242-2383
                                Fax: 410-468-1808
                         e-mail: admin@afud.org
                                      www.afud.org

Organization that helps the prevention and cure of urologic diseases with its research and educating health care professionals.

3138 National Kidney and Urologic Diseases Information Clearinghouse
9000 Rockville Pike
Bethesda, MD 20892   301-651-4415
                                     800-891-5390
                                Fax: 301-907-8906
                                www.niddk.nih.gov

Web Sites

3139 American Enuresis Foundation
galaxy.galstar.com/~aef/

3140 Dr. Koop
drkoop.com/adam/peds/top/001556.htm

3141 National Enuresis Foundation
www.peds.umn.edu/Centers/NES

3142 Sleep Home Pages
bisleep.medsch.ucla.edu/

DESCRIPTION

3143 NON-HODGKIN'S LYMPHOMA

Synonym: NHL

Disorder Type: Neoplasm: Benign or Malignant Tumor

Covers these related disorders: Non-Hodgkin's lymphoma, large cell type, Non-Hodgkin's lymphoma, lymphoblastic type, Non-Hodgkin's lymphoma, small noncleaved cell (SNC, Lymphatic System

Non-Hodgkin's lymphoma is a group of diseases characterized by malignant tumors of lymphoid tissue (lymphoma). These cancerous tumors usually develop due to uncontrolled growth of certain white blood cells (B and T lymphocytes) that are components of the lymphatic and immune systems. The lymphatic system includes a network of vessels that collect lymphatic fluid (lymph) from the different areas of the body and drain this fluid into the bloodstream. As lymph moves through the lymphatic system, it is filtered by a network of lymph nodes, which are relatively small structures located along the course of the lymphatic vessels. Lymph nodes store certain white blood cells (lymphocytes) and are thought to play a role in producing antibodies, thus functioning as part of the body's immune system. Some of the white blood cells known as T lymphocytes (i.e., helper cells) assist in the recognition of foreign proteins and help to activate other T lymphocytes (killer cells), which bind to cells invaded by viruses or other microorganisms and destroy them (cell-mediated immunity). The white blood cells known as B lymphocytes produce antibodies, which recognize and help to neutralize or destroy invading microorganisms (humoral-mediated immunity).

Malignancies of lymph tissue, known as lymphomas, are the third most common form of childhood cancer in the United States, affecting about 13 per one million children annually. There are two major categories of lymphoma, including non-Hodgkin's lymphoma (NHL) and Hodgkin's disease. Although NHL most often affects individuals over age 50, these malignancies may develop in children, particularly those with impaired immune systems. These include patients with acquired immune deficiency syndrome (AIDS) or certain genetic immunodeficiency disorders that are present at birth (primary immunodeficiencies), such as Wiskott-Aldrich syndrome, X-linked lymphoproliferative syndrome, or ataxia-telangiectasia. About 50,000 patients are diagnosed with NHL in the U.S. each year. Although the cause of the disease is unknown, researchers suggest that immune mechanisms play an important role.

A common feature of the various non-Hodgkin's lymphomas is the absence of a particular cancerous cell type that is seen in patients with Hodgkin's disease. These cancerous cells, known as Reed-Sternberg cells, are relatively large, abnormal white blood cells that have more than one nucleus and a distinctive appearance under a microscope. Children with NHL typically have highly malignant forms of lymphoma that rapidly infiltrate entire, affected lymph nodes (diffuse, high-grade tumors). There are several classification systems used to categorize the different forms of non-Hodgkin's lymphoma. However, the high-grade lymphoid tumors typically seen in children with the disease are often classified based upon their cellular structure and composition, including the type of white blood cells from which the tumor cells are derived (e.g., B or T lymphocytes). Primary, high-grade subtypes of NHL include small noncleaved cell (SNCC) NHL, including Burkitt's and non-Burkitt subtypes; large cell NHL; and lymphoblastic NHL.

In children with NHL, initial symptoms and findings vary and depend upon the specific location and extent of the disease. Most forms of NHL arise from lymph nodes in the head and neck region, the space in the chest cavity between the lungs (mediastinum), or the abdomen. Rarely, NHL may develop in other lymph nodes or affect the skin, bone, thyroid gland, or other areas. There is a close association between specific NHL subtypes and initial disease sites. For example, SNCC NHL usually initially develops in the head and neck or abdominal region. Lymphoblastic NHL tends to arise in the head and neck region or in the front of the chest cavity between the lungs (anterior mediastinum). Large cell NHL may develop in any area of the body.

Depending on disease location, associated findings often include painless swelling of lymph nodes in the neck, the groin area, or deep within the abdominal or chest region. Tumor development in the area of the mediastinum may result in abnormal accumulations of fluid between layers of the membrane lining the lungs and the chest cavity (pleural effusion), difficulties breathing, and abnormal swelling of tissues of the face, neck, and arms. Involvement of the tonsils may cause difficulty swallowing. Children with abdominal involvement typically experience nausea, vomiting, lack of appetite (anorexia), abdominal pain and swelling (distension), severe constipation, or other digestive symptoms. In those with NHL that affects the skin, associated findings include dark, thickened, itchy patches of skin. Tumor infiltration of the bone marrow may result in abnormally low levels of circulating red blood cells (anemia) or platelets (thrombocytopenia). In advanced cases, involvement of the brain may cause increased fluid pressure around the brain, severe headache, paralysis of certain nerve pairs arising from the brain (cranial nerve palsies), or other findings. In addition, advancing disease may cause progressive impairment of the body's immune system, leading to potentially severe or life-threatening complications due to certain infections.

NHL is classified into different stages, based upon the number and location of lymphatic tumors or affected node-like areas (nodules), the degree that the disease may have spread , and other factors. The treatment of children with NHL varies, depending on the stage of the disease and other factors. Therapy with certain anticancer drugs (combination chemotherapy), such as with a cyclophosphamide-based COMP or LSA2L2 regimen, is effective for many children. Radiation therapy is not used as a primary treatment in most children with NHL. In those with advanced disease, treatment may include measures to prevent brain involvement and potentially associated neurologic symptoms. Bone marrow transplantation has been shown to be an effective treatment for some children with NHL who experience relapses or have advanced disease that is unresponsive to combination chemotherapy.

The following organizations in the General Resources Section can provide additional information: Candlelighters Childhood Cancer Foundation, Candlelighters Childhood Cancer Foundation Canada, National Childhood Cancer Foundation, NIH/National Cancer Institute

National Associations & Support Groups

3144 Cure for Lymphoma Foundation
215 Lexington Avenue
New York, NY 10016   212-213-9595
                              Fax: 212-213-1987
                              e-mail: infocfl@aol.com
                              www.cfl.org

3145 Leukemia Society of America, Inc.
600 Third Avenue, 4th Floor
New York, NY 10016   212-573-8484
                              800-955-4572
                              Fax: 212-856-9686
                    e-mail: infocenter@leukemia.org
                              www.leukemia.org

The Leukemia Society will give the caller the address and phone number for the nearest local chapter. Application for financial aid is made to the local chapter. It is important to apply as soon as possible after diagnosis.

3146 Lymphoma Association (UK)
P.O. Box 275, Haddenham, Aylesbury
Bucks Intl,
England
                              www.lymphoma.org.uk

3147 Wellness Community
2716 Ocean Park Blvd., #1040
Santa Monica, CA 90405   310-314-2555

Research Centers

3148 Lymphoma Research Foundation Canada
2100-1075 West Georgia Street
Vancouver, BC,
Canada
                              Fax: 604-631-3232
                    e-mail: pmanson@lymphoma.ca
                              www.lymphoma.ca

3149 Lymphoma Research Foundation of America
8800 Venice Boulevard, Suite 207
Los Angeles, CA 90034   310-204-7040
                                  800-500-9976
                             Fax: 310-204-7043
                        e-mail: LRFA@aol.com
                            www.lymphoma.org

Web Sites

3150 CancerCare
www.cancercare.org/faq/cancer_faq.html

3151 Children's Cancer Web
www.ncl.ac.uk/~nchwww/guides/guide2n.htm

DESCRIPTION

3152 NOONAN SYNDROME

Synonyms: Female Pseudo-Turner syndrome, Male Turner syndrome, NS

Disorder Type: Birth Defect, Genetic Disorder

May involve these systems in the body (see Section III):

Cardiovascular System, Skeletal System

Noonan syndrome is a genetic disorder that is usually apparent at birth (congenital). The symptoms and findings associated with the disorder may be extremely variable, differing in range and severity from case to case. However, children with Noonan syndrome often have short stature, webbing of the neck (pterygium colli), and characteristic abnormalities of the head and facial (craniofacial) area, such as downwardly slanting eyelid folds (palpebral fissures), drooping of the upper eyelids (ptosis), a small jaw (micrognathia), and prominent, low-set ears that are rotated toward the back of the head. In addition, in many affected males, the testes fail to descend into the scrotum (cryptorchidism) before birth or during the first year of life. Therefore, in some cases, the male reproductive cells (sperm) may fail to develop appropriately within the testes, potentially causing infertility. Many children with Noonan syndrome also have distinctive skeletal malformations, such as abnormal depression of the lower portion of the breastbone (pectus excavatum) and protrusion of the upper portion of the breastbone (pectus carinatum); outward deviation of the elbows upon extension (cubitus valgus); sideways curvature of the spine (scoliosis); or front-to-back curvature of the spine (kyphosis). Affected children may also have structural heart abnormalities that are present at birth (congenital heart defects), particularly obstruction of the normal blood flow from the lower right chambr (ventricle) of the heart to the lungs (pulmonary valvular stenosis). During infancy, there may also be an abnormal accumulation of lymph fluid in and associated swelling of body tissues (lymphedema) due to lymphatic system malformations. Additional symptoms and findings may include deficient functioning of certain blood cells known as platelets that play an essential role in preventing or stopping bleeding, abnormally low levels of circulating platelets (thrombocytopenia), or blood clotting (coagulation factor) deficiencies, potentially causing abnormal bleeding and susceptibility to bruising. In some cases, affected children may also have mental retardation or experience delays in acquiring certain skills that require the coordination of physical and mental activities (psychomotor retardation). The treatment of children with Noonan syndrome includes symptomatic and supportive measures, such as certain medications or surgical intervention for those with congenital heart defects; surgery to move undescended testes into the scrotum (orchiopexy) in males with cryptorchidism; possible hormone replacement therapy (i.e., human growth hormone therapy); appropriate preventive or supportive measures for those with platelet dysfunction, thrombocytopenia, coagulation deficiences, or lymphedema; special education; and other treatment measures as required.

In most cases, Noonan syndrome appears to occur randomly (sporadically) due to spontaneous genetic changes (mutations). In other cases, the disorder may be inherited as an autosomal dominant trait. A gene responsible for Noonan syndrome has been located on the long arm (q) of chromosome 12 (12q24). Most estimates in the literature indicate that the disorder may affect approximately one in 1,000 to 2,500 newborns. However, due to the wide variablity of associated symptoms and findings, it may be difficult to determine the true frequency of Noonan syndrome in the general population.

The following organizations in the General Resources Section can provide additional information: National Organization for Rare Disorders, Inc., (NORD), NIH/Office of Rare Diseases, March of Dimes Birth Defects Foundation, Genetic Alliance, Online Mendelian Inheritance in Man:

www3.ncbi.nlm.nih.gov/Omim/searchomim.html

National Associations & Support Groups

3153 Human Growth Foundation
7777 Leesburg Pike, Ste 202 S.
Falls Church, VA 22043   703-883-1773
                               800-451-6434
                          Fax: 703-883-1776
               e-mail: hgfound@erols.com
                    www.genetic.org/hgf/

Devoted to the dispersion of medical knowledge
of this and similar disorders, along with providing suport for the sufferers and their families.

3154 MAGIC Foundation for Children's Growth
1327 North Harlem Ave
Oak Park, IL 60302   708-383-0808
                               800-362-4423
                          Fax: 708-383-0899
        e-mail: mary@magicfoundation.org
               www.magicfoundation.org

Support and education provided to families of
children with growth related disorders. Specialty divisions include: Growth Hormone Defiency; Precocious Puberty; Congenital Adrenal
Hyperplasia; McCune Albright Syndrome; Congenital Hypothyroidism; Down Syndrome with
Growth Failure; Russell-Silver Syndrome; Tuners Syndrome.

3155 TNSSG Noonan Syndrome Support Group, Inc
P.O. Box 145
Upperco, MD 21155   410-374-5245
                               888-686-2224
          e-mail: wandar@bellatlantic.net
                 www.noonansnydrome.org

Sharing of information and encouragement
among individuals who have been affected by
the syndrome. The organization offers forums
where physicians and other professionals can
provide information on living with the daily challenges.

Web Sites

3156 AGSA Newsletter
www.icondata.com/health/ped-
base/files/NOONANSY.HTM

3157 Congenital Heart Resource Page
www.csun.edu/~hcmth011/heart/
              e-mail: sheri.berger@csun.edu
              www.csun.edu/~hcmth011/heart/

3158 Family Village
www.familyvillage.wisc.edu/lib_noon.htm

3159 Noonan Syndrome Society
www.paston.co.uk/users/maygurney/ns1.html

3160 Pedbase
www.icondata.com/health/ped-
base/files/NOONANSY.HTM

DESCRIPTION

3161 NYSTAGMUS

Disorder Type: Vision
Covers these related disorders: Jerky nystagmus,
Pendular nystagmus

Nystagmus is a condition characterized by involuntary, rhythmic movements of the eyes. These movements may be vertical, horizontal, circular, or a mixture of two varieties (mixed). Nystagmus may be present at birth (congenital) or develop later in life (acquired). There are two general categories or types of nystagmus: jerky nystagmus and pendular nystagmus.

Jerky nystagmus is the most common form of the condition. It is characterized by relatively slow movements of the eyes in one direction followed by rapid, corrective movements or jerks in the opposite direction. In many patients with jerky nystagmus, head movements accompany the eye movements. These unusual head movements are thought to represent so-called compensatory posturing, that is, turning of the head to bring the eyes to a position in which the nystagmus lessens and vision is best (null positioning) In pendular nystagmus, movements of the eyes are approximately equal in rate in both directions. The different forms of nystagmus result due to abnormalities in certain mechanisms that regulate the movements and positioning of the eyes. These include conjugate gaze, fixation, and vestibular mechanisms. Conjugate gaze is the normal movement of both eyes in the same direction to bring objects into view. Fixation describes the direction of the gaze so that visual images fall on a certain area of the retina, which is the nerve-rich membrane at the back of the eye (fovea centralis). The vestibular mechanism is the balancing mechanism of the inner ear.

In some affected individuals, pendular or jerky nystagmus is present at birth or develops during early infancy or childhood. Pendular nystagmus often occurs in association with eye and visual defects (e.g., congenital glaucoma, congenital cataract, albinism, etc.). In other patients, pendular nystagmus may be an isolated finding that occurs in the absence of such conditions. Jerky nystagmus is usually unassociated with other eye or visual defects, and its cause is unknown. Familial cases of isolated pendular or jerky nystagmus are reported in which the condition appears to be transmitted as an autosomal dominant, autosomal recessive, or X-linked trait.

A specific, acquired form of pendular nystagmus, known as spasmus nutans, may also affect some infants or children. This condition typically develops at approximately four months to two years of age. In spasmus nutans, nystagmus is accompanied by head nodding and, in some children, abnormal tightness or contractions of the neck muscles, resulting in twisting of the neck and abnormal positioning of the head (torticollis). In most children with spasmus nutans, pendular nystagmus is limited to or more pronounced in one eye. Symptoms usually spontaneously resolve within months or a few years.

Some infants or children may also have a form of nystagmus in which there is repetitive jerking of the eyes toward each other or backward into the eye sockets (convergent nystagmus). This form of nystagmus often occurs with impaired vertical gaze in association with certain underlying syndromes (e.g., Parinaud syndrome, sylvian aqueduct syndrome, etc.).

The development of persistent nystagmus later in life may occur in association with certain disorders of the nervous system (e.g., brain tumors, multiple sclerosis) or disorders affecting the balancing (vestibular) mechanism of the inner ear (labyrinthine-vestibular disease). Individuals with acquired nystagmus should receive immediate, thorough evaluations to diagnose the underlying cause and ensure prompt, appropriate treatment.

In infants and children with nystagmus, diagnostic evaluations typically include the use of a specialized imaging technique (electronystagmography) that records eye movements and helps to determine or confirm the type of nystagmus present. Treatment of patients with nystagmus includes appropriate therapies for any diagnosed, underlying causes of the condition. Other treatment includes symptomatic and supportive measures.

The following organizations in the General Resources Section can provide additional information: National Organization for Rare Disorders, Inc. (NORD), Genetic Alliance, March of Dimes Birth Defects Foundation, Online Mendelian Inheritance in Man: www3.ncbi.nlm.nih/gov/Omim/searchomim.html

National Associations & Support Groups

3162 NIH/National Eye Institute (NEI)
9000 Rockville Pike
Bethesda, MD 20892   301-496-5248
                           www.nei.nih.gov/

3163 National Eye Research Foundation
910 Skokie Boulevard
Northbrook, IL 60062

Devoted to the enhancement of care and study of eye related diseases.

Web Sites

3164 American Nystagmus Network
www.nystagmus.org

3165 National Association for Visually Handicapped
www.navh.org/

3166 Nystagmus Information Page
www.btinternet.com/~lynest/nystag01.htm

3167 Nystagmus Network
www.btinternet.com/~lynest/nystag01.htm

3168 Royal National Institute for the Blind
www.rnib.org.uk/info/eyeimpoi/congen.htm

DESCRIPTION

3169 OBESITY

Obesity refers to a condition in which there is an excessive accumulation of fat in subcutaneous and other tissues of the body. Being obese and being overweight are not necessarily synonymous, as people who are overweight may have an increased body size as a result of increased muscle or skeletal tissue mass. Obesity in children may develop at any age, but peak development periods occur during the first 12 months of life, between the ages of five and six years, and during the adolescent years. Obesity may result from an increase in the actual number of fat cells or from an increase in the size of the individual fat cells. Researchers believe that fat cells increase in number in proportion to caloric intake increase and that this increase is particularly evident in the first 12 months of life. As children grow, increases in fat cell populations continue at a slower rate. Because the number of fat cells cannot be decreased, except surgically, later weight loss must result from the reduction of fat in individual cells.

Obesity usually results when caloric intake exceeds the energy demands of the body, thus increasing the storage of body fat. Fat accumulation is usually a progressive process, resulting from repeated episodes of food intake exceeding the body's demand for energy (calories). Many factors may influence appetite or obesity. Such factors may include environmental influences; psychologic disturbances that may be induced by stress or emotional upset or trauma; brain lesions that may involve certain areas of the brain such as the hypothalamus or the pituitary gland (both essential to hormone production); an overabundance of insulin in the body (hyperinsulinism); and genetic influences. In addition, in rare instances, obesity may be a feature of certain genetic disorders.

Complications of childhood obesity may include respiratory difficulties such as shortness of breath and increased cardiovascular risk factors such as high blood pressure, elevated total cholesterol levels as well as increased bad or LDL cholesterol and decreased good or HDL cholesterol, and increased levels of fatty acid and glycerol compounds (triglycerides). In addition, childhood obesity may be associated with a resistance to the hormone insulin that aids in the metabolism of glucose, fats, carbohydrates, and proteins. This resistance may lead to excessive levels of circulating insulin in the body (hyperinsulinism); however, the body is not able to appropriately use insulin. The symptoms associated with insulin resistance may include hunger, weight loss, sweating, and tremor.

The diagnosis of obesity in children and adolescents is usually determined through the use of certain screening methods such as measurement of the body mass index (BMI) as well as the triceps skinfold thickness. In addition, special consideration may be given to certain criteria in determining differential diagnosis and possible treatment. These criteria may include elevated blood pressure; high total cholesterol levels; regular and consecutive increases in annual body mass index screenings; psychologic or emotional weight concerns; and a family history of heart disease, elevated cholesterol levels, and diabetes.

Patterns of behavior that may lead to obesity may be established as early as infancy. For example, if parents or caregivers persistently use a bottle to pacify a crying baby, the baby may learn that food is equivalent to relief of stress. Treatment for childhood and adolescent obesity should include the cooperation and support of the entire family and may be directed toward psychologic considerations, as well as proper exercise and nutrition to avoid complications. Treatment for psychologic and emotional needs may include behavior modification, as well as individual and family counseling.

The following organizations in the General Resources Section can provide additional information: NIH/National Digestive Diseases Information Clearinghouse

National Associations & Support Groups

3170 Obesity: National Eating Disorders Organization
National Eating Disorders Organization
6655 South Yale Ave
Tulsa, OK 74136
918-481-4044
Fax: 918-481-4076
e-mail: lpchnedo@IDNET.NET
www.laureate.com

Web Sites

3171 Obesity Information
www.quantumhcp.com/obesity.htm

3172 Obesity Online
www.obesity-online.com/

3173 Obesity.com
www.obesity.com/

3174 UCLA
www.ccon.com/uclarfo/

Books

3175 Feed Your Kids Well: How to Help You Child Lose Weight and Get Healthy

Fred Pescatore, author

John Wiley & Sons, INC.
605 Third Avenue
New York, NY 10158
212-850-6000
Fax: 212-850-6088
www.wiley.com

Aimed toward parents, this book offers advice and tips to help their children lose excess weight. It also examines the popular fat-free diet fads and advises diets containing the small amounts of fat that are crucial to human growth.

304 pages
ISBN: 0-471248-55-X

3176 Understanding Childhood Obesity

J.Clinton Smith, M.D., author

University Press of Mississippi
3825 Ridgewood Road
Jackson, MS 39211
601-432-6205
800-737-7788
Fax: 601-432-6217
e-mail: press@ihl.state.ms.us
www.upress.state.ms.us

A clear explanation of causes, diagnosis, and treatment of childhood obesity.

120 pages Hardcover
ISBN: 1-578061-33-4

Miriam Bloom, Ph.D, Editor

Pamphlets

3177 Childhood Obesity
Natl Institute of Child Health & Human Development
9000 Rockville Park, Bldg 31
Bethesda, MD 20892
301-496-5133

Free government publication which describes approaches for solving childhood obesity.

DESCRIPTION

3178 OBSESSIVE-COMPULSIVE DISORDER
Synonyms: Obsessive-compulsive neurosis, OCD
Disorder Type: Genetic Disorder, Mental,
Emotional or Behavioral Disorder

Obsessive-compulsive disorder (OCD) is characterized by the performance of repetitive actions, rituals, or compulsions in response to recurrent, persistent thoughts or obsessions. These actions and thoughts may significantly interfere with personal, social, or occupational functioning. OCD may affect approximately two to three percent of the general population worldwide. In most cases, the onset of OCD is gradual and typically becomes apparent during adolescence or early adulthood. However, onset of the disorder during childhood is not rare. Males and females are thought to be affected equally.

Many children have minor compulsions that result in little or no distress, such as avoiding cracks while walking on the sidewalk. Most such compulsions typically subside later in life. However, some rituals may continue through adulthood, such as repeatedly checking that the stove is turned off. Children who develop obsessive-compulsive disorder may initially have repetitive, persistent thoughts that constantly invade their consciousness. They may conduct a repetitive action or a series of actions during certain situations, particularly during times of stress, such as preparing to go to school. Performing compulsive actions or rituals may temporarily relieve a feeling of anxiety, whereas resisting such compulsions may serve to increase their tension. Obsessions may consist of certain ideas, phrases, or strong images; impulses to perform objectionable acts; or impulses to perform objectionable acts; or impulses to repeatedly analyze certain acts before carrying them out. Some obsessions may concern bodily secretions or wastes or a need for routine or sameness. Compulsions often include repetitive hand washing, touching certain objects in a particular sequence, or checking and rechecking door locks.

Attempts may be made to involve parents or other family members in the performance of certain compulsive actions or rituals. Children with OCD are usually aware of the irrationality of their obsessive thoughts and compulsive behaviors but are unable to control them. The symptoms associated with OCD often periodically decrease or increase in intensity over time. However, in some patients, a progressive worsening of the condition may result in gradual deterioration of personal and social functioning. Treatment of OCD may include therapy with certain medications, such as fluoxetine, fluvoxamine, or clomipramine, and behavioral therapy, including gradually increased exposure to situations that typically trigger compulsive behaviors.

OCD may occur as an isolated condition or in association with other underlying disorders or conditions, such as Tourette syndrome, epilepsy, or anorexia nervosa. Although the exact cause of obsessive-compulsive disorder is not known, studies suggest that the disorder may result from biochemical abnormalities affecting particular areas of the brain. There are also reports of multiple cases of isolated OCD in a multigenerational family (kindred), suggesting autosomal dominant inheritance in these patients. In addition, the occurrence of OCD in several kindreds affected by Tourette syndrome also indicates that changes (mutations) of certain genes may result in or contribute to OCD.

The following organizations in the General Resources Section can provide additional information: Federation of Families for Children's Mental Health, National Alliance for Research on Schizophrenzia/Depression, National Alliance for the Mentally Ill, (NAMI) National Mental Health Association, National Mental Health Consumer Self-Help Clearinghouse, NIH/National Institute of Mental Health, Genetic Alliance

National Associations & Support Groups

3179 Center for Family Support
1049 5th Ave.
New York, NY 10028   212-629-7939
                            Fax: 212-239-2211
                            e-mail: www.cfsny.org

Provides comprehensive answers to the most commonly asked questions and situations.

Steven Vernickofs, Executive Director

3180 Center for Mental Health Services Knowledge Exchange Network
U.S. Department of Health and Human Services
P.O. Box 42490
Washington, DC 20015
                            800-789-2647
                            Fax: 301-984-8796
                            e-mail: ken@mentalhealth.org
                            www.mentalhealth.org

Supplies the public with responses to their commonly asked questions.

3181 National Mental Health Consumer's Self-Help Clearinghouse
311 S. Juniper St., Ste. 1000
Philadelphia, PA 19107   215-751-1810
                                800-553-4539
                                Fax: 215-735-0275
                                e-mail: thekey@delphi.com
                                www.liberty.net

Goal of the organization is to support the expansion of self-help groups.

Alex Morrsey, Information/Referral

3182 Obsessive Compulsive Foundation
P.O. Box 9573
New Haven, CT 06535   203-315-2190
                            Fax: 203-315-2196
                            e-mail: info@ocfoundation.org
                            www.ocfoundation.org

An international, not-for-profit organization with more than 10,000 members. Its mission is to increase research, treatment and understanding of obsessive-compulsive and related disorders. Membership dues are $45; $75 for professionals.

11M Members

3183 Obsessive-Compulsive Information Disorder Center
Madison Institute of Medicine, Inc.
7671 Mineral Point Rd., Ste 300
Madison, WI 53717   608-827-2470
                          Fax: 608-827-2479
                          www.healthytechsys.com

Supplies resources both visual and by the telephone.

3184 Obsessive Compulsive Foundation
P.O. Box 70, 9 Depot St
Milford, CT 06460   203-315-2190
                          Fax: 203-874-2826

Geared towards people burdened with obsessive-compulsive disorder and the people in their lives.

Research Centers

3185 Lithium Infomation Center
7617 Mineral Point Rd., Ste 300
Madison, WI 53717   608-827-2470
                          Fax: 608-827-2479
                          e-mail: mim@healthsys.com
                          www.healthtechsys.com

Staffed by medical librarians. Provides access to the published literature and alternative treatment for bipolar disorder.

3186 Obsessive-Compulsive Information Center
Oc Information Center
2711 Allen Blvd.
Middleton, WI 53562   608-827-2470
                            Fax: 608-827-2479
                            e-mail: mim@healthsys.com
                            www.healthtechsys.com

Staffed by medical librarians. Provides access to the published literature on OCD and publishes very useful guides.

Audio Video

3187 Hope and Solutions for Obsessive Compulsive Disorder, Part III
Awareness Foundation for OCD
3N374 Limberi Lane
St. Charles, IL 60175   630-513-9234

An educational psychologist offers educators effective classroom strategies that school personnel may implement with students who have obsessive compulsive disorder and addresses federal law as it pertains to students with disabilities.

3188 Touching Tree
Obsessive-Compulsive Foundation
P.O. Box 70
Milford, CT 06460   203-878-5669

This video will foster awareness of early onset obsessive-compulsive disorder and demonstrate the symptoms and current therapies that are most successful. Typical ritualistic compulsions of children and adolescents such as touching, hand washing, counting, etc. are explained.

Web Sites

3189 Anxiety Disorders Association of America
www.adaa.org/4_info/4e_ocd/4e_01.htm

3190 CyberPsych
www.cyberpsych.com

3191 National Anxiety Foundation
www.lexington-on-line.com/naf.html

3192 National Institute of Health
www.nimh.nih.gov

3193 OCD Resource Center
www.ocdresource.com/ocdresource.nsf

3194 OCD Web Server
www.fairlite.com/ocd/

3195 OCD Web Sites
www.interlog.com/~calex/ocd/

3196 PlanetPsych
www.planetpsych.com

3197 Psych Central
www.psychcentral.com

Books

3198 Boy Who Couldn't Stop Washing, The The Experience and Treatment of OCD
Penguin Group
375 Hudson St.
New York, NY 10014

A comprehensive treatment of obsessive-compulsive disorder that summarizes evidence that the disorder is neurobiological. It also describes the effect of medication combined with behavioral therapy.

1991 292 pages

3199 Childhood Obsessive Compulsive Disorder
Sage Publications, Inc.
2455 Teller Rd.
Thousand Oaks, CA 91320   805-499-0721
Fax: 805-499-0871
e-mail: info@sagepub.com
www.sagepub.com

1996

3200 OCD in Children and Adolescents: A Cognitive-Behavioral Treatment Manual
John S. March and Karen Mulle, author
Guilford Publications
72 Spring St.
New York, NY 10012   212-431-9800
800-365-7006
Fax: 212-966-6708
e-mail: info@guilford.com
www.guilford.com

Written for clinicians, the book includes tips for parents, and treatment guidelines. The cognitive-behavioral approach to OCD has been problematic for many to understand because patients with symptoms of increased anxiety are told that their treatment initially involves further increases in their anxiety levels. The authors provide this in a modified and developmentally appropriate approach.

1998 298 pages

3201 Obsessive Compulsive Disorder in Children and Adolescents: A Guide
Hugh F. Johnson and J. Jay Fruelhing, author
Madison Institute of Medicine
7617 Mineral Point Rd, Ste 300
Madison, WI 53717   608-827-2470
Fax: 608-827-2479
e-mail: mim@healthtecgsys.com
www.healthtechsys.com

The guide is a comprehensive introduction to obsessive-compulsive disorder for parents who are learning about the illness. Discuss treating symptoms by a combination of behavorial therapy and medication and describes various drugs that can be used with children and adolescents in terms of their effects on brain functioning, symptom control, and side effects. The book is attuned to the difficulties families of OCD children face.

3202 Obsessive Compulsive Disorder: Helping Children and Adolescants

Mitzi Waltz, author

O'Reilly and Associates, Inc.
101 Morris Street
Sebastopol, CA 95472

800-998-9938
Fax: 707-829-0104
e-mail: patientsguide@oreilly.com
www.patientsguide.com

This book helps parents secure an accurate and complete diagnosis, and live with OCD children using effective parenting techniques. Offers support systems, medical interventions and explore therapeutic and other interventions, such as cognitive therapy; helps to secure care with an existing health plan even with no coverage of mental disorders, navigate the special education system and find resources.

3203 Obsessive-Compulsive Disorder in Children and Adolescents

Judith L. Rapaport, MD, author

American Psychiatric Press, Inc.
1400 K St. NW
Washington, DC 20005

202-682-6262
800-368-5777
Fax: 202-789-2648
e-mail: order@appi.org
www.appi.org

Examines the early development of obsessive-compulsive disorder and describes to effective treatments.

1989 360 pages

3204 School Personnel: A Critical Link in the Identification and Management of OCD

Gail Adams and Marcia Torchia, author

Obsessive-Compulsive Foundation, Inc.
P.O. Box 70
Milford, CT 06460

203-878-5669

Recognizing OCD in the school setting, current treatments, the role of school personnel in identification, assessment, and educational interventions, are thoroughly covered in this brief, but informative booklet especially targeted to educators and guidance counselors.

1996 24 pages

Pamphlets

3205 Obsessive-Compulsive Disorder
National Institute of Mental Health
5600 Fishers Lane
Rockville, MD 20857

301-443-4513
Fax: 301-443-4279
www.nimh.nih.gov

This pamphlet encourages persons suffering from OCD to receive help from a mental health professional. Between 1 and 3 percent of the population suffers from OCD which usually begins in the teenage or young adult years.

DESCRIPTION

3206 OMPHALOCELE

Disorder Type: Birth Defect
May involve these systems in the body (see Section III):
Digestive System

An omphalocele is a birth defect characterized by bulging or protrusion of a portion of the intestines through an abnormal opening in the abdominal wall near the navel, the region where the umbilical cord meets the abdomen during fetal growth and development. The bulging area of the intestines is covered by a thin, membrane-like sac consisting of part of the amnion and peritoneum. The amnion is the inner layer of membrane that forms the amniotic sac, the fluid-filled sac within which a fetus grows and develops. The peritoneum is the thin membrane that lines the abdominal cavity and covers the internal abdominal organs.

Depending upon the size of the abdominal wall defect in an affected newborn, varying amounts of intestine or, in severe cases, other abdominal organs, may protrude through the navel. Associated complications may include rupture of the protruding, membranous sac, damage to body tissues due to drying, or onset of infection. Because these complications may be life-threatening, an omphalocele is usually surgically repaired immediately after birth.

An omphalocele is thought to affect approximately one in 4,000 newborns. In many infants, omphaloceles occur in association with other birth defects, such as abnormalities of the urinary and reproductive systems, central nervous system, or cardiovascular system. This condition may also occur in association with certain rare malformation syndromes that are apparent at birth. These include Beckwith-Wiedemann syndrome, also known as exomphalos-macroglossia-gigantism, and Shprintzen omphalocele syndrome, also called pharynx and larynx hypoplasia with omphalocele.

In other cases, omphaloceles may occur as isolated findings for unknown reasons. There have been reports of multiple cases of isolated omphaloceles within certain families (kindreds). In these families, the condition may be caused by abnormal changes (mutations) in a gene or genes that may be inherited as an autosomal recessive or X-linked trait. It is also possible that the interaction of several different genes in association with certain environmental factors (multifactorial inheritance) may play a role in the development of some omphaloceles.

The following organizations in the General Resources Section can provide additional information: NIH/Office of Rare Diseases, National Organization for Rare Disorders, Inc., (NORD), March of Dimes Birth Defects Foundation, Online Mendelian Inheritance in Man: www3.ncbi.nlm.nih.gov/Omim/searchomim.html

Research Centers

3207 University of California, San Francisco
1001 Portero Road
San Francisco, CA 94110   415-206-8313

Research done into traumatic brain and head injuries.

Lawrence H. Pitts, MD
Pitts, MD

Web Sites

3208 Harvard University
www.brighamrad.harvard.edu/Cases/bwh/hcache/30/full

3209 Pedbase
www.icondata.com/health/pedbase/files/OMPHALOC.HTM

3210 Pediatric Surgery Update
www.home.coqui.net/titolugo/PSU11.htm#1152

3211 University of California, San Francisco
ultrasound.ucsf.edu/Default6.html

Lawrence H. Pitts, MD
Pitts, MD

DESCRIPTION

3212 OSTEOGENESIS IMPERFECTA

Synonyms: Brittle bone disease, OI

Disorder Type: Birth Defect, Genetic Disorder

Covers these related disorders: Osteogenesis imperfecta Type I (OI Type I), Osteogenesis imperfecta Type II (OI Type II), Osteogenesis imperfecta Type III (OI Type III), Osteogenesis imperfecta Type IV (OI Type IV)

May involve these systems in the body (see Section III):

Connective Tissue, Prenatal & Postnatal Growth & Development, Skeletal System

Osteogenesis imperfecta (OI) is an inherited collagen disorder characterized by abnormally brittle, fragile bones that are prone to fracture. Collagen is a protein that forms connective tissue such as bone. This disorder is subdivided into Types I, II, III, and IV. Symptoms of this disorder are widely variable and may include a deep blue appearance of the whites of the eyes (sclerae), loose joints, multiple fractures that may result in stunted or abnormal growth, and deafness resulting from irregular development of the bones in the inner ears (otosclerosis).

Osteogenesis imperfecta Type I is the least severe and most common form of OI. It occurs in approximately one in every 30,000 live births. Common characteristics associated with Type I include bowing of the lower limbs, knock knees (genu valgum), flat feet, short stature, and irregularities of the teeth. As affected children reach adolescence, the frequency of bone fractures may be dramatically reduced. OI Type I is inherited as an autosomal dominant trait.

OI Type II is incompatible with life and is characterized by low birth weight; crumpled bones; and other skeletal abnormalities of the limbs, ribs, and face. As many as 50 percent of Type II births are stillborn, while defects in the rib cage cause death in the others soon after birth. Approximately one in 60,000 infants is affected with OI Type II. This form of the disorder is inherited as an autosomal recessive trait, an autosomal dominant trait, or represents a new spontaneous genetic mutation.

Osteogenesis imperfecta Type III is a progressive form of this disorder characterized in the newborn by multiple fractures and severely fragile bones, progressing to deformity of the skeleton and skull. Although many children reach adolescence, adulthood is rarely attained. Type III is inherited as an autosomal recessive trait or occurs as a result of a new mutation.

OI Type IV is characterized by bone mass reduction (osteoporosis) resulting in fragile bones; however, other symptoms typical of Type I may be absent or less severe. Bone fractures may be present at birth or at any time up to adulthood. Although most individuals will be short of stature, other symptoms of this disorder often improve during early puberty. Osteogenesis Type IV is inherited as an autosomal dominant trait.

Treatment for osteogenesis Types I, III, and IV may include immediate orthopedic intervention for management of bone fractures and deformity correction or surgical intervention as necessary.

The following organizations in the General Resources Section can provide additional information: NIH/National Information Center for Children & Youth with Disabilities, NIH/Office of Rare Diseases: rarediseases.info.nih.gov/ord/, Online Mendelian Inheritance in Man: www3.ncbi.nlm.gov/Omim/searchomim.html, Genetic Alliance, March of Dimes Birth Defects Foundation

---

National Associations & Support Groups

3213 Canadian Osteogenesis Imperfecta Society
128 Thronhill Crescent
Chatham, On N7L4M3,
Canada
519-436-0025
Fax: 519-351-4043
e-mail: marylouk@usa.net

Aims to provide emotional support to parents and people with Osteogenesis Imperfecta. Maintain and up-to-date library of literature both medical and general, promote and understand awareness of brittle bones.

3214 Little People of America
P.O. Box 745
Lubbock, TX 79408   360-636-0276
                          888-572-2001
            e-mail: lpadatabase@juno.com
                    www.lpaonline.org

To assist dwarfs with their physical and developmental concerns resulting from short stature. LPA offers information on, employment, education, disability rights, adoption of short statured children, medical issues, clothing, adaptive devices and parenting tips. Information is provided through hundreds of dedicated volunteers throughtout the U.S., LPA also provides opportunities for social interaction at chapter, district, regional meetings, national conferences, and participation in events.

Robert Jacobson, National Parent Coordinator
Betty Jacobson, National Parent Coordinator

3215 Osteogenesis Imperfecta Foundation

Heller An Shapiro, Executive Director, author

804 West Diamond Avenue, Suite 204
Gaithersburg, MD 20878   301-947-0083
                                800-981-2663
                   Fax: 301-947-0456
            e-mail: bonelink@oif.org
            www.members.aol.com/bonelink

This foundation serves the needs of people afflicted with Osteogenesis Imperfecta, a brittle bone disorder. Offers information, support, resources, bi-annual conference and publishes medical professionals.

1,000 members

3216 Osteoporosis and Related Bone Diseases National Resource Center
1232 22nd Street NW
Washington, DC 20037   202-223-0344
                              800-624-2663
                   Fax: 202-293-2356
                   TTY: 301-565-2966
            e-mail: orbdnrc@nof.org
                    www.osteo.org

Devoted to the dissemination of knowledge regarding the disease along with several helpful medias to explore.

Jessica Branch, Health Information Specialist

3217 UK O.I. Foundation
Enbrook Valley
Folkeston CT20 3NE Eng,   130-322-0447
            e-mail: ukoif@aol.com
            www.ukoifoundation.org

Osteogenesis Imperfecta (OI) is a genetic disorder characterized by bones that break easily, often from little or no apparent cause. There are at least four distinct forms of the disorder, representing extreme variation in severity. The Foundation supports those with the disease and conduct research.

Audio Video

3218 Going Places: A Day in the Life of A Teenager with Osteogenesis Imperfecta
Osteogenesis Imperfecta Foundation
804 W. Diamond Avenue Suite 204
Gaithersburg, MD 20878   301-947-0083
                                800-981-2663
                   Fax: 301-947-0456
            e-mail: bonelink@oif.org
                    www.oif.org

Follow Blair Smith a ninth grade student through a day of classes, shopping at the mall, and spendingtime at home with her family.

15 minutes Audiocassette

3219 Plan for Success: An Educator's Guide to Studentts with Osteogenesis Imperfecta
Osteogenesis Imperfecta Foundation
804 W. Diamond Avenue Suite 204
Gaithersburg, MD 20878   301-947-0083
                                800-981-2663
                   Fax: 301-947-0456
            e-mail: bonelink@oif.org
                    www.oif.org

Information for parents and educators on planning steps that will help children with Osteogenesis Imperfecta to fully participate in school activities.

15 minutes

3220 You Are Not Alone
Osteogenesis Imperfecta Foundation
804 W. Diamond Avenue Suite 204
Gaithersburg, MD 20878   301-947-0083
                                800-981-2663
                   Fax: 301-947-0456
            e-mail: bonelink@oif.org
                    www.oif.org

Explores the emotional turmoil of dealing with the diagnosis of OI and offers practical and uplifting solutions for caring for infants with Type II to severe Type III OI. Also valuable for new families with the more mild forms of OI. Available open captioned or with Spanish subtitles.

Web Sites

3221 Shriner's Hospital Research Study Report
www.osteo.org/

3222 UK Osteogenesis Imperfecta Foundation
www.ukoifoundation.org

3223 Usenet
alt.support.osteogenesis.imperfecta

3224 Wheeless' Textbook of Orthopaedics
medmedia.com/o14/81.htm

Books

3225 Living with Osteogenesis Imperfecta - A Guidebook for Families

Heidi Galuser, author

Osteogenesis Imperfecta Foundation
804 West Diamond Avenue Suite 210
Gaithersburg, MD 20878

800-981-2663
Fax: 301-947-0456
e-mail: bonelink@oif.org
www.oif.org

This book offers people with OI and their caregivers encouragement, comfort, knowledge, and a store of practical advice.

Heidi Glauser, Editor

3226 Managing Osteogenesis Imperfecta: A Medical Manual

Priscilla Wacaster, MD, author

Osteogenesis Imperfecta Foundation
804 West Diamond Avenue Suite 210
Gaithersburg, MD 20878

800-981-2663
Fax: 301-947-0456
e-mail: bonelink@oif.org
www.oif.org

The manual is designed for physicians, physical and occupational therapists, orthopedic technologists, early intervention providers and others who come in contact with persons with OI. It covers a broad range of topics including genetics, diagnosis, pregnancy, arthritis, and osteoperosis.

1997

Newsletters

3227 Breakthrough

Osteogenesis Imperfecta Foundation
804 W. Diamond Avenue Suite 204
Gaithersburg, MD 20878

800-981-2663
Fax: 301-947-0456
e-mail: bonelink@oif.org
www.oif.org

Newsletter of the Osteogenesis Imperfecta Foundation that provides information on current research and OIF fundraising activities, as well as support features.

15 pages Bi-Monthly

Pamphlets

3228 Caring for Infants and Children with Osteogenesis Imperfecta

Osteogenesis Imperfecta Foundation
804 W. Diamond Avenue Suite 204
Gaithersburg, MD 20878

301-947-0083
800-981-2663
Fax: 301-947-0456
e-mail: bonelink@oif.org
www.oif.org

A companion to the videotape You Are Not Alone. Presents some basic information and unique tips on caring for a baby or toddler with OI. Available in Spanish.

3229 We're Growing Stronger

Osteogenesis Imperfecta Foundation
804 W. Diamond Avenue Suite 204
Gaithersburg, MD 20878

301-947-0083
800-981-2663
Fax: 301-947-0456
e-mail: bonelink@oif.org
www.oif.org

Describes OI and introduces the Osteogenesis Imperfecta Foundation, Inc.

DESCRIPTION

3230 OTITIS MEDIA

Synonym: Tympanitis

Disorder Type: Hearing, Infectious Disease

Covers these related disorders: Acute otitis media, Chronic otitis media, Secretory otitis media

Otitis media refers to an infection or inflammation of the middle ear, which is an irregularly-shaped cavity that lies in the temporal bone on each side of the skull. This type of inflammation is one of the most common disorders of childhood, especially in children from the ages of six months to three years.

Acute otitis media usually occurs in conjunction with or as a complication of upper respiratory tract infections such as those caused by the common cold. Infections of the respiratory tract commonly involve the eustachian tube that extends from the rear of the nasal area to the middle ear and, in infants and young children, is narrow, short, and positioned somewhat horizontally, thus making these young patients more susceptible to the backward flow of infectious secretions into the middle ear and subsequent infection. In addition, adenoids that are swollen or enlarged from upper respiratory tract infection may block the eustachian tube, thus impairing its ability to drain pus-filled secretions resulting in an accumulation of these infection-causing substances in the middle ear.

Symptoms associated with acute otitis media often develop within a few days of the onset of a respiratory tract infection and include sudden and severe ear pain (otalgia), ringing in the ears (tinnitus), fever, temporary hearing loss, and discomfort. Infants and young children may be irritable, nauseated, and may vomit and have diarrhea. The eardrum (tympanic membrane) may rupture, thus releasing fluid, which leads to relief of pain. In the absence of further complications, the eardrum may heal within a short period of time. The development of symptoms such as dizziness, headache, sudden and significant hear-

ing loss or deafness, chills, and fever may suggest the presence of severe complications including inflammation of the membranes surrounding the brain and spinal cord (meningitis), infection of the inner ear canals (labyrinthitis) or the mastoid bone behind the ear (mastoiditis). Treatment for acute otitis media is dependent upon the causative agent. For example, if the infection is bacterial, antibiotics may be administered. Some children may require surgical intervention through the use of a procedure called myringotomy during which an incision is made in the eardrum to relieve pressure and allow the release of pus and other secretions or through tympanocentesis, a procedure during which the eardrum is surgically punctured to release fluid. Other treatment is symptomatic and supportive. For example, pain relief may be accomplished through the use of analgesic medications.

Some children may develop secretory otitis media (otitis media with effusion), which is a condition that occurs subsequent to eustachian tube blockage or successful resolution of acute otitis media and is characterized by the escape of thin (serous), thick (mucoid), or pus-like fluid from the ear. Associated symptoms may include dizziness and a ringing or buzzing (tinnitus) in the ears. Although this condition may sometimes resolve spontaneously, treatment is often indicated in some infants and children to prevent possible hearing loss and subsequent difficulties in speech and language development. In addition, surgical incision of the eardrum along with insertion of tubes into the eardrum may allow for drainage of fluid. Children who do not respond to these medications and procedures may benefit from the removal of their adenoids (adenoidectomy). Other treatment is symptomatic and supportive.

Chronic otitis media is a persistent infection of the middle ear that is caused by perforation of the eardrum resulting from acute otitis media, eustachian tube blockage, or various injuries. Drainage of pus-filled fluid may occur subsequent to upper respiratory tract infections or after swimming or bathing. Chronic flare-ups may result in the development of relatively small growths (polyps) in the ear and in damage to the small bones (ossicles) of the middle ear, resulting in the impaired ability to conduct sound and subsequent conductive hearing loss. If the perforation is located on the perimeter of the eardrum, complications may include facial paralysis, inflammations involving other ear structures and the brain, and the formation of skinlike growths (cholesteatomas) that may damage or destroy adjacent bones. Treatment may include cleansing of the ear in conjunction with the installation of a hydrocortisone/acetic acid solution, the administration of antibiotics, and surgical removal of cholesteatomas. Surgical intervention may also be indicated to restore the mechanism of the middle ear by establishing the continuity of the small bones and repairing the eardrum through a procedure called tympanoplasty. Other treatment is symptomatic and supportive.

The following organizations in the General Resources Section can provide additional information: National Organization for Rare Disorders, Inc., (NORD), March of Dimes Birth Defects Foundation, NIH/National Institute of Allergy and Infectious Disease, World Health Organization (WHO), Centers for Disease Control (CDC)

Web Sites

3231 Baylor
www.bcm.tmc.edu/oto/grand42194.html

3232 Group Health Cooperative
www.bcm.tmc.edu/oto/grand/42194.html

3233 PDR.net
www.pdr.net/gettingwell/otitismedia/disease.html

3234 PedBase
www.icondata.com/health/pedbase/files/OTISME.HTM

3235 UTMB
www.utmb.edu/oto/Grnds.dir/om-comp.html

3236 Wayne State University Scool of Medicine
biochem.genetics.wayne.edu/diseases.htm

Books

3237 Otitis Media: Coping with the Effects in the Classroom
Dorinne S. Davis, MA, CCC-A, author

Alexander Graham Bell Association for the Deaf
3417 Volta Place N.W.
Washington, DC 20007   202-337-5220
                              800-432-7543
                         Fax: 202-337-8314
                         TTY: 202-337-5220
                    e-mail: agbell2@aol.com
                         www.agbell.org

This unique book alerts classroom teachers and specialists to educational problems for children who have otitis media and are experiencing difficulties with communication, listening, and/or learning. Enhancement of the auditory environment, teaching strategy modifications, and curriculum adaptations can provide substantial benefit to children with recurrent and/or presistent otitis media and those with residual effects of earlier infections.

1989 137 pages

Pamphlets

3238 Otitis Media
Deafness Research Foundation
15 West 39th Street
New York, NY 10018   212-768-1181

Offers information on otitis media, prevention, causes, treatments and symptoms.

DESCRIPTION

3239 PASSIVE-AGGRESSIVE BEHAVIOR

Disorder Type: Mental, Emotional or Behavioral Disorder

Passive-aggressive behavior refers to a type of disruptive conduct that is apparent in approximately 20 percent of children and adolescents. Although seemingly compliant, affected individuals usually harbor negative, aggressive, or hostile feelings, but are unable to directly express them. These negative, hostile feelings are typically manifested indirectly and nonviolently through procrastination, forgetfulness, inefficiency, pouting or sullenness, stubbornness, obstructionism, and resistance to requests or demands. When infants and toddlers, passive-aggressive children and adolescents may have manifested their negativistic personalities through difficulties with feeding and toilet training.

Passive-aggressive individuals may be unaware that they are using their behavior to counteract or offset certain frustrations (e.g., feelings of inadequacy). They may persist in these behaviors in an attempt to regain control of a situation or to punish and retaliate. These stubbornly compliant behaviors are apparent in other situations that typically provoke direct displays of assertiveness, hostility, or other forms of aggression. Parents may be overly, but inconsistently, demanding and critical; conversely, affected individuals may, in some cases, be reared by parents or caregivers who are overly permissive and tolerant.

Treatment for passive-aggressive behavior includes the cooperation of parents or caregivers who are often in the best position to provide motivation for children to learn to appropriately express their assertiveness. Such motivation may be further supported by the establishment of firm rules and guidelines, the setting of realistic goals, and the prioritizing of responsibilities. Some parents or caregivers may benefit from direct management training that teaches the necessary skills to facilitate proper behavior and other social skills. Individual, group, and family psychotherapy may also be indicated. Other treatment is supportive.

The following organizations in the General Resources Section can provide additional information: National Alliance for the Mentally Ill (NAMI), Federation of Families for Children's Mental Health, National Mental Health Association, National Mental Health Consumer Self-Help Clearinghouse, NIH/National Institute of Mental Health

National Associations & Support Groups

3240 American Mental Health Foundation (AMNF)
1049 5th Avenue
New York, NY 10028
USA
212-639-1561
Fax: 212-737-9027

Researches the theories and techniques of treatment of emotional illness and to the implementation of reforms in the mental health system. Efforts have resulted in development of better and less expensive treatment methods. Findings are disseminated in English and other major languages.

Monroe W. Spero, MD

3241 Association for Persons with Mental and Developmental Disabilities
132 Fair St.
Kington, NY 12401
914-334-4336
800-331-4569
Fax: 914-331-4596
e-mail: nadd@mhv.net

Geared to supply families and medical personel with the information that will help individuals deal with mental retardation.

3242 Center for Family Support (CFS)
333 7th Avenue
New York, NY 10001
USA
212-629-7939
Fax: 212-239-2211
www.cfsny.org

Devoted to the physical well-being and development of the retarded child and the sound mental health of the parents. Helps families with retarded children with all aspects of home care including counseling, referrals, home aide service and consultation. Offers intervention for parents at the birth of a retarded child with in-home support, guidance and infant stimulation. Pioneered training of nonprofessional women as home aides to provide supportive services in homes.

Steven Vernickofs, Executive Director

3243 Christian Horizons, Inc.
P.O. Box 334
Williamstown, MI 48895   517-655-3463

Devoted to assisting individuals, with mental disabilities, on a day-to-day basis.

Adonna Jory, Executive Secretary
Noel Churchman, Board President

3244 Mental Illness Foundation
772 W 168th Street
New York, NY 10032   212-682-4699
                          Fax: 212-682-4896

Supports community housing, treatment, research, outreach and public-awareness efforts for people with mental illness. Publications: Mental Illness Foundation, quarterly newsletter. Directory that lists mental illnesses and provides information on how to contact related associations. Annual meeting.

3245 National Alliance for the Mentally Ill
200 North Glebe Road #1015
Arlington, VA 22203   703-524-7600
                          800-950-6264
                     TDD: 703-516-7991
          e-mail: membership@nami.org
                          www.nami.org

Aids families and individuals find the emotional and physical answers to the habitual forming disorders through several media resources.

Web Sites

3246 Borderline Personality Disorder Sanctuary
www.navicom.com

3247 CyberPsych
www.cyberpsych.com

3248 I.D. Weeks Library
www.usd/library/extension/persondis.html

3249 National Anxiety Foundation
www.lexington-on-line.com/naf.html

3250 New York Online Access to Health Borderline Pages
www.noah.cuny.edu/
          e-mail: webmaster@noah.cuny.edu
                          www.noah.cuny.edu/

Provides high quality, full-text health information for condsumers that is accurate, timely, relevant and unbiased. NOAH currently supports English and Spanish.

3251 PlanetPsych
www.planetpsych.com

3252 Psych Central
www.psychcentral.com

Books

3253 Challenging Behavior
Emerson, author

Cambridge University Press
40 W 20th St
New York, NY 10011   212-924-3900
                          800-872-7423
                     Fax: 914-937-4712
                          www.cup.org

3254 Clinical Assessment and Management of Severe Personality Disorders
Paul S. Links, MD, author

American Psychiatric Press, Inc.
1400 K St NW
Washington, DC 20005   202-682-6262
                          800-368-5777
                     Fax: 202-789-2648
          e-mail: order@appi.org
                          www.appi.org

Focuses on issues relevant to the clinician in private practice, including the diagnosis of a wide range of personality disorders and alternative management approaches.

1995 260 pages

Paul S. Links, Editor

3255 Personality and Psychopathology

C. Robert Cloninger, MD, author

American Psychiatric Press, Inc.
1400 K St. NW
Washington, DC 20005   202-682-6262
                            800-368-5777
                       Fax: 202-789-2648
                e-mail: order@appi.org
                        www.appi.org

Compiles the most recent findings from more
than 30 internationaly recognized experts. Analyzes the association between personality and
psychopthology from several interlocking perspectives, descriptive, developmental, etiologi-
cal, and theraputic.

1999 496 pages

3256 Type A Behavior

Michael J. Strube, Washington University, author

Sage Publications, Inc.
2455 Teller Rd.
Thousand Oaks, CA 91320   805-499-0721
                          Fax: 805-499-0871
                e-mail: info@sagepub.com
                        www.sagepub.com

This important book brings together leading
scholars to answer questions about enviromental
and genetic factors role in the development of
Type A behavior, whether or not gender has an
effect and if Type A parents raise Type A children. Presents current Type A research and discusses issues including theoretical advances,
hostility, special populations, measurement and
prediction refinements, work settings, medical
and psychological refinements and extensions,
and interventions.

1991 436 pages Hardcover

DESCRIPTION

3257 PATENT DUCTUS ARTERIOSUS

Synonym: PDA

Disorder Type: Birth Defect, Heart

Patent ductus arteriosus is a heart defect that is present at birth (congenital) and characterized by the persistence of a fetal vessel that maintains a passageway between the major artery that carries oxygen-rich blood to the tissues of the body (descending aorta) and the artery that carries deoxygenated blood to the lungs (pulmonary artery). Before birth, fetal blood receives oxygen from the mother's blood rather than from its own lungs, making it unnecessary for fetal blood to pass from the right side of the heart to the lungs to be oxygenated. To accommodate this fetal blood flow, blood passes through an opening (foramen ovale) in the wall (septum) between the two upper chambers of the heart (atria). Fetal blood is diverted away from the lungs through a vessel known as the ductus arteriosus that connects the pulmonary artery and the aorta. Normally, both the foramen ovale and ductus arteriosus close soon after birth. The persistence of the opening (patency) of the ductus arteriosus causes some blood from the aorta to flow into the pulmonary artery to the lungs instead of moving away from the heart to nourish the tissues of the body.

Symptoms and physical findings associated with patent ductus arteriosus depend upon the size of the opening and the volume of the diverted blood. A small defect may result in no symptoms while a larger opening may result in difficulty in breathing (dyspnea), rapid heartbeat (tachycardia), failure to gain weight, inflammation of the lining of the heart (bacterial endocarditis), and inefficient pumping by the heart (heart failure). Physical findings may include enlargement of the heart (cardiomegaly); characteristic heart sounds; a machinery-like heart murmur; and, if left untreated, abnormally high pressure in the lung's circulatory system (pulmonary hypertension).

Premature infants may require early intervention through restriction of fluid intake, certain drug therapy, or surgery to prevent malfunctioning of the heart or lungs. However, if no immediate surgical or medicinal intervention is required or administered, this defect may spontaneously close in many premature newborns.

In full-term infants and children, a patent ductus arteriosus may require intervention (surgical or catheter closure). Such treatment may be helpful in preventing or alleviating associated complications. The exact cause of patent ductus arteriosus in the full-term infant is unknown. It is thought to result from different genetic and environmental factors (multifactorial). For example, this irregularity is often associated with maternal German measles (rubella) infection. In addition, patent ductus arteriosus is often accompanied by other congenital heart defects. This defect appears in approximately 60 of 100,000 births and is more prevalent in females than males by a ratio of about two to one.

The following organizations in the General Resources Section can provide additional information: Genetic Alliance, March of Dimes Birth Defects Foundation, National Organization for Rare Disorders, Inc. (NORD), NIH/National Heart, Lung & Blood Institute, NIH/National Institute of Child Health and Human Development

National Associations & Support Groups

3258 American Heart Association
7272 Greenville Avenue
Dallas, TX 75231

214-373-6300
800-242-8721
Fax: 214-706-1341
e-mail: inquire@amhrt.org
www.amhrt.org

Supports research, education and community service programs with the objective of reducing premature death and disability from cardiovascular diseases and stroke; coordinates the efforts of health professionals, and other engaged in the fight against heart and circulatory disease.

Web Sites

3259 Children's Health Information Network
www.ohsu.edu/cliniweb/C14.240.400.html

3260 Congenital Heart Disease Resource
www.csun.edu
e-mail: sheri.berger@csun.edu
www.csun.edu

3261 Pediatric Database (PEDBASE)
www.icondata.com/health/pedbase/files/PATEN-TDU.HTM

3262 Southern Illinois University School of Medicine
www.siumed.edu/peds/teaching/patient%20edu-cation.htm

DESCRIPTION

3263 PEMPHIGUS

Disorder Type: Autoimmune Disease
May involve these systems in the body (see Section III):
Dermatologic System

Pemphigus refers to a group of chronic skin disorders that are characterized by the appearance of blisters on the skin and delicate mucous membranes that line the mouth, for example. Pemphigus most often occurs among the adult population, but may appear at any age. Associated findings include a phenomenon known as Nikolsky's sign, characterized by the tendency of the upper layer of the skin to separate or slough off from the lower layer upon rubbing or other minor trauma. Pemphigus is thought to result from an autoimmune reaction during which the body mistakenly attacks healthy cells. In this case, antibodies attack the cells that glue skin together, resulting in disruptions in contact between the cells.

Benign familial pemphigus is a relatively mild form of this disorder that is inherited as an autosomal dominant trait and is characterized by the persistent and recurrent formation of blisters mainly in the groin area, the armpit (axillary) region, the sides of the neck, and on the bending surfaces of the arms and legs. These localized or widespread lesions rupture, erode, and then crust over and heal. This form of pemphigus is also known as Hailey-Hailey disease.

Pemphigus foliaceus is a rare, usually mild form of the disorder that is characterized by small blisters that are usually localized and rupture easily, erode, and then heal by crusting over or scaling. These lesions most commonly appear on the scalp, neck, face, and trunk. The blisters may cause itching, pain, or burning in the affected areas. Affected individuals may also experience the sloughing off of the upper skin layer (Nikolsky's sign). Some affected individuals may develop a more generalized pattern of eruptions characterized by excessive shedding or peeling of the skin. Treatment for pemphigus foliaceus may include therapy with corticosteriod drugs. In some cases, topical application of corticosteroid ointments, salves, or creams proves beneficial.

Pemphigus vulgaris is a very severe form of disease that is manifested by eruptions of painful, ulcerative lesions in the delicate mucous membranes that line the mouth. Later findings include the appearance of large blisters on previously unaffected areas of the face, chest, abdomen, armpit region, groin area, and the various pressure points of the body. These lesions enlarge and rupture, leaving raw areas that may partially crust over, but have little or no tendency to heal. These raw or denuded areas sometimes give rise to wart-like granulations that emit a strong, offensive odor. This stage of pemphigus vulgaris is sometimes referred to as pemphigus vegetans. The folds of the skin are particularly susceptible to the development of these wart-like lesions. Individuals with pemphigus vulgaris also exhibit Nikolsky's sign. Life-threatening complications associated with pemphigus vulgaris may include secondary bacterial infections such as sepsis or debilitating conditions such as malnutrition and the loss of essential elements, known as electrolytes, in the fluid portion of the blood (e.g., sodium, potassium, and calcium). For this reason, early diagnosis and treatment of pemphigus vulgaris is essential to its successful management. Positive diagnosis may be determined through microscopic examination of a skin sample, obtained through biopsy, that indicates the presence of certain antibody deposits. Initial treatment may include high-dose corticosteroid therapy, followed by long-term administration of corticosteroid or other immunosuppressive drugs to control the disease. Antibiotic therapy may be indicated for treatment of skin or secondary bacterial infections.

Neonatal pemphigus vulgaris develops in the unborn fetus of an affected mother by transmission of the mother's antibodies through the placenta. In most cases, the severity of disease in the fetus is related to the severity of the mother's disease. If the mother is severely affected, the placental transmission of antibodies may potentially threaten the life of the unborn child.

The following organizations in the General Resources Section can provide additional information: National Organization for Rare Disorders, Inc. (NORD), NIH/Office of Rare Diseases, March of Dimes Birth Defects Foundation, Genetic Alliance, NIH/National Institute of Child Health and Human Development, American Autoimmune Related Diseases Association, Inc., NIH/National Institute of Arthritis and Musculoskeletal and Skin Diseases

National Associations & Support Groups

3264 National Pemphigus Foundation
PO Box 9606, 1098 Euclid Avenue
Berkeley, CA 94709   510-527-4970
                              Fax: 510-527-8497
                         e-mail: PVnews@aol.com
                              www.pemphigus.org

Web Sites

3265 Pemphigus fAQ
www.geocities.com/HotSprings/7445/

DESCRIPTION

3266 PERTUSSIS
Synonym: Whooping cough
Disorder Type: Infectious Disease

Pertussis is a highly contagious infectious disease in which inflammation of the respiratory tract occurs as the result of infection with the bacterium Bordetella pertussis (B. pertussis). Transmission of the disease usually occurs through inhalation of airborne bacteria-containing droplets that are spread through coughing or sneezing. Pertussis primarily affects infants and children, although the disease may occur at any age.

Approximately 60 million cases of pertussis occur each year worldwide. Before the pertussis vaccine was introduced in the United States in the 1950s, pertussis was the leading cause of death from infectious disease in children younger than 14 years of age. Widespread administration of the pertussis vaccine in the U.S. and other countries contributed to a rapid decline of the disease. However, pertussis remains widespread in countries where vaccination is unavailable. In addition, in the 1980s and early 1990s in the United States, incomplete implementation of pertussis childhood vaccination programs contributed to increased frequency of the disease as well as epidemics in certain states.

Pertussis infection usually lasts approximately six weeks and occurs in three main stages: catarrhal, paroxysmal, and convalescent stages. Disease progression is typically characterized by moderate, cold-like symptoms (catarrhal stage); severe coughing episodes (paroxysmal stage); and a gradual cessation of symptoms (convalescent stage). The catarrhal stage begins approximately one to two weeks after initial infection. Associated symptoms may include a slight fever, irritability, listlessness, a runny nose (rhinorrhea), sneezing, and a dry cough. In about a week or two, the paroxysmal stage begins, which is characterized by a series of short, quick coughs that may end with long, high-pitched, deep intakes of breath (whooping).

During such episodes, infants and young children may experience abnormal redness of the face, choking, bluish discoloration of the skin and mucous membranes (cyanosis), flailing of the arms and legs, bulging of the eyes, protruding of the tongue, and the release of large amounts of mucus. Vomiting often occurs after coughing subsides due to gagging on mucus. In some affected infants, coughing episodes may be precipitated by seemingly insignificant stimuli, such as changes in light or sound, and may be characterized by choking rather than forceful whooping. During the convalescent stage of pertussis, which lasts approximately two weeks, coughing episodes become less forceful and frequent and gradually subside. Many children may continue to experience periodic coughing episodes during the following year or so. In some patients, complications may occur due to pertussis infection, such as cessation of breathing (apnea) during coughing episodes; secondary infections causing inflammation of the middle ear (otitis media) or the lungs (pneumonia); or other abnormalities. In some cases, without appropriate treatment, life-threatening complications may result. Although infection with the B. pertussis bacterium usually results in future immunity, some patients may experience a second, usually more mild episode of the disease.

The treatment of pertussis typically includes bedrest and measures to ensure proper nutrition and adequate fluid intake. Erythromycin or other antibiotics may be administered to help treat pertussis, reduce disease transmission, and control secondary infections. Hospitalization may be required for infants or for children with severe coughing episodes or complications. Treatment measures may include suctioning of mucus from air passages, intravenous therapy to ensure appropriate intake of nutrients, or oxygen therapy to help alleviate difficulties breathing or abnormal bluish discoloration of the skin and mucous membranes. Affected infants are often kept in a quiet, darkened room to prevent unnecessary disturbances that may provoke coughing episodes. As mentioned above, pertussis vaccination is routinely provided during childhood in the United States. Such vaccination typically consists of combined immunization with the DPT (diphtheria, pertussis, tetanus) vaccine and booster shots as required.

The following organizations in the General Resources Section can provide additional information: National Organization for Rare Disorders, Inc., (NORD), March of Dimes Birth Defects Foundation, NIH/National Institute of Allergy and Infectious Disease, World Health Organization

Web Sites

3267 About.com
babyparenting.miningco.com/library/blillness5.htm

3268 Centers for Disease Control
www.edc.gov/epo/mmwr/other/case_def/pertus97.html

3269 Pedbase
www.icondata.com/health/pedbase/files/PERTUSSI.htm

DESCRIPTION

3270 PHENYLKETONURIA (PKU)
Synonyms: Classic phenylketonuria, PKU
Disorder Type: Genetic Disorder, Metabolism

Phenylketonuria (PKU) is an inherited metabolic disorder characterized by the absence or deficiency of phenylalanine hydroxylase, an enzyme that assists in the metabolism of phenylalanine. This enzyme normally converts phenylalanine into tyrosine. The absence of phenylalanine hydroxylase results in the accumulation of excessive phenylalanine in the blood. This may lead to severe mental retardation that is frequently accompanied by seizures and other neurologic problems.

Initially, affected newborns usually have no symptoms; however, early symptoms may include severe vomiting and poor eating. Mental retardation develops slowly but progressively and may become apparent within the first few months of life. Untreated or undiagnosed children may develop neuromuscular irregularities such as involuntary, continuous, slow movements of the arms and legs (athetosis). Other findings may include seizures and hyperactivity, sometimes accompanied by rhythmic behaviors such as rocking. Affected infants usually have light-colored skin, blonde hair, and blue eyes. In addition, an eczema-type rash may develop that eventually disappears with age. Children with PKU often produce an unpleasant, musty odor that results from the presence of phenylacetic acid in the sweat and urine. Other findings in untreated children may include a small head (microcephaly), irregularities of the teeth and upper jaw (maxilla), and delayed growth.

Phenylketonuria is diagnosed by a blood test known as the Guthrie or PKU test. A small amount of blood is withdrawn from the newborn's heel. If blood levels of phenylalanine are elevated, further testing is done to confirm the presence of this disorder. Treatment for PKU is aimed toward reducing dietary intake of phenylalanine in order to prevent or lessen the effects of damage to the brain. This diet is administered and monitored under close supervision. Phenylalanine is not manufactured by the body and is obtained solely through diet. Certain levels of phenylalanine must be maintained to prevent life-threatening complications. Immediate dietary management is initiated upon diagnosis. It is recommended that pregnant women with PKU or affected women who are planning to become pregnant maintain a low phenylalanine diet to avoid the risk of miscarriage. In addition, infants born to women with PKU who are not on a special diet are at high risk of such irregularities as mental retardation, microcephaly, and congenital heart defects.

Phenylketonuria is transmitted as an autosomal recessive trait. In the United States, approximately one in 16,000 is affected by this disorder.

The following organizations in the General Resources Section can provide additional information: NIH/Office of Rare Diseases, National Organization for Rare Disorders, Inc., (NORD), March of Dimes Birth Defects Foundation, Online Mendelian Inheritance in Man: www3.ncbi.nlm.nih.gov/Omim/searchomim.html

---

National Associations & Support Groups

3271 Association for Neuro-Metabolic Disorders
5223 Brookfield Ln
Sylvania, OH 43506   419-885-1497

Organization that is comprised of families of children with disorders that affect the nervous system and the brain. It provides assistance and information through conferences, meetings and phone calls.

3272 Children Phenylketonuria PKU Network
1520 State Street, Suite 110
San Diego, CA 92101   619-233-3202
Fax: 619-233-0838
e-mail: pkunetwork@aol.com

3273 Childrens PKU Network
3790 Via de la Valle Suite 116E
Del Mar, CA 92014   858-509-0767
800-377-6677
Fax: 858-509-0768
e-mail: pkunetwork@aol.com

Provides support services and treatment products to families afflicted with Phenylketonuria (PKU), a rare metabolic disorder which, when left untreated can cause brain damage. Services include referal, newborn express packages, digital scale sales, crisis intervention aid.

1981

3274 Metabolic Disorders National PKU News
6869 Woodland Avenue NE, Suite 116
Seattle, WA 98115   206-525-8140
Fax: 206-525-5023
e-mail: schuett@pkunews.org
www.pkunews.org

3275 National Phenylketonuria (PKU) News
6869 Woodlawn Avenue NE, Suite 116
Seattle, WA 98115

www.wolfenet.com/~kronmal/

Research Centers

3276 National Phenylketonuria (PKU) Foundation
6301 Tejas Drive
Pasadena, TX 77503   713-487-4802

International

3277 Research Trust for Metabolic Diseases in Children
Goldengates Lodge Weston Rd., Crewe
Cheshire,
United Kingdom

Dedicated to providing the most up-to-date medical knowledge for the families and friends of people suffering from this and related diseases.

Web Sites

3278 National Society for Phenylketonuria (UK)
www.ukonline.co.uk.nspku/mornspku.htm

3279 PKU Kid's Zone
www.pkuil.org/kidzone.htm

3280 PKU of Illinois
www.pkuil.org/

Pamphlets

3281 PKU Information Sheet
March of Dimes
P.O. Box 1657
Wilkes-Barre, PA 18703   717-820-8104
800-367-6630
Fax: 717-825-1987

Phenylketonuria (PKU) is an inherited disorder that affects the way the body is able to process food, which, if untreated, causes mental retardation. This pamphlet outlines how PKU is passed on and how it is treated.

pkg of 50
ISBN: 0-927400- -

DESCRIPTION

3282 PHOBIAS

Disorder Type: Mental, Emotional or Behavioral Disorder

A phobia is a persistant, exaggerated, unreasonable fear or dread of certain activities, situations, or objects. These feelings typically provoke a state of panic or horror. Most children are fearful of particular things as they reach certain age plateaus. For example, young children are often afraid of monsters or of being alone in the dark. Older children may be fearful of death or other distressing situations. Children may become fearful of events or situations that they view on television. Others may have fear or dread related to conflicts in the home. These fears are not unusual and may often be alleviated by reassurances and comforting by parents and caregivers. However, a fear or phobia that interferes with normal, day-to-day functioning is considered pathologic.

Simple or specific phobias include fear of certain animals and insects or particular situations (e.g., fear of flying, etc.). Social phobias, often appearing in late childhood or adolescence, include fear and avoidance of certain social situations such as using public bathroom facilities or eating, speaking, performing, or writing in public. Researchers believe that some simple phobias may result from an associated, traumatic childhood experience or from the existence of a similar fear in a parent or caregiver. More complicated specific phobias (e.g., fear of attending school, etc.) may be associated with such conflicts as a hostile-dependent relationship between the parent or caregiver and the child. Exposure to the activity, situation, or object that arouses fear elicits signs of anxiety or panic reaction. Such symptoms may include nausea, abdominal pain, irregular pulsation or racing of the heart (palpitations), sweating, and dizziness.

Treatment for phobias is dependent upon the specific fear, the extent of the fear, and the effect of the phobias on day-to-day living. Parents or caregivers are counseled to remain calm and patient when confronted with a phobic episode. Behavioral therapy may be indicated and may include the training of parents or caregivers in the use of supportive measures and techniques. Slow and orderly exposure to the activity, situation, or object of fear (desensitization) may help to alleviate the fear. Older children and adolescents with social phobias may learn to overcome their particular fear through social skills training. Other treatment is symptomatic and supportive.

The following organizations in the General Resources Section can provide additional information: National Alliance for the Mentall Ill (NAMI), National Mental Health Association, National Mental Health Consumer Self-Help Clearinghouse, NIH/National Institute of Mental Health, Federation of Families for Children's Mental Health

National Associations & Support Groups

3283 American Mental Health Foundation
1049 5th Avenue
New York, NY 10028   212-639-1561
                                         Fax: 212-737-9027

Organization dealing with medical theory of emotional illness.

3284 Anxiety Disorders Association of America
11900 Parklawn Dr, Ste 100
Rockville, MD 20852   301-231-9350
                                       Fax: 301-231-7392
                             e-mail: anxdis@adaa.org
                                              www.adaa.org

Organization provides an in-depth and personal outlook at this illness.

3285 Anxiety Disorders Institute
2150 Peachford Rd., Ste B
Atlanta, GA 30338   770-395-6845

3286 Anxiety and Phobia Treatment Center
Davis Ave at E. Post Rd.
White Plains, NY 10601   914-681-1038
                                          Fax: 914-681-2284
                              e-mail: www.phobia-anxiety.com

Gatherings to help the phobic understand their fear in a life-like setting.

3287 Center for Family Support
333 7th Ave.
New York, NY 10001   212-629-7939
Fax: 212-239-2211
e-mail: www.cfsny.org

Gives simple, but thorough answers to the most commonly asked questions of families with retarded children; provides many services, including training and referrals.

3288 Center for Mental Health Services Knowledge Exchange Program
U.S. Department of Health and Human Services
P.O. Box 42490
Washington, DC 20015
800-789-2647
Fax: 301-984-8796
e-mail: ken@mentalhealth.org
www.mentalhealth.org

Supplies the public with expert responses to commonly asked questions about various mental health disorders, and directs the caller to appropriate resources.

3289 Center for Self-Help Research
1918 University Ave, Ste 3D
Berkeley, CA 94704   510-849-0731
Fax: 510-849-3402

Unites various groups to examine the different features of the public health care systems.

Steven P. Segal, Director
Carol J. Silverman, Program Director

3290 Phobia Society of America
133 Rollins Ave, Ste 4B
Rockville, MD 20852   301-231-9350
Fax: 301-231-7392
www.adaa.org

Offers support for those suffering from phobia and panic attacks.

3291 Selective Mutism Foundation
P.O. Box 450632
Sunrise, FL 33345   305-748-7714
Fax: 305-748-7714
e-mail: www.personal.mia.bellsouth.net

Raises consciousness regarding the illness, and provides answers to commonly asked questions.

Sue Leszczyk

3292 Special Interest Group on Phobias and Related Anxiety Disorders
245 E. 87th St.
New York, NY 10028   212-860-5560
Fax: 212-744-5751
e-mail: lindy@interport.net

Various organizations gather to communicate about the modern treatment techniques and how to improve diagnosis procedures.

Carol Lindemann, PhD, CEO

3293 Territorial Apprehensiveness Programs
932 Evelyn St.
Menlo Park, CA 94025
800-274-6242

Founded to distribute knowledge regarding phobias and offer various services and referrels.

Crucita V. Hardy, Director

Audio Video

3294 Acquiring Courage: An Audio Cassette Program for the Fast Treatment of Phobia

Zev Wanderer, PhD, author

New Harbinger Publications, Inc.
5674 Shattuck Ave
Oakland, CA 94609   610-652-2002
800-748-6273
e-mail: customerservice@newharbinger.com
www.newharbinger.com

1991

Web Sites

3295 About.com
About.com, Inc.
www.panicdisorder.minigco.com   212-849-2000
800-517-9020
Fax: 212-849-2121
e-mail: robh@about.com
www.panicdisorder.minigco.com

3296 Anxiety Panic Internet Resource
www.algy.com

3297 CyberPsych
www.cyberpsych.org

3298 National Anxiety Foundation
www.lexington-on-line.com/naf.html

3299 Panic Support

www.alt.support.anxiety-panic

3300 Planetpsych

www.planetpsych.com

3301 Recovery Panic Anxiety

www.alt.recovery.panic.anxiety.self-help

Books

3302 Anxiety and Phobia Workbook

Edmund J. Bourne, PhD, author

New Harbinger Publications, Inc.
5674 Shattuck Ave.
Oakland, CA 94609   510-652-2002
                                     800-748-6273
        e-mail: customerservice@newharbinger.com
                        www.newharbinger.com

This comprehensive guide is recommended to
those who are struggling with anxiety disorders.
Includes step-by-step instructions for the crucial
cognitive-behavioral techniques that have given
real help to hundreds of thousands of readers
struggling with anxiety disorders.

1995 448 pages

3303 Encyclopedia of Phobias, Fears, and Anxieties

Ronald M. Doctor, PhD and Ada P. Kahn, author

Facts On File
11 Penn Plaza, Rm M274
New York, NY 10001   212-290-8090
                                      800-322-8755

500 pages

3304 Perfectionism: What's Bad About Being Too Good
Free Spirit Pub

With help for superkids, workaholics, type A's.
straight A's, procrastinators, overacheivers, and
caring adults, this book explains the difference
between healthy ambition and unhealthy perfectionism and gives straight strategies for getting
out of the perfectionist trap- from recognizing
the symptoms to rewarding yourself for who you
are, not what you do. It explains why some people become perfectionists, what it does to the
body, and why girls are more prone to it, and
more.

1999 144 pages

Miriam Adderholt, PhD, Author
Miriam Elliot, Author

3305 Psychological Trauma

Rachel Yehuda, PhD, author

American Psychiatric Press, Inc.
1400 K St, NW
Washington, DC 20005   202-682-6262
                                      800-368-5777
                               Fax: 202-789-2648
                            e-mail: order@appi.org
                                     www.appi.org

Epidermiology of trauma and post-traimatic
stress disorder. Evaluation, neuroimaging,
neuroendocrinology and pharmacology.

1998 206 pages

**3306 Shy Children, Phobic Adults: Nature and Treatment
of Social Phobia**

Deborah C. Beidel and Samual M. Turner, author

American Psychological Press, Inc.
1400 K St, NW
Washington, DC 20005   202-682-6262
                                      800-368-5777
                               Fax: 202-789-2648
                           e-mail: orders@appi.org
                                     www.appi.org

Describes the similiarities and differences in the
syndrome across all ages. Draws from the clinical, social and developmental literatures, as well
as from extensive clinical experience. Illustrates
the impact of developmental stage on pheon-
menology, diagnosis and assessment and treatment of social phobia.

1998 321 pages

DESCRIPTION

3307 PHOTOSENSITIVITY

Covers these related disorders: Photoallergic reaction, Phototoxic reaction
May involve these systems in the body (see Section III):
Dermatologic System

Photosensitivity is an abnormal reaction of the skin to sunlight or artificial light that is usually characterized by the rapid development of redness, swelling, tenderness, peeling, blistering, hives, or other skin irregularities. The skin reactions associated with photosensitivity are often induced by the interaction of light and certain substances known as photosensitizers that are ingested or applied directly to the skin. Such photosensitizers may include antibodies, antifungal agents, and other drugs as well as some perfumes, soaps, dyes, and plants (e.g., buttercups, parsley, parsnips, mustard, etc.).

Particular wavelengths of light interact with photosensitizers to produce skin inflammations (dermatitis) that may be considered photoallergic or phototoxic. A photoallergic reaction is a delayed immune or allergic response of the skin that results from having been previously exposed to a photosensitizer and light. Such photosensitizers may include barbiturates, certain antibiotics such as tetracycline, and other medications as well as certain topical agents such as coal tar derivatives, perfume oils such as bergamot, etc. A phototoxic reaction is a nonimmune response to the accumulation of certain chemicals in the skin. This type of skin reaction may be similar in appearance to a severe sunburn; some individuals may develop hives or blisters. The initial inflammation is usually followed by abnormally increased skin pigmentation (hyperpigmentation). Phototoxic reactions result from high doses of certain photosensitizers that may cause photoallergic reactions in lower doses, as well as from additional chemical substances. Treatment includes the withdrawal of offending medications and other photosensitizers and sunlight avoidance. In addition, administration of antihistamines and topical corticosteroids may be effective in eliminating associated itching.

Photosensitivity is also associated with certain disorders in children. Such disorders may include congenital erythropoietic porphyria (EPP), an autosomal recessive disorder that results from a deficiency of an enzyme. This particular enzyme is necessary for the synthesis of heme, which is the oxygen-carrying component of a certain protein (hemoprotein) found in the tissues of the body. Congenital erythropoietic porphyria develops within a few months of birth and is characterized by a severe sensitivity to light that may cause blistering eruptions on the skin, leading to severe scarring, abnormally increased skin pigmentation, and other skin irregularities. Children with this disorder may also have numerous other abnormalities. Erythropoietic protoporphyria is an autosomal dominant disorder that results from a deficiency of an enzyme that is also essential to the proper synthesis of heme. This disorder appears during early childhood and is characterized by pain, tingling, and a burning feeling upon exposure to sunlight. The skin may redden, swell, and form blisters or hives. In addition to nail irregularities, children may develop fever and chills. Repeated exposure to sunlight may result in skin thickening and other chronic associated irregularities; however, some children experience improvement after the age of 10 years. Treatment for these types of disorders includes the avoidance of direct sunlight and the use of protective clothing and appropriate sunscreens. In addition, the administration of sufficient quantities of beta-carotene to cause a light yellowing of the skin may be effective in reducing sensitivity to sunlight. Photosensitivity is a feature of many other disorders that may include Cockayne syndrome, xeroderma pigmentosum, hydroa vacciniforme, Rothmund-Thomson syndrome, and other diseases.

Occasionally, some individuals experience photosensitive reactions to sunlight in the absence of any apparent photosensitizer or associated disease. This type of photosensitivity is called polymorphous light eruption and is characterized by the appearance of hives or other itchy, rash-type reactions on exposed areas. Polymorphous light eruption usually occurs after a prolonged initial sun exposure in the spring or summer. The eruption may occur within hours or days of the exposure and may remain for hours, days, or weeks. Treatment may include oral or topical corticosteroid therapy. In addition, susceptible people are counseled to avoid the sun, wear protective clothing, and use sunscreen.

Individuals with certain types of photosensitivity may benefit from the cautious administration of photosensitizing drugs that enhance pigmentation of the skin (psoralens). In addition, certain types of phototherapy may be effective. Other treatment is symptomatic and supportive.

The following organizations in the General Resources Section can provide additional information: National Organization for Rare Disorders, Inc., (NORD), March of Dimes Birth Defects Foundation, Genetic Alliance, NIH/National Institute of Child Health and Human Development, NIH/National Institute of Arthritis and Musculoskeletal and Skin Diseases, NIH/National Eye Institute, NIH/Office of Rare Diseases

DESCRIPTION

3308 PICA

Disorder Type: Mental, Emotional or Behavioral Disorder

Pica is a type of eating disorder characterized by the recurrent or chronic ingestion of nonfood or nonnutritive substances such as dirt, flaking paint or plaster, clay, charcoal, ashes, wool, and other nonfoods. Although this psychological disorder usually commences during the first or second year of life, some children are affected during infancy. Pica is often self-limiting with resolution occurring during the childhood years; however, sometimes it may persist into adolescence or adulthood. If the symptoms associated with pica occur initially in older children or adults (e.g., pregnant women), this is usually indicative of a nutritional deficiency rather than a psychological disorder.

Children who are mentally retarded are particularly susceptible to development of this unusual disorder. Other factors that may influence the evolution of pica include environmental influences such as family discord, lack of or ineffective nurturing, and nutritional and emotional neglect. In addition, pica is sometimes associated with certain psychiatric disorders.

Children who eat nonfood or nonnutritive substances may be at risk of developing certain types of parasitic infections. For example, the ingestion of dirt (geophagia) may result in toxocariasis, an infection resulting from the spread of the larvae of the common roundworm (Toxocara canis) throughout the body. Symptoms of toxocariasis are often mild and may include fever, weakness, and discomfort. Other children may develop a cough, wheezing, enlarged liver (hepatomegaly), and eye lesions. In addition, another parasitic infection known as toxoplasmosis may develop from dirt ingestion. This common parasitic infection is caused by Toxoplasma gondii and may produce no symptoms or may sometimes be characterized by rash, fever, and other mononu-

cleosis-type symptoms. In individuals with compromised immune systems, toxoplasmosis may result in more serious, widespread disease. Children who eat paint, paint dust, or paint flakes are at risk of developing lead poisoning that may damage the central nervous system, red blood cells, and digestive system.

Treatment for pica is symptomatic and supportive. Nutritional supplements may be considered.

The following organizations in the General Resources Section can provide additional information: National Organization for Rare Disorders, Inc., (NORD), NIH/Office of Rare Diseases, National Alliance for the Mentally Ill (NAMI), NIH/National Mental Health Association, National Mental Health Consumer Self-Help Clearinghouse, NIH/National Institute of Mental Health

Web Sites

3309 Pica Information Page
www.tobacco.org/Misc/pica.html

DESCRIPTION

3310 PINWORM (ENTEROBIUS VERMICULARIS)
Synonyms: Enterobiasis, Oxyuriasis, Threadworm
Disorder Type: Infectious Disease

Pinworm infection (enterobiasis) refers to a common condition in which small, white, parasitic worms (Enterobius vermicularis) infect the human intestinal tract. Such infection results due to ingestion of parasitic eggs. The eggs hatch in the stomach, and the larvae then typically migrate to and grow within the upper part of the large intestine (cecum). On rare occasions, pinworms may migrate to the vagina of affected girls, potentially causing such symptoms as vaginal irritation or itching. Pinworms have also been recovered from other areas of the body, such as the appendix and a certain region of the abdominal cavity (peritoneal cavity).

At night, pinworms migrate from the intestines to the anal region where they deposit their eggs, potentially causing itching (pruritus), irritation, and sleeplessness (insomnia). Scratching often results in reinfestation from ingestion of eggs that become imbedded under the fingernails and are inadvertently deposited in the mouth. Parasitic eggs are also often deposited from the anal area onto clothing, bedding, furniture, or toys, where they may then be transferred from the fingers to the mouth, causing reinfection or infection of others. In addition, in some cases, eggs may be inhaled from the air and swallowed. Parasitic eggs may remain viable for up to three weeks at regular room temperature.

The diagnosis of enterobiasis is made by detecting parasitic eggs or pinworms. The eggs or worms may be obtained by pressing sticky tape against the perianal region of affected children during early morning hours before the children awaken. The tape is then examined under a microscope by a physician or other medical technician to verify the presence of pinworms or eggs. In addition, pinworms may sometimes be detected by the naked eye. Treatment may include the administration of drugs that destroy pinworms (anthelmintic drugs), such as pyrantel pamoate or mebendazole, and, in some patients, topical anti-itch ointments that help relieve itching and irritation. Anthelmintic medications may also be prescribed to all other members of the household.

Enterobiasis is a very common infection that may occur in individuals of all ages. However, children between the ages of five to 14 years are most commonly affected.

The following organizations in the General Resources Section can provide additional information: NIH/National Institute of Child Health and Human Development, NIH/National Institute of Allergy and Infectious Disease, National Organization for Rare Disorders, Inc., (NORD), World Health Organization (WHO), Centers for Disease Control (CDC)

Web Sites

3311 CDC Pinworm Fact Sheet
www.cdc.gov/health/pinworm.htm

3312 Pediatric Database (PEDBASE)
www.icondata.com/health/pedbase/files/PIN-WORM.HTM

DESCRIPTION

3313 PITYRIASIS ROSEA

May involve these systems in the body (see Section III):
Dermatologic System

Pityriasis rosea is an inflammatory skin condition that may develop at any age but mostly commonly affects children and young adults. In some cases, the onset of the condition may be preceded by certain generalized symptoms, such as fever, inflammation of the throat (pharyngitis), and muscle and joint pain (myalgia and arthralgia). Pityriasis rosea typically begins with the development of a single oval or round patch known as a herald patch. This patch is usually red, pink, or light brown with a raised border and is covered with fine scales. A herald patch varies in diameter from one to 10 centimeters and may occur anywhere on the body. About five to 10 days after the appearance of the herald patch, there is a widespread eruption of similar, smaller patches (lesions), particularly on the torso and upper arms and thighs. These lesions, which are less than one centimeter in diameter, are usually slightly raised, oval or round, and red, pink, or light brown. In addition, they may be scaly and tend to peel. Lesions may continue to appear over several days and develop on other areas of the body, such as the forearms and calves, face, and scalp. The lesions are typically distributed along the subtle lines in the skin that indicate the direction of skin fibers (Langer's or cleavage lines). Some individuals with the condition may experience no associated symptoms (asymptomatic). Others may experience mild to severe itching (pruritus). Pityriasis rosea is a self-limited condition that has a duration of approximately two to 12 weeks, with an average of approximately four to five weeks. As skin lesions heal, affected areas may have abnormally increased or diminished pigmentation (postinflammatory hyperpigmentation or hypopigmentation) that gradually resolves after several weeks or months.

If individuals with pityriasis rosea experience no associated symptoms, treatment may not be necessary. Those with widespread lesions and scaling may benefit from using a cream that softens the skin (emollient). Associated itching may be relieved by lubricating lotions that contain the natural compounds camphor or menthol or medicated skin creams, such as a nonfluorinated topical corticosteroid. Certain medications taken by mouth such as oral antihistamines may help those who experience bothersome itching while attempting to sleep. Antihistamines, which are medications that often induce drowsiness, reduce the effects of histamine, a chemical that is released during allergic inflammatory reactions.

The cause of pityriasis rosea is unknown. However, many researchers speculate that the condition results from infection with a viral agent.

The following organizations in the General Resources Section can provide additional information: NIH/National Institute of Arthritis and Musculoskeletal and Skin Diseases

National Associations & Support Groups

3314 National Psoriasis Foundation
6600 SW 92nd Avenue Suite 300
Portland, OR 97223   503-244-7404
800-723-9166
Fax: 503-245-0626
e-mail: getinfo@npsusa.org
www.psoriasis.org

Offers information, support and referrals for victims of psoriasis and their families.

Gail M. Zimmerman, Executive Director

Web Sites

3315 DermNet:
www.dermnet.org.nz/dna.pitros.html

3316 Indiana University
www.pathology.iupui.edu/drhood/pityriasis-rosea.html

Pamphlets

3317 Pityriasis Rosea
American Academy of Dermatology
930 N Meacham Road
Schaumberg, IL 60173   847-330-0230
                             Fax: 847-330-0050
                             www.aad.org

Discusses the appearance, symptoms, and causes
of this common rash. Diagnosis and treatment
are also explained.

DESCRIPTION

3318 PNEUMONIA

Disorder Type: Infectious Disease

Pneumonia refers to a group of disorders characterized by an acute inflammation of the lungs. The causes of pneumonia are many and may include infection by certain bacteria, viruses, bacteria-like organisms, fungi, yeasts, and protozoa. In addition, noninfectious causes include the inhalation (aspiration) of food or other substances into the airway and lungs, an abnormal response of the immune system to certain substances (hypersensitivity reaction), and an inflammatory response to radiation or certain drugs. Pneumonia may also result as a complication of surgery or injury, due to the impaired ability to cough, breathe deeply, or expel mucus.

Pneumonia in very young children is most commonly caused by certain respiratory viruses, such as RSV, or respiratory syncytial virus; influenza; parainfluenza; and adenoviruses. Symptoms and findings associated with this type of pneumonia in infants and young children may include cough, nasal discharge, fever, rapid breathing (tachypnea), or a bluish color to the skin and mucous membranes (cyanosis). Antibiotics do not treat viral infections, though some viruses are susceptible to new antiviral therapies. Most infants and children recover from viral pneumonia with no complications. However, some may develop subsequent lung irregularities.

Although bacterial pneumonia is not common among children, certain conditions (e.g., viral respiratory illnesses, immune deficiency disorders, certain congenital defects, blood irregularities, etc.) may put them at increased risk for developing this type of pneumonia. The most common types of bacteria that cause pneumonia in children include Streptococcus pneumoniae (pneumococcus), Streptococcus pyogenes, Staphylococcus aureus, and Haemophilus influenzae type b. Symptoms associated with bacterial pneumonia vary according to age, type of bacteria involved, and other factors. Infants and young children may develop a stuffy nose and other signs of upper respiratory infection, loss of appetite, sudden onset of fever, restlessness, respiratory distress, and cyanosis. In addition, infants with Staphylococcus aureus infection, a more serious type of disease, may develop lethargy, increased irritability, difficulty breathing (dyspnea), vomiting, or diarrhea. Abscesses may form in the lungs and may lead to the development of air-containing cysts (pneumatoceles). Accumulation of pus, or empyema, may occur in the space surrounding the lungs. Older children and adolescents with bacterial pneumonia may develop symptoms commonly associated with mild upper respiratory tract infection followed by chills, shaking, fever, drowsiness, rapid breathing, coughing, or chest pain. Infection with Haemophilus influenzae type b may be prevented by the administration of Haemophilus vaccine. Treatment for bacterial pneumonia includes the use of appropriate antibiotics. In the case of Staphylococcus aureus infection, drainage of pus accumulations may be indicated. Other treatment is symptomatic and supportive.

Atypical pneumonias include those resulting from infection by bacteria-like microorganisms such as Mycoplasma pneumoniae and Chlamydia pneumoniae. Symptoms associated with these types of infections include fatigue, sore throat, cough, joint pain, or rash. Treatment may include the use of certain antibiotics.

Children with compromised immune systems are at risk for developing certain types of pneumonia infections caused by fungi (e.g., histoplasmosis, coccidioidomycosis, cryptococcosis, etc.) and other common organisms such as Pneumocystis carinii. Pneumocystis pneumonia is particularly prevalent among individuals with AIDS. Choice of drug therapy relates to the appropriate identification of the causative organism. Other treatment is symptomatic and supportive.

The following organizations in the General Resources Section can provide additional information: National Organization for Rare Disorders, Inc., (NORD), March of Dimes Birth Defects Foundation, NIH/National Institute of Allergy and Infectious Disease, World Health Organization (WHO)

Web Sites

3319 American Lung Association
www.lungssa.org/diseases/lungpneumoni.html

3320 Department of Health and Human Services
www.ahcpr.gov/consumer/pneucons.htm

3321 Kid's Health
http://kidshealth.org/parent/common/pneumonia.html

3322 Mayo Clinic
http://www.mayohealth.org/mayo/9311/htm/cold-flu.htm

3323 National Jewish & Medical Research Center
http://www.njc.org/MFhtml/PNE MF.html

DESCRIPTION

3324 POLIO

Synonyms: Heine-Medin disease, Infantile Paralysis, Medin's disease, Poliomyelitis
Disorder Type: Infectious Disease

Polio, or poliomyelitis, is an acute infectious disease that is caused by one of three polioviruses transmitted through fecal contamination or, occasionally, through the air. In some patients, polio may produce no symptoms (asymptomatic poliomyelitis), but will grant immunity to those infected. In most patients, especially young children, polio is accompanied by only mild symptoms (abortive poliomyelitis). These symptoms usually appear three to five days after infection and may include fever, headache, sore throat, vomiting, weakness, and abdominal discomfort. Recovery is often complete in one to three days. However, in some cases there is only a brief recovery period before symptoms reappear, accompanied by additional findings related to involvement of the brain and spinal cord such as stiffness of the neck and back and skin sensitivity. This reappearance is designated as major illness and, in some cases, may develop directly after abortive poliomyelitis, with no recovery period between. Major illness, more common in older children and adults, may be further categorized as nonparalytic or paralytic. In nonparalytic polio, symptoms progress no further and there is complete recovery; however, in paralytic polio, brain and spinal cord involvement progresses to include paralysis of certain muscles, especially of the lower trunk and legs. Infection may involve a portion of the brain stem (medulla oblongata), possibly resulting in difficulties with swallowing and breathing. In rare cases, symptoms and findings associated with this disease may be potentially life-threatening. Approximately 50 percent of those affected with paralytic polio recover with no residual effects of the disease. Approximately 25 percent may experience minor, but permanent, muscle weakness. Those remaining may experience severe and permanent disability. In addition, two to three decades after infection, some individuals who had paralytic polio may experience renewed muscle weakness and pain (post-polio syndrome).

Immunization to prevent polio is routinely administered in a series of vaccination doses active against all three types of the poliovirus. Oral vaccine (Sabin vaccine), containing live but harmless virus, is most commonly given to children. In very rare cases, live vaccine may cause polio in the person vaccinated or in those with close contact. For this reason, children with compromised immune systems and those in direct contact with these children are usually given inactivated polio vaccine (Salk vaccine). Treatment for those with mild disease or nonparalytic polio may include bedrest and the administration of pain relievers. Paralysis usually necessitates the use of physical therapy to prevent damage and enhance function of the affected muscles. In addition, ventilators or surgical methods (i.e., tracheostomy) may be employed in those with impaired respiratory function. Other treatment is symtomatic and supportive.

The following organizations in the General Resources Section can provide additional information: National Organization for Rare Disorders, Inc., (NORD), March of Dimes Birth Defects Foundation, NIH/National Institute of Allergy and Infectious Disease, World Health Organization (WHO), Centers for Disease Control (CDC)

National Associations & Support Groups

3325 International Polio Network
Gazette International Networking Institute
4207 Lindell Blvd., #110
St.Louis, MO 63108
314-534-0475
Fax: 314-534-5070
e-mail: gini_intl@msn.com
www.post-polio.org

Dedicated to supporting the independant living, self direction, and personal acheivement of people with disabilities worldwide. Promotes patient and professional education, has a network of support groups, conducts workshops and conferances, and offer a networking program.

Joan L. Headley, Executive Director

3326 Polio Society
4200 Wisconsin Ave NW, PMB #106-273
Washington, DC 20016   301-897-8180
                              Fax: 202-466-1911
                              e-mail: jsh1@mhg.edu

Created for the purpose of providing educational resources and support group services to people who had polio and are now experiencing the late effects of polio. We are a chartered non-profit organization governed by a board of directors composed primarily of polio survivors and family members of polio survivors. Our programs and services are funded by membership dues, gifts and private contributions. Staffed chiefly by volunteers, donations go toward programming and outreach efforts.

5000 members

3327 Polio Survivors Association
12720 La Reina Avenue
Downey, CA 90242   213-923-0034

Web Sites

3328 PBS on Jonas Salk
www.pbs.org/wgbh/aso/databank/entries/bmasalk.html

3329 Polio Connection of America
www.village.ios.com/~w1066/

3330 Polio Experience Network
www.polionet.org/

3331 Polio Information Center Online
www.cumicro2.cpmc.columbia.edu/PICO/PICO.html

3332 Polio Remember Your Strength Foundation
www.prys.net/home.htm

3333 Polio Survivors' Page
www.eskimo.com/~dempt/polio.html

3334 Polio.com
www.polio.com/

Books

3335 IVUN Resource Directory
Gazette International Networking Institute
4207 Lindell Blvd., #110
St.Louis, MO 63108   314-534-0475
                            Fax: 314-534-5070
                            e-mail: gini_intl@msn.com
                            www.post-polio.org

A networking tool for heatlh professionals and both long-term and new ventilator users. Sections include health professionals, ventilaro users, equipment and mask manufacturers, service and repair, organizations, etc. Published annually in October.

Joan L. Headley, Executive Director

3336 Post-Polio Directory
Gazette International Networking Institute
4207 Lindell Blvd., #110
St.Louis, MO 63108   314-534-0475
                            Fax: 314-534-5070
                            e-mail: gini_intl@msn.com
                            www.post-polio.org

Lists self-identified clinics, health professionals, and support groups knowledgeable about the late effects of polio. The Directory contains over 500 entries including an international section. Published annually in March

Joan L. Headley, Executive Director

Newsletters

3337 Polio Network News
Gazette International Networking Institute
4207 Lindell Blvd., #110
St. Louis, MO 63108   314-534-0475

12 pages Quarterly

Joan L. Headley, Executive Director

DESCRIPTION

3338 POLYDACTYLY

Synonyms: Polydactylia, Polydactylism
Disorder Type: Birth Defect, Genetic Disorder

Poldactyly refers to an abnormality that is present at birth (congenital) in which an infant has more than the usual number of fingers or toes (supernumerary digits) or, in some cases, extra fingers and toes. Defects associated with this abnormality may range from simple skin tags or stumps of flesh to extra fingers or toes that are completely developed. In some families polydactyly is passed from generation to generation.

Polydactyly involving the toes is somewhat common, occurring in approximately two out of every 1,000 births. Although the fifth toe is the digit most often duplicated, polydactyly sometimes affects the great or big toe. Before treatment is initiated, careful evaluation is indicated so that treatment of possible associated abnormalities may be appropriately coordinated. However, if the extra digit is small or rudimentary, it may be tied off (ligated) at birth or soon thereafter. This method allows for the digit to spontaneously detach itself after a period of time. In those cases where the digit is jointed, treatment usually involves surgical amputation of the extra digit and repair of other associated structures and tissues. Surgical intervention of this type is usually performed at approximately one year of age.

Duplication of a finger usually appears near teh small finger (pinky) or thumb. As in polydactyly of the toes, small, rudimentary digits may be tied off, while more complex deformities typically require surgical intervention at about one year of age.

Polydactyly may also occur in association with several genetic disorders. These disorders include acrocephalopolysyndactyly type II (Carpenter's syndrome), characterized by mental retardation and irregularities involving the head, hand, and genitalia; trisomy 13 syndrome (Patau's syndrome), characterized by cleft lip and palate, polydactyly, mental retardation, and irregularities of the central nervous system, heart, genitalia, and internal organs; chondroectodermal dysplasia (Ellis-van Creveld syndrome), a bone growth disorder characterized by short stature, cardiac defects, polydactyly, and developmental defects of the teeth, and nails (hypoplastic). The efficacy of treating polydactyly associated with these and other disorders depends upon the exact nature of the disorder in question.

The following organizations in the General Resources Section can provide additional information: National Organization for Rare Disorders, Inc. (NORD), Genetic Alliance, NIH/National Institute of Child Health and Human Development, March of Dimes Birth Defects Foundation, NIH/National Institute of Arthritis and Musculoskeletal and Skin Diseases

National Associations & Support Groups

3339 CHERUB—Association of Families and Friends of Children with Limb Disorders
936 Delaware Avenue
Buffalo, NY 14209

Offers support to families of juveniles diagnosed with a limb disorder.

3340 Shriners Hospitals for Children
P.O. Box 31356
Tampa, FL 33613
813-281-0300
800-237-5055
Fax: 813-281-8496
www.shrinershq.org

Network of 22 hospitals that provide expert, no-cost orthopaedic and burn care to children under 18.

Web Sites

3341 CliniWeb
www.ohsu.edu/cliniweb/c5/c5.660.585.600.html

3342 Superkids, Inc.
www.super-kids.org

DESCRIPTION

3343 PRADER-WILLI SYNDROME
Synonym: PWS
May involve these systems in the body (see Section III):
 Genetic Disorder

Prader-Willi syndrome is a genetic disorder characterized by severely diminished muscle tone (hypotonia) during early infancy, short stature, unusually small hands and feet, obesity, genital abnormalities, and mental retardation. The disorder is thought to affect approximately one in 15,000 individuals. In most cases of Prader-Willi syndrome, there is decreased fetal activity during the last months of pregnancy. After birth, most affected infants experience severe loss of muscle tone (hypotonia), have feeding difficulties due to decreased swallowing and sucking reflexes, and fail to grow and gain weight at the expected rate (failure to thrive). Starting at approximately six months to six years of age, affected infants or children begin to have an excessive appetite, become obsessed with eating, or lack a sense of satisfaction after a meal and often engage in binge-type eating. As a result, patients develop an abnormally increased body weight (progressive obesity) due to an excessive accumulation of body fat, particularly over the thighs, buttocks, and lower abdomen.

Infants and children with Prader-Willi syndrome also may have characteristic abnormalities of the head and face (craniofacial area), such as almond-shaped eyes, upslanting eyelid folds (palpebral fissures), abnormal deviation of one eye in relation to the other (strabismus), a thin, tented upper lip, and full cheecks. In addition, affected males and females may have insufficient secretion of certain hormones that stimulate the gonads (hypogonadotropic hypogonadism). The gonads are the reproductive glands, such as the testes or ovaries, within which the reproductive cells (sperm or ova) are produced. Affected males typically have an abnormally small penis (micropenis) and unde-

scended testes (cryptorchidism), potentially delayed or incomplete development of secondary sexual charateristics, insufficient production of the male sex hormone testosterone, decreased or absent sperm production, and infertility. Affected females often have abnormally small underdeveloped external genitalia (i.e., hypoplastic labia minor and clitoris), absence or abnormal cessation of menstrual cycles (primary or secondary amenorrhea), and infertility. Development of female secondary sexual characteristics may be normal or incomplete. Most children with Prader-Willi syndrome also have mild to moderate mental retardation; however, in some cases, severe mental retardation may be present. Many affected children also experience difficulties with speech articulation and may have an abnormally high-pitched, nasal voice. Although children with Prader-Willi syndrome may often be cheerful and good natured, behavioral problems may become apparent during later childhood, including outbursts of anger, rage-like episodes, and stubbornness.

Some individuals with Prader-Willi syndrome may develop diabetes mellitus during or soon after puberty. Diabetes mellitus is characterized by impaired fat, protein, and carbohydrate metabolism due to insufficient production of the hormone insulin or the body's inability to appropriately utilize insulin. Associated symptoms may include excessive thirst and urination. In addition, adolescents and young adults may be prone to experiencing cardiac insufficiency, potentially resulting in life-threatening complications during the second or third decade of life.

In children with Prader-Willi syndrome, treatment typically includes measures to help prevent progressive obesity or to ensure strict weight control, such as a low-calorie diet and a proper exercise program under a physician's direction. In addition, nutritional behavioral modification methods may be implemented that require the cooperation and support of all family members, such as ensuring regular feeding habits (e.g., having meals at the same time and location on a daily basis) and the inaccessibility of food between meals. In young males with Prader-Willi syndrome, testosterone replacement therapy may result in enlargement of micropenis; in addition, testosterone therapy during adolescence or young adulthood may have beneficial effects on the development of secondary sexual characteristics. Treatment of children with Prader-Willi syndrome also may include special education and behavioral therapies to help manage behavioral problems.

Prader-Willi syndrome is caused by deletion or disruption of certain genes (contiguous gene syndrome) located on the long arm of chromosome 15 (15q11-13). Most affected individuals have missing genetic material or deletion of 15q11-13 that affects the chromosome received from the father (paternally derivwed chromosome).

The following organizations in the General Resources Section can provide additional information: National Organization for Rare Disorders, Inc., (NORD), NIH/Office of Rare Diseases, March of Dimes Birth Defects Foundation, Genetic Alliance, Online Mendelian Inheritance in Man:

www3.ncbi.nlm.nih.gov/Omim/searchomim.html

National Associations & Support Groups

3344 Prader-Willi Connection
40 Holly Lane
Roslyn Heights, NY 11577   516-621-2445
                                  800-358-0682
                            Fax: 516-484-7154
        e-mail: foundation@prader-willi.inter.net
                            www.prader-willi.org

24 hour fax hotline and the information forum on the internet.

3345 Prader-Willi Foundation
223 Main Street
Port Washington, NY 11050   516-944-8136
                                   800-926-4797
                             Fax: 516-944-3173
        e-mail: foundation@prader-willi.inter.net
                             www.willi.inter.net

A major non-profit public charity that works for the benefit of individuals with Prader-Willi syndrome and their families, as well as professionals who work with the PWS population.

Janalee Heinmenn, Executive Director

3346 Prader-Willi Syndrome Association
5700 Midnight Pass Road, Suite 6
Sarasota, FL 34242   941-312-0400
                                 800-926-4797
                           Fax: 941-312-0142
                 e-mail: pwsausa@aol.com
                            www.pwsausa.org

Provides to parents and professionals a national and international network of information, support services and research endeavors to expressly meet the needs of affected children and adults and their families. Offers 31 state chapters and published materials on numerous topics ranging from family stress to wills.

Janalee Heinemann, Executive Director

International

3347 Prader-Willi Syndrome Association (UK)
33 Leopold St.
Derby Intl.,
United Kingdom
                e-mail: roger@pwsa-uk.demon.co.uk
                          www.pwsa-ukdemon.co.uk

Provides to parents and professionals a national and international network of information, support services and research endeavors to exspressly meet the needs of affected children and adults and their families. Offers 31 state chapter and published materials ranging from family stress to wills.

State Agencies & Support Groups

Alabama

3348 PWSA of Alabama
Prader-Willi Syndrome Association
117 Pavillion Drive
Meridianville, AL 35759   256-828-6889

Cheryl Couch, President

Arizona

3349 PWSA of Arizona
Prader-Willi Syndrome Association
7725 E 33rd St.
Tuscan, AZ 85710   520-296-9172

Teresa Kellerman, President

Arkansas

3350 PWSA of Arkansas
Prader-Willi Syndrome Association
2504 South Drive
North Little Rock, AR 72118   501-753-8715

Jim Patton, President

California

3351 PWS Foundation of California
Prader-Willi Foundation
360 Mobil Ave, Ste 205C
Camarillo, CA 93010

Fran Moss, Executive Director

3352 PWS Foundation of California (Solana Beach)
Prader-Willi Foundation
616 Ridgeline Road
Solana Beach, CA 92705   858-509-0741
                                805-389-3484
                           Fax: 858-509-0728
                      e-mail: pwcf@msn.com

Paul Paolini, President

3353 PWSA of California
Prader-Willi Syndrome Association
805 El Toro Drive
Bakersfield, CA 93304   805-831-7627

Wesley Crawford

Colorado

3354 PWSA of Colorado
Prader-Willi Syndrome Association
6477 W. Nova Dr.
Littleton, CO 80128   303-973-4780

Lynette Hosler, President

Connecticut

3355 PWSA of Connecticut
Prader-Willi Syndrome Association
5 Sunset Drive
Danbury, CT 06811   203-744-4189

Barbara Farmer, President

3356 PWSA of Connecticut (North Haven)
Prader-Willi Syndrome Association
35 Ansonia Drive
North Haven, CT 06473   203-744-4189
                      e-mail: bmaf@juno.com

Barb Farmer, President

Delaware

3357 PWSA of Delaware
Prader-Willi Syndrome Association
455 Granger Drive
Bear, DE 19701   302-836-6213
                   Fax: 302-428-4548
              e-mail: swede455@aol.com

Karen Swanson, President

Florida

3358 PWSA of Florida
Prader-Willi Syndrome Association
2246 19th Court NE
Jensen Beach, FL 34957   561-334-7389

Dan Krauer, President

3359 PWSA of Florida (Tampa)
Prader-Willi Syndrome Association
1914 West Carmen Street
Tampa, FL 33606   813-251-1259
                  e-mail: PWFA2000@aol.com

Debbie Peaton, President
Keith Peaton, President

Georgia

3360 PWSA of Georgia
Prader-Willi Syndrome Association
111 Chestnut St.
Roswell, GA 30075   770-518-4795

Hope M. Mays, Executive Director

Hawaii

3361 PWSA of Hawaii
Prader-Willi Syndrome Association
269 Kaha Street
Kailua, HI 96734   808-263-8177
                          e-mail: Oncpa@pixi.com

Tarni Ho, President

Idaho

3362 PWSA of Idaho
Prader-Willi Syndrome Association
RR 1 Box 31N
Athol, ID 83801   208-683-2993

Gene Todhunter

Illinois

3363 PWSA of Illinois
Prader-Willi Syndrome Association
14107 Catherine Dr.
Orland Park, IL 60462   708-460-2535

Karen Engelhardt, President

3364 PWSA of Illinois Group
Prader-Willi Syndrome Association
200 East Delaware Place, Apt 15E
Chicago, IL 60611   312-664-3090
                          e-mail: Kengelz@uic.edu

Karen Englhardt, President

Indiana

3365 PWSA of Indiana
Prader-Willi Syndrome Association
4912 Cayman Court
Columbus, IN 47203   812-372-1901
                          e-mail: jacmac@in.net

Jacque McGuire, President

Iowa

3366 PWSA of Iowa
Prader-Willi Syndrome Association
15554 226th Street
Zwingle, IA 52079   319-686-4270
                          e-mail: Ktcaeday@netins.net

Tammy Davis, President

Kansas

3367 PWSA of Kansas
Prader-Willi Syndrome Association
117 S. Topeka Avenue
Scranton, KS 66537   785-793-2539

Mike Hamblin
Carolyn Hamblin

Kentucky

3368 PWSA of Kentucky
Prader-Willi Syndrome Association
P.O. Box 18132
Louisville, KY 40261   502-968-2626

Willie Lacy, President

Louisiana

3369 PWSA of Region Gulf Coast (Louisiana, Mississippi)
Prader-Willi Syndrome Association
333 Wilkinson
Shreveport, LA 71104   318-222-4689
                          e-mail: KKPWS616198@aol.com

Serving patients and familes with Prader-Willi syndrome of the Louisanna and Mississippi region.

Velma Jones, President

Maryland

3370 PWSA of Maryland & Metro Washington DC Inc
Prader-Willi Syndrome Association
14608 Stonewall Drive
Silver Spring, MD 20905   301-384-4955
                          Fax: 301-384-4955
                          e-mail: Keder@erols.com

Linda Keder, President

Massachusetts

3371 PWSA of Massachusetts
Prader-Willi Syndrome Association
377 Cross Road
North Dartmouth, MA 02747   508-991-6705

Kim Silva, President

3372 PWSA of Region New England
Prader-Willi Syndrome Association
377 Cross Road
North Dartmouth, MA 02747   508-991-6705
          e-mail: Pwsane@aol.com

Kim Howlett-Silva, President

Michigan

3373 PWSA of Michigian
Prader-Willi Syndrome Association
2213 Cross Country Drive
Kalamazoo, MI 49009   616-353-7556
          Fax: 616-353-7556
          e-mail: Carolynloker@yahoo.com

Jim Loker, President
Caroline Loker, President

Minnesota

3374 PWSA of Minnesota
Prader-Willi Syndrome Association
8131 Westbend Road
Minneapolis, MN 55427   612-546-4926
          e-mail: Nshapiro@bernick-lifson.com

Neal Shapiro, President

Missouri

3375 PWSA of Missouri
Prader-Willi Syndrome Association
219 Paddlewheel Drive
Florussant, MO 63033   314-839-0644
          e-mail: Prespwsamo@aol.com

Mark Floretta, President

Nebraska

3376 PWSA of Nebraska
Prader-Willi Syndrome Association
1441 S. 167th Ave.
Omaha, NE 68130   402-333-8400

Roger Rhoads, President

Nevada

3377 PWSA of Nevada
Prader-Willi Syndrome Association
1671 Heather Ridge Road
North Las Vegas, NV 89031   702-486-1548

Mary Jackson, President

New Jersey

3378 PWSA of New Jersey
Prader-Willi Syndrome Association
16 Gettysburg Way
Lincoln Park, NJ 07035   973-628-6945
          e-mail: maaemba@bellatlantic.net

Doug Taylor, President

New York

3379 PWSA of New York
Prader-Willi Syndrome Association
190 Lincoln Place
Brooklyn, NY 11217   718-783-0181

Henry Singer, President

3380 PWSA of New York Alliance
Prader-Willi Syndrome Association
267 Oxford Street
Rochester, NY 14607   716-442-1655

Henry Singer, President

North Carolina

3381 PWSA of North Carolina
Prader-Willi Syndrome Association
10001 Windrift Road
Charlotte, NC 28215   704-537-3656

Patricia Spitler, President

North Dakota

3382 PWSA of North Dakota
Prader-Willi Syndrome Association
8501 435th Avenue NE
Regan, ND 58477   701-286-6228
e-mail: shellysivak@yahoo.com

Michelle Sivak, President

Ohio

3383 PWSA of Ohio
Prader-Willi Syndrome Association
1763 Hickory Hill Drive
Columbus, OH 43228   614-876-1732
e-mail: pwsaohio@aol.com

Tom Guisti, President

Oklahoma

3384 PWSA of Oklahoma
Prader-Willi Syndrome Association
3820 SE 89th Street
Oklahoma City, OK 73135   405-677-8089
e-mail: Rdmosley@swbell.net

Daphne Mosley, President

Oregon

3385 PWSA of Oregon
Prader-Willi Syndrome Associtaion
P.O. Box 204
Fairview, OR 97024   503-661-5146
e-mail: Jamesmw@hevenet.com

Kim Wingler, President

Pennsylvania

3386 PWSA of Pennsylvania
Prader-Willi Syndrome Association
102 Timberlane Drive
Pittsburgh, PA 15229   412-369-4433
e-mail: kahlanrule@aol.com

Maria Silvia, President

South Carolina

3387 PWSA of South Carolina
Prader-Willi Syndrome Association
1817 Pickens Street
Columbia, SC 29201   803-788-0544
e-mail: Kengel2@uic.edu

Rhett Eleazer, President

Tennessee

3388 PWSA of Tennessee
Prader-Willi Syndrome Association
105 Foxwood Lane
Franklin, TN 37065   615-790-6659
e-mail: Tebo333@aol.com

Terry Bolander, President

Texas

3389 PWSA of Texas
Prader-Willi Syndrome Association
11205 El Salido Parkway
Austin, TX 78750   512-219-7966
e-mail: smiley99@flash.net

Diane Smiley, President

Utah

3390 PWSA of Utah
Prader-Willi Syndrome Association
5295 South Cobble Creek Road, Apt. #26J
Holladay, UT 84121   801-277-9266

Pam Rauch

3391 PWSA of Utah (Orem)
Prader-Willi Syndrome Association
235 South Palisade Drive
Orem, UT 84097   801-221-5964

Brent Tobler, President
Tobler Pamela, Tobler

Virginia

3392 PWSA of Virginia
Prader-Willi Syndrome Association
3022 Fox Den Lane
Oakton, VA 22124   703-620-0330

Stacey Diaz, President

Washington

3393 PWSA of Region Northwest
Prader-Willi Syndrome Association
3706 29th Avenue West
Seattle, WA 98199
          e-mail: slundh@ips.net

Serving patients and families with Prader-Willi
syndrome in the Washington, Oregon, Idaho,
Alaska, and Hawaii regions.

Billie McSwan, Presidents

3394 PWSA of Washington
Prader-Willi Syndrome Association
8130 382nd Avenue Southeast
Snoqualmie, WA 98065

Janet Pearson, President

West Virginia

3395 PWSA of West Virginia
Prader-Willi Syndrome Association
717 Morgan Avenue
Morgantown, WV 26305   304-296-6412
          e-mail: Lee@be.wvu.edu

Henry Lee, President
Margaret Lee, President

Wisconsin

3396 PWSA of Wisconsin
Prader-Willi Syndrome Association
305 Amanda Way
Verona, WI 35393   608-238-6757
          Fax: 608-238-9597
          www.athenet.net/~pwsa-usa/WI/

Pat Bellan, President

3397 PWSA of Wisconsin - Madison
Prader-Willi Syndrome Association
115 Marinette Trail
Madison, WI 53593   608-238-6757

Pat LaBella, President

Web Sites

3398 Pedbase
www.icondata.com/health/ped-
base/files/PRADER-W.HTM

3399 Prader Willi Syndrome Chat
www.pwsausa.org/pwchat.htm

Books

3400 An Early Prader-Willi Syndrome Diagnosis & How to Make it Easier on Parents
Mary Patterson, author

Prader-Willi Foundation
223 Main Street
Port Washington, NY 11050   516-944-8136
          800-253-7993
          Fax: 516-944-3173
          e-mail: foundation@prader-willi.inter.net
          www.prader-willi.org

A parent of a child with PWS and an advocate
for others with the afflication speaks.

3401 Educational Choices for Children with PWS
Barry Margolis and Meg Comeau, author

Prader-Willi Foundation
223 Main Street
Port Washington, NY 11050   516-944-8136
          800-253-7993
          Fax: 516-944-3173
          e-mail: foundation@prader-willi.inter.net
          www.prader-willi.org

Parents of young children with Prader-Willi syndrome discuss their individual philosophies of
educational choice - inclusion vs. specialized setting.

3402 Handbook for Parents

Shirley Neason, author

Prader-Willi Syndrome Association
5700 Midnight Pass Road, Suite 6
Sarasota, FL 34242   941-312-0400
800-926-4797
Fax: 941-312-0142
e-mail: pwsausa@aol.com
www.pwsausa.org

Parent-to-parent handbook for understanding and managing issues related to PWS.

1999 75 pages

3403 Management of Prader-Willi Syndrome

Louise R. Greenwag, author

Prader-Willi Syndrome Association
5700 Midnight Pass Road, Suite 6
Sarasota, FL 34242   941-312-0400
800-926-4797
Fax: 941-312-0142
e-mail: pwsausa@aol.com
www.pwsausa.org

Comprehensive textbook on PWS.

1995 393 pages
ISBN: 0-387943-73-0

3404 Ongoing Research on Family Functioning & Behavior Problems in Prader-Willi

Elisabeth M. Dykens, PhD & Robert M. Hodapp, PhD, author

Prader-Willi Foundation
223 Main Street
Port Washington, NY 11050   516-944-8136
800-253-7993
Fax: 516-944-3173
e-mail: foundation@prader-willi.inter.net
www.prader-willi.org

Discusses the results of a survey conducted by the authors among families of individuals with PWS.

3405 Overview of PWS

Lota Mitchell, M.S.W., author

Prader-Willi Syndrome Association
5700 Midnight Pass Road, Suite 6
Sarasota, FL 34242   941-312-0400
800-926-4797
Fax: 941-312-0142
e-mail: pwsausa@aol.com
www.pwsausa.org

Offers information to parents and professionals on Prader-Willi Syndrome.

1994 13 pages

3406 Sometimes I'm Mad, Sometimes I'm Glad

Janalee Heinemann, author

Prader-Willi Syndrome Association
5700 Midnight Pass Road, Suite 6
Sarasota, FL 34242   941-312-0400
800-926-4797
Fax: 941-312-0142
e-mail: pwsausa@aol.com
www.pwsausa.org

Explains family relationships and how they are affected by PWS.

32 pages

3407 Supporting the Student/PWS for Teachers

Prader-Willi Syndrome Association
5700 Midnight Pass Road, Suite 6
Sarasota, FL 34242   941-312-0400
800-926-4797
Fax: 941-312-0142
e-mail: pwsausa@aol.com
www.pwsausa.org

Offers educational information for the professional dealing with a child who has PWS. Contains a worksheet, brochure, and 27-minute audiotape.

Newsletters

3408 Gathered View

Prader-Willi Syndrome Association
5700 Midnight Pass Road, Suite 6
Sarasotas Park, FL 34242   941-312-0400
800-926-4797
Fax: 941-312-0142
e-mail: pwsausa@aol.com
www.pwsausa.org

Offers current research findings, behavior and weight management techniques, educational news and more.

16+ pages BiMonthly

Linda Keder, Editor
Lota Mitchell, Editor

Pamphlets

3409 Directions: Help for Parents of Young Children with Prader-Willi Syndrome
Prader-Willi Syndrome Association
5700 Midnight Pass Road, Suite 6
Sarasota, FL 34242   941-312-0400
800-926-4797
Fax: 941-312-0142
e-mail: pwsausa@aol.com
www.pwsausa.org

Handbook for managing PWS from infancy through the age of five years.

1991 39 pages

3410 Gathered View Articles

Prader-Willi Syndrome Association
5700 Midnight Pass Road, Suite 6
Sarasota, FL 34242
941-312-0400
800-926-4797
Fax: 941-312-0142
e-mail: pwsausa@aol.com
www.pwsausa.org

A series of Association Newsletter reprints.

3411 Medical Alert: Prader-Willi Syndrome

Prader-Willi Syndrome Association
5700 Midnight Pass Road, Suite 6
Sarasota, FL 34242
941-312-0400
800-926-4797
Fax: 941-312-0142
e-mail: pwsausa@aol.com
www.pwsausa.org

A diagnosis and reference guide for physicians and other health professionals.

3412 Personal Reflections of a Mother

Prader-Willi Syndrome Association
5700 Midnight Pass Road, Suite 6
Sarasota, FL 34242
941-312-0400
800-926-4797
Fax: 941-312-0142
e-mail: pwsausa@aol.com
www.pwsausa.org

A collection of 15 articles.

3413 Physical Therapy Intervention in Prader- Willi Syndrome

Maria Fragala, PT, author

Prader-Willi Syndrome Association
5700 Midnight Pass Road, Ste 6
Sarasota, FL 34242
914-312-0400
800-926-4797
Fax: 941-312-0142
e-mail: pwsausa@aol.com
www.pwsausa.org

3414 Prader-Willi Syndrome: A Guide for Families & Others

Moris A. Angulo, MD, author

Prader-Willi Foundation
223 Main Street
Port Washington, NY 11050
516-944-8136
800-253-7993
Fax: 516-944-3173
e-mail: foundation@prader-willi.inter.net
www.prader-willi.org

Diagnostician and clinician gives a brief, non-technical introduction to PWS and its components.

3415 Prader-Willi Syndrome: Some Reflections on Behavior

Terrance N. James, PhD, author

Prader-Willi Foundation
223 Main Street
Port Washington, NY 11050
516-944-8136
800-253-7993
Fax: 516-944-3173
e-mail: foundation@prader-willi.inter.net
www.prader-willi.org

3416 Psychiatric Medicine & Prader-Willi Syndrome

Ivy Boyle, MD, author

Prader-Willi Foundation
223 Main Street
Port Washington, NY 11050
516-944-8136
800-253-7993
Fax: 516-944-3173
e-mail: foundation@prader-willi.inter.net
www.prader-willi.org

Child/adolescent psychiatrist and mother of a child with Prader-Willi syndrome speaks as an advocate of the use of psychiatric medicine in the treatment of certain aspects of PWS behaviors.

DESCRIPTION

3417 PRECOCIOUS PUBERTY

Synonym: Pubertas praecox

Covers these related disorders:

Gonadotropin-dependent precocious puberty,

Gonadotropin-independent precocious puberty

May involve these systems in the body (see Section III):

Endocrine System

Precocious puberty refers to a condition in which the onset of sexual maturation occurs before the age of eight years in girls and nine years in boys. True precocious puberty refers to the premature sexual development of the sex glands (i.e., ovaries and testes) as well as the outward appearance of the child. Precocious pseudopuberty refers to the early development of only the secondary sex characteristics with no involvement of the sex glands.

True precocious puberty results from the premature production and secretion by the pituitary gland of gonadotropin, a hormone that stimulates the ovaries and the testes. Because the release of hormones from the pituitary is controlled by another gland known as the hypothalamus, functional abnormalities of or growth of a tumor in the pituitary or the hypothalamus may also result in premature sexual development. These abnormalities may include hormone-secreting tumors of the pituitary gland, brain lesions such as a hypothalamic hamartoma, and other lesions of the central nervous system that may activate the hypothalamus. True precocious puberty may also result from an underactive thyroid gland (hypothyroidism). However, for most children with precocious puberty, the exact cause is not known. More girls are affected by precocious puberty than boys. Although most cases appear sporadically, some patients have a family history of this condition. Sexual characteristics associated with true precocious puberty are always consistent with the sex of the affected child (isosexual characteristics). Such characteristics may include the early appearance of underarm and pubic hair, facial hair in boys, and breasts and menstrual cycles in girls. The penis, testes, and ovaries enlarge and acne may develop. Although height and weight may increase rapidly, advanced bone growth may result in premature closure of the growing ends of the bone (epiphyses) and, thus, slower linear growth leading to short stature.

Precocious pseudopuberty may be caused by a tumor of the ovary, testis, or adrenal gland. Such tumors may cause excessive production of sex hormones. This form of the disorder may also be inherited as an autosomal dominant trait. In addition, precocious pseudopuberty may be associated with other disorders such as McCune-Albright syndrome, which is a condition resulting from the overproduction of hormones of multiple glands. This syndrome is characterized by premature sexual development in girls, irregularities of skin color (pigmentation) and the skeletal system, and abnormalities of various glands. Physical characteristics associated with precocious pseudopuberty are similar to those of true precocious puberty, although the testes and ovaries are not usually involved. However, children affected with this form of the disorder may develop secondary sexual characteristics associated with those of the opposite sex (heterosexual characteristics). In addition, precocious pseudopuberty may prompt early maturation of the hormonal cycle that results in true precocious puberty.

Treatment for true precocious puberty may include the administration of gonadotropin-releasing hormones. These hormones work by diminishing the stimulatory response of the pituitary gland to the gonadotropin-releasing hormones produced naturally within the body. Treatment for precocious pseudopuberty may include the use of certain medications that reduce the levels of male and female sex hormones (i.e., testosterone and estrogen). In addition, surgery may be indicated in those patients who have precocious puberty as a result of certain types of tumors. Other treatment is symptomatic and supportive.

The following organizations in the General
Resources Section can provide additional
information: National Organization for Rare
Disorders, Inc., (NORD), Genetic Alliance, March of
Dimes Birth Defects Foundation, NIH/National
Institute of Child Health and Human Development,
NIH/Office of Rare Diseases

National Associations & Support Groups

3418 Magic Foundation for Children's Growth
1327 N. Harlem Ave
Oak Park, IL 60302   708-383-0808
                                    800-362-4423
                         www.magicfoundation.org/

Provides assistance and education for individuals with growth related diseases through several
helpful medians.

Web Sites

3419 Johns Hopkins/InteliHealth
www.intelihealth.com/IH/ihtIH?t=6862

3420 Online Mendelian Inheritance in Man
www3.ncbi.nlm.nih.gov/Omim/searchomim.html

3421 Pediatric Database (PEDBASE)
www.icondata.com/health/pedbase/files/PRE-
COCI1.HTM

3422 Society for Endocrinology
www.endocrinology.org/

3423 University of Pittsburg Medical Center
path.upmc.edu/cases/cases71.html

Pamphlets

3424 Precocious Puberty
Human Growth Foundation
7777 Leesburg Pike Suite 202S
Falls Church, VA 22043   703-883-1773
                                800-451-6434

DESCRIPTION

3425 PREMATURITY

Prematurity refers to the birth of an infant before the 37-week gestational period. Although at least 40 percent of premature births occur for unknown reasons, prematurity may result from many different factors including a condition in which the mother develops high blood pressure, large quantities of protein in the urine, and an abnormal accumulation of fluid in the body (preeclampsia); maternal heart disease, kidney disease, or diabetes; acute infection; trauma; uterine irregularities (e.g., bicornate uterus); and placental abnormalities (e.g., placenta previa). Other contributing factors may include multiple pregnancy, maternal drug use, and fetal distress. Poor nutrition and lack of appropriate prenatal care may also put the unborn child at risk for premature birth.

Premature infants usually have a characteristic appearance in addition to their small size. For example, their heads often appear too large for their bodies and their skin may be very pink, smooth, translucent, and covered with downy hair (lanugo). They may have sparse hair and very little subcutaneous fat. In girls, the genitals may be incompletely developed such that the labia majora do not cover the labia minora. In affected boys, the testes may not fully descend into the scrotum. Other findings may include the absence of the creases on the palms and soles, incomplete development of the ear, and other irregularities. In addition, the survival or health of a premature infant may be compromised as a result of the incomplete development of certain body systems. The earlier the delivery, the more immature the organs. Common irregularities associated with prematurity include inadequate development of the lungs and subsequent deficiency in the production of a substance that allows the air sacs in the lungs to remain open (surfactant). This condition may lead to respiratory distress syndrome and associated life-threatening oxygen deficiency in the blood. Immature organ development may affect the brain, resulting in deficiencies in spontaneous breathing, inadequate sucking, and difficulty in swallowing. There is also an increased risk of bleeding in the brain (intraventricular hemorrhage). Premature infants are also particularly susceptible to serious infection resulting from incomplete placental transfer of maternal antibodies. Immature liver function may result in a temporary increase in blood levels of bilirubin causing yellowing of the eyes, skin, and mucous membranes (jaundice). Other complications of prematurity may include poor body temperature regulation, small stomach capacity, inadequacy of the intestinal tract that may result in injury or decreased blood flow to the intestines (necrotizing enterocolitis), immature kidney function, fluctuations in blood sugar levels, reduced levels of calcium in the blood, and other irregularities related to underdevelopment of body systems.

Treatment for premature infants depends upon the maturity of the various organ systems at the time of birth. In many cases, these infants are cared for around the clock in a neonatal care unit where body temperature may be regulated in an incubator and respiration may be maintained through artificial ventilation, if necessary. Feeding may be accomplished through the use of intravenous feeding or through a feeding tube directly into the stomach. Nutritional supplementation may include the administration of iron and vitamins. In addition, liquids may be given to maintain fluid levels in the body. Antibiotics may be administered to help treat infection. Discharge from the hospital takes place once the infant has reached appropriate weight and certain functional criteria have been established. In addition, before discharge, parents or caregivers of these infants are given complete instructions in their proper care. Other treatment is symptomatic and supportive.

The following organizations in the General Resources Section can provide additional information: March of Dimes Birth Defects Foundation, NIH/National Institute of Child Health and Human Development

DESCRIPTION

3426 PROTEIN C DEFICIENCY

Synonyms: PC deficiency, PROC deficiency

Disorder Type: Genetic Disorder

Covers these related disorders: Protein C deficiency Type I, Protein C deficiency Type II

May involve these systems in the body (see Section III):

Blood (Hematologic)

Protein C deficiency is a blood clotting (thrombotic) disorder characterized by the recurrent formation of blood clots within the veins of the body (venous thrombosis). Protein C, which is formed in the liver, is a specialized protein that helps to prevent the formation of blood clots. When activated, protein C helps to dissolve fibrin, the semisolid portion of blood clots, thus inhibiting the formation of a clot. A deficiency of this protein, therefore, results in abnormal clot formation. Some signs of this disorder may become apparent during adolescence. Associated symptoms depend upon the organ or tissue affected by clot formation that leads to reduced or absent blood flow. Affected individuals may develop blood clots and inflammation in the veins of the legs (thrombophlebitis). In some patients, these clots may dislodge from the vein and travel through the blood stream (embolus). These clots may travel to different parts of the body including the heart, lungs, or brain, potentially leading to life-threatening complications. However, not all patients with protein C deficiency experience all the signs associated with this disorder.

In the event of a blood clotting episode, the antithrombin factor heparin may be administered through injection into a vein (intravenous) or under the skin (subcutaneous). Other treatment may include continuing oral administration of the anticoagulant drug warfarin to prevent a recurrence of thrombotic activity.

Two types of protein C deficiency have been described in the general population. The more common form is Type I in which both protein C levels and activity are deficient. In the less common Type II, the amount of protein is normal but its activity or performance is impaired. The inherited form of protein C deficiency may be transmitted as an autosomal dominant trait. The gene for this disorder is located on the long arm of chromosome 2 (2q13-14). Protein C deficiency may also be acquired in connection with infection.

The following organizations in the General Resources Section can provide additional information: NIH/National Heart, Lung & Blood Institute, Online Mendelian Inheritance in Man: www3.ncbi.nlm.nih.gov/Omim/searchomim.html, Genetic Alliance, March of Dimes Birth Defects Foundation, National Organization for Rare Disorders, Inc., (NORD)

Web Sites

3427 Factor V Leiden
fvleiden.org

e-mail: debsmith@fvleiden.org
fvleiden.org

Factor V Leiden is the most common hereditary blood coagulation disorder in the US. It is present in 3-7% of the population in Europe and America. It is associated with Venous thrombosis, DVT, unexplained miscarriage, blood clots in the lungs, gall bladder dysfunction, preeclampsia and/or eclapsia, stroke and/or heart attack.

DESCRIPTION

3428 PSORIASIS

May involve these systems in the body (see Section III):
Dermatologic System

Psoriasis is a common, chronic skin disease characterized by red patches of skin that are covered by dry, thick, silvery scales. This disorder may occur at any age, but most commonly appears from the ages of 10 to 40 years. Although males and females are affected equally, females are more prone to development of this disorder when it appears during childhood. In addition, approximately half of those individuals who develop psoriasis in childhood have a family history of the disorder, but the pattern of transmission has not been determined. Individuals with psoriasis appear to produce new skin cells at a greatly accelerated rate while shedding their old cells at a normal rate. The subsequent buildup of new cells produces thickened areas of new skin that are covered by old skin, thus forming the characteristic dry, thickened, silvery patches associated with psoriasis.

Psoriatic lesions may appear anywhere on the body, but most commonly form on the scalp, elbows, knees, back, buttocks, navel area, and genitalia. In addition, relatively smaller lesions may appear on the face and pitting may develop on the nails. On rare occasions, severe psoriasis may develop in newborns, accompanied by lesion formation in the diaper area.

There are different types of psoriasis. The most common form is called discoid psoriasis and is characterized by patches that form mainly on the elbows, knees, scalp, and other areas of the arms, legs, and trunk. Other findings may include nail irregularities such as pitting, thickening, and separation from the nail beds. In addition, psoriasis is sometimes accompanied by painful swelling of the joints (arthritis). Guttate psoriasis occurs primarily in children and young adults and is characterized by the sudden appearance of small, oval, drop-like lesions on the trunk and upper portions of the arms and legs. Guttate psoriasis often develops following a streptococcal infection, viral infection, or sunburn. In addition, this form of the disorder sometimes follows the conclusion or withdrawal of corticosteroid treatment. Pustular psoriasis may be localized or generalized. In its localized form, eruptions of pustules develop over individual reddish patches that are present, usually, on the palms of the hands and the soles of the feet. Psoriasis is usually apparent on other parts of the body. Affected individuals may also experience localized discomfort. Generalized pustular psoriasis is an acute, severe, sometimes life-threatening form of the disorder that is characterized by the widespread eruption of small pustules in individuals with mild, moderate, or other types of psoriasis. Generalized pustular psoriasis is sometimes accompanied by high fever, pain in the joints, elevated levels of white blood cells (leukocytosis), low levels of blood calcium (hypocalcemia), and other irregularities.

Treatment of psoriasis is dependent upon age, area of involvement, and the type and severity of the disease. Many treatment protocols that are effective for adults may be too toxic for children; therefore, most treatment for children with psoriasis is conservative and mainly directed toward comfort and alleviation of pain. Such treatment may include the use of tar preparations in the form of gels, ointments, or bath emulsions. Additional topical treatments may include the cautious use of corticosteroid preparations, vitamin D analogs, and other ointments. Treatment for scalp lesions may include the use of a phenol and saline solution followed by tar shampoo and, when lesions are reduced, the application of a corticosteroid preparation. Severe psoriasis in children may indicate the use of various drugs such as methotrexate and certain oral retinoids; however, this therapy may be accompanied by severe side effects. Other treatment is symptomatic and supportive.

The following organizations in the General Resources Section can provide additional information: NIH/National Institute of Arthritis and Musculoskeletal and Skin Diseases

National Associations & Support Groups

3429 Canadian Psoriasis Foundation
824 Meath Street
Ottawa, K1Z
Canada
613-728-4000
800-265-0926
Fax: 613-728-8913
e-mail: cpf-fcp@psoriasis.ca
www.psoriasis.ca

3430 National Psoriasis Foundation
6600 SW 92nd Avenue Suite 300
Portland, OR 97223
503-244-7404
800-723-9166
Fax: 503-245-0626
e-mail: getinfo@npsusa.org
www.psoriasis.org

Offers information, support and referrals for
victims of psoriasis and their families.

Gail M. Zimmerman, Executive Director

Research Centers

3431 Psoriasis Research Institute
600 Town & Country Center
Palo Alto, CA 94301
650-326-1848
Fax: 650-326-1262

Studies the causes, symptoms and treatments of
psoriasis.

Web Sites

3432 AAD
www.aad.org/aadpamphrework/Psoriasis.html

3433 DermInfoNet
tray.dermatology.uiowa.edu/PIPs/Psoriasis.html

3434 Newsgroup
alt.support.psoriasis

3435 Psoriasis Help Group
marsonearth.freeservers.com/

Books

3436 Managing Your Psoriasis
Nicholas Lowe, author

MasterMedia, Ltd.
16 East 72nd Street
New York, NY 10021
212-260-5600

1993 Softcover
ISBN: 0-942361-83-0

3437 Psoriasis
Harry Clements, author

HarperCollins Canada Limited/Order Department
1995 Markham Road
Scarborough, ON, M1B 5M8, IT
800-387-0117
Fax: 800-668-5788

This book offers an effective four week treatment program for psoriasis and address such issues as danger foods, and the importance of a
low protein, toxin-free diet.
96 pages
ISBN: 0-722529-29-5

3438 Psoriasis,
Charles Camisa, author

Blackwell Scientific Publications
350 Main Street
Malden, MA 02148
781-388-8250
Fax: 781-388-8255
www.blackwellscience.com

1994
ISBN: 0-865422-47-8

3439 Psoriasis: Questions and Anwers
NAMSIC, National Institutes of Health
1 AMS Circle
Bethesda, MD 20892
301-495-4484
Fax: 301-587-4352
TTY: 301-565-2966
www.nih.gov/niams/

Offers various information for the psoriasis patient and their family regarding treatments,
risks, nutrition and more.
24 pages

Newsletters

3440 National Psoriasis Foundation Bulletin
National Psoriasis Foundation
6600 SW 92nd Avenue Suite 300
Portland, OR 97223   503-244-7404
                           800-723-9166
                           Fax: 503-245-0626
                           e-mail: getinfo@npfusa.org
                           www.psoriasis.org

Offers members updated, legislative news, medical news and more for the psoriasis patient.
BiMonthly

3441 Psoriasis Newsletter
Psoriasis Research Institute
600 Town & Country Center
Palo Alto, CA 94301   650-326-1848
                             Fax: 650-326-1262

Offers information and medical updates on the disease of psoriasis, events, fundraising and more.
Quarterly

Pamphlets

3442 Overview of Psoriasis Treatments
National Psoriasis Foundation
6600 SW 92nd Avenue Suite 300
Portland, OR 97223   503-244-7404
                           800-723-9166
                           Fax: 503-245-0626
                           e-mail: getinfo@npfusa.org
                           www.psoriasis.org

3443 PUVA
National Psoriasis Foundation
6600 SW 92nd Avenue Suite 300
Portland, OR 97223   503-244-7404
                           800-723-9166
                           Fax: 503-245-0626
                           e-mail: getinfo@npfusa.org
                           www.psoriasis.org

3444 Psoriasis Research
National Psoriasis Foundation
6600 SW 92nd Avenue Suite 300
Portland, OR 97223   503-244-7404
                           800-723-9166
                           Fax: 503-245-0626
                           e-mail: getinfo@npfusa.org
                           www.psoriasis.org

3445 Psoriasis on Specific Skin Sites
National Psoriasis Foundation
6600 SW 92nd Avenue Suite 300
Portland, OR 97223   503-244-7404
                           800-723-9166
                           Fax: 503-245-0626
                           e-mail: getinfo@npfusa.org
                           www.psoriasis.org

The disease affecting nails, ears, eyelids, face, mouth and lips, hands and feet.

3446 Psoriasis: Common Questions & Their Answers
National Psoriasis Foundation
6600 SW 92nd Avenue Suite 300
Portland, OR 97223   503-244-7404
                           800-723-9166
                           Fax: 503-245-0626
                           e-mail: getinfo@npfusa.org
                           www.psoriasis.org

3447 Psoriasis: How it Makes You Feel
National Psoriasis Foundation
6600 SW 92nd Avenue Suite 300
Portland, OR 97223   503-244-7404
                           800-723-9166
                           Fax: 503-245-0626
                           e-mail: getinfo@npfusa.org
                           www.psoriasis.org

3448 Psoriatic Arthritis
National Psoriasis Foundation
6600 SW 92nd Avenue Suite 300
Portland, OR 97223   503-244-7404
                           800-723-9166
                           Fax: 503-245-0626
                           e-mail: getinfo@npfusa.org
                           www.psoriasis.org

3449 Scalp Psoriasis
National Psoriasis Foundation
6600 SW 92nd Avenue Suite 300
Portland, OR 97223   503-244-7404
                           800-723-9166
                           Fax: 503-245-0626
                           e-mail: getinfo@npfusa.org
                           www.psoriasis.org

3450 Skin Cancer Risks from Psoriasis Treatments
National Psoriasis Foundation
6600 SW 92nd Avenue Suite 300
Portland, OR 97223   503-244-7404
                           800-723-9166
                           Fax: 503-245-0626
                           e-mail: getinfo@npfusa.org
                           www.psoriasis.org

3451 Specific Forms of Psoriasis
National Psoriasis Foundation
6600 SW 92nd Avenue Suite 300
Portland, OR 97223   503-244-7404
                            800-723-9166
                       Fax: 503-245-0626
            e-mail: getinfo@npfusa.org
                       www.psoriasis.org

Pustular, Guttate, Inverse, and Erythrodermic.

3452 Sunlight & Psoriasis
National Psoriasis Foundation
6600 SW 92nd Avenue Suite 300
Portland, OR 97223   503-244-7404
                            800-723-9166
                       Fax: 503-245-0626
            e-mail: getinfo@npfusa.org
                       www.psoriasis.org

3453 Young People and Psoriasis
National Psoriasis Foundation
6600 SW 92nd Avenue Suite 300
Portland, OR 97223   503-244-7404
                            800-723-9166
                       Fax: 503-245-0626
            e-mail: getinfo@npfusa.org
                       www.psoriasis.org

Infancy through adolescence.

3454 Your Diet & Psoriasis
National Psoriasis Foundation
6600 SW 92nd Avenue Suite 300
Portland, OR 97223   503-244-7404
                            800-723-9166
                       Fax: 503-245-0626
            e-mail: getinfo@npfusa.org
                       www.psoriasis.org

DESCRIPTION

3455 PTOSIS

Synonym: Blepharoptosis

Disorder Type: Birth Defect, Vision

Covers these related disorders: Acquired ptosis, Congenital ptosis

Ptosis, or blepharoptosis, refers to a condition in which one or both of the upper eyelids droop or sag as a result of an irregularity that is present at birth or an acquired weakness in the muscles of the upper eyelid that are responsible for movement. This condition may also be the result of irregularities of the nerve response for regulating muscle movements of the upper eyelids (third cranial nerve or oculomotor nerve). Congenital ptosis varies in severity; therefore, treatment depends upon the extent of the defect. If the eyelid droop is sufficient to cover the pupil, the ability to see is impaired by the drooping eyelid. In some infants and children, the development of the affected eye may be slowed, resulting in reduced or lost vision (amblyopia) in that eye. In such cases, early intervention through surgery may aid in preventing the development of impaired vision. However, surgery to correct ptosis strictly for cosmetic reasons is often postponed until the affected child reaches the age of three or four years.

In some cases, ptosis is accompanied by an abnormality of certain eye muscles, resulting in irregular movements of the eyes. Other ocular irregularities often associated with congenital ptosis include misalignment of the eyes in relation to each other (strabismus) or an imbalance in the way each eye deflects light (anisometropia). Medical specialists recommended early treatment of any accompanying abnormalities to avert complications. Ptosis may also occur as a characteristic feature of several syndromes including congenital fibrosis syndrome, Horner syndrome, or Sturge-Weber syndrome. Congenital ptosis is transmitted as an autosomal dominant trait.

Acquired ptosis may develop secondary to several disorders or conditions including myasthenia gravis, a muscular disorder; botulism, a severe type of food poisoning; progressive lesions within the skull that impact on the third cranial nerve; inflammation or growths that impact the eye orbit or lid. Treatment for acquired ptosis depends upon and may be directed toward the underlying cause.

The following organizations in the General Resources Section can provide additional information: National Organization for Rare Disorders, Inc., (NORD), Genetic Alliance, March of Dimes Birth Defects Foundation, Online Mendelian Inheritance in Man: www3.ncbi.nlm.nih.gov/Omim/searchomim.html

National Associations & Support Groups

3456 NIH/National Eye Institute (NEI)
9000 Rockville Pike
Bethesda, MD 20892   301-496-5248
www.nei.nih.gov/

3457 National Eye Research Foundation
910 Skokie Boulevard
Northbrook, IL 60062

Devoted to the enhancement of care and study of eye related diseases.

Web Sites

3458 EyeNet (AAO)
www.eyenet.org/public/faqs/ptosis_faq.html

3459 National Association for Visually Handicapped
www.navh.org

3460 Royal National Institute for the Blind
www.rnib.org.uk/info/eyeimpoi/congen.htm

3461 Sleep Tight Encyclopedia
www.sleeptight.com/encymaster/p/ptosis.html

3462 University of Minnesota
www.med.umn.edu/opthalmology/ptosis.html

3463 UseNet
www.sci.med.vision

DESCRIPTION

3464 PULMONARY HYPERTENSION, PRIMARY

Disorder Type: Heart
Covers these related disorders: Persistent fetal circulation (PFC)
May involve these systems in the body (see Section III):
Cardiovascular System, Respiratory System

Primary pulmonary hypertension is a heart condition in which blood pressure within the pulmonary artery is abnormally high (hypertension). The pulmonary artery arises from the base of the lower right chamber of the heart (ventricle) and carries oxygen-poor blood to the lungs, where the exchange of oxygen and carbon dioxide occurs. The term primary pulmonary hypertension may be used to refer to a condition in newborns known as persistent fetal circulation as well as a congenital heart abnormality in which pulmonary hypertension occurs for unknown reasons (idiopathic).

Persistent fetal circulation (PFC) is a condition in newborns in which blood continues to circulate through certain fetal openings or channels. These include the fetal opening between the left and right upper chambers of the heart (foramen ovale) and the fetal channel that joins the major artery of the body (aorta) and the pulmonary artery (ductus arteriosus). These openings usually close shortly after birth. However, in newborns with PFC, fetal circulation persists due to abnormal narrowing of the pulmonary blood vessels as well as unusually high blood pressure in these vessels. PFC may occur in newborns for unknown reasons (idiopathic) or may result from a lack of oxygen during the birth process (birth asphyxia); certain abnormalities during pregnancy (e.g., amniotic fluid lead); certain birth defects (e.g., underdevelopment of the lungs seen in a diaphragmatic hernia); or other conditions, such as meconium aspiration, polycythemia, etc. PFC affects approximately one in 500 to 700 newborns.

Newborns with PFC often experience symptoms immediately after birth or within the first 12 hours of life. Some may have bluish discoloration of the skin and mucous membranes (cyanosis) and increasing difficulties breathing (respiratory distress). Symptoms associated with respiratory distress may include rapid breathing (tachypnea), grunting upon exhalation, drawing in of the chest wall during inhalation, and a rapid heart rate (tachycardia).

In newborns with PFC, immediate measures may be necessary to prevent or treat potentially life-threatening complications. Additional therapy is directed toward treating the underlying cause of the condition and providing ongoing supportive measures to increase the supply of oxygen to bodily tissues. Oxygen therapies may include the use of measures to mechanically assist breathing (mechanical ventilation), administration of certain medications (e.g., surfactant therapy; inhalation of nitric oxide to help widen pulmonary blood vessels), or use of a device known as an extracorporeal membrane oxygenator (ECMO). This device delivers oxygen to an infant's blood and returns the oxygenated blood to the body.

In contrast to PFC, primary pulmonary hypertension is a progressive condition that often becomes apparent between the ages of 10 to 20 years. Females appear to be slightly more affected than males. Researchers suspect that the condition may be the result of the interactions of different genes, possibly in association with the involvement of certain environmental factors (multifactorial inheritance).

In patients with primary pulmonary hypertension, abnormal thickening and loss of elasticity of pulmonary arterial walls may cause abnormal obstruction and increased resistance of the blood flow from the right ventricle to the lungs. Consequently, the heart muscle must pump harder and at a higher pressure to adequately propel blood through the pulmonary artery, leading to enlargement of the right ventricle. Affected individuals may experience exercise intolerance, easy fatigability, and, in some cases, dizziness, fainting episodes (syncope), headaches, and chest pain. In addition, as the right ventricle begins to weaken in its ability to pump blood efficiently (right ventricular failure), patients may experience bluish discoloration of the skin of the arms and legs, coldness of the affected limbs, enlargement of the liver (hepatomegaly), and an abnormal accumulation of fluid in body tissues (edema). Patients with severe pulmonary hypertension may experience sudden abnormalities in the rhythm or rate of the heartbeat (arrythmias), resulting in life-threatening complications. Supportive therapies for the treatment of primary pulmonary hypertension may include intravenous administration of the medication prostacyclin to help widen pulmonary arteries (vasodilation) and increase blood flow. In adition, in some patients, the administration of calcium channel blocking agents by mouth may be beneficial. In many patients with severe primary pulmonary hypertension, heart-lung or lung transplantation may be required.

The following organizations in the General Resources Section can provide additional information: Genetic Alliance, National Organization for Rare Disorders, Inc., (NORD), March of Dimes Birth Defects Foundation, American Lung Association, National Child Health and Human Development, NIH/Office of Rare Diseases, NIH/National Heart, Lung & Blood Institute

National Associations & Support Groups

3465 American Heart Association
7272 Greenville Avenue
Dallas, TX 75231
214-373-6300
800-242-8721
Fax: 214-706-1341
e-mail: inquire@amhrt.org
www.amhrt.org

Supports research, education and community service programs with the objective of reducing premature death and disability from cardiovascular diseases and stroke; coordinates the efforts of health professionals, and other engaged in the fight against heart and circulatory disease.

3466 Foundation for Pulmonary Hypertention, Inc
PO Box 61540
New Orleans, LA 70161
504-533-5888
Fax: 504-533-2447

3467 Pulmonary Hypertention Association
PO Box 463
Ambler, PA 19002
215-591-9016
800-748-7274
Fax: 212-542-5692
e-mail: admin@phassociation.org
www.phassociation.org

Web Sites

3468 Geocities
www.geocities.com/ResearchTriangle/2006/pph5html

3469 Thrive Online
www.thriveonline.com/health/Library/CAD/

DESCRIPTION

3470 PULMONARY VALVE STENOSIS

Disorder Type: Birth Defect, Heart
Covers these related disorders: Critical pulmonic stenosis

Pulmonary valve stenosis is a heart defect characterized by abnormal narrowing (stenosis) of the opening between the lower right-sided, pumping chamber of the heart (right ventricle) and the pulmonary artery at the level of the pulmonary valve. Situated where the pulmonary artery arises from the base of the right ventricle, the pulmonary valve enables blood to flow from the right ventricle to the lungs while preventing the backward flow of blood. The pulmonary artery carries oxygen-depleted (deoxygenated) blood to the lungs, where the exchange of oxygen and carbon dioxide occurs. In infants and children with pulmonary valve stenosis, narrowing of the pulmonary valve opening increases resistance of the blood flow from the right ventricle to the pulmonary artery. As a result, the heart muscle must pump harder and at a higher pressure to propel blood to the pulmonary artery, potentially leading to thickening of the heart muscle (hypertrophy) of the right ventricle. Pulmonary valve stenosis affects approximately one in 1,250 individuals in the general population, comprising approximately 10 percent of all heart defects that are present at birth (congenital heart defects). Less commonly, abnormal narrowing of the opening between the pulmonary artery and the right ventricle (pulmonary stenosis) may be due to structural abnormalities other than a restricted valvular opening, such as narrowing within the upper region of the right ventricle or a portion of the pulmonary artery (e.g., isolated infundibular stenosis, branch pulmonary artery stenosis).

In infants and children with pulmonary valve stenosis, the severity of associated symptoms may vary, depending on the size of the restricted valvular opening and, in some patients, the presence of additional heart defects. For example, some af-
fected children may also have relatively small septal defects, such as an abnormal opening in the fibrous partition (septum) that divides the ventricles or the two upper chambers (atria) of the heart (ventricular or atrial septal defects). Infants and children with mild pulmonary valve stenosis usually have no associated symptoms (asymptomatic), do not experience hypertrophy of heart muscle, and have normal growth and development. In such patients, the condition is usually initially suspected due to detection of characteristic, abnormal heart sounds (heart murmurs) during a physician's examination with a stethoscope. In patients with moderate pulmonary valve stenosis, the right ventricle may be of normal size or mildly thickened. Although most such patients are asymptomatic, others may experience some symptoms, such as easy fatigability and exercise intolerance.

In newborns or young infants with severe pulmonary valve stenosis, the right ventricle may be unable to pump blood adequately (right ventricular failure) and become moderately or severely enlarged. Findings associated with right ventricular failure may include poor feeding, enlargement of themegaly), an abnormal accumulation of fluid in body tissues (edema) or other abnormalities. In addition, blood may begin to circulate through a previously closed fetal opening in the heart (foramen ovale). The foramen ovale is a fetal opening between the left and right upper chambers of the heart (atria) that closes shortly after birth. Abnormal opening of the foramen ovale in those with pulmonary valve stenosis may cause oxygen-depleted blood to pass from the right to the left side of the atria (right-to-left shunting), into the left ventricle and into the aorta for transport to the body's tissues. Because this oxygen-depleted blood bypasses the lungs and instead recirculates throughout the body, bodily tissues receive less oxygenated blood (hypoxia). In such cases, affected newborns or infants are said to have critical pulmonic stenosis. In addition, in some infants, certain associated heart (cardiac) defects, such as atrial or ventricular septal defects, may also allow some mixing of oxygen-poor and oxygen-rich blood. Due to recirculation of oxygen-poor blood to the body's tissues, affected newborns or infants may experience mild to moderate bluish discoloration of the skin and mucous membranes (cyanosis), shortness of breath, and other serious symptoms and findings.

In newborns or infants with critical pulmonic stenosis, emergency procedures are performed to widen the restricted valvular opening. Such procedures may include inflation of a balloon-tipped catheter (valvuloplasty) or surgical correction or resection of the valve (valvotomy). Although corrective measures may not be required in those with mild or moderate stenosis, such patients should receive regular evaluations. Such monitoring is necessary to ensure appropriate intervention for patients who may potentially experience increasing obstruction across the pulmonary valve or increasing hypertrophy of the right ventricle. In severe, untreated cases of pulmonary valve stenosis, associated symptoms may suddenly worsen due to inability of the right ventricle to pump blood effectively (right ventricular failure). Intervention for patients with moderate or severe stenosis includes balloon valvuloplasty or, in some cases, valvotomy. Other treatment is symptomatic and supportive.

Pulmonary valve stenosis may occur as a spontaneous, isolated finding; with other congenital heart defects; or in association with certain underlying disorders (e.g., Noonan syndrome). In some patients, the condition is thought to be determined by the interactions of several different genes, possibly in association with the involvement of certain environmental factors (multifactorial inheritance).

The following organizations in the General Resources Section can provide additional information: Genetic Alliance, March of Dimes Birth Defects Foundation, NIH/National Heart, Lung & Blood Institute, NIH/National Institute of Child Health and Human Development

National Associations & Support Groups

3471 American Heart Association
7272 Greenville Avenue
Dallas, TX 75231
214-373-6300
800-242-8721
Fax: 214-706-1341
e-mail: inquire@amhrt.org
www.amhrt.org

Supports research, education and community service programs with the objective of reducing premature death and disability from cardiovascular diseases and stroke; coordinates the efforts of health professionals, and other engaged in the fight against heart and circulatory disease.

Web Sites

3472 Children's Health Information Network/ Congenital Heart Defects
www.ohsu.edu/cliniweb/C14/C14.240.400.html

3473 Congenital Heart Disease Resource
www.csun.edu/~hcmth011/heart/

3474 Southern Illinois University School of Medicine
www.siumed.edu/peds/teaching/patient%20education.htm

DESCRIPTION

3475 PYLORIC STENOSIS

Synonym: Infantile pyloric stenosis

May involve these systems in the body (see Section III):

Digestive System

Pyloric stenosis refers to a condition in which the passageway (pyloric canal) that leads from the stomach to the first part of the small intestine known as the duodenum is narrowed or obstructed due to the thickening of the muscle that surrounds this opening (pyloric sphincter). Although the specific cause for this thickening is not known, many factors may be responsible, including breast-feeding, irregularities in nerve distribution to the muscle, and certain disorders such as Turner syndrome, Cornelia de Lange syndrome, trisomy 18 syndrome, and eosinophilic gastroenteritis. Pyloric stenosis is also commonly associated with certain birth defects of the gastrointestinal tract such as tracheoesophageal fistula.

Symptoms and findings associated with this disorder may develop as early as the first week of life; however, in some infants, this abnormality does not cause noticeable symptoms until the fourth or fifth month. At about the third week of life, episodes of forceful and explosive vomiting (projectile vomiting) may occur. After eating, rhythmic, wave-like movements (peristalsis) may be visible in the infant's abdominal area. Prolonged vomiting may result in excessive fluid loss (dehydration) and loss of essential elements known as electrolytes in the fluid portion of the blood (e.g., sodium, potassium, and calcium).

Treatment for infantile pyloric stenosis includes the administration of fluids to counteract the effects of dehydration. Once body fluids and electrolytes stabilize, a surgical procedure known as a pyloromyotomy may be performed. During this procedure, a lengthwise incision is made along the thickened pyloric muscle to correct the defect.

Pyloric stenosis affects approximately three in every 1,000 infants in the United States. Boys are more often affected than girls by a ratio of four to one. Children of parents who had pyloric stenosis are approximately 10 to 20 percent more likely to be affected. Infants with types B or O blood develop this defect more often than those with other blood types.

The following organizations in the General Resources Section can provide additional information: NIH/Office of Rare Diseases, National Organization for Rare Disorders, Inc., (NORD), March of Dimes Birth Defects Foundation, Online Mendelian Inheritance in Man.: www3.ncbi.nlm.nih.gov/Omim/searchomim.html, NIH/National Digestive Diseases Information Clearinghouse

National Associations & Support Groups

3476 National Association for Visually Handicapped
22 West 21st Street-6th Floor
New York, NY 10010   212-889-3141
                            Fax: 212-727-2931
                            e-mail: staff@navh.org
                            www.navh.org

Serves the partially seeing (not totally blind) with informational literature, newsletters for adults and children, educational outreach, referrals, counsel and guidance. Works with eye care professionals and the business community regarding abilities for the partially seeing. Also has a large print lending library program available to persons within the U.S.A.

Lorraine Marchi, Founder/CEO

3477 National Retinoblastoma Parent Group
P.O. Box 317
Watertown, MA 02272
                            800-562-6265

Dedicated to providing information and support to parents of children with Retinoblastoma, a malignant tumor appearing in one or both eyes. Provides a variety of educational and support materials including a regular newsletter and medical journal article reprints concerning Retinoblastoma.

Web Sites

3478 Dr. Koop
drcoop.com/adam/mhc/top/000970.htm

3479 Southern Illinois University School of Medicine
www.siumed.edu/peds/teaching/patient%20education.htm

3480 Vanderbilt University
www.mc.vanderbilt.edu/peds/pidl/gi/pylorstn.htm

DESCRIPTION

3481 REFRACTION ABNORMALITIES
    Synonym: Ametropia
    Disorder Type: Vision
    Covers these related disorders: Anisometropia, Astigmatism, Hyperopia (Farsightedness), Myopia (Nearsightedness)

Refraction abnormalities are defects in the cornea and the lens of the eye to focus visual images appropriately on the nerve-rich membrane at the back of the eye (retina). The cornea is the convex, transparent area in front of the eye. The lens, which is located behind the pupil, is held in place by a circular muscle that changes the shape of the lens to make appropriate adjustments in focus (ciliary muscle). As light passes through the cornea and the lens, it is bent (refracted) so that it is properly focused on the retina, which contains millions of tiny nerve cells that respond to light (photoreceptors). However, in individuals with refraction defects, light rays are not properly focused on the retina (ametropia) due to abnormalities of the cornea, the lens, or the size of the eye. These refraction defects lead to visual abnormalities.

There are three primary types of refraction abnormalities: namely, farsightedness (hyperopia), nearsightedness (myopia), and astigmatism. In farsightedness, parallel light rays come to focus behind rather that on the retina. This may be due to shortness of the eyeball from front to back, abnormally reduced refractive power of the cornea or lens, or backward displacement of the lens. If farsightedness is mild or moderate, affected children may be able to clearly visualize near and far objects due to accommodation, a process by which the shape of the lens changes and brings the area of focus forward. The range and extent of accommodation is highest durign childhood and gradually decreases with age. With greater degrees of farsightedness, affected children may experience blurring of vision, eyestrain, fatigue, and recurrent headaches. They may also engage in repeated eye rubbing and squinting and appear uninterested in reading or schoolwork. Children with farsightedness may achieve clear vision with glasses or contact lenses with convex lenses.

In children with nearsightedness (myopia), parallel light rays come to focus in front of the retina due to increased length of the eyeball from front to back, abnormally increased refractive power of the cornea or lens, or forward displacement of the lens. Affected children experience blurring of vision when focusing on distant objects, tend to hold reading material and other objects close to their face, and often squint in an effort to improve clearness and clarity of vision. Nearsightedness usually becomes apparent during school age, particularly in the years prior to and up to adolescence. The degree of nearsightedness typically becomes more severe until early adulthood, when it tends to stabilize. Many affected children have a hereditary predisposition for nearsightedness; in addition, the condition may occur in association with the other eye abnormalities (e.g., glaucoma, keratoconus) or other underlying disorders. Clear vision may be attained with glasses or contact lenses with concave lenses. Until the degree of nearsightedness stabilizes, prescriptions may need to be periodically increased in strength (e.g., varying from every few months to once every one or two years).

In children with astigmatism, parallel light rays are not clearly focused in a point on the retina due to unequal curvature of refractive surfaces of the eye. Astigmatism may result from irregularities in curvature of the cornea or, in some cases, abnormalities of the lens. Many individuals have minor degrees of astigmatism and have no associated symptoms. With more severe degrees of astigmatism, affected children may experience blurring and distortion of vision, fatigue, eyestrain, and recurrent headaches. In many cases, they may also engage in frequent eye rubbing, squint in an attempt to improve clearness and clarity of vision, hold reading materials and other objects close, and appear uninterested in schoolwork. In children with astigmatism, visual correction may be achieved with the part-time or ongoing use of glasses with cylindric or spherocylindric lenses. In some cases, contact lenses may be used to help correct vision.

Some children may also have a visual condition known as anisometropia in which the refractive or focusing ability of one eye significantly differs from the other. For example, one eye may have normal focusing ability, whereas the other may be affected by nearsightedness, farsightedness, and astigmatism. For proper vision to develop during infancy and early childhood, corresponding visual images must form on both retinas to ensure the transmission of compatible nerve impulses (via the optic nerves) to the brain. If the images from one eye differ dramatically from the other, one may be suppressed, causing impaired visual development in one eye (amblyopia). Therefore, in infants and children with anisometropia, prompt detection and appropriate visual correction is essential to ensure proper visual development in both eyes.

National Associations & Support Groups

3482 Division on Visual Impairments
The Council for Exceptional Children
1920 Association Drive
Reston, VA 20191 703-620-3660
Fax: 703-264-9474
TTY: 703-264-9446
www.cec.spec.org

Advances the education of youth who have visual impairments that impede their educational progress.

3483 Lighthouse National Center for Vision and Child Development
111 East 59th Street
New York, NY 10022 212-821-9200
800-821-9713
Fax: 212-821-9705

Provides for the needs of children who are visually impaired and their families through professional training, technical assisance, and research.

3484 National Alliance of Blind Students
American Council of the Blind
1155 15th Street NW Suite 720
Washington, DC 20005 202-467-5081
800-424-8666
Fax: 202-467-5085

Works to facilitate progress toward full accessibility of college programs and facilities, provides opportunities for discussion of issues important to students and assists with National Student Seminars.

3485 National Association for Parents of the Visually Impaired
National Office
P.O. Box 317
Watertown, MA 02272
800-562-6265
Fax: 781-972-7444

National organization that strives to serve families of children of all ages and ranges with visual loss; whose members include parents, parent organizations, agencies and other persons who support and service parents of children with visual impairments.

3486 National Association for Visually Handicapped
22 West 21st Street-6th Floor
New York, NY 10010 212-889-3141
Fax: 212-727-2931
e-mail: staff@navh.org
www.navh.org

Serves the partially seeing (not totally blind) with informational literature, newsletters for adults and children, educational outreach, referrals, counsel and guidance. Works with eye care professionals and the business community regarding abilities for the partially seeing. Also has a large print lending library program available to persons within the U.S.A.

Lorraine Marchi, Founder/CEO

DESCRIPTION

3487 RESPIRATORY DISTRESS SYNDROME OF THE NEWBORN

Synonyms: Hyaline membrane disese (HMD), RDS

May involve these systems in the body (see Section III):

Respiratory System

Respiratory distress syndrome of the newborn (RDS) is a breathing disorder characterized by insufficient production of surfactant, which consists of substances produced by certain cells in the lungs. Surfactant contributes to the elasticity of lung (pulmonary) tissue and enables the air sacs (alveoli) of the lungs to remain open between breaths. The exchange of oxygen and carbon dioxide takes place across the thin walls of the air sacs. Due to insufficient surfactant in newborns with RDS, greater pressure is required to expand the lungs' airways and air sacs. As a result, the air sacs may collapse and the lungs may become unable to properly provide oxygenated blood to the body.

Surfactant is produced as the lungs mature during fetal development. Sufficient levels of surfactant are often present after approximately 35 weeks of pregnancy (gestation). RDS primarily occurs in newborns who are born prior to 37 weeks of gestation (premature newborns), affecting up to 80 percent of those who are born before 28 weeks' gestation and up to 30 percent of infants born between 32 and 36 weeks' gestation. The condition also occurs with increased frequency in infants who are born to mothers with diabetes or those who are delivered by Cesarean section. In other newborns, RDS may occur in the absence of known predisposing factors or may be due to certain birth defects or other conditions, such as underdevelopment of the lungs seen in diaphragmatic hernia, meconium aspiration syndrome, or persistent fetal circulation. Respiratory distress syndrome of the newborn is sometimes referred to as hyaline membrane disease, because insufficient surfactant production may cause the formation of a fibrous membrane known as hyaline membrane lining the lungs' small airways (bronchioles), ducts (alveolar ducts), and air sacs (alveoli).

Symptoms associated with RDS usually occur within minutes of birth, although they may not be recognized for several hours. These symptoms may vary in severity, depending upon the degree of prematurity or other underlying causes responsible for the condition. Newborns may experience increasing difficulty breathing (dyspnea), characterized by rapid, labored, shallow breaths (tachypnea); grunting upon exhalation; drawing in of the chest wall during inhalation; and bluish discoloration of the skin and mucous membranes (cyanosis) due to lack of sufficient oxygen supply to bodily tissues (hypoxia). Air may leak into the chest cavity surrounding the lungs (pneumothorax), causing collapse of the lungs and further breathing difficulties. Without appropriate treatment, cyanosis and breathing difficulties may progressively worsen and body temperature and blood pressure may fall. As infants with severe RDS tire, grunting upon exhalation may subside, breathing becomes irregular, and life-threatening complications may result. Depending upon the severity of the condition, infants with RDS may begin to gradually improve in about three days or may experience life-threatening symptoms within approximately two to seven days after birth.

If physicians suspect that a newborn may be born prematurely, steps may be taken to delay delivery in order to help decrease the risk of RDS. If delivery cannot be delayed, some women may be given certain corticosteroid medications (e.g., dexamethasone or betamethasone) approximately 48 to 72 hours before the delivery of premature newborns to help stimulate the production of surfactant before birth. In addition, an artificial surfactant may be administered into the windpipe (trachea) of affected newborns immediately after birth or within the first 24 hours of life to help reduce the severity of RDS and associated symptoms or complications. Additional treatment may include symptomatic and supportive measures, such as use of an oxygen hood or support with a ventilator.

The following organizations in the General Resources Section can provide additional information: Genetic Alliance, National Organization for Rare Disorders, Inc., (NORD), March of Dimes Birth Defects Foundation, NIH/Office of Rare Diseases, NIH/National Child Health and Human Development, NIH/National Heart, Lung & Blood Institute, American Lung Association

DESCRIPTION

3488 RESPIRATORY SYNCYTIAL VIRUS INFECTION
Synonym: RSV infection
Disorder Type: Infectious Disease

The respiratory syncytial virus (RSV) is the most common cause of lower respiratory tract infections in infants and young children. RSV is primarily spread by the inhalation of virus-containing airborne droplets. The virus is present worldwide and causes annual epidemics of RSV infection in late autumn, winter, or as late as May or June. Such outbreaks typically peak from January through March. Nearly every child is affected by RSV infection by age two, and many experience recurrent reinfection throughout childhood.

In older children and adults, RSV infection may cause no apparent symptoms (asymptomatic) or may result in mild to moderate lung infection and associated cold-like symptoms. However, RSV infection may be severe in others, particularly infants, young children, children with heart or lung disease, or individuals with compromised immune systems. In such patients, RSV infection may lead to inflammation of the lungs' small airways (bronchiolitis), inflammation of the airways and lung tissue (bronchopneumonia), or, in extremely severe cases, potentially life-threatening complications. RSV infection is known to be the leading cause of bronchiolitis or bronchopneumonia in children younger than one year of age.

In infants and young children with RSV infection, symptoms typically begin approximately four days after infection. Initial symptoms include a runny nose (rhinorrhea) and sore throat (pharyngitis). Patients may then develop a low fever, begin to cough and sneeze, and soon experience wheezing, which is the production of a whistling sound during breathing due to inflammation and associated narrowing of the airways. If RSV infection progresses, patients may develop additional symptoms, including increasing wheezing and coughing, an abnormally rapid rate of breathing

(tachypnea), drawing in of the chest wall during inhalation, and bluish discoloration of the skin and mucous membranes (cyanosis). Patients with extremely severe disease progression may develop increasingly rapid breathing, temporary cessation of breathing (apnea), listlessness, and potentially life-threatening complications. In other infants or young children with RSV infection, initial running of the nose and coughing may be followed by poor feeding, listlessness, and difficulties breathing (dyspnea) with little or no wheezing.

As mentioned above, many children experience reinfection with RSV. Reinfection usually causes less severe symptoms than those associated with initial disease. However, depending upon the age of patients and other factors, secondary infections may also sometimes be associated with severe lower respiratory tract infections. Older children who experience reinfection with RSV generally have more mild symptoms.

In children with mild or moderate RSV infection without associated bronchiolitis or bronchopneumonia, treatment typically includes symptomatic and supportive measures. Affected infants, young children, children with heart or lung disease, or those with compromised immune systems may require hospitalization. Treatment may include providing respiratory therapy with humidified air to help supply adequate oxygen to bodily tissues; ensuring an adequate intake of fluids; or administering certain medications to relax the smooth muscles of the small airways (bronchodilators). Certain infants and children are at high risk for severe RSV disease, such as those with lung disease, congenital heart disease, or immunodeficiency. In these children, certain preventive or prophylactic therapies such as RSV-specific antibodies (immune globulin) may be recommended to help reduce (or even prevent) the severity of RSV infection in these at-risk infants and young children.

The following organizations in the General Resources Section can provide additional information: NIH/National Institute of Child Health and Human Development, NIH/National Institute of Allergy and Infectious Disease, World Health Organization, (WHO), Centers for Disease Control (CDC)

Web Sites

3489 American Lung Association
www.lungusa.org/diseases/rsvfac.html

3490 KidsHealth
http://kidshealth.org/parent/common/rsv.html

3491 MediConsult
www.mediconsult.com/kids/shareware/rsv/

3492 RSV Center
www.rsvinfo.com/

DESCRIPTION

3493 RETINITIS PIGMENTOSA
Synonym: RP
Disorder Type: Genetic Disorder, Vision

Retinitis pigmentosa (RP) refers to a group of inherited disorders in which changes occur in the light-sensitive, nerve-rich tissue membrane (retina) at the rear of the eye. This process is a slow, progressive degeneration leading to blindness. Changes in the retina include clumping (aggregation) or scattering (dispersion) of the retinal pigment, thinning or weakening of the vessels that supply the retina with oxygen-rich blood, and shrinking of the retina and the area where the optic nerve enters the retina (optic disk). Characteristic findings and symptoms of RP include difficulty in seeing at night or in dim light (night blindness; nyctalopia), a progressive reduction in the visual field with gradual loss of central vision, tunnel vision associated with loss of the peripheral visual field, and accompanying reduction of retinal function. Retinitis pigmentosa usually becomes apparent in childhood, progressing to blindness during middle age. However, the onset, severity, and rate of this progressive degeneration are widely variable.

Leber congenital retinal amaurosis (amaurosis congenita; congenital amaurosis) is a form of retinitis pigmentosa that occurs at birth or shortly thereafter and is characterized by shrinking of the optic disk (optic atrophy), thinning or weakening of the blood vessels of the retina, and widespread irregularities of retinal pigmentation. Leber congenital retinal amaurosis is transmitted as an autosomal recessive trait. In addition, retinitis pigmentosa-like degenerative changes may be associated with several metabolic, neurodegenerative, and multifold disorders.

Treatment for retinitis pigmentosa is supportive and may include the use of visual devices to enhance remaining vision. This disorder may appear as a sporadic occurrence or may be inherited, usually as an autosomal dominant disorder.

There is also evidence of autosomal recessive and X-linked genetic transmission.

The following organizations in the General Resources Section can provide additional information: National Organization for Rare Disorders, Inc., (NORD), Genetic Alliance, March of Dimes Birth Defects Foundation, Online Mendelian Inheritance in Man: www3.ncbi.nlm.nih.gov/Omim/searchomim.html

National Associations & Support Groups

3494 Association of Retinitis Pigmentosa
P.O. Box 8388
Corpus Christi, TX 78468   512-852-8515

A nonprofit organization based in Texas serving as a national information-sharing center to provide human services to persons with progressive vision loss from Retinitis Pigmentosa and other retinal degenerative disorders.

Dorothy H. Stiefel, AAS, Executive Director

3495 Foundation Fighting Blindness
Executive Plaza, Suite 800
11350 McCormick Road
Hunt Valley, MD 21031   301-785-7770
                              TTY: 800-683-551
                              www.blindness.org

Provides information, referral services, and support networks for individuals with retinitis pigmentosa and their families. Funds research on the causes, cures, and prevention of Retinitis Pigmentosa, Usher syndrome, and related retinal degenerations.

3496 National Eye Health Education Program
1855 West Taylor Street
Chicago, IL 60612   312-996-4356

Offers information and support for persons with vision disorders, including Retinitis Pigmentosa.

3497 National Eye Institute
9000 Rockville Pike
Bethesda, MD 20892   301-496-5248
                          www.nei.nih.gov/

3498 National Eye Research Foundation
910 Skokie Blvd
Northbrook, IL 60062

Devoted to the enhancement of care and study of eye related diseases.

3499 National Retinitis Pigmentosa Foundation Helpline

800-638-2300

Provides information and referral services to persons suffering from Retinitis Pigmentosa.

3500 Retinitis Pigmentosa International
23241 Ventura Blvd
Woodland Hills, CA 91364   818-992-0500
                                  800-344-4877
                             Fax: 818-992-3265
                     e-mail: RPINT@pacbell.net
                        www.rpinternational.org

Dedicated to promoting and supporting research to find effective treatments and cures for Retinitis Pigmentosa, Macular Degeneration, and other degenerative diseases. Provides referrals to genetic counselors and support groups and offers a variety of educational materials including a regular newsletter and brochures.

Research Centers

3501 Department of Ophthalmology/Eye and Ear Infirmary
1855 West Taylor Street
Chicago, IL 60612   312-996-6582

Offers help, support, information and research for persons with vision problems, including Retinitis Pigmentosa.

Web Sites

3502 British Retinitis Pigmentosa Association
www.brps.demon.co.uk/

3503 Foundation Fighting Blindness
www.blindness.org

3504 International Retinitis Pigmentosa Association
www/irpa.org/

3505 National Association for Visually Handicapped
www.navh.org

3506 National Retinitis Pigmentosa Foundation
http://kumchttp.mc.ukans.edu

3507 Retinitis Pigmentosa of South Africa
www.rpsa.org.za/retinitis.htm

3508 Royal National Institute for the Blind
www.rnib.org.uk/info/eyeimpoi/congen.htm

3509 UseNet
www.sci.med.vision

Newsletters

3510 RP Messenger
Texas Association of Retinitis Pigmentosa
P.O. Box 8388
Corpus Christi, TX 78468   512-852-8515

A bi-annual newsletter offering information on Retinitis Pigmentosa.

BiAnnual

DESCRIPTION

3511 RETINOBLASTOMA

Disorder Type: Neoplasm: Benign or Malignant Tumor, Vision

Retinoblastoma is a malignant tumor of the nerve-rich membrane at the back of the eye known as the retina. This membrane converts light waves into nerve impulses and transmits them to the brain via the optic nerve (the second cranial nerve), resulting in vision. Retinoblastoma occurs in approximately one in 18,000 live births. In most cases, one eye is affected (unilateral). However, both eyes may be involved (bilateral) in about 30 percent of affected children. In some severe cases, the tumor may spread to other parts of the body (metastasize), particularly when there is tumor invasion of the middle layer of the eye (choroid) or the optic nerve. If tumor growth occurs along the optic nerve, the brain may be affected. However, in most children with retinoblastoma, metastasis rarely occurs before the tumor is detected.

Unilateral retinoblastoma is usually detected at approximately 21 months to two years of age, whereas bilateral retinoblastoma is typically diagnosed at about 11 to 12 months. Rarely, the tumor may be detected at birth, during later childhood or adolescence, or adulthood. In most cases, the first sign associated with retinoblastoma is the appearance of a yellowish-white mass in the pupil area (leukokoria) due to the presence of the tumor behind the lens of the eye and reflection of light off the tumor. Additional symptoms and findings often include abnormal deviation of the affected eye in relation to the other (strabismus) and impaired or absent vision. In some cases, affected children experience secondary complications, such as detachment of the retina or abnormally increased pressure of the fluid of the eye (glaucoma). Children who have more advanced retinoblastoma may also experience bleeding (hemorrhaging) within the chamber of the eye in front of the iris (hyphema), irregularities of the pupil, pain, or other symptoms. In cases of severely advanced disease or metastasis, associated findings may include protusion of the eye ball (proptosis) and abnormally increased pressure within the skull (intracranial pressure).

A gene responsible for retinoblastoma (RB gene) has been located on the long arm chromosome 13 (13q14). Many cases of unilateral retinoblastoma are thought to be due to deletions or abnormal changes (mutations) of the gene that occur randomly, for unknown reasons (sporadic). In familial cases, the exact mechanisms of inheritance are not understood. However, bilateral retinoblastoma and some cases of unilateral disease are thought to result from deletion of the gene from one chromosome and inheritance of one mutated disease gene (hemizygous state) or inheritance of two mutated RB genes (homozygous state of RB gene). Individuals with familial retinoblastoma may also have an increased risk for other malignancies. About one percent of children treated for familial retinoblastoma eventually develop a malignant bone tumor (osteosarcoma) by 10 years of age. In addition, estimates in the literature indicate that about 30 percent of those with familial retinoblastoma are affected by a second malignancy within 30 years after their initial diagnosis.

In some rare cases, affected children may have retinoblastoma in association with an underlying chromosomal deletion syndrome (chromosome 13, monosomy 13q syndrome) that is characterized by deletion (monosomy) of a portion of chromosome 13q including the RB gene at band 13q14. Although associated symptoms and findings may vary, affected children may have characteristic abnormalities of the head and facial (craniofacial) area including a high forehead, prominent eyebrows, a rounded (bulbous) tip of the nose and broad nasal bridge, prominent earlobes, a large mouth, and a thin upper lip.

The treatment of children with retinoblastoma is directed toward preserving vision. In children with unilateral retinoblastoma, treatment typically includes surgical removal of the affected eye and a portion of the optic nerve. However, if the tumor is very small, other measures may be indicated, such as the use of radiation or extremely cold temperatures (cryotherapy) to destroy the tumor. In children with bilateral retinoblastoma, treatment is directed toward preserving useful vision in at least one eye. Therefore, initial therapy may include cryotherapy or radiotherapy of one or both eyes. Bilateral therapy may be recommended since there have been cases in which the more severely affected eye has responded more dramatically to such measures. When one eye has no remaining vision or is affected by painful complications, removal of the eye may be advised. If tumor growth has begun to extend beyond the eye, radiation therapy may also be conducted. Therapy with anticancer drugs, such as cyclophosphamide and doxorubicin, may be considered with radiation therapy. Children and adults who have been affected by familial retinoblastoma should be carefully monitored for secondary malignancies. In addition, family members of affected children should be examined by an eye specialist to detect or help rule out the presence of retinoblastoma.

The following organizations in the General Resources Section can provide additional information: National Organization for Rare Disorders, Inc., (NORD), NIH/Office of Rare Diseases, NIH/National Cancer Institute, Genetic Alliance, NIH/National Eye Institute, National Childhood Cancer Foundation, Candlelighters Childhood Cancer Foundation, NIH/National Institute of Neurological Disorders & Stroke, Online Mendelian Inheritance in Man: www3.ncbi.nlm.nih.gov/Omim/searchomim.html

National Associations & Support Groups

3512 Division on Visual Impairments
The Council for Exceptional Children
1920 Association Drive
Reston, VA 20191   703-620-3660
Fax: 703-264-9474
TTY: 703-264-9446
www.cec.spec.org

Advances the education of youth who have visual impairments that impede their educational progress.

3513 Lighthouse National Center for Vision and Child Development
111 East 59th Street
New York, NY 10022   212-821-9200
800-821-9713
Fax: 212-821-9705

Provides for the needs of children who are visually impaired and their families through professional training, technical assistance, and research.

3514 National Alliance of Blind Students
American Council of the Blind
1155 15th Street NW Suite 720
Washington, DC 20005   202-467-5081
800-424-8666
Fax: 202-467-5085

Works to facilitate progress toward full accessibility of college programs and facilities, provides opportunities for discussion of issues important to students and assists with National Student Seminars.

3515 National Association for Parents of the Visually Impaired
National Office
P.O. Box 317
Watertown, MA 02272
800-562-6265
Fax: 781-972-7444

National organization that strives to serve families of children of all ages and ranges with visual loss; whose members include parents, parent organizations, agencies and other persons who support and service parents of children with visual impairments.

3516 National Association for Visually Handicapped
22 West 21st Street-6th Floor
New York, NY 10010   212-889-3141
Fax: 212-727-2931
e-mail: staff@navh.org
www.navh.org

Serves the partially seeing (not totally blind) with informational literature, newsletters for adults and children, educational outreach, referrals, counsel and guidance. Works with eye care professionals and the business community regarding abilities for the partially seeing. Also has a large print lending library program available to persons within the U.S.A.

Lorraine Marchi, Founder/CEO

3517 National Retinoblastoma Parent Group
P.O. Box 317
Watertown, MA 02272

800-562-6265

Dedicated to providing information and support
to parents of children with Retinoblastoma, a
malignant tumor appearing in one or both eyes.
Provides a variety of educational and support
materials including a regular newsletter and
medical journal article reprints concerning Retinoblastoma.

Web Sites

3518 Children's Cancer Web
www.ncl.ac.uk/~nchwww/guides/guide2n.htm

3519 Retinoblastoma Fact Sheet
www.rnib.org.uk/info/eyeimpoi/retino.htm

DESCRIPTION

3520 RETINOPATHY OF PREMATURITY
Synonym: ROP
Disorder Type: Birth Defect, Vision
May involve these systems in the body (see Section III):
Prenatal & Postnatal Growth & Development

Retinopathy of prematurity (ROP) is a condition characterized by improper development of blood vessels within the retinas of both eyes. The retinas are the nerve-rich membranes at the back of the eyes that contain specialized, light-sensitive nerve cells (rods and cones). The rods and cones convert visual images into nerve impulses that are transmitted to the brain via the optic nerve (second cranial nerve). ROP primarily occurs in newborns of low birth weight who are born at less than 37 weeks after conception (premature newborns). Premature infants who weigh less than approximately three pounds, are delivered before 33 weeks of pregnancy, and develop abnormally high levels of oxygen in the blood (hyperoxia) as a result of oxygen therapy for breathing difficulties are considered to be particularly at risk for retinopathy of prematurity. Less commonly, other factors may play some role in contributing to the condition, such as heart disease, infection, abnormally low levels of circulating red blood cells (anemia), or other conditions. Generally, the lower an infant's birthweight and the greater the degree of prematurity, the higher the risk for the development of ROP.

During fetal development, the blood vessels that will supply the retinas grow from the center of the retinas, gradually extending to their outer edges shortly after birth. However, in premature newborns, the retinal blood vessels are incompletely developed, potentially causing abnormalities in subsq uent retinal growth and function. In infants with ROP, associated findings may range from mild or temporary changes of the outer edges of the retina to severe abnormalities affecting the entire retina. During the active or acute stage of ROP, which typically occurs within the first month or so of life, associated findings may include abnormal narrowing of certain retinal blood vessels and subsequent widening or abnormal twisting of other retinal vessels. In addition, there is an apparent lack of blood vessel growth in certain areas of the retina, particularly of the outer rim. There may also be a gradual development of new blood vessels outside the normal area of retinal blood vessel growth, such as over the surface of the retina or into the jelly-like fluid behind the lens of the eye (vitreous humor). These vessels may tend to bleed (hemorrhage) into the retina, and some patients may develop retinal scarring as well as the formation of retinal folds or breaks or detachment of the outer portion of the retina. In severe cases, patients may undergo chronic disease progression, leading to complete retinal detachment and progressive retinal degeneration. The retina may eventually appear as an abnormal whitish membrane behind the lens of the eye (leukokoria). As the condition continues to progress, infants may develop increased fluid pressure within the eye (glaucoma), gradual degeneration and shrinkage of the eye (phthisis bulbi), and associated visual impairment leading to blindness.

In many infants with ROP, the condition spontaneously subsides and regresses. Such children may have an increased risk of progressive nearsightedness (myopia) or other eye abnormalities. However, in fewer than 10 percent, there may be ongoing disease progression, potentially causing total retinal detachment and severe visual impairment or blindness.

The prevention of ROP depends upon proper prenatal care and other measures to help prevent premature births. In addition, infants who are born prematurely are monitored closely to ensure prompt detection of ROP and appropriate treatment as required. In severe cases of ROP, a technique that freezes affected areas of the retina (cryotherapy) may help to reduce potentially severe complications. In addition, in patients with total retinal detachment, surgical techniques may be used to help reattach the retina.

The following organizations in the General Resources Section can provide additional information: NIH/National Eye Institute, NIH/National Institute of Child Health and Human Development, National Eye Research Foundation

National Associations & Support Groups

3521 Division on Visual Impairments
The Council for Exceptional Children
1920 Association Drive
Reston, VA 20191 703-620-3660
Fax: 703-264-9474
TTY: 703-264-9446
www.cec.spec.org

Advances the education of youth who have visual impairments that impede their educational progress.

3522 Lighthouse National Center for Vision and Child Development
111 East 59th Street
New York, NY 10022 212-821-9200
800-821-9713
Fax: 212-821-9705

Provides for the needs of children who are visually impaired and their families through professional training, technical assistance, and research.

3523 National Alliance of Blind Students
American Council of the Blind
1155 15th Street NW Suite 720
Washington, DC 20005 202-467-5081
800-424-8666
Fax: 202-467-5085

Works to facilitate progress toward full accessibility of college programs and facilities, provides opportunities for discussion of issues important to students and assists with National Student Seminars.

3524 National Association for Parents of the Visually Impaired
National Office
P.O. Box 317
Watertown, MA 02272
800-562-6265
Fax: 781-972-7444

National organization that strives to serve families of children of all ages and ranges with visual loss; whose members include parents, parent organizations, agencies and other persons who support and service parents of children with visual impairments.

3525 National Association for Visually Handicapped
22 West 21st Street-6th Floor
New York, NY 10010 212-889-3141
Fax: 212-727-2931
e-mail: staff@navh.org
www.navh.org

Serves the partially seeing (not totally blind) with informational literature, newsletters for adults and children, educational outreach, referrals, counsel and guidance. Works with eye care professionals and the business community regarding abilities for the partially seeing. Also has a large print lending library program available to persons within the U.S.A.

Lorraine Marchi, Founder/CEO

3526 National Retinoblastoma Parent Group
P.O. Box 317
Watertown, MA 02272
800-562-6265

Dedicated to providing information and support to parents of children with Retinoblastoma, a malignant tumor appearing in one or both eyes. Provides a variety of educational and support materials including a regular newsletter and medical journal article reprints concerning Retinoblastoma.

DESCRIPTION

3527 REYE'S SYNDROME

Reye's syndrome is a potentially life-threatening disease of childhood characterized by rapid accumulation of fat in the liver and inflammation and swelling of the brain (acute encephalopathy) following certain viral infections, such as respiratory tract infections (e.g., influenza) or chickenpox (varicella). Studies suggest that administration of aspirin as a treatment for viral infections plays a role in causing Reye's syndrome. Therefore, it is essential that aspirin or aspirin-containing medications are avoided in patients with a cold, flu, or chickenpox.

Reye's syndrome was initially reported in the early 1960s. In the decade from 1974 to 1984, approximately 200 to 550 children were affected in the United States each year. Beginning in the mid to late 1980s, the frequency of Reye's syndrome decreased dramatically and fewer than approximately 20 children are now affected annually in the U.S. This decrease is thought to be due to an increased awareness of the association between Reye's syndrome and the administration of aspirin-containing preparations. Reye's syndrome is most frequently seen in rural and suburban populations and typically affects children between the ages of four to 12 years.

Patients with Reye's syndrome initially experience a viral infection, such as a cold or flu in approximately 90 percent and chickenpox in about five to seven percent of affected children. Approximately five to seven days after the viral infection, patients suddenly experience severe nausea and prolonged, uncontrollable vomiting. A few hours after the onset of vomiting, patients may experience confusion, agitation, and delirium, which is characterized by disorganized thinking, reduced levels of consciousness, disorientation, memory impairment, and restlessness. These symptoms may be rapidly followed by episodes of abnormally increased electrical activity in the brain (seizures), a state of unconsciousness

(coma), and potentially life-threatening complications. Patients also have mild to moderate enlargement of the liver (hepatomegaly) and abnormalities of liver (hepatic) functioning (e.g., elevated serum transaminase levels). With severe liver involvement, there may be abnormal yellowish discoloration of the whites of the eyes, the mucous membranes, and the skin (jaundice). The severity of the disease may vary greatly from case to case, with most patients experiencing mild illness without progression.

Reye's syndrome should be suspected in any children with severe, uncontrollable vomiting and sudden swelling of the brain. Certain underlying metabolic disorders, such as defects in fatty acid metabolism, organic acidurias, or urea cycle disorders, or particular liver diseases may cause symptoms and findings similar to those seen in Reye's syndrome. Therefore, if young children have abnormally decreased concentrations of the sugar glucose in the blood (hypoglycemia), for example, thorough screening should be conducted to detect the possible presence of metabolic disease. In addition, removal and microscopic examination of small samples of liver tissue (liver biopsies) may help to differentiate certain underlying disorders from Reye's syndrome. Testing to help confirm a diagnosis of Reye's syndrome may include specialized laboratory studies, such as measures of liver function (i.e., demonstrating elevated transaminase levels), and evaluation of cerebrospinal fluid (which may demonstrate abnormally increased pressure within the brain). Treatment of affected children may vary, depending upon the severity of the disease. Although observation alone may be appropriate in those with very mild disease, aggressive therapies are typically required for patients with associated neurologic deterioration. Such measures may include ongoing monitoring and support of vital functions including proper blood circulation and breathing; continual assessment of pressure in the brain; administration of intravenous glucose; measures to reduce pressure in the brain (e.g., with corticosteroids, mannitol, glycerol), to manage blood clotting abnormalities (e.g., with vitamin K, platelet transfusions, fresh frozen plasma), and to ensure proper oxygenation (e.g., endotracheal intubation); and other therapies as required (e.g., phenobarbital). In children with mild disease, recovery is usually complete. However, patients with severe Reye's syndrome mya show residual effects due to associated brain damage, such as mental retardation and difficulties with visual and motor integration.

The following organizations in the General Resources Section can provide additional information: National Organization for Rare Disorders, Inc., (NORD), March of Dimes Birth Defects Foundation, NIH/National Institute of Allergy and Infectious Disease, World Health Organization, Centers for Disease Control

National Associations & Support Groups

3528 National Reye's Syndrome Foundation
P.O. Box 829, 426 North Lewis
Bryan, OH 43506   419-636-2679
                                800-233-7393
                           Fax: 419-636-9897
              e-mail: reyessyn@mail.bright.net
                       www.bright.net/~reyessyn

This group informs and educates the public, supports research, and provides services to victims of Reye's syndrome, a fatal disease whose cause is unknown. Although a major cause of death in children age 1-10, Reye's does affect adults and is often misdiagnosed. The organization responds to questions, sends literature and offers local referrals.

Susan Landversicht, Director of Development

3529 National Subacute Sclerosing Panencephalitis Registry
University of Alabama School of Medicine
Department of Neurology, 2451 Fillingim
Mobile, AL 36617   205-471-7834

Libraries & Resource Centers

3530 Children's Hospital Research Foundation
700 Children's Drive
Columbus, OH 43205   614-722-2000

Offers research activities into Reye's Syndrome, genetics and children's cancer chemotherapy.

Dr. Grant Morrow, III, Medical Director

Research Centers

3531 Clinical Research Center, Pediatrics
Children's Hospital Research Foundation
Elland & Bethesda Avenues
Cincinnati, OH 45229   513-559-4412
                           Fax: 513-559-7431

Studies of pediatric acquired diseases including liver disease and Reyes Syndrome.

Dr. James Heubi, Director

Web Sites

3532 American Lung Foundation
http://sadieo.ucsf.edu/alf/alffinal/inforeyes.html

3533 Canadian Pediatric Society
www.cps.ca/english/statements/ID/id85-08.htm

3534 Kid's Health.org
www.kidshealth.org/parent/common/reye.html

3535 National Reye's Syndrome Foundation
www.bright.net/~reyessyn/

DESCRIPTION

3536 SARCOIDOSIS

Synonyms: Sarcoid of Boeck, Schaumann's disease

Sarcoidosis is a multisystem disorder that is characterized by the abnormal development of inflammatory growths or nodules (i.e., epithelioid granulomas) in various organs in the body. The cause of this inflammatory disorder is unknown; however, it is believed that granuloma formation associated with sarcoidosis may result from infection or an exaggerated immune response to specific agents (antigens). In addition, researchers believe that some people may be genetically predisposed to sarcoidosis and develop the disease only if triggered by environmental or other factors. Although this disorder most commonly occurs during young adulthood, it may occur in children and in the elderly. Symptoms and physical findings associated with sarcoidosis are dependent upon the organ(s) involved and, in children, the age of onset. Most affected children, however, share the common symptoms of fatigue, weight loss, cough, pain in the bones and joints, and abnormally low levels of circulating red blood cells (anemia).

The nodules or granulomas associated with sarcoidosis may develop in almost any organ of the body, but most commonly affect the lungs, upper respiratory tract, lymph nodes, skin, eyes, liver, bones, joints, bone marrow, skeletal muscles, heart, liver, spleen, or the central and peripheral nervous systems. In older children and adults, the lungs are most often affected, while younger children experience less lung involvement. Characteristic findings in older children may include swelling of the lymph nodes near the blood vessels that enter and exit the lungs (hilar lymphadenopathy) as well as the lymph nodes near the windpipe (paratracheal lymphadenopathy) and those under the skin (peripheral lymphadenopathy). In addition, nodule formation may cause inflammations in the eye (e.g., uveitis and iritis) and other eye lesions, skin lesions, and liver changes.

Younger children may develop a reddish, combination-type rash consisting of waxy pimples and flat, discolored lesions (maculopapular erythematous rash) as well as inflammation of the joints (arthritis).

Diagnosis of sarcoidosis is usually a challenge as it is often difficult to distinguish from other disorders with similar symptoms and findings. Therefore, differential diagnosis often involves a physical examination, medical and environmental history, and the comprehensive evaluation of laboratory tests and chest x-rays, biopsy of tissue samples, and specialized testing. Laboratory findings may show excessive levels of calcium in the blood (hypercalcemia) and in the urine (hypercalciuria), abnormally high levels of protein in the blood (hyperproteinemia), excessive levels of certain granular white cells in the blood (eosinophilia), and other blood irregularities. For example, the cells of the nodules secrete a substance called angiotensin-converting enzyme, which, in some patients, is elevated to detectable levels in the blood. Testing for this enzyme may also be employed to measure disease activity. In addition, pulmonary function tests may be used to measure progress of the disease in those children with lung involvement, and repeat chest x-rays may also be indicated to monitor progress.

In some children, sarcoidosis may resolve spontaneously within a period of months or years; however, some children may have a more chronic form of the disease that may result in progressive lung involvement, eye disease that may cause blindness, and other prolonged symptoms and findings. Treatment for sarcoidosis may include the use of corticosteroid drops or ointments to alleviate eye inflammations and oral corticosteroids to alleviate acute symptoms such as resistant inflammatory lesions of the eyes, joint pain, fever, shortness of breath, and other symptoms. If no symptoms are present, corticosteroid treatment is usually not advised. Other treatment is symptomatic and supportive.

The following organizations in the General Resources Section can provide additional information: American Autommune Related Diseases Association, Inc., National Organization for Rare Disorders, Inc., (NORD), NIH/Office of Rare Diseases, Online Mendelian Inheritance in Man: www3.ncbi.nlm.nih.gov/Omim/searchomim.html

National Associations & Support Groups

3537 National Sarcoidosis Family Aid and Research Foundation
268 Martin Luther King Blvd.
Newark, NJ 07108   973-624-4703
                               800-223-6429
                               Fax: 973-877-2850

Provides information on a rare disease involving inflammation in lymph nodes and other body tissues, usually in young adults.

3538 National Sarcoidosis Resource Center
P.O. Box 1593
Piscataway, NJ 08855   732-699-0733
                                Fax: 732-699-0882
                                www.nsrc-global.net

Formed to heighten public awareness and to educate people about this often chronic and disabling disease; offers information and support. The center serves the United States, Canada, Europe and has a registry of over sixty thousand patients. The center recieves patient referrals from the American Lung Association, national Organization for Rare Diseases, National Institute of Health and physicians.

Sandra Conroy, President

3539 Sarcoid Networking Association
13925 80th St E.
Puyallup, WA 98372   253-845-3108
                               Fax: 253-845-3108
                               e-mail: VBKR29A@prodigy.com

National, non-profit self-help organization providing information and support to those affected by sarcoidosis.

3540 Sarcoidosis Network Foundation, Inc.
13337 E. South St, Ste 420
Cerritos, CA 90703   714-739-1398
                               Fax: 714-739-1398

Non-profit organizated supporting research to find a cause, cure and prevention of sarcoisosis. It promotes education and awareness and improves the lifes of those with affected by sarcoidosis.

State Agencies & Support Groups

Delaware

3541 Sarcoidosis Support Group - Delaware
4th & Walnut Street
Wilmington, DE   302-655-7258

Beth Yoncha, Facilitator

District of Columbia

3542 Sarcoidosis Support Group - Washington DC
475 H Street NW
Washington, DC 20001   202-682-5864

Illinois

3543 Sarcoidosis Support Group - Illinois
Let's Breathe
2225 Foster Street
Evanston, IL 60201   847-328-9410

Brenda Harris, Facilitator

New Jersey

3544 Sarcoidosis Support Group - Central New Jersey
National Sarcoidosis Resource Center
P.O. Box 1593
Piscataway, NJ 08855   732-699-0733
                               Fax: 732-699-0882

Jean Curlin, Facilitator

3545 Sarcoidosis Support Group - New Jersey
Newark Sarcoidosis Support Group
268 Martin Luther King Blvd.
Newark, NJ 07102   973-624-4703
                               800-223-6429

Jean Curlin, Facilitator

Virginia

3546 Sarcoidosis Self-Help Group - Virginia
9735 Main Street
Fairfax, VA 22031   703-591-4131

Carolyn Thomas, Facilitator

Washington

3547 NW Sarcoidosis Support Group
TACID Center, TCC Campus
6315 South 19th Street
Tacomna, WA   253-845-3108

Dolores O'Leary, Facilitator

3548 Pacific NW Support Group
Providence Hospital
Casey Room 500 17th Avenue
Seattle, WA   206-784-9365

Ed Girvan, Facilitator

Research Centers

3549 Sarcoidosis Research Institute
c/o Baptist Hospital East
3475 Central
Memphis, TN 38111   901-766-6951
Fax: 901-774-7294
e-mail: soskelnt@netten.net
www.netten.ent/~soskelnt/

A non-profit, tax-exempt organization dedicated to increasing knowledge of the disease sarcoidosis. This broad goal encompasses three main areas: (1) Disseminating information to professionals who assist with treatment of the disease (2) Obtaining and dispersing funds to assist with investigation into the cause and treatment of the disease and (3) providing support for individuals afflicted with the disease.

Audio Video

3550 Dialogue with Doris
PC Publications
P.O. Box 1593
Piscataway, NJ 08855   732-699-0733
800-223-6429
Fax: 732-699-0882

3551 Help with a Hidden Disease Update
PC Publications
P.O. Box 1593
Piscataway, NJ 08855   732-699-0733
800-223-6429
Fax: 732-699-0882

3552 Of Their Own - Person To Person Show
PC Publications
P.O. Box 1593
Piscataway, NJ 08855   732-699-0733
800-223-6429
Fax: 732-699-0882

3553 Sarcoidosis - What's That?
PC Publications
P.O. Box 1593
Piscataway, NJ 08855   732-699-0733
800-223-6429
Fax: 732-699-0882

3554 Sarcoidosis Conference 2
PC Publications
P.O. Box 1593
Piscataway, NJ 08855   732-699-0733
800-223-6429
Fax: 732-699-0882

3555 Sarcoidosis Conference 3
PC Publications
P.O. Box 1593
Piscataway, NJ 08855   732-699-0733
800-223-6429
Fax: 732-699-0882

3556 XIV International World Conference on Sarcoidosis - Patient Symposium
PC Publications
P.O. Box 1593
Piscataway, NJ 08855   732-699-0733
800-223-6429
Fax: 732-699-0882

Cassette.

Web Sites

3557 Sarcoidosis Online Sites: A Comprehensive Source for Sarcoidosis Information
http://members.aol.com/jaysjob/sar-
coid/sos1.html#TOP

e-mail: JaysJob@aol.com
http://members.aol.com/jaysjob/sarcoid/sos1.html#TO
P

3558 Sarcoidosis Research Institute
3475 Central Ave
Memphis, TN 38111   901-766-6951
Fax: 901-774-7294
e-mail: sosklnt@netten.net
www.netten.net/~soskelnt/

Books

3559 Sarcoidosis Resource Guide and Directory
Sandra Conroy, author

PC Publications
P.O. Box 1593
Piscataway, NJ 08855   732-699-0733
Fax: 732-699-0882

1993 304 pages Softcover
ISBN: 0-963122-25-8

Newsletters

3560 Online Sarcoidosis Newsletter
National Sarcoidosis Resource Center
P.O. Box 1593
Piscataway, NJ 08855   732-699-0733
Fax: 732-699-0882

Offers information on the center's activities and events, medical and legislative updates for the patients and their families.

Quarterly

Pamphlets

3561 A Sarcoidosis Questionnaire: Demographics and Symptomatology-Patients Respond
PC Publications
P.O. Box 1593
Piscataway, NJ 08855   732-699-0733
800-223-6429
Fax: 732-699-0882

3562 Anemia of Sarcoidosis
PC Publications
P.O. Box 1593
Piscataway, NJ 08855   732-699-0733
800-223-6429
Fax: 732-699-0882

3563 Bronchoalveolar Lymphocytes in Sarcoidosis
PC Publications
P.O. Box 1593
Piscataway, NJ 08855   732-699-0733
800-223-6429
Fax: 732-699-0882

3564 Case Report - MR Imaging of Myocardial Sarcoidosis
PC Publications
P.O. Box 1593
Piscataway, NJ 08855   732-699-0733
800-223-6429
Fax: 732-699-0882

3565 Case Report - Osseous Sarcoidosis and Chronic Polyarthritis
PC Publications
P.O. Box 1593
Piscataway, NJ 08855   732-699-0733
800-223-6429
Fax: 732-699-0882

3566 Coping with Sarcoidosis
National Sarcoidosis Resource Center
P.O. Box 1593
Piscataway, NJ 08855   732-699-0733
800-223-6429
Fax: 732-699-0882

A pamphlet offering information on how to manage and live with sarcoidosis.

3567 Drugs That Have Been Used for the Treatment of Sarcoidosis
PC Publications
P.O. Box 1593
Piscataway, NJ 08855   732-699-0733
800-223-6429
Fax: 732-699-0882

3568 Effects of Sarcoid and Steroids on Angiotensin-Converting Enzyme
PC Publications
P.O. Box 1593
Piscataway, NJ 08855
732-699-0733
800-223-6429
Fax: 732-699-0882

3569 Masqueraders of Sarcoidosis
PC Publications
P.O. Box 1593
Piscataway, NJ 08855
732-699-0733
800-223-6429
Fax: 732-699-0882

3570 Multidisciplinary Clinico-Pathologic Conference
PC Publications
P.O. Box 1593
Piscataway, NJ 08855
732-699-0733
800-223-6429
Fax: 732-699-0882

3571 National Sarcoidosis Resource Center
PC Publications
P.O. Box 1593
Piscataway, NJ 08855
732-699-0733
Fax: 732-699-0882
www.nsrc-global.net

A booklet offering a brief introduction to the illness and offers information on finding a cure and educating the public on Sarcoidosis.

3572 Neurosarcoidosis
PC Publications
P.O. Box 1593
Piscataway, NJ 08855
732-699-0733
800-223-6429
Fax: 732-699-0882

3573 Neurosarcoidosis or Multiple Sclerosis?
National Sarcoidosis Resource Center
P.O. Box 1593
Piscataway, NJ 08855
732-699-0733
800-223-6429
Fax: 732-699-0882

3574 Paranoid Psychosis Due to Neurosarcoidosis
PC Publications
P.O. Box 1593
Piscataway, NJ 08855
732-699-0733
800-223-6429
Fax: 732-699-0882

3575 Patient Information Package
National Sarcoidosis Resource Center
P.O. Box 1593
Piscataway, NJ 08855
732-699-0733
800-223-6429
Fax: 732-699-0882

Contains various brochures and pamphlets offering information about Sarcoidosis.

3576 Presidential Proclamation - National Sarcoidosis Awareness Day
PC Publications
P.O. Box 1593
Piscataway, NJ 08855
732-699-0733
800-223-6429
Fax: 732-699-0882

3577 Psychological Factors in Sarcoidosis
PC Publications
P.O. Box 1593
Piscataway, NJ 08855
732-699-0733
800-223-6429
Fax: 732-699-0882

3578 Pulmonary Sarcoidosis: Evaluation with High Resolution
PC Publications
P.O. Box 1593
Piscataway, NJ 08855
732-699-0733
800-223-6429
Fax: 732-699-0882

3579 Pulmonary Sarcoidosis: What We Are Learning
PC Publications
P.O. Box 1593
Piscataway, NJ 08855
732-699-0733
800-223-6429
Fax: 732-699-0882

3580 Right & Left Ventricular Function at Rest in Patients with Sarcoidosis
PC Publications
P.O. Box 1593
Piscataway, NJ 08855
732-699-0733
800-223-6429
Fax: 732-699-0882

3581 Sarcoidosis
PC Publications
P.O. Box 1593
Piscataway, NJ 08855   732-699-0733
       800-223-6429
      Fax: 732-699-0882

Offers information on the illness, causes, symptoms and treatments.

3582 Sarcoidosis - International Review
PC Publications
P.O. Box 1593
Piscataway, NJ 08855   732-699-0733
       800-223-6429
      Fax: 732-699-0882

3583 Sarcoidosis - Pleural Involvement Mimicking a Coin Lesson
PC Publications
P.O. Box 1593
Piscataway, NJ 08855   732-699-0733
       800-223-6429
      Fax: 732-699-0882

3584 Sarcoidosis Patient Questionnaire
PC Publications
P.O. Box 1593
Piscataway, NJ 08855   732-699-0733
       800-223-6429
      Fax: 732-699-0882

3585 Sarcoidosis and Other Granulatomous
PC Publications
P.O. Box 1593
Piscataway, NJ 08855   732-699-0733
       800-223-6429
      Fax: 732-699-0882

3586 Sarcoidosis and You - A Listing of Possible Symptoms
PC Publications
P.O. Box 1593
Piscataway, NJ 08855   732-699-0733
       800-223-6429
      Fax: 732-699-0882

3587 Sarcoidosis: A Multisystem Disease
PC Publications
P.O. Box 1593
Piscataway, NJ 08855   732-699-0733
       800-223-6429
      Fax: 732-699-0882

Explains the effects of the illness on the lungs and joints.

3588 Sarcoidosis: Usual and Unusual Manifestations
PC Publications
P.O. Box 1593
Piscataway, NJ 08855   732-699-0733
       800-223-6429
      Fax: 732-699-0882

3589 Seasonal Clustering of Sarcoidosis
National Sarcoidosis Resource Center
P.O. Box 1593
Piscataway, NJ 08855   732-699-0733
       800-223-6429
      Fax: 732-699-0882

3590 Successful Treatment of Myocardial Sarcoidosis with Steriods
PC Publications
P.O. Box 1593
Piscataway, NJ 08855   732-699-0733
       800-223-6429
      Fax: 732-699-0882

DESCRIPTION

3591 SCLERODERMA

Covers these related disorders: Linear scleroderma, Morphea, Systemic sclerosis
May involve these systems in the body (see Section III):
Connective Tissue, Dermatologic System

Scleroderma is a connective tissue disease characterized by thickening and hardening of the skin and underlying tissues or, in some forms of scleroderma, other organs of the body. In patients with morphea, a form of the disease that primarily affects the skin and its underlying (subcutaneous) tissues, lesions appear as limited or localized patches. In linear scleroderma, lesions appear in a band-like pattern. In other patients, particularly in adults, scleroderma may occur as a generalized, systemic disease affecting the skin and subcutaneous tissues, blood vessels, and internal organs, such as the heart, lungs, kidneys, and certain parts of the digestive tract. Although the underlying cause of scleroderma is not known, some researchers speculate that it may be an autoimmune disease in which there is an abnormal immune response against the body's own tissues. During childhood, scleroderma is more common in girls than boys.

Children with scleroderma are primarily affected by morphea or linear scleroderma. Associated symptoms and findings usually become apparent at age two or older. Patients initially develop patchy skin lesions that are dry, red or violet, and shiny in appearance. These lesions may cause associated pain or unusual sensations, such as prickling feelings in affected areas. In some children, the lesions may have a linear distribution and develop primarily on one side of the body. The lesions gradually become hard (indurated) and develop waxy, pale centers and elevated borders. As the disease continues to progress, the lesions become larger and merge, potentially involving a large area, such as an entire arm or leg. Affected areas may eventually develop deep scar tissue and firmly bind to underlying tissues, potentially resulting in pain and permanent bending of affected joints in fixed postures (joint contractures). In children with morphea or linear scleroderma, active disease may spontaneously subside over months or years or may slowly progress over many years.

Rarely, children may develop generalized, systemic scleroderma (systemic sclerosis). In such cases, associated symptoms and findings usually become apparent at age four or older. Children with systemic sclerosis often initially experience Raynaud's phenomenon, a condition characterized by sudden contraction of blood vessels supplying the fingers or toes, causing an interruption of blood flow and a subsequent excess of blood in affected areas following the restoration of blood flow (reactive hyperemia). Such episodes are usually triggered by exposure to cold temperatures and are characterized by numbing, tingling, and bluish or whitish discoloration of the fingers or toes due to lack of blood flow and subsequent reddening and pain.

Children with systemic sclerosis also often develop skin lesions on the hands and feet and, in some cases, the torso and facial area. These lesions may include groups of permanently widened (dilated) blood vessels (telangiectasias). As the disease progresses, skin lesions typically become hard, develop unusually light or dark pigmentation, and gradually bind to underlying tissues and structures. Children may also experience joint swelling, discomfort, and inflammation (arthritis) as well as degenerative changes of various organs, including those of the digestive tract, particularly the esophagus; the heart; the lungs and the kidneys. Associated symptoms may be extremely variable, depending upon the rate of disease progression and the specific bodily tissues and organs affected. In some patients, such abnormalities may include difficulties swallowing (dysphagia); chronic inflammation of the lungs due to inhalation of foreign matter into the airways (aspiration pneumonia); high blood pressure (hypertension); or respiratory, heart, or kidney failure. Active disease may be gradually progressive or include periods during which symptoms temporarily subside (remit).

The treatment of children with scleroderma is symptomatic and supportive. Such measures may include the use of medicated skin creams, such as topical corticosteroids, for skin lesions; early physical therapy to help prevent or minimize the development of joint contractures; systemic therapy with penicillamine or other medications (e.g., cytotoxic drugs), if appropriate; careful control of high blood pressure in those with systemic disease; and other measures as required. In addition, patients with Raynaud's phenomenon should avoid cold temperatures whenever possible and dress warmly before such exposure.

The following organizations in the General Resources Section can provide additional information: National Organization for Rare Disorders, Inc., (NORD), NIH/Office of Rare Diseases, American Autoimmune Related Diseases Association, Inc., NIH/National Institute of Arthritis and Musculoskeletal and Skin Diseases, Online Mendelian Inheritance in Man: www3.ncbi.nlm.nih.gov/Omim/searchomim.html

National Associations & Support Groups

3592 Raynaud's & Scleroderma Association
112 Crewe Road, Alsager
Cheshire,
United Kingdom
e-mail: webmaster@raynauds.demon.co.uk
www.raynauds.demon.co.uk

3593 Scleroderma Foundation
89 Newbury Street, Suite 201
Danvers, MA 01923
978-750-4499
800-722-4673
Fax: 978-750-9902
e-mail: sclerofed@aol.com
www.scleroderma.com

Non-profit organization providing educational and emotional support for individuals and families affected by scleroderma. Increase awareness and support research to find the cause, treatment and cure of the disease.

3594 Scleroderma Info Exchange
Group Coordinator
150 Hines Farm Road
Cranston, RI 02921
401-943-3909
Fax: 401-946-5666
e-mail: bmst77b@prodigy.com

A nonprofit voluntary organization for individuals with scleroderma, their families, friends, and other interested persons. The Exchange (formerly The Scleroderma Information Exchange) serves both as a support group and a clearinghouse for scleroderma information. Provides referrals to self-help and support groups throughout the country, and also answers inquiries from the general public concerning scleroderma and related diseases.

Research Centers

3595 Scleroderma Research Foundation
The Scleroderma Research Foundation
2320 Bath Street, Suite 307
Santa Barbara, CA 93105
805-563-9133
800-441-2873
www.srfcure.org/

Mission is to find a cure for scleroderma, a life-threatening and degenerative illness, by funding and facilitating the most promising, highest quality research and placing the disease and its need for a cure in the public eye.

Web Sites

3596 Scleroderma A to Z
www.scerlo.org//

3597 Scleroderma Message Board
disc.server.com/Indices/7571.html

3598 Scleroderma Support
clubs.yahoo.com/clubs/sclerodermasupport

Books

3599 Scleroderma
NAMSIC, National Institutes of Health
1 AMS Circle
Bethesda, MD 20892
301-495-4484
Fax: 301-587-4352
TTY: 301-565-2966
www.nih.gov/niams/

143 pages

3600 Scleroderma: Caring for Your Hands & Face

Jeanne L. Melvin, author

American Occupational Therapy Association
P.O. Box 31220
Bethesda, MD 20824   301-652-2682
                          Fax: 301-652-7711
                          www.aota.org

1994 32 pages Softcover
ISBN: 1-569000-06-9

DESCRIPTION

3601 SCOLIOSIS

Synonym: Rachioscoliosis

Disorder Type: Birth Defect

Covers these related disorders: Compensatory scoliosis, Congenital scoliosis, Idiopathic scoliosis, Neuromuscular scoliosis, Syndrome-associated scoliosis

May involve these systems in the body (see Section III):
Prenatal & Postnatal Growth & Development, Skeletal System

The term scoliosis refers to a condition characterized by a sideward (lateral) curvature of the spine. Idiopathic scoliosis is the most common form of this disorder and occurs for no known reason in otherwise healthy individuals who range in age from infancy to adolescence. Adolescent scoliosis is the most common form and accounts for 80% of idiopathic scoliosis. Approximately 20 percent of people with scoliosis report at least one other affected family member. Therefore, in these cases, scoliosis is thought to have a genetic component. Idiopathic scoliosis that develops during infancy often corrects itself, but it may become progressive in older children. Treatment is dependent upon age and the degree of curvature progression. Mild curvatures may require little or no treatment, while more severe involvement may require surgery or the use of braces, etc. (orthotics). Although men and women are affected in about equal numbers, women are more at risk for more significant curvature progression.

Congenital scoliosis, apparent at birth or soon thereafter, results from the improper or incomplete development of the vertebrae during the first trimester of pregnancy. This condition may appear singularly or in association with abnormalities of other systems of the body including the heart (i.e., congenital heart disease) and genitourinary tract (e.g., absence of one kidney, duplication of the tubes that carry urine, horseshoe kidney, and other malformations). Congenital scoliosis is often accompanied by other spinal cord defects (spinal dysraphism) that may range from mild to severe. In addition, children born with certain genetic disorders such as Klippel-Feil syndrome may experience associated scoliosis. The progression of the curvature is dependent upon the specific underlying vertebral malformation, its particular growth potential, and its location. About one quarter of affected children experience no progression of the curvature and, therefore, require no treatment. Approximately half of those remaining may require early treatment, such as spinal fusion of the affected area, to stop progression of the curvature.

Neuromuscular scoliosis is associated with certain childhood diseases (e.g., cerebral palsy, Duchenne muscular dystrophy, polio, and other disorders). This type of scoliosis tends to be progressive, with the degree of deformity dependent upon many factors. Those affected children who are unable to walk (nonambulatory) often develop additional skeletal irregularities involving the pelvis and spine. In severe cases, respiratory difficulties may develop. Early evaluation and intervention through surgery and other means help to alter the progression of the spinal deformity and its associated complications.

Certain syndromes (e.g., Marfan syndrome, neurofibromatosis) place affected children at risk for spinal irregularities such as scoliosis. Treatment for these children includes regular orthopedic examination and intervention to prevent progression of the irregularity.

Scoliosis sometimes results from unequal leg length resulting from an irregular tilt (obliquity) of the pelvis. Treatment for this compensatory scoliosis may include the use of special orthopedic shoes.

The following organizations in the General Resources Section can provide additional information: March of Dimes Birth Defects Foundation, NIH/National Institute of Arthritis and Musculoskeletal and Skin Diseases, NIH/National Information Center for Children & Youth with Disabilities, Online Mendelian Inheritance in Man: www3.ncbi.nlm.nih.gov/Omim/searchomim.html

National Associations & Support Groups

3602 National Scoliosis Foundation
5 Cabot Place
Stoughton, MA 02072   781-341-6333
800-673-6922
Fax: 781-341-8333
e-mail: scoliosis@aol.com
www.scoliosis.com

Promotes school screening, offers public awareness materials to promote public education,
maintains a resource center for professional information, conducts scoliosis conferences, and offers support groups.

Joseph P. O'Brien, President

3603 Scoliosis Association, Inc.
P.O. Box 811705
Boca Raton, FL 33481   561-994-0669
800-800-0669
Fax: 561-994-2455
e-mail: normlipin@aol.com
www.scoliosis-assoc.org/

A non-profit, volunteer non-medical organization established in 1974. The association provides information, support groups and
information lines about scoliosis. It also publishes a newsletter for members called BACKTALK,
written by patients and medical professionals.

International

3604 International Federation of Spine Associations
c/o Howard M. Shulman
9908 Cape Scott Court
Raleigh, NC 27614   919-846-2204
www.ifosa.org

IFOSA is a federation of various national Spine
Associations from countries in North America,
Europe and Australia. These organizations prin-
cipally represent the spine patients and their
families. At the annual meetings of IFOSA, representatives from each of these member organizations are invited to attend and discuss the
emotional and social problems which face the
spine patient and his or her family.

Libraries & Resource Centers

3605 Johns Hopkins Department of Orthopaedics Surgery
601 N. Caroline Street
Baltimore, MD 21287   410-955-1830
Fax: 410-955-1719
med.jhu.edu/ortho/peds/kyphosis/

Scoliosis is a three-dimensional curvature of the
spine, best appreciated on an anteroposterior ra-
diograph and physical examination. Many different causes have been identified. The most
common type is idiopathic scoliosis. Kyphosis, a
curvature in the sagittal plane only. Physical deformity is often confused.

3606 Shriners Hospital for Children
Chicago Unit
2211 North Oak Park Avenue
Chicago, IL 60707   773-622-5400
Fax: 773-385-5453
TDD: 773-385-5419
e-mail: vlwalter@earthlink.net
www.shrinerschicago.org

Providing orthopedic treatment (especially for
scoliosis, osteogenesis imperfecta, clubfoot, cerebral palsy and limb deficiencies), plastic and craniofacial surgery (including orthognathic and
cleft lip and palate), and comprehensive spinal
cord injury rehabilitation at no charge for children under age 18. Combines quality family-centered care with innovative education and
research.

A. James Spang, Administrator
Paula Canham, Admissions Coordinator

Research Centers

3607 International Scoliosis Research Center
104 East Summit Avenue
Wales, WI 53183
800-554-8806
Fax: 414-968-5214
e-mail: dpmolloydc@scoliosishelp.org
www.scoliosishelp.org/

The International Scoliosis Research Center is
committed to furthering the levels of health care
for those affected with scoliosis. It also promtoes
educational programs and offers assistance to
doctors, educators, schools and victims of
scoliosis as well as to their families.

3608 Scoliosis Research Society
Information
6300 N. River Road
Rosemont, IL 60018   847-803-3550

This society provides an international forum for
those interested in the management of scoliosis.
It holds a yearly meeting at which health professionals share observations and results, and explore new avenues of research.

Audio Video

3609 Dealing with Scoliosis: A Patient Guide to Diagnosis and Treatment
National Scoliosis Foundation
5 Cabot Place
Stoughton, MA 02072   781-341-6333
                               800-673-6922
                          Fax: 781-341-8333
                     e-mail: scoliosis@aol.com

An upbeat video features Miss North Carolina Michelle Mauney and explains diagnosis and treatment of scoliosis through the experience of several teenagers and young adults.

3610 Ellie's Back
National Scoliosis Foundation
5 Cabot Place
Stoughton, MA 02072   781-341-6333
                               800-673-6922
                          Fax: 781-341-8333
                     e-mail: scoliosis@aol.com

An eight year old, and her mother team up together to produce a film that portrays life with scoliosis through the eyes of a young child.

3611 Growing Straighter and Stronger
National Scoliosis Foundation
5 Cabot Place
Stoughton, MA 02072   781-341-6333
                               800-673-6922
                          Fax: 781-341-8333
                     e-mail: scoliosis@aol.com

A presentation for the pre-screening education of students in grades 5 through 7.

15 Minutes

3612 Preparing Yourself for Spinal Surgery for Teenagers with Severe Scoliosis
National Scoliosis Foundation
5 Cabot Place
Stoughton, MA 02072   781-341-6333
                               800-673-6922
                          Fax: 781-341-8333
                     e-mail: scoliosis@aol.com

Patient educational video helping to reduce the anxiety for teenagers facing surgery by giving a sense of what to expect before, during, and after surgery.

3613 School Screening with Dr. Robert Keller
National Scoliosis Foundation
5 Cabot Place
Stoughton, MA 02072   781-341-6333
                               800-673-6922
                          Fax: 781-341-8333
                     e-mail: scoliosis@aol.com

A training video that teaches the proper technique for doing spinal screening. Defines scoliosis and kyphosis. Four teenagers, three with curves and one without, are examined and the findings explained.

Videotape

3614 Taking the Mystery Out of Spinal Deformities
Children's Hospital of LA, Div. of Orthopaedics
4650 Sunset Blvd., Mail Stop #69
Los Angeles, CA 90027   213-660-2450
                               800-841-7439

Answers questions most often asked by screeners, patients and parents.

Videotape

3615 Understanding Scoliosis
National Scoliosis Foundation
5 Cabot Place
Stoughton, MA 02072   781-341-6333
                               800-673-6922
                          Fax: 781-341-8333
                     e-mail: scoliosis@aol.com

Kaiser Permanente's educational video clearly and positively addresses the patient community. In this video four teenagers at various stages of treatment talk about their life with scoliosis.

3616 You Are Not Alone
Minnesota Spine Center
913 East 26th Street
Minneapolis, MN 55454   612-332-3843
                          Fax: 612-775-6222
                     e-mail: informat@mr.net

A video presenting two women's experiences with surgery. Personal life, concerns, hospital experience, recovery and improved lifestyle are openly discussed.

Videotape

Web Sites

3617 John Hopkins Department of Orthopaedics Surgery
www.med.jhu.edu/ortho/peds/scoliosis/

3618 Scoliosis Mailing List
www.ai.mit.edu/extra/scoliosis//scoliosis.html

3619 Scoliosis Research Society
www.srs.org/

3620 Wheeless' Textbook of Orthopaedics
www.medmedia.com/o11/47.htm

Books

3621 Adult Scoliosis Surgery...It Can be Done
St. Luke's Spine Center
11311 Shaker Blvd.
Cleveland, OH 44104   216-368-7000

Describes various types of surgery and procedures used in adult scoliosis patients.

21 pages

3622 Handbook of Scoliosis
Scoliosis Research Society
6300 N. River Road, Suite 727
Rosemont, IL 60018   847-698-1627

3623 Textbook of Scoliosis & Other Spinal Deformities
David S. Bradford, author

W.B. Saunders Company
Independence Square West
Philadelphia, PA 19106   215-238-7800

1994
ISBN: 0-721655-33-5

3624 Tina's Story...Scoliosis and Me
Alfred I. DuPont Institute
P.O. Box 269
Wilmington, DE 19899   302-651-4000

Suggested for parents of children anticipating surgery. This outstanding book, written as an eighth grade project by a thirteen year old scoliosis patient, relates her experiences and emotions while wearing a brace for three years prior to surgery.

3625 What Can I Give You?
Mary Mahony, author

National Scoliosis Foundation
5 Cabot Place
Stoughton, MA 02072   781-341-6333
                                        800-673-6922
                                        Fax: 781-341-8333
                                        e-mail: scoliosis@aol.com

A wounderful story of a loving mother's care for her daughter. The medical saga of Erin and Mary offers insight and inspiration to families living with congenital scoliosis and vauable guidance to the physicians who treat them.

3626 What Young People and Parents Need to Know About Scoliosis
American Physical Therapy Association
111 N. Fairfax Street
Alexandria, VA 22314   703-684-2782
                                        Fax: 703-706-8578
                                        www.apta.org

A physical therapist's perspective, about what coliosis is and what parents and young people should look for to detect scoliosis.

Children's Books

3627 Deenie
Judy Blume, author

Bradbury Press
866 Third Avenue
New York, NY 10022   212-702-2000
                                        800-257-5755

Deenie, a beautiful thirteen-year-old girl, had a mother who was pushing her to become a model. The agency told Deenie she had the looks but walked differently. Deenie's main wish was to become a cheerleader, but didn't make the finalist list. Her gym teacher noticed her posture and called her family, and the diagnosis of adolescent idiopathic scoliosis was made.

159 pages Hardcover
ISBN: 0-027110-20-6

3628 Nothing Hurts but My Heart
Linda Barr, author

National Scoliosis Foundation
5 Cabot Place
Stoughton, MA 02072   781-341-6333
                                        800-673-6922
                                        Fax: 781-341-8333
                                        e-mail: scoliosis@aol.com

For every boy, girl, and their parents who learn that bracing may be needed to treat their scoliosis. The story is of a young gymnast dealing with the issues of wearing a brace.

3629 There's an S on My Back: S is for Scoliosis

Mary Mahony, author

National Scoliosis Foundation
5 Cabot Place
Stoughton, MA 02072
781-341-6333
800-673-6922
Fax: 781-341-8333
e-mail: scoliosis@aol.com

The medical journy of a fifth grader diagnosised with idiopathic scoliosis at a school screening. A realistic fiction, the story gives us a day-by-day account of what a preadolescent experiances.

3630 Twenty Years At Hull House

Jane Addams, author

New American Library
375 Hudson Street
New York, NY 10014
212-366-2000

Book dealing with scoliosis.

Grades 7-12

Magazines

3631 Scoliosis, Me?

North Dallas Scoliosis Center
1910 N. Collins Blvd.
Richardson, TX 75080
972-644-1930

Detailed answers to questions most asked by parents and teens.

Newsletters

3632 Backtalk

Scoliosis Association
P.O. Box 811705
Boca Raton, FL 33481
561-994-4435
800-800-0669
Fax: 561-994-2455
e-mail: scolioassn@aol.com
scoliosis-assn.org

Information for families, patients and health care professionals.

3633 Spinal Connection

National Scoliosis Foundation
5 Cabot Place
Stoughton, MA 02072
781-341-6333
800-673-6922
Fax: 781-341-8333
e-mail: scoliosis@aol.com

Offers updated information and the latest medical advances in the area of spinal cord injury and spina bifida. Includes resources, reviews, support group and meeting information.

8 pages BiAnnual

Pamphlets

3634 1 in Every 10 Persons Has Scoliosis

National Scoliosis Foundation
5 Cabot Place
Stoughton, MA 02072
781-341-6333
800-673-6922
Fax: 781-341-8333
e-mail: scoliosis@aol.com

Explains what scoliosis is, and how to screen for it. Also contains facts about the Foundation.

3635 Adolescent Idiopathic Scoliosis-Prevalence Natural History, Treatments

Stuart L. Weinstein, MD, author

National Scoliosis Foundation
5 Cabot Place
Stoughton, MA 02072
781-341-6333
800-673-6922
Fax: 781-341-8333
e-mail: scoliosis@aol.com

3636 Boston Bracing System for Idiopathic Scoliosis

National Scoliosis Foundation
5 Cabot Place
Stoughton, MA 02072
781-341-6333
800-673-6922
Fax: 781-341-8333
e-mail: scoliosis@aol.com

3637 Brace & Her Brace is No Handicap

National Scoliosis Foundation
5 Cabot Place
Stoughton, MA 02072
781-341-6333
800-673-6922
Fax: 781-341-8333
e-mail: scoliosis@aol.com

Contains two illustrated short stories, each about a teenage girl coping successfully with scoliosis.

3638 Getting a Second Opinion
National Scoliosis Foundation
5 Cabot Place
Stoughton, MA 02072   781-341-6333
                             800-673-6922
                        Fax: 781-341-8333
               e-mail: scoliosis@aol.com

Reprinted from Health Tips.

3639 Going Home
University Hospital Spine Center
2074 Abington Road
Cleveland, OH 44106   216-844-1616

Instructions for pediatric and adult patients who have had a spinal fusion.

3640 Medical Update Column
National Scoliosis Foundation
5 Cabot Place
Stoughton, MA 02072   781-341-6333
                             800-673-6922
                        Fax: 781-341-8333
               e-mail: scoliosis@aol.com

Reprints from past issues of the Spinal Connections Medical Update Column available on various topics.

3641 NSF Packets
National Scoliosis Foundation
5 Cabot Place
Stoughton, MA 02072   781-341-6333
                             800-673-6922
                        Fax: 781-341-8333
               e-mail: scoliosis@aol.com

Contains information for parents and young people, adults, and healthcare professionals.

3642 Patient with Scoliosis
Educational Services, Division of AJV Company
555 57th Street
New York, NY 10019   212-996-6473

A reprint from the American Journal of nursin.

3643 Postural Screening Program
National Scoliosis Foundation
5 Cabot Place
Stoughton, MA 02072   781-341-6333
                             800-673-6922
                        Fax: 781-341-8333
               e-mail: scoliosis@aol.com

Guidelines for physicians and school nurses.

3644 Questions Most Often Asked the NSF
National Scoliosis Foundation
5 Cabot Place
Stoughton, MA 02072   781-341-6333
                             800-673-6922
                        Fax: 781-341-8333
               e-mail: scoliosis@aol.com

Answers the most frequently asked questions about scoliosis.

3645 Scoliosis Detecting and Treating Scoliosis
Consumer Info Ctr, Dept 554B
Pueblo, CO 81009

This disorder involves a curvature of the spine that can eventually become crippling. It is imperative that scoliosis be detected and treated early in children.

3646 Scoliosis - a Handbook for Patients
National Scoliosis Foundation
5 Cabot Place
Stoughton, MA 02072   781-341-6333
                             800-673-6922
                        Fax: 781-341-8333
               e-mail: scoliosis@aol.com

Information on detection and treatment of adolescent scoliosis, kyphosis and lordosis and adult scoliosis.

3647 Scoliosis Research Society
6300 N. River Road, Suite 727
Rosemont, IL 60018   847-698-1627
                        Fax: 847-823-0536
               e-mail: goulding@aaos.org
                             www.srs.org/

The Scoliosis Research Society has prepared a booklet to provide patients, and in the case of children, their parents, with a better understanding of scoliosis, its diagnosis and management, using idiopathic scoliosis-the most common type-as a model. This information in intended as a supplement to the information your physician will provide you.

Courtney W Brown, President
Harry L Shufflebarger, President-Elect

3648 Scoliosis Road Map
University Hospital Spine Center
2074 Abington Road
Cleveland, OH 44106   216-844-1616

Written for teenagers affected by this illness.

3649 Scoliosis Screening, the Carlsbad Program

Win Van Cleave, RN, author

National Scoliosis Foundation
5 Cabot Place
Stoughton, MA 02072   781-341-6333
800-673-6922
Fax: 781-341-8333
e-mail: scoliosis@aol.com

Exceptional scoliosis screening program.

3650 Scoliosis Surgery, What's it All About?

University Hospital Spine Center
2074 Abington Road
Cleveland, OH 44106   216-844-1616

This pamphlet answers many of the questions patients ask before having surgery.

3651 Scoliosis and Kyphosis

Scoliosis Research Society
6300 N. River Road, Ste. 727
Rosemont, IL 60018   847-698-1627

Information and advice from parents.

3652 What If You Need An Operation For Scoliosis?

St. Luke's Spine Center
11311 Shaker Blvd.
Cleveland, OH 44104   216-368-7000

3653 What Young People & Their Parents Need To Know About Scoliosis

American Physical Therapy Association
1111 N. Fairfax Street
Alexandria, VA 22314   703-684-2782

A physical therapists' perspective.

3654 When the Spine Curves

National Scoliosis Foundation
5 Cabot Place
Stoughton, MA 02072   781-341-6333
800-673-6922
Fax: 781-341-8333
e-mail: scoliosis@aol.com

3655 You and Your Brace

University Hospital Spine Center
2074 Abington Road
Cleveland, OH 44106   216-844-1616

DESCRIPTION

3656 SEIZURES

Synonym: Convulsions

Covers these related disorders: Absence (petit mal) seizures, Complex partial seizures, Generalized tonic-clonic seizures, Simple partial seizures

May involve these systems in the body (see Section III):

Central Nervous System, Nervous System

Seizures are a neurologic condition characterized by sudden episodes of uncontrolled electrical activity in the brain. These electrical disturbances may cause abnormal motor activities, lost or impaired consciousness, impaired control of certain involuntary functions (autonomic dysfunction), or sensory or behavioral abnormalities. Seizures are a common neurologic condition of childhood, affecting approximately six in 1,000 children. Approximately 70 percent of children who experience one seizure never experience another, whereas about 30 percent develop recurring seizures, which is referred to as epilepsy. Seizures may result from many different causes, including fever, head injury, infection or inflammation of the brain, insufficient oxygen supply to the brain, or certain metabolic imbalances. Seizures may also be caused by brain tumors, particular degenerative metabolic or neurological diseases, abnormal reactions to certain medications, or drug intoxication. There are also a number of syndromes and genetic disorders in which seizures are a primary feature. In many children, the exact underlying cause of recurrent seizures cannot be determined and the disorder is termed idiopathic epilepsy.

The specific form that a seizure takes and its associated symptoms may depend upon a number of factors, including the region of the brain in which the electrical disturbance arises and how widely it spreads from its point of origin. Epileptic seizures may be broadly classified into two groups: partial and generalized seizures. Partial seizures often result due to damage or impairment of a limited area of the brain, whereas generalized seizures may affect a wide area of the brain. In addition, some partial seizures may begin in a particular brain region but spread to affect most of the brain, ultimately becoming a generalized seizure. Because different seizure types may cause similar symptoms, specialized techniques that record brain wave activity (electroencephalography or EEG) and other neurologic imaging tests (such as MRI or CT scans) may play an important role in classifying certain seizure disorders.

Partial seizures, which may account for up to 40 percent of childhood seizures, may be subdivided into simple partial seizures, during which consciousness is retained, and complex partial seizures, during which consciousness is impaired. Simple partial seizures are characterized by abnormal, rhythmic muscle contractions and relaxations (clonic seizures) and increased muscle tone and rigidity (tonic seizures), particularly affecting muscles of the neck, face, arms, and legs. These seizures, which usually last about 10 to 20 seconds, are frequently associated with abnormal eye movements and head turning. In many children, simple partial seizures may be preceded by an aura consisting of headache, chest discomfort, and a feeling of anxiety, fear, or dread.

Complex partial seizures are characterized by a sudden pause in activity and a blank stare and may be preceded by an aura that consists of a vague feeling of fear or unpleasantness, headache, and chest discomfort. Most patients also perform certain involuntary actions following loss of consciousness. In infants, such actions may include lip smacking, swallowing, or chewing, whereas older children may conduct incoordinated, semipurposeful actions, such as rubbing objects or pulling at clothing. Such seizures may last approximately one to two minutes.

Generalized seizures may be subdivided into absence (petit mal) seizures and generalized tonic-clonic seizures. Absence seizures, which rarely occur before the age of five, usually last from a few seconds up to half a minute. During an episode, children experience a momentary loss of consciousness during which they cease speaking or performing other motor activities. They typically have a blank facial expression, their eyelids may flicker, and the head may fall forward. Patients typically have no awareness of the episode and resume the activity they were performing before the seizure.

Generalized tonic-clonic seizures may be preceded by an aura and occasionally begin with a shrill cry as patients lose consciousness. During an episode, the eyes roll back, muscles of the entire body stiffen, and all muscle groups begin to rhythmically contract and relax. If temporary cessation of breathing (apnea) occurs, patients may quickly develop an abnormal, bluish discoloration of the skin and mucous membranes (cyanosis). Bladder and bowel control may be temporarily lost. After an episode, patients are typically semiconscious and disoriented and may remain in a deep sleep for up to two hours (postictal state). During such a seizure episode, patients should be placed on one side, tight clothing around the neck should be loosened, and the jaw should be gently extended to enhance breathing. However, the mouth should not be forcibly opened nor should an object be placed between the teeth.

Generalized seizures also include a form of epilepsy known as infantile spasms, which typically begin between the ages of four and eight months and continue to approximately 18 months. Infantile spasms are characterized by sudden, brief, symmetric contractions of the arms and legs, neck, and torso. Spasms may occur for several minutes with brief intervals between each spasm. Episodes tend to occur when children are drowsy or immediately upon awakening. Depending upon the underlying cause, the condition may evolve into different forms of epilepsy later in life and may be associated with an increased risk of mental retardation.

Seizures that occur in association with a rapidly rising fever, known as febrile seizures, are the most common seizure disorder of childhood. Febrile seizures most commonly occur between nine months to five years of age and may affect up to four percent of all children. This type of seizure rarely develops into epilepsy. In many cases, there is a history of such seizures among siblings and parents, indicating that genetic factors may play some causative role. Febrile seizures often occur in association with certain upper respiratory infections and acute inflammation of the middle ear (otitis media). However, because convulsions may result from serious infections of the brain (e.g., meningitis), a thorough medical evaluation must be conducted to determine the cause of the fever. Febrile seizures are typically characterized by muscle rigidity followed by abnormal, rhythmic contractions and relaxations of muscle groups (generalized tonic-clonic seizures). The seizure may last from seconds up to about 10 minutes and is often followed by a brief period of drowsiness.

Generalized or partial seizures that continue for more than 30 minutes without a return to consciousness are known as status epilepticus. Such seizures may occur due to underlying metabolic abnormalities, neurologic disorders, congenital brain malformations, or inflammation of the brain. They may also represent prolonged febrile seizures, develop due to sudden withdrawal of antiseizure (anticonvulsant) medication, or result from unknown causes. Status epilepticus may result in life-threatening complications and is considered a medical emergency, requiring hospitalization. Treatment may include supplemental oxygen, intravenous fluids, physical and neurologic evaluations, intravenous medications including appropriate antiseizure drugs, and other measures as required. Children affected by the condition before one year of age are more likely to have mental retardation and other long-term effects, secondary to an underlying CNS disorder.

The treatment of seizures depends on the underlying cause, the type of seizure present, and other factors. If a treatable condition or disorder is identified, such as a fever, abnormal blood sugar levels, or certain tumors, measures are taken as required to treat the underlying cause. For example, in the case of febrile seizures, thorough evaluations are conducted to determine the fever's cause and measures are then taken as necessary to control the fever. If an underlying cause cannot be identified or adequately treated or controlled, treatment typically includes the administration of antiseizure (anticonvulsant) medications to help prevent, reduce, or control seizures. The specific anticonvulsant medication prescribed may depend on several factors, including the classification of the seizure, patient history, and possible side effects. Anticonvulsant drugs used to treat certain types of seizures may include carbamazepine, phenobarbital, primidone, phenytoin, gabapentin, or valproate. In addition, adrenocorticotropic hormone (ACTH) is often used to treat children with infantile spasms. If seizure control is not obtained with a particular medication, other anticonvulsants may be substituted. In some patients, combination drug therapy may be necessary to adequately control seizures. If seizure control is not obtained with anticonvulsant medications, surgery may be considered. Additional treatment is symptomatic and supportive.

The following organizations in the General Resources Section can provide additional information: Genetic Alliance, NIH/National Institute of Neurological Disorders & Stroke, March of Dimes Birth Defects Foundation

National Associations & Support Groups

3657 American Epilepsy Society
342 North Main Street
West Hartford, CT 06117
860-586-7505
Fax: 860-586-7550
e-mail: info@aesnet.org
www.aesnet.org

Fosters treatment of epilepsy in its biological, clinical and social phases.

Sue Barry, Executive Director

3658 C.A.N.D.L.E.
4414 McCampbell Drive
Montgomery, AL 36106
334-271-3947
Fax: 334-271-3947

3659 Cleveland Clinic Children's Hospital
9500 Euclid Avenue
Cleveland, OH 44195
216-444-5437
800-223-2273
Fax: 216-445-7792
TTY: 216-444-7991
www.clevelandclinic.org/pediatrics

Provides innovative care for infants, children, and adolescents with complex medical problems. Includes medical, surgical, rehabilitation, psychiatric and intensive care, latest technology, including a computerized epilepsy monitoring unit, a consolidated pediatric intensive care unit and operating suites. Physicians are known for their expertise in treating major medical problems, such as cardiovascular disease, cancer, digestive disorders, musculoskeletal problems and neurosensory disorders.

Douglas S. Moodle, M.D., M.S., Chairman and Director

3660 Epilepsy Canada
1470 Peel Street, Suite 745
Montreal, Quebec H3A1T1,
Canada
514-845-7855
800-860-5499
Fax: 514-845-7866
e-mail: epilepsy@epilepsy.ca
www.epilepsy.ca

Non-profit organizated dedicating to improving the quality of life for those affected by epilepsy.

3661 Epilepsy Education Association, Inc.
4335-1C Irish Hills Dr
South Bend, IN 46614
219-273-4050
www.iupui.edu/~epilepsy/

Dedidcated to promoting education about epilepsy. Educational programs directed to patients and their families including information about epilepsy, its history, causes and treatment.

3662 Epilepsy Foundation
Epilepsy Foundation of America
4351 Garden City Drive
Landover, MD 20785
301-459-3700
800-332-1000
Fax: 301-377-9056

A toll free information and referral service staffed by specially trained people who will answer questions and discuss concerns about seizure disorders and their treatment. Staff will direct callers to local affiliates of the foundation and tell about a brand range of services that respond to the needs of people with seizure disorders.

18,000 members

3663 National Association of Epilepsy Centers
5775 Wayzata Blvd.
Minneapolis, MN 55416
612-525-4526
Fax: 612-525-1560

A nonprofit organization that encourages and supports professional and technical education in the treatment of epilepsy. Over 50 centers nationwide are members of the trade association, which will make referrals to its member centers.

Robert J. Gumnit, MD, President
Gumnit, MD Timothy A., Pedley, MD

State Agencies & Support Groups

California

3664 Epilepsy Foundation of Northern California
1624 Franklin Street Suite 900
Oakland, CA 94612   510-893-6272
                                 800-632-3532
                            Fax: 510-893-8608
                        www.efnc.com.index.html

Florida

3665 Collier, Hendy, and Glades Counties Epilepsy Foundations of Florida
852 First Avenue, South Room 1
Naples, FL 33919   941-649-7430
                            Fax: 941-649-7680

Alissa Wallace, MA

3666 Epilepsy Association of Big Bend
1108-B East Park Avenue
Tallahassee, FL 32301   850-222-1777
                            Fax: 850-222-7440
                e-mail: bigbend@floridaepilepsy.org

Services include: Case management, prevention education, counseling and advocacy, information and referral.

3667 Epilepsy Foundation of South Florida
7300 N. Kendal Dr.,#700
Miami, FL 33156   305-670-4949
                            Fax: 305-670-0904
            e-mail: information@epilepsysofla.org

The Epilepsy Foundation of South Florida, is a twenty-five year old non profit community based organization dedicated to enhancing the personal and social adjustments of individuals with seizure disorders and their families.

3668 Epilepsy Services of North Central Florida
1010 N.W. 8th Avenue, Suite B
Gainesville, FL 32601   352-392-6449
                                 800-330-9746
                            Fax: 352-392-5792
            e-mail: jlyons@college.med.ufl.edu

3669 Epilepsy Services of Northeast Florida
6028 Chester Ave, #106
Jacksonville, FL 32217   904-731-3751
                e-mail: efnefjohn@aol.com

Services include : Program case management, program prevention and education, employment services, children's summer camp, counseling and advocacy, and information and referrals.

3670 Epilepsy Services of West Central Florida
4023 N. Armenia Ave., #100
Tampa, FL 33607   813-870-3414
                            Fax: 813-870-1321
            e-mail: tampa@floridaepilepsy.org

3671 Lee County Epilepsy Foundations of Florida
1436 Royal Palm Square Blvd.
Fort Myers, FL 33919   941-275-4838
                            Fax: 941-275-7022

Nanette Frankel, Lead Social Worker
Frankel Robert, Perkins

3672 Manattee County Office Epilepsy Foundations of Florida
1701 - 14th Street West, Room 6
Bradenton, FL 34205   941-746-6488
                            Fax: 941-746-8382

Brian Larocque, Social Worker

3673 Sarasota and Desoto Counties Epilepsy Foundation of Florida
1900 Main Street, Suite 212
Sarasota, FL 34236   941-953-5988
                            Fax: 941-366-5890

Kela Miller, MSE
Miller Sarah, Gorman

New Jersey

3674 Epilepsy Foundation of New Jersey
429 River View Plaza
Trenton, NJ 08611   609-392-4900
                                     800-335-6843
                                Fax: 609-392-5621
                                TDD: 800-852-7899
                                     www.egnj.com

3675 Epilepsy Foundation New Jersey
429 River View Plaza
Trenton, NJ 08611   609-392-4900
                                Fax: 609-392-5621
                                TDD: 800-852-7899
                                     www.efnj.com

Non-profit agency dedicated to improving the
lives of those affected by epilepsy and their families. The EFNJ provides a variety of programs
such as support groups, counseling, emergency
medication assistance, scholarships and family
support services. Financial stipend assistance is
also available.

New York

3676 Epilepsy Foundation of Long Island
506 Stewart Avenue
Garden City, NY 11530   516-739-7733
                                Fax: 516-739-1860
                                e-mail: info@efli.org
                                     www.efli.org

Provides education counseling, residential care,
and day programs to Long Island residents with
epilepsy and related conditions.

Richard Daly, Executive Director

Pennsylvania

3677 Epilepsy Foundation of Southeastern Pennsylvania
7 Benjamin Franklin Parkway 6th Floor
Philadelphia, PA 19103   215-232-9180
                                Fax: 215-627-4741

3678 Epilepsy Foundation of Western Pennsylvania
1323 Forbes Ave, Suite 102
Pittsburgh, PA 15219   412-261-5880

Washington

3679 Epilepsy Association of Washington
3800 Aurora Ave. N. #370
Seattle, WA 98103   206-547-4551
                                     800-752-3509
                                Fax: 206-547-4557
                                e-mail: epilepsy@juno.com
                                www.cyberspace.con/~epilepsy/

Research Centers

Illinois

3680 University of Illinois At Chicago Consultation Clinic for Epilepsy
912 S. Wood Street
Chicago, IL 60612   312-996-5461

Dr. John R. Hughes, Director

New York

3681 Neurology Research Center
Helen Hayes Hospital
Route 9W
West Haverstraw, NY 10993   914-947-3000
                                Fax: 914-947-3000

Robert S. Slociter, Research Director

North Carolina

3682 Duke University Epilepsy Research Center
401 Bryan Research Bldg.
Durham, NC 27710   919-684-4241
                                Fax: 919-684-8219

Dr. James McNamara, Director

3683 Duke University, Center for the Advanced Study of Epilepsy
Medical Center
Box 2905
Durham, NC 27710   919-286-6811
                                Fax: 919-286-4662

Clinical and research unit that experiments in
limbic epilepsy.

Dr. James McNamara, Director

3684 Wake Forest University Comprehensive Epilepsy Program
300 S. Hawthorne Road
Winston Salem, NC 27103   336-716-8010
Fax: 336-748-4480

Dr. Kiffin Penry, Director

Ohio

3685 Case Western Reserve University Applied Neural Control Laboratory
Charles B. Bolton Bldg., #3480
Cleveland, OH 44106   216-368-3200
Fax: 216-368-4872

Specializes in research and development of technology based stimulation of the central nervous system in epilepsy treatment.

J. Thomas Mortimer, Director

Pennsylvania

3686 Medical College of Pennsylvania Mid Atlantic Regional Epilepsy Center
3200 Henry Avenue
Philadelphia, PA 19129   215-842-6990
Fax: 215-849-0820

Epileptic seizure detection including apparatus studies.

Dr. Richard Harner, Director

Tennessee

3687 University of Tennessee, Center For Neuroscience
875 Monroe Avenue
Memphis, TN 38163   901-528-5956
Fax: 901-528-7193

Epilepsy research and studies.

Dr. Stephen Kitai, Director

Texas

3688 Baylor College of Medicine Epilepsy Research Center
Texas Medical Center

Houston, TX 77030   713-797-0100

Dr. Peter Kellaway, Director

Wisconsin

3689 University of Wisconsin - Madison Neuropsychology Laboratory
600 N. Highland Avenue
Madison, WI 53792   608-263-1530

Epilepsy research.

Dr. Charles Matthews, Director

Audio Video

3690 Comprehensive Clinical Management of The Epilepsies
Epilepsy Foundation of America
4351 Garden City Drive
Landover, MD 20785   301-459-3700
800-332-1000
Fax: 301-577-9056
TDD: 800-332-2070

Excellent reference on the treatment of epilepsy.
17 minutes

3691 Epilepsy
Fanlight Productions
47 Halifax St
Boston, MA 02130   617-469-4999
Fax: 617-469-3379
e-mail: fanlight@tiac.net
www.fanlight.com

This program examines new surgical techniques which may offer help.
28 minutes

3692 How to Recognize and Classify Seizures
Epilepsy Foundation of America
4351 Garden City Drive
Landover, MD 20785   301-459-3700
800-332-1000
Fax: 301-577-9056
TDD: 800-332-2070

Discusses the classification of seizures and epileptic syndromes.
25 minutes

3693 Just Like You and Me
TASH
11201 Greenwood Avenue North
Seattle, WA 98133   206-361-8870
                          Fax: 206-523-9495

A video/print package on successful living with epilepsy.

25 Minutes

3694 Rest of the Family
Epilepsy Foundation of America
4351 Garden City Drive
Landover, MD 20785   301-459-3700
                          800-332-1000
                          Fax: 301-577-9056
                          TDD: 800-332-2070

Presents the feelings and concerns of other family members including siblings, of children with epilepsy.

3695 Seizure First Aid
Epilepsy Foundation of America
4351 Garden City Drive
Landover, MD 20785   301-459-3700
                          800-332-1000
                          Fax: 301-577-9056
                          TDD: 800-332-2070

This video combines footage of real seizures with reenactments to demonstrate proper first aid procedures. In addition, people with epilepsy talk about how they feel when they have a seizure, discuss how they would like friends, family and the general public to react when a seizure occurs.

10 minutes

3696 Understanding Seizure Disorders
Epilepsy Foundation of America
4351 Garden City Drive
Landover, MD 20785   301-459-3700
                          800-332-1000
                          Fax: 301-577-9056
                          TDD: 800-332-2070

Provides an explanation of seizure disorders in everyday language and dispels many misconceptions about epilepsy with medically accurate information.

Web Sites

3697 Seizures.net
www.seizures.net/

3698 Usenet
alt.support.epilepsy

Books

3699 A Bomb In the Brain: A Heroic Tale Of Science, Surgery and Survival
Steve Fishman, author

MacMillan Publishing Co.
866 Third Avenue
New York, NY 10022   212-702-2000

The autobiographical account of this author's struggle with epilepsy and the debilitating effects it has on health, emotions, and mental stability.

Grades 10-12

3700 Americans with Disabilities Act
Epilepsy Foundation of America
4351 Garden City Drive
Landover, MD 20785   301-459-3700
                          800-332-1000
                          Fax: 301-577-9056
                          TDD: 800-332-2070

Learn how the Americans With Disabilities Act of 1990 can benifit you. Excellent comprehensive resource for individuals with seizure disorders.

46 pages Softcover
ISBN: 0-802774-65-2

3701 Children with Epilepsy
Helen Reisner, author

Epilepsy Foundation of America
4351 Garden City Drive
Landover, MD 20785   301-459-3700
                          800-332-1000
                          Fax: 301-577-9056
                          TDD: 800-332-2070

Offers direction and support to parents of a child with epilepsy, by first educating them about epilepsy and then helping them cope with the effects this disorder will have on their child and family.

314 pages Softcover
ISBN: 0-933149-19-0

3702 Does Your Child Have Epilepsy?

James E. Jan, author

Epilepsy Foundation of America
4351 Garden City Drive
Landover, MD 20785   301-459-3700
                            800-332-1000
                       Fax: 301-577-9056
                       TDD: 800-332-2070

This book establishes Ten Basic Rules for parents of children with epilepsy.

201 pages Softcover

3703 Educator's Guide to Students with Epilepsy

Robert J. Michael, author

Charles C. Thomas Publishing, Ltd.
2600 South First Street
Springfield, IL 62704   217-789-8980
                               800-258-8980
                          Fax: 217-789-9130
                 e-mail: books@ccthomas.com
                          www.ccthomas.com

Presents relevant knowledge about epilepsy for the educator, creates an awareness of and sensitivity to students with epilepsy, focuses attention on the role of education with such students, presents the major educational issues, defines the educator's responsibility to afflicted students, and presents useful resources.

1995 174 pages Softcover
ISBN: 0-398065-38-1

3704 Epilepsies of Childhood

Niall V. Donohue, author

Butterworth-Heinemann
225 Wildwood Avenue
Woburn, MA 01801   617-928-2500
                          800-366-2665

1994 320 pages
ISBN: 0-750615-98-2

3705 Epilepsy Surgery

Hans Otto Luders, author

Raven Press
1185 Avenue of the Americas
New York, NY 10036   212-930-9500

The most complete and current references on surgical treatments of the epilepsies.

880 pages
ISBN: 0-881678-21-0

3706 Epilepsy-I Can Live with That

Writings By People with Epilepsy, author

Epilepsy Foundation of America
4351 Garden City Drive
Landover, MD 20785   301-459-3700
                            800-332-1000
                       Fax: 301-577-9056
                       TDD: 800-332-2070

The experience of epilepsy as recorded by a group of ordinary men and women living in Australia. Each story focuses on personal growth, triumph over disability and emphasizes individual courage and hope.

Softcover
ISBN: 0-802774-65-2

3707 Epilepsy: A Behavior Medicine Approach to Assessment & Treatment in Children

JoAnne C. Dahl, author

Hogrefe & Huber Publications
Box 51
Lewiston, NY 14092   716-282-1610
                       Fax: 716-484-4200

1993 200 pages
ISBN: 0-889371-06-7

3708 Epilepsy: Current Approaches to Diagnosis and Treatment

Raven Press
1185 Avenue of the Americas
New York, NY 10036   212-930-9500

288 pages
ISBN: 0-881676-15-2

3709 Epilepsy: Diagnosis, Management & Quality of Life

Kiffin J. Penry, author

Raven Press
1185 Avenue of the Americas
New York, NY 10036   212-930-9500

1994 64 pages Softcover
ISBN: 0-881671-92-6

3710 Epilepsy: Models, Mechanisms & Concepts

Phillip A. Schwartzkroin, author

Cambridge University Press
40 W. 20th Street
New York, NY 10011   212-924-3900
                       Fax: 212-691-3239

1993 400 pages
ISBN: 0-521392-98-5

3711 Equal Partners

Jody Heymann, author

Epilepsy Foundation of America
4351 Garden City Drive
Landover, MD 20785   301-459-3700
         800-332-1000
       Fax: 301-577-9056
      TDD: 800-332-2070

This book tells the story of a young Harvard-trained doctor whose experiences with seizures, brain surgery and subsequent epilepsy turns her from physician to patient.

257 pages Hardcover
ISBN: 0-802774-65-2

3712 Finding Out About Seizures: A Guide To Medical Tests

Epilepsy Foundation of America
4351 Garden City Drive
Landover, MD 20785   301-459-3700
         800-332-1000
       Fax: 301-577-9056
      TDD: 800-332-2070

Introduces adults and children with epilepsy to the types of tests they have to undergo.

3713 Guide to Understanding and Living with Epilepsy

Orrin Devinsdy, author

Epilepsy Foundation of America
4351 Garden City Drive
Landover, MD 20785   301-459-3700
         800-332-1000
       Fax: 301-577-9056
      TDD: 800-332-2070

Easy-to-understand resource for people with epilepsy and their families. Covers a wide range of medical, social and legal issues. Topics include expanation of seizures and epilepsy; information about medication, side effects and risks; and getting the best medical care.

3714 Living Well with Epilepsy

Robert J. Gumnit, MD, author

Epilepsy Foundation of America
4351 Garden City Drive
Landover, MD 20785   301-459-3700
         800-332-1000
       Fax: 301-577-9056
      TDD: 800-332-2070

Designed to help both health-care professionals and patients to understand all aspects of diagnosis and of pharmacologic and surgical management; to enable patients to participate more knowledgeably in interactions with their health care team and to help steer them toward a more normal, fulfilling life.

1990 166 pages Softcover
ISBN: 1-888799-11-0

3715 Managing Seizure Disorder

Nancy Santilli, author

Epilepsy Foundation of America
4351 Garden City Drive
Landover, MD 20785   301-459-3700
         800-332-1000
       Fax: 301-577-9056
      TDD: 800-332-2070

Provides health professionals with detailed information, on a variety of subjects, designed to help them help people with epilepsy live the kind of life they desire.

276 pages softcover
ISBN: 0-802774-65-2

3716 Moments That Disappear - Children Living With Epilepsy

Thomas Bergman, author

Gareth Stevens Publishing
1555 North River Center Drive
Milwaukee, WI 53212   414-225-0333
       Fax: 414-225-0377

Twelve-year-old Joakim has recently discovered that he has epilepsy. Joakim and his family must make changes as they learn to live with this condition and accommodate the limitations that imposes on his life.

ISBN: 0-836807-39-1

3717 School Planning

Epilepsy Foundation of America
4351 Garden City Drive
Landover, MD 20785   301-459-3700
         800-332-1000
       Fax: 301-577-9056
      TDD: 800-332-2070

This guide describes some epilepsy-related problems that children and youth may face in the areas of academics, school achievement and social development. Suggests ways parents can take a proactive approach to ensure appropriate testing, placement and achievement of educational goals for their children.

125 pages Hardcover
ISBN: 0-802774-65-2

3718 Seizures & Epilepsy In Childhood

John M. Freeman, author

Epilepsy Foundation of America
4351 Garden City Drive
Landover, MD 20785   301-459-3700
                            800-332-1000
                        Fax: 301-577-9056
                       TDD: 800-332-2070

Written for parents who want to understand as much as possible about the causes, mechanisms, treatment and social aspects of epilepsy. Encouages parents ot become active partners in their children's care and gives them the background information to do so.

1995 238 pages Softcover
ISBN: 0-802774-65-2

3719 Seizures and Epilepsy In Childhood

John M. Freeman, M.D., author

Johns Hopkins University Press
2715 North Charles Street
Baltimore, MD 21218   410-516-6900
                            800-537-5487
                        Fax: 410-516-6998

This book has already become the standard resource for parents in need of comprehensive medical information about their child with epilepsy.

1997 352 pages Hard Bound
ISBN: 0-801854-97-0

3720 Students with Seizures: A Manual For School Nurses

Epilepsy Foundation of America
4351 Garden City Drive
Landover, MD 20785   301-459-3700
                            800-332-1000
                        Fax: 301-577-9056
                       TDD: 800-332-2070

A professional text with the sole purpose of creating a more accepting and understanding school environment for children with seizure disorders.

131 pages Manual

3721 Your Child and Epilepsy

Robert J. Gumnit, MD, author

Demos Vermande
386 Park Avenue South, #201
New York, NY 10016   212-683-0072
                            800-532-8663
                        Fax: 212-683-0118

Provides information to help parents understand their childrens' epilepsy, suggestions on how to evaluate health care, to find better care if necessary and advice on how to help children with epilepsy to develop self-confidence and self-motivation.

1995 248 pages
ISBN: 0-939957-76-0

Children's Books

3722 A Season of Secrets

Alison Herzig, author

Little, Brown & Company
34 Beacon Street
Boston, MA 02108   617-227-0730

Grades 4-6

3723 Dotty the Dalmatian has Epilepsy

Tim Peters & Company, author

Epilepsy Foundation of America
4351 Garden City Drive
Landover, MD 20785   301-459-3700
                            800-332-1000
                        Fax: 301-577-9056

This is the story of Dotty the Dalmatian who discovers she has epilepsy.

16 pages Softcover
ISBN: 0-802774-65-2

3724 Epilepsy

Tom McGowen, author

Franklin Watts c/o Grolier
90 Old Sherman Tpke
Danbury, CT 06816   203-797-3500
                           800-621-1115
                       Fax: 203-797-3197
                       www.grolier.com

This book explains what epilepsy is, causes of epileptic seizures, diagnosis and treatments.

96 pages Grades 7-12
ISBN: 0-531108-07-4

Magazines

3725 Brainstorms: Epilepsy in Our Words
Steven C. Schachter, author

Lippincott Raven
4351 Garden City Drive
Landover, MD 20785   301-459-3700
                          800-332-1000
                          Fax: 301-459-3700

Patients describe their experiences with seizures. Sixty-eight in-depth personal accounts of actual seizures are followed by a short section on how epilepsy affects the lives of patients.

197 pages Softcover
ISBN: 0-802774-65-2

3726 Epilepsy Foundation
Epilepsy Foundation of America
4351 Garden City Drive
Landover, MD 20785   301-459-3700
                          800-332-1000
                          Fax: 301-377-9056

Catalog of epilepsy information materials, including pamphlets, books, manuals, video tapes and other items is available upon request.

3727 Epilepsy USA
Epilepsy Foundation
4351 Garden City Drive
Landover, MD 20785   301-459-3700
                          800-332-1000
                          Fax: 301-577-9056
                          TDD: 800-332-2070
                          e-mail: postmaster@efa.org
                          www.epilepsyfoundation.org

Information on concerns about seizure disorders and their treatment, responds to the needs of people with seizure disorders.

24 pages

Judith O'Toole, Editor

3728 Lee the Rabbit with Epilepsy
Deborah M. Moss, author

Epilepsy Foundation of America
4351 Garden City Drive
Landover, MD 20785   301-459-3700
                          800-332-1000
                          Fax: 301-557-9056

Written for children ages 3-6, this illustrated picture book follows the adventures of a small rabbit who has seizures during a fishing trip with her Grandpa.

21 pages Hardcover

Newsletters

3729 Epilepsia: Journal of the International League Against Epilepsy
Timothy A. Pedley, MD, Editor-in-Chief, author

Lippincott-Raven Publishers
P.O. Box 1600
Hagerstown, MD 21741   301-714-2300
                          800-638-3030
                          Fax: 301-824-7390
                          e-mail: lrorders@phl.lrpub.com
                          www.lrpub.com

The leading international journal on the epilepsies for more than 30 years, Epilepsia provides comprehensive coverage of current clinical and research results.

12 issues/year
ISBN: 0-013958-0 -

3730 THRESHOLD
2150 Highway 35 North Suite 207c
Sea Grit, NJ 08750   732-974-1144
                          800-336-5843
                          TTY: 800-852-7889
                          e-mail: fscnj@aol.com
                          www.efnj.com

Provides information and supports to parents of children with uncontrolled seizure disorders. Also provides parent-to-parent support information.

Pamphlets

3731 A Patient's Guide to Everyday Life
Epilepsy Foundation of America
4351 Garden City Drive
Landover, MD 20785   301-459-3700
                          800-332-1000
                          Fax: 301-577-9056
                          TDD: 800-332-2070

Provides information for the newly diagnosed individual with epilepsy.

3732 Child with Epilepsy At Camp
Epilepsy Foundation of America
4351 Garden City Drive
Landover, MD 20785   301-459-3700
                          800-332-1000
                          Fax: 301-577-9056
                          TDD: 800-332-2070

Helps to explain why the child with epilepsy should be included in the camping experience.

14 pages

3733 Children and Seizures: Information For Babysitters
Epilepsy Foundation of America
4351 Garden City Drive
Landover, MD 20785
301-459-3700
800-332-1000
Fax: 301-577-9056
TDD: 800-332-2070

Explains seizures, routine and special care, emergency aid and first aid to babysitters. Also offers a graph to write down important information about the child with seizure disorders for a quick reference.

3734 Epilepsy Medicines and Dental Care
Epilepsy Foundation
4351 Garden City Drive
Landover, MD 20785
301-459-3700
800-332-1000
Fax: 301-677-9056

Explains dental care and includes instructions for brushing and flossing.

3735 Epilepsy: Legal Rights, Legal Issues
Epilepsy Foundation of America
4351 Garden City Drive
Landover, MD 20785
301-459-3700
800-332-1000
Fax: 301-577-9056
TDD: 800-332-2070

Offers persons diagnosed with epilepsy information on their legal rights in employment, education, insurance and general disability benefits.

9 pages

3736 Epilepsy: Part of Your Life Series
Epilepsy Foundation of America
4351 Garden City Drive
Landover, MD 20785
301-459-3700
800-332-1000
Fax: 301-577-9056
TDD: 800-332-2070

Provides information for staying healthy, describes various tests and diagnostic procedures, includes information for parents of children with epilepsy and provides general answers to questions about epilepsy.

Series of 4

3737 Epilepsy: You and Your Child, a Guide For Parents
Epilepsy Foundation of America
4351 Garden City Drive
Landover, MD 20785
301-459-3700
800-332-1000
Fax: 301-577-9056
TDD: 800-332-2070

This instructional booklet offers information on emotional aspects of epilepsy, how to handle seizures, medication, diet and nutrition, and offers referral organizations for parents.

3738 Epilepsy: You and Your Treatment
Epilepsy Foundation of America
4351 Garden City Drive
Landover, MD 20785
301-459-3700
800-332-1000
Fax: 301-577-9056
TDD: 800-332-2070

Reviews medical tests and diagnostic procedures used by physicians in diagnosing epilepsy.

3739 Facts About Epilepsy
W. Allen Hauser, MD, author

Epilepsy Foundation of America
4351 Garden City Drive
Landover, MD 20785
301-459-3700
800-332-1000
Fax: 301-577-9056
TDD: 800-332-2070

Designed for use by physicians and other health professionals with an interest in or who deal with the problems of people with epilepsy.

16 pages Softcover

3740 Management by Common Sense
Epilepsy Foundation of America
4351 Garden City Drive
Landover, MD 20785
301-459-3700
800-332-1000
Fax: 301-577-9056
TDD: 800-332-2070

Promotes the employability of people with seizure disorders. Provides employers with information about epilepsy, customer/client reactions, workers' compensation issues, side effects of medication and other information relevant to employing a person with epilepsy.

46 pages
ISBN: 0-802774-65-2

3741 Me and My World Packet for Children

Epilepsy Foundation of America
4351 Garden City Drive
Landover, MD 20785

301-459-3700
800-332-1000
Fax: 301-577-9056
TDD: 800-332-2070

Collection of pamphlets designed for children with epilepsy.

3742 Medicines for Epilepsy

Epilepsy Foundation of America
4351 Garden City Drive
Landover, MD 20785

301-459-3700
800-332-1000
Fax: 301-577-9056
TDD: 800-332-2070

Offers information on medication and treatments, generic drugs, side effects, drug abuse and more.

3743 Mom I Have a Staring Problem

Marian Carla Buckel and Tiffany Buckel, author

Epilepsy Foundation of America
4351 Garden City Drive
Landover, MD 20785

301-459-3700
800-332-1000
Fax: 301-577-9056
TDD: 800-332-2070

Tiffany, a seven-year-old, describes her experience with petit mal seizures; her feelings, wishes and fears. Written to help adults recognize a hidden problem that could be occuring with a child who has learning problems.

24 pages Softcover
ISBN: 0-802774-65-2

3744 Mom I Have a Starting Problem

Marian Carla Buckel and Tiffany Buckel, author

Epilepsy Foundation of America
4351 Garden City Drive
Landover, MD 20785

301-459-3700
800-332-1000
Fax: 301-577-9056

Tiffany, a seven-year old, describes her experiences with petit mal seizures; her feelings, wishes and fears. Written to help adults recognize a hidden problem that could be occuring with a child who has learning problems.

24 pages Softcover
ISBN: 0-802774-65-2

3745 My Brother Matthew

Mary Thompson, author

Epilepsy Foundation of America
4351 Garden City Drive
Landover, MD 20785

301-459-3700
800-332-1000
Fax: 301-577-9056

A picture and text book for children who have a brother or sister with developmental delay.

25 pages Hardcover
ISBN: 0-802774-65-2

3746 My Friend Emily

Susanne M. Swanson, author

Epilepsy Foundation of America
4351 Garden City Drive
Landover, MD 20785

301-459-3700
800-332-1000
Fax: 301-577-9056
TDD: 800-332-2070

A story about Emily and her best friend Katy. Emily, a self confident child who enjoys life, shows that kids with epilepsy are just like other kids.

35 pages Softcover
ISBN: 0-802774-65-2

3747 Preventing Epilepsy

Epilepsy Foundation of America
4351 Garden City Drive
Landover, MD 20785

301-459-3700
800-332-1000
Fax: 301-577-9056
TDD: 800-332-2070

Examines some known causes of seizures and suggests precautionary measures which may prevent the occurrence of epilepsy.

16 pages

3748 Recognizing the Signs of Childhood Seizures

Epilepsy Foundation of America
4351 Garden City Drive
Landover, MD 20785

301-459-3700
800-332-1000
Fax: 301-577-9056
TDD: 800-332-2070

Explains what seizures are and what to look for in your child.

3749 Seizure Recognition and First Aid
Epilepsy Foundation of America
4351 Garden City Drive
Landover, MD 20785   301-459-3700
                                  800-332-1000
                             Fax: 301-577-9056
                             TDD: 800-332-2070

Helps you recognize a seizure when it happens
and give basic first aid.

3750 Surgery for Epilepsy
Epilepsy Foundation of America
4351 Garden City Drive
Landover, MD 20785   301-459-3700
                                  800-332-1000
                             Fax: 301-577-9056
                             TDD: 800-332-2070

Describes current surgical treatment and the
testing that precedes it.

    12 pages

3751 Talking to Your Doctor About Seizure Disorders
Epilepsy Foundation of America
4351 Garden City Drive
Landover, MD 20785   301-459-3700
                                  800-332-1000
                             Fax: 301-577-9056
                             TDD: 800-332-2070

Designed to help the patient talk with medical
personnel about treatment of epilepsy.

3752 Teacher's Role, A Guide for School Personnel
Epilepsy Foundation of America
4351 Garden City Drive
Landover, MD 20785   301-459-3700
                                  800-332-1000
                             Fax: 301-577-9056
                             TDD: 800-332-2070

Provides tips on recognizing seizures and handling a seizure in the classroom.

    14 pages

DESCRIPTION

3753 SICKLE CELL DISEASE

Synonyms: Homozygous Hb S, Sickle cell anemia
Disorder Type: Genetic Disorder
May involve these systems in the body (see Section III):

Blood (Hematologic)

Sickle cell disease is an inherited blood disorder that affects blacks primarily and is characterized by the presence of crescent or sickle-shaped red cells in the blood and the chronic premature destruction of red blood cells (hemolytic anemia). In this disorder, the red blood cells contain an abnormal form of the oxygen-carrying protein (hemoglobin) called hemoglobin S. This abnormality reduces the level of available oxygen in the blood cells and results in their characteristic sickle shape. These irregular cells tend to block the tiny blood vessels of various tissues and organs; they may cause restricted or obstructed blood flow resulting in tissue or organ damage. In addition, their unusual shape renders them fragile, leading to their premature destruction and thus anemia.

The symptoms of sickle cell disease tend to appear at or around six months of age and may include headaches; shortness of breath (dyspnea); paleness; fatigue; and a yellowish hue of the eyes, skin, and mucous membranes (jaundice). Any activity that would normally reduce the blood oxygen levels (e.g., exercise, exertion, illness, or high-altitude flying) may induce a sickle cell crisis or sudden worsening of the anemic condition accompanied by abdominal and bone pain, dyspnea, and vomiting. Infection or a blocked blood vessel may also result in sickle cell crisi with the affected child experiencing chest pain and increased dyspnea. By adolescence most of those affected develop an enlarged spleen (splenomegaly) that is no longer capable of assisting in fighting infections, leaving the body more vulnerable to certain types of infections. Other symptoms may include skin changes resulting from poor circulation, stroke resulting from nervous system damage, or blood in the urine (hematuria) resulting from kidney damage. As the affected child grows to adulthood, the liver and heart may enlarge and a heart murmur may develop. The lungs, intestines, and gall bladder may also be affected. In addition, affected children may develop such distinct characteristics as a short torso with long extremities, fingers, and toes.

Because there is no known cure for sickle cell disease, treatment is geared toward prevention, control, and pain management. Such treatment may include the avoidance of activities that reduce blood oxygen levels, a full immunization regimen, and prompt medical intervention for any illness or viral infection. Other treatment may include folic acid supplementation, antibiotic medication for treatment and prevention of infection, oxygen therapy to improve the level of oxygen in the blood, and acetaminophen or other medication to relieve pain. To manage a sickle cell crisis, as well as the pain associated with it, affected children may be given intravenous fluids, pain-relieving drugs, and possibly blood transfusions. Other treatments being studied include certain drugs, gene therapy, and bone marrow transplantation.

Sickle cell disease is inherited as an autosomal recessive trait. In this case, the defective gene for hemoglobin S is transmitted by both parents. If a child inherits this gene from only one parent, that child will usually be symptom-free, but will be a carrier of the sickle cell trait. The incidence of this disorder in the United States is approximately 150 black children in 100,000; however, approximately one in 12 black children carries the sickle cell trait.

The following organizations in the General Resources Section can provide additional information: Genetic Alliance, March of Dimes Birth Defects Foundation, NIH/National Heart, Lung & Blood Institute, Online Mendelian Inheritance in Man: www3.ncbi.nlm.nih.gov/Omim/searchomim.html, NIH/National Institute of Child Health and Human Development

National Associations & Support Groups

3754 American Sickle Cell Anemia
P.O. Box 1971, 10300 Carnegie Ave.
Cleveland, OH 44106   216-229-8600
                            Fax: 216-229-4500
                    e-mail: irabragg@ascaa.org
                            ascca.org

Provides education, testing, counseling, supportive services to the population at risk for sickle cell anemia and its hemoglobin variants. Bilingual educator on staff, educational materials and distribution of literature is provided by AS-CAA. Referrals for children and families with special needs.

Ira Bragg-Grant, Executive Director

3755 Center for Sickle Cell Disease
2121 Georgia Avenue NW
Washington, DC 20059   202-806-7930
                            Fax: 202-806-4517

3756 International Association of Sickle Cell Nurses and Physician Assistants
IASCNAPA \ Duke University Medical Center
Box 3939 DUMC
Durham, NC 27710   919-572-6714
                    www.emory.edu/PEDS/SICKLE/

IASCNAPA recognizes its responsibility to maintain high standards in the provision of quality and accessible health care services for individuals with sickle cell disease. IASCNAPA is committed to strengthening the relationship between nurses and physician assistants that care for patients with sickle cell disease.

3757 National Association for Sickle Cell Disease, Inc.
200 Corporate Point Suite 495
Culver City, CA 90230   310-216-6363
                            800-421-8453
                            Fax: 310-215-3722
                    www.sicklecelldisease.org

Provides programs and services for individuals and families affected by sickle cell disease through its network of affiliated members. Provides education, advocacy and other initiatives which promote awareness and support for sickle cell programs and patients.

3758 Sickle Cell Disease Association of America
200 Corporate Pointe, Suite 495
Culver City, CA 90230   310-216-6363
                            800-421-8453
                            Fax: 310-215-3722
                    www.sicklecelldisease.org

Purpose is to promote leadership on a national level in order to create awareness in all circles of the impact of sickle cell disease on emotional and economic well-being of families and the individual.

Lynda K. Anderson, Executive Director

3759 Triad Sickle Cell Anemia Foundation
1102 East Market Street
Greensboro, NC 27401   336-274-1507
                            800-733-8297
                            Fax: 336-275-7984
                    e-mail: SCDAP@aol.com
                    www.greensboro.com/sickle

Community based organization that provides education counseling, case management and support services for persons with sickle cell disease and their families. Addresses and provides education relative to HIV/AIDS and teenage pregnency prevention. Services are provided in six area counties in North Carolina.

Gladys A. Robinson, Executive Director
Kathy M. Norcott, Program Director

International

3760 Canadian Sickle Cell Society
6999 Cote-des-Neiges, Suite 33
Montreal, Quebec,
Canada

Non-profit organization educating the at-risk population, recruiting and training volunteers, and providing counseling for those affected by sickle cell disease.

3761 Sickle Cell Association of Ontario
55 Gateway Boulevard
Don Mills, ON,
Canada

State Agencies & Support Groups

California

3762 Sickle Cell Disease Foundation of California
5110 West Goldleaf Circle, Suite 150
Los Angeles, CA 90056   323-299-3600
                            877-288-2873
                            Fax: 323-299-3605
                    www.scdfc.org

Georgia

3763 Sickle Cell Foundation of Georgia, Inc.
Sickle Cell Foundation of Georgia, Inc.
2391 Benjamin E. Mays Dr. SW
Atlanta, GA 30311   404-755-1641
                              Fax: 404-755-7955
e-mail: sicklefg@mindspring.com
www.mindspring.com/~sicklefg/

Provides education, screening, and counseling programs for sickle cell and other abnormal hemoglobins. The Foundation has a deep-rooted commitment to making strides in monitoring the occurrence of sickle cell, improving the quality of life for those with the disease and cooperating with individuals conducting research.

3764 Sickle Cell Information Center .
c/o Grady Memorial Hospital
P.O. Box 109 80 Butler Street
Atlanta, GA 30335   404-616-3572
                              Fax: 404-616-5998
e-mail: aplatt@emory.edu
www.emory.edu/PEDS/SICKLE/

New York

3765 Sickle Cell Disease Foundation of Greater New York
127 W. 127, Room 421
New York, NY 10027   212-865-1500

A voluntary health organization formed to support and conduct research and educational programs aimed at the control of sickle cell anemia.

Dick Campbell, Executive Director

North Carolina

3766 Sickle Cell Disease Association of the Piedmont
1102 East Market Street
Greensboro, NC 27401   336-274-1507
                                 800-733-8297
                              Fax: 336-275-7984
e-mail: scdap@aol.com

Dedicated to educating the public and providing support to people affected by Sickle Cell Disease. The Association seeks to educate the public about sickle cell disease and the sickle cell trait and develp educational materials on these conditions for extensive circulation.

Research Centers

California

3767 University of California, Northern Comprehensive Sickle Cell Center
San Francisco General Hospital
1001 Potrero Avenue
San Francisco, CA 94110   415-206-3504

Sickle cell disease research.

William C. Mentzer, MD, Director

3768 University of Southern California Comprehensive Sickle Cell Center
2025 Zonal Avenue, Room 204
Los Angeles, CA 90033   213-342-1259

Dr. Cage S. Johnson, Director

District of Columbia

3769 Howard University Center for Sickle Cell Disease
2121 Georgia Avenue NW
Washington, DC 20059   202-806-7930

Dr. Oswaldo Castro, Director

Georgia

3770 Medical College of Georgia, Sickle Cell Center
1435 Laney-Walker Blvd.
Augusta, GA 30912   404-724-1388
                              Fax: 404-721-6611

Offers research into sickle cell disease.

Dr. Titus Huisman, Director

Massachusetts

3771 Boston Sickle Cell Center
Boston Medical Center
One Boston Medical Center Place
Boston, MA 02118   617-414-7437
                             800-641-7437
                          Fax: 614-414-5555
www.bmc.org/pedi/bostonchildhealth/

Dr. Lillian E.C. McMahon, Director

Michigan

3772 Wayne State University Comprehensive Sickle Cell Center
Curricular Affairs Office
Scott Hall, Room 1206
Detroit, MI 48201   313-577-1546
                                     Fax: 313-577-8777

Charles F. Whitten, M.D., Director

New York

3773 Columbia University Comprehensive Sickle Cell Center
Harlem Hospital
506 Lenox Avenue
New York, NY 10037   212-939-1426

Research into sickle cell disease.

Dr. Jeanne Smith, Director

3774 SUNY Health Science Center at Brooklyn Sickle Cell Center
450 Clarkson Avenue, Box 20
Brooklyn, NY 11203   718-270-1000

Dr. R.F. Rieder, Program Director

North Carolina

3775 Duke University Comprehensive Sickle Cell Center
Medical Center
Box 3934
Durham, NC 27710   919-684-3724
                                     Fax: 919-681-8477

Research into sickle cell disease including molecular and organ studies.

Wendell F. Rossee, MD, Director

Ohio

3776 Comprehensive Sickle Cell Center
Children's Hospital Research Foundation
Elland & Bethesda Avenues
Cincinnati, OH 45229   513-559-4412
                                     Fax: 513-559-7431

Offers research and statistical information in the area of sickle cell disease.

Donald Rucknagel, MD, Director

Texas

3777 Pediatric Sickle Cell Disease Program University of Texas Southwestern Medical
1935 Motor St,Childrens Medical Ctr
Dallas, TX 75235   214-450-6102
                                     Fax: 214-456-2382

A comprehensive program for diagnosis, patient/family education and management of sickle cell diseases in childhood and adolesance. Offers access to state-of-the art research projects and clinical management.

George R. Buchanan, Medical Director
Lora R. Rogers, M.D., Associate Medical Director

Books

3778 Sickle Cell Anemia
George Beshore, author
Franklin Watts c/o Grolier
90 Old Sherman Tpke
Danbury, CT 06816   203-797-3500
                                     800-621-1115
                                     Fax: 203-797-3197
                                     www.grolier.com

1994 76 pages
ISBN: 0-531125-10-6

3779 Sickle Cell Disease: Basic Principles & Clinical Practice
Stephen H. Embury, author
Raven Press
1185 Avenue of the Americas
New York, NY 10036   212-930-9500

1994 928 pages
ISBN: 0-781701-42-2

3780 Understanding Sickle Cell Disease
Miriam Bloom, Ph.D, author
University Press of Mississippi
3825 Ridgewood Road
Jackson, MS 39211   601-432-6205
                                     800-737-7788
                                     Fax: 601-432-6217
                                     e-mail: press@ihl.state.ms.us
                                     www.upress.state.ms.us

For general readers, a guide to understanding a debilitating genetic disease that affects tens of thousands who are of African heritage.

128 pages Softcover
ISBN: 0-878057-45-5

Pamphlets

3781 Sickle Cell Anemia Disease
March of Dimes Resource Center
1275 Mamaroneck Avenue
White Plains, NY 10605   **888-663-4637**
                               Fax: 914-997-4763

DESCRIPTION

3782 SLEEPWALKING

Synonym: Somnambulism

Disorder Type: Sleep

Sleepwalking, also known as somnambulism, is a condition that occurs most commonly in children, particularly those from approximately four to six years of age. About 10 to 15 percent of children experience at least one episode of sleepwalking during childhood. In addition, approximately one in five children who sleepwalk has a family history of the condition. In many patients, sleepwalking occurs in association with bed-wetting (nocturnal enuresis) or night terrors. Bed-wetting is an involuntary discharge of urine during sleep. Night terrors are sleep disturbances that typically occur shortly after the onset of sleep. Affected children abruptly awaken and experience intense fright, may moan or scream, and have an abnormally increased heart rate (tachycardia) and rapid, labored breathing. In some cases, a stressful event may lead to an episode of sleepwalking.

In children, sleepwalking occurs during stage four of NREM (nonrapid eye movement) sleep. NREM sleep consists of four progressively deeper stages of sleep that are typically characterized by slow, deep brain waves, muscle relaxation and slowed breathing rate, slowed heart rate, and lowered blood pressure. In contrast, REM (rapid eye movement) sleep, which is associated with dreaming, is characterized by increased levels of brain activity, rapid eye movements, and involuntary muscle jerks.

During an episode of sleepwalking, affected children may simply sit up in bed or move to the edge of the bed, without engaging in actual sleepwalking. In other cases, however, children may get out of bed and walk through their home. They may also perform certain routine acts, such as turning on a hallway light. Unless children are simultaneously experiencing night terrors, they usually do not have associated anxiety. During an episode, most children have their eyes open and are guided by their vision. Therefore, they typically move around familiar obstacles; however, some children may make no effort to avoid certain objects in their path, potentially resulting in injury. In addition, some children may mumble simple words or phrases or repeatedly perform certain acts, such as turning a doorknob back and forth. If children are urged to return to bed during such an episode, they may sometimes follow such instruction; however, they usually must be gently steered back to their beds. Sleepwalking episodes typically last only a few minutes, and children usually have little or no memory of the experience. In children, sleepwalking is rarely associated with psychologic abnormalities, and the number of episodes usually decreases by early adolescence. However, the persistence of sleepwalking episodes into adulthood is thought to be associated with a significant risk of psychiatric disease. Parents or caregivers of children who sleepwalk should take precautions to help protect them against injury. Possible obstacles or breakable objects should be removed from their paths. It may be advisable to block staircases and to have children sleep on the ground floor of the house, if possible.

The following organizations in the General Resources Section can provide additional information: Federation of Families for Children's Mental Health, National Sleep Foundation, National Mental Health Association, National Mental Health Consumer Self-Help Clearinghouse, NIH/National Institute of Mental Health, Online Mendelian Inheritance in Man: www3.ncbi.nlm.nih.gov/Omim/searchomim.html

National Associations & Support Groups

3783 American Mental Health Foundation (AMNF)
1049 5th Avenue
New York, NY 10028
USA

212-639-1561
Fax: 212-737-9027

Dedicated to the extensive and intensive research in the theories and techniques of treatment of emotional illness and to the implementation of reforms in the mental health system. Efforts have resulted in development of better and less expensive treatment methods. Findings are disseminated in English and other major languages.

Monroe W. Spero, MD

3784 Association for Persons with Mental and Developmental Disabilities
132 Fair Street
Kingston, NY 12401
USA
    914-334-4336
    800-331-5362
    Fax: 914-331-4569
    e-mail: nadd@mhv.net

Non-profit organization designed to promote interest of professional and parent development with resources for individuals who have the co-existence of mental illness and mental retardation. Provides conference, educational services and training materials to professionals, parents, concerned citizens and service organizations. Formerly known as the National Association for the Dually Diagnosed.

Robert Fletcher, Executive Director

3785 Center for Family Support
333 7th Ave.
New York, NY 10001
    212-629-7939
    Fax: 212-239-2211
    www.cfsny.org

Provides comprehensive answers to the most commonly asked questions and situations.

Steven Vernickofs, Executive Director

3786 Center for Mental Health Services Knowledge Exchange Program
U.S. Department of Health and Human Services
P.O. Box 42490
Washington, DC 20015
    800-789-2647
    Fax: 301-984-8796
    e-mail: ken@mentalhealth.org
    www.mentalhealth.org

Supplies the public with responses to their commonly asked questions.

3787 Center for Self-Help Research
1918 University Ave, Ste 3D
Berkeley, CA 94704
    510-849-0731
    Fax: 510-849-3402

Unites various groups to examine the different features of the public health care systems.

Steven P. Segal, Director
Carol J. Silverman, Program Director

3788 Christian Horizons, Inc.
P.O. Box 334
Williamstown, MI 48895
    517-655-3463

Devoted to assisting individuals, with mental disabilities, on a day-to-day basis.

Adonna Jory, Executive Secretary
Noel Churchman, Board President

3789 Mental Illness Foundation
772 W 168th Street
New York, NY 10032
    212-682-4699
    Fax: 212-682-4896

Supports community housing, treatment, research, outreach and public-awareness efforts for people with mental illness. Publications: Mental Illness Foundation, quarterly newsletter. Directory that lists mental illnesses and provides information on how to contact related associations. Annual meeting.

3790 National Alliance for the Mentally Ill
200 North Glebe Road #1015
Arlington, VA 22203
    703-524-7600
    800-950-6264
    TDD: 703-516-7991
    e-mail: membership@nami.org
    www.nami.org

Aids families and individuals find the emotional and physical answers to the habitual forming disorders through several media resources.

Web Sites

3791 Cyber Psych
www.cyberpsych.org/

3792 Mental Health Net
borderline.mentalhelp.net/disorders/sx93.htm

3793 Planetpsych
www.planetpsych.com

3794 Psych Central

www.psychcentral.com

3795 Sleep Home Pages

bisleep.medsch.ucla.edu

Books

3796 American Academy of Somnology-Membership Directory

David L. Hopper, PhD, author

P.O. Box 29124
Las Vegas, NV 89126   702-450-5353
                              800-513-5833
                           Fax: 702-450-5833
                    e-mail: drdavelv@aol.com

Covers about 75 physcians, dentists, nurses, psychologists, technicians, and students and sponsoring organizations, including associations, institutions, and corporations, with a special interest in sleep.

3797 Concise Guide to Evaluation and Management of Sleep Disorders

American Psychiatric Press, Inc.
1400 K St., NW
Washington, DC 20005   202-682-6262
                              800-368-5777
                           Fax: 202-789-2648
                    e-mail: order@appi.org
                           www.appi.org

Over view of sleep disorders medicine, sleep physiology and pathology, insomnia complaints, excessive sleepiness disorders, parasomnias, medical and psychiatric disorders and sleep, medications with sedative-hypnotic properties, special problems and populations.

1997 304 pages Softcover

3798 Depression and Sleep

American Psychiatric Press, Inc.
1400 K St., NW
Washington, DC 20005   202-682-6262
                              800-368-5777
                           Fax: 202-789-2648
                    e-mail: order@appi.com
                           www.appi.com

Contents include normal sleep, neurochemistry of sleep, sleep in depression, neurochemistry of depression, antidepressent drugs and sleep, and clinical management of sleep disorders in depression.

1996 64 pages

3799 Sleep Disorders Diagnosis and Treatment: Current Clinical Practice Series

American Psyciatric Publishing Group.
1400 K St., NW
Washington, DC 20005   202-682-6262
                              800-368-5777
                           Fax: 202-789-2648
                    e-mail: order@appi.com
                           www.appi.com

1998 250 pages

3800 Snoring From A to Zzzz

Spencer Press
2525 NW Lovejoy St, Ste 402
Portland, OR 97210   503-223-4959
                           Fax: 503-223-1608
                    e-mail: reallip@aol.com
                 www.foxcontent.com/snoring/htm

Covers organizations, associations, support groups, and manufactorers of sleep-related medical products relevant to sleep disorders. Discussess every aspect of snoring abd sleep apnea from causes to cures.

1999 248 pages

DESCRIPTION

3801 SPEECH IMPAIRMENT

Synonym: Speech dysfunction

Disorder Type: Hearing, Mental, Emotional or Behavioral Disorder

May involve these systems in the body (see Section III):

Central Nervous System, Muscular System

Speech impairment refers to the decreased ability or inability to effectively communicate through vocalizations or uttered sounds. Difficulty speaking or more profound dysfunctions of speech may result from many different factors that include neurologic influences; muscular defects, injuries, or paralysis; structural irregularities of the vocal cords; psychologic influences; mental retardation; and other factors.

In some children, speech impairment may be classified as a dysfunction of articulation characterized by the inability to articulate or produce words properly (dysarthria) as a result of damage to the part of the brain responsible for regulation of the muscles that control the speech apparatus (e.g., mouth, lips, and voice box or larynx). Such damage may result from head or brain injuries, tumors, strokes, and certain diseases. Characteristic speech patterns of children with dysarthria are varied and may be described as unintelligible, slow, slurred, halting, tremulous, hoarse, or possessing a nasal quality. Additional causes of articulation dysfunction or delay include structural defects such as cleft lip or palate, hearing impairment or deafness, and other nervous system irregularities. In addition, speech impairment may result from irregularities directly related to the vocal cords that may affect the quality of the voice.

Impaired ability to communicate (aphasia or dysphasia) may also result from injury to the part of the brain responsible for language comprehension, resulting in the reduced ability or inability to express, write, or understand language. Such injury may be caused by head trauma, brain lesions, infection, or other factors. This type of impairment may be present in many different variations such as garbled sentences, extremely slow and difficult speech, absence of speech (mutism), and other irregularities. In addition, children with behavioral, emotional, or psychologic irregularities as well as those with hearing impairment may also experience delays in language comprehension and development.

It is important to identify the underlying cause of any dysfunction of speech or delay in speech development in order to allow for the most favorable educational and social outcome. Specialists in the diagnosis and treatment of these types of disorders (e.g., otolaryngologists and speech therapists) may base their treatment plans on the evaluation of family and medical histories, physical examination of essential speech structures, and specialized testing that may include speech, language, and hearing assessments. Treatment is directed toward the specific cause of impairment and may include exercises tailored to the specific patient's needs, as well as the cooperation of parents or caregivers, pediatricians, educators, and others to provide a supportive environment.

National Associations & Support Groups

3802 American Speech-Language-Hearing Association
10801 Rockville Pike
Rockville, MD 20852   301-897-5700
                            800-638-8255

A professional and scientific organization for speech-language pathologists and audiologists concerned with communication disorders. Provides informational materials and a toll-free HELPLINE number for consumers. Also provides referrals to audiologists and speech-language pathologists in the United States.

Frederick T. Spahr, Ph.D., Executive Director

3803 Auditory-Verbal International, Inc.
2121 Eisenhower Avenue, Ste. 402
Alexandria, VA 22314   703-739-1049
                        Fax: 703-739-0395
                        TTY: 703-739-0874
                  e-mail: avi@csgi.com
                  www.digitalnation.com/avi

Dedicated to helping children who have hearing losses learn to listen and speak. Promotes the Auditory-Verbal Therapy approach, which is based on the belief that the overwhelming majority of these children can hear and talk by using their residual hearing and hearing aids.

Fran Price, Executive Director

State Agencies & Support Groups

Colorado

3804 University of Colorado, Boulder Communication Disorders Clinic
Communication Disorders & Speech

Boulder, CO 80309   303-492-5375

Focuses on communication disorders including speech and hearing impairments.

Susan M. Moore, Director

District of Columbia

3805 Scottish Rite Center for Childhood Language Disorders
1630 Columbia Road NW
Washington, DC 20009   202-939-4703
                                  Fax: 202-939-4717

Association offering speech-language evaluations and treatment, hearing screening and consultation and referrals to children ages birth to 18 years with hearing or speech disorders.

Martin Fischer

Illinois

3806 David T. Siegel Institute For Communicative Disorders
Humana Hospital-Michael Reese
3033 S. Cottage Grove Avenue
Chicago, IL 60616   773-791-2900
                                  Fax: 773-791-4014

Conducts behavioral research on language development and sign language for the deaf.

Edward Applebaum, Chief of Service

Michigan

3807 University of Michigan, Communicative Disorders Clinic
1111 E. Catherine Street
Ann Arbor, MI 48109   734-764-8440
                                  Fax: 734-747-2489
                                  www.umich.edu/~comdis

Focuses on communicative disorders including hearing impairments and speech disorders. Provides intensive language intervention for adults with aphasia as well as children with language disorders. Clinic offers residential program for adults and school liaon for children.

Dr. Holly Craig, Director

Nevada

3808 University of Nevada, Reno Speech And Language Pathology Department

Reno, NV 89557   702-784-4887
                                  Fax: 702-784-4889

Communication disorders research pertaining to hearing and speech impairments.

Dr. Stephen McFarlane, Chairman

New York

3809 Brooklyn College of City University of New York - Speech & Hearing Center
Boylan Hall, Room 4400
Brooklyn, NY 11210   718-780-5186

Research activities include normal communications and communication disorders, studies relating to language, hearing and speech disorders.

Dr. Oliver Bloodstein, Director

3810 City University of New York Center for Research in Speech and Hearing
33 W. 42nd Street
New York, NY 10036   212-642-2352
                                  Fax: 212-642-2379

Programmable research of digital and auditory hearing aids and sensory aids for the speech and hearing impaired person.

Dr. Irving Hochberg, Director

3811 International Center for Hearing and Speech Research
1 Lomb Memorial Drive
Rochester, NY 14623
716-475-6403
Fax: 716-475-6677

Focuses on prevention, early detection and treatment of hearing impaired people.

Dr. Robert Firisina, Sr., Director

3812 National Cued Speech Association
Nazareth College-Speech & Language Department
4245 East Avenue
Rochester, NY 14618
716-389-2525
800-459-3529
Fax: 716-586-2456
e-mail: cuedspdic@aol.com
www.cuedspeech.org

Provides instruction, support services and information pertaining to deafness and the application of Cued Speech. The center provides classes and workshops in Cued Speech, maintains a speakers bureau and provides counseling and support for hearing-impaired adults and their families.

Mary Elsie Daisey, Executive Director

3813 State University College at Fredonia Youngerman Center
Thompson Hall
Fredonia, NY 14063
716-673-3203

Studies communications disorders including hearing and speech.

Dr. Robert Manzella, Director

North Carolina

3814 University of North Carolina at Chapel Hill, Division of Speech & Hearing
Medical School, Wing D
CB 7190
Chapel Hill, NC 27599
919-966-1006

Dr. Thomas Layton, Director

Ohio

3815 Cleveland Hearing and Speech Center
11206 Euclid Avenue
Cleveland, OH 44106
216-231-8787

Offers research and studies into speech, language and hearing disorders.

Bernard P. Henri, Executive Director

3816 Kent State University, Speech and Hearing Clinic
Kent, OH 44242
330-672-2672

Mary Eleise Jones, PhD, Contact

3817 Ohio University School of Hearing and Speech Sciences
Lindley Hall, Room 201
Athens, OH 45701
740-593-1407

Focuses on hearing and speech impairments.

Dr. Edwin Leach, Director

Oklahoma

3818 University of Oklahoma, Speech & Hearing Center
P.O. Box 26901
Oklahoma City, OK 73190
405-271-4214

Dr. Glenda Ochaner, Director

Pennsylvania

3819 Temple University Speech and Hearing Science Laboratories
13th & Cecil B. Moore Aves.
Philadelphia, PA 19122
215-787-7543

Speech and hearing studies.

Dr. Aquilles Iglesias, Director

Tennessee

3820 Memphis State University, Center for the Communicatively Impaired
807 Jefferson Avenue
Memphis, TN 38105
901-678-2009
Fax: 901-525-1282

Offers research into hearing loss, deafness, and speech impairments.

Maurice I. Mendel, Director

Texas

3821 Texas Tech University Speech-Language- Hearing Clinic

Lubbock, TX 79409   806-742-3907

Sherry Sancribian, Director

3822 University of Texas Health Science Center at Houston - Speech & Hearing
1343 Moursund
Houston, TX 77030   713-792-4500
                          Fax: 713-792-4513

Provides rehabilitation services for children and adults with hearing and speech disorders.

Louise Kent-Udolf, Director

3823 University of Texas at Dallas, Callier Center for Communication Disorders
1966 Inwood Road
Dallas, TX 75235   214-905-3000
                          Fax: 214-905-3022
                          TDD: 214-905-3012
                          e-mail: elloyce@callier.utdallas.edu
                          www.callier.utdallas.edu

Multidisciplinary center serving infants through adults with all types of communcation disorders: diagnostic and treatment; hearing aid services; cochlear implant evelation and follow-up; North Texas Cochlear Implant Summer Listening Camp; aural (re) habilitation services; assistive listening device program; tinnitus and hyperacusis clinic; speech-language pathology and psychological diagnostic and therapy services; research.

Eloycess J. Newman, Head of Public Information

Virginia

3824 Speech Simulation Research Foundation
Cedar Hall, Box 824
Nassawadox, VA 23413   757-442-2755

Focuses on hearing and speech disorders.

Monte Penney, Director

Washington

3825 University of Washington Department of Speech & Hearing Sciences
1417 NE 42nd Street
Seattle, WA 98105   206-685-4702
                          Fax: 206-543-1093
                          www.depts.washington.edu/sphsc/

Committed to understanding the basic processes and mechanisms involved in human speech, hearing, language, their disorders and to improving the quality of life for individuals affected by communication disorders across the life span.

Carol Stoel-Gammon, Ph.D, Professor, Chair

3826 University of Washington Speech and Hearing Clinic
4131 15th Avenue NE
Seattle, WA 98105   206-543-5440
                          Fax: 206-616-1185
                          depts.washington.edu/sphsc/

A center of excellence in education, research, and clinical practice serving speech, language, and hearing needs within the university and the community. Serves as a teaching facility in the fields of Speech-language pathology and Audiology. With state of the art technology, innovative diagnostic and treament methods, and internationally and nationally recognized areas of research. Meeting the needs of individuals with speech, language, hearing and related communication disorders.

Nancy Alarcon, M.S., CCC-SLP, Director

Wisconsin

3827 University of Wisconsin, Auditory Physiology Center
273 Medical Sciences Bldg.
Madison, WI 53706   608-262-0818

Activities include studies in hearing loss and deafness.

Dr. John Brugge, Director

Research Centers

3828 Boys Town National Research Hospital
555 N. 30th Street
Omaha, NE 68131   402-498-6511
                         Fax: 402-498-6638
                         TTY: 402-498-6543

An internationally recognized center for state-of-the-art research, diagnosis, treatment of patients with ear diseases, hearing and balance disorders, cleft lip and palate, and speech/language problems. Also includes programs such as Parent/Child Workshops, Center for Childhood Deafness, Register for Heredity Hearing Loss, Center for Hearing research, Center for Abused Handicapped, and summer programs for gifted deaf teens and college students.

Patrick E. Brookhouser, M.D., Director

3829 Gallaudet University, Cued Speech Team
800 Florida Avenue NE
Washington, DC 20002   202-651-5000

Transmission of spoken languages are researched.

Elizabeth L. Kiplia, Coordinator

Books

3830 Is My Child's Speech Normal?
Jon Eisenson, author

Pro-Ed
8700 Shoal Creek Boulevard
Austin, TX 78757   512-451-3246
                          800-897-3202
                          Fax: 512-451-8542
                          www.proedinc.com

Physicians and clinicians who need to share information with parents about child language will find the text very useful. Answers commonly asked questions and concerns.

158 pages
ISBN: 0-890797-04-8

3831 Language Intervention: Beyond the Primary Grades for Clinicians by Clinicians
Edited by Donald F. Tibbits, author

Pro-Ed
8700 Shoal Creek Boulevard
Austin, TX 78757   512-451-3246
                          800-897-3202
                          Fax: 512-451-8542
                          www.proedinc.com

Programming and procedures for students 10 years and older who are receiving services for language disabilities in school settings with an emphasis on actual treatment procedures.

528 pages
ISBN: 0-890796-24-6

3832 Management of Motor Speech Disorders in Children and Adults
Yorkston, Beukelman, Strand, Bell, author

Pro-Ed
8700 Shoal Creek Boulevard
Austin, TX 78757   512-451-3246
                          800-897-3202
                          Fax: 512-451-8542
                          www.proedinc.com

Second edition of this popular text incorporates information about both dysarthria and apraxia of speech in children and adults and reviews techniques for physical and motor speech examination and treatment techniques.

618 pages
ISBN: 0-890797-84-6

3833 Traumatic Brain Injury In Children and Adolescents: A Sourcebook
Janet S. Tyler, Mary P. Mira, author

Pro-Ed
8700 Shoal Creek Boulevard
Austin, TX 78757   512-451-3246
                          800-897-3202
                          Fax: 512-451-8542
                          www.proedinc.com

New and updated invaluable information for all educators who are serving students with TBI. Describes causes and consequences (both short-term and long-term) of TBI and presents techniques and procedures to successfully return the child to school following an injury.

150 pages
ISBN: 0-890798-05-2

3834 Visible Speech
SRC Software Research Corp.
Box 4277, Station A
Victoria, BC, V8X 3X8, IT   250-727-3744

Computerized speech culture, analysis and computer-based speech training.

6 pages

A.E. Wright, Publisher

Journals

3835 American Journal of Speech-Language Pathology
American Speech-Language-Hearing Association
10801 Rockville Pike
Rockville, MD 20852   301-897-5700
800-638-8255

Russell L. Malone, Ph.D., Editor

Pamphlets

3836 Set-Ups for Speeches
Self Help for Hard of Hearing People, Inc.
7910 Woodmont Avenue Suite 1200
Bethesda, MD 20814   301-657-2248
Fax: 301-913-9413
TTY: 301-657-2249
e-mail: national@shhh.org
www.shhh.org

3837 Speech and Voice Impairment

Manfred D. Muenter, MD, author

United Parkinson Foundation
833 West Washington Boulevard
Chicago, IL 60607   312-733-1893

1983

Camps

Nebraska

3838 Boys Town National Research Hospital
555 N. 30th Street
Omaha, NE 68131   402-498-6511
Fax: 402-498-6638
TTY: 402-498-6543

An internationally recognized center for state-of-the-art research, diagnosis, treatment of patients with ear diseases, hearing and balance disorders, cleft lip and palate, and speech/language problems. Also includes programs such as Parent/Child Workshops, Center for Childhood Deafness, Register for Heredity Hearing Loss, Center for Hearing research, Center for Abused Handicapped, and summer programs for gifted deaf teens and college students.

Patrick E. Brookhouser, M.D., Director

Texas

3839 University of Texas at Dallas, Callier Center for Communication Disorders
1966 Inwood Road
Dallas, TX 75235   214-905-3000
Fax: 214-905-3022
TDD: 214-905-3012
e-mail: elloyce@callier.utdallas.edu
www.callier.utdallas.edu

Multidisciplinary center serving infants through adults with all types of communcation disorders: diagnostic and treatment; hearing aid services; cochlear implant evalution and follow-up; North Texas Cochlear Implant Summer Listening Camp; aural (re) habilitation services; assistive listening device program; tinnitus and hyperacusis clinic; speech-language pathology and psychological diagnostic and therapy services; research.

Eloycess J. Newman, Head of Public Information

DESCRIPTION

3840 SPINA BIFIDA

Disorder Type: Birth Defect, Genetic Disorder
Covers these related disorders: Encephalocele,
Meningocele, Myelocele (Myelomeningocele;
Meningomyelocele), Spina bifida occulta
May involve these systems in the body (see Section III):
Central Nervous System, Prenatal & Postnatal
Growth & Development, Nervous System, Skeletal
System

Spina bifida is a congenital abnormality, known as a neural tube defect, that is characterized by the failure during embryonic development of one or more of the developing vertebrae to develop completely or fuse. This frequently results in the exposure of part of the spinal cord. Spina bifida occulta, the most common and least severe form of this defect, is characterized by a dimpling, dark tufts of hair, spider-like fine lines (telangiectasia), or a benign fatty tumor (lipoma) on the lower back or lumbosacral area. There is no protrusion or exposure of the spinal cord and it rarely involves problems with the nervous system. Some affected children, however, may experience weakness in the legs and feet and difficulty in bladder and bowel control resulting from an adhesion of the spinal cord to the area of the abnormality.

Meningocele occurs when the three membranes (meninges) surrounding the spinal cord protrude through the vertebral defect. Most meningoceles are covered by skin and contain cerebrospinal fluid. Although most affected children have no apparent neurologic involvement, some children may experience nerve involvement and associated irregularities (e.g., tethered spinal cord, diastematomyelia, and syringomyelia). If cerebrospinal fluid is leaking from the meningocele, immediate surgery is usually required to avoid infection or inflammation of the meninges (meningitis). Surgery to correct the meningocele may be performed

at a later date in those children who are not at risk for such infection.

Myelocele is a severe form of spina bifida that affects one in 1,000 newborns. This form of the disorder is characterized by a protrusion of the spinal cord and meninges through the vertebral canal, covered by a raw swelling. Most myeloceles are located in the lower back (lumbosacral region). This abnormality may result in impaired function of the skeletal system, the skin, the genitourinary tract, and the peripheral and central nervous systems. Physical findings associated with myelocele are widely variable and depend upon the portion of the spinal cord affected. These findings may include the inability to control the bladder and bowel functions, lack of muscle tone in the legs, and other irregularities of the lower extremities. Some children with myelocele develop an unusual accumulation of cerebrospinal fluid in the skull, resulting in enlargement of the head and associated symptoms that may include choking and difficulty in feeding and breathing. The insertion of a tube or shunt is often indicated to relieve fluid buildup. Treatment of myelocele often involves a team of medical specialists working closely to manage care for the affected child. This care usually involves surgery to repair the myelocele. Other approaches to treatment are geared toward correction, alleviation, or management of symptoms. For example, training children or their parents how to empty the bladder through catheterization may help to avoid urinary tract infections and kidney disease. Also, laxatives or enemas may be used to relieve the constipation often associated with this abnormality. Other treatment may include the use of braces and canes or crutches and physical therapy to maintain joint mobility and to strengthen muscular function. Further treatment is supportive. The exact cause of myelocele is unknown; however, it is thought that environmental and nutritional influences may be contributing factors.

Encephalocele, a very severe and rare type of spina bifida, is characterized by the protrusion of the brain through a defect in the cranium. Affected children often experience visual difficulties, mental retardation, and seizures.

Research has shown that supplementation with folic acid, starting before pregnancy, reduces the risk of neural tube defects. Women of child-bearing age are encouraged to take these supplements as directed by their physician.

The following organizations in the General Resources Section can provide additional information: Genetic Alliance, Online Mendelian Inheritance in Man: www3.ncbi.nlm.nih.gov/Omim/searchomim.html, March of Dimes Birth Defects Foundation, NIH/National Information Center for Children & Youth with Disabilities, NIH/National Institute of Arthritis and Musculoskeletal and Skin Diseases

National Associations & Support Groups

3841 National Center for Education in Maternal and Child Health
Information Services Department
2000 15th Street North Suite 701
Arlington, VA 22201   703-524-7802
                                Fax: 703-524-9335
        e-mail: ncemch01@gumedlib.dml.georgeto

Provides information services and technical assistance to organizations, agencies, and individuals with an interest in maternal and child health (MCH), public health policy, and systems of care.

3842 National Rehabilitiation Information
8455 Colesville Road, Suite 935
Silver Spring, MD 20910   301-588-9284
                                Fax: 800-227-0216

3843 Spina Bifida - Spina Bifida Association of Canada
220-388 Donald Street
Winnipeg,
Canada   204-452-7580

Dedicated to promoting the rights and well-being of individuals with spina bifida. The Association supports research into the causes, treatment, and prevention of the disease and seeks to increase public awareness of spina bifida and its prevention.

3844 Spina Bifida Association of America
4590 MacArthur Blvd., Suite 250
Washington, DC 20007   202-944-3285
                                 800-621-3141
             e-mail: spinabifida@aol.com
             www.infohiway.com/spinabifida

Serves as the national office representing approximately 80 chapters of parents and other members of families having children born with Spina Bifida, individuals with Spina Bifida, and health professionals who work with them. Operates a national information clearinghouse, an information and referral toll-free number, periodic public awareness, scholarships and related efforts and an annual meeting.

International

3845 Association for Spina Bifida and Hydrocephalus
ASBAH House, 42 Park Road
Peterborough,
United Kingdom

             http://www.asbah.demon.co.uk/

Provides services to people with spina bifida and/or hydrocephalus, and their care providers. Professionals develop and maintain expertise in spina bifida and hydrocephalus so that they may inform and assist other professionals in giving the best possible service.

3846 International Federation for Hydrocephalus and Spina Bifida
Attn. David Bagares
c/o RBU Gata 3
Stockholm,
Sweden

             www.asbah.demon.co.uk

Provides information, assistance, and support to individuals affected by hydrocephalus and their family members. Offers patient referrals, engages inpatient advocacy, offers networking services, and promotes research.

State Agencies & Support Groups

Alabama

3847 Spina Bifida Association of Alabama
P.O. Box 130538
Birmingham, AL 35213   205-978-7287

Arizona

3848 Spina Bifida Association of Arizona
1001 E. Fairmount Avenue
Phoenix, AZ 85014   602-274-3323
                                Fax: 602-274-7632
                      e-mail: rlwsbaz@aol.com

3849 Spina Bifida Association of Bay Area
P.O. Box 6015
Marage, CA 94570   925-210-6006
Fax: 925-377-0906
e-mail: randyb@sfo.harbinger.com

3850 Spina Bifida Association of Oakdale California
1040 West H Street
Oakdale, CA 95361   209-847-7035
e-mail: servan1@hisnet.org

3851 Spina Bifida Association of the Central Coast
1190 Margarita Way
Grover Beach, CA 93433   805-481-3510
Fax: 805-481-1745
e-mail: caprice@june.com

Arkansas

3852 Spina Bifida Association of Arkansas
P.O. Box 24663
Little Rock, AR 72221   501-851-3351
e-mail: vstefans@oz.ach.uams.edu

California

3853 Spina Bifida Association of East Bay
P.O. Box 6015
Moraga, CA 94570   415-210-6006

3854 Spina Bifida Association of Greater Rialto
1014 W. Jackson Street
Rialto, CA 92376   909-875-1650
e-mail: wmonlg6997@aol.com

3855 Spina Bifida Association of Greater San Diego
P.O. Box 232272
San Diego, CA 92193   619-491-9018
Fax: 619-534-7383
e-mail: mwreynolds@home.com

3856 Spina Bifida Association of Sacramento Valley
P.O. Box 60083
Sacramento, CA 95860   916-927-7146
e-mail: sbasvc@aol.com

3857 Spina Bifida Association of Stanford
1921 Clairemont
San Bruno, CA 94066   650-589-2992

Colorado

3858 Spina Bifida Association of Colorado
10351 E. Berry Drive
Englewood, CO 80228   303-790-3338
Fax: 303-770-3346
e-mail: kithovey@aol.com

3859 Spina Bifida Association of Florida
24 Beach Walker Road
Fernandine Beach, FL 32034
800-722-6355
Fax: 904-277-8678
e-mail: psabadie@net-magic.net

3860 Spina Bifida Association of Southwest Florida
P.O. Box 2684
Fort Meyers, FL 33902   941-332-7904

Connecticut

3861 Spina Bifida Association of Connecticut
P.O. Box 2545
Hartford, CT 06146   860-874-2339
800-574-6274
e-mail: dmaloney03@snet.net

Delaware

3862 Spina Bifida Association of Delaware
P.O. Box 807
Wilmington, DE 19899   302-478-4805
e-mail: sbaold@earthlink.net

55 Families

Florida

3863 Spina Bifida Association of Central Florida
P.O. Box 547970
Orlando, FL 32854   407-263-8350
Fax: 407-333-3662
e-mail: sbacf7970@aol.com

3864 Spina Bifida Association of Florida Space Coast
3685 Starlight Ave
Merrill Island, FL 32953   407-454-9737
                                 Fax: 407-454-9737
                        e-mail: sbafc@castlegate.net

3865 Spina Bifida Association of Jacksonville
P.O. Box 5720
Jacksonville, FL 32247   904-390-3686
                                 Fax: 904-390-3466
                        e-mail: sjking@nemours.org

3866 Spina Bifida Association of Southeast Florida
10060 S.W. 2nd St.
Plantation, FL 33324   954-472-4089
                                 Fax: 954-472-7252
                        e-mail: amcdds@aol.com

3867 Spina Bifida Association of Tampa
P.O. Box 151038
Tampa, FL 33684   813-933-4827
                                 Fax: 813-872-9845

Georgia

3868 Spina Bifida Association of Georgia
3355 NE Expressway, Suite 207
Atlanta, GA 30341   770-454-7600
                                 Fax: 770-454-7676
                        e-mail: sbag@mindspring.com

3869 Spina Bifida Program at the Shepherd Spinal Center
2020 Peachtree Road NW
Atlanta, GA 30309   404-352-2020

Provides referrals, evaluation, treatment and
therapeutic activities for children and teens afflicted with Spina Bifida. The goal of this center
is to help children or teenagers prepare for life.

Illinois

3870 Spina Bifida Association of Illinois
3080 Ogden Avenue, Ste. 103
Lisle, IL 60532   630-637-1050
                                 800-969-4722
                                 Fax: 630-637-1066
                        e-mail: ilsba@aol.com
                        www.illinoissba.org

Dedicated to improving the quality of life of people with spina bifida through direct services, information, referral and public awareness.
Services include a family Outreach program,
quarterly newsletter, Education Advocacy, and
a residential camp for people over age 7.

Indiana

3871 Spina Bifida Association of Central Indiana
P.O. Box 19814
Indianapolis, IN 46219   317-592-1630
                                 Fax: 317-577-2568
                        e-mail: pjwyman@gateway.com

118 members

3872 Spina Bifida Association of Northeast Indiana
919 S. Harrison St. #400/Art
Fort Wayne, IN 46802   219-423-1423
                                 Fax: 219-423-1425
                        e-mail: artjukev@aol.com

3873 Spina Bifida Association of Northern Indiana
P.O. Box 1935
South Bend, IN 46634   219-234-6260
                        e-mail: tabaldyod@michgantoday.com

Iowa

3874 Spina Bifida Association of Iowa
P.O. Box 1456
Des Moines, IA 50305   515-967-9229
                                 Fax: 515-279-1606

Kansas

3875 Spina Bifida Association of Kansas
4421 W. Harry
Wichita, KS 67209   316-945-0890
                        e-mail: tntwolker@email.msn.com

Kentucky

3876 Spina Bifida Association of Kentucky
Kosair Charities Center
982 Eastern Parkway, Box 16
Louisville, KY 40217   502-637-7696
                                 Fax: 502-637-1010
                        e-mail: sbak@sbak.org

Louisiana

3877 Spina Bifida Association of Greater New Orleans
P.O. Box 1346
Kenner, LA 70063   504-737-5181
Fax: 504-737-5181
e-mail: sbagno@email.com

Maryland

3878 Spina Bifida Association of Chesapeake- Polomac
P.O. Box 1750
Annapolis, MD 21404   888-733-0988
Fax: 410-295-9744
e-mail: shumate@kennedykrieger.org

3879 Spina Bifida Association of Maryland
600 W. Baker Avenue
Abingdon, MD 21009   410-833-5059
Fax: 410-833-1700

3880 Spina Bifida Association of the Eastern Shore
316 Prospect Avenue
Easton, MD 21601   410-822-8609
Fax: 410-822-5455

Massachusetts

3881 Spina Bifida Association of Massachusetts
456 Lowell St.
Peabody, MA 01960   978-531-6789
e-mail: apbcon@mindspring.com

Michigan

3882 Spina Bifida Association of Grand Rapids
235 Wealthy Street SE
Grand Rapids, MI 49503   616-796-6735
e-mail: amberg14@webtv.com

3883 Spina Bifida Association of Southeastern Michigan
1000 John R. Rd., Suite 101
Troy, MI 46083   248-359-1545
Fax: 734-487-1808
e-mail: kimph@quix.net

3884 Spina Bifida Association of Upper Peninsula Michigan
1220 North Third Street
Ishpeming, MI 49849   906-485-5127
Fax: 906-225-7230
e-mail: cbengson@nmu.edu
sba-up.8m.com

Support information for parents and people with Spina Bifida.

Lois Bergon, President

3885 Spina Bifida and Hydrocephalus Association of Southwestern Michigan
P.O. Box 212
Mattawan, MI 49071   616-385-3959
Fax: 616-381-3687

Dedicated to improving the quality of life of individuals with spina bifida and/or hydrocephalus and their families through awareness, education, and research. Offers a variety of educational guides and materials for schools, professionals, parents, and the general public.

Minnesota

3886 Spina Bifida Association of Minnesota
P.O. Box 29323
Brooklyn Center, MN 55429   651-222-0914
Fax: 651-226-0914
e-mail: juliaw@excite.com

Mississippi

3887 Spina Bifida Association of Mississippi
1511 Tracewood Drive
Jackson, MS 39211   601-957-2410
Fax: 601-957-2410
e-mail: spbranson@juno.com

Missouri

3888 Spina Bifida Association of Greater St. Louis
5609 Hampton Ave
St. Louis, MO 63109   314-353-7079
Fax: 314-353-1446
e-mail: c.guzdial@cwixmall.com
www.members.aol.com/sbastl

Nebraska

Spina Bifida/State Agencies & Support Groups

3889 Spina Bifida Association of Nebraska
7101 Newport Avenue.
Omaha, NE 68152   402-572-3570
                                Fax: 402-572-3002
                  e-mail: jbhuskar@home.com

New Jersey

3890 Spina Bifida Association of Bergen and Passaic Counties
181 Glen Avenue
Midland Park, NJ 07432   201-670-0590
                                Fax: 201-670-6361
                  e-mail: tja84@aol.com

Family support group, of parents of children with Spina Bifida.

25 Members

Shirl Cichewicz, President

3891 Spina Bifida Association of New Jersey
84 Park Avenue
Flemington, NJ 08822   908-782-7475
                                Fax: 908-782-6102
                  e-mail: sbanj@sbanj.org

New Mexico

3892 Spina Bifida Association of New Mexico
1127 University Boulevard NE
Albuquerque, NM 87102   505-242-1184
                                Fax: 505-242-1184
                  e-mail: sbanm@aol.com

New York

3893 Spina Bifida Association of Albany/Capital District
109 Spring Road
Scotia, NY 12302   518-399-9151
                  e-mail: rexdar109@aol.com

3894 Spina Bifida Association of Greater Rochester
P.O. Box 3
Fairport, NY 14601   716-381-5471
                                Fax: 716-361-2006
                  e-mail: wdddep@aol.com

3895 Spina Bifida Association of Nassau County
15 Linden Street
Garden City, NY 11530   516-294-4420
                                Fax: 516-562-8909
                  e-mail: dewkow@worldnet.alt.net

3896 Spina Bifida Association of Western New York
P.O. Box 50
Williamsville, NY 14231   716-446-5595
                                Fax: 716-735-7661
                  e-mail: slack@pcorn.net

3897 Spina Bifida Association of the Niagara Frontier
P.O. Box 50
Williamsville, NY 14231   716-691-3768

North Carolina

3898 Spina Bifida Association Lipomysiomeningcele Family Support
415 Webster St
Cary, NC 27511   610-404-1338
                                Fax: 610-582-1262
                  e-mail: bborchert@mindspring.com

3899 Spina Bifida Association of North Carolina
5632 Ebley Lane
Charlotte, NC 28227
                            800-847-2262
                                Fax: 910-424-7589
                  e-mail: sbanc@mindspring.com

Ohio

3900 Spina Bifida Association of Canton
P.O. Box 9089
Canton, OH 44711   330-966-9208
                                Fax: 330-499-6263
                  e-mail: tucker@wg.essnet.com

3901 Spina Bifida Association of Central Ohio
5569 Ulry Road
Westerville, OH 43081   614-695-6963
                                Fax: 614-891-1633
                  e-mail: danrake@coll.com

3902 Spina Bifida Association of Cincinnati
3245 Deborah Lane
Cincinnati, OH 45239   513-923-1378
                    e-mail: mclisms@aol.com

3903 Spina Bifida Association of Cleveland
P.O. Box 347385 - Edgewater Br
Parma, OH 44134   440-826-0551

3904 Spina Bifida Association of Greater Dayton
1631 Harshman Road
Dayton, OH 45424   937-236-1122
                    Fax: 937-434-4899
                    e-mail: fouresh@arinst.com

3905 Spina Bifida Association of Northwest Ohio
145 Water St.
Waterville, OH 43532   419-533-6212
                    Fax: 419-533-3952
                    e-mail: lorilindau@aol.com

3906 Spina Bifida Association of Tri-County Ohio
P.O. Box 8701
Warren, OH 44484   330-856-7228
                    Fax: 330-837-8435
                    e-mail: vamerine@lung.com

Oklahoma

3907 Spina Bifida Association of Oklahoma
P.O. Box 2117
Oklahoma City, OK 73101   405-789-7056
                    e-mail: sbaq@nstar.net

Pennsylvania

3908 Spina Bifida Association of Central Pennsylvania
c/o Dennis Carney
1360 Swope Drive
Boiling Springs, PA 17007   717-258-6402
                    Fax: 717-258-0350

3909 Spina Bifida Association of Delaware Valley
P.O. Box 289
Glenolden, PA 19036   856-858-6555
                    800-223-0222
                    Fax: 610-872-9294
                    e-mail: president@sbadv.org

3910 Spina Bifida Association of Greater Pennsylvania
205 West View Road
Ligonier, PA 15688   724-238-7579
                    e-mail: verne@sgl.net

3911 Spina Bifida Association of Lancaster County
209 East State, Suite B
Quarryville, PA 17566   717-786-9280
                    Fax: 717-766-8821
                    e-mail: sbaoflc@aol.com

3912 Spina Bifida Association of Pennsylvania, Central
University Hospital Rehabilitation Center
P.O. Box 850
Hershey, PA 17033   717-531-8521

3913 Spina Bifida Association of Western Pennsylvania
134 Shanot Road
Wexford, PA 15090   724-934-9600
                    Fax: 724-934-9610
                    e-mail: alkwood@brads.net

3914 Spina Bifida Coalition of Pennsylvania
209 East State Street, Ste. B
Quarryville, PA 17566   717-786-9280
                    888-770-7272
                    Fax: 717-786-8821
                    e-mail: sbaoflc@aol.com

Serves as a clearing house of information and referral services, dedicated to finding services in all areas of PA.

Patricia Folvio, Executive Director

Rhode Island

3915 Spina Bifida Association of Rhode Island
P.O. Box 6948
Warwick, RI 02887   401-732-7862
                    Fax: 401-732-7862
                    e-mail: dahliadebz@aol.com

Tennessee

3916 Spina Bifida Association of Mid-Tennessee
546 Hopewood Court
Franklin, TN 37064　　　　616-791-1518
　　　　　　　　　　　　Fax: 615-791-1518
　　　　　　　　e-mail: spinabifin@aol.com

Texas

3917 Spina Bifida Association of Austin
8710 Tailwood Drive
Austin, TX 78759　　　　512-794-8156

3918 Spina Bifida Association of Dallas
705 W Avenue B
Garland, TX 75040　　　　972-238-8755
　　　　　　　　　　　　Fax: 972-474-3772
　　　　　　　　e-mail: sbad@aol.com
　　　　　　　　　　　　www.sbad.org

Carol Barrett, Office Manager

3919 Spina Bifida Association of Texas
705 West Avenue B Suite 300
Garland, TX 75040　　　　972-238-8755

3920 Spina Bifida Association of Texas, Gulf Coast
2340 Albans Road
Houston, TX 77005　　　　409-849-6864
　　　　　　　　　　　　Fax: 520-752-5018
　　　　　　　　e-mail: tabtytamon@aol.com

**3921 Spina Bifida Association of Texas/Alamo Area
Support Group**
2935 Thousand Oaks #6-124
San Antonio, TX 78247　　　210-690-1780

Utah

3922 Spina Bifida Association of Utah
P.O. Box 27601
Salt Lake City, UT 84127　　435-245-7894

Virginia

3923 Spina Bifida Association of the National Capital Area
9079 Tiffany Park Court
Springfield, VA 22152　　　703-455-4900

Washington

3924 Spina Bifida Association of Evergreen
9826 18th Street, Ct. E
Puyallup, WA 98371　　　　253-927-2188
　　　　　　　　e-mail: rhenry0001@aol.com

Wisconsin

3925 Spina Bifida Association of Northeastern Wisconsin
1813-21st Street
Two Rivers, WI 54476　　　715-359-9674

3926 Spina Bifida Association of Northern Wisconsin
P.O. Box 421
Schofield, WI 54476　　　　715-359-9674
　　　　　　　　e-mail: mary139@aol.com

3927 Spina Bifida Association of Southeastern Wisconsin
W300 N1725 Timberbrook Road
Pewaukee, WI 53072　　　　414-367-6226
　　　　　　　　　　　　Fax: 414-781-5144

3928 Spina Bifida Association of Wisconsin
830n. 109th St, Suite #6
Wauwatosa, WI 53226　　　414-607-9061
　　　　　　　　　　　　Fax: 414-607-9061
　　　　　　　　e-mail: sbawis@aol.com

3929 Spina Bifida Association of the Greater Fox Valley
418 E. Handcock Street
New London, WI 54961　　　920-962-3783
　　　　　　　　　　　　Fax: 920-962-3783
　　　　　　　　e-mail: fus1234@aol.com

Audio Video

3930 Challenge
Spina Bifida Association of America
4590 MacArthur Blvd. N.W. Suite 250
Washington, DC 20007　　　202-944-3285
　　　　　　　　　　　　800-621-3141
　　　　　　　　　　　　Fax: 202-944-3295
　　　　　　　　e-mail: spinabifida@aol.com
　　　　　　　　www.infohiway.com/spinabifida

A human look of how people come to grips with
and overcome the challenges related to living
with Spina Bifida.
1992 14 minutes

3931 How to Guide Your Child Through Special Education
Spina Bifida Association of America
4590 MacArthur Blvd. N.W. Suite 250
Washington, DC 20007   202-944-3285
800-621-3141
Fax: 202-944-3295
e-mail: spinabifida@aol.com
www.infohiway.com/spinabifida

Enlightens and encourages viewers, and informs parents on special education, planning for the future, and laws designed to protect children with disabilities.

3932 Raising a Child with Spina Bifida: An Introduction
Ajn Company

New York, NY 10019
800-225-5256
Fax: 212-586-5462

Offers information for parents: clear explanations to define spina bifida; implications for the child; procedures the child may face, such as a ventricular shunt; early intervention; footage of happy and healthy children and interviews with parents.

29 min.

3933 Teaching the Student with Spina Bifida
Paul H. Brookes Publishing Company
P.O. Box 10624
Baltimore, MD 21285   410-337-8539
800-638-3775

A compelling companion to the book by the same name, this heartening videotape draws viewers into the inclusive classroom for a first-hand look.

Video

Web Sites

3934 Children with Spina Bifida: A Resource Page for Parents
www.waisman.wisc.edu/~rowley/sb-kids/ind

3935 Harvard Web Forum for Spina Bifida
www.disabilities.miningco.com/msub128

3936 Wheeless' Textbook of Orthopaedics
www.medmedia.com/o11/91.htm

Books

3937 Answering Your Questions About Spina Bifida
Dr. Catherine Shaer, et al., author
Spina Bifida Association of America
4590 MacArthur Blvd. N.W. Suite 250
Washington, DC 20007   202-944-3285
800-621-3141
Fax: 202-944-3295
e-mail: spinabifida@aol.com
www.infohiway.com/spinabifida

Provides information to help people understand the basic medical, educational and social issues which commonly affect people with Spina Bifida.

3938 Clinic Directory
Spina Bifida Association of America
4590 MacArthur Blvd. N.W. Suite 250
Washington, DC 20007   202-944-3285
800-621-3141
Fax: 202-944-3295
e-mail: spinabifida@aol.com
www.infohiway.com/spinabifida

A directory of health care clinics throughout the United States for children and adults with Spina Bifida.

200 pages 3-Ring Binder

3939 Confronting the Challenges of Spina Bifida
Spina Bifida Association of America
4590 MacArthur Blvd. N.W. Suite 250
Washington, DC 20007   202-944-3285
800-621-3141
Fax: 202-944-3295
e-mail: spinabifida@aol.com
www.infohiway.com/spinabifida

A group curriculum addressing self-care, self-esteem, and social skills in 8 to 13 year olds.

3940 SBAA General Information Brochure
David McLone M.D., author
Spina Bifida Association of America
4590 MacArthur Blvd. N.W. Suite 250
Washington, DC 20007   202-944-3285
800-621-3141
Fax: 202-944-3295
e-mail: spinabifida@aol.com
www.infohiway.com/spinabifida

3941 Social Development and the Person With Spina Bifida

Donald J. Lollar, Ed.D., author

Spina Bifida Association of America
4590 MacArthur Blvd. N.W. Suite 250
Washington, DC 20007   202-944-3285
                              800-621-3141
                              Fax: 202-944-3295
                              e-mail: spinabifida@aol.com
                              www.infohiway.com/spinabifida

20 pages

3942 Taking Charge

Kay H. Kriegsman, Ph.D., et al, author

Spina Bifida Association of America
4590 MacArthur Blvd. N.W. Suite 250
Washington, DC 20007   202-944-3285
                              800-621-3141
                              Fax: 202-944-3295
                              e-mail: spinabifida@aol.com
                              www.infohiway.com/spinabifida

Teenagers talk about life and physical disabilities.

3943 Teaching the Student with Spina Bifida

F.L. Rowley-Kelly, author

Books On Special Children
P.O. Box 305
Congers, NY 10920   914-638-1236
                           Fax: 914-638-0847

Discusses health care needs, how to tailor academic programs with special testing and evaluating, social and family issues and school outreach programs.

470 pages Softcover
ISBN: 1-557660-64-6

Children's Books

3944 COLT

N. Springer, author

Association for the Care of Children's Health
8701 Hartsdale Avenue
Bethesda, MD 20817   301-493-5113

An adolescent boy with Spina Bifida becomes involved in a therapeutic riding program and uses skills learned there to cope with the challenges of everyday life.

Hardcover

3945 Margaret's Moves

Bernice Rabe, author

Dutton Children's Books
375 Hudson Street
New York, NY 10014   212-366-2000

This story deals with all the nuances and impairments that children afflicted with Spina Bifida must encounter and succeed in overcoming.

Grades 4-6

3946 You Are Special - You Are the One

Barbara Pence & Gloria Nelson, author

Spina Bifida Association of America
4590 MacArthur Blvd. N.W. Suite 250
Washington, DC 20007   202-944-3285
                              800-621-3141
                              Fax: 202-944-3295
                              e-mail: spinabifida@aol.com
                              www.infohiway.com/spinabifida

A coloring storybook about Holly, a little girl with Spina Bifida.

Newsletters

3947 INSIGHTS

Spina Bifida Association of America
4590 MacArthur Blvd. N.W. Suite 250
Washington, DC 20007   202-944-3285
                              800-621-3141
                              Fax: 202-944-3295
                              e-mail: spinabifida@aol.com
                              www.infohiway.com/spinabifida

Includes articles on the latest research, legislation, features, emotional aspects, educational information, and information on the Association's national conference.

Bi-Monthly

3948 NASS News

222 S. Prospect Avenue
Park Ridge, IL 60068   847-698-1628

Association activities newsletter.

Pamphlets

3949 Educational Issues Among Children With Spina Bifida

Donald Lollar, Ed.D., author

Spina Bifida Association of America
4590 MacArthur Blvd. N.W. Suite 250
Washington, DC 20007   202-944-3285
                              800-621-3141
                    Fax: 202-944-3295
          e-mail: spinabifida@aol.com
          www.infohiway.com/spinabifida

3950 Urologic Care of the Child with Spina Bifida

Stuart B. Bauer, MD, author

Spina Bifida Association of America
4590 MacArthur Blvd. N.W. Suite 250
Washington, DC 20007   202-944-3285
                              800-621-3141
                    Fax: 202-944-3295
          e-mail: spinabifida@aol.com
          www.infohiway.com/spinabifida

DESCRIPTION

3951 SPINAL MUSCULAR ATROPHIES

Synonym: SMA

Disorder Type: Genetic Disorder, Neuromuscular

Covers these related disorders: Fazio-Londe disease (Progressive bulbar palsy of childhood), SMA type I (Werdnig-Hoffmann disease; Acute SMA), SMA type II (Intermediate SMA), SMA type III (Kugelberg-Welander disease;Wohlfart-Kugelberg-Wela)

The spinal muscular atrophies (SMAs) refer to a group of progressive, inherited neuromuscular disorders characterized by the progressive degeneration of motor neurons. Motor neurons are nerves that originate in the spinal cord and stimulate and control muscle movement (motor neurons). Spinal muscular atrophy type I, also called Werdnig-Hoffmann disease, usually becomes apparent between the second and fourth month of life; however, some infants may have symptoms at birth, including difficult breathing and the inability to feed. Other characteristic symptoms and findings include lack of muscle tone (hypotonia), muscle weakness, the inability to control head movements, absence of tendon stretch reflexes, and uncontrollable twitching or small movements (fasciculations) of the tongue and possibly other muscles. Within two to three years of age, continued breathing and feeding difficulties, along with other progressive problems, may lead to life-threatening complications. Treatment is symptomatic and supportive.

Children with SMA type II usually show signs of progressive muscle weakness of the legs and, to a lesser degree, the arms during the first or second year of life. As the disease progresses, many affected children develop side-to-side curvature of the spine (scoliosis), difficulty swallowing, and a nasal quality to their speech. Children with SMA type II may be severely physically handicapped and are usually of average or above average intelligence. Affected chidren are prone to repeated respiratory infections and breathing difficulties.

Life-threatening complications may occur during adolescence or early adulthood.

SMA type III or chronic spinal muscular atrophy may become apparent between the ages of two to 17 years. This is the mildest form of SMA. Progressive weakness associated with chronic SMA is most apparent in the trunk area of the body, especially in the muscles of the shoulder girdle area. There is muscle weakness and loss of muscle mass (atrophy). In addition, deep tendon reflexes may be decreased or absent and muscle twitching (fasciculations) may be present. Some affected children may also have a tremor when the hands are outstretched. Repeated respiratory infections are common.

Fazio-Londe disease, also called progressive bulbar palsy of childhood, is a rare type of spinal muscular atrophy that results from degeneration of motor neurons located, for the most part, in the brain stem. This rare disorder is characterized by progressive palsy or paralysis of the nerves that emerge from the skull (cranial nerves). Symptoms and physical findings associated with Fazio-Londe disease include progressive loss of muscle mass (atrophy) and paralysis of the muscles of the tongue, mouth, lips, throat (pharynx), and voice box (larynx).

A team approach involving specialists such as neurologists, orthopedists, and physical therapists, in cooperation with parents or caregivers, may be helpful in providing care for children with spinal muscular atrophies. Other treatment is symptomatic and supportive.

SMA is usually inherited as an autosomal recessive trait, although some cases of autosomal dominant transmission have been reported. This disorder occurs in approximately one out of every 25,000 births. The genes for SMA types I, II, and III seem to be related and are located on the long arm of chromosome 5 (5q11-13).

The following organizations in the General Resources Section can provide additional information: National Organization for Rare Disorders, Inc., (NORD), NIH/Office of Rare Diseases, Genetic Alliance, March of Dimes Birth Defects Foundation, Online Mendelian Inheritance in Man:

www3.ncbi.nlm.nih.gov/Omim/searchomim.html, NIH/National Institute of Neurological Disorders & Stroke

National Associations & Support Groups

3952 Association for Neuro-Metabolic Disorders
5223 Brookfield Lane
Sylvania, OH 43506   419-885-1497

Organization that is comprised of families of children with disorders that affect the nervous system and the brain. It provides assistance and information through conferences, meetings and phone calls.

3953 Muscular Dystrophy Association
3300 E Sunrise Dr
Tucson, AZ 85718

800-572-1717
www.mdausa.org/

Dedicated to supplying the general public with the knowledge to properly assess and choose their doctors and medical facilities.

International

3954 Jennifer Trust for Spinal Muscular Atrophy
296 Avon House
New Broad Street, Stratford-Upon-Avon
Warwick,
United Kingdom
e-mail: jennifer@jtsma.demon.co.uk
www.jtsma.demon.co.uk

Research Centers

3955 Families of SMA
P.O. Box 196
Libertyville, IL 60048   847-367-7620
800-886-1762
Fax: 847-367-7623
e-mail: sma@fsma.org
www.fsma.org

Families of SMA was founded for the purpose of encouraging support and raising funds to promote research into the causes and cure of spinal muscular atrophy. Funds are specifically directed to scientific, educational, or literary purposes in keeping with a charitable organization.

Web Sites

3956 SMA Net
fortuna.italia.com/smanet/index.html

3957 UseNet Newsgroup
alt.support.musc-dystrophy

Pamphlets

3958 Facts About Spinal Muscular Atrophy
Muscular Dystrophy Association
3300 E. Sunrise Drive
Tucson, AZ 85718   520-529-2000
Fax: 520-529-5300

Covers the four forms of the disease and outlines the characteristics and genetic patterns of the SMAs. Research efforts aimed at finding the causes, treatments, and cures are also described.

DESCRIPTION

3959 STRABISMUS

    Synonyms: Heterotropia, Manifest deviation, Squint
    Disorder Type: Genetic Disorder, Vision
    Covers these related disorders: Accommodation strabismus, Nonparalytic strabismus, Paralytic strabismus

Strabismus refers to a condition in which the eyes are not aligned properly in relation to each other and are focused on different objects simultaneously. Approximately four percent of all children under six years of age are affected by some form of strabismus. The eye deviations associated with this condition are classified according to the direction of the deviation. An eye that is turned inward is considered esotropic or convergent; an eye turned outward is exotropic or divergent; an eye turned upward is hypertropic; and an eye turned downward is hypotropic. In normal vision, both eyes focus as a unit to produce a single, three-dimensional image. In children with strabismus, the divergent images sent to the brain from the eyes may produce double vision (diplopia). In many cases, the brain will compensate for this error by blocking the image from the deviated eye, often resulting in poor vision or loss of vision in that eye (suppression amblyopia).

The most common type of strabismus is nonparalytic, in which this often-inherited ocular deviation is constant and results from a defect in the actual positioning of the eyes. Approximately 50 percent of individuals with nonparalytic strabismus have one eye turned inward. These inward-turned or esotropic deviations that appear before six months of age are classified as congenital or infantile esotropia. Outward-turned or exotropic deviations, the second most common type of strabismus, usually occur in children between six months and four years of age. Some outward deviations may result from neurologic disorders and craniofacial abnormalities.

Paralytic strabismus results from dysfunction of an eye muscle as the result of ocular muscle paralysis or a deficit of the nerves that supply the muscles. This resultant muscular imbalance causes the degree of deviation in the affected eye to vary as the eyes move.

Farsighted children are at particular risk for developing accommodative strabismus (accommodative esotropia), in which the lens of the eye tries to compensate for blurred images received by the brain by focusing the eyes inward (converging). If the compensation or accommodation demands are too great, some children may develop this additional eye abnormality.

Strabismus may result from many different factors; therefore, medical specialists make every effort to determine and treat the underlying cause as soon as possible after diagnosis. Such factors may include hereditary influences; trauma; neurologic abnormalities resulting from intracranial tumors or weaknesses in the walls of blood vessels in the brain (aneurysms); infection; systemic disorders; blood vessel malformations; structural abnormalities; and association with certain syndromes such as Duane syndrome.

Early treatment for nonparalytic strabismus may prevent a permanent loss of sight and may include wearing a patch over the normal eye in order to compel the brain to receive images from the affected eye. Patching often improves the vision in the deviating eye. Upon improvement, surgery may be performed to equalize the pull of the eye muscles. Children affected with paralytic strabismus may also benefit from wearing glasses with special lenses (prisms) that deflect light, thus altering positioning of objects seen through the lenses. In addition, children with paralytic strabismus with significant ocular deviation may benefit from eye muscle surgery to improve alignment. Farsighted children with accommodative strabismus may be treated with prescription glasses that lessen the need for ocular accommodation when focusing on objects that are far away. Certain medications in the form of eye drops may also aid in focusing on objects that are nearby. Other treatment is aimed toward the underlying cause of the ocular deviation.

The following organizations in the General Resources Section can provide additional information: National Organization for Rare Disorders, Inc., (NORD), Genetic Alliance, Online Mendelian Inheritance in Man: www3.ncbi.nlm.nih.gov/Omim/searchomim.html

National Associations & Support Groups

3960 NIH/National Eye Institute (NEI)
9000 Rockville Pike
Bethesda, MD 20892   301-496-5248
                           www.nei.nih.gov/

3961 National Eye Research Foundation
910 Skokie Boulevard
Northbrook, IL 60062

Devoted to the enhancement of care and study of eye related diseases.

Web Sites

3962 American Association for Pediatric Ophthalmology and Strabismus
med-aapos.bu.edu/

3963 Eye Net (AAO)
www.eyeynet.org/public/faqs/strabis-mus_faq.html

3964 Karolista Institute
www.mic.ki.se/diseases/c11.html

3965 National Association for Visually Handicapped
www.navh.org

3966 Pedbase
www.icondata.com/health/ped-base/files/STRABISM.HTM

3967 Royal National Institute for the Blind
www.rnib/org.uk/info/eyeimpoi/congen.htm

3968 Strabismus Web Book
www.smbs.buffalo.edu/oph/ped/webbook.htm

DESCRIPTION

3969 STUTTERING

Disorder Type: Neuromuscular, Mental, Emotional or Behavioral Disorder
May involve these systems in the body (see Section III):
Central Nervous System

Stuttering refers to a type of speech dysfunction that interferes with the flow of speech (dysfluency). This dysfunction is characterized by difficulty in uttering certain sounds, letters, syllables, words, or phrases and is usually manifested by frequent hesitations, stumbling, or delay in enunciation, as well as prolongation of certain sounds. As young children develop language skills, they typically experience hesitations in speech as a result of still-developing muscle coordination and limited vocabulary. If excessive attention is given to these temporary speech deficiencies, some children may become self-conscious, anxious, and fearful of speaking. These types of emotional reactions may be manifested as persistent and compulsive movements of certain muscle groups that interfere with the normal flow of speech. Children who stutter may have difficulty with only particular letters, sounds, or words. In addition, the severity of the stutter is often related to the amount of stress evoked by the particular situation. Some affected children and adults may have associated tremors or tics. Stuttering is a relatively common condition that develops in approximately five percent of children.

Although most stuttering results from psychological causes, this speech dysfunction may sometimes occur as a result of certain disorders of the central nervous system, neuromuscular abnormalities, or injury to organs related to speech. Stuttering that results from behavioral influences is often self-limited and, in 80 percent of those affected, resolves during childhood.

In young children, treatment for stuttering is mainly supportive. Parents or caregivers are often counseled not to place undue emphasis on speech irregularities. Additional supportive care may include recognition of accomplishments and other gestures that will contribute to the development of self-worth. If stuttering persists beyond early childhood or into adulthood, speech therapy is usually indicated.

The following organizations in the General Resources Section can provide additional information: Genetic Alliance, NIH/National Institute on Deafness and Other Communication Disorders Clearinghouse, Online Mendelian Inheritance in Man:
www3.ncbi.nlm.nih.gov/Omim/searchomim.html

National Associations & Support Groups

3970 Canadian Association for People Who Stutter
P.O. Box 2274 Square One
Mississauga Ontario, L5B   905-252-8255
                                  888-788-8837
                        e-mail: caps@webcon.net
                               caps.webcon.net

3971 National Center for Stuttering
200 E 33rd St
New York, NY 10016
                                  800-221-2483
                            Fax: 212-683-1372
          e-mail: executivedirector@stuttering.com
                              www.stuttering.com

Distributes information for parents of young children showing early signs of stuttering. For older children and adults, free information is available on treatment programs nationwide.

3972 National Stuttering Project
5100 E. La Palma Ave, Ste 208
Anaheim Hills, CA 92807   714-693-7554
                                 800-364-7554
                            Fax: 714-693-7554
                        e-mail: NSPmail@aol.com

Dedicated tp the improved treatment and the prevention of stuttering. Also maintains a toll-free Hotline on stuttering and a nationwide resource list for individuals seeking a speech-language pathologist who specializes in stuttering. Several publications are also directed toward medical professionals who serve the stuttering community.

3973 Ontario Association for Families of Children with Communication Disorders
13 Segal Drive
Tillsonburg Ontario, N4G   519-842-9506
Fax: 519-842-3228
e-mail: oafccd@cyberus.ca
www.cuberus.ca/oafccd

3974 Speak Easy International Foundation
233 Concord Dr
Paramus, NJ 07562   201-262-0895

Dedicated to support those individuals who are burdened with the speech dysfluency commonly known as stuttering. Acts as an advocate group and encourages family and friends of stutterers to become cognizant of the speech dysfluent individual's plight and problems.

3975 Stuttering Foundation of America
P.O. Box 11749
Memphis, TN 38111   901-452-7343
800-992-9392
Fax: 901-452-3931
e-mail: stutter@vantek.net
www.stutterhelp.org

Dedicated to people affected by stuttering. Also maintains a toll-free Hotline on stuttering and a nationwide resource list for individuals seeking a speech-language pathologist who specializes in stuttering. Several publications are also directed toward medical professionals who serve the stuttering community.

3976 Stuttering Resource Foundation
123 Oxford
New Rochelle, NY 10804
800-232-4773

International

3977 British Stammering Association
15 Old Ford Rd.
London Intl.,
United Kingdom
e-mail: mail@stammer.demon.co.uk
www.bss.org

Aims to prevent stammering in young children, promoting a wider understanding of stammering and helping stammerers help themselves. Runs a free information service, advice, counseling and a parents network.

Web Sites

3978 Parent Pals
www.parentpals.com
e-mail: superpal@parentpals.com
www.parentpals.com

Books

3979 Adolescent Psychotherapy Treatment Planner
Courage*To*Change
P.O. Box 1268
Newburgh, NY 12551
800-440-4003
Fax: 800-772-6499

Focuses on adolescent behavioral and psychological problems, this edition provides treatment planning guidelines and pre-written treatment plan components for 30 main presenting problems including anger management, blended family conflicts, self-esteem, chemical dependence, eating disorders, sexual acting out and more.

288 pages Softcover

3980 Child Psychotherapy Treatment Planner
Courage*To*Change
P.O. Box 1268
Newburgh, NY 12551
800-440-4003
Fax: 800-772-6499

Provides treatment planning guidelines and pre-written treatment plan components for 30 child behavioral and psychological problems, including blended family problems, divorce, communication disorder, attachment disorder, academic problems, stuttering, underachievement and more.

288 pages Softcover

3981 Straight Talk on Stuttering: Information, Encouragement, and Counsel
Lloyd M. Hulit, author
Charles C. Thomas Publishing, Ltd.
2600 South First Street
Springfield, IL 62704   217-789-8980
800-258-8980
Fax: 217-789-9130
e-mail: books@ccthomas.com
www.ccthomas.com

Written for stutterers and those who interact with stutterers, including parents, caregivers, teachers, and speech-language pathologists. The author dispels myths, corrects the misperceptions and creates a message of hope for all people who have this fascinating communication disorder.

278 pages $37.95 paper
ISBN: 0-398065-91-8

3982 Stuttering

C. Woodruff Starkweather, Janet Givens-Ackerman, author

Pro-Ed
8700 Shoal Creek Boulevard
Austin, TX 78757   512-451-3246
                                      800-897-3202
                                      Fax: 512-451-8542
                                      www.proedinc.com

Written by a practicing clinician and a recovering stutterer, this text supplies a detailed description of the development of the disorder in school-age children and a description of the demands and capacities model that has proven so useful in planning therapy for preschool children.

233 pages
ISBN: 0-890796-99-8

3983 Stuttering Intervention Program

Rebekah H. Pindzola, author

Pro-Ed
8700 Shoal Creek Boulevard
Austin, TX 78757   512-451-3246
                                      800-897-3202
                                      Fax: 512-451-8542
                                      www.proedinc.com

A complete package consisting of a four-part approach which provides the speech pathologist with a normed, thorough evaluation protocol that easily differentiates normal disfluency from incipient stuttering. A valuable clinical resource.

3984 Stuttering Prediction Instrument for Young Children

Glyndon D. Riley, author

Pro-Ed
8700 Shoal Creek Boulevard
Austin, TX 78757   512-451-3246
                                      800-897-3202
                                      Fax: 512-451-8542
                                      www.proedinc.com

The SPI is designed for children ages 3 to 8 years and assesses a child's history, reactions, part-word repititions, prolongations, and frequency of stuttered words to assist in measuring severity and predicting chronicity.

3-8 pages

3985 Stuttering Severity Instrument for Children and Adults

Glyndon D. Riley, author

Pro-Ed
8700 Shoal Creek Boulevard
Austin, TX 78757   512-451-3246
                                      800-897-3202
                                      Fax: 512-451-8542
                                      www.proedinc.com

Measures the stuttering severity of both children and adults for clinical and research use. Complete SSI-3 kit includes examiner's manual and picture plates and 50 test record and frequency computation forms all in a sturdy storage box.

DESCRIPTION

3986 SUBACUTE SCLEROSING PANENCEPHALITIS (SSPE)

Synonyms: Dawson's encephalitis, Van Bogaert's encophalitis

Disorder Type: Infectious Disease

Subacute sclerosing panencephalitis (SSPE) is a rare, life-threatening, slow viral infection of the brain caused by a measles-like virus. SSPE appears months or years after a typical mild or severe measles infection and occurs most frequently in children and adolescents between the ages of five and 15 years. This disease occurs more often in children who develop measles before 18 months of age and is twice as prevalent in boys as it is in girls. Symptoms develop gradually and may commence with subtle behavioral changes such as forgetfulness or outbursts of temper, deterioration in school performance, sleeplessness, and hallucinations. These symptoms are often followed by more bizarre behavior, seizures, repetitive muscular jerks (myoclonic jerks) and other abnormal movements, eye irregularities, and mental deterioration (dementia). Late findings may include muscular rigidity or, in some patients, weak muscles, difficulty swallowing, blindness, or coma. In addition, due to generalized weakness and impaired muscle control associated with SSPE, life-threatening complications such as pneumonia may occur. Subacute sclerosing panencephalitis is incompatible with life; its usual duration is from one to three years.

The diagnosis of SSPE may be confirmed through laboratory tests that detect the presence of antibodies to the measles virus in the cerebrospinal fluid and the presence of large numbers of measles antibodies in the serum. In most cases, subacute sclerosing pnencephalitis may be prevented by immunization with attenuated measles virus vaccine.

Treatment of SSPE is geared toward chronic care. In addition, certain medications (e.g., antiviral drugs) may aid in symptomatic improvement. Studies of other therapeutic programs are ongoing. Other treatment is symptomatic and supportive.

The following organizations in the General Resources Section can provide additional information: Genetic Alliance, March of Dimes Birth Defects Foundation, NIH/National Child Health and Human Development, National Organization for Rare Disorders, Inc., (NORD), NIH/National Institute of Allergy and Infectious Disease, World Health Organization

Web Sites

3987 Centers for Disease Control
www.cdc.gov/epo/mmwr/preview/mmwrhtml/00001185.htm

3988 Dr. Koop
drkoop.net/adam/peds/top/001419.htm

3989 Encephalitis Support Group
glaxocentre.merseyside.org/esgindex.html

DESCRIPTION

3990 SUDDEN INFANT DEATH SYNDROME
Synonyms: Cot death, Crib death, SIDS

Sudden infant death syndrome (SIDS) refers to the sudden, unexpected, and unexplained death of an apparently healthy infant. This syndrome may occur from the ages of two weeks to one year, but most commonly occurs between the ages of two to four months. Approximately 75 to 95 percent of all deaths related to SIDS occur by the age of six months. Sudden infant death syndrome is responsible for approximately half of all infant deaths that occur between the ages of 1 month and one year and, in the United States, affects approximately 1.3 of every 1,000 infants in that age group. SIDS is somewhat more common in boys and in infants born to individuals of African-American or Native American descent as well as to women of certain other backgrounds. In addition, sudden infant death syndrome occurs more often during the winter months.

Although the cause of SIDS is unknown, researchers believe that certain brain stem abnormalities may be a contributing factor to its occurrence. Such irregularities may affect the regulation of body temperature, cardiorespiratory function, and associated sleep and arousal mechanisms. Although the relationship is not fully understood, brain stem abnormalities, especially sleep and arousal deficit, may interact with certain other influencing factors (epidemiologic risk factors) to put infants at risk for SIDS. Such epidemiologic risk factors may include prematurity, low birth weight, bottle feeding, exposure to smoking, recent illness with fever and previous near death episodes requiring resuscitation. Also, mothers with abnormally low levels of circulating red blood cells (anemia) or those who smoke or use drugs during pregnancy may be at increased risk for having an infant with SIDS. Other factors may include insufficient prenatal care and low socioeconomic status. In addition, recent studies have shown that putting infants to sleep on their stomachs is a significant risk factor, as is the use of soft bedding or extra linens and toys (e.g., comforters, quilts, stuffed animals, etc.) in the crib.

To alleviate certain risk factors, appropriate prenatal care is essential in the possible prevention of SIDS. Also, after birth, parents are counseled to be alert to any respiratory changes or distress and to closely observe infants during and after any illness. In addition, new guidelines recommend that infants be placed in the crib on their backs, as statistics have shown declines in SIDS rates among those who have complied with this recommendation. Other guidelines include the advice that crib mattresses should be firm and should fit tightly within the crib frame; that comforters, quilts, pillows, toys, etc. should be removed from the crib; that, if possible, sleeper-type pajamas be used instead of blankets; that if a blanket must be used, it should be thin, should reach no further than the infant's chest, and should be tucked around the infant's chest and mattress; and that the baby's head should be uncovered at all times during sleep. In the event of the death of an infant from SIDS, counseling by trained specialists is strongly advised for parents and remaining siblings. In addition, support groups composed of families who have been affected by SIDS may be comforting and helpful.

The following organizations in the General Resources Section can provide additional information: Online Mendelian Inheritance in Man: www3.ncbi.nlm.nih.gov/Omim/searchomim.html

National Associations & Support Groups

3991 American SIDS Institute
2480 Windy Hill Road, Suite 380
Marietta, GA 30067   770-612-1030
                                                     800-232-7437
                                            Fax: 770-612-8277
                              e-mail: prevent@sids.org
                                                          sids.org/

Dedicated to the prevention of sudden infant death and the promotion of infant health through research, clinical services, education and family support.

Betty McEntire, Executive Director

3992 Canadian Foundation for the Study of Infant Deaths
586 Eglinton Ave E, Ste 308, Toronto
Ontario M4P 1P2,
Canada
                                    416-488-3864
                                    800-363-7437
                              Fax: 416-488-3864
            e-mail: sidscanada@inforamp.net
            http://www.sidscanada.org.sids.html

**3993 Clearinghouse National Sudden Infant Death
Syndrome**
2070 Chain Bridge Road, #3450
Vienna, VA 22182
                                    703-821-8955
                              Fax: 703-821-2098
                 e-mail: sids@circsol.com

A clearinghouse that supplies fact sheets, bibliographies, directories, booklets, Information Exchange, which is a national forum for sharing SIDS-related news, and a catalog listing its publications.

**3994 National Sudden Infant Death Syndrome Resource
Center**
8201 Greensboro Drive #600
McLean, VA 22102
                                    703-821-8955
                              Fax: 703-821-2098
            http://www.circsol.com/sids

3995 National Sudden Infant Death Syndrome Foundation
31 Center Dr, Rom 2A32
Bethesda, MD 20892
                                    301-496-5133
                              Fax: 301-496-7101

3996 SIDS Alliance
1314 Bedford Avenue, Suite 210
Baltimore, MD 21208
                                    410-653-8226
                                    800-221-7437
                              Fax: 410-653-8709
                 e-mail: sidsha@charm.net
                 www.sidsalliance.org

The SIDS Alliance operates a national referral program to respond to questions and concerns about SIDS. This organization can identify local resources available to SIDS families, interested health professionals, and the public.

3997 SIDS Educational Services, Inc.
2905 64th Avenue
Cheverly, MD 20785
                                    301-773-9671
                              Fax: 301-322-2620
                 e-mail: SIDSES@aol.com

State Agencies & Support Groups

Alabama

**3998 Bureau of Family Health Services Alabama
Department of Public Health**
434 Monroe Street
Montgomery, AL 36130   334-242-5766

Alaska

**3999 SIDS Information & Counseling Program Alaska
Department of Health**
1231 Gambell Street, Ste. 302
Anchorage, AK 99501   907-279-4711

Linda D. Vlastuin, RN, MPH, Program Consultant

Arizona

**4000 Office of Maternal & Child Health Arizona
Department of Health**
1740 West Adams St, Rm 200
Phoenix, AZ 85007   602-542-1875

Jane Pearson, RN, Chief

Arkansas

**4001 Arkansas Department of Health - SIDS Information
& Counseling Program**
4815 West Markham
Little Rock, AR 72205   501-661-2321

Deborah Frazier, RN, Project Coordinator

California

4002 California SIDS Program
P.O. Box 11447
Berkeley, CA 94701   510-849-4111
                             800-369-7437

Sally Jacober, MSW, MPH, Program Director

Colorado

4003 Colorado SIDS Program
6825 E Tennessee Ave
Denver, CO 80224   303-320-7771
     800-332-1018
     Fax: 303-322-8775

Sheila Marquez, RN, Executive Director

Connecticut

4004 SIDS Program Connecticut Department of Health
150 Washington Street
Hartford, CT 06106   860-566-3767

Jann Dalton, MSW

Delaware

4005 SIDS Information & Counseling - Division Of Public Health
501 Ogletown Road
Newark, DE 19711   302-368-6840

Elaine Markell, LCSW, BCD, Program Coordinator

District of Columbia

4006 Division of Community Health Nursing
1905 E. Street, SE
Washington, DC 20003   202-727-5122

Mary Breach, RN, MSN, Nursing Coordinator

Florida

4007 Children's Medical Services Program Florida SIDS Program
1317 Winewood Blvd.
Tallahassee, FL 32399   850-487-2690

Georgia

4008 Georgia Department of Human Resources Children's Health Services
2600 Skyland Drive
Atlanta, GA 30319   404-320-0547

Linette Jackson Hunt, MD, MPH, Chief

Hawaii

4009 Hawaii SIDS Information & Counseling Project
Kapiolani Children's Medical Center
1319 Punahou Street, 7th Fl
Honolulu, HI 96826   808-983-8368

Sharon Morton, RN, Nurse Consultant

Idaho

4010 Child Health Improvement Program Idaho Department of Health
450 West State Street
Boise, ID 83720   208-334-5957

Simonne deGlee, MS, PNP, SIDS Coordinator

Illinois

4011 Region V Office Program Consultants For Maternal and Child Health
105 W. Adams, 17th Floor
Chicago, IL 60603   312-353-1700

Kathryn Vedder, MD, MPH

Indiana

4012 Indiana State Board of Health - SIDS Project
1330 W Michigan St, Rm 232-W
Indianapolis, IN 46206   317-383-6585

Larry Humbert, Project Director

Iowa

4013 Iowa SIDS Program
Iowa Department of Public Health
Lucas State Office Bldg.
Des Moines, IA 50319   515-281-7767

Beverly Richardson, MA, MCH Consultant

Kansas

4014 Kansas Department of Health & Environment
Bureau of Family Health
900 SW Jackson, 10th Floor
Topeka, KS 66612   785-296-1300

Azzie N. Young, PhD, Director

Kentucky

4015 Kentucky Department of Human Resources Bureau
of Health Services
275 East Main Street
Frankfort, KY 40621   502-564-3236

Ida Lyons, RN, SIDS Coordinator

Louisiana

4016 Public Health Services of Louisiana
1772 Woodale Blvd.
Baton Rouge, LA 70806   504-925-7200

Jamie Roques, RNC, SIDS Coordinator

Maine

4017 Department of Human Services
151 Capitol Street
Augusta, ME 04333   207-289-3259

Kathleen Jewett, Program Coordinator

Maryland

4018 Maryland SIDS Information & Counseling Program
630 W Fayette St, Rm 5-684
Baltimore, MD 21201   410-328-5062

Daniel Timmel, MSW, Project Director

Massachusetts

4019 Massachusetts Center for SIDS
Boston Medical Center
One Boston Medical Center Place
Boston, MA 02118   617-414-7437
                         800-641-7437
                    Fax: 617-414-5555
         e-mail: mary.mcclain@bmc.org
         www.bmc.org/pedi/bostonchildhealth/

Mary McClain, RN, MS, Project Coordinator

Michigan

4020 Apnea Identification Program
Children's Hospital of Michigan
3901 Beaubien
Detroit, MI 48201   313-745-5437

Karen Braniff, RN, MSW, Nurse Specialist

Minnesota

4021 Minnesota Sudden Infant Death Center
Minneapolis Children's Medical Center
2525 Chicago Avenue, South
Minneapolis, MN 55404   612-863-6107

Kathleen Farnbach, PHN, Project Coordinator

Mississippi

4022 Mississippi State Department of Health and Child
Health Services
P.O. Box 1700
Jackson, MS 39215   601-960-7441

Geneva Cannon, Nurse Consultant

Missouri

4023 Region VII Office Program Consultants For
Maternal and Child Health
601 East 12th Street
Kansas City, MO 64106   816-426-2924

Bradley Appelbaum, MD, MPH

Montana

4024 Montana Department of Health & Environmental
Sciences
Family & Maternal & Child Health Bureau
Cogswell Building
Helena, MT 59620   406-444-4740

Maxine Ferguson, RN, MN, Bureau Chief

Nebraska

4025 Nebraska SIDS Foundation
University of Nebraska Medical Center
600 South 42nd Street
Omaha, NE 68198   402-935-1911
                e-mail: nesidsathome.com

Valerie Ciciulla, Coordinator

Nevada

4026 Nevada State Division of Health, Maternal & Child Health
505 E King Street, Room 205
Carson City, NV 89710   702-687-4885

Luana Ritch, Health Educator

New Hampshire

4027 New Hampshire SIDS Program
New Hampshire Division of Public Health Services
6 Hazen Drive
Concord, NH 03301   603-271-4477

Audrey Knight, MSN, CPNP, SIDS Coordinator

New Jersey

4028 New Jersey Department of Health - Child Health Program
CN 364, 363 W. State Street
Trenton, NJ 08625   609-292-5616

Judith Hall, BSN, RNC, Evaluator

New Mexico

4029 New Mexico SIDS Information & Counseling Program
University of New Mexico School of Medicine

Albuquerque, NM 87131   505-277-3053

Beverly White, RN, MS, Director

New York

4030 New York City Information & Counseling Program for SIDS
520 First Avenue, Room 506
New York, NY 10016   212-757-1051

Judith Gaines, CSW, PhD, SIDS Program Dir.

North Carolina

4031 North Carolina SIDS Information and Counseling Program
North Carolina Department of Environmental Health
P.O. Box 27687
Raleigh, NC 27611   919-553-6868

Dianne Tyson, BSW, Administrative Asst.

North Dakota

4032 North Dakota SIDS Management Program
600 East Boulevard Avenue
Bismarck, ND 58505   701-328-2227

Bertie Hagberg, RN, Coordinator

Ohio

4033 Perinatal and Infant Health Unit - SIDS Information and Counseling Program
Ohio Department of Health
246 North High Street
Columbus, OH 43266   614-466-4716

Ben Chukwumah, MD, MPH, Project Director

Oklahoma

4034 Oklahoma State Department of Health - Maternal and Child Health Services
1000 NE 10th Street
Oklahoma City, OK 73117   405-271-4200

Edd D. Rhoades, MD, MPH, Director

Oregon

4035 SIDS Resource of Oregon
4035 NE Sandy Blvd, Suite 209
Portland, OR 97212   503-287-8265
                            800-303-7437
                       Fax: 503-287-8693
        e-mail: sidsor@teleport.com
        www.teleport.com/~sidsor

Barbara Brunkow

Pennsylvania

4036 Pennsylvania SIDS Center
321 University Avenue
Philadelphia, PA 19104   215-222-1400
                                800-258-7434

Rosanne English, RN, Executive Director

Rhode Island

4037 Rhode Island Department of Health National SIDS Foundation
3 Capitol Hill
Providence, RI 02908   401-277-2312

Anne M. Roach, RN, SIDS Coordinator

South Carolina

4038 South Carolina Department of Health & Environmental Control - SIDS
2600 Bull Street
Columbia, SC 29201   803-252-9250

Brenda Creswell, ACSW, LMSW, SIDS Coordinator

South Dakota

4039 South Dakota Department of Health
118 West Capitol Street
Pierre, SD 57501   605-773-3737

Nancy Hoyme, SIDs Coordinator

Tennessee

4040 Tennessee SIDS Program
Division of Maternal & Child Health
525 Cordell Hull Bldg.
Nashville, TN 37247   615-741-7353

Judith Womack, RN, Dir. Of Child Health

Texas

4041 Harris County Health Department
2501 Dunstan, P.O. Box 25249
Houston, TX 77265   713-715-2800

Kathleen Ingrando, RN, BSN, Program Coordinator

Utah

4042 Utah Department of Health
Child Health Bureau
288 North 1460 West
Salt Lake City, UT 84116   801-538-6140

Karen Nash, RN, MS, PNP, SiDS Director

Vermont

4043 Vermont Department of Health - SIDS Information and Counseling Program
1193 North Avenue
Burlington, VT 05402   802-863-7333

Cindy Indham, RN, BSN, Director

Virginia

4044 Virginia SIDS Program - Virginia Department of Health
109 Governor Street
Richmond, VA 23219   804-786-3915

Arlethia V. Rogers, RN, Nurse Consultant

Washington

4045 Region X Office Program Consultants for Maternal and Child Health
2201 Sixth Avenue
Seattle, WA 98121   206-553-0215

Kay Girl, RNC, MN, Acting

West Virginia

4046 West Virginia Department of Health and Human Services
Division of Local Health
1411 Virginia Street East
Charleston, WV 25301   304-348-8870

Joan R. Kenny, RN, SIDS Director

Wisconsin

4047 Counseling and Research Center for SIDS
9000 W. Wisconsin Avenue
Milwaukee, WI 53201   414-266-2743

Kathy Geracie, BSW, Program Coordinator

Wyoming

4048 Wyoming Department of Health
Division of Health and Medical Services
Hathaway Building
Cheyenne, WY 82002   307-777-6186

J. Richard Hillman, MD, PhD, Administrator

Research Centers

4049 American SIDS Institute
2480 Windy Hill Road, Suite 380
Marietta, GA 30067   770-612-1030
                                     800-232-7437
                                Fax: 770-612-8277
                           e-mail: prevent@sids.org
                                          sids.org/

A non-profit organization for research into the causes and prevention of SIDS.

Betty McEntire, Executive Director

4050 Canadian Foundation for the Study of Infant Deaths
586 Eglinton Ave E. Ste 308
Toronto Ontario, M4P1   416-488-3260
                                     800-363-7437
                                Fax: 416-488-3864
                    e-mail: sidscanada@inforamp.net
                                www.sidscanada.org

4051 National Sudden Infant Death Syndrome Research Center
8201 Greensboro Drive #600
McLean, VA 22102   703-821-8955
                                Fax: 703-821-2098
                                     www.circsol.com

Provides information services and technical assistance concerning SIDS and related topics in order to promote understanding of SIDS and to comfort those affected by a SIDS loss. Offers its services to parents, family members, caregivers, counselors, medical and legal professionals, and the general public.

4052 USC - Neonatology Research Units
1240 Mission Road
Los Angeles, CA 90033   213-226-3408
                                Fax: 213-226-3440

Focuses on clinical problems of the newborn and premature infant.

Paul Y.K. Wu, MD, Director

Conferences

4053 National Sudden Infant Death Syndrome Alliance Conference

                                     800-221-7437

Unites parents, caregivers, and researchers with government, business, and community service groups in a nationwide movement to advance the support of SIDS families and hasten the elimination of SIDS through medical research. Funds medical research and offers emotional support nationally and locally.

Audio Video

4054 A Cradle Song: The Families of SIDS

Dennis Spalsbury, author

Fanlight Productions
47 Halifax St
Boston, MA 02131   617-469-4999
                                Fax: 617-469-3379
                          e-mail: fanlight@tiac.net
                                     www.fanlight.com

SIDS parents share the pain and anger which have dominated their lives, but they also offer hope to others coping with grief. Provides much-needed information about this mysterious illness.

29 minutes
ISBN: 1-572950-63-3

4055 SIDS: Reducing the Risk
InJoy Videos
1435 Yarmouth, Suite 102
Boulder, CO 80304

800-326-2082
Fax: 303-449-8788
www.injoyvideos.com

An informative video in which leading medical experts explain practical measures parents can take to reduce the risk of Sudden Infant Death Syndrome.

27 minutes

Web Sites

4056 American SIDS Institute
www.sids.org/

4057 SID Network
sids-network.org/net.htm

Books

4058 Apparent Life-Threatening Event and Sudden Infant Death Syndrome
National SIDS Resource Center
2070 Chain Bridge Road, Ste. 450
Vienna, VA 22182
703-821-8955
Fax: 703-821-2098

Provides information about ALTE and its relationship to SIDS.

1992 29 pages

4059 Crib Death: The Sudden Infant Death Syndrome

Warren G. Guntheroth, author

Futura Publishing Company, Inc.
135 Bedford Road
Armonk, NY 10504
914-273-1014
Fax: 914-273-1015

Discusses the theories of SIDS and their implications. Aimed at the medical professional, also provides peoples with a clearer understanding of SIDS.

Pamphlets

4060 After Sudden Infant Death Syndrome
National SIDS Resource Center
2070 Chain Bridge Road, Ste. 450
Vienna, VA 22182
703-821-8955
Fax: 703-821-2098

1993 16 pages

4061 SIDS Prevention
ETR Associates
P.O. Box 1830
Santa Cruz, CA 95061

800-321-4407
Fax: 800-435-8433
www.etr.org

Gives overview, risk factors, prevention of Sudden Infant Death Syndrome.

50 pamphlets

4062 SIDS: Toward Prevention and Improved Infant Health
American SIDS Institute
2480 Windy Hill Road, Suite 380
Marietta, GA 30067
770-612-1030
800-232-7437
Fax: 770-612-8277
e-mail: prevent@sids.org
www.sids.org

Practical guide for those planning a pregnancy, for parents-to-be and for new parents.

DESCRIPTION

4063 SUPERNUMERARY TEETH
Synonyms: Polydontia, Supplementary teeth
Disorder Type: Teeth
Covers these related disorders: Distomolar (retromolar), Mesiodens, Natal teeth, Paramolar, Peridens

Supernumerary teeth refers to the presence of one or more teeth in excess of the normal number that is, more than 20 primary (deciduous) teeth or 32 secondary (permanent) teeth. These teeth are usually abnormal in shape and size and may erupt through the gums or may remain impacted against another tooth, in the soft tissue of the gums, or in the jaw bone. In addition, a primary tooth or a secondary tooth is typically not present to replace the supernumerary tooth. In most affected infants, children, and adults, only one supernumerary tooth is present; however, instances of multiple supernumerary teeth have been reported.

The presence of supernumerary teeth may cause delayed eruption, abnormal positioning, or impaction of nearby teeth. Therefore, early diagnostic confirmation may be helpful in ensuring appropriate preventive measures. These measures include removal or extraction of the extra tooth or, in some cases, ongoing monitoring including regular clinical and dental x-ray examinations to assess the need for possible extraction.

In some cases, supernumerary teeth must be distinguished from prematurely erupted natal teeth. Natal teeth, which are teeth that are present at birth, may be supernumerary teeth or primary teeth that have erupted unusually early. Natal teeth usually have little bony support or root formation and are typically loose and mobile. The presence of natal teeth may cause pain and feeding difficulties in newborns as well as maternal discomfort during nursing. If natal teeth are determined to be supernumerary through examinations such as dental x-rays, they are often extracted; however, if they are primary teeth, attempts may be made to maintain them.

Most supernumerary teeth tend to develop between the central front teeth in the upper jaw (maxillary central incisors). Known as mesiodens, such teeth tend to be unusually small and have short roots and cone-shaped crowns. (The crown is the exposed portion of the tooth). Some supernumerary teeth are termed paramolars, which are usually abnormally small, incompletely formed teeth located between molars in the upper jaw.

Distomolars, also known as retromolars, develop in back of the third molars (wisdom teeth). Peridens are supernumerary teeth that erupt outside the dental arches, such as within the roof of the mouth (palate).

Supernumerary teeth may be the result of abnormalities during embryonic development of the membrane that forms part of the gums. The presence of supernumerary teeth may occur in association with certain conditions that are apparent at birth, such as cleft lip and palate, or may be an isolated finding. There have been reports of several affected individuals within certain families (kindreds) that suggest possible autosomal dominant inheritance. In addition, some researchers suspect that the development of supernumerary teeth may be caused by the interaction of several different genes (polygenic).

The following organizations in the General Resources Section can provide additional information: NIH/National Institute of Child Health and Human Development

National Associations & Support Groups

4064 American Dental Association
211 East Chicago Avenue
Chicago, IL 60611
312-440-2500
www.ada.org

Professional association of dentists dedicated to serving both the public and the profession of dentistry. Promotes the profession of dentistry by enhancing the integrity and ethics of the profession and strengthening the patient/dentist relationship. Fulfills its mission by providing services and through its initiatives in education, research, advocacy and the development of standards.

4065 National Institute of Dental Research
31 Cntr Dr.,Msc 2290,Bldg31,Rm2c35
Bethesda, MD 20892   301-496-4261
                              Fax: 301-496-9988
                              www.nidr.nih.gov/

Provides leadership for a national research program designed to understand, treat and prevent the infectious and inherited craniofacial-oral-dental diseases and disorders.

Web Sites

4066 American Academy of Pediatric Dentistry
www.aapd.org/

4067 American Association of Orthodontics
www.aaortho.org/

4068 Dental Consumer Advisory
www.toothinfo.com/

4069 Dental Resources on the Web
www.dental-resources.com/

4070 Straight Talk about Orthodontics
www.oao.on.ca/faq.htm

DESCRIPTION

4071 SYNDACTYLY

Synonyms: Syndactylia, Syndactylism
Disorder Type: Birth Defect, Genetic Disorder

Syndactyly refers to an abnormality that is present at birth (congenital) and characterized by the joining together (fusing) of two or more fingers or toes. This relatively common abnormality seems to occur more frequently in boys than in girls. It is often inherited as an autosomal dominant trait. Syndactyly often results from incomplete or abnormal embryonic development of the fingers or toes. In some infants, it occurs spontaneously as the hands or feet of the developing fetus may be unnaturally constricted within the uterus. Defects associated with syndactyly may range from a simple or incomplete joining or webbing of the skin between two digits to fusion from the base to the tip of the digits, complete with fusion of the bones and nails.

Syndactyly of the foot may involve complete or incomplete webbing that usually affects the second and third toes. This simple condition is referred to as zygosyndactyly and often requires no treatment. Syndactyly may also involve webbing and bone fusion (synostosis) of the fourth and fifth toes with duplication of the fifth toe in a condition called syndactyly/polysyndactyly. Treatment for polysyndactyly may include surgical intervention.

As in the foot, syndactyly of the hand may involve a simple webbing. However, in some cases, the fusion of certain fingers may be more complex and involve shared nerves and blood supply. Syndactyly of the fingers should be carefully evaluated to determine the best method of treatment, allowing for growth and dexterity of the fingers.

Syndactyly may also occur in association with several genetic disorders. Such disorders include acrocephalopolysyndactyly type II (Carpenter's syndrome), characterized by mental retardation and irregularities involving the head, hand, and genitalia; acrocephalosyndactyly type I (Apert's syndrome), characterized by craniofacial irregularities and syndactyly of the hands and feet; trisomy 18 syndrome, a chromosomal abnormality characterized by multiple craniofacial abnormalities, irregularities of the hands and feet, and severe mental retardation; and other inherited diseases. Treatment of syndactyly associated with these and other inherited disorders depends upon the nature of the underlying disorder.

The following organizations in the General Resources Section can provide additional information: National Organization for Rare Disorders, Inc., (NORD), Genetic Alliance, NIH/National Institute of Child Health and Human Development, NIH/National Institute of Arthritis and Musculoskeletal and Skin Diseases, Online Mendelian Inheritance in Man: www3.ncbi.nlm.nih.gov/Omim/searchomim.html

National Associations & Support Groups

4072 CHERUB—Association of Families and Friend of Children with Limb Disorders
936 Delaware Avenue
Buffalo, NY 14209

Answers the questions and problems that families of juveniles diagnosed with a disorder may be experiencing.

4073 Shriners Hospitals for Children
P.O. Box 31356
Tampa, FL 33613

813-281-0300
800-237-5055
Fax: 813-281-8496
www.shrinershq.org

Network of 22 hospitals that provide expert, no-cost orthopaedic and burn care to children under 18.

Web Sites

4074 CliniWeb
www.ohsu.edu/cliniwebC5/C5.660.585.html

4075 Eaton Hand Links
www.eatonhand.com/ccc/ccc26562.htm

DESCRIPTION

4076 SYSTEMIC LUPUS ERYTHEMATOSUS
Synonyms: Lupus, SLE
May involve these systems in the body (see Section III):
Connective Tissue

Systemic lupus erythematosus (SLE) is a chronic, inflammatory, multisystem disorder of connective tissue that may affect many organ systems in the body including the skin, joints, membranes that line the walls of certain bodily cavities (serosal membranes), or kidneys. In children with the disorder, associated symptoms are often progressive and, without appropriate treatment, may result in life-threatening complications. However, in some patients, symptoms may spontaneously subside and periodically recur with varying levels of severity (relapsing-remitting). SLE usually becomes apparent during late adolescence or during a patient's 20s or 30s. However, in up to 20 percent of patients, symptoms may begin during childhood, usually after the age of eight. Females are more commonly affected than males in all age groups.

The specific underlying cause of SLE is unknown. However, the disorder is thought to result from abnormalities in the regulating mechanisms of the immune system that normally prevent it from attacking the body's own cells and tissues. In addition, researchers speculate that certain microorganisms or other environmental factors may play some role in causing SLE. Familial cases have also been reported, suggesting potential genetic mechanisms. In some individuals, SLE-like symptoms may also occur after exposure to certain medications, such as particular antiseizure drugs or certain antibiotics known as sulfonamides. Drug-induced symptoms are usually relatively mild and subside when the responsible medication is removed.

The range and severity of associated symptoms and findings may vary. Although associated symptoms may begin suddenly or gradually, most children with SLE tend to have more acute, severe symptoms than adults. In some children, symptoms may tend to recur or worsen in association with certain infections. In addition, exposure to sunlight may worsen associated skin or other symptoms. Many children with SLE initially experience generalized symptoms, such as a fever, a general feeling of ill health (malaise), joint swelling and inflammation (arthritis) or pain (arthralgia), loss of appetite (anorexia), and weight loss. Most children also have associated skin abnormalities, including a scaly, reddish or bluish rash that is in a distinctive butterfly distribution across the cheeks and the bridge of the nose (butterfly rash). The affected area may be abnormally sensitive to sunlight (photosensitive), and the rash may gradually spread to other facial areas, the neck, scalp, chest, and arms. Additional skin symptoms may include flat, reddish, dot-like spots (punctate lesions) on the fingertips, palms, soles, arms, legs, and torso; abnormal changes of the tissues beneath the fingernails and toenails (nail beds); tender, reddish-purple swellings or nodules on the legs (erythema nodosum); and itchy, reddish, flat or raised lesions of the skin and mucous membranes (erythema multiforme). Patients may also develop painless sores of the mucous membranes of the mouth and nose. The hair may be abnormally coarse and dry, and some children may have patchy areas of baldness on the scalp (alopecia).

Many children with SLE may also experience joint stiffness; inflammation of muscles (myositis), causing muscle pain and weakness; abnormal changes and localized loss of bone in certain areas (aseptic necrosis), particularly the head of the thigh bone (femur); and Raynaud's phenomenon. This condition is characterized by sudden contraction of the relatively small blood vessels supplying the fingers and toes (digits), causing an interruption of blood flow to the digits and a subsequent excess of blood in affected areas following restoration of blood flow (reactive hyperemia). Such episodes are usually triggered by exposure to cold temperatures and are characterized by numbing, tingling, and bluish or whitish discoloration of the digits due to lack of blood flow and subsequent reddening and pain as blood flow is reestablished.

Many children with SLE may also develop inflammation of the membranes that line the lungs and chest cavity (pleurisy), surround the heart (pericarditis), and line the wall of the abdomen and cover the abdominal organs (peritonitis). Additional heart abnormalities may also be present, such as abnormal heart murmurs, inflammation of heart muscle (myocarditis), enlargement of the heart (cardiomegaly), a decreased ability of the heart to pump blood effectively to the lungs and the rest of the body (heart failure), and, in some severe cases, heart attacks (myocardial infarctions), potentially causing life-threatening complications.

Kidney involvement is common among children with SLE and may be the only disease manifestation. Associated inflammation of the filtering units of the kidneys (glomerulonephritis) may be mild, moderate, or severe. Symptoms and findings may range from small amounts of blood in the urine (hematuria) of mildly increased levels of protein in the urine (proteinuria) to kidney failure that causes potentially life-threatening complications. Some children with SLE may also experience symptoms due to involvement of the brain and spinal cord (central nervous system). Associated neurologic abnormalities may include personality changes, episodes of abnormally increased electrical activity in the brain (seizures), or other findings. In addition, in some children, disease progression may also affect other tissues and organs, causing additional symptoms and findings.

The treatment of SLE is individualized and based upon the severity of the disease and the specific organ systems affected. Episodes of active disease should be considered emergencies that require immediate evaluation and aggressive treatment to help prevent damage to affected tissues and organs. In addition, careful follow-up and ongoing monitoring is required to detect worsening disease and to ensure prompt, appropriate treatment as required. Therapy may include the use of nonsteroidal antiinflammatory medications to help alleviate joint pain and antimalarial agents or topical corticosteroid creams to treat skin symptoms. In severe cases, immunosuppressive drugs may also be administered; however, such agents must be used with great caution in children. Treatment of kidney inflammation may also include the use of certain corticosteroids, such as prednisone, and in some patients, the addition of immunosuppressive agents, such as azathioprine. Children with severe kidney disease may require regular dialysis or kidney transplantation. Dialysis is a medical procedure that removes excess fluid from the body and waste products from the blood. Additional treatment is symptomatic and supportive.

The following organizations in the General Resources Section can provide additional information: National Organization for Rare Disorders, Inc., (NORD), NIH/Office of Rare Diseases, March of Dimes Birth Defects Foundation, American Juvenile Arthritis Organization, NIH/National Child Health and Human Development, Genetic Alliance, American Autoimmune Related Diseaes Association, Inc., NIH/National Institute of Neurological Disorders & Stroke

National Associations & Support Groups

4077 European Lupus Erythematosus Federation
1 Eastern Road, Romford
Essex Intl,
United Kingdom

e-mail: elef@rheumanet.org
www.elef.rheumanet.org/

4078 Lupus Canada
PO Box 64034
Calgary, Alberta, T2K
Canada

430-274-5599
800-661-1468
Fax: 403-274-5599
e-mail: lupuscan@cadvision.com
www.lupuscanada.org

4079 Lupus Foundation of America, Inc.
1300 Piccard Drive Suite 200
Rockville, MD 20850

301-670-9292
800-558-0121
Fax: 301-670-9486
www.lupus.org/lupus

The LFA mission is to educate and support those affected by lupus. It supports research into the cause and cure of lupus. Information resources are available on request including free pamphlets, brochures (English/Spanish), and articles for people seeking an understanding of lupus. Seeral books and materials on lupus are also available through the LFA.

4080 Lupus Network
230 Ranch Drive
Bridgeport, CT 06606   203-372-5795

Seeks to foster better understanding of the disease among patients and the general public, educators and professionals through the distribution of educational materials.

Linda Rosinsky, President

4081 Lupus UK
1 Eastern Road, Romford
Essex Intl,
United Kingdom
          e-mail: strathclyde.lupus-uk@usa.net
          www.geocities.com/HotSprings/2911/

Research Centers

4082 Hahnemann University Lupus Study Center
221 N. Broad Street
Philadelphia, PA 19107   215-854-8100

Raphael J. DeHoratius, Director

4083 SLE Foundation, Inc.
149 Madison Avenue
New York, NY 10016   212-685-4118
          Fax: 212-545-1843

Purpose is to raise funds for research grants, provide information and services to lupus patients, and educate the public about lupus. Patient services include self-help groups, orientation meetings, referrals, publications, and counseling on personal and financial problems related to the disease.

4084 Terri Gotthelf Lupus Research Institute
3 Duke Place
South Norwalk, CT 06854   203-852-0120
          Fax: 203-852-9720

Founded to help millions of lupus victims in the world and to encourage, coordinate and direct future progress in the etiology, diagnosis and treatment of this disease.

Theodore Gotthelf, President

Books

4085 Coping with Lupus
Robert H. Phillips, PhD, author

Lupus Foundation of America
1300 Piccard Drive Suite 200
Rockville, MD 20850   301-670-9292
          800-558-0121
          www.lupus.org

A practicing psychologist offers sound, meaningful and compassionate advice to individuals who mlust deal with lupus.

4086 Disability Workbook for Social Security Disability Applicats
Douglas Smith, author

Lupus Foundation of America
1300 Piccard Drive Suite 200
Rockville, MD 20850   301-670-9292
          800-558-0121
          www.lupus.org

Helps people get their disability benefits promptly, without unnecessary appeals. Tells what you have to prove and how to prove it.

4087 Get to Sleep! How To Sleepwell...Despite Lupus
Robert H. Phillips, author

Lupus Foundation of America
1300 Piccard Drive Suite 200
Rockville, MD 20850   301-670-9292
          800-558-0121
          www.lupus.org

Written in a simple, straightforward style, this easy-to-follow action guide teaches you the most effective strategies for enabling you to get the steep you want and need.

ISBN: 0-895294-75-3

4088 Lupus Book
Daniel J. Wallace, M.D., author

Lupus Foundation of America
1300 Piccard Drive Suite 200
Rockville, MD 20850   301-670-9292
          800-558-0121
          www.lupus.org

Packed with usful, easy-to-understand information and practical guidance for people with lupus, their family members, friends and physicians. This hardcover book explains virtually every aspect of the disease and will help people better manage their day-to-day fight with lupus

ISBN: 0-195084-43-8

4089 Lupus Erythematosus: A Handbook for Physicians, Patients & Families

Ronald Carr, MD, author

Lupus Foundation of America, Inc.
1300 Piccard Drive, Suite 200
Rockville, MD 20850   301-670-9292
                              800-558-0121
                              www.lupus.com

Written for physicians, people with lupus, their families and friends, this is LFA's most popular publication. The handbook provides a brief, but detailed, overview of the disease and guide for living well with lupus.

27 pages

4090 Lupus: Everything You Need To Know

Robert G. Lahita, MD, author

Lupus Foundation of America, Inc.
1300 Piccard Drive, Suite 200
Rockville, MD 20850   301-670-9292
                              800-558-0121
                              www.lupus.com

Resource written for patients that want to learn more about lupus than what their doctors may of may not tell them.

27 pages

4091 Sick and Tired of Feeling Sick and Tired

Paul J. Donoghue, author

Lupus Foundation of America
1300 Piccard Drive Suite 200
Rockville, MD 20850   301-670-9292
                              800-558-0121
                              www.lupus.org

Written in simple terms, the authors offer all readers - people with invisible chronic illness (ICI's), spouses, friends, family memebers, employers or health care providers, both understanding and practical guidance. This is a very useful resource for all those who live with ICI's and those who care for and about them.

288 pages

Children's Books

4092 Embracing the Wolf: A Lupus Victim and Her Family Learn to Live

Joanna Baumer Permut, author

Cherokee Publishing Company
PO Box 1730
Marietta, GA 30061   770-438-7366
                              800-653-3952

This book gives a very detailed accout of the effects of the disease that include emotions and moods for the victim and the way in which these attributes affect loved ones.

192 pages
ISBN: 0-877971-66-8

Kenneth W. Boyd, Publisher

4093 In Search of the Sun: A Woman's Courageous Victory Over Lupus

Scribner
866 3rd Ave
New York, NY 10022   212-702-2000
                              800-257-5755

This book is a revision of Henrietta Aladjem's book, The Sun Is My Enemy. In this bvook, with Peter Schur she discusses her fight with this deadly and widspread disease.

4094 When Mom Gets Sick

Rebecca Samuels, author

Lupus Foundation of America, Inc.
1300 Piccard Drive, Suite 200
Rockville, MD 20850   301-670-9292
                              800-558-0121
                              www.lupus.com

Written and illustrated by a 9-year-old, this is a compelling story based on the experiences of a sensitive and insightful yough girl who makes the best from what could be a devastating situation.

27 pages

DESCRIPTION

4095 TAY-SACHS DISEASE

Synonyms: GM2 gangliosidosis, type I, Hexa deficiency, Hexosaminidase A deficiency, Tay-Sachs disease, infantile type, TSD
Disorder Type: Genetic Disorder, Metabolism
Covers these related disorders: Tay-Sachs disease, juvenile type (GM2 gangliosidosis, type III)

Tay-Sachs disease, also known as GM2 gangliosidosis type I or infantile type, is a progressive degenerative metabolic disorder that occurs when two copies of the disease gene are inherited from the parents (autosomal recessive trait). The disorder, which belongs to a group of diseases known as lysosomal storage disorders, results from deficiency of the enzyme hexosaminidase A. Enzymes within lysosomes, which are the major digestive units of cells, break down particles of nutrients such as certain fats and carbohydrates. In individuals with Tay-Sachs disease, deficiency of the enzyme hexosaminidase A causes an abnormal accumulation of particular fats (i.e., gangliosides) in certain tissues of the body, particularly nerve cells of the brain. Tay-Sachs disease affects approximately one in 3,500 to 4,000 newborns. The disease occurs predominantly in people of Ashkenazi Jewish (i.e., northeastern European Jewish) descent. About one in 30 individuals of Ashkenazi Jewish ancestry carries a single copy of the disease gene (heterozygous carrier).

Infants with Tay-Sachs disease appear to develop as expected until approximately four to six months of age, except for a marked startle reaction to sudden noises (hyperacusis) that may be apparent soon after birth. From four to six months of age, affected infants may begin to have decreased focusing and eye contact and appear listless and irritable. As the disease progresses, infants have delays in the acquisition of skills requiing the coordination of mental and physical activities (psychomotor delays) and lose previously acquired skills. By about one year of age, most affected children lose the ability to roll over, sit, stand, or vocalize sounds. In addition, muscle tone is severely diminished (hypotonia). With continuing disease progression, children experience increasing muscle rigidity and associated restrictions of movement (spasticity); uncontrolled electrical disturbances in the brain (seizures) that may be accompanied by prolonged contractions and relaxations of certain muscles (tonic-clonic convulsions); development of abnormal red circular areas of the middle layer of the eyes (cherry-red spots or Tay's sign); blindness; deafness; and loss of cognitive abilities (dementia). In many affected children, there is also enlargement of the brain (metabolic megalencephaly) due to abnormal accumulation of gangliosides in brain cells. Life-threatening complications often develop by approximately two to four years of age.

There are also variants of Tay-Sachs disease in which the onset of symptoms occurs later in life. For example, in children with the variant known as Tay-Sachs disease, juvenile type (GM2 gangliosidosis, type III), symptoms typically become apparent during mid-childhood although they may sometimes develop as early as the second year of life. This disease variant, which is characterized by varying levels of hexosaminidase deficiency, is also inherited as an autosomal recessive trait. Associated symptoms may include progressive impairment of voluntary movements (ataxia); involuntary movements characterized by rapid, jerking or slow, repetitive, writhing movements (choreoathetosis); loss of speech; seizures; and visual loss. Patients may experience life-threatening complications by approximately 15 years of age.

The disease gene responsible for Tay-Sachs disease is located on the long arm of chromosome 15 (15q23-24). Several distinct changes (mutations) in this disease gene have been identified in individuals with Tay-Sachs disease. In addition, different mutations are responsible for the infantile and juvenile forms of the disorder. Tests have been developed to help confirm carrier status in individuals who may carry a single copy of the disease gene (e.g., serum or leukocyte hexosaminidase A testing). In addition, genetic counseling is provided for those individuals who are heterozygous carriers and desire to start a family or have additional children. Specialized testing is also available that may confirm a diagnosis of Tay-Sachs disease before birth (e.g., chorionic villus sampling). The treatment of infants and children with Tay-Sachs disease includes symptomatic and supportive measures.ampling). The treatment of infants and children with Tay-Sachs disease includes symptomatic and supportive measures.

The following organizations in the General Resources Section can provide additional information: NIH/Office of Rare Diseases, National Organization for Rare Disorders, Inc., (NORD), Genetic Alliance, Online Mendelian Inheritance in Man:

www3.ncbi.nlm.nih.gov/Omim/searchomim.html, NIH/National Institue of Child Health and Human Development, NIH/National Institute of Neurological Disorders & Stroke

National Associations & Support Groups

4096 Association for Neuro-Metabolic Disorders
5223 Brookfield Lane
Sylvania, OH 43506   419-885-1497

4097 Home Care of Children with Progressive Neurological Diseases
2001 Beacon Stret,Suite 204
Brookline, MA 02146   617-277-4463

The National Tay-Sachs and Allied Diseases Association can provide a publication, The Home Care Book, and offers home care support.

4098 National Foundation for Jewish Genetic Diseases
250 Park Ave, Ste 1000
New York, NY 10017   212-371-1030

Provides the information regarding this and related disorders for the people suffering from them.

4099 National Tay-Sachs and Allied Diseases Association, Inc.
2001 Beacon Street, Suite 204
Brighton, MA 02135   617-277-4463
                                      Fax: 617-277-0134
e-mail: ntsad_boston@worldnet.att.net
                                      www.ntsad.org

Tay-Sachs is a degenerative disease occuring in infants, children, and adults. This organization sponsors massive screening programs to detect the disease. It provides educational materials on this disorder and parent support groups.

International

4100 Tay-Sachs and Allied Diseases Association
17 Sydney Rd
Barkingside, Ilford Essex,
United Kingdom

Research Centers

4101 Research Trust for Metabolic Diseases in Children
Golden Gate Lodge
Weston Rd
Crewe, Cheshire CW1 1XN,
United Kingdom

Web Sites

4102 Healthfinder.com
www.healthfinder.gov/text/docs/Doc0793.htm

4103 Kansas University Medical Center
www.kumc.edu/gec/support/tay-sach.html

4104 National Institute of Neurological Disorders & Stroke
www.ninds.nih.gov

4105 National Tay-Sachs and Allied Disease Foundation (Delaware Valley)
www.tay-sachs.org/

DESCRIPTION

4106 TEETH GRINDING

Synonyms: Bruxism, Bruxomania
Disorder Type: Mental, Emotional or Behavioral Disorder

Teeth grinding or bruxism refers to compulsive, involuntary, rhythmic, and nonfunctional grinding, clenching, or gnashing of the teeth. This habitual grinding is most evident during sleep; however, affected individuals may unconsciously grind their teeth during the daytime as well. Daytime teeth grinding is known as bruxomania. In some individuals, teeth grinding may be considered a habit or a habit disorder, depending upon the degree of severity and its impact upon daily functioning. The prevalance of bruxism is not known.

Children and adults may grind, clench, or gnash their teeth in an unconscious attempt to release tension. Bruxism most often results from unresolved or unexpressed anger, aggression, fear, frustration, resentment, or other negative emotions. Teeth grinding that occurs during sleep exerts more force than that of normal, daytime chewing or grinding. For this reason, bruxism may cause muscle pain or tightness in the jaw area as well as irregularities in the surface contact between the upper and lower teeth (dental occlusion). In addition, bruxism may wear down or loosen the teeth.

Treatment for teeth grinding is directed toward teaching children effective methods of expressing anger or other negative feelings, thus relieving tension. Such supportive treatment may include the setting aside of quiet time before bedtime, during which children are encouraged to talk about the day's events, including anything that may have precipitated fear, anger, etc. Reading at bedtime may also have a calming effect on these children. In addition, emotional support that offers positive reinforcement and encouragement may be beneficial. Other treatment is symptomatic. A dental appliance such as a biteplate may be worn at night to help reduce associated dental injury.

National Associations & Support Groups

4107 American Dental Association
211 East Chicago Avenue
Chicago, IL 60611   312-440-2500
                                      www.ada.org

Professional association of dentists dedicated to serving both the public and the profession of dentistry. Promotes the profession of dentistry by enhancing the integrity and ethics of the profession and strengthening the patient/dentist relationship. Fulfills its mission by providing services and through its initiatives in education, research, advocacy and the development of standards.

4108 National Institute of Dental Research
31 Cntr Dr.,Msc 2290,Bldg31,Rm2c35
Bethesda, MD 20892   301-496-4261
                                      Fax: 301-496-9988
                                      nidr.nih.gov/

Provides leadership for a national research program designed to understand, treat and prevent the infectious and inherited craniofacial-oral-dental diseases and disorders.

Web Sites

4109 International Association for Dental Research
www.iadr.com/

DESCRIPTION

4110 TELANGIECTASIA

Synonym: Telangiectasis

May involve these systems in the body (see Section III):

Dermatologic System

Telangiectasia refers to the permanent widening or dilation of small blood vessels near the surface of the skin (superficial capillaries, arterioles, and venules). This results in the appearance of relatively small, red, well-defined skin lesions that have fine or coarse red lines or a spider-like network of red lesions that radiate from a central point (spider telangiectasia). Telangiectasias may develop as the result of an underlying disorder such as lupus erythematosus, dermatomyositis, rosacea, or psoriasis. These skin lesions may also result from exposure to sunlight, x-rays, or other forms of radiation.

Ataxia-telangiectasia (AT) is a rare, inherited, progressive disorder of the nervous system involving degenerative changes in the central nervous system along with defects in the immune system. AT is transmitted as an autosomal recessive trait and is characterized by the appearance during early childhood of telangiectasias involving the ears, face, the membranes that line the white outer coat of the eyes (bulbar conjunctiva), or other areas. Affected children are at risk for recurrent respiratory infections. Degeneration of the cerebellum, which is the part of the brain responsible for the regulation and coordination of voluntary movement and other vital functions, also occurs as children with AT age.

Congenital generalized phlebectasia, sometimes called cutis marmorata telangiectatica congenita, is a benign telangiectasia that is apparent at birth and is characterized by red or purple-hued net-like lesions that may have a somewhat marbled appearance. These telangiectasias may be localized to an arm or leg or the trunk of the body; however, sometimes these skin lesions are more widely spread. In addition, the lesions may be-

come more prominent with changes in outside temperature, crying, or exertion. This condition often resolves spontaneously by adolescence. Treatment is supportive.

Generalized essential telangiectasia is a rare condition that may affect children or adults and is characterized by the appearance of solitary or convergent patches of network-like telangiectasias. These lesions may appear on large but localized areas of the body such as the arms or legs or may sometimes involve or progress to the entire body. This disorder is limited to the skin with no health-associated irregularities. Treatment is supportive.

Hereditary benign telangiectasia is a rare, genetic disorder that is inherited as an autosomal dominant trait and is characterized by the appearance of telangiectasias on the skin of the face, arms, and upper portion of the trunk. This progressive disorder is limited to the skin.

Hereditary hemorrhagic telangiectasia, also called Rendu-Osler-Weber disease, is an inherited disorder that is transmitted as an autosomal dominant trait and is characterized by recurrent nosebleeds and the development of small telangiectasias of the skin and mucous membranes. These lesions range in color from red to purple and most often appear on the face, lips, and the membranes of the nose and mouth. In addition, the gastrointestinal tract, genitourinary tract, liver, brain, lungs, throat, voice box (larynx), and the membrane that lines the eyelids and whites of the eyes (conjunctiva) may be involved. Because the affected blood vessels may be fragile, they often break resulting in bleeding or hemorrhage from the gastrointestinal and genitourinary tracts, lungs, mouth, and nose.

Spider angioma, sometimes called spider nevus, is a telangiectasia characterized by the central, elevated, red lesion that is surrounded by a radiating, spider-like network of small blood vessels. Although these types of telangiectasias are often associated with conditions in which levels of circulating estrogen are elevated (e.g., pregnancy and liver disease), spider angiomas may also occur in preschool and school-age children. These lesions usually appear on the face, ears, forearms, and hands and often resolve on their own. Treatment is directed toward the removal of persistent angiomas and may include various methods such as freezing with liquid nitrogen (cryotherapy), the use of electric current to promote coagulation (electrocoagulation), or certain laser techniques.

Unilateral nevoid telangiectasia refers to the appearance of telangiectasias on one side of the body in conjunction with an increase in the levels of circulating estrogen. These lesions sometimes develop in adolescet girls when they begin menstruation. Pregnancy and liver disease may also prompt their development. If this condition results from pregnancy, the lesions often fade or resolve during the postpartum period.

The following organizations in the General Resources Section can provide additional information: NIH/National Institute of Arthritis and Musculoskeletal and Skin Diseases, Online Mendelian Inheritance in Man: www3.ncbi.nlm.nih.gov/Omim/searchomim.html

National Associations & Support Groups

4111 American Academy of Dermatology
930 North Meacham Road, P.O.Box4014
Schaumburg, IL 60168   708-330-0230
www.aad.org

Largest, most influential and most representative of all dermatologic associations. Committed to the highest quality standards in continuing medical education. Developed a platform in which to promote and advance the science and art of medicine and surgery related to the skin; promote the highest possible standards in clinical practice, education and research in dermatology and related disciplines; and support and enhance patient care and promote the public interest relating to dermatology.

4112 American Skin Association
150 East 58th Street, 33rd Floor
New York, NY 10155   212-753-8260
800-499-7546
Fax: 212-688-6547
e-mail: AmericanSkin@compuserve.com

4113 Ataxia-Telangiectasia Children's Project
1 West Camino Real, Suite 212
Boca Raton, FL 33432   561-395-2621
800-543-5728
Fax: 561-395-2640
e-mail: bradmargus@delphi.com
www.atcp.org

The purpose of the Project is to raise funds to accelerate scientific research aimed at finding a cure or a therapy that would improve the lives of children affected by Ataxia-Telangiectasia. The Project's activities also include the establishment and maintenance of a cell-bank for unlimited access by research scientists.

4114 Hereditary Hemorrhagic Telangiectasia (HHT) Foundation Internation, Inc.
P.O. Box 8087
New Haven, CT 06530   914-887-5844
800-448-6389
Fax: 914-887-5844
e-mail: hhtinfo@hht.org
www.htt.org

Dedicated to increasing public and professional awareness and understanding of Hereditary Hemorrhagic Telangiectasia (HHT). Supports ongoing medical research into the cause, prevention, and treatment of HHT; and offers a variety of materials including informational brochures and a quarterly newsletter.

DESCRIPTION

4115 TETANUS

Disorder Type: Infectious Disease
Covers these related disorders: Generalized tetanus, Localized tetanus, Neonatal tetanus

Tetanus is an infectious disease of the central nervous system caused by a poison (toxin) produced by the bacterium Clostridium tetani (tetanospasmin). Once the bacterium enters the body through wound sites, dead tissue that is low in oxygen within such wounds enables the bacterium's spores to multiply and produce the toxin tetanospasmin. The toxin then acts on nerves that control muscle activity, causing the symptoms associated with tetanus. Clostridium tetani is a common bacterium that resides in soil and in the intestinal tracts of certain mammals, such as cows and horses.

Although tetanus occurs worldwide, its frequency varies widely in different countries. The disease primarily occurs in certain developing countries in Asia and Africa. Approximately 50 to 100 cases of tetanus occur in the United States each year, primarily in people over age 60; however, some newborns and infants are also affected.

The C. tetani bacterium typically enters puncture wounds caused by dirty objects, such as nails, wood splinters, of fragments of glass. The bacterium may also enter the body via drug injection sites, surgical wounds, burns, animal bites, or the fetal umbilical cord stump after birth (neonatal tetanus). Although associated symptoms usually become apparent approximately two to 14 days after initial infection, some patients may not experience symptoms for several months.

Tetanus is often classified into two major categories: generalized and localized tetanus. Initial symptoms associated with generalized tetanus often include prolonged spasms of muscles of the jaw (trismus or lockjaw); associated difficulties keeping the mouth open, chewing, and swallowing (dysphagia); irritability; headaches; and restlessness. Patients may also experience prolonged spasms of facial muscles, causing a fixed, grinning expression (risus sardonicus); profuse sweating; a mild fever; and a rapid pulse. As the disease progresses, patients may have repeated episodes of sudden, severe, prolonged muscle contractions (tetanic seizures), causing clenching of the fists, inward bending of the arms (adduction), and overextension (hyperextension) of the legs. These episodes may initially range from seconds to minutes and eventually become more sustained. Prolonged contractions of abdominal, hip, thigh, and lower back muscles may result in a characteristic arched posture in which the heels and the head are bent backward (opisthotonos). If spasms affect muscles of the voice box (larynx) or the chest wall, airway obstruction and an inability to breathe (asphyxiation) may result, potentially causing life-threatening complications. In individuals with generalized tetanus, associated muscle spasms typically stabilize approximately two weeks after onset and eventually subside over the following one to four weeks.

As mentioned above, newborns may develop a severe form of tetanus due to unsterile conditions that result in infection of the umbilical stump after birth. Known as neonatal tetanus, this form of the disease occurs in newborns whose mothers have not been vaccinated against tetanus. Infants with this generalized form of tetanus typically develop symptoms within three to 12 days after birth. These symptoms include feeding problems, stiffness to the touch, diminished movements or paralysis, muscle spasms, a characteristic arched posture in which the heels and the head are bent backward (opisthotonos), and potentially life-threatening complications.

Localized tetanus is considered less common than generalized tetanus. In mild cases, localized tetanus is characterized by muscle contractions, spasms, and twitching near the wound site. However, in some patients, localized tetanus may progress to generalized tetanus.

The treatment of tetanus includes administration of human antibodies against tetanus toxins (tetanus immune globulin) and antibiotic medications; immediate surgical cleaning of and removal of foreign material and infected, dead, or damaged tissue from the wound site to expose healthy tissue (debridement); and the use of muscle relaxants. In severe cases, supportive measures may include insertion of a tube into the windpipe to assist breathing (tracheostomy) or maintenance of breathing through use of a ventilator. Combined immunization with DPT (diphtheria, pertussis, tetanus) vaccine is routinely provided in the United States during childhood to prevent tetanus. Booster shots are required every five to 10 years. A booster shot should also be provided to patients with any wound if they have an incomplete or unknown tetanus booster status.

The following organizations in the General Resources Section can provide additional information: National Organization for Rare Disorders, Inc., (NORD), March of Dimes Birth Defects Foundation, NIH/National Institute of Allergy and Infectious Disease

Web Sites

4116 Centers for Disease Control
www.babybag.com/articles/cdc tetn.htm

4117 New York State Department of Health
www.medhelp.org/lib/tetanus.htm

4118 Parent Zone
www.parentzone.com/health/tetanus.htm

4119 World Health Organization
www.paho.org/english/svi/svi-vptt.htm

DESCRIPTION

4120 TETRALOGY OF FALLOT
Synonym: Fallot's syndrome
Disorder Type: Birth Defect, Heart

Tetralogy of Fallot is a combination of four specific heart malformations that are present at birth (congenital heart defects). Normally, oxygen-poor blood that has circulated throughout the body enters the right upper chamber of the heart (right atrium), is pumped into the right lower chamber (right ventricle), and is then pumped into the pulmonary artery and on to the lungs, where the exchange of oxygen and carbon dioxide occurs. Oxygen-rich blood returns to the heart via the left atrium, is pumped into the left ventricle, and is subsequently pumped into the major artery of the body (aorta) for circulation to the body's tissues. However, newborns with tetralogy of Fallot typically have four coexisting cardiac defects: i.e., (1) obstruction of the normal outflow of blood from the right ventricle due to abnormal narrowing (stenosis) of the opening between the right ventricle and the pulmonary artery (pulmonary stenosis); (2) an abnormal opening in the partition (septum) that separates the ventricles of the heart (ventricular septal defect or VSD); (3) displacement or override of the aorta, allowing oxygen-poor blood to flow directly from the right ventricle into the aorta; and (4) abnormal thickness of the right ventricle (right ventricular hypertrophy). Tetralogy of Fallot is thought to affect approximately one in 1,000 infants and children.

In patients with tetralogy of Fallot, the onset and severity of associated symptoms depend, in part, upon the degree of right ventricular outflow obstruction. Primary symptoms and findings in mild cases may be only a murmur. In other cases, there may be a bluish discoloration of the skin and mucous membranes (cyanosis) due to decreased levels of oxygen in the blood; an insufficient supply of oxygen to bodily cells (hypoxia); and difficulties feeding. In infants with tetralogy of Fallot, cyanosis is typically most apparent in the nail beds of the fingers and toes and in the mucous membranes of the mouth and lips. In severe cases, cyanosis may be apparent soon after birth. In such newborns, pulmonary blood flow may primarily depend upon the fetal vascular channel that joins the pulmonary artery and the aorta (ductus arteriosus). Because this fetal vascular channel closes shortly after birth, severe cyanosis may develop within the first hours or days after birth. In other patients, cyanosis may not become apparent until later during the first year of life. In addition, affected infants and toddlers may experience difficult or labored breathing (dyspnea) upon exertion. Infants and toddlers may lie down or sit after short periods of playing, whereas older children may assume a characteristic squatting position to obtain relief.

Some affected infants and children experience periodic attacks or spells during which cyanosis worsens (hypoxic or blue spells). Such spells appear to be most prevalent during the first two years of life. Patients may become restless; develop extreme shortnessh deep, rapid, gasping respirations; and potentially lose consciousness (syncope). Although the onset of these attacks is unpredictable, they may tend to occur after severe crying episodes or upon awakening. The duration of the spells may range from a few minutes to a few hours, and they should be considered life-threatening and an indication for surgical repair.

Tetralogy of Fallot may be diagnosed based upon a complete clinical examination and patient history, detection of distinctive heart murmurs, and various specialized tests (e.g., x-ray studies, echocardiogram, electrocardiogram, cardiac catheterization). In infants and children who experience hypoxic spells, treatment measures may include placing the affected child on the abdomen in a knee-chest position after removing any constrictive clothing; administering oxygen; administering morphine; providing intravenous fluids or medications; or taking other additional measures. Surgery is usually performed in the first year of life depending upon the severity of right ventricular outflow obstruction. In some cases, a procedure may initially be performed during which a temporary artificial duct is created between the pulmonary artery and the aorta to divert some blood pumped into the aorta toward the lungs (palliative systemic-to-pulmonary artery shunt). Corrective open-heart surgery is then performed later in the first year to patch the ventricular septal defect, widen the opening between the pulmonary artery and right ventricle, and close any artificial connection between the pulmonary artery and the right ventricle. In many cases, corrective open-heart surgery may be recommended during the neonatal or infant period as opposed to an initial palliative shunt and later surgical correction. Before and after palliative or corrective open-heart surgery, patients may be susceptible to bacterial infection of certain areas of the heart (e.g., bacterial endocarditis). Therefore, patients should be provided with antibiotic medication (antibiotic prophylaxis) with dental visits and certain surgical procedures. Additional treatment is symptomatic and supportive.

Tetralogy of Fallot may occur as an isolated condition, with other congenital heart defects, or in some cases, in association with certain chromosomal abnormalities (e.g., DiGeorge syndrome). Researchers indicate that, in some patients, tetralogy of Fallot may be due to the interaction of one or more genes v(zzq11) and possibly in association with certain environmental factors (multifactorial inheritance).

The following organizations in the General Resources Section can provide additional information: Genetic Alliance, March of Dimes Birth Defects Foundation, NIH/National Heart, Lung & Blood Institute, National Organization for Rare Disorders, Inc., (NORD), NIH/National Institute of Child Health and Human Development

National Associations & Support Groups

4121 American Heart Association
7272 Greenville Avenue
Dallas, TX 75231   214-373-6300
                                    800-242-8721
                                Fax: 214-706-1341
                        e-mail: inquire@amhrt.org
                                www.amhrt.org

Supports research, education and community service programs with the objective of reducing premature death and disability from cardiovascular diseases and stroke; coordinates the efforts of health professionals, and other engaged in the fight against heart and circulatory disease.

Web Sites

4122 Children's Health Information Network
www.ohsu.edu.cliniweb/c14/c14.240.400.html

4123 CliniWeb: Congenital Heart Defects
www.ohsu.edu/cliniweb/c14/c14.240.400.html

4124 Congenital Heart Disease Resource Page
www.csun.edu/~hcmth011/heart/
                    e-mail: sheri.berger@csun.edu
                    www.csun.edu/~hcmth011/heart/

4125 Southern Illinois University School of Medicine
www.siumed.edu/peds/teaching/patient%20education.htm

DESCRIPTION

4126 THALASSEMIAS

Disorder Type: Genetic Disorder
Covers these related disorders: Alpha-thalassemia,
Beta-thalassemia, Beta-thalassemia minor,
Beta-thalassemia major
May involve these systems in the body (see Section III):
Blood (Hematologic)

The term thalassemia refers to a group of inherited blood disorders that includes the alpha-thalassemias and the more common beta-thalassemias. The thalassemias are characterized by the faulty production of hemoglobin, the protein that carries oxygen within the red blood cells. Hemoglobin is composed of two pairs of amino acid chains (globins), the alpha chains and the beta chains. The improper synthesis of hemoglobin is caused by a defect within the globin genes and results in abnormal, fragile red blood cells. Beta-thalassemia minor, a less severe form of the disease, is inherited when the defective gene is transmitted by one parent, while beta-thalassemia major is inherited through the defective genes of both parents.

A mild anemia is usually present in individuals with beta-thalassemia minor; however, it is not unusual for affected individuals to be symptom-free. Symptoms of beta-thalassemia major include fatigue; shortness of breath (dyspnea); and yellowing of the skin, eyes, and mucous membranes (jaundice). Other symptoms, usually associated with the premature destruction of red blood cells (hemolytic anemia) and subsequent release of iron, may include bronzed or freckled skin and enlargement of the spleen (splenomegaly). In severe cases, iron deposits in the heart, liver, and pancreas may eventually lead to impaired function. In addition, expanding bone marrow may result in thickened and enlarged bones in the skull and face, while normal growth may be retarded.

Alpha-thalassemia, far less common than beta-thalassemia, ranges in severity from a carrier state with no symptoms to the most severe form that is incompatible with life. The severity of symptoms is dependent upon the level of alpha-chain involvement. The most severe form of alpha-thalassemia involves the complete absence of alpha-chain production.

Treatment for symptomatic thalassemias includes blood transfusion therapy to ensure normal growth. However, repeated blood transfusions may exacerbate iron deposition into the internal organs (hemosiderosis), necessitating treatment with iron-chelating drugs that increase iron excretion. Other treatment may include bone marrow transplantation.

Thalassemia is inherited as an autosomal recessive trait and is most prevalent among people living in or originating from the Mediterranean, the Middle East, and Southeast Asia.

The following organizations in the General Resources Section can provide additional information: Online Mendelian Inheritance in Man: www3.ncbi.nlm.nih.gov/Omim/searchomim.html, Genetic Alliance, NIH/National Heart, Lung & Blood Institue, National Organization for Rare Disorders, Inc., (NORD), NIH/Office of Rare Diseases: rarediseases.info.nih.gov/ord/

National Associations & Support Groups

4127 AHEPHA Cooley's Anemia Foundation
1909 Q Street Nw
Washington, DC 20009   513-339-6033

Dedicated to advancing the treatment and cure of Cooley's Anemia, an inherited blood disorder. Provides information, referrals to local medical sources, medical supplies to people in need, and listings of informational materials available from the Foundation.

4128 Cooley's Anemia Foundation
129-09 26th Avenue
Flushing, NY 11354   718-321-2873
                            800-522-7222
                       Fax: 718-321-3340
                    e-mail: ncaf@aol.com
                       www.thalassemia.org

The CAF is the only U.S.-based voluntary health organization that aids in patient services, medical research, education and public information to fight Thalassemia, a blood disease also known as Cooley's Anemia. Members of CAF work alongside the Thalassemia Action Group (TAG) to provide national support, encouragement and friendship to other patients and families.

1954 32 pages 2x year

Frank Somma, National President
Gina Cioffi, National Executive Director

4129 Sickle Cell Disease Association of America
200 Corporate Pointe, Suite 495
Culver City, CA 90230   310-216-6363
                              800-421-8453
                              Fax: 310-215-3722
                              www.sicklecelldisease.org

Provides programs and services for individuals and families affected by sickle cell disease through its network of affiliated members. Provides education, advocacy and other initiatives which promote awareness and support for sickle cell programs and patients.

4130 Thalassemias Action Group (TAG)
129-09 26th Avenue
Flushing, NY 11354   718-321-2873
                           800-522-7222
                           Fax: 718-321-3340
                           e-mail: ncaf@aol.com
                           www.thalassemia.org

4131 X-Linked Aalpha Thalassemia Family Support Network
1437 Cool Springs Drive
Mesquite, TX 75181   972-222-0050
                           e-mail: nordtx@earthlink.net

State Agencies & Support Groups

California

4132 Cooley's Anemia Foundation-California
PO Box 1201
Costa Mesa, CA 92628   562-496-8517

Alisa DiLorenzo, President

Illinois

4133 Cooley's Anemia Foundation-Illinois
Oakbrook Towers
40 North Tower Road #2A
Oakbrook, IL 60521   630-268-8775

Pat Matarrese, President

Massachusetts

4134 Cooley's Anemia Foundation - Massachusetts Chapter
44 Joseph Road
Newton, MA 02160   617-332-5952

Rudi Viscomi

New Jersey

4135 Cooley's Anemia Foundation - New Jersey Chapter
1 Engle Street
Englewood, NJ 07631   201-569-2193
                            Fax: 201-569-2613

Vincent D'Elia Esq

New York

4136 Cooley's Anemia Foundation - Rochester
19 Devenwood Lane
Pittsford, NY 14534   716-248-3385

Peter Paradiso, President

4137 Cooley's Anemia Foundation - Staten Island
2136 East 4th Street
Brooklyn, NY 11223   718-627-7469

Terri DiFilippo, President

4138 Cooley's Anemia Foundation - Suffolk Chapter Office
738 Smithtown Bypass
Smithtown, NY 11787   516-863-0532

Edward Martella, President

4139 Cooley's Anemia Foundation - Westchester
3 Sammuel Purdy Lane
Katonah, NY 10536 914-232-1808
Fax: 914-232-1808

Peter Chieco, President

4140 Cooley's Anemia Foundation-Buffalo
135 Wellington Road
Buffalo, NY 14216 716-832-3055

Dennis Locurto, President

4141 Cooley's Anemia Foundation-Queens
92-02 Sutter Avenue
Ozone Park, NY 11416 718-848-6868
Fax: 718-848-6866

John Mancino, President

Texas

4142 Cooley's Anemia Foundation - Texas
1004 Field Trail
Mesquite, TX 75150 214-324-6147
Fax: 214-324-0612

Mateen Shah, President

Audio Video

4143 Tag Surfing
Cooley's Anemia Foundation
129-09 26th Avenue
Flushing, NY 11354 718-321-2873
800-522-7222
Fax: 718-321-3340
e-mail: ncaf@aol.com
www.thalassemia.org

Video

Gina Cioffi, Esq, National Executive Director

4144 Wish
Cooley's Anemia Foundation
129-09 26th Avenue
Flushing, NY 11354 718-321-2873
800-522-7222
Fax: 718-321-3340
e-mail: ncaf@aol.com
www.thalassemia.org

Video

Gina Cioffi, Esq, National Executive Director

Web Sites

4145 Pedbase
www.icondata.com/health/pedbase/files/THA-
LASSE.HTM

Books

4146 Genes, Blood & Courage
David Nathanas, author

Cooley's Anemia Foundation
129-09 26th Avenue
Flushing, NY 11354 718-321-2873
800-522-7222
Fax: 718-321-3340
e-mail: ncaf@aol.com
www.thalassemia.org

Teresa Piropato, Executive Director

4147 Mom, I'll Stop Crying, If You Stop Crying
Robert Samaras, author

Cooley's Anemia Foundation
129-09 26th Avenue
Flushing, NY 11354 718-321-2873
800-522-7222
Fax: 718-321-3340
e-mail: ncaf@aol.com
www.thalassemia.org

A courageous battle against a deadly disease.

4148 What is Cooley's Anemia
Cooley's Anemia Foundation
129-09 26th Avenue
Flushing, NY 11354 718-321-2873
800-522-7222
Fax: 718-321-3340
e-mail: ncaf@aol.com
www.thalassemia.org

Patient and family handbook.

Gina Cioffi, National Executive Director

4149 What is Thalassemia?
Cooley's Anemia Foundation
129-09 26th Avenue
Flushing, NY 11354 718-321-2873
800-522-7222
Fax: 718-321-3340
e-mail: ncaf@aol.com
www.thalassemia.org

A guide to help thalassemics and their parents understand thalassemia, the reasons for treatment and hope for the future.

Rino Vullo
Bernadette Modell

Children's Books

4150 Coloring Book on Thalassemia
Cooley's Anemia Foundation
129-09 26th Avenue
Flushing, NY 11354   718-321-2873
                                        800-522-7222
                                   Fax: 718-321-3340
                              e-mail: ncaf@aol.com
                              www.thalassemia.org

Available in English, Italian, Greek and Chinese.

Gina Cioffi, National Executive Director

Newsletters

4151 Lifeline
Colley's Anemia Foundation
129-09 26th Avenue
Flushing, NY 11354   718-321-2873
                                        800-522-7222
                                   Fax: 718-321-3340
                              e-mail: ncaf@aol.com
                              www.thalassemia.org

Cooley's anemia Foundation, Inc.
   BiAnnually

Teresa Piropato, Executive Director

Pamphlets

4152 All You Need to Know About Being a Carrier of Cooley's Anemia
Cooley's Anemia Foundation
129-09 26th Avenue
Flushing, NY 11354   718-321-2873
                                        800-522-7222
                                   Fax: 718-321-3340
                              e-mail: ncaf@aol.com
                              www.thalassemia.org

This booklet offers information on the thalassemia trait.
   1995 13 pages

4153 Desferal
Cooley's Anemia Foundation
129-09 26th Avenue
Flushing, NY 11354   718-321-2873
                                        800-522-7222
                                   Fax: 718-321-3340
                              e-mail: ncaf@aol.com
                              www.thalassemia.org

Guidelines for home infusion.

Gina Cioffi, Esq, National Executive Director

DESCRIPTION

4154 THROMBOCYTOPENIAS

Covers these related disorders: Idiopathic thrombocytopenia purpura (ITP)
May involve these systems in the body (see Section III):
 Blood (Hematologic)

Thrombocytopenia is a term that describes a condition in which the level of circulating platelets in the blood is reduced, resulting in a tendency to bleed. By changing shape and adhering to each other and the walls of broken blood vessels, platelets, also known as thrombocytes, play an essential role in the clotting process. Normal blood levels usually demonstrate 150,000 to 350,000 platelets per microliter. When the platelet count is reduced to 30,000 per microliter or lower, abnormal bleeding under the skin may occur and result in purple bruising or spots (purpura). Nosebleeds (epistaxis), bleeding in the mouth, and blood in the urine (hematuria) are also common. In a few patients, bleeding or hemorrhaging into the brain may occur. This may be heralded by headache and dizziness.

Thrombocytopenia may result from a slowdown in platelet production or the rapid destruction of these cells. Certain diseases such as anemias, leukemia, lymphoma, bone marrow disorders, or autoimmune diseases may cause thrombocytopenia. Other causes include enlargement of the spleen (splenomegaly), cirrhosis, certain drugs, viral infection, and x-ray or radiation exposure.

The treatment of thrombocytopenia is based upon its underlying cause. For example, if the low platelet count is caused by a specific underlying disease, treatment is geared toward that disease. Low platelet counts caused by a specific drug necessitate the withdrawal of that drug. If bleeding is severe, platelet transfusions may be administered.

Idiopathic thrombocytopenia purpura (ITP) is a term used to describe thrombocytopenia of un-known origin. This condition often follows a viral affection and, in children, usually disappears within a month or so with no treatment. The duration of ITP in adolescents and adults is often more prolonged.

The following organizations in the General Resources Section can provide additional information: Genetic Alliance, Online Mendelian Inheritance in Man: www3.ncbi.nlm.nih.gov/Omim/searchomim.html, National Organization for Rare Disorders, Inc. (NORD), NIH/National Heart, Lung & Blood Institute, NIH/Office of Rare Diseases: rarediseases.info.nih.gov/ord/

National Associations & Support Groups

4155 ITP Society Children's Blood Foundation
333 East 38th Street
New York, NY 10016
212-297-4340
800-487-7010

Promotes the welfare of and addresses the issues that affect people with Immune or Idiopathic Thrombocytopenic Purpura. Goals are to provide patient support ongoing medical research to advance the knowledge and treatment; and educate the public and medical communities about the disorder. Provides educational and support materials including fact sheets, brochures, and a booklet entitled 'What's It Called Again?'

Web Sites

4156 Web site for ITP People
www.itppeople.com

DESCRIPTION

4157 THUMBSUCKING

Disorder Type: Mental, Emotional or Behavioral Disorder

Thumbsucking is a common habit that is prevalent among infants and young children. This behavior is usually used as a device for providing pleasure, amusement, comfort, oral gratification, and release of stress or tension. In most children, thumbsucking reaches a plateau between the ages of 18 months to two years and then slowly but steadily decreases until it disappears at about five to six years of age. Thumbsucking in older children or adults may indicate the presence of some type of emotional disturbance.

Although it is generally thought that thumbsucking does not cause any long-term developmental irregularities, thumbsucking that continues beyond age six may lead to acquired problems with the bones and tissues of the thumb and an abnormal bite or contact pattern between upper and lower teeth (malocclusion). The longer the habit persists, the more likely affected children are to develop these types of problems. Conversely, the earlier this habit comes to an end, the more likely that irregular positioning of the teeth will improve without intervention.

Many physicians agree that, as a general rule, the best treatment for thumbsucking is to ignore the behavior and wait patiently for the children to outgrow the habit or to discontinue the behavior on their own. Treatment is generally supportive as punishing or reprimanding often adds to stress levels and may actually worsen the problem. Other treatment may include the use of certain appliances that are fitted with small projections that alert children to their behavior when they attempt to suck their thumbs. Older children may require the use of orthodontic appliances to correct irregularities associated with malocclusion.

National Associations & Support Groups

4158 National Institute of Dental and Craniofacial Research
31 Ctr Dr MSC 2290, Bldg 31, Rm 2C35
Bethesda, MD 20892   301-496-4261
Fax: 301-496-9988
www.nidr.nih.gov/

4159 National Oral Health Information Clearinghouse
1 NOHIC Way
Bethesda, MD 20892   301-402-7364
Fax: 301-907-8830
TDD: 301-656-7581
e-mail: nidr@aerie.com
www.aerie.com/nohicweb/

4160 Thumbsucking
Nat'l Institute of Dental & Craniofacial Research
31 Center Dr MSC 2290
Bethesda, MD 20892   301-496-4261
Fax: 301-496-9988
www.nidr.nih.gov/

DESCRIPTION

4161 TICS

Disorder Type: Genetic Disorder, Neuromuscular, Mental, Emotional or Behavioral Disorder
Covers these related disorders: Chronic motor tic disorder, Tourette syndrome, Transient tics of childhood
May involve these systems in the body (see Section III):
Nervous System

Tics are repetitive or stereotypical, compulsive, abrupt (spasmodic) movements of a muscle or muscle groups. Although any muscle may be affected, tics most commonly involve muscles of the eyes, face, neck, or shoulders. Movements may include blinking, sniffing, facial grimacing, lip smacking, tongue thrusting, or shoulder shrugging. Tics may begin as intentional movements to relieve perceived tension. However, they may rapidly become unintentional or involuntary in nature. Although tics are extremely difficult to suppress, most patients are able to do so for short periods. Tics are often worsened by stress or any perceived attention to the condition; in contrast, they typically disappear during sleep.

In most patients, tics become apparent between approximately five to 10 years of age. According to some estimates, as many as 25 percent of children may be affected. Most children may experience a spontaneous disappearance of tics within a few weeks or less than one year after onset. In such patients, the condition is referred to as transient tics of childhood. Supportive measures that may be helpful in alleviating transient tics include providing children with a tranquil environment as well as additional rest.

Some children may experience chronic motor tics that persist throughout adult life. In such patients, the condition is known as chronic motor tic disorder. Chronic motor tics may simultaneously affect muscles in up to three different muscle groups.

In contrast to transient tics of childhood and chronic motor tics, which are considered relatively benign, restricted tic disorders, a genetic, neurologic disorder known as Tourette syndrome is characterized by multiple, chronic, complex tics. Tourette syndrome usually becomes apparent in children between the ages of two to 14 years. Initial symptoms typically include motor tics of the face, eyelids, shoulders, and neck. Movements may include grimacing, excessive eye blinking, or stretching of the neck. Vocal tics, such as involuntary coughing, grunting, barking, or throat clearing, are also common. Additional symptoms may include involuntary repetition of obscene words (coprolalia) or words spoken by other individuals (echolalia); aggressive behaviors; the performance of repetitive actions or impulses in response to recurrent, persistent thoughts (obsessive-compulsive behaviors); and secondary learning, emotional, or social difficulties. Researchers suggest that variable expression of the disease gene responsible for Tourette syndrome may cause transient tics of childhood or chronic motor tics in other individuals, indicating possible overlap between the conditions. Several studies have demonstrated that immediate (first-degree) relatives of patients with Tourette syndrome have an increased frequency of such tic conditions.

In some patients with severe chronic motor tic disorder, treatment may include therapy with certain medications (e.g., certain benzodiazepines or haloperidol). The treatment of Tourette syndrome is symptomatic and supportive and may include therapy with certain medications, such as haloperidol, pimozide, clonidine, clonazepam, or carbamazepine. In addition, for those with learning, behavioral, and social difficulties, multidisciplinary management and the provision of special social, academic, and vocational services may be important in helping patients achieve their potential. (Please refer to the section entitled Tourette Syndrome for further information on this disorder.)

The following organizations in the General Resources Section can provide additional information: National Organization for Rare Disorders, Inc., (NORD), Genetic Alliance, March of Dimes Birth Defects Foundation, NIH/Office of Rare Diseases, Online Mendelian Inheritance in Man: www3.ncbi.nlm.nih.gov/Omim/searchomim.html

National Associations & Support Groups

4162 Tourette Syndrome Association, Inc.
42-40 Bell Blvd
Bayside, NY 11361   718-224-2999
                          888-486-8738
                     Fax: 718-279-9596
          e-mail: tourette@ix.netcom.com
www.neuro-www2.mgh.harvard.edu/tsa/tsamain.nclk

4163 Tourette Syndrome Foundation of Canada
194 Jarvis St, Ste 206
Toronto, Ontario M5B 1M6,   416-861-8398
                            800-361-3120
                       Fax: 416-861-2472
          e-mail: tsfc.org@sympatic.org
                        www.tourette.ca

4164 We Move: Worldwide Education and Advocacy for Movement Disorders
204 East 84th Street
New York, NY 10024   212-241-8567
                           800-437-6682
                      Fax: 212-987-7363
          e-mail: wemove@wemove.org
                        www.wemove.org

Gives the general public the knowledge that they desire regarding any disorder involving movement difficulties.

Web Sites

4165 MHG Neurology Web Forums
http://neuro-www.mgh.harvard.edu/forum

4166 NewsGroup
www.Alt.support.tourette

4167 Parents Helping Parents
http://php.com/tourette.htm

4168 Tourette Spectrum Disorder Association
www.discover.net/~cwangtsa

4169 Tourette Syndrome Online
http://members.tripod.com/~tourette_syndrome/

DESCRIPTION

4170 TOURETTE SYNDROME
Synonyms: Gilles de la Tourette syndrome, GTS
Disorder Type: Genetic Disorder
May involve these systems in the body (see Section III):
 Nervous System

Tourette syndrome is a neurologic disorder that typically becomes apparent in children between the ages of two to 14 years, with approximately 50 percent of cases occurring before seven years of age. The disorder, which is thought to affect about one in 2,000 individuals, is approximately three times more prevalent in males than females and is more common among Caucasians than other populations. In children with Tourette syndrome, associated symptoms and findings vary greatly in range and severity. Initial symptoms may include involuntary, repetitive (stereotypical) muscle movements (motor tics) of the face, eyelids, shoulders, and neck, such as grimacing, abrupt head turning, excessive eye blinking, or stretching of the neck. In some patients with severe symptoms, motor tics may evolve to include self-mutilating behaviors, such as nail biting, lip biting, or facial punching. Children with Tourette syndrome may also develop vocal tics, such as involuntary coughing, grunting, barking, sniffling, or throat clearing. As the disease progresses, additional symptoms may develop including involuntary repetition of obscene words (coprolalia), words spoken by other individuals (echolalia), or one's own words (palilalia) or imitation of other individuals' behaviors (echokinesis or echopraxia). The symptoms associated with Tourette syndrome may periodically decrease or increase in intensity; may subside during high levels of concentration, such as when reading or studying; and may worsen with stress. Tourette syndrome is considered a life-long disorder; however, in approximately 50 to 66 percent of patients, symptoms significantly decrease about 10 to 15 years after initial diagnosis and treatment.

Children with Tourette syndrome may also experience associated behavioral abnormalities, such as aggressive behavior or the performance of repetitive actions or impulses in response to recurrent, persistent thoughts (obsessive-compulsive behaviors). Obsessive-compulsive behaviors are typically performed to help neutralize obsessive thoughts and relieve anxieties. Many affected children may also develop learning, emotional, or social difficulties. The treatment of Tourette syndrome is symptomatic and supportive and may include therapy with certain medications, such as haloperidol, pimozide, clonidine, clonazepam, or carbamazepine. In addition, for those with learning, behavioral, and social difficulties, multidisciplinary management and the provision of special social, academic, and vocational services may be important in helping patients achieve their potential.

Although the exact cause of Tourette syndrome is unknown, studies suggest that the disorder may result due to abnormalities of neurotransmitter (dopamine) activity within a certain area of the brain (basal ganglia). In most cases, Tourette syndrome is thought to be inherited as an autosomal dominant trait that occurs as the result of changes (mutations) in a gene located on the long arm (q) of chromosome 18 (18q22.1). Some children with mutations of this disease gene may not have symptoms associated with the disorder (incomplete penetrance). In addition, in those children with the defective gene who do have symptoms associated with Tourette syndrome, such symptoms may vary in range and severity from case to case (variable expressivity). Such variability of gene expression and penetrance may be suggested by the fact that immediate (first-degree) relatives of patients have an increased frequency of Tourette syndrome, tic conditions, and obsessive-compulsive disorder. In addition, some researchers suspect that Tourette syndrome may result from inheritance of a disease gene in combination with certain environmental factors that may trigger the gene's expression (multifactorial inheritance). Research suggests that individuals who have two copies of a disease gene for Tourette syndrome (homozygotes) typically express the disorder, whereas some who inherit one disease gene (heterozygotes) may not develop the disorder unless particular environmental factors (e.g., infection, such as due to exposure to Group A beta-hemolytic streptococcus) trigger its expression.

The following organizations in the General Resources Section can provide additional information: National Organization for Rare Disorders, Inc., (NORD), Genetic Alliance, March of Dimes Birth Defects Foundation, NIH/Office of Rare Diseases, NIH/National Institute of Neurological Disorders & Stroke, Online Mendelian Inheritance in Man:

www3.ncbi.nlm.nih.gov/Omim/searchomim.html

National Associations & Support Groups

4171 American Academy of Neurology: Tourette Syndrome
1080 Montreal Avenue
St. Paul, MN 55116   320-695-1940
                    www.aan.com/public/tour.html

4172 Tourette Syndrome Association
42-40 Bell Boulevard
Bayside, NY 11361   718-224-2999
                          888-486-8738
                      Fax: 718-279-9596
                e-mail: tourette@ix.netcom.com
neuro.www2.mgh.harvard.edu/tsa/tsamain.

This disorder is characterized by tic-like muscular movements and involuntary utterances. This organization assists individuals and families with many services, including maintaining a library and a list of doctors familiar with this disorder.

4173 Tourette Syndrome Foundation of Canada
194 Jarvis St
Toronto, Ontario M5B 1M6,
Canada   416-861-8398
                          800-361-3120
                      Fax: 416-861-2472
                e-mail: tsfc.org@sympatico.ca
                          www.tourette.ca

4174 Worldwide Education and Advocacy for Movement Disorders
204 E 84th St
New York, NY 10024   212-241-8567
                          800-437-6682
                      Fax: 212-987-7363
                e-mail: wemove@wemove.org
                          www.wemove.org

Research Centers

4175 Tourette Syndrome Clinic
Yale Child Study Center
230 S Frontage Rd, PO 3333
New Haven, CT 06510   203-785-3492

Largest clinical care center offering research solely into the causes, symptoms and treatments for persons with Tourette Syndrome.

James F. Leckman, MD

Audio Video

4176 Gift of Hope
Tourette Syndrome Association, Inc.
42-40 Bell Blvd.
Bayside, NY 11361   718-224-2999
                      Fax: 718-279-9596

The cause of Tourette Syndrome lies in the brain. This video offers five people who have TS explaining their reasons for agreeing to register with TSA's Brain Bank Program.

14 minutes

Web Sites

4177 MHG Neurology Web Forums
http://neuro-www.mgh.harvard.edu/forum

4178 NewsGroup
www.Alt.support.tourette

4179 Parents Helping Parents
http://php.com/tourette.htm

4180 Tourette Spectrum Disorder Association
www.discover.net/~cwangtsa

Newsletters

4181 Tourette Syndrome Association Newsletter
42-40 Bell Blvd.
Bayside, NY 11361   718-224-2999

Offers information, articles and news on the latest technology and advancements for persons with Tourette Syndrome.

Pamphlets

4182 Just Right

J.F. Leckman, MD, author

Tourette Syndrome Association, Inc.
42-40 Bell Blvd.
Bayside, NY 11361   718-224-2999
                                  Fax: 718-279-9596

Details data gathered about the awareness and perceptions their subjects had immediately prior to the onset of tic and obsessive-compulsive symptoms, which are important to the implication of certain brain regions that may be involved in processing sensorimotor information in tic disorder pathology.

1997 6 pages

4183 Peer Problems in Tourette's Disorder

A. Stokes, MD, author

Tourette Syndrome Association, Inc.
42-40 Bell Blvd.
Bayside, NY 11361   718-224-2999
                                  Fax: 718-279-9596

Detailed research findings of peer problems in children with TS. Includes statistical results obtained from these studies.

1991 7 pages

DESCRIPTION

4184 TOXOPLASMOSIS

Disorder Type: Infectious Disease
Covers these related disorders: Congenital toxoplasmosis

Toxoplasmosis is a common infection caused by the single-celled parasite Toxoplasma gondii. This parasite multiplies in the intestines of cats, and its eggs (oocysts) are shed in cat feces. Humans may acquire toxoplasmosis due to contact with cat feces (e.g., in litter boxes), from exposure to contaminated soil, or by eating undercooked or raw meat that contains a form of the parasite (tissue cysts). In addition, if a woman acquires toxoplasmosis during pregnancy, the developing fetus may be affected (congenital toxoplasmosis) due to transmission via the placenta.

Most children who acquire toxoplasmosis after birth and have normally functioning immune systems do not have any apparent symptoms (asymptomatic). However, some children may experience enlargement of one or more lymph nodes (lymphadenopathy). More rarely, such patients may also have other, variable symptoms and findings, such as fever; joint or muscle pain; enlargement of the liver (hepatomegaly); or inflammation of the lungs (pneumonia), the liver (hepatitis), or the middle layer of and the nerve-rich membrane at the back of the eyes (chorioretinitis). Most children with normal immune systems who acquire toxoplasmosis after birth recover spontaneously. However, others may require treatment with certain medications.

Toxoplasmosis is typically more severe in children who acquire the disease during fetal development or who have compromised immune systems. When the infection is transmitted via the placenta during pregnancy (or, in some cases, during vaginal delivery), patients are said to have congenital toxoplasmosis. The disease is typically more severe if the infection is acquired during early pregnancy (first trimester), but the risk of disease

transmission is greatest during later pregnancy (third trimester). Approximately 50 percent of women who acquire toxoplasmosis during pregnancy and do not receive treatment transmit the infection to the developing fetus. In the United States, congenital toxoplasmosis affects approximately one in 1,000 newborns.

Newborns who contract toxoplasmosis during early fetal development may have severe symptoms, whereas those affected later during fetal growth may have mild or no apparent symptoms. However, without treatment, almost all patients demonstrate certain findings associated with toxoplasmosis by adolescence, particularly inflammation of the middle layer of and the nerve-rich membrane at the back of the eye (chorioretinitis). Chorioretinitis may cause blurred vision, abnormal sensitivity to light (photophobia), and possible visual impairment. In some affected infants, certain findings may be present, such as short height and low weight at birth (intrauterine growth retardation); persistent yellowish discoloration of the skin, whites of the eyes, and mucous membranes (jaundice); retinal scarring; skin rash; lymph node enlargement (lymphadenopathy); decreased levels of circulating blood platelets (thrombocytopenia); inflammation of the liver (hepatitis); hearing loss; or other findings. Severely affected infants may have an abnormally small head (microcephaly), an abnormal accumulation of cerebrospinal fluid around the brain (hydrocephalus), inflammation of membranes of the eyes (chorioretinitis), episodes of abnormally increased electrical activity in the brain (seizures), delays in the acquisition of skills requiring the coordination of physical and mental activities (psychomotor retardation), and calcium deposits in the brain (brain calcifications). Life-threatening complications may occur shortly after birth.

In children who have compromised immune systems, such as those with acquired immunodeficiency syndrome (AIDS), toxoplasmosis often occurs suddenly and is extremely severe (fulminant). In such patients, infection may rapidly affect the lungs, heart, and brain. In fulminant toxoplasmosis, the most common symptoms are often neurological and may include headache, impaired thinking, episodes of abnormally increased electrical activity in the brain (seizures), and impaired control of voluntary movement (ataxia). Without treatment, life-threatening complications result.

The treatment of newborns with congenital toxoplasmosis, affected children with compromised immune systems, and other patients with acquired toxoplasmosis may include the use of combination drug therapies with such medications as pyrimethamine, folinic acid, sulfadiazine or triple sulfonamides, leukovorin, or spiramycin. Additional treatment is symptomatic and supportive. It is important to note that all newborns with congenital toxoplasmosis should receive appropriate drug therapy, regardless of whether they have severe, mild, or no associated symptoms. Appropriate drug therapy for women who contract toxoplasmosis any time during pregnancy may reduce the risk of congenital toxoplasmosis by approximately 60 percent. Such therapy may include spiramycin and pyrimethamine combined with triple sulfonamides or sulfadiazine. Pyrimethamine is not given during early pregnancy since it may increase the risk of birth defects during early fetal development. In addition, certain measures may be helpful in preventing toxoplasmosis, such as thoroughly cooking all meat, washing hands after handling raw meat, and avoiding direct contact with cat feces.

The following organizations in the General Resources Section can provide additional information: Centers for Disease Control (CDC), World Health Organization (WHO), NIH/National Institute of Allergy and Infectious Disease

National Associations & Support Groups

4185 ARC
500 East Border Street, Suite 300
Arlington, TX 76010   817-261-6003
                             800-433-5255
                    TDD: 817-277-0553

This national organization for retarded citizens offers parent to Parent (P-P) programs that provide informational and emotional support to parents who have a child, adolescent, or adult family member with special needs. P-P programs offer an important connection for a parent who is seeking support for special disability issue, by matching him or her with a trained veteren parent

Web Sites

4186 Academica Home Page for Toxoplasmosis
www2.uic.edu/~mczartl/

4187 Toxoplasmosis Fact Sheet
www.thebody.com/treat/toxo.html

4188 University Graz, Austria
www-ang.kfunigraz.ac.at/~trojovsk/toxo/

4189 University of Florida
nersp.nerdc.ufl.edu/~iacue/Toxoplasmosis/index.ntm

Pamphlets

4190 Toxoplasmosis
March of Dimes Resource Center
1275 Mamaroneck Avenue
White Plains, NY 10605   888-663-4637
                          Fax: 914-997-4763

DESCRIPTION

4191 TRANSPOSITION OF THE GREAT ARTERIES
Synonym: Transposition of the great vessels
Disorder Type: Birth Defect, Heart

Transposition of the great arteries is a heart defect that is present at birth (congential) in which the major blood vessels that transport blood away from the heart (aorta and pulmonary artery) are transposed or in one another's normal positions. The pulmonary artery normally arises from the base of the lower right-sided pumping chamber (right ventricle) of the heart and carries oxygen-poor blood to the lungs, where the exchange of oxygen and carbon dioxide occurs. The aorta, the main artery of the body, normally arises from the base of the left ventricle and carries oxygen-rich (oxygenated) blood to the body's tissues. However, in infants with transposition of the great arteries, the aorta arises from the right ventricle and the pulmonary artery arises from the left ventricle. As a result, oxygenated blood recirculates to the lungs, while the oxygen-poor blood recirculates throughout the body, and bodily tissues receive insufficient levels of oxygenated blood (hypoxia).

Transpositon of the great arteries is not compatible with life unless there is some communication between the pulmonary and systemic circulation, thus allowing for some mixing of deoxygenated and oxygenated blood. Certain fetal shunts may provide such mixing. These include persistance of the fetal chanel that joins the pulmonary artery and the aorta (ductus arteriosus), an opening in the fibrous partition (septum) between teh upper chambers (atria) of the heart (patent foramen ovale). Some patients with transposition have mixing of blood between the ventricles (VSD).

In newborns with transposition of the great arteries, associated symptoms vary in severity, depending upon the amount of oxygenated blood that is able to reach the aorta and systemic circulation. Shortly after birth, affected infants may experience abnormally rapid and deep breathing (tachypnea, hyperpnea) and an abnormal bluish discoloration of the skin and mucous membranes (cyanosis). Without treatment, life-threatening complications may result. Medical treatment includes a medication called prostaglandin E to open the ductus arteriosus and allow mixing. A cardiac catheterization to place a balloon catheter across the atrial septum (balloon septostomy) may be done to allow for mixing of blood. The treatment of infants with transposition of the great arteries includes surgery to switch the aorta and coronary arteries and pulmonary artery back to their normal positions (arterial switch operation). This operation is done in the first weeks of life and is corrective.

Transposition of the great arteries is most common in males than females and affects approximately one in 2,000 newborns. Infants are most often normal - sized, full - term, and otherwise healthy. The condition is thought to result from the interactions of several different genes, possibly in association with the involvement of environmental factors (multifactorial inheritance). Although the exact underlying cause of this hert defect is unknown, researchers suggest that it may result from an error during the development of an embryonic structure that later divides the aorta and pulmonary artery.

The following organizations in the General Resources Section can provide additional information: Genetic Alliance, March of Dimes Birth Defects Foundation, NIH/National Heart, Lung & Blood Institute, NIH/National Institute of Child Health and Human Development

National Associations & Support Groups

4192 American Heart Association
7272 Greenville Avenue
Dallas, TX 75231
                        214-373-6300
                        800-242-8721
                        Fax: 214-706-1341
                        e-mail: inquire@amhrt.org
                        www.amhrt.org

Supports research, education and community
service programs with the objective of reducing
premature death and disability from cardiovascular diseases and stroke; coordinates the efforts of health professionals, and other engaged
in the fight against heart and circulatory disease.

Web Sites

4193 Children's Health Information Network
www.ohsu.edu.cliniweb/C14/C14.240.400.html

4194 Congenital Heart Disease Resource Page
www.csun.edu/~hcmth011/heart/
e-mail: sheri.berger@csun.edu
www.csun.edu/~hcmth011/heart/

4195 Southern Illinois University School of Medicine
www.siumed.edu/peds/teaching/patient%20edu-
cation.htm

DESCRIPTION

4196 TRIPLO X SYNDROME

Synonyms: 47,XXX syndrome, 47,XXX chromosome constitution, Triple X syndrome, Trisomy X, XXX syndrome

Disorder Type: Chromosomal Disorder, Developmental Milestones

Covers these related disorders: 47,XXX/48,XXXX mosaicism, 47,XXX/48,XXXX/49,XXXXX mosaicism

Triplo X syndrome, also known as 47,XXX syndrome, is a chromosomal disorder that affects females. Although females usually have two X chromosomes, those with triplo X syndrome have three X chromosomes (trisomy) in cells of the body. Some children with triplo X syndrome may have no or few apparent symptoms; however, others may have developmental delays, learning disabilities, behavioral abnormalities, and/or, in some cases, physical abnormalities.

According to some reports in the medical literature, most females with triplo X syndrome tend to have an intelligence quotient (I.Q.) lower than that of their sisters and brothers (siblings), potentially experiencing a mild intellectual deficit. Per certain studies, affected females have demonstrated an I.Q. ranging from 115 (normal range = 80-120) to 55 (considered mild mental retardation), with a majority in the range of approximately 85 to 90. Individuals with mild mental retardation have an I.Q. of approximately 50 to 70. Many children with triplo X syndrome may have language and speech delays and difficulties with verbal learning, potentially requiring special education classes. Affected children may also be prone to early delays in motor development, have diminished muscle tone (hypotonia), and experience awkwardness and poor coordination. In addition, some children with triplo X syndrome may have behavioral problems including poor social skills and mild depression; however, they may tend to adapt during early adulthood without severe difficulties.

Most females with triplo X syndrome usually attain tall stature. Affected adolescents typically develop female secondary sexual characteristics as expected (e.g., breast development, menstruation, etc.); in addition, fertility is thought to be normal in most cases.

Rarely, in some affected females, some cells of the body have three X chromosomes and others have four or five X chromosomes (e.g., 47,XXX 48,XXXX/ or 47,XXX/ 48, XXXX/ 49,XXXXX mosaicism). The risk of mental retardation, developmental and behavioral abnormalities, and physical malformations may increase depending upon the number of additional X chromosomes and the percentage of cells affected.

Triplo X syndrome results from errors during the division of a parent's reproductive cells (meiosis). Researchers suspect that the extra X chromosome is received from the mother in most cases (i.e., nondisjunction at maternal meiosis I). Triplo X syndrome is thought to affect approximately one in 1,000 newborn females. However, because many affected females may have few or no apparent symptoms, it may be difficult to estimate the true frequency of triplo X syndrome in the general population.ent symptoms, it may be difficult to estimate the true frequency of triplo X syndrome in the general population.

The following organizations in the General Resources Section can provide additional information: National Organization for Rare Disorders, Inc., (NORD), Genetic Alliance, NIH/Office of Rare Diseases, National Center for Learning Disabilities, NIH/National Information Center for Children & Youth with Disabilities (NICHCY), Learning Disabilities Association of America (LDA)

National Associations & Support Groups

4197 ARC
500 East Border Street, Suite 300
Arlington, TX 76010

817-261-6003
800-433-5255
TDD: 817-277-0553

Provides informational and emotional support to parents who have a child, adolescent, or adult family member with special needs. P-P programs offer an important connection for a parent who is seeking support for special disability issue, by matching him or her with a trained vetern parent who has already been there.

4198 Support Organization for Trisomy 18, 13, and Related Disorders
2982 South Union Street
Rochester, NY 14624

716-594-4621
800-716-7638
Fax: 716-594-1507
e-mail: barbsoft@aol.com
www.trisomy.org

SOFT is an international organization. SOFT is a network of families and professionals dedicated to providing support and understanding to families involved in the issue and decision surrounding the diagnosis and cure 718113 and related chromosome disorders, support is provided during pre-natal diagnosis, the childs life and after their childs passing. SOFT is committed to support the family's personal decision in alliance with a parent-professional partnership.

28-40 pages Bi-Monthly

Web Sites

4199 Pedbase
www.icondata.com/health/ped-base/files/XXXSYNDR.HTM

4200 Triplo X Web page
www.triplo-x.org/index.htm

Books

4201 Support Organization for Trisomy 18, 13, and Related Disorders
2982 South Union Street
Rochester, NY 14624

716-594-4621
800-716-7638
Fax: 716-594-1507
e-mail: barbsoft@aol.com
www.trisomy.org

Information related to chromosome disorders, support is provided during pre-natal diagnosis, the childs life and after their childs passing. SOFT is committed to support the family's personal decision in alliance with a parent-professional partnership.

28-40 pages Bi-Monthly

DESCRIPTION

4202 TRISOMY 18 SYNDROME
Synonyms: Chromosome 18, trisomy 18, Edwards syndrome
Disorder Type: Birth Defect, Chromosomal Disorder, Developmental Milestones
Covers these related disorders: Trisomy 18 mosaicism

Trisomy 18 syndrome is a chromosomal disorder that affects about one in 300 newborns. With the exception of reproductive cells, cells of the body normally have 23 pairs of chromosomes that are numbered from 1 to 22 (with a 23rd pair consisting of one X chromosome from the mother and an X or a Y chromosome from the father). However, in infants with trisomy 18 syndrome, all or a portion of chromosome 18 is present three times (trisomy) rather than twice in cells of the body. In some affected infants, only a percentage of cells may contain the trisomy 18 chromosomal abnormality (mosaicism).

The symptoms and physical findings associated with trisomy 18 syndrome are variable and depend upon the exact location of and the percentage of body cells containing the additional chromosomal material from chromosome 18. However, most infants with trisomy 18 syndrome experience development delays, usually severe mental retardation, low birth weight, difficulties feeding and breathing, and a failure to gain weight and grow at the expected rate (failure to thrive). In addition, associated abnormalities may include structural heart defects, failure of one or both testes to descend into the scrotum (cryptorchidism) in affected males, malformations of the hands and feet, additional skeletal abnormalities, and characteristic malformations of the head and facial (craniofacial) area.

In infants with trisomy 18 syndrome, defects of the hands and feet often include closed fists with overlapping, abnormally bent fingers; underdeveloped or absent thumbs; and webbing between certain fingers or toes (syndactyly). Affected infants also often have additional skeletal abnor-

malities, such as a small pelvis, narrow hips with limited movements, fusion of certain bones of the spinal column (vertebrae), or sideways curvature of the spine (scoliosis). Characteristic craniofacial abnormalities associated with trisomy 18 syndrome typically include an abnormally small head (microcephaly); a prominent back portion of the head (occiput); a small mouth (microstomia) and a small jaw (micrognathia); malformed, low-set ears; and short, narrow eyelid folds (palpebral fissures). Additional craniofacial malformations may be present, such as incomplete closure of the roof of the mouth (cleft palate), an abnormal groove in the upper lip (cleft lip), and drooping of the upper eyelids (ptosis). In addition, some infants may have kidney malformations. In many patients, life-threatening complications may develop during the first year of life. Treatment includes symptomatic and supportive measures. Although the exact cause of trisomy 18 syndrome is unknown, it is thought to result from errors during division of a parent's reproductive cells (meiosis) and, in some cases of mosaicism, errors during cellular division after fertilization (e.g., postzygotic nondisjunction).cells (meiosis) and, in some cases of mosaicism, errors during cellular division after fertilization (e.g., postzygotic nondisjunction).

The following organizations in the General Resources Section can provide additional information: National Organization for Rare Disorders, Inc., (NORD), Genetic Alliance, March of Dimes Birth Defects Foundation, NIH/National Institute of Child Health and Human Development, NIH/Office of Rare Diseases

National Associations & Support Groups

4203 ARC
500 East Border Street, Suite 300
Arlington, TX 76010   817-261-6003
                             800-433-5255
                        TDD: 817-277-0553
         e-mail: thearc@metronet.com
                 thearc.org/welcome.html

Parent to Parent (P-P) programs provide informational and emotional support to parents who have a child, adolescent, or adult family member with special needs. P-P programs offer an important connection for a parent who is seeking support for special disability issue, by matching him or her with a trained vetern parent who has already been there. Because the two parents share so many common concerns and interests, the support given and received is often uniquely meaningful.

4204 Chromosome 18 Registry & Research Society
6302 Fox Head
San Antonio, TX 78247   210-657-4968
Fax: 210-657-4968
e-mail: cody@chromosome18.org
hhp://www.chromosome18.org

The purpose of the Chromosome 18 Registry & Research Society is to offer support to patients and families, to educate the public about different available treatments and to connect families and doctors to the research community.

500 Members

4205 Congenital Heart Anomalies, Support, Education & Resources
James H. Myers, author

2112 North Wilkins Road
Swanton, OH 43558   419-825-5575
Fax: 419-825-2880
e-mail: chaser@compuserve.com
www.csun.edu/~hfmth006/ch

National organization for support, education and resources for families, patients and psionals who deal with children born with congenital heart malformations. Informafdjkdhospitalls

5000+ Members

4206 Support Organization for Trisomy (S.O.F.T.) Canada, Inc.
760 Brant Street, Suite 420
Burlington, On L7R4B8,
Canada   905-632-7755
800-668-0696
Fax: 905-632-5997

SOFT is a group of families and professionals providing information, support, and understanding to thoith Trisomy 18 or 13. Support is offered continuously during the diagnosis, lifespan, and after the pasing .

4207 Support Organization for Trisomy 18, 13, and Related Disorders
2982 South Union Street
Rochester, NY 14624   716-594-4621
800-716-7638
Fax: 716-594-1507
e-mail: barbsoft@aol.com
www.trisomy.org

SOFT is an international organization. SOFT is a netowrk of families and professional dedication to providing support and undrstanding to families involved in the issue and decision surrounding the diagnosis and care in 718113 and related chromosome disorders. Support is provided during pre-natal diagnosis, to child'd life and after their passing. SOFT is committed to the support of families personal decision in alliance with a parent-professional partnership.

28-40 pages Bi-Monthly

International

4208 In Touch Trust
10 Norman Road, Sale
Cheshire,
United Kingdom

Dedicated to bringing together parents of children with similar special needs such as learning and/or physical disabilities, a particular interest in assisting those affected by rare and complex conditions. Also provides information concerning a wide range of support groups for specific disorders, many of which help families come together for the purpose of mutual support.

Web Sites

4209 Pediatric Database
www.icondata.com/health/ped-base/files/TRISOMY2.HTM

4210 Trisomy 18 WWW Bulletin Board
www.chr18.uthscsa.edu/WWWboard/

DESCRIPTION

4211 TRISOMY 13 SYNDROME
Synonyms: Chromosome 13, trisomy 13, D1 trisomy syndrome, Patau syndrome
Disorder Type: Birth Defect, Chromosomal Disorder, Developmental Milestones
Covers these related disorders: Trisomy 13 mosaicism

Trisomy 13 syndrome is a chromosomal disorder that is thought to affect approximately one in 5,000 newborns. With the exception of reproductive cells, cells of the body normally have 23 pairs of chromosomes that are numbered from 1 to 22. The 23rd pair includes one X chromosome from the mother and an X or a Y chromosome from the father. In infants with trisomy 13 syndrome, all or a portion of chromosome 13 is present three times (trisomy) rather than twice. In some affected infants, a certain percentage of cells contain the extra chromosome 13, whereas other cells have the normal two. This finding is known as chromosomal mosaicism.

In infants with trisomy 13 syndrome, associated symptoms and physical findings are variable and depend upon the specific length and location of the duplicated portion of chromosome 13 as well as the percentage of the body cells containing the abnormality. For example, in some infants with trisomy 13 mosaicism, associated symptoms and findings may be less severe.

Abnormalities associated with trisomy 13 syndrome include severe developmental delays, profound mental retardation, incomplete closure of the roof of the mouth (cleft palate), an abnormal groove in the upper lip (cleft lip), and unusually small eyes (microphthalmia). Additional characteristic symptoms and findings include abnormal bending of the fingers, the presence of extra fingers and toes (polydactyly), failure of the testes to descend into the scrotum (cryptorchidism) in affected males, and malformation of the uterus in affected females (i.e., bicornuate uterus). Many infants have severe feeding difficulties, abnor-mally diminished muscle tone (hypotonia), and episodes of temporary cessation of breathing (apnea).

Most infants with trisomy 13 syndrome also have additional physical malformations, including an abnormally small head (microcephaly) with a sloping forehead; widely set eyes (ocular hypertelorism); a broad, flat nose; low-set, malformed ears; and a small jaw (micrognthia). Reddish, purplish benign growths (hemangiomas) may be present on the forehead or other areas due to an abnormal distribution of minute blood vessels (capillaries). Many affected infants may also have additional skeletal abnormalities, heart defects, and brain malformations. Life-threatening complications may develop within the first month of life. Treatment includes symptomatic and supportive measures. The exact cause of trisomy 13 syndrome is unknown.

The following organizations in the General Resources Section can provide additional information: National Organization for Rare Disorders, Inc. (NORD), Genetic Alliance, March of Dimes Birth Defects Foundation, NIH/National Institute of Child Health and Human Development, NIH/National Information Center for Children & Youth with Disabilities (NICHCY)

National Associations & Support Groups

4212 ARC
500 East Border Street, Suite 300
Arlington, TX 76010   817-261-6003
                             800-433-5255
                        TDD: 817-277-0553
          e-mail: thearc@metronet.com
                   thearc.org/welcome.html

Provides informational and emotional support to parents who have a child, adolescent, or adult family member with special needs. P-P programs offer an important connection for a parent who is seeking support for special disability issue, by matching him or her with a trained vetern parent who has already been there.

4213 Congenital Heart Anomalies, Support, Education & Resources

James H. Myers, author

2112 North Wilkins Road
Swanton, OH 43558
419-825-5575
Fax: 419-825-2880
e-mail: chaser@compuserve.com
www.csun.edu/~hfmth006/ch

National organization for support, education and resources for families, patients and professionals who deal with children born with congenital heart malformations. Information on hospitals, medical assistance, and schooling. Offers Chaser News, an international newsletter and Chaser's Pediatric Heart Surgeons Facility Directory.

5000+ Members

4214 Support Organization for Trisomy 18, 13, and Related Disorders

2982 South Union Street
Rochester, NY 14624
716-594-4621
800-716-7638
Fax: 716-594-1507
e-mail: barbsoft@aol.com
www.trisomy.org

SOFT is an international organization. SOFT is a netowrk of families and professional dedication to providing support and undrstanding to families involved in the issue and decision surrounding the diagnosis and care in 718113 and related chromosome disorders. Support is provided during pre-natal diagnosis, to child'd life and after their passing. SOFT is committed to the support of families personal decision in alliance with a parent-professional partnership.

28-40 pages Bi-Monthly

International

4215 In Touch Trust

10 Norman Road, Sale
Cheshire,
United Kingdom

Dedicated to bringing together parents of children with similar special needs such as learning and/or physical disabilities, a particular interest in assisting those affected by rare and complex conditions. Also provides information concerning a wide range of support groups for specific disorders, many of which help families come together for the purpose of mutual support.

4216 Support Organization for Trisomy (S.O.F.T.) Canada, Inc.

760 Brant Street, Suite 420
Burlington, Ontario,
Canada
800-668-0696

Provides support, assistance, and information for families in many different situations and stages of diagnosement, caregiving, and for some, grief. Offers informational packets, booklets, a link-list networking service, newsletters, support groups, patient education, advocacy, journals, a database, and a variety of audio-visual aids.

4217 Support Organization for Trisomy 13/18 and Related Disorders, UK

Tudor Lodge, Redwood, Ross-on-wye
Herefordshire,
United Kingdom

Provides support, assistance, and information for families in many different situations and stages of diagnosement, caregiving, and for some, grief. Offers informational packets, booklets, a link-list networking service, newsletters, support groups, patient education, advocacy, journals, a database, and a variety of audio-visual aids.

Web Sites

4218 Pediatric Database
www.icondata.com/health/ped-base/files/TRISOMY1.HTM

DESCRIPTION

4219 TUBERCULOSIS
Synonym: TB
Disorder Type: Infectious Disease

Tuberculosis is an infectious disease that is most often caused by the bacterium Mycobacterium tuberculosis, but may sometimes result from infection with Mycobacterium bovis or Mycobacterium africanum. As a result of improvements in living conditions, the number of people in the United States infected with this disease declined dramatically throughout most of the twentieth century. However, tuberculosis rates once again began to rise in the mid-1980s in association with such factors as immigration of individuals from countries that had high incidence rates of TB, poverty, poor access to health care among groups at high risk, the increase in AIDS infections, overcrowded and sometimes unsanitary conditions in certain institutional settings, and the development of antibiotic-resistant strains of tuberculosis bacteria. This disease is most prevalent among the elderly, people with compromised immune systems, and those of low socioeconomic status.

Tuberculosis is usually transmitted through airborne droplets coughed or sneezed into the air by an infected person. The droplets are inhaled into the lungs where the bacteria multiply and travel to the lymph nodes that are responsible for draining the lungs; however, in the vast majority of cases, the immune system either destroys or seals off the bacteria. If this primary pulmonary tuberculosis infection is not completely resolved, the bacteria may becomre dormant within certain white blood cells called macrophages and be latr reactivated. This reemergence of symptoms at a later date may be due to influences such as an impaired immune system, corticosteroid drug usage, or advancing age. In addition to the lungs, the tuberculosis bacteria may sometimes spread throughout the body via the bloodstream and affect other parts of the body (extrapulmonary tuberculosis). This type of disseminated disease may infect the lymph nodes, upper respiratory tract, skin, liver, spleen, kidneys, gastrointestinal tract, bones, joints, brain, spine, the sac surrounding the heart (pericardium), and other organs.

Symptoms and physical findings associated with primary pulmonary tuberculosis in children may include enlargement of the lymph nodes and the subsequent compression and obstruction of the large air passages of the lungs (bronchial tubes). This obstruction may result in lung collapse, cough, and less commonly wheezing, rapid breathing (tachypnea), and respiratory distress. Other symptoms may be absent or mild, but more pronounced in infants, and may include moderate difficulty in breathing (dyspnea), a nonproductive cough, and occasionally fever, loss of appetite, and night sweats. In addition, some infants may fail to thrive. Pneumonia may develop and, in rare instances, blister-type lesions may develop in the lungs that sometimes rupture, resulting in the presence of air between the lungs and the chest wall (pneumothorax) and possible associated lung collapse. Complications of progressive primary pulmonary disease may include extensive lung involvement and associated symptoms such as a severe productive cough, high fever, night sweats, and weight loss.

On rare occasions, tuberculosis may be transmitted from mother to fetus through a placental lesion or by the inhalation or swallowing of infected amniotic fluid by the baby before or during birth. Congenital tuberculosis more commonly occurs soon after birth, usually through inhalation of airborne droplets from an infected person. Symptoms and findings associated with congenital tuberculosis may not develop for two or three weeks and may include drowsiness, fever, difficulty in breathing, poor feeding, drainage from the ears, enlarged lymph glands, enlarged liver and spleen (hepatosplenomegaly), abdominal swelling, skin lesions, and failure to thrive.

Diagnosis of tuberculosis may be established through evaluation of family and medical history, physical examination, skin and sputum testing, chest x-ray, and sometimes testing of cerebrospinal and other fluids as well as microscopic examination of tissue samples (biopsy).

Treatment for tuberculosis includes the prolonged administration of at least two different types of antibodies to assure that all bacteria are destroyed. The abtibiotics most often used for children with this disease include combinations of isoniazid, rifampin, pyrazinamide as well as streptomycin, ethambutol, and ethionamide that are especially effective for drug-resistant disease. The antibiotics most often used for children with this disease include combinations of isoniazid, rifampin, pyrazinamide as well as streptomycin, ethambutol, and ethionamide that are especially effective for drug-resistant disease. Children who take these medications are carefully monitored for possible toxic side effects. Corticosteroids may also be administered, especially in children with associated inflammatory irregularities that adversely affect organ function. In addition, the medication isoniazid may sometimes be preventively administered to those at high risk of tuberculosis infection or to those with positive skin test results but no symptomatic or x-ray evidence of disease. Other treatment is symptomatic and supportive.

The following organizations in the General Resources Section can provide additional information: National Organization for Rare Disorders, Inc., (NORD), March of Dimes Birth Defects Foundation, NIH/National Institute of Allergy and Infectious Disease, World Health Organization

National Associations & Support Groups

4220 American Lung Association
1740 Broadway
New York, NY 10019   212-315-8700
                            800-586-4812
                   e-mail: info@lungusa.org
                        www.lungusa.org

Offers research, medical updates, fund-raising, educational materials and public awareness campaigns relating to lung disease and related disorders. Focuses on asthma, tobacco control, and environmental issues.

4221 Centers for Disease Control and Prevention Division: Tuberculosis Elimination
National Center for Prevention Services
1600 Clifton Road NE, MS E-10
Atlanta, GA 30333   404-639-2503
               www.cdc.gov/diseases/diseases.html

4222 National Tuberculosis Center at New Jersey Medical School
Executive Office, Ste GB1, 65 Bergen St
Newark, NJ 07107   973-972-3270

Dr. Lee Rushman

Federal Agencies

4223 New York City Department of Health Bureau of Tuberculosis Control
125 Worth Street
New York, NY 10012   212-788-4204
                  www.cpmc.columbia.edu/hocpp

Web Sites

4224 American Lung Association
www.lungusa.org

4225 Centers for Disease Control
www.cdc.gov/nchstp/tb/default.htm

4226 Columbia University
www.cpmc.columbia.edu/resources/tbcpp/

4227 NOAH
www.noah.cuny.edu/tb/nycdoh/nycdohtb1.html

4228 National Tuberculosis Center
www.nationaltbcenter.edu/

4229 Tuberculosis and Airborne Disease Weekly
www.newsfile.com/xlt.htm

Books

4230 Forgotten Plague: How the Battle Against Tuberculosis Was Won & Lost
Frank Ryan, author

Little Brown & Company, Inc.
34 Beacon Street
Boston, MA 02108   617-227-0730
                     Fax: 617-227-4633

1994 Softcover
ISBN: 0-316763-81-0

Pamphlets

**4231 Classification of Tuberculosis and Other
Mycobacterial Diseases**
American Lung Association
1740 Broadway
New York, NY 10017   212-315-8700

Chart listing different classes of tuberculosis
and other mycobacterial diseases.

DESCRIPTION

4232 TUBEROUS SCLEROSIS
    Synonyms: Epiloia, TS
    Disorder Type: Genetic Disorder
    May involve these systems in the body (see Section III):
    Central Nervous System, Dermatologic System

Tuberous sclerosis (TS) is a hereditary multisystem disorder that may affect the skin, brain, heart, kidneys, or other tissues and organs of the body. The disorder is characterized by multiple, wart-like, raised areas (papules) on the skin of the face (adenoma sebaceum); benign, tumor-like nodules (hamartomas) of the brain, the heart, the kidneys, the nerve-rich membrane at the back of the eyes (retinas), or other organs; episodes of abnormally increased, uncontrolled electrical activity in the brain (seizures); and mental retardation. Associated symptoms and findings may vary greatly from patient to patient, including among members of the same family. TS is caused by abnormal changes (mutations) in a gene or genes. These mutations may occur randomly for unknown reasons (sporadically) or may be inherited as an autosomal dominant trait. At least two genes have been identified that may cause TS. One disease gene, known as TSC1 gene, is located on the long arm (q) of chromosome 9 (9q34). A second gene, called the TSC2 gene, is on the short arm (p) of chromosome 16 (16p13.3). Tuberous sclerosis affects approximately one in 30,000 individuals.

TS is often apparent shortly after birth and presents as distinctive skin abnormalities and the development of either infantile spasms or partial seizures. Infantile spasms are a seizure disorder characterized by sudden, repeated flexion or extension of the muscles of the neck, torso, arms, and legs. Seizures may later take the form of myoclonic epilepsy, in which there are sudden, shock-like contractions of a muscle or muscle groups. As many as 90 percent of infants with TS also have sharply defined areas of abnormally diminished skin coloration (hypopigmentation) on the torso, face, arms, or legs. These areas typically have an ashleaf-like appearance.

Seizures that begin during later childhood are often characterized by prolonged muscle contractions and alternating relaxation and contraction of muscles (generalized tonic-clonic seizures). Seizures tend to become progressively more severe and are often difficult to treat. In addition, approximately 60 to 70 percent of children with TS experience mental retardation, almost all of whom also have seizure disorders. However, seizures also occur in most of those without mental retardation. Generally, the younger a patient experiences symptoms associated with TS, the greater the risk for mental retardation.

Beginning at about age two to six, about 80 percent of children with TS also develop red, shiny nodules (lesions) over the cheeks and nose. These nodules gradually become larger and assume a wart-like, fleshy appearance (adenoma sebaceum). Similar nodules may also develop on the forehead. Many children have additional, distinctive skin lesions. These may include raised, knobby, skin-colored lesions with an orange-peel consistency (shagreen patches) primarily located on the lower back; firm, skin-colored nodules that develop around the nails of the fingers and toes during puberty, and rarely, coffee-colored discolorations of the skin (cafe-au-lait spots).

In patients with TS, the characteristic tumor-like nodules (hamartomas) that develop in the brain are known as tubers. These growths often become hardened due to an abnormal accumulation of calcium salts (calcification). In addition, depending upon their size and location, tubers may block the normal flow of cerebrospinal fluid (CSF), causing an abnormal accumulation of CSF in the brain (hydrocephalus). The severity of neurologic impairment typically increases with the number of tubers within the brain. Rarely, a tuber may differentiate into a malignant brain tumor (astrocytoma).

Approximately 50 percent of affected children also have benign tumors of the heart muscle (rhabdomyoma). Although rhabdomyomas may disrupt the normal rhythm or rate of the heartbeat (arrythmias), these tumors tend to gradually re-solve on their own. Benign, tumor-like nodules or multiple cysts may also develop in the kidneys, causing blood in the urine (hematuria), pain, or, in severe cases, kidney failure. Hamartomas may also develop in other tissues and organs of the body, such as the retinas and the lungs. In patients with severe TS, life-threatening complications may occur by adulthood.

The management of patients with TS is sympto-matic and supportive, including therapy with an-ticonvulsant medications to help control seizures. In addition, physicians may regularly monitor pa-tients to detect certain serious conditions poten-tially associated with TS, such as abnormal accumulations of cerebrospinal fluid or malignant transformation of hamartomas in the brain. If such conditions are confirmed, immediate surgical intervention or other measures are performed as required.

The following organizations in the General Resources Section can provide additional information: National Organization for Rare Disorders, Inc., (NORD), NIH/Office of Rare Diseases, Genetic Alliance, March of Dimes Birth Defects Foundation, Online Mendelian Inheritance in Man: www3.ncbi.nlm.nih.gov/Omim/searchomim.html, NIH/National Institute of Neurological Disorders & Stroke

National Associations & Support Groups

4233 ARC
500 East Border Street, Suite 300
Arlington, TX 76010   512-454-6694
800-433-5255
Fax: 817-277-3491
TDD: 817-277-0553
e-mail: thearc@metronet.com
thearc.org/welcome.html

The ARC of the United States works through education, research and advocacy to improve the quality of life for children and adults with mental retardation and their families and works to prevent both the causes and the effects of men-tal retardation.

4234 National Tuberous Sclerosis Association
8181 Professional Place Suite 110
Landover, MD 20785   301-459-9888
800-225-6878
Fax: 301-459-0394
e-mail: ntsa@ntsa.org
www.ntsa.org

TS is a rare genetic disorder that may affect a number of organs and result in mental retarda-tion. The National Tuberous Sclerosis Associa-tion, Inc., offers referrals, support groups and literature.

Holly Knorr, Managing Editor

4235 Tuberous Sclerosis (NTSA)
8181 Professional Pl
Landover, MD 20785   301-459-9888
800-225-6872
Fax: 301-459-0394

A voluntary, non-profit organization that is dedi-cated: to fostering and supporting tuberous scle-rosis research: providing education of the public, educators and health care professionals providing support of individuals with tuberous sclerosis and their families.

4236 Tuberous Sclerosis Canada
2443 New Wood Drive
Oakville Ontario, L6H
Canada   905-257-1997
800-347-0252
e-mail: jillian.dasilvia@ablelink.org

International

4237 Tuberous Sclerosis Association
Little Barnsley Farm, Catshill, Bromsgrove
Worcesterhire,
United Kingdom
e-mail: tsassn@compuserve.com
ourworld.compuserve.com/homepages/tsassn

Dedicated to providing support to individuals and their families, increasing awareness of the disorder, and promoting fundraising to support research into the causes and management of TS. Also advises on where to obtain assistance con-cerning social services, benefits, and educational concerns and has a Family Care Worker who en-gages in patient and family advocacy. offers a va-riety of materials.

Web Sites

4238 AGSA Newsletter
www.dirsca.org.au/pub/docs/facttube.txt

4239 TS International
www.stsn.nl/tsi/tsi.htm

4240 TS Pages
ourworld.compuserve.com/homepages/Tom_Carter/ts.htm

4241 Tuberous Sclerosis
www.icondata.com/health/pedbase/files/TUBEROUS.HTM

Books

4242 Tuberous Sclerosis

M.R. Gomez, author

Raven Press
1185 Avenue of the Americas
New York, NY 10036   212-930-9500

A revision offering up-to-date medical information to researchers and professionals on TS.

Newsletters

4243 Perspective
National Tuberous Sclerosis Association
8181 Professional Place Suite 110
Landover, MD 22265   301-459-9888
                                        800-225-6872
                                 Fax: 301-459-0394
                            e-mail: ntsa@ntsa.org
                                         www.ntsa.org

Offers the latest research and medical information on tuberous sclerosis to physicians and health care professionals.

Bimonthly

Holly Knorr, Managing Editor

Pamphlets

4244 Living with Tuberous Sclerosis
National Tuberous Sclerosis Association
8181 Professional Place Suite 110
Landover, MD 20785   301-459-9888
                                        800-225-6872
                                 Fax: 301-459-0394
                            e-mail: ntsa@ntsa.org
                                         www.ntsa.org

True stories of people living with Tuberous Sclerosis.

Softcover

DESCRIPTION

4245 TURNER SYNDROME
Synonyms: Chromosome 45,X syndrome, XO syndrome
Disorder Type: Birth Defect, Chromosomal Disorder
May involve these systems in the body (see Section III):
Cardiovascular System, Skeletal System

Turner syndrome is a chromosomal disorder that affects females. In most cases, females have two X chromosomes and males have one X and one Y chromosome in cells of the body. However, in females with Turner syndrome, one of the X chromosomes is deleted (missing) from cells or is functionally defective; some cells have the normal pair of X chromosomes whereas others do not (mosaicism). Although associated symptoms and findings may be variable, the most consistent abnormalities associated with the disorder include short stature and defective development of the ovaries (gonadal dysgenesis).

Many newborns with Turner syndrome have an abnormal accumulation of fluid in and associated swelling of the backs of the hands and the tops of the feet (peripheral lymphedema). Additional features that may be apparent at birth include short stature; an abnormally short, webbed neck (pterygium colli) with a low hairline; a narrow roof of the mouth (palate) or a small jaw (micrognathia); abnormal outward deviation of the elbows upon extension (cubitus valgus); a broad chest with widely spaced, underdeveloped, and/or inverted nipples; or deeply set, narrow, and/or outwardly curved (convex) nails. In most cases, females with Turner syndrome also have kidney (renal) malformations (e.g., horseshoe kidney and/or cleft or double renal pelvis). In addition, in some cases, heart (cardiac) defects may be present, such as abnormalities affecting the major artery (aorta) that arises from the lwer left chamber (ventricle) of the heart (e.g., bicuspid aortic valve, coarctation of the aorta). In almost all affected females, there is also defective development of the ovaries (ovarian dysgenesis), i.e., the paired glands within which the female reproductive cells are produced (ova or eggs) and from which certain female hormones are secreted. Consequently, in most cases, female secondary sexual characteristics fail to develop (e.g., breast development, appearance of hair in the pubic area and under the arms, menstruation) and most affected females are infertile. In addition, although intelligence is typically normal, some females with Turner syndrome may experience learning disabilities (e.g., difficulty with visual-spacial relationships) and may have poor coordination. The treatment of children with Turner syndrome may include hormone replacement therapy (e.g., estrogen therapy, human growth hormone therapy); surgical intervention for congenital heart defects, renal malformations, webbing of the neck, or other abnormalities; special education for those with learning disabilities; and other treatment measures as required. Turner syndrome is thought to result from errors during the division of a parent's reproductive cells (meiosis). According to estimates in the medical literature, the disorder may affect from approximately one in 2,000 to one in 4,000 female newborns.

The following organizations in the General Resources Section can provide additional information: Genetic Alliance, March of Dimes Birth Defects Foundation, NIH/Office of Rare Diseases, Online Mendelian Inheritance in Man: www3.ncbi.nlm.nih.gov/Omim/searchomim.html, National Organization for Rare Disorders, Inc., (NORD), NIH/National Institute of Child Health and Human Development

National Associations & Support Groups

4246 American Society for Reproductive Disorders
1209 Montgomery Highway
Birmingham, AL 35216   205-987-5000
                                                    Fax: 205-978-5005
                                    e-mail: asrm@asrm.org
                                    www.asrm.org/mainpati.html

The ASRM provides patient understanding and involvement in reproduction medicine and health care decision making.

4247 Human Growth Foundation
7777 Leesburg Pike-#202 S
Falls Church, VA 22043   703-883-1773
                               800-451-6434
                    e-mail: hgfound@erols.com
                               www.genetic.org

Devoted to the dissemination of medical knowledge of this and similar disorders, along with providing support for the sufferes and their families.

4248 Turner Syndrome Society
7777 Keele Street, 2nd Floor
Concord, ON L4K 1Y7,
Canada   905-660-7766

Provides support services for individualsand their families and disseminates up-to-date medical information to affected families, physicians and other health care professionals, and the general public. Also provides educational newsletter, brochures, and booklets, and a video documentary. Offers support groups and holds an annual conference.

4249 Turner's Syndrome Society
1313 South East 5th Street,Suite327
Minneapolis, MN 55414   612-379-3607
                               800-365-9944
                          Fax: 612-379-3619
                    www.turner-syndrome-us.org

More than 38 chapters across the country. Goals are to promote public awareness of the disease, support those affected by the condition and aid in continuing research. Membership dues for a single person is $40, a family is $60, and for professionals is $60.

2,500 members

Michelle Allen, Chapter Membership Director

State Agencies & Support Groups

Alaska

4250 Turner's Syndrome Society of Alaska
1334 N Street
Anchorage, AK 99501   907-279-3202

Mary Tullius

Arizona

4251 Turner's Syndrome Society of Arizona
8151 East Smokehouse Trail
Scottsdale, AZ 85264   480-443-3805

Keith Edwards

California

4252 Turner's Syndrome Society of Bay Area
89 Breaker Drive
Bay Point, CA 94565   925-458-1658

Rosemary Morris

Colorado

4253 Turner's Syndrome Society of Rocky Mountain
2292 Fallview Drive
Pueblo, CO 81006   719-542-6706

Lisa Mawson

Connecticut

4254 Turner's Syndrome Society of Connecticut
11 Fallview Drive
Wethersfield, CT 06109   860-529-9985

Choong Morelli

Florida

4255 Turner's Syndrome Society of Northern Florida
8054 S.W. 108th Loop
Ocala, FL 34481   352-854-4898

Carol Larson

Georgia

4256 Turner's Syndrome Society of Atlanta
1113 Sandy Lane Drive
Alpharetta, GA 30202   770-642-2165

Shelly McClain

Iowa

4257 Turner's Syndrome Society of Iowa/New Found Friends
4775 Sharon Center Road S.W.
Iowa City, IA 52240   319-683-2626

Cathie Berglund

Kentucky

4258 Turner's Syndrome Society of Kentucky
380 Bob-O-Link Drive
Lexington, KY 40503   606-278-5935

Elizabeth Howard

Louisiana

4259 Turner's Syndrome Society of Gulf Coast
7731 Butterfield Road
New Orleans, LA 70126   504-241-2368

Donna Baudier

Maryland

4260 Turner's Syndrome Society of Maryland
2206 229th Street
Pasadena, MD 21122   410-360-5571

Kathy Mattson

Massachusetts

4261 Turner's Syndrome Society of New England
60 Joy Street #303
Boston, MA 02115   617-557-4837

Geralyn Dwyer

Minnesota

4262 Turner's Syndrome Society of Minnesota
1313 SE 5th Street, Suite 327
Minneapolis, MN 55414   612-379-3607
                         Fax: 612-379-3619
                         www.turner-syndrome-us.org

Becky Mobarry

Mississippi

4263 Turner's Syndrome Society of Southeastern Michigan
731 Watersedge
Ann Arbor, MI 48105   734-663-6493

Carol Collins

Missouri

4264 Turner's Syndrome Society of West Illinios
1514 Azalea Drive
St. Louis, MO 63119   314-351-9416

Cheryl Jost

Nevada

4265 Turner's Syndrome Society of Nevada
4683 Monterey Circle
Las Vegas, NV 89109   702-736-3958

Jackie LeDuc

New Hampshire

4266 Turner's Syndrome Society of Northern New England
38 Beaman
Laconia, NH 03246   603-524-6011

Lori Ann Pawlowski

New Jersey

4267 Turner's Syndrome Society of New Jersey
22 Shadylawn Drive
Madison, NJ 07940   973-377-5639

Julia Rickert

New York

4268 Turner's Syndrome Society of Long Island and New York City
49 Cliff Road
Hicksville, NY 11801   516-822-9438

Jessica Fitzgibbon

North Carolina

4269 Turner's Syndrome Society of North Carolina
111 Weatherly Place
Cary, NC 27511 919-859-1133

Pam Gorman

Ohio

4270 Turner's Syndrome Society of Southwestern Ohio
8530 Gateview Court
Dayton, OH 45424 937-667-5276

Barb Schwandner

Oklahoma

4271 Turner's Syndrome Society of Oklahoma
2207 Fairway Drive
Duncan, OK 73533 580-252-4510

David Laurel

Pennsylvania

4272 Turner's Syndrome Society of Philadelphia
601 Ferris Lane
New Britain, PA 18901 215-348-3005

Barbara Flink

Rhode Island

4273 Turner's Syndrome Society of Rhode Island
311 Crestwood Road
Warwick, RI 02886 401-884-8382

Lynne Zelonis

South Carolina

4274 Turner's Syndrome Society of South Carolina
1002 Madrid Avenue
Port Royal, SC 29935 843-521-0713

Rebecca Kreps

Texas

4275 Turner's Syndrome Society of Houston
3000 Greenridge #1412
Houston, TX 77057 281-784-4303

Jennifer Chumas

Utah

4276 Turner's Syndrome Society of Salt Lake City
4084 South 300 East #B
Salt Lake City, UT 84107 801-281-0980

Sarah Stevenson

Virginia

4277 Turner's Syndrome Society of National Capitol Area
9826 Hampton Lane
Fairfax, VA 22030 703-591-8442

Gena Norquist

Washington

4278 Turner's Syndrome Society of Inland Northwest
N 5317 Washington
Spokane, WA 99205 509-326-3703

Nancy Owen

Wisconsin

4279 Turner's Syndrome Society of Southeastern Wisconsin
4572 S 14th
Milwaukee, WI 53221 414-871-5930

Lynn Holland

Web Sites

4280 American Society of Reproductive Medical Fertility Fact Sheet
www.asrm.org/mainpati.html

4281 Endocrine Society
www.endo-society.org/pubaf-
fai/factshee/turner.htm

4282 Pediatric Database
www.icondata.com/health/ped-
base/files/TURNERSY.HTM

4283 Usenet
alt.support.turner-syndrom

Newsletters

4284 Turner's Syndrome News
Turner's Syndrome Society of the United States
1313 S.E. 5th Street-Suite 327
Minneapolis, MN 55414

800-365-9944
Fax: 612-379-3619
www.turner-syndrome-us.org

Includes articles addressing current issues in
Turner's Syndrome, updates on national and local activities and letters from girls and women
with Turner's Syndrome and their families.

Quarterly

Pamphlets

4285 Answers to Some Commonly Asked Questions
Turner's Syndrome Society of the United States
1313 S.E. 5th Street-Suite 327
Minneapolis, MN 55414

800-365-9944
Fax: 612-379-3619
www.turner-syndrome

Offers information on the Society's activities
and the role they play in supporting people with
Turner's Syndrome.

4286 Turner's Syndrome
Human Growth Foundation
7777 Leesburg Pike Suite 202S
Falls Church, VA 22043

703-883-1773
800-451-6434

DESCRIPTION

4287 ULCERATIVE COLITIS

May involve these systems in the body (see Section III):

Digestive System

Ulcerative colitis is an inflammatory bowel disease (IBD) characterized by chronic inflammation and ulceration of the lining of the colon, the major part of the large intestine. The disease initially affects the lowest region of the large intestine (rectum) and gradually progresses to involve varying lengths or all of the colon. The range and severity of associated symptoms is extremely variable and may depend in part on the amount of the colon that is affected. Ulcerative colitis usually becomes apparent during adolescence or young adulthood. However, in some patients, associated symptoms may occur as early as the first year of life. The frequency of the disorder varies greatly in different countries and is thought to be higher in urban areas. In the United States and northern Europe, ulcerative colitis affects approximately 100 to 200 per 100,000 individuals in the general population. In developed countries, inflammatory bowel disease, including ulcerative colitis, is the most common cause of chronic intestinal inflammation during mid-childhood. The exact cause of ulcerative colitis is unknown. However genetic, immune, and environmental factors are thought to be contributing factors.

In patients with ulcerative colitis, the onset of symptoms may be gradual (insidious) or sudden, rapid, and severe (fulminant). Most patients experience episodes of watery diarrhea with varying amounts of blood, mucus, or pus. Associated findings may include abdominal cramping and pain; persistant, ineffectual spasms of the rectum (tenesmus); and an urgent, compelling urge to defecate. Fulminant colitis is characterized by over six daily bowel movements, a high fever, chills, abnormally low levels of iron or the protein albumin in the blood, an increase in certain circulating white blood cells (leukocytosis), and other findings. In some children, additional findings include failure to grow and gain weight at the expected rate and lack of appetite (anorexia). The frequency of episodes may vary greatly. Most patients experience periods of remission during which symptoms subside and eventual, periodic recurrences (exacerbations). However, some patients may have infrequent episodes and others may experience severe, ongoing symptoms.

Certain complications may occur in association with ulcerative colitis. For example, because of blood loss during episodes, there may be inadequate levels of iron and abnormally reduced levels of the oxygen-carrying protein of the blood (iron-deficiency anemia). Some individuals with ulcerative colitis may develop sudden massive enlargement of the colon (toxic megacolon). Without prompt, appropriate treatment, toxic megacolon may result in tearing or perforation of the colon, potentially causing life-threatening complications. In addition, patients who have ulcerative colitis for more than 10 years have an increased risk of colon cancer. Regular examination of the colon (colonoscopies) and biopsies are recommended beginning at eight to 10 years after disease onset to help ensure prompt detection and treatment. During a colonoscopy, tissue inside the colon is examined using a flexible viewing instrument. During a biopsy, small samples of tissue are removed from the colon for examination under a microscope.

Many patients with ulcerative colitis may also eventually experience more generalized, systemic symptoms. By the third decade of life, some patients may develop ankylosing spondylitis (AS), a chronic, progressive, inflammatory disease that affects joints of the spine and results in pain, stiffness, and possible loss of spinal mobility. In patients with ulcerative colitis, AS most commonly affects joints of the back and the hips and may cause lower back pain and stiffness, particularly in the morning. Some patients with ulcerative colitis may also develop a chronic skin condition characterized by irregular, bluish-red skin sores (pyoderma gangrenosum); chronic inflammation of the liver (chronic active hepatitis); and inflammation of the bile ducts (primary sclerosing cholangitis).

The treatment of ulcerative colitis is directed at managing symptoms and preventing future episodes. In patients with mild colitis, treatment often includes administration of the drug sulfasalazine, which may alleviate symptoms and potentially prevent recurrences. Patients with moderate to severe colitis who do not respond to such treatment may receive corticosteroid therapy, such as with the drug prednisone. If affected individuals have fulminant colitis or colitis that is unresponsive to drug therapy, treatment may include surgical removal of the colon (colectomy). Additional treatment is symptomatic and supportive.

The following organizations in the General Resources Section can provide additional information: Genetic Alliance, National Organization for Rare Disorders, Inc., (NORD), March of Dimes Birth Defects Foundation, Online Mendelian Inheritance in Man: www3.ncbi.nlm.nih.gov/Omim/searchomim.html, NIH/National Digestive Diseases Information Clearinghouse

National Associations & Support Groups

4288 Center for Digestive Disorders
Central Dupage Hospital
225 N Winfield Rd
Winfield, IL 60190

4289 Crohn's & Colitis Foundation of America
386 Park Avenue South, 17th Fl.
New York, NY 10016   212-685-3440
                             800-932-2423
                        Fax: 212-779-4098
                             www.ccfa.org

Supports basic and clinical research into a cure and treatment for Crohn's disease and ulcerative colitis; conducts professional education activities; produces public service programs and a wide variety of literature about inflammatory bowel disease for patients and their families, professionals and the public; and sponsors more than 97 chapters and satellite groups.

Barbara T. Boyle, Executive Director

4290 Crohn's and Colitis Foundation of Canada
21 St. Clair Ave E, Ste 301
Toronto, Ontario M4T 1L9,   416-920-5035
                                 800-387-1479
                   e-mail: ccfc@netcoma.ca
                             www.ccfc.ca

4291 Digestive Disease National Coalition
507 Capitol Ct, Ste 200
Washington, DC 20002   202-544-7497
                            Fax: 202-546-7105

Promotes federal investment in biomedical research. Serves as a research for consumer-directed educational information and has local support groups. Offers a toll-free hotline, and provides patient networking services.

4292 United Ostomy Association Hotline
19772 MacArthur Blvd.-Suite 200
Irvine, CA 92612   949-660-8624
                                 800-826-0826
                            Fax: 949-660-9262
                                 www.uoa.org

An advocate for ostomy and alternative procedure patients answering questions from employment issues to insurability practices.

Web Sites

4293 Colitis Cookbook
www.colitiscookbook.com/

4294 Crohn's and Colitis Foundation of Canada
www.ccfc.ca

4295 IBS Self-help group
www.ibsgroup.org/

4296 NewsGroup
www.altsupport.crohns-colitis

4297 Thrive Online
www.thriveonline.com/health/Library/

Books

4298 Alive and Kicking

Rolf Benirschke, author

Rolf Benirschke Enterprises
P.O. Box 9922
Rancho Santa Fe, CA 92067

800-560-9700
Fax: 858-755-8597
e-mail: jhedges@iexpres.com
www.greatcomebacks.com

Football star writes of his struggle with ulcerative colitis, and hepatitis C, providing encouragement and inspiration to patients, and others who are interested in an incrediable story.

Softcover
ISBN: 1-885553-40-4

Judy Hedges, Assistant to President

Newsletters

4299 Inner Circle

Reach Out for Youth with Ileitis and Colitis
15 Chemung Place
Jericho, NY 11753   516-822-8010

Newsletter for youth with ileitis and colitis.

Pamphlets

4300 Bleeding in the Digestive Tract

Nat'l Digestive Diseases Information Clearinghouse
9000 Rockville Pike
Bethesda, MD 20892   301-496-3583

Informational fact sheet.

DESCRIPTION

4301 URTICARIA

Synonym: Hives

May involve these systems in the body (see Section III):

Dermatologic System

Urticaria, more commonly known as hives, is a skin condition characterized by the development of raised, usually itchy (pruritic), white or reddish lesions (wheals). The wheals associated with urticaria vary in size and may sometimes blend together to form large, patchy skin lesions. Although individual lesions may disappear within minutes, hours, or days, new eruptions may continue to appear for weeks. Urticaria is considered to be a chronic skin disorder if wheals continue to appear for six weeks or longer.

Although the cause of urticaria is sometimes unknown, it often results as an immune or allergic response during which histamine or other substances are released causing small blood vessels in the upper skin layer to widen and release fluid, thus producing the characteristic wheals associated with hives. These allergic reactions may be caused by ingestion of certain foods such as shellfish, strawberries, nuts, eggs; drugs such as aspirin, penicillin, or codeine; and food dyes or other additives. In addition, allergic responses may be triggered by contact with certain plant substances, insects, animals or animal saliva, or topical skin preparations. Other causative agents may include injection of certain drugs, blood transfusions, insect bites or stings, and inhalation of pollen and other allergens.

Urticaria may also develop in association with certain viral infections such as infectious mononucleosis or hepatitis, certain bacterial or parasitic infections, or in response to the cold, the sun, or exercise. Hives are also associated with many other disorders. For example, hives may develop in conjunction with swelling of certain areas of soft tissue (angioedema or angioneurotic edema). Angioedema involves deeper layers of the skin as well as the upper respiratory tract, the gastrointestinal tract, the face and neck, the hands and feet, and genitalia. A distinct disorder known as urticaria pigmentosa may develop during early childhood and is characterized by reddish-brown skin lesions that are spread over the body and change into hive-like lesions when stroked, rubbed, or scratched. Hives may be associated with other systemic disorders and with certain inherited disorders such as amyloidosis, familial cold urticaria, and hereditary angioedema, which is a severe and potentially life-threatening form of angioedema.

Hives often disappear quickly with no intervention; however, the application of calamine lotion or the administration of antihistamines may be helpful in relieving associated itching and swelling. Children with acute, severe urticaria or those who experience difficulty in breathing or swallowing require immediate medical attention. Other treatment for urticaria is often dependent upon the underlying cause. For example, the administration of two specific types of antihistamines is often indicated for the control of chronic urticaria, while sunscreen protection is the treatment of choice for those individuals with urticaria resulting from sun exposure (solar urticaria). Stress reduction is often effective in reducing symptoms associated with hives. In addition, if a causative agent can be found, the permanent removal of that agent often precludes recurrent episodes. Other treatment is symptomatic and supportive.

The following organizations in the General Resources Section can provide additional information: Genetic Alliance, March of Dimes Birth Defects Foundation, NIH/National Child Health and Human Development, NIH/National Institute of Arthritis and Musculoskeletal and Skin Diseases, NIH/National Institute of Allergy and Infectious Diseases

National Associations & Support Groups

4302 Allergy Information Association
25 Ponynter Drive Suite 7
Weston, Ontario, M9R
Canada

Web Sites

4303 AAD
www.aad.org/aadpamphrework/Urticaria.html

4304 Allergy Web
www.allergyweb.com/articles/ChronicUrticaria-
MD.html

4305 InteliHealth
www.intelihealth.com/IH/ihtIH?t=8210&p=~b

DESCRIPTION

4306 VENTRICULAR SEPTAL DEFECTS
Synonym: VSDs
Disorder Type: Birth Defect, Heart

Ventricular septal defects (VSDs) are considered the most common structural heart malformations, comprising approximately 25 to 30 percent of all heart defects that are present at birth (congenital). VSDs are characterized by the presence of an abnormal opening in the fibrous muscular partition (septum) that separates the two lower pumping chambers (ventricles) of the heart. The ventricles are the chambers that pump blood out of the heart via large blood vessels (arteries). The pulmonary artery arises from the base of the right ventricle and carries oxygen-poor (deoxygenated) blood to the lungs, where the exchange of oxygen and carbon dioxide occurs. The aorta, the main artery of the body, arises from the base of the left ventricle and carries oxygen-rich (oxygenated) blood to the body's tissues.

In infants with ventricular septal defects, the abnormal opening in the septum between the two ventricles allows oxygenated blood in the left ventricle to flow into the right ventricle and recirculate to the lungs rather than to the rest of the body's tissues. Symptoms and findings may vary, depending upon the size and location of the ventricular septal defect and the associated effects on pulmonary blood pressure and flow. If the VSD is large, it may result in significantly increased blood flow through the lungs blood vessels.

Small VSDs usually cause no associated symptoms and, in up to 50 percent of patients, may close spontaneously before school age. Small ventricular septal defects may be detected during a routine physical examination based upon characteristic heart sounds (heart murmurs) heard with a stethoscope. In infants with larger VSDs, too much blood is pumped to the lungs. This may result in persistent elevation of blood pressure in the pulmonary circulation (pulmonary hypertension), enlargement of the heart (cardiomegaly), and abnormally rapid breathing (tachypnea). Additional symptoms and findings may include increased susceptibility to lower respiratory tract infections, increased sweating, difficulties feeding, and failure to grow and gain weight at the expected rate (failure to thrive). When these symptoms and findings occur, the infant is said to have congestive heart failure (CHF). Large VSDs may be diagnosed upon a complete clinical examination, detection of distinctive heart murmurs, and various specialized tests, such as x-ray studies, echocardiogram (ultrasound of the heart), electrocardiogram, or cardiac catheterization.

Children and adolescents with VSDs may be at an increased risk of bacterial infection of the lining of the heart (endocarditis). Such infection is rare before the age of two years. Due to the increased risk of bacterial endocarditis, affected individuals are cautioned to take antibiotic medication before dental visits and surgical procedures. Depending upon the size and severity of the VSD, treatment may include the use of certain medications (e.g., diuretics, digitalis medications)supportive measures to ensure proper nutrition and help maintain normal growth (e.g., increasing caloric intake, nasogastric feedings); or early surgical correction, such as between six to 12 months of age or earlier if necessary. Small VSDs often require no therapy.

Ventricular septal defects may occur as isolated conditions or with other congenital heart defects or other birth defects. In some patients, VSDs may occur in association with certain underlying genetic syndromes, chromosomal abnormalities, or malformation syndromes that are caused by exposure to certain infectious agents, medications, or other environmental factors (teratogenic syndromes).

The following organizations in the General Resources Section can provide additional information: Genetic Alliance, March of Dimes Birth Defects Foundation, National Organization for Rare Diseases, Inc., (NORD), NIH/National Heart, Lung & Blood Institute, NIH/National Institute of Child Health and Human Development

National Associations & Support Groups

4307 American Heart Association
7272 Greenville Avenue
Dallas, TX 75231
214-373-6300
800-242-8721
Fax: 214-706-1341
e-mail: inquire@amhrt.org
www.amhrt.org

Supports research, education and community service programs with the objective of reducing premature death and disability from cardiovascular diseases and stroke; coordinates the efforts of health professionals, and other engaged in the fight against heart and circulatory disease.

Web Sites

4308 Children's Health Information Network
www.ohsu.edu.cliniweb/C14/C14.240.400.html

4309 Congenital Heart Disease Resource Page
www.csun.edu/~hcmth011/heart/
e-mail: sheri.berger@csun.edu
www.csun.edu/~hcmth011/heart/

4310 Southern Illinois University School of Medicine
www.siumed.edu/peds/teaching/patient%20education.htm

DESCRIPTION

4311 VIRAL HEPATITIS

Disorder Type: Infectious Disease

Hepatitis refers to an inflammatory condition of the liver that may result from viral, bacterial, or parasitic infection; certain blood disorders; or exposure to certain drugs, toxins, or alcohol. However, viral infection is most frequently the cause of hepatitis. Liver inflammation may develop in association with certain viral infections such as German measles (rubella), chickenpox (varicella), or HIV. In addition, there are at least five infectious agents known as hepatotropic viruses that specifically target the liver.

Hepatitis A virus is thought to be the most common cause of hepatitis in children, with an extremely high prevalence rate in underdeveloped countries. In addition, approximately 30 percent of adults in the United States show evidence of an earlier infection with hepatitis A. This form of hepatitis is usually spread by fecal-oral contamination through drinking water, food, or direct contact. Children under five years of age often have no symptoms, but still acquire immunity to future hepatitis A infection. When symptoms become evident in children, they are often mild and may include fever, weakness, general discomfort, loss of appetite, nausea and vomiting, diarrhea, and abdominal distress. Occasionally, some children develop a very slight yellowing of the eyes, skin, and mucous membranes (jaundice). Hepatitis A is an acute, self-limited form of this disease, with a return to general health typically within one month, although relapses may occur. Life-threatening complications associated with this type of hepatitis are extremely rare. Prevention of hepatitis A transmission is directed toward the teaching of good hygiene (e.g., frequent hand washing) in hospitals, child-care facilities, etc. In addition, the administration of recently developed vaccines or immunoglobulin is recommended for children and adults who plan to travel to countries with a high incidence of hepatitis A. Young children are at risk for becoming carriers of this disease while older travelers may be at risk for more significant disease involvement. Early administration of immunoglobulin is also recommended for children and adults who may have been exposed to the virus. Other treatment is symptomatic and supportive.

Hepatitis B infection in children and adolescents may be transmitted through intravenous injection of blood, blood products, or drugs; sharing of needles or razors; ear piercing with contaminated equipment; and other carrier-contact modes of transmission. For example, the hepatitis B virus may be spread by apparently healthy people who are chronic carriers. Symptoms usually develop six to seven weeks after exposure, persist for six to eight weeks, and are similar to those of hepatitis A, but are often more severe. Additional manifestations may include tenderness and enlargement of the liver (hepatomegaly), enlargement of the spleen (splenomegaly), swollen lymph glands, accumulation of fluid within the abdomen (ascites), skin lesions, or joint pain (arthralgia). Newborns of infected mothers are at high risk for infection during delivery, possibly through infected amniotic fluid, blood, or fecal material. Although infected newborns usually do not manifest symptoms, if left untreated, most develop a chronic form of hepatitis that may result in potentially life-threatening liver disease during adulthood. Prevention of hepatitis B infection in newborns is first directed toward testing for infection in pregnant women. If a mother is positive for infection, her newborn is given a hepatitis B immune globulin injection within the first day of life, followed by immunization with hepatitis B vaccine. The American Academy of Pediatrics as well as the United States Public Health Service advocate administration of a series of hepatitis B and immunoglobulin vaccinations to all infants in order to prevent transmission and subsequent complications. Immunizations are also recommended to anyone who may have been exposed to hepatitis B. Treatment is symptomatic and supportive.

Hepatitis C may be transmitted among the general population through intravenous drug use, transfusions of blood or blood products, sexual contact, and other, unknown causes. Although transmission from an infected mother to her infant is possible, it is rare except in instances where the mother also has HIV or other contributing factors. The onset of disease is approximately seven to nine weeks after exposure and symptoms associated with hepatitis C are similar to those of other types of viral hepatitis. In addition, hepatitis C is the most likely of all the hepatotropic viruses to cause chronic hepatitis. Complications may also include cirrhosis and cancer of the liver, but rarely fulminant hepatitis. Because infection with the hepatitis C virus may occur more than once in the same person, a preventive vaccine is not effective. Treatment is symptomatic and supportive.

The hepatitis D virus cannot replicate itself without the help of the hepatitis B virus; therefore, hepatitis D only occurs in people with prior or simultaneous infection with hepatitis B. The most common mode of transmission in the United States is through intimate contact and needle sharing; therefore, this form of hepatitis is relatively rare in children in this country. Symptoms and findings may be similar to but more severe than those of hepatitis B infection. There is no vaccine for hepatitis D; therefore, prevention is directed toward prevention of hepatitis B infection. Treatment is symptomatic and supportive.

Hepatitis E is the cause of epidemic-associated infection and is spread by fecal-oral transmission, usually through contaminated water or food. The symptoms and findings of this form of disease are similar to but more severe than those associated with hepatitis A. However, this acute, self-limited infection may pose a life-threatening risk to pregnant women. Hepatitis E is extremely rare in the United States, thus far occurring only in people who have traveled to or emigrated from indigenous countries. No vaccine is available. Treatment is symptomatic and supportive.

The following organizations in the General Resources Section can provide additional information: National Organization for Rare Disorders, Inc., (NORD), March of Dimes Birth Defects Foundation, NIH/National Institute of Allergy and Infectious Disease, World Health Organization (WHO)

National Associations & Support Groups

4312 American Liver Foundation
75 Maiden Lane Suite 603
New York, NY 10038   212-668-1000
800-465-4837
Fax: 212-483-8179
e-mail: info@liverfoundation.org
www.liverfoundation.org

Organization provides several different medias for answering questions and to help clarify any uncertainties the individual may be experiencing.

4313 Hepatitis B Foundation
700 East Butler Avenue
Doylestown, PA 18901   215-489-4900
Fax: 215-489-4920
e-mail: info@hepb.org
www.hepb.org

4314 Hepatitis Foundation International
30 Sunrise Terr
Cedar Grove, NJ 07009   973-239-1035
800-891-0707
Fax: 973-857-5044
e-mail: hfi@intac.com
www.hepfi.org

Thelma King Theil

4315 National Headquarters Hepatitis C Foundation
1502 Russett Dr
Warminster, PA 18974   215-672-2606
Fax: 215-672-1518
e-mail: hepatitis_c_foundation@msn.com
www.hepcfoundation.org

Web Sites

4316 Centers for Disease Control
www.cdc.gov/epo/mmwr/other/case_def/hep_a1.html

4317 Columbia University
http://cpmcnet.columbia.edu/dept/gi/autoimmume.html

4318 Hepatitis United
www.hepu.org/

4319 PedBase
www.icondata.com/health/pedbase/files/HEPA-
TITI.HTM

Pamphlets

4320 Chronic Viral Hepatitis Backgrounder
Schering Corporation

Kenilworth, NJ 07033   908-298-4000

Offers information and statistics on viral hepatitis.

4321 Viral Hepatitis: Everybody's Problem?
American Liver Foundation
1425 Pompton Avenue
Cedar Grove, NJ 07009   973-857-2626
                               800-223-0179

Covering a broad range of topics including: a
definition of the disease, descriptions of types of
infections, transmission, symptoms, treatment
options and prevention.

DESCRIPTION

4322 WILLIAMS SYNDROME

Synonyms: WBS, Williams-Beuren syndrome, WMS, WS

Disorder Type: Developmental Milestones, Genetic Disorder

Williams syndrome is a genetic disorder characterized by mild growth delays before birth (prenatal growth retardation); growth delays after birth (postnatal growth retardation); mild short stature; characteristic abnormalities of the head and face (craniofacial area); and variable levels of mental deficiency. Unusual features of the head and face may result in a distinctive appearance that becomes more pronounced with advancing age. Characteristic features include a rounded face with full cheeks; full, thick lips and a large mouth that is typically in an open position, prominent ears; flared eyebrows; short eyelid folds (palpebral fissures); and a broad nasal bridge with a wide tip and nostrils that flare forward (anteverted). Dental abnormalities are often present, such as small teeth (hypodontia) with underdeveloped (hypoplastic) tooth enamel. Distinctive abnormalities of the eyes may also occur, including divergence of one eye in relation to the other (strabismus) and an unusual star-like (stellate) pattern in the colored portions of the eyes (irides).

Most children and adults with Williams syndrome also have mild to moderate mental retardation. Affected individuals may have an intelligence quotient (I.Q.) ranging from 80, which is considered the low end of average, to 40, which is considered moderate mental retardation. The average I.Q. is approximately 56, which is considered at the lower end of the range for mild mental retardation. Other findings associated with Williams syndrome may include a short attention span, easy distractibility, a poor relationship between visual stimuli and resultant movements (motor-visual integration skills), and strong general language skills as opposed to general cognitive abilities. Most affected children and adults have a friendly personality and a talkative, outgoing manner of speech.

Some infants and children with Williams syndrome may also have additional physical abnormalities, such as heart defects, musculoskeletal abnormalities, unusually increased blood calcium levels during infancy (transient infantile hypercalcemia), or other abnormalities. For example, affected infants may develop narrowing in the area above the valve leading from the lower left-sided pumping chamber (ventricle) of the heart to the main artery (aorta) of the body (supravalvular aortic stenosis); obstruction of normal blood flow from the right ventricle of the heart to the lungs (branch pulmonary stenosis); high blood pressure (hypertension); or other cardiovascular abnormalities. Musculoskeletal defects may include limited movements of certain joints; abnormal curvature of the spine (e.g., scoliosis, kyphosis, lordosis); and an awkward gait. Some individuals with Williams syndrome also have abnormalities affecting the urinary tract, such as the return flow of urine from the urinary bladder back into a ureter (vesicoureteral reflux), recurrent urinary tract infections, and other findings (e.g., nephrocalcinosis, bladder diverticula). Digestive problems may also occur, including chronic constipation. Depending upon the specific abnormalities present, treatment may include limitation of calcium in and elimination of vitamin D from the diet in those with high levels of calcium in the blood; heart surgery for those with certain structural cardiac defects; and special educational and supportive services, such as physical therapy, individualized educational programs, speech therapy, and occupational therapy. Other treatment is symptomatic and supportive.

Most cases of Williams syndrome appear to occur randomly (sporadically) for unknown reasons; however, some familial cases have been reported. Sporadic and inherited cases of the disorder appear to occur due to missing genetic material (deletion) from genes located next to one another (contiguous genes) on the long arm (q) of chromosome 7 (7q11.23). The syndrome is thought to affect approximately one in 10,000 newborns.

The following organizations in the General Resources Section can provide additional information: NIH/National Institute of Child Health and Human Development, Genetic Alliance, ARC, National Organization for Rare Disorders, Inc., (NORD), NIH/Office of Rare Diseases, Online Mendelian Inheritance in Man: www3.ncbi.nlm.nih.gov/Omim/searchomim.html

National Associations & Support Groups

4323 Canadian Association for Williams Syndrome
P.O. Box 2115
Vancouver, BC V6B
Canada   604-853-0231
                        e-mail: sev@uniserve.com
                        www.bmts.com/~williams/caws.htm

CAWS is dedicated to providing support and assistance to families with affected children and supporting research into educational, behavioral, social, and medical aspects of this syndrome. Committed to locating affected families who are unaware of the association; becoming a visible group in the medical, scientific, educational, and professional communities in order to facilitate referrals of newly diagnosed individuals; and provides a variety of educational materials.

4324 Cincinnati Center for Developmental Disorders
3333 Burnet Avenue, Pavilion Building
Cincinnati, OH 45229   513-636-4688
                        Fax: 513-636-7361
                        www.chmcc.org

4325 Williams Syndrome Association
1312 North Campbell, Ste 33
Royal Oak, MI 48067   248-541-3630
                        e-mail: TMonkaba@aol.com
                        www.williams-syndrome.org

4326 Williams Syndrome Association
P.O. Box 297
Clawson, MI 48017   248-541-3630
                        Fax: 248-541-3631
                        e-mail: WSAoffice@aol.com
                        members.aol.com/BobHazard/wsc.html

Devoted to improving the lives of individuals with Williams Syndrome and their families.

4327 Williams Syndrome Foundation
University of California
Irvine, CA 92679   949-824-7259
                        e-mail: wsfmail@prodigy.net
                        www.williamssyndrome.org/

The WSF offers support for those affected with the condition through opportunities in education, housing, employment and recreation.

Research Centers

**4328 Patient Recruitment & Public Liaison Office
Clinical Center**
10 Cloister Court, Building 61
Bethesda, MD 20892
                        800-411-1222
                        Fax: 301-480-9793
                        e-mail: prpl@cc.nih.gov
                        www.cc.nih.gov

The NIH Clinical Center is a Federally funded biomedical research facility that supports clinical investigations conducted by the institutes of the National Institute of Health.

Web Sites

4329 Congenital Heart Disease Resource Page Web Site
www.csun.edu/~hcmth011/heart/
                        e-mail: sheri.berger@csun.edu
                        www.csun.edu/~hcmth011/heart/

4330 Healthfinder
www.haelthfinder.gov

4331 Kansas University Medical Center
www.kumc.edu

4332 Lili Claire Foundation
www.liliclairefoundation.org/

4333 Pedbase
www.icondata.com/health/pedbase/files/WILLIAMS.HTM

4334 Rare Genetic Diseases in Children
mcrcr2.med.nyu.edu

4335 Williams Syndrome E-mail List
www.geocities.com/HotSprings/8172/listserve.html

4336 Williams Syndrome Foundation Home Page
www.williamssyndrome.org/

4337 Williams Syndrome Monthly Medline Alert
www.geocities.com/HotSprings/8172/
                        e-mail: shue@ix.netcom.com
                        www.geocities.com/HotSprings/8172/

DESCRIPTION

4338 WILMS TUMOR

Synonym: Nephroblastoma

Disorder Type: Neoplasm: Benign or Malignant Tumor

Wilms tumor is a malignant tumor of the kidney that accounts for about eight percent of childhood cancers. It occurs with equal frequency among males and females. Wilms tumor may develop in any region of either kidney. In most cases, tumor development occurs in one kidney (unilateral). However, both kidneys may be involved (bilateral) in about five to 10 percent of affected children. In some severe cases, the tumor may spread to other parts of the body (metastasize), particularly the lungs.

Wilms tumor typically becomes apparent by approximately three to five years of age. The most common sign is the presence of a smooth, firm mass in the abdominal area. Approximately 50 percent of affected children experience associated abdominal pain or vomiting (emesis) and about 10 to 25 percent have blood in their urine (microscopic or gross hematuria). In addition, up to 60 percent of children with Wilms tumor have high blood pressure (hypertension) due to the tumor's pressure on an artery near the kidney (renal artery). In severe cases, long-term hypertension may result in the inability of the heart to pump blood effectively throughout the body (cardiac failure).

In children with Wilms tumor in one kidney, treatment typically includes immediate surgical removal of the affected kidney (nephrectomy). During surgery, the remaining kidney is examined to exclude tumor development. After surgery, therapy may include the use of certain anticancer drugs (chemotherapy). According to the National Wilms Tumor Study Group, the preferred chemotherapy regimen consists of therapy with dactinomycin and vincristine that may be combined with doxorubicin. Those with advanced disease may also receive radiation therapy through the use of x-rays or other sources of radioactivity. In children with Wilms tumor in both kidneys, chemotherapy and radiation therapy may be considered before surgery.

The exact cause of Wilms tumor is not understood. However, missing genetic material (deletion) from one of at least three different chromosomal locations has been noted in affected individuals. Such deletions have been located on the short arm of chromosome 11 (at 11p13 or 11p15.5) and on the long arm of chromosome 16 (16q). These genetic changes may appear to occur randomly for unknown reasons (sporadic) or may be inherited as an autosomal dominant trait. In rare cases, deletions at one of these locations (i.e., 11p13) may be associated with two rare disorders that are characterized by Wilms tumor. These include Denys-Drash syndrome and WAGR syndrome. Denys-Drash syndrome is characterized by Wilms tumor, abnormal kidney function (nephropathy leading to renal failure), and severe malformations of the reproductive and urinary tracts (e.g., pseudohermaphroditism). WAGR syndrome is characterized by Wilms tumor, absence of all or a portion of the pigmented area (iris) of the eyes at birth (aniridia), genitourinary malformations, and mental retardation.

The following organizations in the General Resources Section can provide additional information: National Organization for Rare Disorders, Inc., (NORD), NIH/Office of Rare Diseases, Candlelighters Childhood Cancer Foundation Canada, NIH/National Cancer Institute, National Childhood Cancer Foundation, Candlelighters Childhood Cancer Foundation, NIH/National Institute of Neurological Disoders & Stroke, Online Mendelian Inheritance in Man: www3.ncbi.nlm.nih.gov/Omim/searchomim.html

Web Sites

4339 CancerCare:
www.cancercare.org/faq/cancer_faq.html

4340 Children's Cancer Web
www.ncl.ac.uk/child-health/guides/guide2w.htm

**4341 OncoLink: The University of Pennslyvania Cancer
Center Resource**
www.oncolink.upenn.edu/disease/ped_wilms

DESCRIPTION

4342 WILSON DISEASE

Synonyms: Hepatolenticular degeneration, WD, WND

Disorder Type: Genetic Disorder, Metabolism

Wilson disease is a genetic disorder in which a defect in copper metabolism causes an abnormal accumulation of copper in the liver, brain, kidneys, corneas, and other tissues of the body. The disorder is often characterized by progressive liver disease, degenerative changes of the brain, kidney failure, and the presence of characteristic grayish-green or reddish-gold rings at the outer margins of the corneas (Kayser-Fleischer rings). Wilson disease is a progressive disorder in which the age at onset may vary from patient to patient. Symptoms and findings may not become apparent until five or six years of age and most commonly begin during mid-adolescence. However, in some patients, the disease may not become apparent until adulthood. Wilson disease is thought to have a prevalence of approximately one in 30,000 individuals worldwide.

In individuals with Wilson disease, copper progressively accumulates in the liver and is released into other organs and tissues of the body, particularly the brain, corneas, and kidneys. Associated symptoms and findings may be variable; however, individuals within certain multigenerational families typically have similar clinical presentations. Affected children under 10 years of age tend to have associated liver abnormalities. Neurologic symptoms rarely affect those under 10 years of age; however, young adults tend to have neurologic involvement. In individuals with Wilson disease, liver disease is characterized by enlargement of the liver (hepatomegaly) with or without enlargement of the spleen (splenomegaly); acute or chronic inflammation of the liver (hepatitis); and internal scarring (fibrosis) and impaired functioning of the liver (cirrhosis). Those with cirrhosis may have yellowish discoloration of the skin, mucous membranes, and whites of the eyes (jaundice); unusually high blood pressure (hypertension) in certain veins near the liver (portal hypertension); an abnormal accumulation of fluid in certain body tissues (edema) and the abdominal cavity (ascites); and enlargement of blood vessels in the wall of the esophagus (esophageal varices), potentially causing them to rupture and bleed. In severe cases, affected individuals may develop fulminant hepatitis, a severe form of liver disease characterized by localized loss of liver tissue (necrosis), defects of blood clotting (coagulation), coma (hepatic encephalopathy), and potentially life-threatening complications.

Neurologic symptoms associated with Wilson disease may appear to develop suddenly or may occur gradually. Many such symptoms are thought to result from progressive involvement of a region of the brain that assists in regulating muscular movements (basal ganglia). Neurologic symptoms often initially include abnormalities of muscle tone (progressive dystonia), muscle stiffness and rigidity, muscle addition, patients may experience involuntary, rhythmic, quivering movements of the extremities on one side of the body (unilateral) that may eventually become generalized. Additional neurologic symptoms include difficulties speaking (dysphonia), drooling, a fixed smile due to drawing back of the upper lip, and involuntary, rapid, jerky movements in association with slow, writhing movements (choreoathetosis). Wilson disease may also result in the premature breakdown of red blood cells (hemolysis). This condition may progress to a chronic condition known as hemolytic anemia. In this form of anemia, premature destruction of red blood cells causes reduced levels of the protein that enables red blood cells to transport oxygen to cells (hemoglobin). In addition, the kidneys may become unable to regulate the appropriate balance between water and salt content, filter waste products from the blood and excrete them in urine, and perform other vital functions (progressive renal failure). In some patients, other symptoms and findings may be present.

Wilson disease is an autosomal recessive disorder that results from changes (mutations) of a gene on the long arm of chromosome 13 (13q14.3-q21.1).

Although the exact nature of the disease is not liver cells, causing decreased excretion of copper into a fluid secreted by the liver (bile).

The treatment of individuals with Wilson disease often consists of administration of penicillamine, a medication that binds with copper and enables it to be excreted from the body. This treatment is accompanied by supplementation of vitamine B6. If affected individuals are unable to tolerate penicillamine, the medication triethylene tetramine dihydrochloride may be an appropriate substitute. Physicians and other health care professionals may also recommend a diet that is low in copper intake (less than one mg/day), suggesting avoidance of such foods as chocolate, liver, shellfish, and nuts. Liver transplantation may be considered in those with fulminant hepatitis. Other treatment for individuals with Wilson disease is symptomatic and supportive.

The following organizations in the General Resources Section can provide additional information: Genetic Alliance, March of Dimes Birth Defects Foundation, NIH/Office of Rare Diseases, National Organization for Rare Disorders, Inc., (NORD), NIH/National Digestive Diseases Information Clearinghouse, NIH/National Institute of Neurological Disorders and Stroke

National Associations & Support Groups

4343 American Liver Foundation
75 Maiden Lane Suite 603
New York, NY 10038　　212-668-1000
800-465-4837
Fax: 212-483-8179
e-mail: info@liverfoundation.org
www.liverfoundation.org

Organization provides several different medias for answering questions and to help clarify any uncertainties the individual may be experiencing.

4344 Children's Liver Alliance
3835 Richmond Avenue, Suite 190
Staten Island, NY 10312　　718-987-6200
Fax: 718-987-6200
e-mail: livers4kids@earthlink.net
www.livertx.org

Aides in easing the physical and emotional strains that the child is experiencing, so they can better deal with the disorder through different media resources that are also available to family and friends.

10,000 members

Lisa Carroccio, Chairwoman and Founder

4345 WE MOVE (Worldwide Education and Awareness for Movement Disorders)
Mt. Sinia Medical Center
1 Gustave L. Levy Place Box 1052
New York, NY 10029　　212-241-8567
e-mail: wemove@wemove.org
www.wemove.org

4346 Wilson's Disease Association
4 Navaho Drive
Brookfield, CT 06804　　203-775-9666
800-399-0266
Fax: 203-775-9666
TTY: 540-743-1415
e-mail: hasellner@worldnet.att.net
www.wilsonsdisease.org

Provides patients and their families with a membership list, e-mail correspondence, meetings for support and education, and a newsletter. Supports patients with financial assistance for medication and travel, and develops centers of excellence.

800 Members

Research Centers

4347 National Center for the Study of Wilson's Disease, Inc
St. Luke's/Roosevelt Hospital
432 West 58th Street, Suite 614
New York, NY 10019　　212-523-8717
Fax: 212-523-8708

Web Sites

4348 Wilson Disease Association International
www.wilsondisease.org/

4349 Wilson Disease Patient Information Exchange
www.isd.net/gourmand/histories/

Newsletters

4350 Children's Liver Alliance Newsletter
3835 Richmond Avenue, Suite 190
Staten Island, NY 10312   718-987-6200
                    Fax: 718-987-6200
          e-mail: livers4kids@earthlink.net
                    www.livertx.org

Aides in easing the physical and emotional
strains that the child is experiencing, so they can
better deal with the disorder through differant
media resources that are also available to both
friends and family.

4-12 pages

JoLayna Arndt, Editor

Pamphlets

4351 Wilson's Disease
Nat'l Digestive Diseases Information Clearinghouse
2 Information Way
Bethesda, MD 20892   301-654-3810
                    Fax: 301-907-8906
          e-mail: nddic@info.niddk.nih.gov
                    www.niddk.nih.gov

DESCRIPTION

4352 XYY SYNDROME

Synonyms: Chromosome XYY, Chromosome XYY, 47, XYY males, Chromosome XYY males

Disorder Type: Chromosomal Disorder, Developmental Milestones

Covers these related disorders: 46, XY/47, XYY mosaicism

XYY syndrome is a chromosomal disorder that affects males. Although males usually have one X and one Y chromosome, those with XYY syndrome have an extra Y chromosome in cells of the body. Most children, adolescents, and adults with XYY syndrome have no associated clinical abnormalities. However, certain variable physical abnormalities may be present in some affected males. The most consistent feature associated with XYY syndrome is unusually tall stature. Some affected infants may be long at birth; however, in most cases, the tendency toward tall stature usually does not become apparent until approximately five or six years of age. Some males with XYY syndrome may also have long hands and feet; unusually large primary and secondary teeth; long ears and a relatively long face; and mild depression of the breastbone (pectus excavatum). In addition, males with XYY syndrome may be prone to experiencing severe acne in which the oily substance (sebum) secreted by certain skin glands (sebaceous glands) obstructs hair follicles, causing overgrowth of bacteria, associated inflammation of hair follicles, and the development of firm swellings (cysts) and solid, node-like structures (nodules) of the skin. In individuals with severe acne, scars appearing as depressed, pitted areas may remain once acne has healed.

Occasional findings seen in males with XYY syndrome may include abnormal joining of the bones of the forearm (radioulnar synostosis); abnormalities of the heart's electrical activities that regulate rhythmic, pumping action of the heart (i.e., prolonged PR interval), a small penis, or abnormal placement of the urinary opening on the underside of the penis (hypospadias). However, in most males with XYY syndrome, genital development is normal. In addition, although the onset of puberty may be delayed approximately six months in many affected males, fertility is usually normal.

Although most males with XYY syndrome have an intelligence quotient (I.Q.) within average ranges, their I.Q.s tend to be lower than those of their sisters and brothers. Reports indicate that affected males have demonstrated an I.Q. ranging from 140 (above average range) to 80 (low end of average range). Approximately 50 percent of children with XYY syndrome have learning disabilities. Speech delays and language difficulties are common, potentially requiring special education classes. Affected children may also have muscle weakness, poor fine motor coordination, and poor development of certain muscles, such as those of the shoulders and chest. In addition, males with XYY syndrome tend to have behavioral problems during childhood and early adolescence. These include easy distractibility, impulsive behavior, temper tantrums, poor social skills, and a low self-image.

XYY syndrome results from an early spontaneous error during the division of a father's reproductive cells. The syndrome is thought to affect approximately one in 840 to 1,000 newborn males. However, because many affected males have few or no apparent symptoms, it may be difficult to estimate the true frequency of XYY syndrome in the general population.

The following organizations in the General Resources Section can provide additional information: March of Dimes Birth Defects Foundation, Genetic Alliance, National Organization for Rare Disorders, Inc., (NORD)

National Associations & Support Groups

4353 National Alliance for the Mentally Ill
200 North Glebe Road, #1015
Arlington, VA 22203
703-524-7600
800-950-6264
Fax: 703-524-9094
TTY: 703-516-7991
e-mail: membership@nami.org
www.nami.org

Aids families and individuals find the emotional and physical answers to the habitual forming disorders through several media resources.

4354 National Institute of Menetal Health
5600 Fishers Lane
Rockville, MD 20857   301-443-4513
www.nimh.nih.gov/

4355 National Mental Health Consumer Self-Help Clearinghouse
311 S. Juniper Street
Philadelphia, PA 19107   215-751-1810
800-553-4539

Offers information, support, and appropriate referrals; and promotes public and professional education. Provides networking for those with spedial interest related to albinism and management of albinism and hypopigmentation.

Associations & Government Agencies

4357 52 Association for the Handicapped
350 5th Avenue, Suite 3304
New York, NY 10118
212-868-1217
Fax: 212-868-1219

Information on adaptive sports and recreation activities for people of many abilities. Includes local chapters, referrals, fun and social interaction and support groups.

4358 A Wish with Wings
917 W Sanford St
Arlington, TX 76012
817-469-9474
Fax: 817-275-6005
e-mail: wish@startext.net
www.awishwithwings.org

Grants wishes for children 3 to 18 years of age with life-threatening diseases. The organization primarily serves children living in or being treated in Texas, but will grant out-of-state wishes if there is no wish-granting organization in client's area.

Pat Skaggs, Founder

4359 AASK: Adopt A Special Kid
287 17th Street, Suite 207
Oakland, CA 94612
510-451-1748
Fax: 510-451-2023
e-mail: andrea@adoptaspecialkid.org
www.adoptaspecialkid.org

Information and advocacy resources for families and professionals. Includes listings of organizations providing general information and organizations focusing on more specific areas of concern to families and young adults who have disabilities.

4360 ABLEDATA
8455 Colesville Road, Suite 935
Silver Spring, MD 20910
301-608-8998
800-227-0216
Fax: 301-608-8958
TTY: 301-608-8912
e-mail: abledata@macroint.com
www.abledata.com

Information and advocacy resources for families and professionals. Includes listings of organizations providing general information and organizations focusing on more specific areas of concern to families and young adults who have disabilities.

4361 AIM for the Handicapped Adventures in Movement
945 Danbury Road
Dayton, OH 45420
937-294-4611
800-332-8210
Fax: 937-294-3783

Information on adaptive sports and recreation activities for people of many abilities. Includes local chapters, referrals, fun and social interaction and support groups.

4362 ARC National Organization Mental Retardation
500 East Border St, Ste 300
Arlington, TX 76010
817-261-6003
800-433-5255
Fax: 817-277-3491
TTY: 817-277-0553
e-mail: thearc@metronet.com
www.thearc.org/welcome

National organization on mental retardation and related disabilities that provides organizational support to affiliated chapters. Parent to Parent (P-P) programs provide informational and emotional support to parents who have a child, adolescent, or adult family member with special needs. P-P programs offer an important connection for a parent who is seeking support for special disability issue, by matching him or her with a trained veteren parent.

4363 AbiliTech
4040 Market Street
Philadelphia, PA 19104
215-243-2033
Fax: 215-243-3631
TTY: 215-243-2443
www.abilitech.org

Provides technical support to families and young adults who have disabilities.

4364 Academy for Guided Imagery
P.O. Box 2070
Mill Valley, CA 94942
800-726-2070

This organization can assist in locating a professional in your area to help your child learn visualization.

4365 Access Board
1331 F Street, NW #1000
Washington, DC 20004
800-872-2253
Fax: 202-272-5447
TTY: 800-993-2822
e-mail: info@access-board.gov

Information and advocacy resources for families and professionals. Includes listings of organizations providing general information.

4366 Administration on Developmental Disabilities
US Department of Health and Human Services

Washington, DC 20201   202-690-6590
Fax: 202-690-6904
TTY: 202-690-6415
www.acf.dhs.gov/programs/ada

Information and advocacy resources for families and professionals. Includes listings of organizations providing general information and organizations focusing on more specific areas of concern to families and young adults who have disabilities.

4367 Adoptive Families of America
2309 Como Avenue
St. Paul, MN 55108   651-645-9955
800-372-3300
Fax: 651-645-0055
www.adoptivefam.org

Information and advocacy resources for families and professionals interested in adoption.

4368 Advocates Across America
P.O. Box 754
Chandler, AZ 85244   480-917-0955
Fax: 480-814-9404
e-mail: support@axa.org
www.axa.org

Information and advocacy resources for families and professionals. Includes listings of organizations providing general information and organizations focusing on more specific areas of concern to families and young adults who have disabilities.

4369 Agency for Health Care Research
P.O. Box 8547
Silver Spring, MD 20907

800-358-9295
Fax: 410-290-3841
www.ahrq.gov

Healthcare information and advocacy resources for families and professionals.

4370 Alliance for Technology Access (ATA)
2173 East Francisco Boulevard
San Rafael, CA 94901   415-455-4575

National organization dedicated to providing access to technology for people with disabilities through its coalition of 45 community-based resource centers in 34 states and the Virgin Islands. Each center provides information, awareness, and training for professionals, and provides guided problem solving and technical assistance for individuals with disabilities and family members.

4371 Ambulatory Pediatric Association
6728 Old McLean Village Drive
McLean, VA 22101   703-556-9222
Fax: 703-556-8729
e-mail: ambpeds@aol.com

4372 American Academy of Child & Adolescent Psychiatry (AACAP)
P.O. Box 96106
Washington, DC 20090

Fax: 212-364-5947
www.aacap.org/

4373 American Academy of Dermatology
930 N. Meacham Rd.
Schaumburg, IL 60168   888-462-3376
www.aad.org

With a membership of over 900, the Academy is committed to the highest quality standards in continuing medical education and plays a major role in formulating socioeconomic policies that can influence the quality of dermatologic care. Promotes and advances the science and art of medicine and surgery related to the skin, promotes the highest possible standards in clinical practice, education and research.

4374 American Academy of Pediatrics
141 Northwest Point Blvd.
Elk Grove Village, IL 60007   847-228-5005
Fax: 847-228-5097
e-mail: pubrel@app.org
www.aap.org

The mission of the Academy is to acheive optimal physical, mental and social health and well-being for infants, children and adolescents through education, research, service and advocacy for children, their families and their communitites.

4375 American Amputee Foundation, Inc
P.O. Box 250218
Little Rock, AR 72225   501-666-2523
Fax: 501-666-8367

Information on adaptive sports and recreation activities for people of many abilities. Includes local chapters, referrals, fun and social interaction and support groups.

4376 American Association for Leisure and Recreation
1900 Association Drive
Reston, VA 20191   703-476-3472
Fax: 703-476-9527
e-mail: aair@aahperd.org
www.aahperd.org/aair

Information on adaptive sports and recreation activities for people of many abilities. Includes local chapters, referrals, fun and social interaction and support groups.

4377 American Association of Children's Residential Centers (AACRC)
122 C Street, NW, Suite 820
Washington, DC 20001   202-628-1816

4378 American Association of University Affiliated Programs
8630 Fenton Street, Suite 410
Silver Spring, MD 20910   301-588-8252
                                 800-424-3410
                          Fax: 301-588-2842
                          TTY: 301-588-3319
              e-mail: AAUAPJONES@aol.com
                          www.aaup.org

Information and advocacy resources for families and professionals. Includes listings of organizations providing general information and organizations focusing on more specific areas of concern to families and young adults who have disabilities.

4379 American Association on Mental Resources
44 N Capitol St, Ste 846
Washington, DC 20001   202-387-1968
                              800-424-3688
                       Fax: 202-387-2193
          e-mail: aamr@access.digex.net
                          www.aamr.org

4380 American Autoimmune Related Diseases Association, Inc.
15475 Gratiot Avenue
Detroit, MI 48205   313-371-8600
              e-mail: aarda@aol.com
                       www.aarda.org

Focused on the dissemination of information to the public of autoimmune and related diseases.

4381 American Blind Bowling Association
315 N Main Street
Houston, PA 15342   412-745-5986

Information on adaptive bowling activities for people of many abilities. Includes local chapters, referrals, fun and social interaction and support groups.

4382 American Blind Skiing Foundation
610 S William Street
Mt. Prospect, IL 60056   847-255-1739

Information on adaptive skiing activities for people of many abilities. Includes local chapters, referrals, fun and social interaction and support groups.

4383 American Board of Dermatology
Henry Ford Hospital

Detroit, MI 48202   313-876-2151
                     Fax: 313-876-2093

Sole mission is to ensure competence for patients with cutaneous diseases through board representation.

4384 American Board of Pediatric Neurological Surgery
930 Madison Avenue
Memphis, TN 38103

                          www.abpns.org

4385 American Board of Pediatrics
111 Silver Cedarcenter
Chapel Hill, NC 27514   919-929-0461
                         Fax: 919-929-9255

4386 American Camping Association
5000 State Road, 67 N
Martinsville, IN 46151   765-342-8456
                                800-428-2267
                         Fax: 765-342-2065
         e-mail: bookstore@aca-campus.org

Information on adaptive camping activities for people of many abilities. Includes local chapters, referrals, fun and social interaction and support groups.

4387 American Cancer Society, Inc.
1599 Clifton Road, NE
Atlanta, GA 30329   404-320-333
                          800-227-2345
              e-mail: www.cancer.org

National voluntary, non-profit organization dedicated to the prevention, treatment and cure of cancer. The foundation offers support groups, advocacy, medical research support and education.

4388 American Canoe Association
7432 Alban Station Blvd, Ste. B-232
Springfield, VA 22150   703-451-0141
                          Fax: 703-451-2245
              e-mail: acadirect@aol.com

Information on adaptive canoe recreation activities for people of many abilities. Includes local chapters, referrals, fun and social interaction and support groups.

4389 American Dermatological Association
University Hospitals BT 2045-1
Dept. of Dermatology
Iowa City, IA 52242   319-356-2274
Fax: 319-356-8317

Professional society of physicians specializing in dermatology. Promotes teaching, practice, public education and research into dermatology.

John S. Strauss, MD, Secretary

4390 American Epilepsy Society
342 North Main Street
West Hartford, CT 06117   860-586-7505
Fax: 860-586-7550
e-mail: info@aesnet.org
www.aesnet.org

The purpose of the American Epilepsy Society is to encourage education and research dedicated to the prevention, treatment and cure of epilepsy.

4391 American Heart Association
7272 Greenville Avenue
Dallas, TX 75231   214-373-6300
800-242-8721
Fax: 214-706-1341
e-mail: inquire@amhrt.org
www.amhrt.org

Supports research, education and community service programs with the objective of reducing premature death and disability from cardiovascular diseases and stroke; coordinates the efforts of health professionals, and other engaged in the fight against heart and circulatory disease.

4392 American Juvenile Arthritis Organization
1330 West Peachtree Street
Atlanta, GA 30309   404-872-7100
e-mail: help@arthritis.org
www.arthritis.org

Caters to the needs of young arthritic sufferers by providing them with the data through a variety of both printed audio and visual mediums.

4393 American Liver Foundation
75 Maiden Lane Suite 603
New York, NY 10038   212-668-1000
800-465-4837
Fax: 212-483-8179
TTY: 123-019-9912
e-mail: info@liverfoundation.org
www.liverfoundation.org

National voluntary, non-profit organization dedicated to the prevention, treatment and cure of liver diseases. The foundation offers support groups, advocacy, medical research support and education.

4394 American Lung Association
1740 Broadway
New York, NY 10019   212-315-8700
800-586-4872
www.lungusa.org

A voluntary organization interested in the prevention and control of lung disease. Promotes and distributes public awareness information on a variety of lung disorders, including allergies.

4395 American Pediatric Surgical Association
Wilshire Park
Neddham, MA 02192   617-482-2915

4396 American Red Cross
2025 E Street NW
Washington, DC 20006   202-728-6492
Fax: 202-728-6649

The American Red Cross provides numerous services, including the coordination of bone marrow testing and donation in association with the National Marrow Donor Program. Local chapters are listed in the white pages of the telephone book.

4397 American Self-Help Clearinghouse
Saint Clare's Health Services
25 Pocono Road
Denville, NJ 07834   973-625-7101
Fax: 973-625-8848
TTY: 973-625-9053
e-mail: ashc@cybernet.net
www.cmhc.com/selfhelpgroups.org

Information and advocacy resources for families and professionals. Includes listings of organizations providing general information and organizations focusing on more specific areas of concern to families and young adults who have disabilities.

4398 American Sled Hockey Association
10933 Johnson Avenue S
Bloomington, MN 55437   612-750-3973
Fax: 612-888-5331
e-mail: janschotzln@aol.com

Information on adaptive sled hockey activities for people of many abilities. Includes local chapters, referrals, fun and social interaction and support groups.

4399 American Wheelchair Table Tennis Association
23 Parker Street
Port Chester, NY 10573   914-937-3932

Information on adaptive table tennis activities for people of many abilities. Includes local chapters, referrals, fun and social interaction and support groups.

4400 Arkenstone, Inc
NASA Ames Moffett Complex, Building 23
P.O. Box 215
Moffett Field, CA 94035   650-603-8880
                                 Fax: 650-603-8887
                                 e-mail: info@arkenstone.org
                                 www.arkenstone.org

Information and advocacy resources for families and professionals. Includes listings of organizations providing general information and organizations focusing on more specific areas of concern to families and young adults who have disabilities.

4401 Association for Education & Rehabilitation of the Blind & Visually Impaired
P.O. Box 22397, 4600 Duke St
Alexandria, VA 22304   703-823-9690
                              Fax: 703-823-9695

Dedicated to the advancement of education and rehabilitation of blind and visually impaired children and adults.

4402 Association for Persons with Severe Handicaps
7010 Roosevelt Way N.E.
Seattle, WA 98115   206-523-8446

Provides information and referral services, and helps chapters to support local and regional concerns. Sponsors an international conference annually and publishes a newsletter and journal.

4403 Association for the Gifted Child
The Council for Exceptional Children
1920 Association Drive
Reston, VA 20191   703-620-3660
                          Fax: 703-264-9474
                          TTY: 703-264-9446
                          www.cec.spec.org

Focuses on the delivery of information to both professionals and parents about gifted and talented children and their needs.

4404 Association of Blind Athletes
33 N Institute Street
Colorado Springs, CO 80903   719-630-0422
                                    Fax: 719-630-0616
                                    e-mail: usaba@usa.net

Information on adaptive sports and recreation activities for people of various degrees of sight. Including local chapters, referrals, fun and social interaction and support groups.

4405 Barbara DeBoer Foundation
2069 S. Busse Road
Mount Prospect, IL 60056
                          800-895-8478

Helps to identify and utilize resources in local community to raise necessary funds for transplants.

4406 Beneficial Designs, Inc
P.O. Box 8317
Santa Cruz, CA 95060   831-429-8447
                              Fax: 831-423-8450
                              e-mail: mail@beneficialdesigns.com

Information on adaptive sports and recreation activities for people of many abilities. Includes local chapters, referrals, fun and social interaction and support groups.

4407 Boundless Playgrounds
Hasbro National Resource Center
One Regency Drivenue
Bloomfield, CT 06002   860-243-8315
                              877-268-6353
                              Fax: 860-243-5854
                              www.boundlessplaygrounds.org

Offers a wide range of services and support and helps communities, scools, parks and hospitals create magical places where all children - both and those with physical, sensory and developmental disabilities - can play together.

Leslyn Clark, Director of Community Prgrams

4408 Boy Scouts of America
1325 W Walnut Hill Lane
Irving, TX 75038   972-580-2000
                          Fax: 972-580-2502

Information on Boy Scout chapters and recreation activities for people of many abilities. Includes local chapters, referrals, fun and social interaction and support groups.

4409 Braille Revival League
American Council of the Blind
1155 15th Street NW, Ste 1004
Washington, DC 20005   202-467-5081
                              800-424-8666
                              Fax: 202-467-5085

Encourages blind people to read and write in braille, advocates for mandatary braille instruction in educational facilities for the blind, strives to make available a supply of braille materials from libraries and printing houses and more.

4410 Brass Ring Society
213 N Washington St
Snow Hill, MD 21863   410-632-4700
                            800-666-9474
                            Fax: 410-632-1811

Society that seeks to fulfill the dreams of children with life-threatening illnesses.

4411 Breckenridge Outdoor Education Center
P.O. Box 697
Breckenridge, CO 80424   970-453-6422
                               800-383-2632
                            Fax: 970-453-4676
                          e-mail: boec@boec.org

Information on adaptive outdoor sports and educational activities for people of many abilities. Includes local chapters, referrals, fun and social interaction and support groups.

4412 Canadian Organization for Rare Disorders
P.O. Box 814, Coaldale
Alberta, Canada T1M 1M7,   403-345-4544
                            Fax: 403-345-3948
                          e-mail: cord@bully.com
                          www.bully.com/~cord

Information and advocacy resources for families and professionals dealing with those diagnosed with a rare disorder. Includes listings of organizations providing general information and organizations focusing on specific areas of concern to families and young adults.

4413 Cancer Information Service
National Cancer Institute, 31 Center Dr, MSC 2580
Building 31, Room 10A16
Bethesda, MD 20892
                            800-422-6237
                          Fax: 301-330-7968
                          TTY: 800-332-8615
                          www.nci.nih.gov

Information and advocacy resources for families and professionals dealing with cancer patients. Includes listings of organizations providing general information and organizations focusing on more specific areas of concern.

4414 Candlelighters Childhood Cancer Foundation
7910 Woodmont Avenue, Suite 460
Bethesda, MD 20814
                            800-366-2223
                          Fax: 301-718-2686
                  e-mail: info@candlelighters.org
                          www.candlelighters.org

Operates a hotline which provides information and services to survivors, families, and medical professionals on all pediatric cancer-related topics. Candlelighters offers many publications (most free), including: Introduction to the Americans with Disabilities Act: A Guide for Families of Children with Cancer and Survivors of Childhood Cancer, Insurance: Your Options and Your Child's; and Tips on Health Insurance for Long Term Survivors.

4415 Center for Best Practices in Early Childhood
College of Education and Human Services
27 Horrabin Hall, W Illinois Univ.
Macomb, IL 61455   309-298-1634
                        Fax: 309-298-2305
                        www.mprojects.wiu.edu

Operates the following: Early Childhood Interactive Technology Literacy Cirriculum Project; Disseminating and Replicating an Effective Early Childhood Comprehensive Technology System; Expressive Arts Outreach; ECCSPLOR-IT; LiTECH Interactive Outreach; STARNET Regions I and III; and Provider Connections.

4416 Center for Literacy and Disability Studies
Duke University Medical Center
Durham, NC 27710   919-684-3740
                        Fax: 919-681-5738
                  e-mail: literacy@acpub.duke.edu
                  www.surgery.mc.duke.edu/hearing/clds

Information and advocacy resources for families and professionals. Includes listings of organizations providing general information and organizations focusing on more specific areas of concern to families and young adults who have disabilities.

4417 Centers for Disease Control (CDC)
1600 Clifton Road
Atlanta, GA 30333   404-639-3311
                        www.cdc.gov

Federal agency that protects America's health and safty, provides information to guide health decisions, and builds strong partnerships to promote health.

4418 Chai Lifeline/Camp Simcha National Office
151 West 30th Street, 3rd Floor
New York, NY 10001   212-465-1300
                        Fax: 212-465-9495
                  e-mail: info@chailife.org
                        www.chailifeline.org

International nonprofit organization dedicated to providing supportservices to Jewish children and their families in medical crisis. All services free of charge and confidential. Some of the many services provided are: visits to hospital and homebound children, information and referrals, socialization and recreational programs, support groups, Grant-a-Wish, respite program, negotiating insurance claims, financial aid, transportation, home tutoring for Judiac studies and many others.

Mrs. Esther Schwartz, MA, Program Director

4419 Child Care Plus+ Rural Institute on Disabilities
Montana University Affiliated Rural Institute
634 Eddy, The University of Montana
Missoula, MT 59812   406-243-6355
                            800-235-4122
                        Fax: 406-243-4730
                        TTY: 406-243-5467
              e-mail: ahill@selway.umt.edu
          www.ruralinstitute.umt.edu/childcareplus

Includes information and resources for child care providers and other professionals: written materials, training/workshops and various resources including techinical assistance.

4420 Children in Hospitals
300 Longwood Avenue
Boston, MA 02115   617-355-6000
                     Fax: 617-355-7429

4421 Children's Cancer Research Institute
2351 Clay Street, Ste 512
San Francisco, CA 94115   415-923-3535

Nonprofit organization specializing in cancer research and care of children with cancer.

Jordan R. Wilbur, MD, Medical Director

4422 Children's Defense Fund
25 E Street NW
Washington, DC 20001   202-628-8787
                            800-233-1200
                        Fax: 202-662-3510
          e-mail: cdfinfo@childrensdefense.org
                www.childrensdefense.org

Information and advocacy resources for families and professionals. Includes listings of organizations providing general information and organizations focusing on more specific areas of concern to families and young adults who have disabilities.

4423 Children's Heart Foundation
200 West Jackson Blvd. Suite 1500
Chicago, IL 60606   312-957-0445
                       Fax: 312-957-0447
                       www.childrenhart.com

A foundation created in 1996 to support methods for diagnosing, treating and preventing congenital heart disease.

4424 Children's Hopes and Dreams
Wish Fulfillment Foundation
280 Route 46
Dover, NJ 07801   973-361-7366
                     Fax: 973-361-6627
           e-mail: chdfdover@juno.com
childrenscharities.org/childrens_wisheso

Four programs: 1)Dream fulfillment program is for children age 4 through 17 with life threatening illness who have not received a dream before; 2)Pen Pal Program matches children 6 through 17 with chronic or life threatening illnesses, conditions, disabilities to other ill children by their age, sex and illness category; 3)Kid's Kare Package program supplies new donated items to children through Pen Pal Program and/or health care professionals; 4)Retreat Home for parents of ill children.

10,000 Members

4425 Children's Hospice International
2202 Mount Vernon Avenue, Suite 3C
Alexandria, VA 22301   703-684-0330
                            800-242-4453
                        Fax: 703-684-0226
              e-mail: chiorg@aol.com
                   www.chionline.org

Provides care and caretaking in a supportive home environment.

4426 Children's Organ Transplant Association
2501 Cota Drive
Bloomington, IN 47403   800-366-2682
                   e-mail: cota@cota.org
                         www.cota.org

Offers guidance and assistance in all aspects of fund-raising for transplants. A COTA staff member will travel to the site of the campaign, help the campaign obtain 501(c)(3) status, provide a toll-free telephone number, and advice on all aspects of fund-raising. Emergency funds available.

4427 Children's Wish Foundation International
8615 Roswell Road
Atlanta, GA 30350   770-393-9474
                        800-323-9474
                    Fax: 770-393-0683
          e-mail: wish@childrenswish.org
                www.childrenswish.org

Children's Wish Foundation International, Inc. is a non-profit organization that fulfills wishes for children with life threatening illnesses. The criteria for wish fulfillment are: the child must be under the age of 18, and have been diagnosed with a life threatening illness.

4428 Circle Solution
2070 Chain Bridge Road, Suite 450
Vienna, VA 22182   703-821-8955
Fax: 703-821-2098
TTY: 703-566-4831
TDD: 703-566-4831
e-mail: info@circsol.comorg
www.circsol.com

Information and advocacy resources for families and professionals. Includes listings of organizations providing general information and organizations focusing on more specific areas of concern to families and young adults who have disabilities.

4429 Compassionate Friends, Inc
P.O. Box 3696
Oak Brook, IL 60522   630-990-0010
Fax: 630-990-0246
e-mail: nationaloffice@compassionatefriends.org
www.compassionatefriends.org

A self-help organization that offers support to families who are grieving the death of a child of any age regardless of cause. Our mission is to assist families in the positive resolution of grief following the death, and to provide information to help others be supportive. Our 600 chapters offer monthly meetings, newsletters and telephone support.

4430 Cooperative Wilderness Handicapped Outdoor Group
P.O. Box 8128
Pocatello, ID 83209   208-236-3912
Fax: 208-236-4600
e-mail: branjeff@isu.edu

Information on adaptive outdoor sports and recreation activities for people of many abilities. Includes local chapters, referrals, fun and social interaction and support groups.

4431 Council for Educational Diagnostic Services (CEDS)
The Council for Exceptional Children
1920 Association Drive
Reston, VA 20191   703-620-3660
Fax: 703-264-9474
TTY: 703-264-9446
www.cec.spec.org

Promotes the highest quality of diagnostic and prescriptive procedures involved in the education of individuals with disabilities and/or who are gifted. Members include educational diagnosticians, psychologists, social workers, speech and language specialists, physcians, and other professionals and related service professionals.

4432 Council for Exceptional Children
1920 Association Drive
Reston, VA 22091   703-620-3660
888-232-7733
Fax: 703-264-9494
TTY: 703-264-9446
e-mail: service@cec.sped.org
www.cec.sped.org

The Council for Exceptional Children (CEC) is the largest international professional organization dedicated to improving educational success for individuals with exceptionalities-student with disabilities and/or gifts. CEC advocates for appropriate governmental policies; sets professional standards; provides continual professional development; advocates for newly and historically underserved individuals with exceptionalities; and helps professionals obtain conditions and resources necessary.

50,000 Members

4433 Council of Administrators of Special Education
The Council for Exceptional Children
1920 Association Drive
Reston, VA 20191   703-620-3660
Fax: 703-264-9474
TTY: 703-264-9446
www.cec.spec.org

Provides special education administrators with oppurtunities for personal and professional advancement. Members include administrators, directors and supervisors of special education programs and services.

4434 Council of Families with Visual Impairments
American Council of the Blind
1155 15th Street NW Suite 720
Washington, DC 20005   202-467-5081
800-424-8666
Fax: 202-467-5085

A network of parents with blind or visually impaired children that offers support and outreach, shares experiences in parent/child relationships, exchanges educational, cultural and medical information about child development and more.

4435 Courage Center
3915 Golden Valley Road
Golden Valley, MN 55422   612-520-0520
                              Fax: 612-520-0577
                      e-mail: sports@courage.com

Information on adaptive sports and recreation activities for people of many abilities. Includes local chapters, referrals, fun and social interaction and support groups.

4436 Department of the Interior Accessibility Management Program
P.O. Box 37127
Washington, DC 20013   202-208-4671
                           Fax: 202-343-3674
                   e-mail: david_park@nps.gov

Information on adaptive sports and recreation activities for people of many abilities. Including local chapters, referrals, fun and social interaction and support groups.

4437 Dermatology Foundation
1560 Sherman Avenue
Evanston, IL 60201   847-328-2256
                          www.dermfind.org

Raises funds for the control of skin diseases through research, improved education and better patient care. Supports basic clinical investigations.

Sandra Rahn Goldman, Executive Director

4438 Developmental Delay Registry
6701 Fairfax Road
Chevy Chase, MD 20815   301-652-2263
                            Fax: 301-229-5005
                            www.devedelay.org

Information and advocacy resources for families and professionals dealing with developmental delay disabilities.

4439 Developmental Disabilities Nurses Associations
228 Grimes Street, Suite 24
Eugene, OR 97402
                            800-888-6733
                       Fax: 541-485-7372
                  e-mail: ddnahq@aol.com
                            www.ddna.org

Specialty nursing organization that certifies nurses in developmental disabilities. Sponsors annual conference and many projects.

4440 Disability Rights Education & Defense Fund
2212 Sixth St
Berkeley, CA 94710   510-664-2555

Nonprofit law and public policy center that specializes in laws affecting more than 45 million Americans with disabilities. DREDF was founded 16 years ago to challenge the barriers that exclude people with disabilities from participating in all aspects of society.

4441 Disabled Shooting Services
National Rifle Association of America
11250 Waples Mill Road
Fairfax, VA 22030   703-267-1000
                    e-mail: info@nrpa.org

Information on adaptive shooting activities for people of many abilities. Includes local chapters, referrals, fun and social interaction and support groups.

4442 Disabled Sports USA
451 Hungerford Drive, Suite 100
Rockville, MD 20850   301-217-0960
                          Fax: 301-217-0968
                   e-mail: dsusa@dsusa.org

Information on adaptive sports and recreation activities for people of many abilities. Includes local chapters, referrals, fun and social interaction and support groups.

4443 Division for Children's Communication Development (DCCD)
The Council for Exceptional Children
1920 Association Drive
Reston, VA 20191   703-620-3660
                       Fax: 703-264-9474
                       TTY: 703-264-9446
                       www.cec.spec.org

Dedicated to improving the education of children with communication delays and disorders, and hearing loss. Members include professionals serving individuals with hearing, speech, and language disorders in the areas of receptive and expressive, verbal and non-verbal, spoken, written, and sign communication.

4444 Division for Early Childhood
The Council for Exceptional Children
1920 Association Drive
Reston, VA 20191   703-620-3660
                       Fax: 703-264-9474
                       TTY: 703-264-9446
                       www.cec.spec.org

Organization designed for individuals who work on behalf of children with special needs, birth through age 8 and their families. Members include early childhood intervention professionals, as well as parents of children who have disabilities, are gifted, or are at risk of future developmental problems.

4445 Division for Physical and Health Disablities
The Council for Exceptional Children
1920 Association Drive
Reston, VA 20191   703-620-3660
                         Fax: 703-264-9474
                         TTY: 703-264-9446
                         www.cec.spec.org

Advocates for quality education for individuals
with physical disabilities and special health care
needs in schools, hospitals, or home settings.

4446 Division of Birth Defects & Developmental Disabilities
National Center for Environmental Health
4770 Buford Highway NE
Atlanta, GA 30341   770-488-7150
                          Fax: 770-488-7156
                          www.cdc.gov

Information and advocacy resources for families
and professionals dealing with children with
birth defects and developmental disabilities.

4447 Division on Career Development and Transition
The Council for Exceptional Children
1920 Association Drive
Reston, VA 20191   703-620-3660
                         Fax: 703-264-9474
                         TTY: 703-264-9446
                         www.cec.spec.org

Focuses on the career development of individuals with disablilities and their transition from school to adult life.

4448 Dream Factory
1218 S Third Street
Louisville, KY 40203   502-637-8700
                             800-456-7556
                             Fax: 502-637-8744

Organization seeking to bring smiles to the faces
of seriously ill children 3-13 by granting their
greatest wish. Sponsors an annual summer camp
for children and supports chapters in 30 states.

4449 ERIC Clearinghouse on Disabilities & Gifted Children
Council for Exceptional Children
1920 Association Drive
Reston, VA 20191
                    TTY: 800-328-0272
        e-mail: ericec@cec.sped.org
        www.cec.sped.org/ericec.htm

Information and advocacy resources for families
and professionals. Includes listings of organizations providing general information and organizations focusing on more specific areas of
concern to families and young adults who have
disabilities.

4450 Educational Help for the Handicapped
Nat'l Info Center for Children and Youth
P.O. Box 1492
Washington, DC 20013
                         800-999-5599

Offers Federal assistance at many levels to enable children, youth and adults to receive education and training. Under the provisions of the
Education for All Handicapped Children Act
(EHA) of 1975, state and local school districts
must provide an appropriate elementary and secondary education for disabled children from age
6 through 21. Presently, some states provide educational and related services for preschool age
children.

4451 Family Voices
P.O. Box 769
Algodones, NM 87001   505-867-2368
                             888-835-5669
                             Fax: 505-867-6517

Information and advocacy resources for families
and professionals. Includes listings of organizations providing general information and organizations focusing on more specific areas of
concern to families and young adults who have
disabilities.

4452 Famous Fone Friends
9101 Sawyer St
Los Angeles, CA 90035   310-204-5683

Offers the ability for a sick child's doctor or
nurse to arrange for a well-known actor, athlete
or other celebrity to call the child.

4453 Federation for Children with Special Needs
1135 Tremont Street, Suite 420
Boston, MA 02116   617-482-2915
                          800-331-0688
                          Fax: 617-572-2094
                          e-mail: fcsninfo@fcsn.org
                          www.fscn.org

A center for parents and parent organizations to
work together on behalf of children with special
needs and their families.

4454 Federation of Families for Children's Mental Health
1021 Prince St.
Alexandria, VA 22314   703-684-7710
                             Fax: 703-836-1040
                             e-mail: ffcmh@crosslink.com
                             www.cals.com/vikings/nami/index.html

Assists young adults with life transitions by offering several support and educational tools.

4455 Foundation for Exceptional Children
1920 Association Dr
Reston, VA 22091   703-620-1054

To encourage, enhance and empower children
and youth with disabilities and/or gifted and talented children to attain their greatest potential.

4456 Freedom's Wings International
1832 Lake Avenue
Scotch Plains, NJ 07076   908-232-6354

Information on adaptive sports and recreation
activities for people of many abilities. Includes
local chapters, referrals, fun and social interaction and support groups.

4457 Friends' Health Connection
P.O. Box 114
New Brunswick, NJ 08903   732-418-1811
                                800-483-7436
                          Fax: 732-249-9897
                e-mail: a48friend@aol.com
                          www.48friends.org

Provide one-to-one support for people with
health problems and their families. Newsletter
published bi-annually.
        1989

Roxanne Black, Executive Director

4458 Genetic Alliance
4301 Connecticut Avenue NW, Ste.404
Washington, DC 20008   202-966-5557
                                800-336-4363
                          Fax: 202-966-8553
            e-mail: info@geneticalliance.org
                      www.geneticalliance.org

A nonprofit tax exempt organization founded in
1986 as a national coalition of consumers, professions and genetic support groups to voice the
common concerns of children and adults and
families living with, and at risk for, genetic conditions. The Alliance builds partnerships among
consumers and professionals and the private and
public sectors to promote optimum healthcare
and enhanced quality of life for individuals identified with genetic conditions.

Mary Davidson, Executive Director
Lois Lander, Resources Coordinator

4459 Girl Scouts of the USA
Membership and Program Group
420 5th Avenue
New York, NY 10018   212-852-8000
                                800-223-0624
                          Fax: 212-852-6515

Information on adaptive Girl Scout activities for
people of many abilities. Includes local chapters,
referrals, fun and social interaction and support
groups.

4460 Give Kids the World
210 S Bass Rd
Kissimmee, FL 34746   407-396-1114

Makes dreams come true for terminally ill children and their families with a six-day, cost-free
visit to Walt Disney World area.

4461 Grant-A-Wish Foundation
P.O. Box 21211
Baltimore, MD 21288   410-242-1549

Variety of programs designed to ease the burden
of long hospital stays and painful treatment programs for children. Grants wishes to individual
children and provides seashore and mountain retreats and in-hospital entertainment programs.
Also manages the Children's House at Johns
Hopkins.

4462 Growth Disorders - Human Growth Foundation
7777 Leesburg Pike, Suite 2025
Falls Church, VA 22043   703-883-1773
                                800-451-6434

Provides referrals to support groups, services,
genetic counseling on its toll-free telephone line.
Encourages communication among support
groups and continuing education.

4463 Handicapped Scuba Association
1104 El Prado
San Clemente, CA 92672   949-498-6128
                                800-673-5084
            e-mail: hsahdq@compuserve.com

Information on adaptive scuba diving activities
for people of many abilities. Includes local chapters, referrals, fun and social interaction and
support groups.

4464 Handle with Care
P.O. Box 1569
Wimberly, TX 78676   512-842-5049
                                888-590-5049
                          Fax: 512-847-6257

Information and advocacy resources for families and professionals. Includes listings of organizations providing general information and organizations focusing on more specific areas of concern to families and young adults who have disabilities.

4465 Helen Keller Center's National Parent Network
111 Middle Neck Road
Sands Point, NY 11050   516-944-8900
                              800-255-0411

Establishes a coalition of state parent organizations to promote the exchange of information among parents of deaf-blind youth. Provides training to parents to develop their legislative advocacy skills, empowers parents and their families to obtain services and ensures parents a meaningful life for their sons and daughters.

4466 Heriditary Disease Foundation
1427 7th Street, Suite 2
Santa Monica, CA 90401   310-458-4183
          e-mail: cures@hdfoundation.org

Conducts interdisciplinary workshop program that recruits scientists to develop and apply new technologies, supports basic research on genetic illness through grant and postdoctural fellowship programs at major universities, and provides research tissue to medical investigators.

4467 Houston Challengers TIRR Sports
1475 West Gray
Houston, TX 77019   713-521-3737

Information on adaptive sports and recreation activities for people of many abilities. Includes local chapters, referrals, fun and social interaction and support groups.

4468 Independent Living Research Utilization Program
2323 S Shepard, Suite 1000
Houston, TX 77019   713-520-0232
                          Fax: 713-520-5785
                          TTY: 713-520-5136

Information and advocacy resources for families and professionals on independent living for people with disabilities.

4469 Indian Health Service
Mental Health/Social Service Programs Branch
5300 Homestead Road NE
Albuquerque, NM 87110   505-248-4245
                              Fax: 505-248-4257

Includes listings of organizations providing general information and organizations focusing on more specific areas of concern to native american families and young adults who have disabilities.

4470 International Society of Dermatology
200 1st Street SW
Rochester, MN 55905   507-284-3736

Promotes interest, education and research in dermatology.

Sigfrid A. Muller, MD, President

4471 International Wheelchair Aviators
1117 Rising Hill Way
Escondido, CA 92029   619-746-5018

Provides information for pilots or future pilots who have a disability.

4472 Iron Overload Diseases Assocation, Inc.
433 Westwind Drive
North Palm Beach, FL 33408   407-840-8512
                              Fax: 407-842-9881
                              www.emi.net/iron iod/iod97.html

Committed to providing information and support to affected individuals and their families, educating the general public, promoting and supporting research, and pressing for earlier diagnosis and more effective treatment. Acts as a clearinghouse for affected individuals and family members, provides telephone consultations, offers referrals to genetic counseling and support groups. Provides a variety of educational and support materials including books, newsletters, pamphlets, and fact sheets.

4473 Jewish Children's Adoption Network
P.O. Box 16544
Denver, CO 80216   303-573-8113
                          Fax: 303-893-1447
                          e-mail: jcan@uswest.net
                          www.users.uswest.net/~jcan

Information and advocacy resources for families and professionals. Includes listings of organizations providing general information.

4474 Job Opportunities for the Blind
1800 Johnson Street
Baltimore, MD 21230   410-659-9314
                          Fax: 410-685-5653
                          e-mail: nfb@iamdigex.net.net
                          www.nfb.org

Information and resources for those with visual impairments.

4475 Just One Break, Inc.
120 Wall Street
New York, NY 10005   212-785-7300
                           Fax: 212-785-4513
                           TTY: 703-907-7422
e-mail: justonebreak@interactive.net
www.justonebreak.com

Information and advocacy resources for families
and professionals dealing with families and
young adults who have disabilities.

**4476 KEN: National Mental Health Knowledge Exchange
Network**
11426-28 Rockville Pike, Suite 405
Rockville, MD 20852
                           800-789-2647
                           Fax: 301-984-8796
www.mentalhealth.org

Information and advocacy resources for families
and professionals. Includes listings of organizations providing general information and organizations focusing on more specific areas of
concern to families and young adults who have
disabilities.

4477 Kids, Inc.
9300-D Old Keene Mill Road
Burke, VA 22015   703-455-KIDS

Grants unfulfilled wishes to gravely ill children
16 and younger anywhere in the U.S.

4478 Learning Disabilities Association of America (LDA)
4156 Library Road
Pittsburgh, PA 15234   412-341-1515
                              888-300-6710
                         Fax: 412-344-0224
e-mail: ldanatl@usaorg.org
www.ldanatl.org

Helps families of the affected individual through
up-to-date technology and further advancement
of the changes in the medical fields related to
this and similar disorders.

4479 MUMS: National Parent to Parent Network
c/o Julie Gordon
150 Cousta Street
Green Bay, WI 54301   920-336-5333
                         Fax: 920-339-0995
e-mail: mums@netnet.net
www.waisman.wisc.edu/~rowley/mums/home.h

Information and advocacy resources for families
and professionals. Includes listings of organizations providing general information and organizations focusing on more specific areas of
concern to families and young adults who have
disabilities.

4480 Make A Wish Foundation of America
100 W Clarendon, Suite 2200
Phoenix, AZ 85013   602-279-9474
                           800-722-9474
                      Fax: 602-279-0855
www.wish.org

Information and advocacy resources for families
and professionals. Includes listings of organizations providing general information and organizations focusing on more specific areas of
concern to families and young adults who have
disabilities.

4481 Make Today Count
101 1/2 South Union St
Alexandria, VA 22314   703-548-9674

An organization that helps patients and their
families cope with cancer and other serious diseases and improve their quality of life.

4482 March of Dimes Birth Defects Foundation
1275 Mamaroneck Avenue
White Plains, NY 10605
                           888-663-4637
                      Fax: 914-997-4763
e-mail: resourcecenter@modimes.org
www.modimes.org

Partnership of volunteers and professionals dedicated to the misson the health of babies by preventing birth defects and infant mortality. Over
100 chapters are located across the country and
can be located through the National Office.

Ann Umemoto, Medical Dir. Office

4483 March of Dimes Nursing Modules
1275 Mamaroneck Ave
White Plains, NY 10605   914-428-7100

Nursing modules are self-directed learning
monographs designed fr registered nurses and
nurse-midwives. Created to help nurses meet the
challenges posed by a rapidly changing world of
technological advances, evolving demographics
and greater cultural diversity, they focus on effective care delivery during the pre-concep-
tional, prenatal, intrapartum, postpartum and
inter-conceptional periods.

4484 Mobility International USA
P.O. Box 10767
Eugene, OR 97440
                           Fax: 541-343-6812
                           TDD: 541-343-1284
e-mail: info@miusa.org
www.miusa.org

Information and advocacy resources for families and professionals dealind with mobility issues of those with disabilities.

4485 NAEYC: National Association for the Education of Young Children
1509 16th Street, NW
Washington, DC 20036   202-232-8777
                            800-424-2460
                            Fax: 202-328-1846
                   e-mail: pubaff@aeyc.org
                            www.naeyc.org

Information and advocacy resources for families and professionals. Includes listings of organizations providing general information and organizations focusing on more specific areas of concern to families and young adults who have disabilities.

4486 NARIC: National Rehabilitation Information Center
1010 Wayne Ave.
Silver Spring, MD 20910   301-562-2400
                            800-346-2742
                       Fax: 301-562-2401
                            www.naric.com.

Resources for families and professionals dealing with the rehabilitation of people with disabilities.

4487 NIH/National Arthritis and Musculoskeletal & Skin Disease Information Clearinghouse
1 AMS Circle
Bethesda, MD 20892   301-495-4484
                       Fax: 301-718-6366
                       TTY: 301-565-2966
                            www.nih.gov/niams

Supports and provides public information and research to increase understanding of skin diseases and related disorders. Provides lists and order forms for resources and materials.

4488 NIH/National Diabetes Information Clearinghouse
2 Information Way
Bethesda, MD 20892   301-654-3810
                       Fax: 301-907-8906
               e-mail: nddic@info.niddk.nih.gov
                            www.niddk.nih.gov

4489 NIH/National Digestive Diseases Information Clearinghouse
2 Information Way
Bethesda, MD 20892   301-654-3810
                       Fax: 301-907-8906
               e-mail: nddic@info.niddk.nih.gov
                            www.niddk.nih.gov

Information and referral service of the National Institute of Diabetes and digestive and kidney diseases, and one of the National Institutes of Health central information resources on the prevention and management of digestive diseases. Responds to written inquiries, develops and distributes publications about digestive diseases, offers referrals to digestive disease organizations, including support groups. Maintains a database of patient and professional education materials.

4490 NIH/National Eye Institute
Building 31, Room 6A32
31 Center Drive, MSC 2510
Bethesda, MD 20892   301-496-5248
                       Fax: 301-402-1065
                  e-mail: 2020@nei.nih.gov

Information and advocacy resources for families and professionals. Includes listings of organizations providing general information and organizations focusing on more specific areas of concern to families and young adults who have disabilities.

4491 NIH/National Heart, Lung & Blood Institute
31 Center Dr, MSC2480, Bldg 31
Bethesda, MD 20892   301-594-1348
                            301-480-4907
                       TTY: 123-019-9912
            www.nhbli.nih.gov/nhlbi/nhlbi.htm

Provides leadership for a national research program in diseases of the heart, blood vessels, lungs, and blood and in transfusion medicine through support of innovative basic, clinical, and population-based and health education research.

4492 NIH/National Heart, Lung and Blood Institute Information Clearinghouse
31 Center Drive Building 31, Room 5A52
Baltimore, MD 20892   301-496-4236
                            www.nhlbi.nih.gov

Primary responsibility of this organization is the scientific investigation of heart, blood vessel, lung and blood disorders. Oversees research, demonstration, prevention, education, control and training activities in these fields and emphasizes the prevention and control of heart diseases.

Dr. Claude Lenfant, M.M., Director

4493 NIH/National Insitute of Allergy and Infectious Diseases
31 Center Drive
Bethesda, MD 20892   301-496-4634
                            www.niaid.nih.gov

Research on allergies and infectious diseases.

4494 NIH/National Institute of Arthritis & Musculoskeletal and Skin Diseases
Information Office-Bldg. 31-Room 4C-05
31 Center Drive - MSC2350
Bethesda, MD 20892   301-496-8188

Handles inquiries on arthritis, bone diseases and skin diseases and offers consumer and professional education materials.

4495 NIH/National Institute of Child Health & Human Development
NICHD Clearinghouse
P.O. Box 3006
Rockville, MD 20847

     800-370-2943
Fax: 301-496-7101
www.nih.gov/nichd

The National Institute for Child Health and Human Development conducts and supports laboratory, clinical and epidemiological research on the reproductive, neurobiologic, developmental, and behavioral processes that determine and maintain the health of children, adults, families, and populations.

4496 NIH/National Institute of Mental Health
5600 Fishers Lane
Rockville, MD 20857   301-443-4513
www.nimh.nih.gov

4497 NIH/National Institute of Neurological Disorders & Stroke
31 Center Dr MSC 2540, Bldg 31, Rm 8806
Bethesda, MD 20892   301-496-5751
800-352-9424
Fax: 301-402-2186
www.ninds.nih.gov

Information and advocacy resources for families and professionals. Includes listings of organizations providing general information and organizations focusing on more specific areas of concern to families and young adults who have disabilities.

4498 NIH/National Institute on Deafness & Other Communication Disorders Clearinghouse
1 Communication Avenue
Bethesda, MD 20892

     800-241-1044
Fax: 301-907-8830
TTY: 800-241-1055
e-mail: nidcdinfo@nidcd.nih.gov
www.nih.gov/nidcd

The National Institute on Deafness and Other Communication Disorders (NIDCD) Information Clearinghouse, a service of NIDCD, is a national resource center for health information about hearing, balance, smell, taste, voice, speech, and language for health professionals, patients, industry, and the public. The clearinghouse collects and disseminates information on normal and disordered process of human communication.

Mia Esserman, Project Manager

4499 NIH/National Kidney & Urologic Diseases Information Clearinghouse
3 Information Way
Bethesda, MD 20892   301-654-4415
Fax: 301-907-8906
e-mail: nddic@info.niddk.nih.gov
www.niddk.nih.gov

Information and referral service, responds to written inquires, develops and distributes publications about kidney and urologic diseases, and provides referrals to kidney and urologic organizations, including support groups. Maintains a database of patient and professional education materials, from which literature searches are generated.

4500 NIH/Office of Rare Diseases (ORD)
31 Center Drive, Room 1B03
Bethesda, MD 20892   301-402-4336
e-mail: sg18b@nih.gov
rarediseases.info.nih.gov/org

Information and advocacy resources for families and professionals. Includes listings of organizations providing general information and organizations focusing on more specific areas of concern to families and young adults who have disabilities.

4501 National Ability Center
P.O. Box 682799
Park City, UT 84068   435-649-3991
Fax: 435-658-3992
TDD: 435-649-3991
e-mail: nac@mission.com

Information on adaptive sports and recreation activities for people of many abilities. Includes local chapters, referrals, fun and social interaction and support groups.

4502 National Academy for Child Development (NACD)
P.O. Box 380
Huntsville, UT 84317   801-621-8606
Fax: 801-621-8389
e-mail: nacdinfo@nacd.org

International organization of parents and professional dedicated to helping children and adults reach their full potential.

4503 National Adoption Center
1500 Walnut Street, Suite 701
Philadelphia, PA 19102   215-735-9988
     800-862-3678
     Fax: 215-735-9410
     e-mail: nac@adopt.org
     www.adopt.org/adopt

Information and advocacy resources for families and professionals interested in or dealing with adoption. Includes listings of organizations providing general information and organizations focusing on specific areas of concern.

4504 National Alliance for the Mentally Ill (NAMI)
200 N Glebe Rd, Ste 1015
Arlington, VA 22203   703-524-7600
     800-950-6264
     Fax: 703-524-9094
     TTY: 703-516-7991
     e-mail: namioffc@aol.com
     www.nami.org

Aids families and individuals find the emotional and physical answers to the habitual forming disorders through several media resources.

4505 National Amputee Golf Association
P.O. Box 23285
Milwaukee, WI 53223   414-376-1268
     800-633-6242
     e-mail: naga@execpc.com

Information on adaptive golf activities for people of many abilities. Includes local chapters, referrals, fun and social interaction and support groups.

4506 National Archery Association
One Olympic Plaza
Colorado Springs, CO 80909   719-578-4576
     Fax: 719-632-4733
     e-mail: naa-ofc@ix.netcom.com
     www.usarchery.org

Information on adaptive archery activities for people of many abilities. Includes local chapters, referrals, fun and social interaction and support groups.

4507 National Arts and Disability Center
300 UCLA Medical Plaza, Suite 3330
Los Angeles, CA 90095   310-794-1141
     Fax: 310-794-1143
     TTY: 310-267-2356
     e-mail: oraynor@mednet.ucla.edu
     www.dcp.ucla.edu/nadc/

Information and advocacy resources for families and professionals. Includes listings of organizations providing general information on art and disabilities.

4508 National Association of Protection and Advocacy Systems
900 2nd Street NE, Suite 211
Washington, DC 20002   202-408-9514
     Fax: 202-408-9520
     TTY: 202-408-9521
     e-mail: NAPAS@earthlink.net
     www.protectionandadvocacy.com

Information and advocacy resources for families and professionals. Includes listings of organizations providing general information and organizations focusing on more specific areas of concern to families and young adults who have disabilities.

4509 National Association of Blind Students
National Federation of the Blind
1800 Johnson Street
Baltimore, MD 21230   410-659-9314
     Fax: 410-685-5653

This national organization of blind students has provided support, information and encouragement to blind college and university students. Leads the way in offering resources in issues such as national testing, accessible textbooks and materials, overcoming negative attitudes about blindness from school personnel, developing new techniques of accomplishing laboratory or field assignments and many other college experiences. Offers strong advocacy and motivational support.

4510 National Association of the Dually Diagnosed
132 Fair St
Kingston, NY 12401   914-331-4336
     800-331-5362
     Fax: 914-331-4569
     e-mail: nadd@ulster.net

Seeks to stimulate the public and professional awareness regarding the dually diagnosed population, and to encourage the exchange of pertinent information, promoting educational and training programs, advocating for appropriate governmental policies, supporting research focusing on indentification, diagnosis, and treatment.

4511 National Birth Defects Center
40 2nd Avenue, Suite 460
Waltham, MA 02154   617-466-9555

4512 National Cancer Institute
Office of Cancer Communications
9000 Rockville Pike Bldg 31 Rm10A16
Bethesda, MD 20892   301-496-5583
                           800-422-6237
                           www.nci.nih.gov/

Leads a national effort to reduce the burden of
cancer morbidity and mortality and ultimately
to prevent the disease. Through basic and clinical biomedical research and training, NCI conducts and supports programs to understand the
causes of cancer; prevent, detect, diagnose,
treat, and control cancer; and disseminate information to the practitioner, patient, and public.

4513 National Center for Education in Maternal & Child Health
2000 15th Street N, Suite 701
Arlington, VA 22201   703-524-7802
                           Fax: 703-524-9335
                           e-mail: info@ncemch.org
                           www.ncemch.org

Information and advocacy resources for families
and professionals. Includes listings of organizations providing general information and organizations focusing on more specific areas of
concern to families and young adults who have
disabilities.

4514 National Center for Health Statistics
6525 Belcrest Road
Hyattsville, MD 20782   301-458-4636
                           e-mail: nchsquery@cdc.gov
                           www.cdc.gov/nchswww

Information and advocacy resources for families
and professionals. Includes listings of organizations providing general information and organizations focusing on more specific areas of
concern to families and young adults who have
disabilities.

4515 National Center for Learning Disabilities
381 Park Ave S, Ste 1401
New York, NY 10016   212-545-7510
                           888-575-7373
                           Fax: 212-545-9665
                           www.ncld.org

Disperses information to the educational community and the general public regarding the disorder through reading and video materials.

4516 National Center for Vision and Child Development
Lighthouse
800 Second Avenue
New York, NY 10017

4517 National Center on Accessbility
University of Indiana
5020 State Road, 67 N
Martinville, IN 46151   765-349-9240
                           800-424-1877
                           Fax: 765-342-6658
                           e-mail: nca@indiana.edu

Information on adaptive activities for people of
many abilities. Includes local chapters, referrals, fun and social interaction and support
groups.

4518 National Childhood Cancer Foundation
440 East Huntington Dr, Ste 300
Arcadia, CA 91066   626-447-1674
                           800-458-6223
                           Fax: 626-447-6359
                           e-mail: nccf-info@ncff.org
                           www.nccf.org

4519 National Children's Cancer Society
1015 Locust Street, Suite 600
St. Louis, MO 63101   314-241-1600
                           800-532-6459
                           Fax: 314-241-6949
                           e-mail: nccs@children-cancer.com
                           www.children-cancer.com

NCCS offers a multifaceted outreach program,
which includes financial assistance, education,
information, and emotional support. They provide financial assistance for bone marrow transplantation, donor harvest, donor search, donor
recruitment, and family emergency expenses
(such as travel, hotel, food). They also have an
active advocacy program to help families with
insurance companies and hospitals.

Mark Stolze, President
Julie Komanetsky, Patient/Family Services, Director

4520 National Christian Resource Center
Bethesda Lutheran Homes
700 Hoffman Drive
Watertown, WI 53094
                           800-369-4636

Information and advocacy resources for families
and professionals. Includes listings of organizations providing general information and organizations focusing on more specific areas of
concern to families and young adults who have
disabilities.

4521 National Clearinghouse on Postsecondary Education
HEATH Resource Center
1 Dupont Cir. NW, Suite 800
Washington, DC 20036
Fax: 202-401-2608
TTY: 202-205-8241
www.ed.gov/offices/osers

Provides information for individuals with disabilities and resources for families and professionals. Includes listings of organizations providing general information and organizations focusing on more specific areas of concern to families and young adults who have disabilities.

4522 National Coalition of Title 1 Chapter 1 Parents
3609 Georgia Ave.
Washington, DC 20010
202-291-8100
Fax: 202-291-8200

Information and advocacy resources for parents and professionals. Includes listings of organizations providing general information and organizations focusing on more specific areas of concern to families and young adults who have disabilities.

4523 National Council on Disability
1331 F Street NW, Suite 1050
Washington, DC 20004
202-272-2004
Fax: 202-272-2022
TTY: 202-272-2074
www.ncd.gov

Information and advocacy resources for families and professionals. Includes listings of organizations providing general information and organizations focusing on more specific areas of concern to families and young adults who have disabilities.

4524 National Early Childhood Technical Assistance System
500 Nation Bank Plaza
137 East Franklin Street
Chapel Hill, NC 27514
919-962-2001

Assists states and other designated governing jurisdictions as they develop multidisciplinary, coordinated and comprehensive services for children with special needs.

4525 National Easter Seals
230 W. Monroe St. Ste 1800
Chicago, IL 60606
312-726-6200
800-221-6827
Fax: 312-726-1494
TDD: 312-726-4258
e-mail: info@easter-seal.org
www.easter-seals.org

Easter Seals mission is to create solutions that change lives for children and adults with disabilities and to provide appropriate developmental and rehabilitation services. Services provided include: early intervention, after-school programs, preschool, tutoring, medical rehabilitation, vocational services, adult and senior day services, respite and in home care, camping and recreation, residential housing, support services, support groups, transportation, and referrals.

4526 National Family Caregivers Association
10605 Concord Street, Suite 50
Kensington, MD 20895
301-942-6430
Fax: 301-942-2302
e-mail: info@nfcacares.org
www.nfcacares.org

The NFCA is the only not-for-profit organization dedicated to making life better for all of America's family caregivers. Services include: information support and validation, public awareness and advocacy; NFCA strives to minimize the dispairity between a caregivers quality of life and that of mainstream Americans.

4527 National Father's Network
Kettering Center
16120 NE 8th Street
Bellevue, WA 98008
425-747-4004
800-224-6827
Fax: 425-284-9664
fathersnetwork.org

Information and advocacy resources for fathers. Includes listings of organizations providing general information and organizations focusing on more specific areas of concern to fathers and young adults who have disabilities.

4528 National Foundation for Facial Reconstruction
317 East 34th Street
New York, NY 10016
212-340-6656

A nonprofit organization whose major purposes are to provide facilities for the treatment and assistance of individuals who are unable to afford private reconstructive surgical care, to train and educate professionals in this surgery, to encourage research in the field; and to carry on public education.

4529 National Foundation for Transplants
1102 Brookfield, Ste 200
Memphis, TN 38119
901-684-1697
800-489-3863
Fax: 901-684-1128
e-mail: notfoundtx@aol.com
www.transplants.org

Non-profit organization that assists transplant canidates and recipients nationwide when public or private insurance does not cover all their transplant related costs. offers a fund raising program for patients who need to raise $10,000 or more, and grant program that helps patients with smaller, one-time needs.

Janice Hill, Manager of Communications
Gary McMahan, Executive Director

4530 National Foundation of Wheelchair Tennis
940 Calle Amanecer, Suite B
San Clemente, CA 92673   714-361-3663
                               Fax: 714-361-6603
                               e-mail: nfwt@aol.com

Information on adaptive tennis for people of many abilities. Includes local chapters, referrals, fun and social interaction and support groups.

4531 National Handicapped Sports
451 Hungerford Drive, Suite 100
Rockville, MD 20850   301-217-0960
                            Fax: 301-217-0968
                            e-mail: dsusa@dsusa.org

Information on adaptive sports and recreation activities for people of many abilities, including local chapters, referrals, fun and social interaction and support groups.

4532 National Health Council
1730 M Street NW, Suite 500
Washington, DC 20036   202-785-3910
                             Fax: 202-785-5923
                             e-mail: info@nhcouncil.org
                             www.healthanswers.com

Information and advocacy resources for families and professionals. Includes listings of organizations providing general information and organizations focusing on more specific areas of concern to families and young adults who have disabilities.

4533 National Health Information Center
P.O. Box 1133
Washington, DC 20013   301-565-4137
                             800-336-4797
                             Fax: 301-984-4256
                             nhicinfo@health.org

The National Health Information Center can put you in touch with organizations that can answer your health-related questions. The National Health Information Center can provide you with names and addresses of appropriate organizations.

4534 National Health Information Center (NHIC)
P.O. Box 1133
Washington, DC 20013
                             800-336-4797
                             Fax: 301-984-4256
                             e-mail: nhicinfo@health.org
                             nhic-nt.health.org

Information and advocacy resources for families and professionals. Includes listings of organizations providing general information and organizations focusing on more specific areas of concern to families and young adults who have disabilities.

4535 National Hospice Organization
1901 North Moore Street Suite 901
Arlington, VA 22209   703-243-5900
                            800-338-8619

The nation's only advocate for terminally ill children, patients and their families. Provides member programs, represents hospice care interests in Congress, regulatory agencies and the public.

4536 National Industries for the Severely Handicapped
2235 Cedar Lane
Vienna, VA 22182   703-560-6800
                         Fax: 703-849-8916

Information and advocacy resources for families and professionals. Includes listings of organizations providing general information and organizations focusing on more specific areas of concern to families and young adults who have disabilities.

4537 National Industries for the Blind
191 N. Beauregard St, Ste 200
Alexandria, VA 22311   703-998-0770
                             Fax: 703-998-8268

A nonprofit organization that represents over 100 associated industries serving people who are blind in thirty-six states. These agencies serve people who are blind or visually impaired and help them to reach their full potential. Services include job and family counseling, job skills training, instruction in Braille and other communication skills, children's programs and more.

4538 National Information Center for Children and Youth with Disabilities (NICHY)
P.O. Box 1492
Washington, DC 20013   202-884-8200
                             800-695-0285
                             Fax: 202-884-8441
                             e-mail: nichey@aed.org
                             www.nichey.org

A clearinghouse that provides free pamphlets and information on disabilities and the rights of disabled children and their parents.

4539 National Institute of Dental Research
31 Ctr Dr Msc 2290, Bldg 31 Rm 2C39
Bethesda, MD 20892   301-496-3571
Fax: 301-402-2185
e-mail: slavkinh@od31.nidcr.nih.gov
www.nidr.nih.gov/discover/welcome.htm

The National Institute of Dental Research promotes the general   health of the American people by improving their oral, dental and craniofacial health. The NIDCR aims to promote health, to prevent diseases and conditions, and to develop new diagonistics and therapeutics.

Harold Slavkin, DDS

4540 National Institute on Deafness and Other Communication Disorders
1 Communication Avenue
Bethesda, MD 20892
800-241-1044
Fax: 301-907-8830
TTY: 800-241-1055
e-mail: nidcdinfo@nidcd.nih.gov
www.nih.gov/nidcd

The National Institute on Deafness and Other Communication Disorders (NIDCD) Information Clearinghouse, a service of NIDCD, is a national resource center for health information about hearing, balance, smell, taste, voice, speech, and language for health professionals, patients, industry, and the public. The clearinghouse collects and disseminates information on normal and disdordered process of human communication.

Mia Esserman, Project Manager

4541 National Library Service for the Blind & Physically Handicapped
Library of Congress Reference Section
1291 Taylor Street NW
Washington, DC 20542   202-707-5100
800-424-8567
Fax: 202-707-0712
TTY: 202-707-0744
TDD: 202-707-0744
e-mail: nis@loc.gov
www.loc.gov/nls

Administers a natural library service that provides recorded and braille reading materials to eligible children and adults who cannot read standard print.

Frank Kurt Cylke, Director

4542 National Maternal & Child Health Clearinghouse
2070 Chain Bridge Road, Suite 450
Vienna, VA 22182   703-821-8955
Fax: 703-821-2098
e-mail: nmchc@circsol.com
www.circsol.com

Information and advocacy resources for families and professionals. Includes listings of organizations providing general information and organizations focusing on more specific areas of concern to families and young adults who have disabilities.

4543 National Mental Health Association
1021 Prince St
Alexandria, VA 22314   703-684-5968
800-969-6642
e-mail: namiofc@aol.com
www.cais.com/vikings/nami/index.html

Notifies the public of the various groups and foundations to answer and assist them with their concerns and questions.

4544 National Mental Health Consumer Self-Help Clearinghouse
1211 Chestnut Street
Philadelphia, PA 19107   215-751-1810
800-553-4539
Fax: 215-636-6310
e-mail: info@mhselfhelp.org
www.mhselfhelp.org

Offers information, support, and appropriate referrals; and promotes public and professional education. Provides networking for those with special interests related to albinism and promotes and supports research and funding that will improve diagnosis and management of albinism and hypopigmentation.

4545 National Oral Health Information Clearinghouse
Institute of Dental and Craniofacial Research
1 NOHIC Way
Bethesda, MD 20892   301-402-7364
Fax: 301-907-8830
TTY: 301-656-7581
e-mail: nidr@aerie.com
www.aerie.com/nohicweb

Produces and distributes patient and professional education materials including fact sheets, brochures, information packets and provides referrals to other organizations dealing with special care in oral health. Special Care is an approach to oral health management that is tailored to the specific needs of persons with a variety of medical, disabling, or mental conditions. Database includes bibliographic citations, abstracts, and availability information for a variety of print and materials.

4546 National Organization for Rare Disorders Inc. (NORD)
P.O. Box 8923
New Fairfield, CT 06812   203-746-6518
                                 800-999-6673
                                 Fax: 203-746-6481
                                 TDD: 203-746-6927
                                 e-mail: orphan@nord-rdb.com
                                 www.nord-rdb.com/~orphan

Federation of voluntary health organizations dedicated to helping people with rare orphan diseases and assisting the organizations that serve them. NORD is committed to the identification, treatment and cure of rare disorders through programs of education, advocacy, research and service.

103,000 Members

Abbey S. Meyers, Ph.D. (Honorary), President

4547 National Organization of Parents of Blind Children
National Federation of the Blind
1800 Johnson Street
Baltimore, MD 21230   410-659-9314
                                 Fax: 410-685-5653
                                 e-mail: nfb@iamdigex.net
                                 www.nfb.org

Support, information and advocacy organization of parents of blind or visually impaired children. Addresses issues ranging from help to parents of a newborn blind infant, mobility and Braille instruction, education, social and community participation, development of self-confidence and other vital factors involved in the growth of a blind child. Strong national network of contacts with other parents offers encouragement and positive philosophical support. Publishes Future Reflections.

Barbara Cheadle, President

4548 National Organization on Disability
910 16th Street NW, Suite 600
Washington, DC 20006   202-293-5960
                                 Fax: 202-293-7999
                                 TTY: 202-293-5968
                                 e-mail: ability@nod.org
                                 www.nod.org

Mission is to promote the full participation of America's men, women and children with physical, sensory or mental disabilities, in all apsects of life, and thus expand their contribution to America. Supports legislation to improve the lives of people with disabilities and is committed to closing the gap between Americans with and without disabilities

4549 National Parent Network on Disabilities, (NPND)
1130 17th Street, NW, Suite 400
Washington, DC 20036   202-463-2299
                                 Fax: 202-463-9403

Information and advocacy resources for families and professionals. Includes listings of organizations providing general information and organizations focusing on more specific areas of concern to families and young adults who have disabilities.

4550 National Parent Resource Center
Federation for Children with Special Needs
1135 Tremont Street, Suite 420
Boston, MA 02116   617-482-2915
                                 800-331-0688
                                 Fax: 617-572-2094
                                 e-mail: fcsninfo@fcsn.org
                                 www.fcsn.org

A parent-run resource system designed to further the needs and goals of family-centered, community-based coordinated care for children with special health needs and their families. Offers written materials, training packages, workshops and presentations for parents and professionals on special education, health care financing and other topics.

4551 National Perinatal Association (NPA)
3500 E Fletcher Avenue, Suite 209
Tampa, FL 33613   813-971-1008
                                 800-638-2229
                                 Fax: 813-971-9306
                                 e-mail: npaonline@aol.com
                                 www.nationalperinatal.org

Information and advocacy resources for families and professionals. Includes listings of organizations providing general information and organizations focusing on more specific areas of concern to families and young adults who have disabilities.

4552 National Prevention Information Network
Center for Disease Control
P.O. Box 6003
Rockville, MD 20849   301-562-1098
                                 800-458-5231
                                 Fax: 888-282-7681
                                 TTY: 800-243-7012
                                 e-mail: info@cdcnac.org
                                 www.cdcnpin.org

Information and advocacy resources for families and professionals. Includes listings of organizations providing general information and organizations focusing on more specific areas of concern to families and young adults who have disabilities.

4553 National Recreation and Park Association
22377 Belmont Ridge Road
Ashburn, VA 20148   703-858-0784
e-mail: info@nrpa.org

Information on adaptive sports and recreation activities for people of many abilities. Includes local chapters, referrals, fun and social interaction and support groups.

4554 National Respite Locator Service
800 Eastowne Drive, Suite 105
Chapel Hill, NC 27514
800-773-5433
Fax: 919-490-4905
e-mail: hn4735@connectinc.com/locator.htm
www.chtop.com

Information and advocacy resources for families and professionals interested in repite care. Includes listings of organizations providing general information and organizations focusing on more specific areas of concern to families and young adults who have disabilities.

4555 National Self-Help Clearinghouse
365 5th Ave.
New York, NY 10016   212-817-1822
www.selfhelpweb.org

Information and advocacy resources for families and professionals. Includes listings of organizations providing general information and organizations focusing on more specific areas of concern to families and young adults who have disabilities.

4556 National Skeet & Sporting Clay Headquarters
5931 Rofp Road
San Antonio, TX 78253   210-688-3371
Fax: 210-688-3014

Information on adaptive skee and sporting clay activities for people of many abilities.

4557 National Sleep Foundation
729 15th Street NW 4th Floor
Washington, DC 20005   202-347-3471
Fax: 202-347-3472
e-mail: natsleep@erols.com
www.sleepfoundation.org

Works to improve the quality of life for millions of Americans who suffer from sleep disorders, and to prevent the catastrophic accidents that are related to poor or disordered sleep through research, education and the dissemination of information towards the cause of Narcolepsy Project. Seeks patients to aid new research project targeting the cause of the disorder.

Allan I. Pack, M.D., Ph.D., Medical Director

4558 National Vaccines Information Center
512 W Maple Avenue, Suite 206
Vienna, VA 22180   703-938-0342
Fax: 703-938-5768
www.909shot.com

Information and advocacy resources for families and professionals. Includes listings of organizations providing general information and organizations focusing on more specific areas of concern to families and young adults who have disabilities.

4559 National Wheelchair Racquetball Association
2380 McGinley Road
Monroeville, PA 15146   412-856-2400
Fax: 412-856-2437

Information on adaptive racquetball activities for people of many abilities.

4560 National Wheelchair Shooting Federation
102 Park Avenue
Rockledge, PA 19046   215-379-2359
Fax: 215-663-0102

Information on adaptive shooting activities for people of many abilities.

4561 National Wheelchair Softball Association
1616 Todd Court
Hastings, MN 55033   651-437-1792
Fax: 612-437-3889

Information on adaptive softball activities for people of many abilities.

4562 North American Riding for the Handicapped
Box 33150
Denver, CO 80233   303-452-1212
800-369-7433
Fax: 303-252-4610
e-mail: narha.org
www.narha.orgs

Information on adaptive riding activities for people of many abilities. Includes local chapters, referrals, fun and social interaction and support groups. NARHA is a membership organization that promotes and supports equine activities for the disabled. Membership dues are $50 - $150.

4563 Office for Fair Housing & Equal Opportunity
Department of Housing & Urban Development

Washington, DC 20002   202-275-0848
Fax: 202-275-2987
TTY: 202-275-0772
e-mail: nis@loc.gov
www.loc.gov/nls

Information and advocacy resources for families and professionals. Includes listings of organizations providing general information and organizations focusing on more specific areas of concern to families and young adults who have disabilities.

4564 Office of Special Education and Rehabilitation Services
330 C St SW, Switzer Bldg, Room 3132
Washington, DC 20202   202-205-8723
Fax: 202-401-2608
TTY: 202-205-8241
www.ed.gov/offices/osers

Information and advocacy resources for families and professionals. Includes listings of organizations providing general information and organizations focusing on more specific areas of concern to families and young adults who have disabilities.

4565 Pathways Awareness Foundation
123 N Wacker Dr
Chicago, IL 60606   312-701-3050
800-955-2445
Fax: 847-729-1116
TTY: 800-326-8154
e-mail: friends@pathwaysawareness.org
http://www.pathwaysawareness.org

Pathways Awareness Foundation provides informational materials to raise awareness of subtle indicators of physical development problems in infants and young children among parents, families, health professionals and others. This foundation advocates for early intervention, including physical, occupational and speech therapy, to prevent or modify a disabling developmental outcome.

Kelli Moore, Director, Marketing

4566 Pharmaceutical Manufacturers Association
1100 15th Street NW
Washington, DC 20005
800-762-4636
www.oncolink.com/specialty/chemo/indigen

Many drug companies have programs to provide free medicines (including chemotherapy) to needy patients. Eligibility requirements vary, but most are available to those not covered by private or public insurance programs. Ask your physician to request, on letterhead, a free copy of the Directory of Pharmaceutical indigent programs.

4567 Pike Institute on Law and Disability
Boston University School of Law
765 Commonwealth Avenue
Boston, MA 02115
Fax: 617-353-2906
TTY: 617-353-2904
e-mail: pikeinst@bu.edu
www.bu.edu/law/pike

Information and advocacy resources for families and professionals. Includes listings of organizations providing general information and organizations focusing on more specific areas of concern to families and young adults who have disabilities.

4568 Pioneers Division of CEC
The Council for Exceptional Children
1920 Association Drive
Reston, VA 20191   703-620-3660
Fax: 703-264-9474
TTY: 703-264-9446
www.cec.spec.org

Promotes activities and programs to increase awareness of the educational needs of children with disablties and/or who are gifted, and the servcies that are available to them.

4569 Planetree Health Information Service
2040 Webster Street
San Francisco, CA 94115   415-923-3680

A nonprofit consumer-oriented resource for health information, including relaxation and visualization techniques. Write or call for a catalog and price list.

4570 President's Committee on Mental Retardation
370 L'Enfant Promenade, S.W.#701
Washington, DC 20447   202-619-0634
Fax: 202-205-9519
e-mail: prma@acp.dhhs.govprograms/pcmr
http://www.acf.dhhs.gov/

Information and advocacy resources for families and professionals. Includes listings of organizations providing general information and organizations focusing on more specific areas of concern to families and young adults who have disabilities. Serves in an advisory capacity to the President of the U.S. and the Secretary of the Dept. of Health and Human Services.

4571 President's Committee on Employment of People with Disabilities
1331 F Street NW, 3rd Floor
Washington, DC 20004   202-376-6200
Fax: 202-376-6219
TTY: 202-376-6205
www.pcepd.gov

Information and advocacy resources for families and professionals. Includes listings of organizations providing general information and organizations focusing on more specific areas of concern to families and young adults who have disabilities.

4572 Resource for Children with Special Needs
200 Park Ave S, Ste 816
New York, NY 10003   212-677-4650
                                Fax: 212-254-4070
                    e-mail: resourcenyc@prodigy.net

4573 Roeher Institute
Kinsmen Building, York University
4700 Keele Street
North York, ON,   M3J
Canada   416-661-9611
                          e-mail: info@roeher.ca
                          www.indie.ca/roeher

Conducts research for various pediatric disabilities.

4574 Ronald McDonald Houses
500 N Michigan Ave, 2nd Floor
Chicago, IL 60611   312-836-7455

Provides national programs, funding and other support to network of 150 local Ronald McDonald Houses, homes-away-from-homes for families of seriously-ill children

4575 Rural Institute on Disabilities
University of Montana
52 Corbin Hall
Missoula, MT 59812

                                800-732-0323
                                Fax: 406-243-4730
                                TTY: 403-243-5467
                    e-mail: muarid@selway.umt.edu
                    www.ruralinstitute.umt.edu

Information and advocacy resources for families and professionals. Includes listings of organizations providing general information and organizations focusing on more specific areas of concern to families and young adults who have disabilities.

4576 Senate Subcommittee on Disability Policy
113 Hart Senate Office Building
Washington, DC 20510   202-224-6265
                                Fax: 202-228-2923
                                TTY: 202-224-3457
                    e-mail: tom_harkin@harkin.senate.gov

Information and advocacy resources for families and professionals. Includes listings of organizations providing general information and organizations focusing on more specific areas of concern to families and young adults who have disabilities.

4577 Sexuality Information and Education Council of the US (SIECUS)
130 W 42nd Street, Suite 350
New York, NY 10036   212-819-9770
                                Fax: 212-819-9776
                          e-mail: siecus@siecus.org
                          www.siecus.org/

Information and advocacy resources for families and professionals. Includes listings of organizations providing general information and organizations focusing on more specific areas of concern to families and young adults who have disabilities.

4578 Sibling Support Project
Children's Hospital and Regional Medical Center
P.O. Box 5371 CL-09
Seattle, WA 98105   206-527-5711
                                Fax: 206-527-5705
                          e-mail: dmeyer@chmc.org
                    www.chmc.org/departmt/sibsupp

Information and advocacy resources for families and professionals. Includes listings of organizations providing general information and organizations focusing on more specific areas of concern to families and young adults who have disabilities.

4579 Ski for Light
5 McAuliffe Drive
North Brunswick, NJ 08902   609-520-8079
                          e-mail: acooke@rfbd.org

Information on adaptive skiing.

4580 Sparrow Foundation
1155 N., 130th, Suite 310
Seattle, WA 98104   206-745-5403

This nonprofit charitable and educational organization was started by the family of a child who needed a bone marrow transplant, for which their insurance carrier refused to pay. The foundation provides seed money to schools, youth organizations, service clubs, and churches which help persons with medical needs.

4581 Spaulding for Children
16250 Northland Drive, Suite 120
Southfield, MI 48075   248-443-7080
                                Fax: 248-443-7099

Information and advocacy resources for families and professionals. Includes listings of organizations providing general information and organizations focusing on more specific areas of concern to families and young adults who have disabilities.

4582 Special Needs Advocate for Parents (SNAP)
1801 Avenue of the Stars #401
Century City, CA 90067   310-201-9614
                               888-310-9889
                          Fax: 310-201-9889
e-mail: info@spapinfo.org
www.spapinfo.org

Non-profit organization with advisors nationwide information and advocacy resources for families and professionals. Includes listings of organizations providing general information and organizations focusing on more specific areas of concern to families and young adults who have disabilities, support groups educational advocates and medical insurance problem solving. Quarterly newsletter with articles of interest.

Marla Kraus, Executive Director

4583 Special Olympics International
1325 G Street NW, Suite 500
Washington, DC 20005   202-628-3630
                          Fax: 202-824-0200
e-mail: specialolympics@msn.com

Information on adaptive sports and recreation activities for people of many abilities. Including local chapters, referrals, fun and social interaction and support groups.

4584 Specialized Training of Military Parents (STOMP)
c/o Washington PAVE
6316 S 12th Street
Tacoma, WA 98465
                               800-298-3543
                          Fax: 253-566-8052
                          TTY: 253-565-2266
e-mail: wapave@washingtonpave.com
www.washingtonpave.org

Information and advocacy resources for families and professionals. Includes listings of organizations providing general information and organizations focusing on more specific areas of concern to families and young adults who have disabilities.

4585 Starbright
1900 S. Bundy Drive, Suite 100
Los Angeles, CA 90025   310-477-9090
                               310-447-9090

This group, led by Steven Spielberg, is composed of pediatric health care professionals, experts in computer technology, and leaders in the field of entertainment. They have developed interactive, virtual-reality playgrounds where kids meet, talk, and play with other sick kids across the country. Starbright's mission is to improve the quality of life of seriously ill children and their families by taking a leadership role in the development of entertainment-oriented therapeutic interventions.

4586 Sunshine Foundation
1041 Mill Creek Drive
Feasterville, PA 19053   215-396-4770
                               800-767-1976
                          Fax: 215-396-4774
e-mail: philly@sunshinefoundation.org
www.sunshinefoundation.org

Grants dreams and wishes of terminally and chronically ill children whose parents are under financial strain due to the child's illness. Original wish granting organization.

Patricia C. Radecke, Executive Assistant

4587 Tech Connection
C/O Family Resource Associates, Inc
35 Haddon Avenue
Shrewsbury, NJ 07702   732-747-5310
                          Fax: 732-747-1896
e-mail: techhorin@aol.com
www.techconnection.org

Tech Connection is a resource center to help children and adults who have disabilities gain access to the benefits of technology. Includes nationwide network of community based assistive technology, resource centers, hands on consultants and product demonstrations and evaluations.

4588 Technology Assistance for Special Consumers
P.O. Box 443
Huntsville, AL 35804   256-532-5996
                          Fax: 256-532-2355
                          TDD: 256-532-5996
e-mail: tasc@travellers.com

Technology group of parents, consumers and professionals; provides resources to help children and adults who have disabilities gain access to the benefits of technology. Includes nationwide network of community-based assistive technology, resource centers, hands on consultants and product demonstrations.

4589 World Health Organization (WHO)
525 23rd Street NW
Washington, DC 20037   202-974-3000
                             Fax: 202-974-3663
                    e-mail: postmaster@paho.org
                              www.paho.org

Acts as the directing and co-ordinating authority on international health work; aids in the prevention and control of epidemic, endemic and other diseases; promotes the improvement of nutrition, housing, sanitation, recreation, economic or working conditions; promotes improved standards of teaching and training in the health, medical and related professions; and fosters activities in the field of mental health.

4590 World Institute on Disability
510 16th Street, Suite 100
Oakland, CA 94612   510-763-4100
                          Fax: 510-763-4109
                          TTY: 510-208-9493
                     e-mail: wid@wid.org
                              www.wid.org

Information and advocacy resources for families and professionals. Includes listings of organizations providing general information and organizations focusing on more specific areas of concern to families and young adults who have disabilities.

4591 Young Adult Institute
460 West 34th Street
New York, NY 10001   212-563-7474

A non-profit professional organization serving developmentally disabled children and adults in many programs throughout the New York metropolitan area. Provides over 50 program sites for thousands of participants.

Joel Levy, Executive Director

State Agencies & Support Groups

Alabama

4592 ARC of Morgan County
2046 Beltline Hwy, Suite 4
Decatur, AL 35601   205-355-6192

Informational and emotional support to parents who have a child, adolescent, or adult family member with special needs.

4593 Alabama Institute for the Deaf & Blind
P.O. Box 698
Talladega, AL 35160   256-761-3200
                            Fax: 256-761-3344
                            www.nectas.unc.edu

Services include central directory, representatives of agencies, service providers, families, and coordinators of infant, toddler, and preschool special education programs.

Joseph Busta, Interagency Coordinating Council

4594 Early Intervention Program
P.O. Box 11586
Montgomery, AL 36111   334-281-8780
                             Fax: 334-613-3541
                  e-mail: oholder@rehab.state.al.us
                              www.nectas.unc.edu

Services include central directory, representatives of agencies, service providers, families, and coordinators of infant, toddler, and preschool special education programs.

Ouidah Holder, Infant/Toodler Program Coor.

4595 Friends for Life Auburn United Methodist Church
137 S Gay Street
Auburn, AL 36830   334-826-8800

Informational and emotional support to parents who have a child, adolescent, or adult family member with special needs.

4596 Magic Moments c/o Children's Hospital of Alabama
1600 7th Avenue South
Birmingham, AL 35233   205-939-9372
                             Fax: 205-939-9189

Grants wishes to children 4 to 19 living or being treated in Alabama, who have chronic, life-threatening diseases, or who have severe trauma (burns, spinal cord, head trauma).

4597 Special Education Action Committee Huntsville Outreach Office
3322 S. Memorial Pkwy, Suite 25
Huntsville, AL 35801   256-882-3911
                             Fax: 256-882-3974
                    e-mail: seach@traveler.com
                          www.hsv.tis.net/~seachsv

Informational and emotional support to parents who have a child, adolescent, or adult family member with special needs.

4598 Special Education Action Committee, Inc.
600 Bel Air Blvd., #210
Mobile, AL 36606   334-478-1208
800-222-7322
Fax: 334-473-7877
e-mail: seacofmobile@zebra.net
www.hsv.tis.net/~seachsv

Parent Training and Information (PTI) programs help parents to: understand their children's specific needs; communicate more effectively with professionals, participate in the educational planning process; and obtain information about relevant programs, services, and resources

4599 Special Education Services

Phyllis Mayfield, author

Department of Education
P.O. Box 302101
Montgomery, AL 36104   334-242-8114
Fax: 334-242-9192
e-mail: jwaid@sdenet.alsde.edu
www.nectas.unc.edu

Services include central directory, representatives of agencies, service providers, families, and coordinators of infant, toddler, and preschool special education programs.

Phyllis Mayfield, Preschool Specialist

4600 Statewide Technology Access & Response System for Alabamians with Disabilities
2125 E South Blvd.
P.O. Box 20752
Montgomery, AL 36120   334-613-3480
800-782-7656
Fax: 334-613-3485
TDD: 334-613-3519
e-mail: tgannaway@rehab.state.al.us
www.mindspring.com/alstar/

State assisted programs and support group information for people of many abilities. Including local chapters, referrals, fun and social interaction and support groups.

Alaska

4601 Alaska Department of Education
801 West 10th Street, Suite 200
Juneau, AK 99801   907-465-2972
Fax: 907-465-2806
e-mail: dbrown@educ.state.ak.us
www.nectas.unc.edu

Individuals with Disabilities Education Act requires early intervention and preschool special education for children with disabilities and special healthcare needs. Services include central directory, representatives of agencies, service providers, families, and coordinators of infant, toddler, and preschool special education programs.

Diann Brown, Preschool Special Ed. Coordinator

4602 Assistive Technologies of Alaska
1016 W 6th Street, Suite 205
Anchorage, AK 99501   907-269-3570
Fax: 907-269-3632
TDD: 907-269-0153
e-mail: atadvr@corecom.net
www.corcom.net/ATA/

State assisted programs and support group information for people of many abilities. Including local chapters, referrals, fun and social interaction and support groups.

4603 Maternal, Child & Family Health, Early Intervention/Infant Learning Program
State of Alaska Department of Health
1231 Gambell Street
Anchorage, AK 99501   907-269-3419
Fax: 907-269-3465
e-mail: jbatuk@health.state.ak.us

Early intervention and preschool special education for children with disabilities and special healthcare needs. Services include administration of statewide early intervention programs for infants and toddlers with developmental delays or disabilities and their families.

Jane Atuk, Part C Coordinator
Karen Martinek, Special Needs Services Unit

4604 PARENTS, Inc.
4743 E. Northern Lights Blvd.
Anchorage, AK 99508   907-337-7678
Fax: 907-337-7671
TDD: 907-337-7678
e-mail: parentsss@alaska.com
www.alaska.net/~parents/

Parent Training and Information (PTI) programs help parents to: understand their children's specific needs; communicate more effectively with professionals, participate in the educational planning process; and obtain information about relevant programs, services, and resources

Arizona

4605 Arizona Early Intervention Program Department of Economic Security
P.O. Box 6123, 801-A-6
Phoenix, AZ 85005 602-532-9960
Fax: 602-200-9820
e-mail: azeip@aztec.asu.edu
www.nectas.unc.edu

Early intervention and preschool special education for children with disabilities and special healthcare needs. Services include central directory, representatives of agencies, service providers, families, and coordinators of infant, toddler, and preschool special education programs.

Diane Renne, Infant/Toodler Program Coordinator

4606 Arizona Technology Access Program Institute for Human Development
NAU Box 5630
Flagstaff, AZ 86011
800-477-9921
Fax: 520-523-9127
TDD: 520-523-1695
e-mail: Daniel.Davidson@nau.edu
www.nau.edu/~ihd/aztap.html

State assisted programs and support group information for people of many abilities. Including local chapters, referrals, fun and social interaction and support groups.

4607 Blake Foundation Children's Achievement Center
3825 East 2nd Street
Tucson, AZ 85716 520-325-0611
Fax: 520-327-5414
www.nectas.unc.edu

Services include central directory, representatives of agencies, service providers, families, and coordinators of infant, toddler, and preschool special education programs.

Annabell Rose, Interagency Coordinating Council

4608 Division of Special Education State Department of Education
1535 West Jefferson
Phoenix, AZ 85007 602-542-3852
Fax: 602-542-5404
e-mail: lbusenb@mail1.ade.state.az.us
www.nectas.unc.edu

Individuals with Disabilities Education Act requires all states and territories to provide early intervention and preschool special education for children with disabilities and special healthcare needs. Services include central directory, representatives of agencies, service providers, families, and coordinators of infant, toddler, and preschool special education programs.

Lynn Busenbark, Preschool Special Ed. Cooridnator

4609 National Association for Parents of the Visually Impaired
1720 E. Hermosa Drive
Tempe, AZ 85282 602-730-8282

Mary Ellen Simmons

4610 Pilot Parent Partnerships
4750 N. Black Canyon Hwy., Suite101
Phoenix, AZ 85017 602-242-4366
Fax: 602-242-4306
TDD: 602-242-4366
www.taalliance.org

Helps parents to: understand their children's specific needs; communicate more effectively with professionals, participate in the educational planning process; and obtain information about relevant programs, services, and resources

4611 Pilot Parents of Southern Arizona
2600 N. Wyatt Drive
Tucson, AZ 85712 520-324-3150
Fax: 520-324-3154
e-mail: ppsa@azstamet.com
www.azstamet.com/~ppsa

Parent Training and Information (PTI) programs help parents to: understand their children's specific needs; communicate more effectively with professionals, participate in the educational planning process; and obtain information about relevant programs, services, and resources

4612 Reaching Harmony: Native American Family Support, Inc.
P.O. Box 1420
Widow Rock, AZ 86515 520-871-6338
Fax: 520-871-7865
e-mail: paulas@dns.nncs.ihs.gov
www.taalliance.org

Programs help parents to: understand their children's specific needs; communicate more effectively with professionals, participate in the educational planning process; and obtain information about relevant programs, services, and resources

4613 Southwest Human Development
202 East Earll #140
Phoenix, AZ 85012   602-266-5976
e-mail: gward@swhd.org
www.nectas.unc.edu

Services include central directory, representatives of agencies, service providers, families, and coordinators of infant, toddler, and preschool special education programs.

Ginger Mach-Ward, Interagency Coordinating Council

Arkansas

4614 Arkansas Disability Coalition
2801 Lee Avenue, Suite 8
Little Rock, AR 72205   501-614-7020
Fax: 501-614-9082
TDD: 501-614-7020
e-mail: adc@cei.net
www.taalliance.org

Parent Training and Information (PTI) programs help parents to: understand their children's specific needs; communicate more effectively with professionals, participate in the educational planning process; and obtain information about relevant programs, services, and resources

4615 DD Services, Department of Human Services
P.O. Box 1437, Slot 2520
Little Rock, AR 72203   501-682-8699
Fax: 501-682-8890
e-mail: dds1@aristotle.net
www.nectas.unc.edu

Individuals with Disabilities Education Act requires all states and territories to provide early intervention and preschool special education for children with disabilities and special healthcare needs. Services include central directory, representatives of agencies, service providers, families, and coordinators of infant, toddler, and preschool special education programs.

Sherry Cobb, Infant/Toodler Program Coordinator

4616 FOCUS, Inc.
305 West Jefferson Avenue
Jonesboro, AR 72401   870-935-2750
Fax: 870-931-3755
e-mail: focusinc@ipa.net
www.taalliance.org

Parent Training and Information (PTI) programs help parents to: understand their children's specific needs; communicate more effectively with professionals, participate in the educational planning process; and obtain information about relevant programs, services, and resources

4617 Increasing Capabilities Access Network
Dept of Education/Arkansas Rehabilitation Services
2201 Brookwood, Suite 117
Little Rock, AR 72202
Fax: 501-666-5319
TTY: 501-666-8868
TDD: 800-828-2799
e-mail: 102503.3602@compuserve.com
www.arkansas-ican.org

State assisted programs and support group information for people of many abilities. Including local chapters, referrals, fun and social interaction and support groups.

4618 Parent to Parent Arc of Arkansas
2000 Main Street
Little Rock, AR 72206   501-375-7770
Fax: 501-372-4621

Informational and emotional support to parents who have a child, adolescent, or adult family member with special needs.

4619 Special Education Section State Department of Education
#4 Capitol Mall, Room 105-C
Little Rock, AR 72201   501-682-4225
Fax: 501-682-4313
e-mail: sreifeiss@arkedu.k12.ar.us
www.nectas.unc.edu

Individuals with Disabilities Education Act requires all states and territories to provide early intervention and preschool special education for children with disabilities and special healthcare needs. Services include central directory, representatives of agencies, service providers, families, and coordinators of infant, toddler, and preschool special education programs.

Sandra Reifeissk, Preschool Special Ed. Cooridnator

California

4620 Bereavement Group for Children
The Center for Attitudinal Healing
19 Main Street
Tiburon, CA   415-331-6161

For children who have suffered the loss of a close loved one. Parent group meets separately at the same time.

Jimmy Pete

4621 CARE Family Resource Center
1350 Arnold Drive, Suite 203
Martinez, CA 94553   925-313-0999
     Fax: 925-370-8651

Informational and emotional support to parents who have a child, adolescent, or adult family member with special needs.

4622 California Assistive Technology System
CA Department of Rehabilitation
830 K Street, Room 102
Sacramento, CA 95814
     Fax: 916-323-0914
     TDD: 916-324-3062
     e-mail: doroa.ccampsisis@hw1.cahwnet.gov
     www.catsca.org

State assisted programs and support group information for people of many abilities. Including local chapters, referrals, fun and social interaction and support groups.

4623 Carolyn Kordich Family Resource Center
P.O. Box 216
Harbor City, CA 90710   310-325-7288
     Fax: 310-325-7288
     e-mail: ckfrc@worldnet.att.net

Informational and emotional support to parents who have a child, adolescent, or adult family member with special needs.

4624 Challenged Family Resource Center
623 W 13st Street
Merced, CA 95340   209-385-8454
     Fax: 209-385-8483
     e-mail: dkuneck@aol.com

Informational and emotional support to parents who have a child, adolescent, or adult family member with special needs.

4625 Comfort Connection Family Resource Center
12361 Lewis Street, Suite 101
Garden Grove, CA 92840   714-748-7491
     Fax: 714-748-8149

Informational and emotional support to parents who have a child, adolescent, or adult family member with special needs.

4626 Early Intervention Program Department of Developmental Services
P.O. Box 944202
Sacramento, CA 95814   916-654-2773
     Fax: 916-654-3255
     e-mail: cflores@dds.ca.gov
     www.nectas.unc.edu

Individuals with Disabilities Education Act requires all states and territories to provide early intervention and preschool special education for children with disabilities and special healthcare needs. Services include central directory, representatives of agencies, service providers, families, and coordinators of infant, toddler, and preschool special education programs.

Carlos Flores, Interagency Coordinating Council

4627 Early Start Family Resource Network
P.O. Box 6127
San Bernadino, CA 92412   909-890-3103
     Fax: 909-890-3371

Informational and emotional support to parents who have a child, adolescent, or adult family member with special needs.

4628 Exceptional Family Resource Center
9245 Sky Park Ct., Suite 130
San Diego, CA 92123   619-292-9092
     Fax: 619-268-4275
     e-mail: efro@cybergate.com

Informational and emotional support to parents who have a child, adolescent, or adult family member with special needs.

4629 Exceptional Family Support, Education and Advocacy Center
6402 Skyway
Paradise, CA 95969   530-876-8321
     Fax: 530-876-0346
     e-mail: sea@sunset.net
     www.taalliance.org

Parent Training and Information (PTI) programs help parents to: understand their children's specific needs; communicate more effectively with professionals, participate in the educational planning process; and obtain information about relevant programs, services, and resources

4630 Exceptional Parents
Family Resource Center
4120 N. First Street
Fresno, CA 93726   559-229-2000
     Fax: 559-229-2956
     e-mail: epu1@cybergate.com

Informational and emotional support to parents who have a child, adolescent, or adult family member with special needs.

4631 Families Caring for Families
Family Resource Center
113 W Pillsbury Street, Suite A1
Lancaster, CA 93534   661-949-1746
                            Fax: 661-948-7266

Informational and emotional support to parents who have a child, adolescent, or adult family member with special needs.

4632 Family First Program Alpha Resource Center
4501 Cathedral Oaks RoadSuite A1
Santa Barbara, CA 93110   805-683-2145
                            Fax: 805-967-3647
                            e-mail: arcofsb@slcom.com

Informational and emotional support to parents who have a child, adolescent, or adult family member with special needs.

4633 Family Focus Resource Center
18111 Nordhoff Street
Northridge, CA 91330   818-677-5675
                            Fax: 818-677-5574
                            e-mail: family.focus@csun.edu
                            www.csun.edu/~ffrc/family-html.html

Informational and emotional support to parents who have a child, adolescent, or adult family member with special needs.

Ann R. Bisno, Ph.D, Project Director
Judith F. Sultan, Coordinator

4634 Family Resource Center
5250 Claremont Avenue
Stockton, CA 95207   209-472-3674
                            Fax: 209-472-3673

Informational and emotional support to parents who have a child, adolescent, or adult family member with special needs.

4635 H.E.A.R.T.S. Connection Family Resource Center
3101 N. Sillect Avenue, Suite 115
Bakersfield, CA 93308   661-328-9055
                            Fax: 661-328-9940

Informational and emotional support to parents who have a child, adolescent, or adult family member with special needs.

4636 Harbor Regional Center Family and Professional Resource Center
21231 Hawthorne Blvd.
Torrance, CA 90503   310-543-0691
                            Fax: 310-316-8843
                            e-mail: familyresourcecntr@hddf.com
                            www.hddf.com

Informational and emotional support to parents who have a child, adolescent, or adult family member with special needs.

4637 MATRIX: Parent Network and Family Resource Center
94 Galli Dr. Suite C
Novato, CA 94949   415-884-3535
                            800-578-2592
                            Fax: 415-884-3555
                            e-mail: matrix@matrixparents.org
                            www.matrixparents.org

Informational and emotional support to parents who have a child, adolescent, or adult family member with special needs.

4638 Matrix Family Resource Center of the North Bay
5440 State Farm Drive, #3
Rohnert Park, CA 94928   707-586-3314
                            Fax: 707-584-3438
                            e-mail: SonomaCo@matrixparents.org
                            www.matrixparents.org

Informational and emotional support to parents who have a child, adolescent, or adult family member with special needs.

4639 Parent Helping Parents of San Francisco
594 Morterey Blvd.
San Francisco, CA 94127   415-841-8820
                            Fax: 415-841-8824

Informational and emotional support to parents who have a child, adolescent, or adult family member with special needs.

4640 Parents Helping Parents of San Francisco
594 Monterey Blvd.
San Francisco, CA 94127   415-841-8820
                            Fax: 415-841-8824
                            www.taalliance.org

Parent Training and Information (PTI) programs help parents to: understand their children's specific needs; communicate more effectively with professionals, participate in the educational planning process; and obtain information about relevant programs, services, and resources

General Resources/State Agencies & Support Groups

4641 Parents Helping Parents of Santa Clara
3041 Olcott Street
Santa Clara, CA 95054   408-727-5775
Fax: 408-727-0182
e-mail: info@php.com
www.php.com

Informational and emotional support to parents who have a child, adolescent, or adult family member with special needs.

4642 Peaks and Valleys Family Resource Center
1145 Acosta Street,c/o Bard Blades
Salinas, CA 93905   891-424-2937
800-400-2937
Fax: 831-771-9132
e-mail: peaks@montereyk12.ca.us

Informational and emotional support to parents who have a child, adolescent, or adult family member with special needs.

4643 Phase One
P.O. Box 219, 2421 Lomitas Avenue
Santa Rosa, CA 95402   707-578-6070
877-694-4335
Fax: 707-578-8610
www.taalliance.org

Parent Training and Information (PTI) programs help parents to: understand their children's specific needs; communicate more effectively with professionals, participate in the educational planning process; and obtain information about relevant programs, services, and resources

4644 Rainbow Connection
500 Esplanade Drive, Suite 500
Oxnard, CA 93030   805-485-9643
800-332-3679
Fax: 805-968-9521
e-mail: jordan@jetlink.net

Informational and emotional support to parents who have a child, adolescent, or adult family member with special needs.

4645 San Gabriel/Pomona Parents' Place
1502 W Covina Pkwy, Suite 108
West Covina, CA 91790   626-856-8861
800-422-2022
Fax: 626-337-2736

Informational and emotional support to parents who have a child, adolescent, or adult family member with special needs.

4646 South Central Los Angeles Regional Center for Devlopmentally Disabled Persons, Inc
2160 W. Adams Blvd.
Los Angeles, CA 90018   562-869-6656
Fax: 213-730-0793

Informational and emotional support to parents who have a child, adolescent, or adult family member with special needs.

4647 Special Connections Family Resource Ctr.
984 Bostwick Lane
Santa Cruz, CA 65062   831-464-0669
Fax: 831-464-0779

Informational and emotional support to parents who have a child, adolescent, or adult family member with special needs.

4648 Special Education Division State Department of Education
P.O. Box 944272
Sacramento, CA 94244   916-327-3696
Fax: 916-327-8878
e-mail: cbourne@mail515a.cde.ca.gov
www.nectas.unc.edu

Individuals with Disabilities Education Act requires all states and territories to provide early intervention and preschool special education for children with disabilities and special healthcare needs. Services include central directory, representatives of agencies, service providers, families, and coordinators of infant, toddler, and preschool special education programs.

Constance J. Bourne, Preschool Special Ed. Coordinator

4649 Starlight Children's Foundation
5900 Wilshire Blvd, Suite 2530
Los Angeles, CA 90036   323-634-0080
800-274-7827
Fax: 323-634-0090

Dedicated to enriching the lives of seriously ill children.

4650 Support for Families of Children with Disabilities
2601 Mission #710
San Francisco, CA 94110   415-282-7494
Fax: 415-282-1226
e-mail: sfcdmiss@aol.com
www.taalliance.org

Parent Training and Information (PTI) programs help parents to: understand their children's specific needs; communicate more effectively with professionals, participate in the educational planning process; and obtain information about relevant programs, services, and resources

4651 Team Advocates for Special Kids, San Diego
3750 Convoy Street, Suite 303
San Diego, CA 92111　　　619-874-2386
Fax: 619-874-2375
www.taalliance.org

Programs help parents to: understand their children's specific needs; communicate more effectively with professionals, participate in the educational planning process; and obtain information about relevant programs, services, and resources

4652 Team Advocates for Special Kids, Anaheim
100 W Cerritos Avenue
Anaheim, CA 92805　　　714-533-8275
Fax: 714-533-2533
e-mail: taskca@aol.com
www.taalliance.org

Programs help parents to: understand their children's specific needs; communicate more effectively with professionals, participate in the educational planning process; and obtain information about relevant programs, services, and resources

4653 Warmline Family Resource Center
9175 Kiefer Blvd., Suite 136
Sacramento, CA 95826　　　916-631-7995
Fax: 916-942-2157

Informational and emotional support to parents who have a child, adolescent, or adult family member with special needs.

4654 Wish Upon a Star
California Law Enforcement
P.O. Box 4000
Visalia, CA 93278　　　209-733-7753

Serves children in the state of California. Nonprofit, law enforcement effort designed to grant wishes of children afflicted with high-risk and terminal illnesses.

Colorado

4655 Colorado Assistive Technology Program
The Pavillion, AO36/B140
1919 Ogden Street, 2nd Floor
Denver, CO 80218　　　303-864-5100
Fax: 303-864-5119
TTY: 303-864-5110
e-mail: cathy.bodine@uCHSC.edu
www.uchsc.edu/catp

State assisted programs and support group information for people of many abilities. Focuses on assitive technology devices and services fro persons with disabilities, training and technical assistance available.

4656 Colorado Consortium of Intensive Care Nurseries United Parents (UP)
1056 E 19th Avenue, B535
Denver, CO 80218　　　303-861-6557
Fax: 303-764-8092
e-mail: McGinley.Pandora@ex.tchden.org

Informational and emotional support to parents who have a child, adolescent, or adult family member with special needs.

4657 Delta/Montrose Parent to Parent
2091 E Locust Road
Montrose, CO 81401　　　970-249-2878
Fax: 970-252-0544
e-mail: children@gi.net

Informational and emotional support to parents who have a child, adolescent, or adult family member with special needs.

4658 Denver Early Childhood Connections
124 East Jewell Avenue
Denver, CO 80204　　　303-744-9193
Fax: 303-744-9502

We provide resource coordination for children eligible for Part C services and referrals to other agencies for children with needs outside of the Part C realm. Parent to parent support, parent education and community playgroups are some of the services that we conduct. We host forums on varied topics relevant to parents of young children as well as inservice and pre-service workshops on child development. IFSP development, parent's rights under IDEA, and other resource packets are available.

Quarter.Newsltr

Judith Persoff, Executive Director

4659 Disability Connection and RAFT, Larimer County's Early Childhood Connection
P.O. Box 270714
Fort Collins, CO 80527   970-229-0224
                               Fax: 970-229-0242
                          e-mail: bstuts@fornet.org

Informational and emotional support to parents who have a child, adolescent, or adult family member with special needs.

4660 Effective Parent Project, Inc
101 South 103rd Street, Suite 350
Grand Junction, CO 81501   970-241-4068
                                Fax: 970-241-3725

Informational and emotional support to parents who have a child, adolescent, or adult family member with special needs.

4661 El Groupo Vida
777 Bannock Mail Code 1701
Denver, CO 80204   303-436-3269

Informational and emotional support to parents who have a child, adolescent, or adult family member with special needs.

4662 Help Parent Spport Group Hope & Education for Loving Parents
378 South Falcon
Pueblo West, CO 81007   719-545-2282
                             Fax: 719-547-1282
                        e-mail: fastgram@aol.com

Informational and emotional support to parents who have a child, adolescent, or adult family member with special needs.

4663 Little People of America Front Range Chapter
7117 East Euclid Drive
Englewood, CO 80111   303-740-8555

Informational and emotional support to parents who have a child, adolescent, or adult family member with special needs.

4664 Mile High Down Syndrome Association
P.O. Box 620847
Littleton, CO 80162   303-797-1699
                           Fax: 303-347-2938
                        e-mail: mhdsa@aol.com

Informational and emotional support to parents who have a child, adolescent, or adult family member with special needs.

4665 Oasis, Inc
1120 North Cicle Drive, Suite 19
Colorado Springs, CO 80909   719-635-8722
                                  Fax: 719-577-9482
                             e-mail: oasis@juno.com

Informational and emotional support to parents who have a child, adolescent, or adult family member with special needs.

4666 PEAK Parent Center, Inc.
6055 Lahman Drive, Suite 101
Colorado Springs, CO 80918   719-531-9400
                                     800-284-0251
                                  Fax: 719-531-9452
                                  TDD: 719-531-9403
                          e-mail: info@peakparent.org
                                www.peakparent.org

Parent Training and Information (PTI) programs help parents to: understand their children's specific needs; communicate more effectively with professionals, participate in the educational planning process; and obtain information about relevant programs, services, and resources

4667 Parent Support Group of Littleton & Auora
7600 East Arapahoe, Suite 219
Englewood, CO 80112   303-773-0044
                           Fax: 303-773-8780

Informational and emotional support to parents who have a child, adolescent, or adult family member with special needs.

4668 Parents Encouraging Parents
96 Gordon Lane
Castle Rock, CO 80112   303-688-4756
                             Fax: 303-688-6387

Informational and emotional support to parents who have a child, adolescent, or adult family member with special needs.

4669 Parents Supporting Parents of Eagle County
P.O. Box 2656
Vail, CO 81658   970-926-6015
                      Fax: 970-926-6015

Informational and emotional support to parents who have a child, adolescent, or adult family member with special needs.

4670 Parents Supporting Parents of Garfield and Pitkin County
P.O. Box 784
Silt, CO 81652   970-876-5768
                      Fax: 970-876-5204

Informational and emotional support to parents who have a child, adolescent, or adult family member with special needs.

4671 Prevention Initiatives State Department of Education
210 East Colfax, Room 301
Denver, CO 80203   303-866-6709
Fax: 303-866-6662
e-mail: smith_s@cde.state.co.us
www.nectas.unc.edu

Provides early intervention and preschool special education for children with disabilities and special healthcare needs. Services include central directory, representatives of agencies, service providers, families, and coordinators of infant, toddler, and preschool special education programs.

Susan Smith, Infant/Toddler Program Coordinator

4672 Prevention Initiatives, Early Childhood Initiative, State Dept. of Education
210 East Colfax, Room 305
Denver, CO 80203   303-866-6712
Fax: 303-866-6662
e-mail: Amundson_J@cde.state.co.us
www.nectas.unc.edu

Individuals with Disabilities Education Act requires all states and territories to provide early intervention and preschool special education for children with disabilities and special healthcare needs. Services include central directory, representatives of agencies, service providers, families, and coordinators of infant, toddler, and preschool special education programs.

Jane L. Amundson, Preschool Special Ed. Coordinator

4673 Resources for Young Children and Families, Inc
1120 North Circle Drive, Suite 19
Colorado Springs, CO 80909   719-577-9190
Fax: 719-577-9482

Informational and emotional support to parents who have a child, adolescent, or adult family member with special needs.

4674 Speech, Language, & Hearing Center University of Colorado
Campus Box 409
Boulder, CO 80309   303-492-5375
Fax: 303-492-3274
e-mail: susan.moore@colorado.edu
www.colorado.edu/slhs

Informational and emotional support to parents who have a child, adolescent, or adult family member with special needs.

4675 Wilderness on Wheels Foundation
3131 S Vaughn Way, #305
Aurora, CO 80014   303-751-3959

State assisted programs and support group information for people of many abilities. Including local chapters, referrals, fun and social interaction and support groups.

Connecticut

4676 Assistive Technology Project
Department of Social Services, BRS
25 Sigourney Street, 11th Floor
Hartford, CT 06106   860-424-4881
800-537-2549
Fax: 860-424-4850
TDD: 860-424-4850
e-mail: cttap@aol./com
www.tachact.uconn.edu

State assisted programs and support group information for people of many abilities. Including local chapters, referrals, fun and social interaction and support groups.

4677 CPAC
338 Main Street
Niantic, CT 06357   860-739-3089
Fax: 860-739-7460
e-mail: cpacino@aol.com
www.members.aol.com/cpacino/cpac.htm

Programs help parents to: understand their children's specific needs; communicate more effectively with professionals, participate in the educational planning process; and obtain information about relevant programs, services, and resources

4678 Department of Mental Retardation
460 Capital Avenue
Hartford, CT 06106   860-418-6147
Fax: 860-418-6003
e-mail: lbgood993@aol.com
www.nectas.unc.edu

Individuals with Disabilities Education Act requires all states and territories to provide early intervention and preschool special education for children with disabilities and special healthcare needs. Services include central directory, representatives of agencies, service providers, families, and coordinators of infant, toddler, and preschool special education programs.

Linda Goodman, Infant/Toddler Program Coor.

4679 Division of Child & Family Studies
National Early Childhood Technical Assistance Ctr
263 Farmington Avenue
Farmington, CT 06030   860-679-1500
                            Fax: 860-679-1571
                    e-mail: bruder@nso1.uchc.edu
                            www.nectas.unc.edu

Individuals with Disabilities Education Act requires all states and territories to provide early intervention and preschool special education for children with disabilities and special healthcare needs. Services include central directory, representatives of agencies, service providers, families, and coordinators of infant, toddler, and preschool special education programs.

Mary Beth Bruder, Interagency Coordinator

4680 Parent to Parent Network of Connecticut the Family Center
Dept. of Connecticut Children's Medical Center
282 Washington
Hartford, CT 06106   860-545-9021
                            Fax: 860-545-9201
                            TTY: 860-545-9002
                    e-mail: mcole@ccmckids.org

Informational and emotional support to parents who have a child, adolescent, or adult family member with special needs.

4681 State Department of Education
25 Industrial Park Road
Middletown, CT 06457   860-807-2036
                            Fax: 860-638-4218
                            www.nectas.unc.edu

Individuals with Disabilities Education Act requires all states and territories to provide early intervention and preschool special education for children with disabilities and special healthcare needs. Services include central directory, representatives of agencies, service providers, families, and coordinators of infant, toddler, and preschool special education programs.

Maria Synodi, Preschool Special Ed. Coordinator

Delaware

4682 Delaware Assisstive Technology Initiative
1600 Rockland Road, Room 117E
P.O. Box 269
Wilmington, DE 19899   302-651-6790
                            800-870-3284
                            Fax: 302-651-6793
                            TDD: 302-651-6794
                    e-mail: dati@asel/udel.edu
                    www.asel.udel.edu/dati/

State assisted programs and support group information for people of many abilities. Including local chapters, referrals, fun and social interaction and support groups.

4683 Department of Public Instruction
P.O. Box 1402
Dover, DE 19703   302-739-4667
                            Fax: 302-739-2388
                    e-mail: mtoomey@state.de.us
                            www.nectas.unc.edu

Individuals with Disabilities Education Act requires all states and territories to provide early intervention and preschool special education for children with disabilities and special healthcare needs. Services include central directory, representatives of agencies, service providers, families, and coordinators of infant, toddler, and preschool special education programs.

Martha Toomey, Preschool Special Ed. Coordinator

4684 Division of Management Services Department of Health & Social Services
1901 North Dupont Highway, Room 204
New Castle, DE 19720   302-577-4647
                            Fax: 302-577-4083
                    e-mail: rcabelli@state.de.us
                            www.nectas.unc.edu

Provides early intervention and preschool special education for children with disabilities and special healthcare needs. Services include central directory, representatives of agencies, service providers, families, and coordinators of infant, toddler, and preschool special education programs.

Rosanne Griff-Cabelli, Infant/Toddler Program Coordinator

4685 Parent Information Center of Delaware
700 Barksdale Road, Suite 3
Newark, DE 19711   302-366-0152
                            Fax: 302-366-0276
                    e-mail: EP700@aol.com
                            www.taalliance.org

Programs help parents to: understand their children's specific needs; communicate more effectively with professionals, participate in the educational planning process; and obtain information about relevant programs, services, and resources

4686 Parent Information Center of Delaware, Inc
700 Barksdale Road, Suite 3
Newark, DE 19711   302-366-0152
                            Fax: 302-366-0276
                    e-mail: PEP700@aol.com

Informational and emotional support to parents who have a child, adolescent, or adult family member with special needs.

District of Columbia

4687 Advocates for Justice and Education
2041 Martin Luther King Jr Avenue
Washington, DC 20020   202-678-8060
                             888-327-8060
                             Fax: 202-678-8062
                             e-mail: aje.qpg.com
                             www.taalliance.org

Programs help parents to: understand their children's specific needs; communicate more effectively with professionals, participate in the educational planning process; and obtain information about relevant programs, services, and resources

4688 DC Arc
900 Vamum Street, NE
Washington, DC 20017   202-636-2950
                             Fax: 202-636-2996
                             www.taalliance.org

Programs help parents to: understand their children's specific needs; communicate more effectively with professionals, participate in the educational planning process; and obtain information about relevant programs, services, and resources

4689 DC-EIP Services
609 H Street Northwest, 5th Floor
Washington, DC 20002   202-727-5930
                             Fax: 202-727-5971
                             www.nectas.unc.edu

Provides early intervention and preschool special education for children with disabilities and special healthcare needs. Services include central directory, representatives of agencies, service providers, families, and coordinators of infant, toddler, and preschool special education programs.

Joan Christopher, Infant/Toddler Program Coordinator

4690 Georgetown University Child Development Center
National Early Childhood Technical Assistance Ctr
3307 M Street Northwest
Washington, DC 20007   202-687-8635
                             Fax: 202-687-8899
                             www.nectas.unc.edu

Individuals with Disabilities Education Act requires all states and territories to provide early intervention and preschool special education for children with disabilities and special healthcare needs. Services include central directory, representatives of agencies, service providers, families, and coordinators of infant, toddler, and preschool special education programs.

Tawara Taylor, Interagency Coordinating Council

4691 Giddings School Special Education Division
National Early Childhood Technical Assistance Ctr
315 G Street Southeast
Washington, DC 20003   202-727-1977
                             Fax: 202-724-5083
                             www.nectas.unc.edu

Services include central directory, representatives of agencies, service providers, families, and coordinators of infant, toddler, and preschool special education programs.

Ann Palmore, Preschool Special Ed. Coordinator

4692 Partnership for Assistive Technology
301 I Street, NE, Suite 202
Washington, DC 20002   202-547-0198
                             Fax: 202-547-2662
                             TDD: 202-547-2657

State assisted programs and support group information for people of many abilities. Including local chapters, referrals, fun and social interaction and support groups.

Florida

4693 Alliance for Assistive Service and Technology (FAAST)
1020 East Lafayette St., Ste. 202
Tallahassee, FL 32301
                             Fax: 850-487-2805
                             TDD: 850-922-5951
                             e-mail: faast@faast.org

State assisted programs and support group information for people of many abilities. Including local chapters, referrals, fun and social interaction and support groups.

2-8 pages Newsletter

4694 Children's Wish Foundation
100 E Sybelia, Suite 300, Joel Jones
Maitland, FL 32751   407-629-8920
                             Fax: 407-629-7206

Orlando-based organization that grants wishes for children with life-threatening illnesses who have not yet reached their 18th birthday. Focuses primarily on children who reside in Florida, but has also granted wishes to children from other parts of the U.S., Canada, England, and Russia.

4695 Early Intervention Unit, Division of Children's Medical Services
1309 Winewood Blvd
Tallahassee, FL 32399   850-488-6005
                         Fax: 850-921-5241
e-mail: Fran_L_Wilber@dcf.state.fl.us
                         www.nectas.unc.edu

Individuals with Disabilities Education Act requires all states and territories to provide early intervention and preschool special education for children with disabilities and special healthcare needs. Services include central directory, representatives of agencies, service providers, families, and coordinators of infant, toddler, and preschool special education programs.

Fran Wilber, Infant/Toddler Program Coordinator

4696 Family Network on Disabilities
2735 Whitney Road
Clearwater, FL 33760   727-523-1130
                         800-825-5736
                         Fax: 727-523-8687
                         TDD: 727-523-1130
                         e-mail: fnd@gate.net
                         www.fndfl.org

Parent Training and Information (PTI) programs help parents to: understand their children's specific needs; communicate more effectively with professionals, participate in the educational planning process; and obtain information about relevant programs, services, and resources

4697 Florida Department of Education
325 West Gaines Street, Suite 754
Tallahassee, FL 32399   850-487-0016
                         Fax: 850-487-0946
e-mail: westc@mail.doe.state.fl.us
                         www.nectas.unc.edu

Individuals with Disabilities Education Act requires all states and territories to provide early intervention and preschool special education for children with disabilities and special healthcare needs. Services include central directory, representatives of agencies, service providers, families, and coordinators of infant, toddler, and preschool special education programs.

Carale West, Preschool Special Ed. Coordinator

4698 Florida's Collaboration for Young Children and their Families Head State
1310 Cross Creek Circle, Suite A
Tallahassee, FL 32301   850-487-8871
                         Fax: 850-487-0045
e-mail: kkamiya@com1.med.usf.edu
                         www.nectas.unc.edu

Provides early intervention and preschool special education for children with disabilities and special healthcare needs. Services include central directory, representatives of agencies, service providers, families, and coordinators of infant, toddler, and preschool special education programs.

Katherine Kamiya, Interagency Coordinator

4699 Teddi Project
Camp Good Days and Special Times
1332 Pittsford-Mendon Road
Memdon, NY 14506   716-624-5555
                         800-785-2135
                         Fax: 716-624-5799

Priority given to children from Central Florida and the upstate New York area, especially Buffalo, Rochester, Syracuse, Albany, and Binghamton. Serves chronically or terminally ill children ages 7 to 17.

4700 US Blind Golfers Association
3094 Shamrock Street N
Tallahassee, FL 32308   904-893-4511
e-mail: nightgolf@concentric.net

State assisted programs and support group information for people of many abilities. Including local chapters, referrals, fun and social interaction and support groups.

Georgia

4701 Babies Can't Wait Program Division of Public Health
2 Peachtree Street NE, 11th Floor
Atlanta, GA 30303   404-657-2726
                         Fax: 404-657-2763
e-mail: wss@ph.dhr.state.ga.us
                         www.nectas.unc.edu

Individuals with Disabilities Education Act requires all states and territories to provide early intervention and preschool special education for children with disabilities and special healthcare needs. Services include central directory, representatives of agencies, service providers, families, and coordinators of infant, toddler, and preschool special education programs.

Wendy Sanders, Infant/Toddler Program Coor.

4702 Department for Exceptional Students Georgia Department of Education
1866 Twin Towers East, 7th Floor
Atlanta, GA 30334   404-657-9955
Fax: 404-651-6457
e-mail: tbowen@doe.k12.ga.us
www.nectas.unc.edu

Provides early intervention and preschool special education for children with disabilities and special healthcare needs. Services include central directory, representatives of agencies, service providers, families, and coordinators of infant, toddler, and preschool special education programs.

Toni Waylor Bowen, Preschool Special Ed. Coordinator

4703 Department of Counseling and Educational Leadership-Columbus State University
4225 University Avenue, Suite 754
Columbus, GA 31907   706-568-2222
Fax: 706-569-3134
www.nectas.unc.edu

Individuals with Disabilities Education Act requires all states and territories to provide early intervention and preschool special education for children with disabilities and special healthcare needs. Services include central directory, representatives of agencies, service providers, families, and coordinators of infant, toddler, and preschool special education programs.

Katherine McCormick, Interagency Coordinating Council

4704 Parent to Parent of Georgia
2900 Woodcock Blvd, Suite 240
Atlanta, GA 30341   770-451-5484
800-229-2038
Fax: 770-458-4091
e-mail: parenttoparent@fga.org

Informational and emotional support to parents who have a child, adolescent, or adult family member with special needs.

4705 Parents Educating Parents and Professional for All Children (PEPPAC)
8318 Durelee Lane, Suite 101
Douglasville, GA 30134   770-577-7771
Fax: 770-577-7774
e-mail: peppac@bellsouth.net
www.taalliance.org

Parent Training and Information (PTI) programs help parents to: understand their children's specific needs; communicate more effectively with professionals, participate in the educational planning process; and obtain information about relevant programs, services, and resources

4706 Southeastern Region - Helen Keller National Center
1005 Virginia Ave Ste 104
Atlant, GA 30354   404-766-9625

4707 Tools for Life Division of Rehabilitation Services
2 Peachtree St. NW, Suite 35-415
Atlanta, GA 30303   404-657-3084
800-578-8665
Fax: 404-657-3086
TDD: 404-657-3085
e-mail: 102476.1737@compuserve.com
www.gatfl.org

State assisted programs and support group information for people of many abilities. Including local chapters, referrals, fun and social interaction and support groups.

Hawaii

4708 AWARE
200 N. Vineyard Blvd., Suite 310
Honolulu, HI 96817   808-536-9684
Fax: 808-537-6780
e-mail: LDAH@gte.net
www.taalliance.org

Parent Training and Information (PTI) programs help parents to: understand their children's specific needs; communicate more effectively with professionals, participate in the educational planning process; and obtain information about relevant programs, services, and resources

4709 Assisstive Technology Training & Services
414 Kuiwii Street, Suite 104
Honolulu, HI 96817
800-532-7110
Fax: 808-532-7120
e-mail: bfi@pixi.com
www.hatts.com

State assisted programs and support group information for people of many abilities. Including local chapters, referrals, fun and social interaction and support groups.

4710 Parents and Children Together (PACT)
1475 Linapuni #117A
Honolulu, HI 96819   808-847-3285
Fax: 808-841-1485
www.nectas.unc.edu

Individuals with Disabilities Education Act requires all states and territories to provide early intervention and preschool special education for children with disabilities and special healthcare needs. Services include central directory, representatives of agencies, service providers, families, and coordinators of infant, toddler, and preschool special education programs.

Ha'Aheo Mansfield, Interagency Coordinating Council

4711 Special Needs Branch Department of Education
637 18th Avenue, Bldg C Room 102
Honolulu, HI 96816   808-733-4840
                           Fax: 808-733-4404
              e-mail: michael_fahley@notes.k12.hi.us
                           www.nectas.unc.edu

Individuals with Disabilities Education Act requires all states and territories to provide early intervention and preschool special education for children with disabilities and special healthcare needs. Services include central directory, representatives of agencies, service providers, families, and coordinators of infant, toddler, and preschool special education programs.

Michael Fahey, Preschool Special Ed. Coordinator

4712 Zero-To-3 Hawaii Project
1600 Kapiolani Blvd, Suite 1401
Honolulu, HI 96814   808-942-8223
                           Fax: 808-946-5222
              e-mail: jeanj@hawaii.edu
                           www.nectas.unc.edu

Services include central directory, representatives of agencies, service providers, families, and coordinators of infant, toddler, and preschool special education programs.

Jean Johnson, Infant/Toddler Program Coordinator

Idaho

4713 Assistive Technology Project
129 W Third Street
Moscow, ID 83844   208-855-3559
                          Fax: 208-855-3628
                          TDD: 208-855-3559
              e-mail: seile861@uidaho.edu
                          www.ets.uidaho.edu

State assisted programs and support group information for people of many abilities. Including local chapters, referrals, fun and social interaction and support groups.

4714 Department of Education
P.O. Box 83720
Boise, ID 83720   208-332-6915
                         Fax: 208-334-4664
              e-mail: jkbrenn@sde.state.id.us
                         www.nectas.unc.edu

Individuals with Disabilities Education Act requires all states and territories to provide early intervention and preschool special education for children with disabilities and special healthcare needs. Services include central directory, representatives of agencies, service providers, families, and coordinators of infant, toddler, and preschool special education programs.

Jane Brennan, Preschool Special Ed. Coordinator

4715 Idaho Parents Unlimited, Inc.
4696 Overland Road, Suite 568
Boise, ID 83705   208-342-5884
                         800-242-4785
                         Fax: 208-342-1408
                         TDD: 208-342-5884
              e-mail: pul@rmci.net
                         www.home.mci.net/PUL

Parent Training and Information (PTI) programs help parents to: understand their children's specific needs; communicate more effectively with professionals, participate in the educational planning process; and obtain information about relevant programs, services, and resources

4716 Infant/Toddler Program
P.O. Box 83720
Boise, ID 83720   208-334-5523
                         Fax: 208-334-6664
              e-mail: jonesm@dhw.state.id.us
                         www.nectas.unc.edu

Services include central directory, representatives of agencies, service providers, families, and coordinators of infant, toddler, and preschool special education programs.

Mary Jones, Infant/Toddler Program Coordinator

4717 Palouse Area Parent To Parent
2714 8th Avenue
Lewiston, ID 83501   208-746-8599
                            TTY: 208-746-8599
              e-mail: irel102w@wonder.em.cdc.gov

Informational and emotional support to parents who have a child, adolescent, or adult family member with special needs.

4718 Parent Reaching Out To Parents
2195 Ironwood Court
Coeur d'Alene, ID 83501   208-769-1409
Fax: 208-769-1430

Informational and emotional support to parents
who have a child, adolescent, or adult family
member with special needs.

Illinois

4719 Archway, Inc
P.O. Box 1180
Carbondale, IL 62903   618-549-4442
Fax: 618-549-0231

Informational and emotional support to parents
who have a child, adolescent, or adult family
member with special needs.

4720 Assistive Technology Project
1 W Old State Capitol Plaza,Ste 100
Springfield, IL 62701   217-522-7985
Fax: 217-522-8067
TDD: 217-522-9966
e-mail: iatp@fgi.net
www.ittech.org

State assisted programs and support group information for people of many abilities. Including local chapters, referrals, fun and social
interaction and support groups.

4721 Child and Family Connections
1757 West 95th Street
Chicago, IL 60643   773-233-1799
Fax: 773-233-2011

Informational and emotional support to parents
who have a child, adolescent, or adult family
member with special needs.

4722 Developmental Services Center
1304 West Bradley
Champaign, IL 61821   217-359-0287
Fax: 217-356-9851

Informational and emotional support to parents
who have a child, adolescent, or adult family
member with special needs.

4723 Family Resource Center on Disabilities
20 E Jackson Blvd., Room 900
Chicago, IL 60604   312-939-3513
Fax: 312-939-7297
TTY: 312-939-3519
TDD: 312-939-3519
www.taalliance.org

Parent Training and Information (PTI) programs help parents to: understand their children's specific needs; communicate more
effectively with professionals, participate in the
educational planning process; and obtain information about relevant programs, services, and
resources

4724 Family T.I.E.S. Network
830 S Spring Street
Springfield, IL 62704   217-544-5809
800-865-7842
Fax: 217-544-6018
e-mail: FTIESN@aol.com
www.taalliance.org

Parent Training and Information (PTI) programs help parents to: understand their children's specific needs; communicate more
effectively with professionals, participate in the
educational planning process; and obtain information about relevant programs, services, and
resources

**4725 Greater Interagency Council Parent to Parent
Support Network**
925 West 175th Street
Homewoodn, IL 60430   708-799-2718
Fax: 708-799-7974

Informational and emotional support to parents
who have a child, adolescent, or adult family
member with special needs.

**4726 National Association for Parents of the Visually
Impaired**
16 Thornfield Lane
Hawthorn Woods, IL 60047   847-438-0705

Kevin O'Connor

4727 National Center for Latinos with Disabilities
1915-17 S Blue Island Avenue
Chicago, IL 60608   312-666-3393
800-532-3393
Fax: 312-666-1787
TTY: 312-666-1788
e-mail: ncld@ncld.com
www.ncld.com

Parent Training and Information (PTI) programs help parents to: understand their children's specific needs; communicate more
effectively with professionals, participate in the
educational planning process; and obtain information about relevant programs, services, and
resources.

Everardo Franco, Executive Director
Nancy Perez, Coordinator of Info and Referral

4728 Next Steps - Parents Reaching Parents
100 West Randolph, Suite 8-100
Chicago, IL 60601 312-814-4042
Fax: 312-814-5849
TTY: 312-814-4042
e-mail: caroldors@aol.com

Informational and emotional support to parents
who have a child, adolescent, or adult family
member with special needs.

4729 North Central Region Helen Keller National Center
35 E. Wacker Drive Suite 772
Chicago, IL 60601 773-726-2090

**4730 Office of Community Health and Prevention Bureau
of Early Intervention, DHR**
P.O. Box 19429
Springfield, IL 62777 217-782-1981
Fax: 217-782-7849
www.nectas.unc.edu

Provides early intervention and preschool special education for children with disabilities and
special healthcare needs. Services include central directory, representatives of agencies, service providers, families, and coordinators of
infant, toddler, and preschool special education
programs.

Mary Miller, Infant/Toddler Program Coordinator

4731 Parent to Parent Network
P.O. Box 587
Charleston, IL 61920 217-348-0127
Fax: 217-348-0740

Informational and emotional support to parents
who have a child, adolescent, or adult family
member with special needs.

4732 Southern IL Child and Family Connections
1108 West Willow
Carbondale, IL 62903
888-340-6702
Fax: 618-549-8137

Informational and emotional support to parents
who have a child, adolescent, or adult family
member with special needs.

**4733 State Board of Education Department of Special
Education**
National Early Childhood Technical Assistance Ctr
100 North 1st Street #233
Springfield, IL 62777 217-782-4835
Fax: 217-782-7849
e-mail: preising@smtp.isbe.state.il.us
www.nectas.unc.edu

Individuals with Disabilities Education Act requires all states and territories to provide early
intervention and preschool special education for
children with disabilities and special healthcare
needs. Services include central directory, representatives of agencies, service providers, families, and coordinators of infant, toddler, and
preschool special education programs.

Pam Reising-Rechner, Preschool Special Ed. Coordinator

Indiana

**4734 ATTAIN: Assistive Technology Through Action in
Indiana**
1815 N Meridan Street, Suite 200
Indianapolis, IN 46202 317-921-8766
800-743-3333
Fax: 317-921-8774
TDD: 800-743-3333
e-mail: cfulford@indian.viru.edu

State assisted programs and support group information for people of many abilities. Including local chapters, referrals, fun and social
interaction and support groups.

**4735 Assistive Technology Training and Information
Center**
3354 Pine Hill Drive, PO Box 2441
Vincennes, IN 47591 812-886-1128
Fax: 812-886-0575
e-mail: inattic1@aol.com

Technology group of parents, consumers and
professionals; provides resources to help children and adults who have disabilities gain access
to the benefits of technology. Includes nationwide network of community-based assistive technology, resource centers, hands on consultants
and product demonstrations.

**4736 Division of Special Education Department of
Education**
State House, Room 229
Indianapolis, IN 46204 317-232-0570
Fax: 317-232-0589
e-mail: cochra@speced.doe.state.in.us
www.nectas.unc.edu

Individuals with Disabilities Education Act requires all states and territories to provide early intervention and preschool special education for children with disabilities and special healthcare needs. Services include central directory, representatives of agencies, service providers, families, and coordinators of infant, toddler, and preschool special education programs.

Sheron Cochran, Preschool Special Ed. Coordinator

4737 Down Syndrome Association of Central Indiana
10792 Downing Street
Carmel, IN 46033   317-574-9757

Provides informational and emotional support to parents who have a child, adolescent, or adult family member with special needs. Program offers an important connection for a parent who is seeking support for special disability issue, by matching him or her with a trained veteran parent.

4738 Down Syndrome Association of NWI
2927 Jewett Avenue
Highland, IN 46322   219-838-3656
                                 Fax: 219-838-6959
                        e-mail: dsa@netnitco.net

Provides informational and emotional support to parents who have a child, adolescent, or adult family member with special needs. Program offers an important connection for a parent who is seeking support for special disability issue, by matching him or her with a trained veteran parent.

4739 Down Syndrome Support Association of Southern Indiana (DSSASI)
P.O. Box 3262
Clarksville, IN 47131   812-948-5182

Provides informational and emotional support to parents who have a child, adolescent, or adult family member with special needs. Program offers an important connection for a parent who is seeking support for special disability issue, by matching him or her with a trained veteran parent.

4740 Family Resource Center of Southeast Indiana
4101 Timberview Road
West Harrison, IN 47060   812-637-1445

Informational and emotional support to parents who have a child, adolescent, or adult family member with special needs.

4741 First Direction
P.O. Box 4234
Lafayette, IN 47903   765-423-1460

Informational and emotional support to parents who have a child, adolescent, or adult family member with special needs.

4742 First Steps
402 West Washington Street, #W-386
Indianapolis, IN 46204   317-232-2429
                                  Fax: 317-232-7948
                     e-mail: mgreer@fssa.state.in.us
                            www.nectas.unc.edu

Individuals with Disabilities Education Act requires all states and territories to provide early intervention and preschool special education for children with disabilities and special healthcare needs. Services include central directory, representatives of agencies, service providers, families, and coordinators of infant, toddler, and preschool special education programs.

Maureen Greer, Infant/Toddler Program Coor.

4743 First Steps for Families
500 8th Avenue
Terre Haute, IN 47804   812-231-8342
                                  Fax: 812-231-8203
                        e-mail: famnetwork@aol.com

Informational and emotional support to parents who have a child, adolescent, or adult family member with special needs.

4744 First Steps, Early Interventions, New Horizons Rehabilitation
P.O. Box 98
Batesville, IN 47006   812-934-4528
                                  Fax: 812-934-2522
                                  TTY: 812-934-4528

Informational and emotional support to parents who have a child, adolescent, or adult family member with special needs.

4745 Future Choices
309 North High Street
Muncie, IN 47305   765-741-3494
                                  Fax: 765-741-8333

Informational and emotional support to parents who have a child, adolescent, or adult family member with special needs.

4746 IN*SOURCE
809 N Michigan Street
South Bend, IN 46601   219-234-7101
                             Fax: 219-234-7279
                    e-mail: insour@speced.doe.state.in.us
                             www.home1.gte.net/insource

Parent Training and Information (PTI) programs help parents to: understand their children's specific needs; communicate more effectively with professionals, participate in the educational planning process; and obtain information about relevant programs, services, and resources

4747 Indiana Parent Information Network (IPIN)
4755 Kingsway Drive, Suite 105
Indianapolis, IN 46205   317-257-8683
                               Fax: 317-251-7488
                    e-mail: familynetw@aol.com

Informational and emotional support to parents who have a child, adolescent, or adult family member with special needs.

4748 Knox County Advocates
1806 Indiana Avenue
Vincennes, IN 47591   812-882-0375
                            Fax: 812-886-1128
                    e-mail: INATTIC1@aol.com

Informational and emotional support to parents who have a child, adolescent, or adult family member with special needs.

4749 NEO Fight
4363 Idlewild Lane
Carmel, IN 46033   317-843-0850

Informational and emotional support to parents who have a child, adolescent, or adult family member with special needs.

4750 Project Special Care
4755 Kinsway Drive, Suite 105
Indianapolis, IN 46205   317-257-8683
                               Fax: 317-251-7488

Informational and emotional support to parents who have a child, adolescent, or adult family member with special needs.

4751 US Rowing Assocation
201 S Capitol Avenue, Suite 400
Indianapolis, IN 46225   317-237-5656
                               Fax: 317-237-5646
                    e-mail: members@usrowing.org

State assisted programs and support group information for people of many abilities. Including local chapters, referrals, fun and social interaction and support groups.

Iowa

4752 ARC of East Central Iowa Pilot Parents
214 First Street, SW
Cedar Rapids, IA 52404   319-365-0487
                               800-843-0272
                               Fax: 319-365-9938

Informational and emotional support to parents who have a child, adolescent, or adult family member with special needs.

4753 Bureau of Childern, Family, and Community Services
Grimes State Office Bldg, 3rd Floor
Des Moines, IA 50319   515-281-5502
                             Fax: 515-242-6019
                    e-mail: dee.gethman@ed.state.ia.us
                             www.nectas.unc.edu

Individuals with Disabilities Education Act requires all states and territories to provide early intervention and preschool special education for children with disabilities and special healthcare needs. Services include central directory, representatives of agencies, service providers, families, and coordinators of infant, toddler, and preschool special education programs.

Dee Gethmann, Preschool Special Ed. Coordinator

4754 Family Educator Connection Program
3706 Cedar Heights Drive
Cedar Falls, IA 50613   319-273-8265
                              Fax: 319-273-8275
                              TTY: 319-273-8291
                    e-mail: dhansen@aea7.k12.ia.us

Informational and emotional support to parents who have a child, adolescent, or adult family member with special needs.

4755 Iowa Program for Assistive Technology
100 Hawkins Drive, Univ Hosp School
Iowa City, IA 52242
                               800-331-3027
                               Fax: 319-356-8284
                               TDD: 800-331-3027
                    e-mail: jane_gay@uiowa.edu
                             www.uiowa.edu/infotech

State assisted programs and support group information for people of many abilities. Including local chapters, referrals, fun and social interaction and support groups.

4756 Iowa's System of EI Services
Grimes State Office Bldg, 3rd Floor
Des Moines, IA 50319   515-281-7145
Fax: 515-242-6019
e-mail: lynda.pletcher@ed.state.ia.us
www.nectas.unc.edu

Individuals with Disabilities Education Act requires all states and territories to provide early intervention and preschool special education for children with disabilities and special healthcare needs. Services include central directory, representatives of agencies, service providers, families, and coordinators of infant, toddler, and preschool special education programs.

Lynda Pletcher, Infant/Toddler Program Coor.

4757 Parent Educator Connection
AEA5 1235 5th Avenue South
Fort Dodge, IA 50501   515-574-5423
Fax: 515-574-5508
e-mail: bjones@aea5.k12.ia.uss

Informational and emotional support to parents who have a child, adolescent, or adult family member with special needs.

4758 Parent Educator Connection Program Resource Center for Issues in Special Ed
Drake Univ, 2507 University Avenue
Des Moines, IA 50311   515-271-3936
Fax: 515-271-4185
e-mail: deb.samson@drake.edu

Provides informational and emotional support to parents who have a child, adolescent, or adult family member with special needs. Program offers an important connection for a parent who is seeking support for special disability issue, by matching him or her with a trained veteran parent.

Kansas

4759 Assistive Technology for Kansas Project
2601 Gabriel, PO Box 738
Parsons, KS 67357   316-421-8367
800-526-3648
Fax: 316-421-0954
TDD: 316-421-0954
e-mail: ssack@parsons.lsi.ukans.edu
www.atk.lsi.ukans.edu

State assisted programs and support group information for people of many abilities. Including local chapters, referrals, fun and social interaction and support groups.

4760 Department of Health & Environment
900 Southwest Jackson
Topeka, KS 66612   913-296-6135
Fax: 913-296-8626
e-mail: uskank86@ibmmail.com
www.nectas.unc.edu

Individuals with Disabilities Education Act requires all states and territories to provide early intervention and preschool special education for children with disabilities and special healthcare needs. Services include central directory, representatives of agencies, service providers, families, and coordinators of infant, toddler, and preschool special education programs.

Jayne Garcia, Infant/Toddler Program Coordinator

4761 Families Together, Inc.
3340 W. Douglas, Suite 102
Witchita, KS 67203   316-945-7747
888-815-6364
Fax: 316-945-7795
e-mail: fmin@feist.com
www.kansas.net/~family

Parent Training and Information (PTI) programs help parents to: understand their children's specific needs; communicate more effectively with professionals, participate in the educational planning process; and obtain information about relevant programs, services, and resources

4762 Families Together/Parent to Parent of KS
501 Jackson, Suite 400
Topeka, KS 66603   785-233-4777
800-264-6343
Fax: 756-233-4787
TTY: 785-233-4777
e-mail: family@inlandnet.net

Informational and emotional support to parents who have a child, adolescent, or adult family member with special needs.

4763 Great Plains Region Helen Keller National Center
430 Shawnee Mission Road Suite 108
Shawnee Mission, KS 66205   913-677-4562

4764 Special Education Administration State Department of Education
120 East 10th Avenue
Topeka, KS 66612   785-296-7454
Fax: 785-296-7933
e-mail: cdermyer@ksbe.state.ks.us
www.nectas.unc.edu

Individuals with Disabilities Education Act requires all states and territories to provide early intervention and preschool special education for children with disabilities and special healthcare needs. Services include central directory, representatives of agencies, service providers, families, and coordinators of infant, toddler, and preschool special education programs.

Carol Dermyer, Preschool Special Ed. Coordinator

Kentucky

4765 Assistive Technology Services Network
8412 Westport Road
Louisville, KY 40242   502-327-0022
                             800-346-2115
                        Fax: 502-327-9974
                        TDD: 502-327-9855
www.state.ky.us/agencies/wforce/vdfblind

State assisted programs and support group information for people of many abilities. Including local chapters, referrals, fun and social interaction and support groups.

4766 College of Education - Western Kentucky University
Interdisciplinary Early Childhood Education
#1 Big Red Way-Western Kentucky University
Bowling Green, KY 42101   270-745-5414
                            Fax: 270-745-6474
e-mail: vicki.stayton@wku.edu
www.nectas.unc.edu

Individuals with Disabilities Education Act requires all states and territories to provide early intervention and preschool special education for children with disabilities and special healthcare needs. Services include central directory, representatives of agencies, service providers, families, and coordinators of infant, toddler, and preschool special education programs.

Vicki Stayton, Interagency Coordinating Council

4767 Division of Preschool Services
500 Mero Street, 16th Floor
Frankfort, KY 40601   502-564-7056
                        Fax: 502-564-6771
e-mail: bsinglet@kde.state.ky.us
www.nectas.unc.edu

Provides early intervention and preschool special education for children with disabilities and special healthcare needs. Services include central directory, representatives of agencies, service providers, families, and coordinators of infant, toddler, and preschool special education programs.

Barbara Singleton, Preschool Special Ed. Coor.

4768 Infant-Toddler Program, Division of Mental Retardation
275 East Main Street
Frankfort, KY 40621   502-564-7722
                        Fax: 502-564-0438
e-mail: jhenson@mail.state.ky.us
www.nectas.unc.edu

Individuals with Disabilities Education Act requires all states and territories to provide early intervention and preschool special education for children with disabilities and special healthcare needs. Services include central directory, representatives of agencies, service providers, families, and coordinators of infant, toddler, and preschool special education programs.

Jim Henson, Infant/Toddler Program Coordinator

4769 Special Parent Involvement Network
2210 Goldsmith Lane, Suite 118
Louisville, KY 40218   502-456-0923
                             800-525-7746
                        Fax: 502-456-0893
e-mail: FamilyTmg@aol.com
www.taalliance.org

Parent Training and Information (PTI) programs help parents to: understand their children's specific needs; communicate more effectively with professionals, participate in the educational planning process; and obtain information about relevant programs, services, and resources

Louisiana

4770 Division of Special Populations
P.O. Box 94064
Baton Rouge, LA 70804   225-342-3631
                          Fax: 225-342-5880
e-mail: edjohnson@mail.doe.state.la.us
www.nectas.unc.edu

Individuals with Disabilities Education Act requires all states and territories to provide early intervention and preschool special education for children with disabilities and special healthcare needs. Services include central directory, representatives of agencies, service providers, families, and coordinators of infant, toddler, and preschool special education programs.

Evelyn Johnson, Infant/Toddler Program Coor.

4771 Families Helping Families of Greater New Orleans
4323 Division Street, Suite 110
Metairie, LA 70002   504-888-9111
                            800-766-7736
                       Fax: 504-888-0246
              e-mail: fhfgno@ix.netcom.com

Informational and emotional support to parents
who have a child, adolescent, or adult family
member with special needs.

4772 Louisiana Assistive Technology Access Network
P.O. Box 14115
Baton Rouge, LA 70898   225-925-9500
                            800-270-6185
                       Fax: 225-925-9560
                       TDD: 225-925-9500
              e-mail: latanstate@aol.com
                            www.latan.org

State assisted programs and support group information for people of many abilities. Including local chapters, referrals, fun and social
interaction and support groups.

4773 Preschool Programs - Division of Special Populations
P.O. Box 94064
Baton Rouge, LA 70804   225-342-1190
                       Fax: 225-342-5880
         e-mail: jzube@mail.doe.state.la.us
                        www.nectas.unc.edu

Individuals with Disabilities Education Act requires all states and territories to provide early
intervention and preschool special education for
children with disabilities and special healthcare
needs. Services include central directory, representatives of agencies, service providers, families, and coordinators of infant, toddler, and
preschool special education programs.

Janice Zube, Preschool Special Ed. Coordinator

4774 Project PROMPT
4323 Division Street, Suite 110
Metairie, LA 70002   504-888-9111
                            800-766-7736
                       Fax: 504-888-0246
              e-mail: thsgno@ix.netcom.com
                        www.taalliance.org

Parent Training and Information (PTI) programs help parents to: understand their children's specific needs; communicate more
effectively with professionals, participate in the
educational planning process; and obtain information about relevant programs, services, and
resources

Maine

4775 CDC Lincoln County
P.O. Box 1114
Damariscotta, ME 04543   207-563-1411
                       Fax: 207-563-6312
                        www.nectas.unc.edu

Individuals with Disabilities Education Act requires all states and territories to provide early
intervention and preschool special education for
children with disabilities and special healthcare
needs. Services include central directory, representatives of agencies, service providers, families, and coordinators of infant, toddler, and
preschool special education programs.

Jean Eaton, Interagency Coordinating Council

4776 Child Department Services
146 State House Station
Augusta, ME 04333   207-287-3272
                       Fax: 207-287-5900
         e-mail: jaci.holmes@state.me.us
                        www.nectas.unc.edu

Provides early intervention and preschool special education for children with disabilities and
special healthcare needs. Services include central directory, representatives of agencies, service providers, families, and coordinators of
infant, toddler, and preschool special education
programs.

Joanne C. Holmes, Infant/Toddler Program Coordinator

4777 Child Department Services, Department of Education
146 State House Station
Augusta, ME 04333   207-287-3272
                       Fax: 207-287-5900
         e-mail: jaci.holmes@state.me.us
                        www.nectas.unc.edu

Provides early intervention and preschool special education for children with disabilities and
special healthcare needs. Services include central directory, representatives of agencies, service providers, families, and coordinators of
infant, toddler, and preschool special education
programs.

Joanne C. Holmes, Preschool Special Ed. Coor.

4778 Children's Dream Factory of Maine
400 U.S. Rt 1, ATTN:Doris Simard
Falmouth, ME 04105   207-781-3406
                            800-639-1492

Grants wishes for chronically or seriously ill
children from Maine.

4779 Consumer Information and Technology Training Exchange (Maine CITE)
46 University Drive
Augusta, ME 04330   207-621-3195
Fax: 207-621-3193
TDD: 207-621-3195
e-mail: powers@maine.maine.edu

State assisted programs and support group information for people of many abilities. Including local chapters, referrals, fun and social interaction and support groups.

4780 Special Needs Parent Info Network
P.O. Box 2067
Augusta, ME 04338   207-582-2504
Fax: 207-582-3638
e-mail: info@mpf.org
www.mpf.org

Parent Training and Information (PTI) programs help parents to: understand their children's specific needs; communicate more effectively with professionals, participate in the educational planning process; and obtain information about relevant programs, services, and resources

4781 York County Parent Awareness. Inc
150 Main Street, Midtown Mall
Sanford, ME 04027   207-324-2337
Fax: 207-324-5621
e-mail: ycpa@mmp.org

Informational and emotional support to parents who have a child, adolescent, or adult family member with special needs.

Maryland

4782 ARC Family Connection Parent to Parent Program
11600 Nebel Street
Rockville, MD 20852   301-984-5777
Fax: 301-816-2429

Informational and emotional support to parents who have a child, adolescent, or adult family member with special needs.

4783 Developmental Pediatrics School of Medicine, University of Maryland
630 West Fayette Street, Room 5686
Baltimore, MD 21201   410-706-3542
Fax: 410-706-0835
www.nectas.unc.edu

Individuals with Disabilities Education Act requires all states and territories to provide early intervention and preschool special education for children with disabilities and special healthcare needs. Services include central directory, representatives of agencies, service providers, families, and coordinators of infant, toddler, and preschool special education programs.

Renee Wachtel, Interagency Coordinating Council

4784 MD Infant/Toddler/Preschool Services Division
200 West Baltimore Street
Baltimore, MD 21201   410-767-0261
Fax: 410-333-2661
e-mail: dmetzger@msde.state.md.us
www.nectas.unc.edu

Individuals with Disabilities Education Act requires all states and territories to provide early intervention and preschool special education for children with disabilities and special healthcare needs. Services include central directory, representatives of agencies, service providers, families, and coordinators of infant, toddler, and preschool special education programs.

Deborah Metzger, Infant/Toddler Program Coordinator

4785 MD Infant/Toddler/Preschool Services
200 West Baltimore Street
Baltimore, MD 21201   410-767-0234
Fax: 410-333-8165
e-mail: nvorobey@msde.state.md.us
www.nectas.unc.edu

Individuals with Disabilities Education Act requires all states and territories to provide early intervention and preschool special education for children with disabilities and special healthcare needs. Services include central directory, representatives of agencies, service providers, families, and coordinators of infant, toddler, and preschool special education programs.

Nancy Vorobey, Preschool Special Ed. Coordinator

4786 Maryland Infant and Toddlers Program Family Support Network
200 W Baltimore 4th Floor
Baltimore, MD 21201   410-767-0652
Fax: 410-333-8165

Informational and emotional support to parents who have a child, adolescent, or adult family member with special needs.

4787 National Organization of Parents of Blind Children
1800 Johnson Street Floor
Baltimore, MD 21230   410-659-9314
                            Fax: 410-685-5653
                    e-mail: nfb@iamdiyrx.net
                                www.nfh.org

Informational and emotional support to parents who have a child, adolescent, or adult family member with blindness or visual impairment.

4788 Parents Place of Maryland, Inc.
7484 Candlewood Rd. Suite S
Hanover, MD 21076   410-859-5300
                          Fax: 410-859-5301
                  e-mail: parplace@aol.com
              www.somerset.net/ParentsPlace

Parent Training and Information (PTI) programs help parents to: understand their children's specific needs; communicate more effectively with professionals, participate in the educational planning process; and obtain information about relevant programs, services, and resources

4789 Partners in Intensive Care, Inc.
P.O. Box 41043
Bethesda, MD 20824   301-681-2708
                          Fax: 202-363-4659

Informational and emotional support to parents who have a child, adolescent, or adult family member with special needs.

4790 Technology Assistance Program Maryland Rehab Center
2301 Argonne Drive
Baltimore, MD 21218
                            800-832-4827
                          Fax: 410-554-9237
                  e-mail: mdtap@clark.net
                                www.mdtap.org

State assisted programs and support group information for people of many abilities. Including local chapters, referrals, fun and social interaction and support groups.

Massachusetts

4791 Bureau of Early Childhood Programs
350 Main Street
Malden, MA 02148   781-388-3300
                          Fax: 781-388-3394
              e-mail: eschaefer@doe.mass.edu
                            www.nectas.unc.edu

Individuals with Disabilities Education Act requires all states and territories to provide early intervention and preschool special education for children with disabilities and special healthcare needs. Services include central directory, representatives of agencies, service providers, families, and coordinators of infant, toddler, and preschool special education programs.

Elisabeth Schaefer, Preschool Special Ed. Coor.

4792 Children's Happiness Foundation
P.O. Box 266
Marshfield, MA 02050   617-837-9609
                              800-424-3543
                            Fax: 617-837-5229

Serves New England children ages 3 to 18 with life-threatening or chronic degenerative diseases.

4793 Early Intervention Services
250 Washington Street
Boston, MA 02108   617-624-5969
                          Fax: 617-624-5992
            e-mail: Ron.Benham@state.ma.us
                            www.nectas.unc.edu

Individuals with Disabilities Education Act requires all states and territories to provide early intervention and preschool special education for children with disabilities and special healthcare needs. Services include central directory, representatives of agencies, service providers, families, and coordinators of infant, toddler, and preschool special education programs.

Ron Benham, Infant/Toddler Program Coordinator

4794 Educational Development Center, Inc (EDC)
55 Chapel Street
Newton, MA 02458   617-969-7100
                          800-225-4276
                        Fax: 617-969-3440
              e-mail: pprintz@edc.org
                          www.edc.org

World's largest nonprofit education and health organizations. Programs for children and families combining research and practice, promoting professional development and systematic change, forging community links, and influencing the policies and legislation that affect the lives of children. The New england RAP for Disabilities Services incorporates proven strategies to enhance the efforts of organizations servicing children disabilities and their families.

Philip Printz, Project Director

4795 Family Ties MA Dept. of Public Health
250 Washington St, DCSHCN 4th Fl
Boston, MA 02108   617-624-5070
                         Fax: 617-624-5990
          e-mail: division.CSHCN@state.ma.us

Informational and emotional support to parents who have a child, adolescent, or adult family member with special needs.

4796 Federation for Children with Special Needs
1135 Tremont St.
Boston, MA 02120   617-236-7210
                         Fax: 617-572-2094
               e-mail: csninfo@csn.org

Informational and emotional support to parents who have a child, adolescent, or adult family member with special needs.

4797 Federation for Children with Special Needs
95 Berkeley Street, Suite 104
Boston, MA 02116   617-482-2915
                         Fax: 617-695-2939
                         TDD: 617-482-2915
              e-mail: fcsninfo@fcsn.org
                    www.fcsn.org/

Parent Training and Information (PTI) programs help parents to: understand their children's specific needs; communicate more effectively with professionals, participate in the educational planning process; and obtain information about relevant programs, services, and resources

4798 Greater Boston Parent to Parent
1505 Commonwealth Avenue
Boston, MA 02135   617-783-3900
                         Fax: 617-783-9190
              e-mail: bostonarc@aol.com

Informational and emotional support to parents who have a child, adolescent, or adult family member with special needs.

4799 Massachusetts Assistive Technology Partnership
1295 Boylston Street, Suite 310
Boston, MA 02215   617-355-7153
                         Fax: 617-355-6345
                         TDD: 617-355-7301
               e-mail: matp@matp.net
                    www.matp.org

State assisted programs and support group information for people of many abilities. Including local chapters, referrals, fun and social interaction and support groups.

4800 New England Region Helen Keller National Center
313 Washington Street Suite 209
Newton, MA 02158   617-630-1580

Michigan

4801 CAUSE
3303 W. Saginaw, Suite F-1
Lansing, MI 48917   517-886-9167
                          Fax: 517-886-9775
                          TTY: 517-886-9167
                          TDD: 517-886-9167
          e-mail: info~cause@voyager.net
                www.cause.home.mi.org

Parent Training and Information (PTI) programs help parents to: understand their children's specific needs; communicate more effectively with professionals, participate in the educational planning process; and obtain information about relevant programs, services, and resources

4802 Early on Michigan
P.O. Box 30008
Lansing, MI 48909   517-335-3888
                          Fax: 517-373-1233
          e-mail: banfieldj@state.mi.us
                www.nectas.unc.edu

Provides early intervention and preschool special education for children with disabilities and special healthcare needs. Services include central directory, representatives of agencies, service providers, families, and coordinators of infant, toddler, and preschool special education programs.

Julie Banfield, Infant/Toddler Program Coordinator

4803 Family Support Network of Michigan Parent Participation Program-MDCH
1200 6th St,3rd Floor,S Tower,St316
Detroit, MI 48226
                          800-359-3722
                          Fax: 313-256-2605
                          TTY: 800-788-7889

Informational and emotional support to parents who have a child, adolescent, or adult family member with special needs.

4804 Livingston County CMH Services
206 South Highlander Way
Howell, MI 48843   517-546-4126
                         Fax: 517-546-1300
               www.nectas.unc.edu

Provides early intervention and preschool special education for children with disabilities and special healthcare needs. Services include central directory, representatives of agencies, service providers, families, and coordinators of infant, toddler, and preschool special education programs.

Mac Miller, Interagency Coordinating Council

4805 Office of Special Education
P.O. Box 30008
Lansing, MI 48909   517-335-3888
                          Fax: 517-373-1233
                          e-mail: banfieldj@state.mi.us
                          www.nectas.unc.edu

Individuals with Disabilities Education Act requires all states and territories to provide early intervention and preschool special education for children with disabilities and special healthcare needs. Services include central directory, representatives of agencies, service providers, families, and coordinators of infant, toddler, and preschool special education programs.

Julie Banfield, Preschool Special Ed. Coordinator

4806 Parents are Experts
23077 Greenfield Road, Suite 205
Southfield, MI 48075   248-557-5070
                             800-827-4843
                             Fax: 248-557-4456
                             TDD: 248-557-5070
                             e-mail: ucp@ameritech.net
                             www.taalliance.org

Parent Training and Information (PTI) programs help parents to: understand their children's specific needs; communicate more effectively with professionals, participate in the educational planning process; and obtain information about relevant programs, services, and resources

4807 TECH 2000 Project Michigan Disability Rights Coalition
740 W Lake Lansing Road, Suite 400
East Lansing, MI 48823   517-333-2477
                               800-760-4600
                               Fax: 517-333-2677
                               TDD: 517-333-2477
                               e-mail: roanne@match.org
                               www.discoalition.org

State assisted programs and support group information for people of many abilities. Including local chapters, referrals, fun and social interaction and support groups.

Minnesota

4808 ARC Suburban
1526 E 122nd Street
Burnsville, MN 56337   612-890-3057
                             Fax: 612-890-3527

Informational and emotional support to parents who have a child, adolescent, or adult family member with special needs.

4809 Department of Children, Family, & Learning
550 Cedar Street
Saint Paul, MN 55101   612-297-3056
                             Fax: 612-296-5147
                             e-mail: michael.eastman@state.mn.us
                             www.nectas.unc.edu

Individuals with Disabilities Education Act requires all states and territories to provide early intervention and preschool special education for children with disabilities and special healthcare needs. Services include central directory, representatives of agencies, service providers, families, and coordinators of infant, toddler, and preschool special education programs.

Michael Eastman, Preschool Special Ed. Coordinator

4810 Family to Family Network ARC of Hennepin County
4301 Hwy 7, Suite 104
Minneapolis, MN 55416   612-920-0855
                              Fax: 612-920-1480

Informational and emotional support to parents who have a child, adolescent, or adult family member with special needs.

4811 Interagency Early Intervention Project
550 Cedar Street
Saint Paul, MN 55101   612-296-7032
                             Fax: 612-296-5076
                             e-mail: jan.rubenstein@state.mn.us
                             www.nectas.unc.edu

Individuals with Disabilities Education Act requires all states and territories to provide early intervention and preschool special education for children with disabilities and special healthcare needs. Services include central directory, representatives of agencies, service providers, families, and coordinators of infant, toddler, and preschool special education programs.

Jan Rubenstein, Infant/Toddler Program Coor.

4812 PACER Computer Resource Center
4826 Chicago Avenue S
Minneapolis, MN 55417
                             Fax: 517-224-0330
                             TTY: 612-827-2966
                             e-mail: crcenter@pacer.org
                             www.pacer.org/crc/crc.htm

Technology group of parents, consumers and professionals; provides resources to help children and adults who have disabilities gain access to the benefits of technology. Includes nationwide network of community-based assistive technology, resource centers, hands on consultants and product demonstrations.

4813 Parents for Parents
290 N Smith Avenue, Suite 245
St. Paul, MN 56102　　　　651-220-6731
　　　　　　　　　　　Fax: 651-220-6707

Informational and emotional support to parents who have a child, adolescent, or adult family member with special needs.

4814 Pilot Parents in Anoka and Ramsey Counties
1201 89th Avenue NE, Suite 305
Blaine, MN 55434　　　　612-783-4958
　　　　　　　　　　　Fax: 612-783-4900

Informational and emotional support to parents who have a child, adolescent, or adult family member with special needs.

4815 Pilot Parents of Northeast Minnesota
201 Ordean Bldg.
Duluth, MN 55802　　　　218-726-4725
　　　　　　　　　　　Fax: 218-726-4722

Informational and emotional support to parents who have a child, adolescent, or adult family member with special needs.

4816 STAR Program
300 Centennial Bldg.,658 Cedar St.
St. Paul, MN 55155　　　　612-296-2771
　　　　　　　　　　　Fax: 612-282-6671
　　　　　　　　　　　TDD: 612-296-8478
　　　　e-mail: rachel.wobscall@state.mn.us
　　　www.state.mn.us/branch/admin/assistivete

State assisted programs and support group information for people of many abilities. Including local chapters, referrals, fun and social interaction and support groups.

4817 Vinland Center
P.O. Box 306, 3675 Ihduhapi Road
Loretto, MN 55357　　　　612-479-3555
　　　　　　　　　　　Fax: 612-479-2605
　　　　　　　　　e-mail: vinland@mtn.org

State assisted programs and support group information for people of many abilities. Including local chapters, referrals, fun and social interaction and support groups.

4818 Voyageur Outward Bound School
111 Third Avenue S, Suite 120
Minneapolis, MN 55401　　　　612-338-0131
　　　　　　　　　　　　800-328-2943
　　　　　　　　　　　Fax: 612-338-3540

State assisted programs and support group information for people of many abilities. Including local chapters, referrals, fun and social interaction and support groups.

4819 Wilderness Inquiry
1313 5th Street SE, Box 84
Minneapolis, MN 55414　　　　612-379-3858
　　　　　　　　　　　　800-728-0719
　　　　　　　　　　　Fax: 612-379-5972
　　　　　　　　　　　TTY: 800-728-0719
　　　　　　　　　e-mail: winquiry@aol.com

State assisted programs and support group information for people of many abilities. Including local chapters, referrals, fun and social interaction and support groups.

4820 Windmill Project
125 W Lincoln Avenue, PO Box 54
Fergus Falls, MN 56538　　　　218-739-3011
　　　　　　　　　　　　800-257-5463
　　　　　　　　　　　Fax: 218-739-3727
　　　　　　　　　e-mail: uwff@prtel.com

Informational and emotional support to parents who have a child, adolescent, or adult family member with special needs.

Mississippi

4821 First Steps Program
P.O. Box 1700
Jackson, MS 39215　　　　601-576-7427
　　　　　　　　　　　Fax: 601-576-7540
　　　　　　　　　　　www.nectas.unc.edu

Individuals with Disabilities Education Act requires all states and territories to provide early intervention and preschool special education for children with disabilities and special healthcare needs. Services include central directory, representatives of agencies, service providers, families, and coordinators of infant, toddler, and preschool special education programs.

Roy Hart, Infant/Toddler Program Coordinator

4822 Office of Special Education
P.O. Box 771
Jackson, MS 39205　　　　601-359-3490
　　　　　　　　　　　Fax: 601-359-2198
　　　　e-mail: dbowman@mdek12.state.ms.us
　　　　　　　　　　　www.nectas.unc.edu

Individuals with Disabilities Education Act requires all states and territories to provide early intervention and preschool special education for children with disabilities and special healthcare needs. Services include central directory, representatives of agencies, service providers, families, and coordinators of infant, toddler, and preschool special education programs.

Dot Bowman, Preschool Special Ed. Coordinator

4823 Parent Partners
1900 North West Street, Suite C 100
Jackson, MS 39202   601-714-5707
Fax: 601-714-4025
e-mail: ptiofms@misnet.com
www.taalliance.org/ptis/ms/

Parent Training and Information (PTI) programs help parents to: understand their children's specific needs; communicate more effectively with professionals, participate in the educational planning process; and obtain information about relevant programs, services, and resources

4824 Project Empower
1427 S. Main, Suite 8
Greenville, MS 38701   601-332-4852
800-337-4852
Fax: 601-332-1622
www.taalliance.org

Parent Training and Information (PTI) programs help parents to: understand their children's specific needs; communicate more effectively with professionals, participate in the educational planning process; and obtain information about relevant programs, services, and resources

4825 Project Start
P.O. Box 1698
Jackson, MS 39215   601-987-4872
Fax: 601-364-2349
e-mail: spower@netdoor.com

State assisted programs and support group information for people of many abilities. Including local chapters, referrals, fun and social interaction and support groups.

Missouri

4826 Assistance Technology Project
4731 S. Cochise, Suite 114
Independence, MO 64055   816-373-5193
Fax: 816-373-9314
TTY: 816-373-9315
e-mail: matpmo@gni.com
www.doir.state.mo.us/matp/

State assisted programs and support group information for people of many abilities. Including local chapters, referrals, fun and social interaction and support groups.

4827 Children's Therapy Center
600 East 14th St.
Sedalia, MO 65301   660-826-4400
Fax: 660-826-4420
www.nectas.unc.edu

Services include central directory, representatives of agencies, service providers, families, and coordinators of infant, toddler, and preschool special education programs.

Roger Garlich, Interagency Coordinating Council

4828 Department of Elementary and Secondary Education
P.O. Box 480
Jefferson City, MO 65102   573-751-0185
Fax: 573-526-4404
e-mail: pgoff@mail.dese.state.mo.us
www.nectas.unc.edu

Individuals with Disabilities Education Act requires all states and territories to provide early intervention and preschool special education for children with disabilities and special healthcare needs. Services include central directory, representatives of agencies, service providers, families, and coordinators of infant, toddler, and preschool special education programs.

Paula Goff, Preschool Special Ed. Coordinator

4829 Disabilities Advocacy & Support Network
The Network 1515 E Pythian
Springfield, MO 65801   417-895-7464
Fax: 417-895-7412
TTY: 417-895-7430

Informational and emotional support to parents who have a child, adolescent, or adult family member with special needs.

4830 Family Resource Network
Park A Plaza
601 Business Loop 70 W, Suite 2161
Columbia, MO 65203   573-449-8663
e-mail: betty@ece.missouri.edu

Informational and emotional support to parents who have a child, adolescent, or adult family member with special needs.

4831 Missouri Parents Act
2100 S. Brentwood, Suite G
Springfield, MO 65804   417-582-7434
                              800-743-7634
                          Fax: 417-882-8413
                          www.taalliance.org

Parent Training and Information (PTI) programs help parents to: understand their children's specific needs; communicate more effectively with professionals, participate in the educational planning process; and obtain information about relevant programs, services, and resources

4832 Parent Act
1 W. Armour, Suite 301
Kansas City, MO 64111   816-531-7070
                          Fax: 816-531-4777
                      e-mail: impactcs@coop.cm.org
                          www.taalliance.org

Parent Training and Information (PTI) programs help parents to: understand their children's specific needs; communicate more effectively with professionals, participate in the educational planning process; and obtain information about relevant programs, services, and resources

4833 Positive Parenting Partners United Services
4140 Old Mill Parkway
St. Peters, MO 63376   636-926-2700
                          Fax: 636-447-4919

Informational and emotional support to parents who have a child, adolescent, or adult family member with special needs.

4834 Positive Solutions for Life Challenges
Route 3, Box 441
Warswaw, MO 65355   660-438-6990

Informational and emotional support to parents who have a child, adolescent, or adult family member with special needs.

4835 Wishing Well Foundation
P.O. Box 717, Jim Reid
St. Louis, MO 63188   314-272-6190

Grants wishes to children in the St. Louis area only who are chronically or terminally ill.

Montana

4836 CO-TEACH/Division of Educational Research and Service
School of Education
University of Montana
Missoula, MT 59812   406-243-5344
                          Fax: 406-243-2797
                      e-mail: coteach@selway.umt.edu

Informational and emotional support to parents who have a child, adolescent, or adult family member with special needs.

4837 Developmental Disabilities Program
P.O. Box 4210
Helena, MT 59604   406-444-2995
                          Fax: 406-444-0230
                      e-mail: jspiegle@mt.gov
                          www.nectas.unc.edu

Individuals with Disabilities Education Act requires all states and territories to provide early intervention and preschool special education for children with disabilities and special healthcare needs. Services include central directory, representatives of agencies, service providers, families, and coordinators of infant, toddler, and preschool special education programs.

Jan Spiegle, Infant/Toddler Program Coordinator

4838 Division of Special Education
P.O. Box 202501
Helena, MT 59620   406-444-4425
                          Fax: 406-444-3924
                      e-mail: dmccarthy@opi.mt.gov
                          www.nectas.unc.edu

Individuals with Disabilities Education Act requires all states and territories to provide early intervention and preschool special education for children with disabilities and special healthcare needs. Services include central directory, representatives of agencies, service providers, families, and coordinators of infant, toddler, and preschool special education programs.

Daniel McCarthy, Preschool Special Ed. Coordinator

4839 MonTECH
634 Eddy Avenue, Rural Inst on Disab
Missoula, MT 59812   406-243-5676
                              800-732-0323
                          Fax: 406-243-4730
                          TDD: 800-732-0323
                      e-mail: montech@selway.umt.edu
                          www.rudi.montech.umt.edu/

State assisted programs and support group information for people of many abilities. Including local chapters, referrals, fun and social interaction and support groups.

4840 Parents Let's Unite for Kids
516 N. 32nd Street
Billings, MT 59101   406-255-0540
e-mail: plukmt@aol.com
www.taalliance.org

Parent Training and Information (PTI) programs help parents to: understand their children's specific needs; communicate more effectively with professionals, participate in the educational planning process; and obtain information about relevant programs, services, and resources

4841 Parents, Let's Unite for Kids
516 N 32nd Street
Billings, MT 59101   406-255-0540
800-222-7585

Support network for parents of children with disabilities and/or chronic illness. Veteran parents offer support to parents who are just learning of their child's diagnosis. Offers support and insight into parenting a child with special needs, as well as referrals to trained veteran parents.

4842 Quality Life Concepts
P.O. Box 2506
Great Falls, MT 59403   406-452-9531
Fax: 406-453-5930

Informational and emotional support to parents who have a child, adolescent, or adult family member with special needs.

Nebraska

4843 Assistive Technology Partnership
5145 S 48th Street
Lincoln, NE 68516   402-471-0734
Fax: 402-471-6052
TDD: 402-471-0734
e-mail: atp@nde4.rde.state.ne.us
www.nde.state.ne.us/atp/ATPECHome.html

State assisted programs and support group information for people of many abilities. Including local chapters, referrals, fun and social interaction and support groups.

4844 Individual and Family Support Arc of Lincoln & Lancaster County
645 M Street, Suite 19
Lincoln, NE 68508   402-477-6925
Fax: 402-477-6927

Informational and emotional support to parents who have a child, adolescent, or adult family member with special needs.

4845 Nebraska Parents Center
1941 S. 42nd Street, #122
Omaha, NE 68105   402-346-0525
800-284-8520
Fax: 402-346-5253
TDD: 402-346-0525
e-mail: npe@uswest.ne.net
www.techlab.esu3k12ne.us/npc/ParentsCent

Parent Training and Information (PTI) programs help parents to: understand their children's specific needs; communicate more effectively with professionals, participate in the educational planning process; and obtain information about relevant programs, services, and resources. The Nebrask Parent Center services families statewide. There is no fee for services. Call for additional information.

Glenda Davis, Project Director

4846 Parent Assistance Network
310 W 24th
Kearney, NE 68847   308-237-6025
Fax: 308-237-6014

Informational and emotional support to parents who have a child, adolescent, or adult family member with special needs.

4847 Parent Support Group
1235 S Webb Road
Grand Island, NE 68803   308-385-5925
Fax: 308-385-5797
e-mail: msheen@genie.esu10.k12.ne.us

Informational and emotional support to parents who have a child, adolescent, or adult family member with special needs.

4848 Parents Encouraging Parents
NE Dept. of Education, 301 Centennial Mall Street
P.O. Box 94987
Lincoln, NE 68509
Fax: 402-471-0117
TTY: 402-471-2471
e-mail: ginny_w@nde4.nde.state.ne.us

Informational and emotional support to parents who have a child, adolescent, or adult family member with special needs.

4849 Special Education Office State Department of Education
P.O. Box 94987
Lincoln, NE 68509   402-471-4319
Fax: 402-471-0117
e-mail: jan_t@nde4.nde.state.ne.us
www.nectas.unc.edu

Individuals with Disabilities Education Act requires all states and territories to provide early intervention and preschool special education for children with disabilities and special healthcare needs. Services include central directory, representatives of agencies, service providers, families, and coordinators of infant, toddler, and preschool special education programs.

Jan Thelen, Preschool Special Ed. Coordinator

Nevada

4850 Assistive Technology Collaborative
711 S. Stewart St., Rehab Division
Carson City, NV 89701   775-687-4452
                              Fax: 775-687-3292
                              TTY: 702-687-3388
                    e-mail: pgowins@govmail.state.nv.us
                              www.state.nv.us.80

State assisted programs and support group information for people of many abilities. Including local chapters, referrals, fun and social interaction and support groups.

4851 Early Intervention Services Division of Child & Family Services
3987 South McCarren Blvd.
Reno, NV 89502   775-688-2284
                        Fax: 775-688-2558
              e-mail: mkwalter@govmail.state.nv.us
                        www.nectas.unc.edu

Provides early intervention and preschool special education for children with disabilities and special healthcare needs. Services include central directory, representatives of agencies, service providers, families, and coordinators of infant, toddler, and preschool special education programs.

Marilyn K. Walter, Infant/Toddler Program Coor.

4852 Educational Equity, Special Education Branch
700 East 5th Street, Suite 113
Carson City, NV 89701   775-687-9171
                              Fax: 775-687-9123
                    e-mail: gdopf@nsn.scs.unr.edu
                              www.nectas.unc.edu

Individuals with Disabilities Education Act requires all states and territories to provide early intervention and preschool special education for children with disabilities and special healthcare needs. Services include central directory, representatives of agencies, service providers, families, and coordinators of infant, toddler, and preschool special education programs.

Gloria Dopf, Preschool Special Ed. Coordinator

4853 Nevada Parent Network
University of Nevada- Reno
COE, REPC/285
Reno, NV 89557   702-784-4921
                        800-216-7988
                  Fax: 702-784-4997
          e-mail: cdinnell@scs.unr.edu
                  www.scs.unr.edu/repc/npn

Informational and emotional support to parents who have a child, adolescent, or adult family member with special needs.

4854 Nevada Parents Encouraging Parents (PEP)
601 S. Ranch Drive, Suite C25
Las Vegas, NV 89106   702-388-8899
                            800-216-5188
                      Fax: 702-388-2966
              e-mail: nvpep@vegas.infi.net
                      www.vegas.infi.net/~nvpep

Parent Training and Information (PTI) programs help parents to: understand their children's specific needs; communicate more effectively with professionals, participate in the educational planning process; and obtain information about relevant programs, services, and resources

New Hampshire

4855 Bureau of Early Learning
101 Pleasant Street
Concord, NH 03301   603-271-2178
                          Fax: 603-271-1953
              e-mail: rlittlefield@ed.state.nh.us
                          www.nectas.unc.edu

Individuals with Disabilities Education Act requires all states and territories to provide early intervention and preschool special education for children with disabilities and special healthcare needs. Services include central directory, representatives of agencies, service providers, families, and coordinators of infant, toddler, and preschool special education programs.

Ruth Littlefield, Preschool Special Ed. Coordinator

4856 Division of Special Education
101 Pleasant Street
Concord, NH 03301   603-271-3776
                          Fax: 603-271-1953
                          www.nectas.unc.edu

Individuals with Disabilities Education Act requires all states and territories to provide early intervention and preschool special education for children with disabilities and special healthcare needs. Services include central directory, representatives of agencies, service providers, families, and coordinators of infant, toddler, and preschool special education programs.

Jane Weisman, Interagency Coordinating Council

4857 Family Center Early Supports & Services
105 Pleasant Street
Concord, NH 03301　　　　　　603-271-5122
　　　　　　　　　　　　Fax: 603-271-5144
　　　　　　　e-mail: cohara@dhhs.state.nh.us
　　　　　　　　　　　　www.nectas.unc.edu

Services include central directory, representatives of agencies, service providers, families, and coordinators of infant, toddler, and preschool special education programs.

Carolyn O'Hara, Infant/Toddler Program Coor.

4858 High Hopes Foundation of New Hampshire Inc
354 North Broadway
Salem, NH 03079　　　　　　603-898-5333
　　　　　　　　　　　　800-639-6804
　　　　　　　　　　　Fax: 603-898-3874
　　　　　　　　　　　www.highhopesnh.org

Volunteer organization dedicated to granting wishes of seriously ill New Hampshire children from three through 18 years old

60+ members

Linda Bennett, President
Patricia Bouley, Director of Marketing

4859 Parent Information Center
P.O. Box 2405
Concord, NH 03302　　　　　　603-224-7005
　　　　　　　　　　　Fax: 603-224-4365
　　　　　　　　　　　TDD: 603-224-7005
　　　　　　　　e-mail: picnh@aol.com
　　　　　　　www.taalliance.org/ptis/nhpic

Parent Training and Information (PTI) programs help parents to: understand their children's specific needs; communicate more effectively with professionals, participate in the educational planning process; and obtain information about relevant programs, services, and resources

4860 Parent to Parent of New Hampshire
12 Flynn St.
Lebanon, NH 03766　　　　　　603-448-6393
　　　　　　　　　　　　800-698-5465
　　　　　　　　　　　Fax: 603-448-6311

Informational and emotional support to parents who have a child, adolescent, or adult family member with special needs.

4861 Technology Partnership Project Institute on Disability/UAP
The Concord Center
#14 10 Ferry Street
Concord, NH 03301　　　　　　603-224-0630
　　　　　　　　　　　　800-238-2048
　　　　　　　　　　　Fax: 603-226-0389
　　　　　　　　　　　TDD: 603-224-0630
　　　　　　e-mail: mipawlek@christa.unh.edu
　　　　　　www.unh.edu/projects/spd.htm

State assistive programs funded by the National Institute on Disability and Rehabilitation Research. Includes directories, support group information, training and project information.

New Jersey

4862 Division of Student Services
Riverview Executive Plaza, Bldg 100
Trenton, NJ 08625　　　　　　609-984-4950
　　　　　　　　　　　Fax: 609-292-5558
　　　　　　　e-mail: btkach@doh.state.nj.us
　　　　　　　　　　www.nectas.unc.edu

Individuals with Disabilities Education Act requires all states and territories to provide early intervention and preschool special education for children with disabilities and special healthcare needs. Services include central directory, representatives of agencies, service providers, families, and coordinators of infant, toddler, and preschool special education programs.

Barbara Tkach, Preschool Special Ed. Coordinator

4863 Early Intervention Program
P.O. Box 364
Trenton, NJ 08625　　　　　　609-777-7734
　　　　　　　　　　　Fax: 609-292-3580
　　　　　　　e-mail: TLH@doh.state.nj.us
　　　　　　　　　　www.nectas.unc.edu

Individuals with Disabilities Education Act requires all states and territories to provide early intervention and preschool special education for children with disabilities and special healthcare needs. Services include central directory, representatives of agencies, service providers, families, and coordinators of infant, toddler, and preschool special education programs.

Terry Harrison, Infant/Toddler Program Coor.

4864 Family Support Center of New Jersey
Lion's Head Office Park
35 Beaverson Blvd. Suite 8 A
Brick, NJ 08723   732-262-8020
                                    800-372-6510
                               Fax: 732-262-4373
                          e-mail: FSCNJ@aol.com
                                    www.efnj.com

Informational and emotional support to parents who have a child, adolescent, or adult family member with special needs.

4865 New Jersey Statewide Parent to Parent
2150 Highway 35, Suite 207C
Sea Girt, NJ 08750
                                    800-372-6510
                               Fax: 973-642-8080

Informational and emotional support to parents who have a child, adolescent, or adult family member with special needs.

4866 Statewide Parent Advocacy Network
35 Halsey Street, 4th Floor
Newark, NJ 07102   973-642-8100
                               Fax: 973-642-8080
                     e-mail: span@bellatlantic.net
                          www.taalliance.org/ptis/nj

Parent Training and Information (PTI) programs help parents to: understand their children's specific needs; communicate more effectively with professionals, participate in the educational planning process; and obtain information about relevant programs, services, and resources

4867 Technology Assistive Resource Program
Protection and Advocacy, Inc.
210 S Broad Street, 3rd Floor
Trenton, NJ 08608   609-292-9742
                                    800-342-5832
                               Fax: 609-777-0817
                               TDD: 609-633-7106
                          e-mail: pauljz@aol.com

State assistive programs for people of many abilities. Including local chapters, referrals, fun and social interaction and support groups.

New Mexico

4868 EPICS Project SW Communication Resources
P.O. Box 788
Bernalilo, NM 87004   505-867-3396
                                    800-765-7320
                               Fax: 505-867-3980
                               TDD: 505-867-3396
                     www.epics@highfiber.com

Parent Training and Information (PTI) programs help parents to: understand their children's specific needs; communicate more effectively with professionals, participate in the educational planning process; and obtain information about relevant programs, services, and resources

4869 Long Term Services Division
P.O. Box 26110
Santa Fe, NM 87502   505-827-2578
                               Fax: 505-827-2455
                               www.nectas.unc.edu

Individuals with Disabilities Education Act requires all states and territories to provide early intervention and preschool special education for children with disabilities and special healthcare needs. Services include central directory, representatives of agencies, service providers, families, and coordinators of infant, toddler, and preschool special education programs.

Cathy Stevenson, Infant/Toddler Program Coor.

4870 Parents Reaching Out
1000-A Main Street NW
Los Lunas, NM 87031   505-865-3700
                                    800-524-5176
                               Fax: 505-865-3737
                               TDD: 505-865-3700
                          e-mail: nmproth@aol.com
                          www.parentsreachingout.org

Provides peer support, technical assistance and information statewide to families in New Mexico who have family member with unique or special needs and professionals who care for them.

4871 Parents Reaching Out (PRO)
1000 A Main Street
Los Lunas, NM 87124
                                    800-524-5176
                               Fax: 505-865-3737
                               TTY: 505-865-3700
                          e-mail: proth@swcp.com

Informational and emotional support to parents who have a child, adolescent, or adult family member with special needs.

4872 Region 5 of the National Association for Parents of the Visually Impaired
P.O. Box 1337
Alamogordo, NM 88310   505-682-2693

4873 Special Education Unit
300 Don Gaspar Avenue
Santa Fe, NM 87501   505-827-6788
Fax: 505-827-6791
e-mail: mlandazuri@sde.state.nm.us
www.nectas.unc.edu

Individuals with Disabilities Education Act requires all states and territories to provide early intervention and preschool special education for children with disabilities and special healthcare needs. Services include central directory, representatives of agencies, service providers, families, and coordinators of infant, toddler, and preschool special education programs.

Maria Landazuri, Preschool Special Ed. Coordinator

4874 Technology Assistance Program
435 St Michael's Drive, Building D
Santa Fe, NM 87505   505-954-8539
800-866-2253
Fax: 505-954-8562
TDD: 800-866-2253
e-mail: nmdvrtap@aol.com

State assisted programs for people of many abilities. Including local chapters, referrals, fun and social interaction and support groups.

New York

4875 Advocacy Center
277 Alexander Street, Suite 500
Rochester, NY 14607   716-546-1700
Fax: 716-546-7069
e-mail: advocacy@frontiernet.net
www.taalliance.org

Parent Training and Information (PTI) programs help parents to: understand their children's specific needs; communicate more effectively with professionals, participate in the educational planning process; and obtain information about relevant programs, services, and resources

4876 Advocates for Children of New York
151 W 30th St. 5th Floor
New York, NY 10001   212-947-9779
Fax: 212-947-9790
e-mail: info@advocatesforchildren.org
www.advocatesforchildren.org

Parent Training and Information (PTI) programs help parents to: understand their children's specific needs; communicate more effectively with professionals, participate in the educational planning process; and obtain information about relevant programs, services, and resources

4877 Early Intervention Program
Corning Tower Rm 208, Empire St Plz
Albany, NY 12237   518-473-7016
Fax: 518-473-8673
e-mail: dmn02@health.state.ny.us
www.nectas.unc.edu

Individuals with Disabilities Education Act requires all states and territories to provide early intervention and preschool special education for children with disabilities and special healthcare needs. Services include central directory, representatives of agencies, service providers, families, and coordinators of infant, toddler, and preschool special education programs.

Donna Noyes, Infant/Toddler Program Coordinator

4878 Friends of Karen
118 Titicus Road P.O. Box 190
Purdys, NY 10578   914-277-4547
800-637-2774

Dedicated to helping terminally and catastrophically ill children and their families in the New York metropolitan area only. They provide assistance with payments for physicians, hospitals and medications, help with extra expenses beyond medical bills, provide home nursing services and equipment, supplies for loans, and offers emotional support.

4879 Marty Lyons Foundation, Inc.
One Penn Plaza, Ste 1824
New York, NY 10119   212-560-9414
877-560-9474
Fax: 212-560-0624
e-mail: mlfhq@earthlink.net
martylyonsfoundation.org

Chapters in New Jersey, New York, Massachussets, Connecticut, Mryland, North Carolina, South Carolina, Georgia, Pennsylvania and Florida provide a special wish to children ages 3 to 17 who are terminally ill or have a chronic life-threatening disease.

300 volunteers

4880 New York Department of Education
1 Commerce Plaza
Albany, NY 12234   518-473-4823
Fax: 518-486-4154
e-mail: mplotzke@mail.nysed.gov
www.nectas.unc.edu

Individuals with Disabilities Education Act requires all states and territories to provide early intervention and preschool special education for children with disabilities and special healthcare needs. Services include central directory, representatives of agencies, service providers, families, and coordinators of infant, toddler, and preschool special education programs.

Michael Plotzker Vesid, Preschool Special Ed. Coordinator

4881 Parent Network Center
250 Delaware Avenue, Suite 3
Buffalo, NY 14202   716-853-1570
                          Fax: 716-853-1574
                          TDD: 716-853-1573
                          www.taalliance.org

Parent Training and Information (PTI) programs help parents to: understand their children's specific needs; communicate more effectively with professionals, participate in the educational planning process; and obtain information about relevant programs, services, and resources

4882 Parent to Parent of New York State
500 Balltown Road
Schenectady, NY 12304   518-381-4350
                               800-305-8817
                          Fax: 518-382-1959
                          e-mail: parent2par@aol.com
                          www.parenttoparentnys.org

Informational and emotional support to parents who have a child, adolescent, or adult family member with special needs.
          1500 Members

Carolyn Schimanski, Executive Director

4883 Resources for Children with Special Needs
200 Park Avenue S., Suite 816
New York City, NY 10003   212-667-4650
                            Fax: 212-254-4070
                          e-mail: resourcenyc@prodigy.net
                          www.epsty.com/resourcenyc

Parent Training and Information (PTI) programs help parents to: understand their children's specific needs; communicate more effectively with professionals, participate in the educational planning process; and obtain information about relevant programs, services, and resources

4884 Sinergia/Metropolitan Parent Center
15 W 65th Street, 6th Floor
New York, NY 10023   212-496-1300
                          Fax: 212-496-5608
                          e-mail: Sinergia@panix.com
                          www.panic.com/~sinergia

Parent Training and Information (PTI) programs help parents to: understand their children's specific needs; communicate more effectively with professionals, participate in the educational planning process; and obtain information about relevant programs, services, and resources

4885 St. Mary's Healthcare System for Children
c/o Rhonda Broden
29-01 216th Street
Bayside, NY 11360   718-281-8750
                          Fax: 718-281-8773
                          www.stmaryskids.org

Information and advocacy resources for families and professionals. Includes listings of organizations providing general information and organizations focusing on more specific areas of concern to families and young adults who have disabilities.

4886 TRIAD Project Advocates for Persons with Disabilities
One Empire State Plaza, Suite 1001
Albany, NY 12223   518-474-2825
                          800-522-4369
                          Fax: 518-473-6005
                          TTY: 518-473-4231
                          e-mail: leffingw@emi.com

State assisted programs and support group information for people of many abilities. Including local chapters, referrals, fun and social interaction and support groups.

4887 Ulster County Social Services
7 Cicero Avenue
New Paltz, NY 12561   914-255-1713
                          Fax: 914-255-3202
                          www.nectas.unc.edu

Individuals with Disabilities Education Act requires all states and territories to provide early intervention and preschool special education for children with disabilities and special healthcare needs. Services include central directory, representatives of agencies, service providers, families, and coordinators of infant, toddler, and preschool special education programs.

Thomas Roach, Interagency Coordinating Council

North Carolina

4888 Assistive Technology Project, Human Resources, Voc. and Rehab. Services
1110 Navaho Drive, Suite 101
Raleigh, NC 27609   919-850-2787
                                       800-852-0042
                                Fax: 919-850-2792
                                TTY: 919-850-2787
                    e-mail: rickic@mindspring.com
                        www.mindspring.com/ncatp

State assisted programs and support group information for people of many abilities. Including local chapters, referrals, fun and social interaction and support groups.

4889 ECAC, Inc.
P.O. Box 16
Davidson, NC 28036   704-892-1321
                                Fax: 704-892-5028
                           e-mail: ECAC1@aol.com
                                www.taalliance.org

Parent Training and Information (PTI) programs help parents to: understand their children's specific needs; communicate more effectively with professionals, participate in the educational planning process; and obtain information about relevant programs, services, and resources

4890 Exceptional Children Division
301 North Wilmington Street
Raleigh, NC 27601   919-715-1598
                                Fax: 919-715-1569
                       e-mail: kbaars@state.nc.us
                                www.nectas.unc.edu

Individuals with Disabilities Education Act requires all states and territories to provide early intervention and preschool special education for children with disabilities and special healthcare needs. Services include central directory, representatives of agencies, service providers, families, and coordinators of infant, toddler, and preschool special education programs.

Kathy Baars, Preschool Special Ed. Coordinator

4891 Family Support Network of North Carolina
CB # 7340
Chase Hall, University of North Carolina
Chapel Hill, NC 27599   919-966-2841
                                       800-852-0042
                                Fax: 919-966-2916
                           e-mail: cdr@med.unc.edu

Family Support Network Carolina serves families of children with developmental disablties, behavorial disorders, and chronic illness and the professionals who serve these families. Information about special needs, North Carolina services and angencies, state and national organizations, support groups, and refferals. Twenty community based programs provide emotional and informational support for the families. Makes referrals for those planning early childhood and early intervention activities.

Mary Tippens, Resource/Referral Director
Karen LeClain, Parent to Parent Director

4892 Partnerships for Inclusion
2415 West Vernon Avenue
Kinston, NC 28501   919-559-5156
                    e-mail: msteele@greenvillenc.com
                                www.nectas.unc.edu

Individuals with Disabilities Education Act requires all states and territories to provide early intervention and preschool special education for children with disabilities and special healthcare needs. Services include central directory, representatives of agencies, service providers, families, and coordinators of infant, toddler, and preschool special education programs.

Sandy Steele, Interagency Coordinating Council

4893 Rockingham County Schools
511 Harrington Highway
Eden, NC 27288   336-627-2615
                                Fax: 336-627-2615
                    e-mail: speele@greenvillenc.com
                                www.nectas.unc.edu

Individuals with Disabilities Education Act requires all states and territories to provide early intervention and preschool special education for children with disabilities and special healthcare needs. Services include central directory, representatives of agencies, service providers, families, and coordinators of infant, toddler, and preschool special education programs.

Susan Peele, Interagency Coordinating Council

North Dakota

4894 Developmental Disabilities Unit
600 South 2nd Street, Suite 1A
Bismarck, ND 58504   701-328-8936
                                Fax: 701-328-8969
                       e-mail: sobald@state.nd.us
                                www.nectas.unc.edu

Individuals with Disabilities Education Act requires all states and territories to provide early intervention and preschool special education for children with disabilities and special healthcare needs. Services include central directory, representatives of agencies, service providers, families, and coordinators of infant, toddler, and preschool special education programs.

Debra Balsdon, Infant/Toddler Program Coor.

4895 Interagency Program Assistive Technology
P.O. Box 743
Cavalier, ND 58220   701-265-4807
                                      Fax: 701-265-3150
                                      TDD: 701-265-4807
                          e-mail: lee@pioneer.state.nd.us
                                      www.ndipat.org

State assisted programs and support group information for people of many abilities. Including local chapters, referrals, fun and social interaction and support groups.

4896 Native American Family Network System
Arrowhead Shopping Center
1600 Second Avenue SW
Minot, ND 58701   701-837-7500
                                      Fax: 701-837-7541
                                      TTY: 701-837-7501
                      e-mail: ndpath01@minot.ndak.net
                                www.ndcd.org/pathfinder

Parent Training and Information (PTI) programs help parents to: understand their children's specific needs; communicate more effectively with professionals, participate in the educational planning process; and obtain information about relevant programs, services, and resources

4897 Special Education Division
600 East Blvd
Bismarck, ND 58505   701-328-2277
                                      Fax: 701-328-2461
                                      www.nectas.unc.edu

Individuals with Disabilities Education Act requires all states and territories to provide early intervention and preschool special education for children with disabilities and special healthcare needs. Services include central directory, representatives of agencies, service providers, families, and coordinators of infant, toddler, and preschool special education programs.

Brenda Oas, Preschool Special Ed. Coordinator
Jeanette Kolberg, Preschool Special Ed. Coordinator

Ohio

4898 Bureau of EI Services
P.O. Box 118
Columbus, OH 43266   614-644-8389
                                      Fax: 614-728-9163
                      e-mail: coser@gw.odh.state.oh.us
                                      www.nectas.unc.edu

Individuals with Disabilities Education Act requires all states and territories to provide early intervention and preschool special education for children with disabilities and special healthcare needs. Services include central directory, representatives of agencies, service providers, families, and coordinators of infant, toddler, and preschool special education programs.

Cindy Oser, Infant/Toddler Program Coordinator

4899 Celebrating Families of Children & Adults with
Special Needs
16 Vassar Drive
Dayton, OH 45406   937-275-0990
                                      Fax: 937-275-0277
                          e-mail: families@erinet.com

Informational and emotional support to parents who have a child, adolescent, or adult family member with special needs.

4900 Child Advocacy Center
1821 Summit Road, Suite 110
Cincinnati, OH 45237   513-821-2400
                                      Fax: 513-821-2442
                                      TDD: 513-821-2400
                          e-mail: CADCCenter@aol.com
                                      www.taalliance.org

Parent Training and Information (PTI) programs help parents to: understand their children's specific needs; communicate more effectively with professionals, participate in the educational planning process; and obtain information about relevant programs, services, and resources

4901 Division of Early Childhood Education
65 South Front Street, Room 309
Columbus, OH 43215   614-466-0224
                                      Fax: 614-728-2338
                                      www.nectas.unc.edu

Individuals with Disabilities Education Act requires all states and territories to provide early intervention and preschool special education for children with disabilities and special healthcare needs. Services include central directory, representatives of agencies, service providers, families, and coordinators of infant, toddler, and preschool special education programs.

Jane Wiechel, Preschool Special Ed. Coordinator

4902 East Central Regional Office
170 West High Avenue
New Philadelphia, OH 44663   330-364-5567
                                   Fax: 330-343-3038
                e-mail: ECE_Greer@ode.ohio.gov@inet
                                   www.nectas.unc.edu

Individuals with Disabilities Education Act requires all states and territories to provide early intervention and preschool special education for children with disabilities and special healthcare needs. Services include central directory, representatives of agencies, service providers, families, and coordinators of infant, toddler, and preschool special education programs.

Edith Greer, Preschool Special Ed. Coordinator

4903 Family Information Network
143 Northwest Avenue, Building A
Tallmadge, OH 44278   330-633-2055
                                  Fax: 330-633-2658

Informational and emotional support to parents who have a child, adolescent, or adult family member with special needs.

4904 Miami Valley Downs Syndrome Association
1444 Beaver Creek Lane
Kettering, OH 45429
                                  Fax: 937-643-1241

Informational and emotional support to parents who have a child, adolescent, or adult family member with special needs.

4905 OCECD
165 W Center Street, Suite 302
Marion, OH 43302   614-382-5452
                                  Fax: 614-383-6421
                                  TDD: 614-382-5452
                        e-mail: ocecd@edu.gte.net
          www.taalliance.org/PTIs/regohio.text.htm

Parent Training and Information (PTI) programs help parents to: understand their children's specific needs; communicate more effectively with professionals, participate in the educational planning process; and obtain information about relevant programs, services, and resources

4906 Ohio Protection and Advocacy Organization
5350 Brookpark Avenue
Cleveland, OH 44134   216-398-5501
                                  800-672-1220
                                  Fax: 216-398-5505

Informational and emotional support to parents who have a child, adolescent, or adult family member with special needs.

4907 Operation Liftoff of Ohio
P.O. Box 1094
Gallipolis, OH 45631

Fulfills a dream for children in Ohio and surrounding states who have a life-threatening illness.

4908 Society for Rehabilitation
9521 Lake Shore Blvd
Mentorck, OH 44060   440-352-8993
                                 Fax: 440-352-6632
               e-mail: society@buckeyeweb.com
                                 www.nectas.unc.edu

Individuals with Disabilities Education Act requires all states and territories to provide early intervention and preschool special education for children with disabilities and special healthcare needs. Services include central directory, representatives of agencies, service providers, families, and coordinators of infant, toddler, and preschool special education programs.

Ann Dietrich, Interagency Coordinating Council

4909 Train Ohio Super Computer Center
1224 Kinnear Road
Columbus, OH 43212   614-292-2426
                                 Fax: 614-292-5866
                                 TDD: 614-292-2426
                                 www.train.state.oh.us

State assisted programs and support group information for people of many abilities. Including local chapters, referrals, fun and social interaction and support groups.

Oklahoma

4910 Oklahoma ABLE Tech Wellness Center
1514 W Hall of Fame
Stillwater, OK 74078   405-744-9748
                                 800-257-1705
                                 Fax: 405-744-7670
                                 TTY: 800-257-1705
               e-mail: mljwell@okway.okstate.edu
             www.okstate.edu/wellness/athome.htm

State assisted programs and support group information for people of many abilities. Including local chapters, referrals, fun and social interaction and support groups.

4911 Parents Reaching Out in Oklahoma
1917 S. Harvard Avenue
Oklahoma City, OK 73128   405-681-9710
                                 Fax: 405-685-4006
                                 TDD: 405-681-9710
                        e-mail: prook@aol.com
                        www.ucp.org/probase.htm

Parent Training and Information (PTI) programs help parents to: understand their children's specific needs; communicate more effectively with professionals, participate in the educational planning process; and obtain information about relevant programs, services, and resources

4912 Special Education Office
2500 North Lincoln Blvd
Oklahoma City, OK 73105   405-521-4880
Fax: 405-521-6205
e-mail: mark_sharp@mail.sde.state.ok.us
www.nectas.unc.edu

Individuals with Disabilities Education Act requires all states and territories to provide early intervention and preschool special education for children with disabilities and special healthcare needs. Services include central directory, representatives of agencies, service providers, families, and coordinators of infant, toddler, and preschool special education programs.

Mark Sharp, Infant/Toddler Program Coordinator

Oregon

4913 Early Childhood CARES Program
1895 East 15th Avenue
Eugene, OR 97403   541-346-2639
Fax: 541-346-2636
e-mail: Judy_Newman@ccmail.uoregon.edu
www.nectas.unc.edu

Individuals with Disabilities Education Act requires all states and territories to provide early intervention and preschool special education for children with disabilities and special healthcare needs. Services include central directory, representatives of agencies, service providers, families, and coordinators of infant, toddler, and preschool special education programs.

Judy Newman, Interagency Coordinating Council

4914 Early Intervention Programs
255 Capitol Street NE
Salem, OR 97301   503-378-3598
Fax: 503-373-7968
e-mail: jane.mulholland@odeexl.ode.state.or.us
www.nectas.unc.edu

Individuals with Disabilities Education Act requires all states and territories to provide early intervention and preschool special education for children with disabilities and special healthcare needs. Services include central directory, representatives of agencies, service providers, families, and coordinators of infant, toddler, and preschool special education programs.

Jane Mulholland, Infant/Toddler Program Coor.

4915 Oregon Cope Project
999 Locust Street NE
Salem, OR 97303   503-581-8156
888-505-2673
Fax: 503-391-0429
e-mail: orcope@open.org
www.open.org/orcope

Informational and emotional support to parents who have a child, adolescent, or adult family member with special needs.

4916 Special Education Programs
255 Capitol Street NE
Salem, OR 97301   503-378-3598
Fax: 503-373-7968
e-mail: nancy.johnson-dorn@state.or.us
www.nectas.unc.edu

Provides early intervention and preschool special education for children with disabilities and special healthcare needs. Services include central directory, representatives of agencies, service providers, families, and coordinators of infant, toddler, and preschool special education programs.

Nancy Johnson-Dorn, Preschool Special Ed. Coor.

4917 Technology Access for Life Needs Project
1257 Ferry Street, SE
Salem, OR 97310   503-361-1201
Fax: 503-378-3599
TDD: 503-361-1201
e-mail: ati@orednet.org

State assisted programs and support group information for people of many abilities. Including local chapters, referrals, fun and social interaction and support groups.

Pennsylvania

4918 Bureau of Special Education
333 Market Street, 7th Floor
Harrisburg, PA 17126   717-783-6882
                              800-874-2301
                         Fax: 717-783-6139
                         TDD: 717-787-7367
                    e-mail: ebeck@state.pa.us
                            rprice@state.pa.us

Services include central directory, representatives of agencies, service providers, families, and coordinators of infant, toddler, and preschool special education programs.

Esther Beck, Educational Supervisor
Rick Price, Division Chief

4919 Division of Early Intervention Services
P.O. Box 2675
Harrisburg, PA 17105   717-783-8302
                         Fax: 717-772-0012
                    e-mail: jackiee@dpw.state.pa.us
                            www.nectas.unc.edu

Individuals with Disabilities Education Act requires all states and territories to provide early intervention and preschool special education for children with disabilities and special healthcare needs. Services include central directory, representatives of agencies, service providers, families, and coordinators of infant, toddler, and preschool special education programs.

Jacqueline Epstein, Infant/Toddler Program Coor.

4920 Montgomery County Intermediate Unit #23
1605 B West Main Street
Norristown, PA 19403   610-539-8550
                         Fax: 610-539-5973
                            www.nectas.unc.edu

Services include central directory, representatives of agencies, service providers, families, and coordinators of infant, toddler, and preschool special education programs.

Dennis Harkin, Interagency Coordinating Council

4921 Parent Education Network
2107 Industrial Highway
York, PA 17402   717-600-0100
                   Fax: 717-600-8101
                   TDD: 717-845-9722
              e-mail: pen@parentednet.org
                   www.homepagecreations.com/pen/

Parent Training and Information (PTI) programs help parents to: understand their children's specific needs; communicate more effectively with professionals, participate in the educational planning process; and obtain information about relevant programs, services, and resources

4922 Parent to Parent ARC Allegheny
711 Bingham Street
Pittsburgh, PA 15203   412-995-5001
                    e-mail: ptparc@arcallegheny.org
                            www.arallegheny.org

Informational and emotional support to parents who have a child, adolescent, or adult family member with special needs.

4923 Parent to Parent of Pennsylvania
150 S Progress Avenue
Harrisburg, PA 17109   717-540-4722
                         Fax: 717-540-7603
                    e-mail: brill134@cdc.gov
                            www.nauticom.net/www/eita

Informational and emotional support to parents who have a child, adolescent, or adult family member with special needs.

4924 Parents Union for Public Schools
311 S Juniper Street, Suite 200
Philadelphia, PA 19107   215-546-1166
                           Fax: 215-731-1688
                      e-mail: Parents@aol.com
                              www.taalliance.org

Parent Training and Information (PTI) programs help parents to: understand their children's specific needs; communicate more effectively with professionals, participate in the educational planning process; and obtain information about relevant programs, services, and resources

4925 Pennsylvania's Initiative on Assistive Technology, Institute on Disabilities
University Affliated Program
423 Ritter Annex, Temple University
Philadelphia, PA 19122   215-204-5966
                                800-204-7428
                           Fax: 215-204-9371
                           TTY: 800-750-7428
                      e-mail: piat@astro.temple.edu
                              www.temple.edu/inst_disabilities

Pennsylvania's Initiative on Assistive Technology (PIAT) is the Commonwealth's) program under the Assistive Technology Act of 1998. Most of PAIT's activities are free to Pennsylvania residents, and are focused on the provision of public awareness of the benefit and scope of assistive technology (AT), information and referral, advocacy and funding, and training. PAIT is the state's contractor for the implementation of Pennsylvania's Assistive Technology Lending library.

4926 US Wheelchair Weightlifting Association
39 Michael Place
Levittown, PA 19057   215-945-1964
                         Fax: 215-946-2574

State assisted programs and support group information for people of many abilities. Including local chapters, referrals, fun and social interaction and support groups.

Rhode Island

4927 Assistive Technology Access Partnership
40 Fountain Street
Providence, RI 02903   401-421-7005
                         Fax: 401-421-9259
                         TTY: 401-421-7016
                         e-mail: reginac@ors.state.ri.us
                         www.atap.state.ri.us

State assisted programs and support group information for people of many abilities. Including local chapters, referrals, fun and social interaction and support groups.

4928 Central Region Early Intervention Program
J. Arthur Trudeau Memorial Center
250 Commonwealth Avenue
Warwick, RI 02886   401-823-1731
                       Fax: 401-823-1849

Informational and emotional support to parents who have a child, adolescent, or adult family member with special needs.

4929 Office Intergrated Social Services
255 Westminister Road
Providence, RI 02903   401-222-4600
                         Fax: 401-222-4979
                         e-mail: abcohen@ride.ri.net
                         www.nectas.unc.edu

Individuals with Disabilities Education Act requires all states and territories to provide early intervention and preschool special education for children with disabilities and special healthcare needs. Services include central directory, representatives of agencies, service providers, families, and coordinators of infant, toddler, and preschool special education programs.

Amy Cohen, Preschool Special Ed. Coordinator

4930 Rhode Island Arc
99 Bald Hill Road
Cranston, RI 02920   401-463-9191
                        Fax: 401-463-9244
                        www.nectas.unc.edu

Individuals with Disabilities Education Act requires all states and territories to provide early intervention and preschool special education for children with disabilities and special healthcare needs. Services include central directory, representatives of agencies, service providers, families, and coordinators of infant, toddler, and preschool special education programs.

James Healey, Interagency Coordinating Council

4931 Rhode Island Department of Health
3 Capitol Hill, Room 302
Providence, RI 02908   401-277-1185
                         www.nectas.unc.edu

Individuals with Disabilities Education Act requires all states and territories to provide early intervention and preschool special education for children with disabilities and special healthcare needs. Services include central directory, representatives of agencies, service providers, families, and coordinators of infant, toddler, and preschool special education programs.

Ron Caldarone, Infant/Toddler Program Coor.

4932 Rhode Island Parent Information Network
500 Prospect Street
Pawtucket, RI 02860   401-727-4144
                         800-464-3399
                         Fax: 401-727-4040

Informational and emotional support to parents who have a child, adolescent, or adult family member with special needs.

South Carolina

4933 Assistive Technology Project
Center for Developmental Disabilities
USC School of Medicine
Columbia, SC 29208

Fax: 803-935-5342
TDD: 803-935-5263
e-mail: scatp@scsn.net
www.scsn.net/users/scatp

State assisted programs and support group information for people of many abilities. Including local chapters, referrals, fun and social interaction and support groups.

4934 BabyNet
Robert Mills Complex, Box 101106
Columbia, SC 29201   803-647-5999
Fax: 803-734-4459
e-mail: hartkf@columbia63.dhec.state.sc.us
www.nectas.unc.edu

Individuals with Disabilities Education Act requires all states and territories to provide early intervention and preschool special education for children with disabilities and special healthcare needs. Services include central directory, representatives of agencies, service providers, families, and coordinators of infant, toddler, and preschool special education programs.

Kathy Hart, Infant/Toddler Program Coordinator

4935 PRO-Parents
2712 Middleburg Drive, Suite 102
Columbia, SC 29204   803-779-3859
800-759-4776
Fax: 803-252-4513
e-mail: pro-parents@aol.com
www.taalliance.org

Parent Training and Information (PTI) programs help parents to: understand their children's specific needs; communicate more effectively with professionals, participate in the educational planning process; and obtain information about relevant programs, services, and resources

3500 Members

4936 Programs for Exceptional Children
1429 Senate Street
Columbia, SC 29201   803-734-8811
Fax: 803-734-4824
e-mail: njenkins@sde.state.sc.us
www.nectas.unc.edu

Individuals with Disabilities Education Act requires all states and territories to provide early intervention and preschool special education for children with disabilities and special healthcare needs. Services include central directory, representatives of agencies, service providers, families, and coordinators of infant, toddler, and preschool special education programs.

Norma Donaldson-Jenkins, Preschool Special Ed. Coordinator

South Dakota

4937 DakotaLink
1925 Plaza Blvd.
Rapid City, SD 57702

605-394-1876
Fax: 605-394-5315
TTY: 800-645-0673
e-mail: rreed@sdtie.sdserv.org
www.tie.net/dakotalink

State assisted programs and support group information for people of many abilities. Including local chapters, referrals, fun and social interaction and support groups.

4938 Office of Special Education
700 Governors Drive
Peirre, SD 57501   605-773-4478
Fax: 605-773-6846
e-mail: barbh@deca.state.sd.us
www.nectas.unc.edu

Individuals with Disabilities Education Act requires all states and territories to provide early intervention and preschool special education for children with disabilities and special healthcare needs. Services include central directory, representatives of agencies, service providers, families, and coordinators of infant, toddler, and preschool special education programs.

Barb Hemmelman, Infant/Toddler Program Coor.

4939 South Dakota Parent Connection
3701 W. 49th, Suite 2008
Souix Falls, SD 57106   605-361-3171
Fax: 605-361-2928
e-mail: bschreck@dakota.net
www.taalliance.org

Parent Training and Information (PTI) programs help parents to: understand their children's specific needs; communicate more effectively with professionals, participate in the educational planning process; and obtain information about relevant programs, services, and resources

4940 University Affiliated Program, School of Medicine
414 East Clark Street
Vermillion, SD 57069   605-677-5311
                             Fax: 605-677-6274
                   e-mail: jwounded@used.edu
                          www.nectas.unc.edu

Individuals with Disabilities Education Act requires all states and territories to provide early intervention and preschool special education for children with disabilities and special healthcare needs. Services include central directory, representatives of agencies, service providers, families, and coordinators of infant, toddler, and preschool special education programs.

Joanne Wounded Head, Interagency Coordinating Council

Tennessee

4941 Center for Early Childhood
E Tennessee State University Box 70434
Johnson City, TN 37614   423-439-7555
                               Fax: 423-439-7561
                                 child.etsu.edu

Individuals with Disabilities Education Act requires all states and territories to provide early intervention and preschool special education for children with disabilities and special healthcare needs. Services include central directory, representatives of agencies, service providers, families, and coordinators of infant, toddler, and preschool special education programs.

Wesley Brown, Interagency Coordinating Council

4942 Office of Special Education, State Department of Education
710 James Robertson Parkway
Nashville, TN 37243   615-532-6319
                            Fax: 615-532-9412
                e-mail: dmattraw@mail.state.tn.us
                          www.nectas.unc.edu

Individuals with Disabilities Education Act requires all states and territories to provide early intervention and preschool special education for children with disabilities and special healthcare needs. Services include central directory, representatives of agencies, service providers, families, and coordinators of infant, toddler, and preschool special education programs.

Doris Mattraw, Preschool Special Ed. Coordinator

4943 Office of Special Education, State Dept of Education
National Early Childhood Technical Assistance Ctr
710 James Robertson Parkway
Nashville, TN 37243   615-741-3537
                            Fax: 615-532-9412
              e-mail: bbledsoe@mail.state.tn.us
                          www.nectas.unc.edu

Individuals with Disabilities Education Act requires all states and territories to provide early intervention and preschool special education for children with disabilities and special healthcare needs. Services include central directory, representatives of agencies, service providers, families, and coordinators of infant, toddler, and preschool special education programs.

Brenda Bledsoe, Infant/Toddler Program Coor.

4944 STEP
424 E Bernard Avenue, Suite 3
Greenvilles, TN 37745   423-639-0125
                              Fax: 423-636-8217
                              TDD: 423-636-8217
                       e-mail: tnstep@aol.com
                           www.taalliance.org

Parent Training and Information (PTI) programs help parents to: understand their children's specific needs; communicate more effectively with professionals, participate in the educational planning process; and obtain information about relevant programs, services, and resources

4945 Technology Access Center of Middle Tennessee
2222 Metrocenter Boulevard, Suite 126
Nashville, TN 37228
                              Fax: 423-947-2194
                              TTY: 615-248-6733
                    e-mail: tactn@nashville.com

Technology group of parents, consumers and professionals; provides resources to help children and adults who have disabilities gain access to the benefits of technology. Includes nationwide network of community-based assistive technology, resource centers, hands on consultants and product demonstrations.

Texas

4946 Grassroads Consortium
6202 Belmark, PO Box 61628
Houston, TX 77208   713-643-9576
                          Fax: 713-643-6291
                 e-mail: SpecKids@aol.com
                     www.taalliance.org

Parent Training and Information (PTI) programs help parents to: understand their children's specific needs; communicate more effectively with professionals, participate in the educational planning process; and obtain information about relevant programs, services, and resources

4947 Office of the Dean, University of Texas at Austin
College of Education; EBB 210
Austin, TX 78712   512-471-7255
Fax: 512-471-0846
www.nectas.unc.edu

Individuals with Disabilities Education Act requires all states and territories to provide early intervention and preschool special education for children with disabilities and special healthcare needs. Services include central directory, representatives of agencies, service providers, families, and coordinators of infant, toddler, and preschool special education programs.

Alba Ortiz, Interagency Coordinating Council

4948 Parent Case Management
4601 Hartford
Abilene, TX 79605   915-793-3500
Fax: 915-793-3549

Support network for parents of children with disabilities and/or chronic illness. Veteran parents offer support to parents who are just learning of their child's diagnosis. Offers support and insight into parenting a child with special needs, as well as referrals to trained veteran parents.

4949 Partners Resource Network
1090 Longfellow Drive, Suite B
Beaumont, TX 77706   409-898-4684
800-866-4726
Fax: 409-898-4869
TTY: 409-898-4816
e-mail: TXPRN@juno.com

Support network for parents of children with disabilities and/or chronic illness. Veteran parents offer support to parents who are just learning of their child's diagnosis. Offers support and insight into parenting a child with special needs, as well as referrals to trained veteran parents.

4950 Project PODER
1017 N. Main Avenue, Suite 207
San Antonio, TX 78212   210-222-2637
Fax: 210-222-2638
e-mail: poder@world-net.com
www.taalliance.org

Parent Training and Information (PTI) programs help parents to: understand their children's specific needs; communicate more effectively with professionals, participate in the educational planning process; and obtain information about relevant programs, services, and resources

4951 South Central Region Helen Keller National Center
4230 LBJ Freeway, LB#31, #340
Dallas, TX 75244   972-490-9677
Fax: 972-490-6054
TTY: 972-490-9677
e-mail: ccfutbol@aol.com

A residential program providing initial assessment, comprehensive evaluation, and rehabilitation for deaf-blind; provides training for workers in services in the field; maintains National Register of Deaf-Blind Persons; provides community education programs; provides technical assistance and training in transition of deaf-blind; maintains a National Parent Network and parent newsletter.

C.C. Davis, Regional Representative

4952 Special Education Programs
1701 North Congress Avenue
Austin, TX 78701   512-463-9414
Fax: 512-463-4934
e-mail: kclayton@tmail.tea.state.tx.us
www.nectas.unc.edu

Early intervention and preschool special education for children with disabilities and special healthcare needs. Services include central directory, representatives of agencies, service providers, families, and coordinators of infant, toddler, and preschool special education programs.

Kathy Clayton, Preschool Special Ed. Coordinator

4953 Texas Assistive Technology Partnership
Texas University Affiliated Program
SZ8252-D5100
Austin, TX 78712   512-471-7621
800-828-7839
Fax: 512-471-7549
TTY: 512-471-1844
e-mail: s.elrod@mail.utexas.edu
www.edb.utexas.edu/coe/depts/sped/tatp/

State assisted programs and support group information for people of many abilities. Including local chapters, referrals, fun and social interaction and support groups.

4954 Texas Interagency Council on Early Childhood Intervention
4900 North Lamar
Austin, TX 78751   512-424-6754
                              Fax: 512-424-6749
              e-mail: mary.edler@eci.state.tx.us
                         www.eci.state.tx.us

Individuals with Disabilities Education Act part C requires all states and territories to provide early intervention to infants and toddlers with disabilities. Services include a full array of infant intervention fields and disciplines.

Mary Elder, Executive Director
Donna Samuelson, Deputy Executive Director

4955 Wish with Wings, Inc.
P.O. Box 3479

                                  817-469-9474
                              Fax: 817-275-6005

Serves children living in or being treated in Texas. Grants wishes for children 3 to 16 with life-threatening diseases.

Pat Skaggs
Kim Clark

Utah

4956 Computer Center for Citizens with Disabilities
C/O UT Center for Assistive Technology
2056 S 1100 E
Salt Lake City, UT 84106   801-485-8675
                              Fax: 801-485-9152
              e-mail: cboogaar@usoe.k12.ut.us

Technology group of parents, consumers and professionals; provides resources to help children and adults who have disabilities gain access to the benefits of technology. Includes nationwide network of community-based assistive technology, resource centers, hands on consultants and product demonstrations.

4957 Early Intervention Program
P.O. Box 144720
Salt Lake City, UT 84114   801-584-8226
                              Fax: 801-584-8496
              e-mail: dsaunder@doh.state.ut.us
                         www.nectas.unc.edu

Individuals with Disabilities Education Act requires all states and territories to provide early intervention and preschool special education for children with disabilities and special healthcare needs. Services include central directory, representatives of agencies, service providers, families, and coordinators of infant, toddler, and preschool special education programs.

Darla Saunders, Infant/Toddler Program Coor.

4958 Special Education Services Unit
250 East 500 South
Salt Lake City, UT 84111   801-538-7708
                              Fax: 801-538-7991
              e-mail: Brenda.Broadbent@usoe.k12.ut.us
                         www.nectas.unc.edu

Individuals with Disabilities Education Act requires all states and territories to provide early intervention and preschool special education for children with disabilities and special healthcare needs. Services include central directory, representatives of agencies, service providers, families, and coordinators of infant, toddler, and preschool special education programs.

Brenda Broadbent, Preschool Special Ed. Coor.

4959 US Disabled Ski Team
Box 100
Park City, UT 84060   435-649-9090
                              Fax: 435-649-3613
                         e-mail: info@usaa.org

State assisted programs and support group information for people of many abilities. Including local chapters, referrals, fun and social interaction and support groups.

4960 Utah Center for Assistive Technology
Center for Persons with Disabilities
UMC 6855
Logan, UT 84322   801-797-3824
                              Fax: 801-797-2355
                              TDD: 801-797-2096
                 e-mail: sharon@cpo2.usu.edu

State assisted programs and support group information for people of many abilities. Including local chapters, referrals, fun and social interaction and support groups.

4961 Utah Parent Center
2290 E. 4500 S, Suite 110
Salt Lake City, UT 84117   801-272-1051
                                  800-468-1160
                              Fax: 801-272-8907
                 e-mail: upc@inconnect.com
                         www.parentcenter.org

Parent Training and Information (PTI) programs help parents to: understand their children's specific needs; communicate more effectively with professionals, participate in the educational planning process; and obtain information about relevant programs, services, and resources. Offers free written materials, workshops, individual consultations, newsletter, statewide volunteer network, parent to parent support.

Helen Post, Director

Vermont

4962 Assistive Technology Project
103 S Main Street
Weeks Building, First Floor
Waterbury, VT 05671

Fax: 802-241-2174
TTY: 802-241-2620
TDD: 801-797-2096
e-mail: lynnec@dad.state.vt.us
www.uvm.edu/uapvt/cats.html

State assisted programs and support group information for people of many abilities. Including local chapters, referrals, fun and social interaction and support groups.

4963 Center on Disabilities and Community Inclusion
5 Burlington Sq. Suite 450
Burlington, VT 05401
802-656-4031
Fax: 802-656-1357
e-mail: wfox@zoo.uvm.edu
www.nectas.unc.edu

Services include central directory, representatives of agencies, service providers, families, and coordinators of infant, toddler, and preschool special education programs.

Wayne L. Fox, Interagency Coordinating Council

4964 Family, Infant, and Toddler Project
P.O. Box 70
Burlington, VT 05402
802-651-1786
Fax: 802-863-7635
e-mail: bmccar@vdh.state.vt.us
www.nectas.unc.edu

Individuals with Disabilities Education Act requires all states and territories to provide early intervention and preschool special education for children with disabilities and special healthcare needs. Services include central directory, representatives of agencies, service providers, families, and coordinators of infant, toddler, and preschool special education programs.

Beverly MacCarty, Infant/Toddler Program Coordinator

4965 Special Education Unit
120 State Street
Montpelier, VT 05620
802-828-5115
Fax: 802-828-3140
e-mail: kandrews@doe.state.vt.us
www.nectas.unc.edu

Individuals with Disabilities Education Act requires all states and territories to provide early intervention and preschool special education for children with disabilities and special healthcare needs. Services include central directory, representatives of agencies, service providers, families, and coordinators of infant, toddler, and preschool special education programs.

Kathy Andrews, Preschool Special Ed. Coordinator

4966 Vermont Parent Information Center
1 Mill Street, Suite A7
Burlington, VT 05401
802-658-5315
800-639-7170
Fax: 802-658-5395
TDD: 802-658-5315
e-mail: vpic@together.net
www.vtpie.com

Parent Training and Information (PTI) programs help parents to: understand their children's specific needs; communicate more effectively with professionals, participate in the educational planning process; and obtain information about relevant programs, services, and resources

Virginia

4967 Assistive Technology System
8004 Franklin Farms Drive
P.O. Box K300
Richmond, VA 23288

Fax: 804-662-9478
TTY: 757-662-9990
e-mail: vatskhk@aol.com

State assisted programs and support group information for people of many abilities. Including local chapters, referrals, fun and social interaction and support groups.

4968 Infant & Toddler Program
P.O. Box 1797
Richmond, VA 23218　　　　804-371-6592
Fax: 804-371-7959
e-mail: alucas@dmhmrsas.state.va.us
www.nectas.unc.edu

Provides early intervention and preschool special education for children with disabilities and special healthcare needs. Services include central directory, representatives of agencies, service providers, families, and coordinators of infant, toddler, and preschool special education programs.

Anne Lucas, Infant/Toddler Program Coordinator

4969 Office of Special Education, State Dept of Education
P.O. Box 2120
Richmond, VA 23218　　　　804-225-2402
Fax: 804-371-8796
e-mail: lbradfor@mail.vak12ed.edu
www.pen.k12.va.us

Individuals with Disabilities Education Act requires all states and territories to provide early intervention and preschool special education for children with disabilities and special healthcare needs. Services include central directory, representatives of agencies and coordinators preschool special education programs.

Linda Bradford, Preschool Special Ed. Coordinator

4970 Parent Education Advocacy Training Center
6320 Augusta Dr. Suite 1200
Springfield, VA 22150　　　　703-923-0010
Fax: 703-923-0030
TDD: 703-923-0030
e-mail: partners@peatc.org
www.peatc.org

Parent Training and Information (PTI) programs help parents to: understand their children's specific needs; communicate more effectively with professionals, participate in the educational planning process; and obtain information about relevant programs, services, and resources

4971 Tidewater Center for Technology Access
960 Windsor Oaks Boulevard
Virginia Beach, VA 23462　　　　757-474-8650
Fax: 757-474-8660
e-mail: tcta@aol.com.vi
www.tcta.ataccess.org

Technology group of parents, consumers and professionals; provides resources to help children and adults who have disabilities gain access to the benefits of technology. Includes nationwide network of community-based assistive technology, resource centers, hands on consultants and product demonstrations.

Washington

4972 Assistive Technology Alliance DSHS/DVR
AT Resource Center, University of Washington
P.O. Box 357920
Seattle, WA 98195　　　　206-685-4181
Fax: 206-543-4779
TDD: 206-616-1396
e-mail: uwat@u.washington.edu
www.wata.org

State assisted programs and support group information for people of many abilities. Including local chapters, referrals, fun and social interaction and support groups.

4973 Infant Toddler Early Intervention Program
P.O. Box 45201
Olympia, WA 98504　　　　360-902-8464
Fax: 360-902-7864
e-mail: LoercSK@dshs.wa.govt
www.nectas.unc.edu

Early intervention and preschool special education for children with disabilities and special healthcare needs. Services include central directory, representatives of agencies, service providers, families, and coordinators of infant, toddler, and preschool special education programs.

Sandy Loerch, Infant/Toddler Program Coordinator

4974 Northwestern Region Helen Keller National Center
2366 Eastlake Avenue E., #209
Seattle, WA 98102　　　　206-324-9120

4975 Office of the Superintendent of Public Instruction
P.O. Box 47200
Olympia, WA 98504　　　　360-753-0317
Fax: 360-586-0247
e-mail: ashureen@inspire.ospi.wednet.edu
www.nectas.unc.edu

Services include central directory, representatives of agencies, service providers, families, and coordinators of infant, toddler, and preschool special education programs.

Anne Shureen, Preschool Special Ed. Coordinator

4976 Rotary Wishing Well, Inc.
10900 NE 8th St#900
Bellevue, WA 98004   206-462-4606
                                      Fax: 206-454-4383

Serves Washington, Oregon, Idaho, Montana, and Arkansas. Provides significant life experiences for children 4 to 19 with life-threatening or chronic diseases.

4977 Washington PAVE
6316 S 12th Street
Tacoma, WA 98465   253-565-2266
                                      800-572-7368
                                      Fax: 253-566-8052
                                      TTY: 800-572-7368
                                      TDD: 253-565-2266
                                      e-mail: washingtonpave.org
www.wapave9@washingtonpave.com

Parent Training and Information (PTI) programs help parents to: understand their children's specific needs; communicate more effectively with professionals, participate in the educational planning process; and obtain information about relevant programs, services, and resources

4978 Wishing Star Foundation
915 West 2nd Avenue
Spokane, WA 99201   509-744-3411
                                      800-685-6956
                                      Fax: 509-744-3414
                                      e-mail: info@wishingstar.org
                                      www.wishingstar.org

Serves Idaho, eastern Washington, and some areas of Oregon and Nevada. Grants wishes to children 3 to 19 with life-threatening diseases.

West Virginia

4979 Early Intervention Program
350 Capitol St. Room 427
Charleston, WV 25301   304-558-1069
                                      Fax: 304-558-2866
                                      www.nectas.unc.edu

Individuals with Disabilities Education Act requires all states and territories to provide early intervention and preschool special education for children with disabilities and special healthcare needs. Services include central directory, representatives of agencies, service providers, families, and coordinators of infant, toddler, and preschool special education programs.

Pam Roush, Infant/Toddler Program Coordinator

4980 Office of Special Education Administration
1900 Kawanha Blvd East
Charleston, WV 25305   304-558-2696
                                      Fax: 304-558-3741
                                      e-mail: pcarte@access.k12.wv.us
                                      www.nectas.unc.edu

Individuals with Disabilities Education Act requires all states and territories to provide early intervention and preschool special education for children with disabilities and special healthcare needs. Services include central directory, representatives of agencies, service providers, families, and coordinators of infant, toddler, and preschool special education programs.

Ginger Huffman, Preschool Special Ed. Coordinator

4981 West Virginia Assistive Technology System
Airport Research and Office Park
955 Hartman Run Road
Morgantown, WV 26505
                                      800-841-8436
                                      Fax: 304-293-7294
                                      TDD: 304-293-4692
                                      e-mail: stewiat@wvnvm.wvnet.edu

State assisted programs and support group information for people of many abilities. Including local chapters, referrals, fun and social interaction and support groups.

4982 West Virginia Parent Training and Information
371 Broaddus Avenue
Clarksburg, WV 26301   304-624-1436
                                      Fax: 304-624-1438
                                      e-mail: WVPTI@aol.com
                                      www.taalliance.org/ptis/wv/index.htm

Parent Training and Information (PTI) programs help parents to: understand their children's specific needs; communicate more effectively with professionals, participate in the educational planning process; and obtain information about relevant programs, services, and resources

Wisconsin

4983 Birth to 3 Program
P.O. Box 7851
Madisonton, WI 53370   608-267-3270
                                      Fax: 608-261-6752
                                      e-mail: kremema@dhfs.state.wi.us
                                      www.nectas.unc.edu

Early intervention and preschool special education for children with disabilities and special healthcare needs. Services include central directory, representatives of agencies, service providers, families, and coordinators of infant, toddler, and preschool special education programs.

Mitchell Kremer, Infant/Toddler Program Coor.

4984 Development and Training Center
2125 3rd Street
Eau Circle, WI 54703   715-833-7755
Fax: 715-833-7757
www.nectas.unc.edu

Individuals with Disabilities Education Act requires all states and territories to provide early intervention and preschool special education for children with disabilities and special healthcare needs. Services include central directory, representatives of agencies, service providers, families, and coordinators of infant, toddler, and preschool special education programs.

Stacy H. Wigfield, Interagency Coordinating Council

4985 Division of Community Services
P.O. Box 7851
Madison, WI 53707   608-267-3270
Fax: 608-267-6752
www.nectas.unc.edu

Individuals with Disabilities Education Act requires all states and territories to provide early intervention and preschool special education for children with disabilities and special healthcare needs. Services include central directory, representatives of agencies, service providers, families, and coordinators of infant, toddler, and preschool special education programs.

Beth Wroblewski, Preschool Special Ed. Coordinator

4986 Early Childhood Handicapped Prgrams
P.O. Box 7841
Madison, WI 53707   608-267-9172
Fax: 608-267-3746
e-mail: langejr@mail.state.wi.us
www.nectas.unc.edu

Services include central directory, representatives of agencies, service providers, families, and coordinators of infant, toddler, and preschool special education programs.

Jenny Lange, Preschool Special Ed. Coordinator

4987 Parent Education Project of Wisconsin, Inc
2192 S. 60th Street
West Allis, WI 53219   414-328-5520
Fax: 414-328-5530
TDD: 414-328-5520
e-mail: pmcolletti@aol.com
www.members.aol.com/pepofwi

Parent Training and Information (PTI) programs help parents to: understand their children's specific needs; communicate more effectively with professionals, participate in the educational planning process; and obtain information about relevant programs, services, and resources

4988 Thurday's Child
P.O. Box 259279
Madison, WI 53725   608-988-4234
Fax: 608-278-4234

Grants wishes to seriously ill children who live in or are being treated in southwest and south central Wisconsin.

4989 WisTech
PO Box 7852
2917 International Lane
Madison, WI 53707
Fax: 608-243-5681
TDD: 608-243-5674

State assisted programs and support group information for people of many abilities. Including local chapters, referrals, fun and social interaction and support groups.

Wyoming

4990 Division of Developmental Disabilities
1413 West 25th Street
Cheyenne, WY 82002   307-777-6972
Fax: 307-777-6047
www.nectas.unc.edu

Provides early intervention and preschool special education for children with disabilities and special healthcare needs. Services include central directory, representatives of agencies, service providers, families, and coordinators of infant, toddler, and preschool special education programs.

Mitch Brauchie, Interagency Coordinating Council

4991 Parent Information Center
5 N Lobban
Buffalo, WY 82834   307-684-2277
                          Fax: 307-684-5314
                          TDD: 307-684-2277
                  e-mail: tdawsonpic@vci.com
                          www.taalliance.org

Parent Training and Information (PTI) programs help parents to: understand their children's specific needs; communicate more effectively with professionals, participate in the educational planning process; and obtain information about relevant programs, services, and resources

4992 Special Education Unit
2300 Cheyenne Avenue, 2nd Floor
Cheyenne, WY 82002   307-777-6236
                          Fax: 307-777-6234
              e-mail: smofie@educ.state.wy.uss
                          www.nectas.unc.edu

Individuals with Disabilities Education Act requires all states and territories to provide early intervention and preschool special education for children with disabilities and special healthcare needs. Services include central directory, representatives of agencies, service providers, families, and coordinators of infant, toddler, and preschool special education programs.

Sara Mofield, Preschool Special Ed. Coordinator

4993 Wyoming's New Options in Technology (WYNOT)
University of Wyoming
1465 North 4th Street, Suite 111
Laramie, WY 82072
                          Fax: 307-721-2084
                          TDD: 307-766-2084
                  e-mail: wynot.uw@uwyo.edu
              www.uwyo.edu/hs/wind/wynot.htm

State assisted programs and support group information for people of many abilities. Including local chapters, referrals, fun and social interaction and support groups.

International

4994 Candlelighters Childhood Cancer Foundation Canada
55 Eglinton Ave E., Ste 401
Toronto Ontario, M4P   416-489-6440
                            800-363-1062
                       Fax: 416-489-9812
               e-mail: staff@candlelighters.org
                       www.candlelighters.org

Operates a hotline which provides information and services to survivors, families, and medical professionals on all pediatric cancer-related topics. Candlelighters offers many publications (most free), including: Introduction to the Americans with Disabilities Act: A Guide for Families of Children with Cancer and Survivors of Childhood Cancer, Insurance: Your Options and Your Child's; and Tips on Health Insurance for Long Term Survivors.

4995 Children's Wish Foundation of Canada
95 Bayly Street, Suite 404
Ajax, On L1S7K8,
Canada   905-426-5656
                            800-267-9474
                       Fax: 905-426-4111
          e-mail: wishesnational@sympatico.ca

Organization devoted to realizing the hopes and dreams of children with life-threatening illnesses.

4996 Easter Seal of Canada
90 Eglinton Avenue East, Suite 511
Toronto, ON,   M4P
Canada
                       TTY: 416-932-9844

Information and advocacy resources for families and professionals. Includes listings of organizations providing general information and organizations focusing on more specific areas of concern to families and young adults who have disabilities.

4997 Guam System for Assistive Service Technology (GSAT)
303 University Drive, University of Guam
UOG Station
Mangilao, Guam, 96923   671-735-2490
                       Fax: 671-734-8378
                       TDD: 671-734-8378
                  e-mail: gsat@ite.net
               uog2.uog.edu/uap/gsat.html

State assisted programs and support group information for people of many abilities. Including local chapters, referrals, fun and social interaction and support groups.

4998 Virgin Island Technology Assistance
University of the Virgin Islands/UAP
#2 John Brewers Bay
St. Thomas, VI, 00801   340-693-1323
                       Fax: 340-693-1325
                  e-mail: yhabtes@uvi.edu

State assisted programs and support group information for people of many abilities. Including local chapters, referrals, fun and social interaction and support groups.

Libraries & Resource Centers

Alabama

4999 Mobile Association for the Blind
2440 Gordon Smith Drive
Mobile, AL 36617   334-473-3585

Offers work adjustment training, activities of daily living, mobility, communication skills and sheltered employment for adults and children who are visually impaired.

Mahlon McCracken, Executive Director

Arizona

5000 Educational Services for the Visually Impaired
P.O. Box 668
Little Rock, AZ 72203   501-371-5710

Offers textbooks, braille books and more to the visually impaired grades K-12 in the Arizona area.

David Beavers, Director

5001 Special Needs Center/Phoenix Public Library
12 East McDowell Road
Phoenix, AZ 85004   602-261-8690

Offers talking books and records, braille books and magazines, large print books, video print enlarger, video magnifier and VersaBraille software with synthetic speech for the blind, visually handicapped, physically/mentally handicapped and speech and hearing impaired children and adults.

Mary Roatch, Supervisor

5002 Technology Access Center of Tucson
P.O. Box 13178
Tucson, AZ 85732   520-745-5588
                               Fax: 520-790-7637
                               e-mail: tactaz@aol.com

Technology group of parents, consumers and professionals; provides resources to help children and adults who have disabilities gain access to the benefits of technology. Includes nationwide network of community-based assistive technology, resource centers, hands on consultants and product demonstrations.

Arkansas

5003 Arkansas Easter Seals Technology Resource Center
3920 Woodland Heights Road
Little Rock, AR 72212   501-227-3602
                               Fax: 501-227-3601
                               e-mail: atrce@aol.com
                               www.arkeasterseals.org

Technology group of parents, consumers and professionals; provides resources to help children and adults who have disabilities gain access to the benefits of technology. Includes nationwide network of community-based assistive technology, resource centers, hands on consultants and product demonstrations.

5004 Arkansas Regional Library for the Blind and Physically Handicapped
One Capitol Mall
Little Rock, AR 72201   501-682-1155
                               Fax: 501-682-1529
                               TDD: 501-682-1002
                               e-mail: jhall@asl.lib.ar.us

Public library books in recorded or braille format. Popular fiction and nonfiction books for all ages, books and players are on free loan, sent to patrons by mail and may be returned postage free. Anyone who cannot see well enough to read regular print with glasses on or who has a disability that makes it difficult to hold a book or turn the pages is eligible.

John D. Hall, Director

5005 CLOC Regional Library
P.O. Box 668
Magnolia, AR 71753   870-234-1991
                               Fax: 870-234-5077

Offers a children's summer reading program and a book collection featuring discs and casettes.

Christine McDonald, Librarian

5006 Crowley Ridge Regional Library
315 West Oak
Jonesboro, AR 72401   870-935-5133

Offers a children's summer reading program, large print and books on cassette.

Ruth Ball

5007 Fort Smith Library for the Blind and Handicapped
61 South 8th Street
Fort Smith, AR 72901   501-783-0229
Fax: 501-782-8571
e-mail: khamlin@fspl.lib.ar.us
www.fspl.lib.ar.us

Children's books on cassette and disc, summer reading programs and large print books.

Kelly Hamlin, Librarian

5008 Northwest Ozarks Regional Library for the Blind and Handicapped
217 East Dickson Street
Fayetteville, AR 72701   501-442-6243
Fax: 501-442-6254
www.vark.edu

Offers a summer reading program, closed-circuit TV, magnifiers, braille writers and large print books.

Rachel Anne Ames, Librarian

California

5009 American Action Fund for Blind Children and Adults
18440 Oxnard Street
Tarzana, CA 91356   818-343-2022

Offers a charitable and educational fund, braille assistive devices and a lending library for the visually impaired.

Kenneth Jernigan, Executive Director

5010 Assistive Technology Center Simi Valley Hospital
Rehabilatation Unit North
P.O. Box 1325
Simi Valley, CA 93062   805-582-1881
Fax: 805-582-2855
e-mail: dssacca@aol.com

Technology group of parents, consumers and professionals; provides resources to help children and adults who have disabilities gain access to the benefits of technology. Includes nationwide network of community-based assistive technology, resource centers, hands on consultants and product demonstrations.

5011 Blind Children's Center
4120 Marathon Street
Los Angeles, CA 90029   213-664-2153
800-222-3566

Offers support and informational groups.

5012 Braille Institute Desert Center
70-251 Ramon Road
Rancho Mirage, CA 92270   760-321-2555

Dedicated to providing blind and visually impaired men, women and children with the training, programs and services they need to enjoy productive lives. Services offered include child development, youth programs, library services and adult education.

5013 Braille Institute Sight Center
741 North Vermont Avenue
Los Angeles, CA 90029   213-663-1111
e-mail: bils@brailib.org

Offers help, programs, services and information to the blind and visually impaired children and adults.

Dr. Henry Chang, Librarian

5014 Braille Institute Youth Center
3450 Cahuenga Blvd. West
Los Angeles, CA 90068   213-851-5695

Offers various youth programs and services for the blind and visually impaired youngster.

5015 Center for Accessible Technology
2547 8th Street, 112-A
Berkeley, CA 94710   510-841-3224
Fax: 510-841-7956
e-mail: cforat@aol.com

Provides resources to help children and adults who have disabilities gain access to the benefits of technology.

5016 Clearinghouse for Specialized Media and Technology
California Department of Education
560 J Street, Suite 390
Sacramento, CA 94244   916-445-5103
Fax: 916-323-9732
e-mail: rbrawley@cde.ca.gov
www.cde.ca.gov

Assists California schools and students in the identification and acquisition of textbooks, reference books and study materials in aural media, braille, large print and electronic media access technology.

Rod Brawley, Director

5017 New Beginnings - The Blind Children's Center
4120 Marathon Street
Los Angeles, CA 90029   213-664-2153
                              800-222-3566

Helps children and their families become independent by creating a climate of safety and trust. Services include an infant stimulation program, educational preschool, interdisciplinary assessment services, family services, correspondence program, toll free national hotline and a publication and research service.

5018 Sacramento Center for Assistive Technology
701 Howe Avenue, Suite E-5
Sacramento, CA 95825   916-927-7228
          e-mail: scatca@quicknet.com
                  www.quicknet.com/~scat

Technology group of parents, consumers and professionals; provides resources to help children and adults who have disabilities gain access to the benefits of technology. Includes nationwide network of community-based assistive technology, resource centers, hands on consultants and product demonstrations.

5019 San Francisco Public Library for the Blind and Print Handicapped
100 Larkin Street
San Francisco, CA 94102   415-557-4293
          e-mail: lbphmgr@sfpl.lib.ca.us

Foreign-language books on cassette, children's books on cassettes and more.

Martin Maqid, Librarian

5020 Technology Access Center
2175 E Francisco Boulevard, Suite L
San Rafael, CA 94901   415-455-4575
                    Fax: 415-455-0654
                    TTY: 415-455-0491
          e-mail: atainfo@ataccess.org
                  www.ataccess.org

Technology group of parents, consumers and professionals; provides resources to help children and adults who have disabilities gain access to the benefits of technology. Includes nationwide network of community-based assistive technology, resource centers, hands on consultants and product demonstrations.

5021 Variety Audio, Inc.
P.O. Box 5731
San Jose, CA 95150   408-277-4839

Summer reading programs, braille writer, magnifiers, closed-circuit T.V., large-print photocopier, cassette books and magazines, children's books on cassette, home visits and other reference materials on blindness and other handicaps.

Louisa Griehshammer

Connecticut

5022 Chapel Haven, Inc.
1040 Whalley Avenue
New Haven, CT 06515   203-397-1714
                    Fax: 203-397-8004
          e-mail: betseypar@aol.com
                  www.chapelhaven.com

An individualized, year-round, transitional independent living program for young adults with a wide range of learning disabilities. The program includes life skills training in an apartment setting, pre-vocational training, vocational placement and support, and practical academics. Participants learn all of the skills necessary to make a smooth entry into independent community living. Comprehensive non-residential, community-based independent living services are also available.

Betsy Farlato, Communications Director

Delaware

5023 Delaware Division of Libraries for the Blind and Physically Handicapped
43 S. Dupont Hwy., P.O. Box 639
Dover, DE 19901   302-736-4748
                    Fax: 302-736-6787
          e-mail: norman@lib.de.us

Braille readers receive service from Philadelphia and Pennsylvania, summer reading program, braille writer and cassettes.

Lee Steele, Librarian

District of Columbia

5024 Georgetown University Child Development Center
3307 M Street NW
Washington, DC 20007   202-687-8635
                                        Fax: 202-687-8899

Florida

5025 Center for Independence Technology and Education, (CITE)
215 E New Hampshire Street
Orlando, FL 32804   407-898-2483
                                    Fax: 407-895-5255
                          e-mail: comcite@aol.com

Technology group of parents, consumers and professionals; provides resources to help children and adults who have disabilities gain access to the benefits of technology. Includes nationwide network of community-based assistive technology, resource centers, hands on consultants and product demonstrations.

5026 Florida Division of Blind Services
Regional Library
420 Platt Street
Daytona Beach, FL 32114   850-254-3824
                                          Fax: 850-239-6069
                                          TDD: 800-226-6079
                          e-mail: weberd@mail.firn.edu

Discs, cassettes, closed-circuit T.V., large-print photocopier, films, children's books on cassettes and more.

Donald John Weber, Librarian

5027 Jacksonville Public Library
2809 Commonwealth Avenue
Jacksonville, FL 32205   904-388-6135

Discs, cassettes, reference materials on blindness and other handicaps and children's books on cassettes.

Gloria Zittrauer, Librarian

5028 Talking Book Service - Mantatee County Central Library
1301 Barcarrota Blvd., West
Bradenton, FL 34205   941-749-7114

Offers children's books on disc and cassette and more reference materials for the blind and physically handicapped.

Debra Kraner, Librarian

5029 University of Miami, Mailman Center For Child Development
P.O. Box 016820
Miami, FL 33101   305-585-2703
                                  Fax: 305-547-6309

Focuses on birth defects and children's illnesses.

Dr. Robert Stempfel, Jr., Director

5030 West Florida Regional Library
200 West Gregory Street
Pensacola, FL 32501   850-435-1760
                                      Fax: 850-432-9582

Offers children's print/braille books.

Martha Lazor, Librarian

Georgia

5031 Albany Talking Book Center
Dougherty County Public Library
300 Pine Avenue
Albany, GA 31701   912-431-2900
                                  Fax: 912-430-4020

Offers discs, cassettes, reference materials on blindness and other handicaps, large-print photocopiers, summer reading programs, cassette books and more.

Kathryn Sinquefield, Librarian

5032 Athens Regional Library Talking Book Center
2025 Baxter Street
Athens, GA 30606   706-613-3650
                                  Fax: 706-613-3660

Discs, cassettes, large print books, reference materials on blindness, films, closed-circuit T.V., magnifiers, braille writer, summer reading programs, cassette books and magazines and more.

Paige Burns, Librarian

5033 Augusta-Richmond County Public Library
425 9th Street
Augusta, GA 30901   706-821-2625
                                  Fax: 706-724-5403
                             e-mail: gswint@csra,net

Discs, cassettes, braille writer, films, large print
books, summer reading program, magnifiers
and reference materials on blindness and other
handicaps.

Gary Swint, Librarian

5034 Bainbridge Subregional Library for the Blind
SW Georgia Regional Library
301 S. Monroe Street
Bainbridge, GA 31717   912-248-2665
                                       800-795-2680
                                  Fax: 912-248-2670

Discs, cassettes, large print books, summer reading programs, closed-circuit T.V., magnifiers
and more.

Susan Whittle, Librarian

5035 CEL Regional Library
2002 Bull Street
Savannah, GA 31499   912-652-3644
                                  Fax: 912-652-3638
                     e-mail: lstokes@cel.co.chatman.ga.us

Summer reading programs, braille writer, magnifiers, closed-circuit T.V., large-print photocopier, cassette books and magazines, children's
books on cassette, home visits and other reference materials on blindness and other handicaps.

Linda Stokes, Librarian

5036 Hay County Public Library
127 North Main Street
Gainesville, GA 30505   770-535-5738
                                  Fax: 770-532-4305

Summer reading programs, braille writer, magnifiers, closed-circuit T.V., large-print photocopier, cassette books and magazines, children's
books on cassette, home visits and other reference materials on blindness and other handicaps.

Sandra Whitmen, Librarian

**5037 La Fayette Subregional Library for the Blind and
Physically Disabled**
301 South Duke Street
La Fayette, GA 30728   706-638-2342
                                  Fax: 706-638-4028

Summer reading programs, braille writer, magnifiers, closed-circuit T.V., large-print photocopier, cassette books and magazines, children's
books on cassette, home visits and other reference materials on blindness and other handicaps.

Charles Stubblefield, Librarian

**5038 Macon Library for the Blind and Physically
Handicapped**
Washington Memorial Library
1180 Washington Avenue
Macon, GA 31201   912-744-0800
                                  Fax: 912-742-3161

Summer reading programs, braille writer, magnifiers, closed-circuit T.V., large-print photocopier, cassette books and magazines, children's
books on cassette, home visits and other reference materials on blindness and other handicaps.

Rebecca Sherrill, Librarian

5039 Oconee Regional Library
P.O. Box 100, Bellave Ave
Dublin, GA 31040   912-275-5382
                                  Fax: 912-272-0524

Summer reading programs, braille writer, magnifiers, closed-circuit T.V., large-print photocopier, cassette books and magazines, children's
books on cassette, home visits and other reference materials on blindness and other handicaps.

Susan Williams, Librarian

5040 Sara Hightower Regional Library
205 Riverside Parkway
Rome, GA 30161   706-236-4611
                                  Fax: 706-236-4631
                   e-mail: floydl@mail.floyd.public.lib.ga.us
                             www.floyd.public.lib.ga.us

Summer reading programs, braille writer, magnifiers, closed-circuit T.V., large-print photocopier, cassette books and magazines, children's
books on cassette, home visits and other reference materials on blindness and other handicaps.

Sue Frazier, Librarian

5041 Subregional Library for the Blind and Physically Handicapped
1120 Bradley Drive
Columbus, GA 31906   706-649-0780
                    Fax: 706-649-1914
                    TDD: 706-649-0974
        e-mail: atbph@mail.muscogee.pub.ga.us

Braille writer, magnifiers, closed-circuit T.V., large-print photocopier, cassette books and magazines, children's books on cassette, home visits and other reference materials on blindness and other handicaps. A free national library service that provides recorded books and Braille materials for people with low-vision, blindness and physical handicaps.

Dorothy Bowen, Librarian

5042 Tech-Able
1112A Brett Drive
Conyers, GA 30094   770-922-6768
                    Fax: 770-922-6769
        e-mail: techable@america.net
                    www.gatfl.org

Technology group of parents, consumers and professionals; provides resources to help children and adults who have disabilities gain access to the benefits of technology. Includes nationwide network of community-based assistive technology, resource centers, hands on consultants and product demonstrations.

Hawaii

5043 Aloha Special Technology Access Center
710 Green Street
Honolulu, HI 96813   808-523-5547
                    Fax: 808-536-3765
        e-mail: stachi@aol.com
                    www.aloha.net/~stachi/

Technology group of parents, consumers and professionals; provides resources to help children and adults who have disabilities gain access to the benefits of technology. Includes nationwide network of community-based assistive technology, resource centers, hands on consultants and product demonstrations.

5044 Library for the Blind and Physically Handicapped of Hawaii
402 Kapahulu Avenue
Honolulu, HI 96815   808-733-8444
                    Fax: 808-733-8449
        e-mail: olbeire@state.lib.hi.us

Summer reading programs, braille writer, magnifiers, closed-circuit T.V., large-print photocopier, cassette books and magazines, children's books on cassette, home visits and other reference materials on blindness and other handicaps.

Fusako Miyashiro, Librarian

Idaho

5045 Idaho State Library
325 West State Street
Boise, ID 83702   208-334-2412
                    Fax: 208-334-2194
        e-mail: ksalmon@isl.state.id.us

Summer reading programs, braille writer, magnifiers, closed-circuit T.V., large-print photocopier, cassette books and magazines, children's books on cassette, home visits and other reference materials on blindness and other handicaps.

Kay Samon, Librarian

Illinois

5046 Chicago Library Service for the Blind
1055 West Roosevelt Road
Chicago, IL 60608   312-746-9210

Summer reading programs, braille writer, magnifiers, closed-circuit T.V., large-print photocopier, cassette books and magazines, children's books on cassette, home visits and other reference materials on blindness and other handicaps.

Carol Pellish, Librarian

5047 Great River Library System
515 York Street
Quincy, IL 62301   217-224-5690
                    Fax: 217-224-9818
        e-mail: eshepard@darkstar.rsa.lib.il

Summer reading programs, braille writer, magnifiers, closed-circuit T.V., large-print photocopier, cassette books and magazines, children's books on cassette, home visits and other reference materials on blindness and other handicaps.

Eileen Sheppard, Librarian

5048 Illinois Regional Library for the Blind and Physically Handicapped
1055 West Roosevelt Road
Chicago, IL 60608
773-746-9210
800-331-2351
Fax: 773-746-9192

Summer reading programs, braille writer, magnifiers, closed-circuit T.V., large-print photocopier, cassette books and magazines, descriptive videos, children's books on cassette, home visits and other reference materials on blindness and other handicaps.

Shawn Thomas, Reference Librarian
Thomas Barbara, Perkins

5049 Mid-Illinois Talking Book Center
845 Brenkman Drive
Pekin, IL 61554
309-353-5444
800-426-0709
Fax: 309-353-8281
e-mail: mitbc@darkstar.rsa.lib.il.us
http://www.rsa.lib.il.us/~mitbe/heart.ht

Summer reading program, braille printer, cassette books and magazines, children's books on cassette, and other reference materials on blindness and other handicaps. Discriptive videos, old-time radio shows on cassette, staff available for programs or exhibits.

Eileen Sheppard, Librarian

5050 National Library of Dermatologic Teaching Slides
American Academy of Dermatology
930 N Meacham Road
Shaumburg, IL 60173
847-330-0230
Fax: 847-330-0050
www.aad.org

A collection of dermatologic teaching slides offering the most comprehensive series ever assembled. Each set offers a realistic presentation of classic clinical skin conditions encountered by the dermatologist.

5051 Northern Illinois Center for Adaptive Technology
3615 Louisana Road
Rockford, IL 61108
815-229-2163
Fax: 815-229-2135
e-mail: ilcat@aol.com

Technology group of parents, consumers and professionals; provides resources to help children and adults who have disabilities gain access to the benefits of technology. Includes nationwide network of community-based assistive technology, resource centers, hands on consultants and product demonstrations.

5052 Parents Alliance Employment Project
Illinois Employment and Training Center
837 S Westmore Drive
Lombard, IL 60148
630-495-4345
Fax: 630-495-0387
TDD: 630-495-6055

Information and advocacy resources for families and professionals. Includes listings of organizations providing general information and organizations focusing on more specific areas of concern to families and young adults who have disabilities.

5053 Professional Assistance Center for Education (PACE)
National-Louis University
2840 Sheridan Road
Evanston, IL 60201
847-475-1100
Fax: 847-256-5190
e-mail: cbur@evan1.nl.edu

A two year, non credit certification program servicing students with learning disabilities. The program provides a rare opportunity for students from all parts of the country to continue their education in an age appropriate environment. Committed to an instructional approach that integrates both group and individual teaching for career preparation, academics, life skills, and socialization. Transitional program offered to qualified graduates.

Carol Burns, Director

5054 Shawnee Library System
607 Greenbriar Road
Carterville, IL 62918
618-985-3711
Fax: 618-985-4211
e-mail: kqurden@shawnet.shawls.lib.il

Summer reading programs, braille writer, magnifiers, closed-circuit T.V., large-print photocopier, cassette books and magazines, children's books on cassette, home visits and other reference materials on blindness and other handicaps.

Kristi Gorden, Librarian

5055 Sulzberger Institute for Dermatologic Education
P.O. Box 4014
Schaumburg, IL 61068
847-330-0230
Fax: 847-330-0050

A nonprofit research center whose sole goal is to enhance patient care through the development and promotion of quality educational programs on the care and disorders of the skin, hair, nails and mucous membranes.

5056 Talking Book Center of North West Illinois
P.O. Box 125
Coal Valley, IL 61240   309-799-3137
                               Fax: 309-353-8281

Subregional library provides Talking Book and Braille Book program to eligible persons unable to use standard print materials due to visual or physical disabilities. Includes cassette books and magazines, and summer reading program.

5057 Technical Aids & Assistance for the Disabled Center
1950 W Roosevelt Road
Chicago, IL 60608   312-421-3464
                              Fax: 312-421-3373
                              e-mail: taad@interaccess.com
                              www.interaccess.com/~taad

Technology group of parents, consumers and professionals; provides resources to help children and adults who have disabilities gain access to the benefits of technology. Includes nationwide network of community-based assistive technology, resource centers, hands on consultants and product demonstrations.

5058 University of Illinois at Chicago, Craniofacial Center
College of Medicine
808 S. Wood Street
Chicago, IL 60680   312-996-6979
                              Fax: 312-413-1526

Dr. Allen Goldman, Director

Indiana

5059 Allen County Public Library
Box 2270
Fort Wayne, IN 46801   219-424-7241

Summer reading programs, braille writer, magnifiers, closed-circuit T.V., large-print photocopier, cassette books and magazines, children's books on cassette, home visits and other reference materials on blindness and other handicaps.

Joyce Misner, Librarian

5060 Assistive Technology Training & Information Center (ATTIC)
3354 Pine Hill Drive
Vincennes, IN 47591   812-886-0575
                              800-962-8842
                              Fax: 812-886-1128
                              TTY: 800-962-8842
                              e-mail: inattic2@aol.com

Informational and emotional support to parents who have a child, adolescent, or adult family member with special needs.

5061 Bartholomew County Public Library
5th at Lafayette
Columbus, IN 47201   812-379-1277
                              Fax: 812-379-1275

Summer reading programs, braille writer, magnifiers, closed-circuit T.V., large-print photocopier, cassette books and magazines, children's books on cassette, home visits and other reference materials on blindness and other handicaps.

Wilma Perry, Librarian

5062 Elkhart Public Library
300 South Second
Elkhart, IN 46516   219-522-2665

Summer reading programs, braille writer, magnifiers, closed-circuit T.V., large-print photocopier, cassette books and magazines, children's books on cassette, home visits and other reference materials on blindness and other handicaps.

Pat Ciancio, Librarian

5063 Northwest Indiana Subregional Library for Blind and Physically Handicapped
1919 West 81st Street
Merrillville, IN 46410   219-769-3541
                              Fax: 219-769-0690

Summer reading programs, braille writer, magnifiers, closed-circuit T.V., large-print photocopier, cassette books and magazines, children's books on cassette, home visits and other reference materials on blindness and other handicaps.

Renee Lewis

5064 Special Services Division - Indiana State Library
140 North Senate Street
Indianapolis, IN 46204   317-232-3684
                              800-622-4970
                              Fax: 317-232-3728

Summer reading programs, braille writer, magnifiers, closed-circuit T.V., large-print photocopier, cassette books and magazines, children's books on cassette, home visits and other reference materials on blindness and other handicaps.

Lissa Shanahan, Librarian

Iowa

5065 Library Commission for the Blind
524 Fourth Street
Des Moines, IA 50309   515-281-1333
                              Fax: 515-281-1378
                    e-mail: iisad@blind.dtate.ia.us

Summer reading programs, braille writer, magnifiers, closed-circuit T.V., large-print photocopier, cassette books and magazines, children's books on cassette, home visits and other reference materials on blindness and other handicaps.

Catherine Ford, Librarian

5066 University of Iowa Birth Defects and Genetic Disorders Unit
2614 JCP
Iowa City, IA 52242   319-335-9901

James M. Smith, Director

Kansas

5067 CKLS Headquarters
1409 Williams
Great Bend, KS 67530   316-792-2393
                              Fax: 316-793-7270
                       e-mail: cenks@ink.org

Summer reading programs, braille writer, magnifiers, closed-circuit T.V., large-print photocopier, cassette books and magazines, children's books on cassette, home visits and other reference materials on blindness and other handicaps.

Jerri Robinson, Librarian

5068 Kansas State Library
ESU Memorial Union
1200 Commercial Street
Emporia, KS 66801   316-341-1200
                            Fax: 316-343-7124
                    e-mail: ksst16lb@ink.org

Summer reading programs, braille writer, magnifiers, closed-circuit T.V., large-print photocopier, cassette books and magazines, children's books on cassette, home visits and other reference materials on blindness and other handicaps.

2aroline Lang, Librarian

5069 Manhattan Public Library
629 Poyntz Ave.
Manhattan, KS 66502   785-776-4741
                              Fax: 785-776-1545
                e-mail: marionr@manhattan.lib.ks.us

Summer reading programs, braille writer, magnifiers, closed-circuit T.V., large-print photocopier, cassette books and magazines, children's books on cassette, home visits and other reference materials on blindness and other handicaps.

Marion Rice, Librarian

5070 Prenatal Diagnostic and Genetic Center
HCA Wesley Medical Center
550 N. Hillside
Wichita, KS 67214   316-688-2362

Sechin Cho, MD

5071 South Central Kansas Library System
901 North Main
Hutchinson, KS 67501   316-663-5441
                              Fax: 316-663-1215
                       e-mail: nwks1lb@ink.org

Summer reading programs, braille writer, magnifiers, closed-circuit T.V., large-print photocopier, cassette books and magazines, children's books on cassette, home visits and other reference materials on blindness and other handicaps.

Karen Socha, Librarian

5072 Technology Resource Solutions for People
1710 W Schilling Road
Salina, KS 67402
                              Fax: 785-323-2015
                              TTY: 913-827-9383
                       e-mail: trspks@midusa.net

Technology group of parents, consumers and professionals; provides resources to help children and adults who have disabilities gain access to the benefits of technology. Includes nationwide network of community-based assistive technology, resource centers, hands on consultants and product demonstrations.

5073 University of Kansas Center for Research on Learning
3061 Dole Center
Lawrence, KS 66045   785-864-4780
                            Fax: 785-864-5728
                            www.ku-crl.org

A research center working to improve learning and performance of adolescants and adults considered to be at risk for failure in today's schools, work places, and communities. Develops products and procedures that can be used to more effectively teach these individuals. Provides support and research-validated instructional materials to an international training network that promotes system change in our schools and institutions. Newsletter for teachers containing tip and advice used in class.

Don Deshler, Director
Jean Schumaker, Associate Director

5074 Wesley Medical Research Institutes
3306 E. Central
Wichita, KS 67208   316-686-7172

Respiratory and birth defects disorders research.

Dr. Sechin Cho, MD, Director

5075 Wichita Public Library
223 South Main
Wichita, KS 67202   316-262-0611
                         Fax: 316-262-4540

Summer reading programs, braille writer, magnifiers, closed-circuit T.V., large-print photocopier, cassette books and magazines, children's books on cassette, home visits and other reference materials on blindness and other handicaps.

Brad Reha, Librarian

Kentucky

5076 Bluegrass Technology Center
169 N Limestone Street
Lexington, KY 40507   606-255-9951
                          Fax: 606-255-0059
                          TTY: 606-255-9951
          e-mail: bluegrass@uky.campus.mci.net

Technology group of parents, consumers and professionals; provides resources to help children and adults who have disabilities gain access to the benefits of technology. Includes nationwide network of community-based assistive technology, resource centers, hands on consultants and product demonstrations.

5077 EnTech: Enabling Technologies of Kentuckiana
301 York Street
Louisville, KY 40203   502-574-1637
                e-mail: entech@iglou.org

Technology group of parents, consumers and professionals; provides resources to help children and adults who have disabilities gain access to the benefits of technology. Includes nationwide network of community-based assistive technology, resource centers, hands on consultants and product demonstrations.

5078 Kentucky Library for the Blind and Physically Handicapped
300 Coffee Tree, PO Box 818
Frankfort, KY 40602   502-564-8300
                          Fax: 502-564-5773
         e-mail: rfeindel@ctr.kdlo.state.ky.us

Summer reading programs, braille writer, magnifiers, closed-circuit T.V., large-print photocopier, cassette books and magazines, children's books on cassette, home visits and other reference materials on blindness and other handicaps.

Richard Feindel, Librarian

5079 Louisville Free Public Library
301 York Street
Louisville, KY 40203   502-574-1600
                          Fax: 502-574-1657

Summer reading programs, braille writer, magnifiers, closed-circuit T.V., large-print photocopier, cassette books and magazines, children's books on cassette, home visits and other reference materials on blindness and other handicaps.

Tom Denning, Librarian

5080 Northern Kentucky Talking Book Library
502 Scott Street
Covington, KY 41011   606-431-4177
                          Fax: 606-655-7960

Summer reading programs, braille writer, magnifiers, closed-circuit T.V., large-print photocopier, cassette books and magazines, children's books on cassette, home visits and other reference materials on blindness and other handicaps.

Jama Rooney, Librarian

5081 Western Kentucky Assistive Technology Consortion
P.O. Box 266, 607 Poplar Street, Suite 211
Murray, KY 42071   270-759-4233
Fax: 270-759-4208
e-mail: wkatc@cablecomm-ky.net

Technology group of parents, consumers and professionals; provides resources to help children and adults who have disabilities gain access to the benefits of technology. Includes nationwide network of community-based assistive technology, resource centers, hands on consultants and product demonstrations.

Louisiana

5082 Louisiana State Library
760 North Fouth Street
Baton Rouge, LA 70802   504-342-4928
Fax: 504-342-3547
e-mail: sbph@pelican. state.lib.la.us

Summer reading programs, braille writer, magnifiers, closed-circuit T.V., large-print photocopier, cassette books and magazines, children's books on cassette, home visits and other reference materials on blindness and other handicaps.

Jennifer Anjier, Librarian

5083 Louisiana State University Genetics Section of Pediatrics
1501 Kings Highway
Shreveport, LA 71130   318-675-5681

T.F. Thurman, MD, Director

Maine

5084 Bangor Public Library
145 Harlow Street
Bangor, ME 04401   207-947-8336

Summer reading programs, braille writer, magnifiers, closed-circuit T.V., large-print photocopier, cassette books and magazines, children's books on cassette, home visits and other reference materials on blindness and other handicaps.

Judith Leighton, Librarian

5085 Cary Library
107 Main Street
Houlton, ME 04730   207-532-3967

Summer reading programs, braille writer, magnifiers, closed-circuit T.V., large-print photocopier, cassette books and magazines, children's books on cassette, home visits and other reference materials on blindness and other handicaps.

Norma Watson, Librarian

5086 Lewiston Public Library
105 Park Street
Lewiston, ME 04240   207-784-0135

Summer reading programs, braille writer, magnifiers, closed-circuit T.V., large-print photocopier, cassette books and magazines, children's books on cassette, home visits and other reference materials on blindness and other handicaps.

Muriel Landry, Librarian

5087 Maine State Library
64 State House Station 64
Augusta, ME 04333   207-287-5650
Fax: 207-287-5624
e-mail: benitad@ursus3.ursus.maine.edu

Summer reading programs, braille writer, magnifiers, closed-circuit T.V., large-print photocopier, cassette books and magazines, children's books on cassette, home visits and other reference materials on blindness and other handicaps.

Benita Davis, Librarian

5088 New England Regional Genetics Group
P.O. Box 682
Gorham, ME 04038   207-839-5324
Fax: 207-839-8637

Human genetic services and educational planning pertaining to birth defects.

Ms. A. Merrill Henderson, Coordinator

5089 Portland Public Library
5 Monument Square
Portland, ME 04101   207-871-1700

Summer reading programs, braille writer, magnifiers, closed-circuit T.V., large-print photocopier, cassette books and magazines, children's books on cassette, home visits and other reference materials on blindness and other handicaps.

Janice Littlefield, Librarian

5090 Waterville Public Library
73 Elm Street
Waterville, ME 04901   207-872-5433

Summer reading programs, braille writer, magnifiers, closed-circuit T.V., large-print photocopier, cassette books and magazines, children's books on cassette, home visits and other reference materials on blindness and other handicaps.

Meta Vigue, Librarian

Maryland

5091 Learning Independence Through Computers
1001 Eastern Avenue, 3rd Floor
Baltimore, MD 21202   410-659-5462
                                       Fax: 410-659-5472
                                       e-mail: lincmd@aol.com

Technology group of parents, consumers and professionals; provides resources to help children and adults who have disabilities gain access to the benefits of technology. Includes nationwide network of community-based assistive technology, resource centers, hands on consultants and product demonstrations.

5092 Maryland State Library for the Blind and Physically Handicapped
415 Park Avenue
Baltimore, MD 21201   410-230-2424
                                       Fax: 410-333-2095
                                       TDD: 800-934-2541
                                       e-mail: recept@lbph.lib.md.us

Summer reading programs, braille writer, magnifiers, large-print photocopier, cassette books and magazines, children's books on cassette, and other reference materials on blindness and other handicaps.

Sharron McFarland, Librarian

5093 Prince George's County Memorial Library Talking Book Center
6530 Adelphi Road
Hyattsville, MD 20782   301-779-9330

Summer reading programs, braille writer, magnifiers, closed-circuit T.V., large-print photocopier, cassette books and magazines, children's books on cassette, home visits and other reference materials on blindness and other handicaps.

Shirley Tuthill, Librarian

Massachusetts

5094 Berkshire Center
18 Park Street Box 160
Lee, MA 01238   413-243-2576

A postsecondary program for young adults with learning disabilities ages 18-26. Services include: Vocational/adacademic preparation, tutoring, college liason, life skills instruction, driver's education, money management, psychotherapy, and more. The program is year-round with two years being the average stay.

5095 Braille and Talking Book Library Perkins School for the Blind
175 North Beacon Street
Watertown, MA 02172   781-972-7240
                                       800-852-3133
                                       Fax: 781-972-7363
                                       e-mail: perkins@bpl.org

Patricia Kirk

5096 Carroll Center for the Blind
770 Centre Street
Newton, MA 02158   617-969-6200
                                    800-852-3131
                                    Fax: 617-969-6204
                                    www.carroll.org

Assists blind and visually impaired adults and adolescents to adjust to loss of vision. The goal of this dynamic program is to help the person become more independent, to restore self-confidence, prepare for employment and improve the quality of life. Programs of individual counseling are offered as part of the program.

Rachel Rosenbaum, President

5097 Talking Book Library at Worcester Public Library
160 Fremont Street
Worcester, MA 01603   508-799-1730
                                       Fax: 508-799-1676
                                       TDD: 508-799-1724
                                       e-mail: talkbook@cwmars.org org
                                       www.worcpublib.org/talkingbook

Summer reading programs, braille writer, magnifiers, closed-circuit T.V., large-print photocopier, cassette books and magazines, children's books on cassette, reference materials on blindness and other disabilities.

James L. Izatt, Librarian

Michigan

5098 Frederick Douglas Branch for Specialized Services and Physically Handicapped
3666 Grand River/Trumbull
Detroit, MI 48226   313-833-5494
                                Fax: 313-833-5597
                                TDD: 313-224-0584
                     e-mail: devans@detroit.lib.mi.us
                                www.detroit.lib.mi.us

Summer reading programs, braille writer, magnifiers, closed-circuit T.V., large-print photocopier, cassette books and magazines, children's books on cassette, home visits and other reference materials on blindness and other handicaps.

Deborah Evans, Librarian
Kenneth Miller, Coordinator

5099 Kent County Library for the Blind and Physically Handicapped
4055 Maple St. Sw
Grandville, MI 49418   616-530-6219
                                Fax: 616-530-6222
                                TDD: 616-530-6219
                          e-mail: lbph@kdl.org
                                www.kdl.org

Audio books and playback equipment to registered borrowers.

Cathy Neis, Librarian

5100 Library of Michigan Service for the Blind
P.O. Box 30007
Lansing, MI 48909   517-373-5614
                                Fax: 517-373-5865
                  e-mail: info@sbph.libomich.lib.mi.us

Summer reading programs, braille writer, magnifiers, closed-circuit T.V., large-print photocopier, cassette books and magazines, children's books on cassette, home visits and other reference materials on blindness and other handicaps.

5101 Macomb Library for the Blind and Physically Handicapped
16480 Hall Road
Clinton Township, MI 48038   810-286-1580
                                Fax: 810-286-0634

Summer reading programs, braille writer, magnifiers, closed-circuit T.V., large-print photocopier, cassette books and magazines, children's books on cassette, home visits and other reference materials on blindness and other handicaps.

Linda Champion, Librarian

5102 Michigan's Assistive Technology Resource
Physically Impaired Association of Michigan
1023 S US 27
St. Johns, MI 48879   517-224-0333
                                800-274-7426
                                Fax: 517-224-0330
                          e-mail: matr@match.org

Technology group of parents, consumers and professionals; provides resources to help children and adults who have disabilities gain access to the benefits of technology. Includes nationwide network of community-based assistive technology, resource centers, hands on consultants and product demonstrations.

5103 Mideastern Michigan Library Co-op
G-4195 West Pasadena Avenue
Flint, MI 48504   810-732-1120
                                Fax: 810-732-1715
                  e-mail: cnash@genesse.freeret.org
                          www.fakon.edu/gdl/talking.htm

Summer reading programs, braille writer, magnifiers, closed-circuit T.V., large-print photocopier, cassette books and magazines, children's books on cassette, home visits and other reference materials on blindness and other handicaps.

Carolyn Nash, Librarian

5104 Muskegon County Library for the Blind
97 East Apple Avenue
Muskegon, MI 49442   231-724-6257
                                Fax: 231-724-6675
                                TDD: 231-722-4103
                     e-mail: mclsm@lakeland.lib.mi.uf
                                www.lakeland.lib.mi.uf

Summer reading programs, braille typewriter, magnifiers, closed-circuit T.V., large-print photocopier, cassette books and magazines, children's books on cassette, home visits and other reference materials on blindness and other handicaps, The Reading Edge, Perkins Brailler & large print books.

Linda Clapp, Librarian

5105 Northland Library Cooperative
316 East Chisholm
Alpena, MI 49707   517-356-1622
                                Fax: 517-354-3939
                     e-mail: nlc.lib.mi.us/lbph.htm

Summer reading programs, braille writer, magnifiers, closed-circuit T.V., large-print photocopier, cassette books and magazines, children's books on cassette, home visits and other reference materials on blindness and other handicaps.

Catherine Glomski, Librarian

5106 Upper Peninsula Library for the Blind
1615 Presque Isle Avenue
Marquette, MI 49855   906-228-7697
                            Fax: 906-228-5627
                    e-mail: uplbph@lib.up.net

Summer reading programs, braille writer, magnifiers, closed-circuit T.V., large-print photocopier, cassette books and magazines, children's books on cassette, home visits and other reference materials on blindness and other handicaps.

Suzanne Dees, Librarian

5107 Washtenaw County Library
P.O. Box 8645
Ann Arbor, MI 48107   734-971-6059
                            Fax: 734-971-3892
                    e-mail: wash@tln.lib.mi.us

Summer reading programs, braille writer, magnifiers, closed-circuit T.V., large-print photocopier, cassette books and magazines, children's books on cassette, home visits and other reference materials on blindness and other handicaps.

Margeret Wolfe, Librarian

5108 Wayne County Regional Library for the Blind & Physically Handicapped
30555 Michigan Avenue
Westland, MI 48186   734-727-7306
                            Fax: 734-727-7333
                            TTY: 734-427-7330
        e-mail: wcrbph@wayneregional.lib.mi.us
                    wayneregional.lib.mi.us

Summer reading programs, braille writer, magnifiers, closed-circuit T.V., large-print photocopier, cassette books and magazines, children's books on cassette, home visits and other reference materials on blindness and other handicaps.

4000 Members

Fred Howkins, Director

Minnesota

5109 KDWB Variety Family Center
University of Minnesota Gateway
200 Oak Street SE, Suite 160
Minneapolis, MN 55455   612-626-3087
                              800-233-1200
                        Fax: 612-626-2134
                www.peds.umn.edu/peds-adol/

A University-Community partnership that provides family-centered services that promote physical, emotional, psychological and social health and well-being for children and youth at risk, including children and youth with disabilities. The center is dedicated to teaching, research, outreach and community services.

5110 Minnesota Library for the Blind & Physically Handicapped
P.O. Box 68 Highway 298
Fairbault, MN 55021   507-333-4828
                            800-722-0550
                      Fax: 507-333-4832
              e-mail: libblnd@state.mn.us

Summer reading programs, braille writer, magnifiers, closed-circuit T.V., large-print photocopier, cassette, large print, braille books and magazines, children's books on cassette, and other reference materials on blindness and other handicaps.

Catherine A. Durivage, Program Director

5111 National Resource Library on Youth With Disabilities
University of Minnesota
Box 721-UMHC
Minneapolis, MN 55455   612-625-5000
                              800-333-6293
                          www.cyfc.umn.edu

Offers comprehensive sources of information related to adolescents, disability and transition. The database contains bibliographic and training/education files for the medical community, families, parents and children with chronic illnesses.

5112 PACER Center, Inc.
4826 Chicago Avenue S
Minneapolis, MN 55417   612-827-2966
                            Fax: 612-827-3065
                            TTY: 612-827-7770
                    e-mail: pacer@pacer.org
                            www.pacer.org

Parent Training and Information (PTI) programs help parents to: understand their children's specific needs; communicate more effectively with professionals, participate in the educational planning process; and obtain information about relevant programs, services, and resources

5113 Star Center for Family Health
University of Minnesota Gateway
200 Oak Street SE, Suite 160
Minneapolis, MN 55455   612-626-4260
Fax: 612-626-2134
www.peds.umn.edu/peds-adol/

Helps children, youth, and families develop new and enhanced ways of coping with stress, learn strategies for adjusting to living with a chronic illness, and discover new ways of finding health, balance and well-being.

Elizabeth Latts, MSW, Resource Coordinator

Mississippi

5114 Mississippi Library Commission
5455 Executive Place
Jackson, MS 39206   601-354-7208
Fax: 601-354-6077
TDD: 601-354-6411
e-mail: tbbs@mls.lib.ms.us
www.mlc.state.me.us/tbbs.htm

Summer reading programs, braille writer, magnifiers, closed-circuit T.V., large-print photocopier, cassette books and magazines, children's books on cassette, home visits and other reference materials on blindness and other handicaps.

Rahya Puckett, Librarian

Missouri

5115 Technology Access Center
12110 Clayton Road
St. Louis, MO 63130   314-569-8404
Fax: 314-569-8449
TTY: 314-569-8446
e-mail: mostltac@aol.com

Technology group of parents, consumers and professionals; provides resources to help children and adults who have disabilities gain access to the benefits of technology. Includes nationwide network of community-based assistive technology, resource centers, hands on consultants and product demonstrations.

5116 Whitney Library for the Blind - Assemblies of God
1445 Boonville Avenue
Springfield, MO 65802   417-862-2781
Fax: 417-863-7276

Offers braille and cassette lending library, braille and cassette Sunday school materials for all ages, braille and cassette periodicals and resource assistance.

Paul Weingariner, Librarian

5117 Wolfner Memorial Library for the Blind
P.O. Box 387
Jefferson City, MO 65102   573-751-8720
Fax: 573-526-2985
TDD: 800-347-1379
e-mail: beckles@mail.sos.state.mo.us

Summer reading programs, braille writer, magnifiers, closed-circuit T.V., large-print photocopier, cassette books and magazines, children's books on cassette, home visits and other reference materials on blindness and other handicaps.

Elizabeth Eckles, Librarian

Montana

5118 Montana State Library
1515 East Sixth Avenue
Helena, MT 59620   406-444-3009
Fax: 406-444-5612
TDD: 406-444-5431

Summer reading programs, braille writer, magnifiers, closed-circuit T.V., large-print photocopier, cassette books and magazines, children's books on cassette, home visits and other reference materials on blindness and other handicaps.

Sandra Jarvie, Librarian

Nebraska

5119 Nebraska Library Commission Talking Book and Braille Service
1200 N Street, Suite 120
Lincoln, NE 68508   402-471-4038
800-742-7691
Fax: 402-471-6244
e-mail: doertii@neon.nk.state.ne.us
www.nlc.state.ne.us/tbbs/tbbs1

Summer reading programs, braille writer, magnifiers, closed-circuit T.V., large-print photocopier, cassette books and magazines, children's books on cassette, home visits and other reference materials on blindness and other handicaps.

David Oertli, Librarian

5120 North Platte Public Library
120 West 4th Street
North Platte, NE 69101　　　　308-535-8036

Summer reading programs, braille writer, magnifiers, closed-circuit T.V., large-print photocopier, cassette books and magazines, children's books on cassette, home visits and other reference materials on blindness and other handicaps.

Brenda Behsman, Librarian

Nevada

5121 Las Vegas-Clark County Library District
1401 East Flamingo Road
Las Vegas, NV 89119　　　　702-453-1180
　　　　　　　　　　　　Fax: 702-733-1567

Summer reading programs, braille writer, magnifiers, closed-circuit T.V., large-print photocopier, cassette books and magazines, children's books on cassette, home visits and other reference materials on blindness and other handicaps.

Mary Anne Morton, Librarian

5122 Nevada State Library and Archives
Capitol Complex
Carson City, NV 89710　　　　702-687-5154
　　　　　　　　　　　　Fax: 702-687-8311
　　　　　　　　　　　　TDD: 702-687-8338
　　　　　　　　　e-mail: putnam@equinox.unr.edu

Summer reading programs, braille writer, magnifiers, closed-circuit T.V., large-print photocopier, cassette books and magazines, children's books on cassette, home visits and other reference materials on blindness and other handicaps.

Kevin E. Putnam, Librarian

New Hampshire

5123 New Hampshire State Library
117 Pleasant Street
Concord, NH 03301　　　　603-271-3429
　　　　　　e-mail: talking@lilac.nhsh.lib.nh.us
　　　　　　　　　　　　www.state.nh.us

Summer reading programs, braille writer, magnifiers, closed-circuit T.V., large-print photocopier, cassette books and magazines, children's books on cassette, home visits and other reference materials on blindness and other handicaps.

Eileen Keim, Librarian

New Jersey

5124 Center for Enabling Technology
622 Route 10 W, Suite 22B
Whippany, NJ 07981　　　　973-428-1455
　　　　　　　　　　　　Fax: 973-560-9751
　　　　　　　　　　　　TTY: 973-428-1450
　　　　　　　　　　　e-mail: cetnj@aol.com

Technology group of parents, consumers and professionals; provides resources to help children and adults who have disabilities gain access to the benefits of technology. Includes nationwide network of community-based assistive technology, resource centers, hands on consultants and product demonstrations.

5125 New Jersey Library for the Blind and Physically Handicapped
2300 Stuyvesant Avenue
Trenton, NJ 08625
　　　　　　　　　　　　800-792-8322
　　　　　　　　　　　　Fax: 609-530-6384
　　　　　　　　　　　　TDD: 609-633-7250

Summer reading programs, braille writer, magnifiers, closed-circuit T.V., large-print photocopier, cassette books and magazines, children's books on cassette, home visits and other reference materials on blindness and other handicaps.

Vianne Connor, Librarian

New Mexico

5126 New Mexico State Library for the Blind And Physically Handicapped
325 Don Gaspar
Santa Fe, NM 87503　　　　505-827-3830
　　　　　　　　　　　　Fax: 505-827-3888
　　　　　　　　e-mail: jbrewstr@stlib.state.nm.us

Summer reading programs, braille writer, magnifiers, closed-circuit T.V., large-print photocopier, cassette books and magazines, children's books on cassette, home visits and other reference materials on blindness and other handicaps.

Glee Wenzel, Librarian

New York

5127 Helen Keller International
90 Washington Street
New York, NY 10006   212-943-0890
                            Fax: 212-943-1220

Nonprofit organization for the blind.

Joh M. Palmer, Executive Director

5128 Helen Keller National Center
111 Middle Neck Road
Sands Point, NY 11050   516-944-8900
                            Fax: 516-944-7302

Provides diagnostic, evaluation, short term comprehensive rehabilitation and personal adjustment training. A technical assistance center is offered providing assistance to public and private agencies and to parent groups who work towards community integration and the enhancement of the quality of life. A national parent network is also provided that develops and shares information about advocacy, legislation, new services and achievements.

5129 Institute for Basic Research In Developmental Disabilities
1050 Forest Hill Road
Staten Island, NY 10314   718-494-0600
                            Fax: 718-494-0837

Conducts research into neurodegenerative diseases, Alzheimer's disease, developmental disabilities, fragile X syndrome, Down Syndrome, autism, epilepsy and basic science issues underlying all developmental disabilities.

Dr. Krystyna Wisniewski

5130 JGB Cassette Library International
15 West 65th Street
New York, NY 10023   212-769-6331

Summer reading programs, braille writer, magnifiers, closed-circuit T.V., large-print photocopier, cassette books and magazines, children's books on cassette, home visits and other reference materials on blindness and other handicaps.

Bruce Massis

5131 Keren-Or, Inc.
3 57th Avenue
New York, NY 10010   212-279-4070
                            Fax: 212-279-4043
                            www.keren-or.org

Maintains the Keren-Or Center for the Multiply Handicapped Blind Child in Jerusalem for rehabilitation and training. Funds acquired through contributions, bequests and legacies.

Paul Goldenberg, Executive Director

5132 Laboratory of Dermatology Research
Memorial Sloane-Kettering Cancer Center
1275 York Avenue
New York, NY 10021   212-639-7766
                            Fax: 212-717-3363

Specific studies on the identification of skin disorders and dermatology.

Biijan Safai, MD, Head

5133 Nassau Library System
900 Jerusalem Avenue
Uniondale, NY 11553   516-292-8920
                            Fax: 516-481-4777
                            e-mail: nls@lilrc.org

Summer reading programs, braille writer, magnifiers, closed-circuit T.V., large-print photocopier, cassette books and magazines, children's books on cassette, home visits and other reference materials on blindness and other handicaps.

Dorothy Pruyear, Librarian

5134 New York State Talking Book & Braille Library
Empire State Plaza, CEC
Albany, NY 12230   518-474-5935
                            800-342-3688
                            Fax: 518-474-5786
                            TDD: 518-474-7121
                            e-mail: jane@mail.nysed.goved.gov
                            www.nysl.nysed.gov

Free books on audio cassette, cassette players, braille books, summer reading programs, braille writer, magnifiers, cassette books and magazines, children's books on cassette, reference materials on blindness and other handicaps.

Jane Somers, Director

5135 Rockefeller University Laboratory for Investigative Dermatology
1230 York Avenue
New York, NY 10021 212-327-7458
Fax: 212-570-8232

Research into skin disorders and the whole specialty of dermatology in general.

D. Martin Carter, MD, PhD, Head

5136 Techspress Resource Center for Independent Living
401-409 Columbia Street, PO Box 210
Utica, NY 13503 315-797-4642
Fax: 315-797-4747
e-mail: lana.gossin@rcil.com

Technology group of parents, consumers and professionals; provides resources to help children and adults who have disabilities gain access to the benefits of technology. Includes nationwide network of community-based assistive technology, resource centers, hands on consultants and product demonstrations.

North Carolina

5137 Carolina Computer Access Center Metro School
700 E 2nd Street
Charlotte, NC 28202 704-342-3004
Fax: 704-342-1513
e-mail: ccacnc@aol.com

Technology group of parents, consumers and professionals; provides resources to help children and adults who have disabilities gain access to the benefits of technology. Includes nationwide network of community-based assistive technology, resource centers, hands on consultants and product demonstrations.

5138 North Carolina Library for the Blind
1811 Capital Blvd.
Raleigh, NC 27635 919-733-4376
Fax: 919-733-6910
TDD: 919-733-1462
e-mail: nclbph@ncsl.der.state.nc

Summer reading programs, braille writer, magnifiers, closed-circuit T.V., large-print photocopier, cassette books and magazines, children's books on cassette, home visits and other reference materials on blindness and other handicaps.

Francine Martin, Librarian

Ohio

5139 American Council of Blind Parents
34400 Cedar Road, Apt. 108
University Heights, OH 44121
800-424-8666

Members are sighted parents of blind or visually impaired children. Offers a forum for support and outreach, sharing of experiences in parent-child relationships, and educational and cultural information about child development. Monitors developments in technical and legislative arenas.

Nola Webb, President

5140 Blick Clinic for Developmental Disabilities
640 W. Market Street
Akron, OH 44303 330-762-5425

Dr. Jane Holan

5141 Cleveland Public Library
525 Superior Avenue
Cleveland, OH 44114 216-623-2800
Fax: 216-623-7015
e-mail: lbphmgr1@library.cpl.org
www.org.cpl

Summer reading programs, braille writer, magnifiers, closed-circuit T.V., large-print photocopier, cassette books and magazines, children's books on cassette, home visits and other reference materials on blindness and other handicaps.

Barbara Mates, Librarian

5142 Ohio Regional Library for the Blind and Physically Handicapped
800 Vine Street, Library Square
Cincinnati, OH 45202 513-369-6999
Fax: 513-369-3111
TDD: 513-369-6072

Summer reading programs, braille writer, magnifiers, closed-circuit T.V., large-print photocopier, cassette books and magazines, children's books on cassette, home visits and other reference materials on blindness and other handicaps.

Donna Foust, Librarian

5143 Technology Resource Center
2049 Harshman Road
Dayton te, OH 45424

Fax: 937-236-3119
TDD: 937-236-6110
e-mail: trcdoh@aol.com
www.trcd.org

Technology group of parents, consumers and professionals; provides resources to help children and adults who have disabilities gain access to the benefits of technology. Includes nationwide network of community-based assistive technology, resource centers, hands on consultants and product demonstrations.

Oklahoma

5144 Oklahoma Library for the Blind & Physically Handicapped
300 NE 18th Street
Oklahoma City, OK 73105   405-521-3514
Fax: 405-521-4582
e-mail: olbph@altn.obl.state.ok.us
www.state.ok.us/library

Summer reading programs, braille writer, magnifiers, closed-circuit T.V., large-print photocopier, cassette books and magazines, children's books on cassette, home visits and other reference materials on blindness and other handicaps.

Geraldine Adams, Librarian

5145 Tulsa City-County Library System
400 Civic Center
Tulsa, OK 74103   918-596-7977

Summer reading programs, braille writer, magnifiers, closed-circuit T.V., large-print photocopier, cassette books and magazines, children's books on cassette, home visits and other reference materials on blindness and other handicaps.

Ellen Ontko, Librarian

Oregon

5146 Oregon State Library, Talking Book and Braille Services
250 Winter Street NW
Salem, OR 97310   503-378-4243
Fax: 503-588-7119
TDD: 503-378-4276
e-mail: tbabs@sparkie.osl.state.or.us

Cassette books and magazines, children's books on cassette, home visits and other reference materials on blindness and other handicaps.

Donna Bensen, Regional Librarian

Pennsylvania

5147 Free Library of Philadelphia
919 Walnut Street
Philadelphia, PA 19107   215-683-3213
800-222-1754
Fax: 215-683-3211
e-mail: flpblind@library.phila.gov

Summer reading programs, braille writer, magnifiers, closed-circuit T.V., large-print photocopier, cassette books and magazines, children's books on cassette, home visits and other reference materials on blindness and other handicaps.

Vickie Lange Collins, Administrator

5148 Library for the Blind & Physically Handicapped, Leonard C. Staisey Building
Carnegie Library of Pittsburgh
4724 Baum Boulevard
Pittsburgh, PA 15213   412-687-2440
800-242-0586
Fax: 412-687-2442
e-mail: clbph@clpgh.org
www.clpgh.org/clp/lbph

Provides on loan recorded books and magazines, large print books, and described videos to Western Pennsylvania residents unable to use standard printed materials due to visual, physically-based reading disabilities. Also loans special cassette and disc machines; does not loan equipment to play described videos. Information about disabilities and related agencies is also available.

Sue Murdock, Agency Head
Kathleen Kappel, Assistant Agency Head

Rhode Island

5149 TechACCESS Center of Rhode Island
100 Jefferson Boulevard
Warwick, RI 02888

Fax: 401-463-3433
TTY: 401-273-0202
e-mail: techaccess@techaccess-ri.org
www.trcd.org

Technology group of parents, consumers and professionals; provides resources to help children and adults who have disabilities gain access to the benefits of technology. Includes nationwide network of community-based assistive technology, resource centers, hands on consultants and product demonstrations.

South Carolina

5150 Children's Center for Cancer and Blood Disorders
University of South Carolina School of Medicine
5 Richland Memorial Park
Columbia, SC 29203

803-540-1000
Fax: 803-253-4637

Joint clinical and basic research of juvenile cancer and blood disorders.

Dr. Robert S. Ettinger, Director

5151 Family Connection of South Carolina
2712 Middleburg Drive, Suite 103-B
Columbia, SC 29204

803-252-0914
800-578-8750
Fax: 803-799-8017
e-mail: famconn@mindspring.org

Support network for parents of children with disabilities and/or chronic illness. Veteran parents offer support to parents who are just learning of their child's diagnosis. Offers support and insight into parenting a child with special needs, as well as referrals to trained veteran parents.

5152 South Carolina State Library
301 Gervais St., P.O. Box 821
Columbia, SC 29202

803-734-0470
Fax: 803-737-9983
TDD: 803-734-7298
e-mail: guynell@leo.scsl.state.sc.us
www.state.sc.us/scsl.bph.html

Summer reading programs, braille writer, magnifiers, closed-circuit T.V., large-print photocopier, cassette books and magazines, children's books on cassette, home visits and other reference materials on blindness and other handicaps.

Guynell Williams, Librarian

South Dakota

5153 South Dakota State Library
800 Governors Drive
Pierre, SD 57501

605-773-3131
Fax: 605-773-4950
TDD: 605-773-4950
e-mail: darn@stlib.state.sd.us

Summer reading programs, braille writer, magnifiers, closed-circuit T.V., large-print photocopier, cassette books and magazines, children's books on cassette, home visits and other reference materials on blindness and other handicaps.

Daniel Boyd, Librarian

Tennessee

5154 East Tennessee Technology Access Center
4918 N.Broadway
Knoxville, TN 37918

423-219-0130
Fax: 423-219-0137
e-mail: etstactn@aol.com
www.korrnet.org/ettac/

Technology group of parents, consumers and professionals; provides resources to help children and adults who have disabilities gain access to the benefits of technology. Includes nationwide network of community-based assistive technology, resource centers, hands on consultants and product demonstrations.

5155 St. Jude Children's Research Hospital
332 North Lauderdale Street
Memphis, TN 38101

901-495-3300

5156 West Tennessee Special Technology Access
60 Lynoak Cove
Jackson, TN 38305

901-668-3888
Fax: 901-668-1666
e-mail: mdoumitt@starcenter.tn.org
www.starcenter.tn.org

Technology group of parents, consumers and professionals; provides resources to help children and adults who have disabilities gain access to the benefits of technology. Includes nationwide network of community-based assistive technology, resource centers, hands on consultants and product demonstrations.

Texas

5157 Baylor College of Medicine Birth Defects Center
6621 Fannin Street
Houston, TX 77030 713-770-3013
Fax: 713-770-4294

Frank Greenberg, M.D., Director

5158 Texas State Library
P.O. Box 12927
Austin, TX 78711 512-463-5460
Fax: 512-463-5436
TDD: 512-463-5449
e-mail: dale.propp@tsl.state.tx.us

Summer reading programs, braille writer, magnifiers, closed-circuit T.V., large-print photocopier, cassette books and magazines, children's books on cassette, home visits and other reference materials on blindness and other handicaps.

Dale Propp, Librarian

Utah

5159 Utah State Library Commission
250 North 1950 West Suite A
Salt Lake City, UT 84116 801-715-6777
Fax: 801-715-6767

Summer reading programs, braille writer, magnifiers, closed-circuit T.V., large-print photocopier, cassette books and magazines, children's books on cassette, home visits and other reference materials on blindness and other handicaps.

Gerald Buttars, Librarian

Vermont

5160 Vermont Department of Libraries
Box 1870, RD #4
Montpelier, VT 05602 802-828-3273
Fax: 802-828-2199
e-mail: ssu@dol.state.vt.us

Summer reading programs, braille writer, magnifiers, closed-circuit T.V., large-print photocopier, cassette books and magazines, children's books on cassette, home visits and other reference materials on blindness and other handicaps.

S. Francis Woods, Librarian

Virginia

5161 Alexandria Library Talking Book Service
826 Slaters Lane
Alexandria, VA 22314 703-838-4295
Fax: 703-838-4614
TDD: 703-838-4568
e-mail: emccaffr@lea.eda
www.aleyandrea.lib.va.vs

Summer reading programs, braille writer, magnifiers, closed-circuit T.V., large-print photocopier, cassette books and magazines, children's books on cassette, home visits and other reference materials on blindness and other handicaps.

Patricia Bates, Librarian

5162 Arlington County Department of Libraries
1015 North Quincy Street
Arlington, VA 22201 703-358-5990
Fax: 703-358-5962
TDD: 703-358-6320

Summer reading programs, braille writer, magnifiers, closed-circuit T.V., large-print photocopier, cassette books and magazines, children's books on cassette, home visits and other reference materials on blindness and other handicaps.

Roxanne Barnes, Librarian

5163 Division on Visual Impairments
1920 Association Drive
Reston, VA 22091 703-620-3660
888-232-7733
Fax: 703-264-9494
http://www.cec.sped.org

Members are teachers, college faculty members, administrators, supervisors and others concerned with enhancing the educational opportunities of children and youth with visual impairments. Publishes the DVI quarterly newsletter.

Stuart Wittenster, President
Robert Brasher, Editor

5164 Fairfax County Public Library
2501 Sherwood Hall Lane
Alexandria, VA 22306 703-660-6943
Fax: 703-765-5893
TDD: 703-660-8524
e-mail: sjapikse@leo.vsla.edu
www.co.fairfax.va.us

Summer reading programs, braille writer, magnifiers, closed-circuit T.V., large-print photocopier, cassette books and magazines, children's books on cassette, home visits and other reference materials on blindness and other handicaps.

Jeanette Studley, Librarian

5165 Hampton Subregional Library for the Blind
4207 Victoria Blvd.
Hampton, VA 23669   757-727-1900
Fax: 757-717-1151
e-mail: swoolard@leo.vsla.edu

Summer reading programs, braille writer, magnifiers, closed-circuit T.V., large-print photocopier, cassette books and magazines, children's books on cassette, home visits and other reference materials on blindness and other handicaps.

Mary Sue Woolard, Librarian

5166 Newport News Public Library System
112 Main Street
Newport News, VA 23601   757-591-4821
Fax: 757-591-7425
e-mail: shalswin@leo.vsla.edu

Summer reading programs, braille writer, magnifiers, closed-circuit T.V., large-print photocopier, cassette books and magazines, children's books on cassette, home visits and other reference materials on blindness and other handicaps.

Sue Balswin, Librarian

5167 Roanoke City Public Library System
2607 Salem Turnpike, NW
Roanoke, VA 24017   540-853-2648
Fax: 540-853-1030

Summer reading programs, braille writer, magnifiers, closed-circuit T.V., large-print photocopier, cassette books and magazines, children's books on cassette, home visits and other reference materials on blindness and other handicaps.

Rebecca Cooper, Librarian

5168 Virginia Beach Public Library
930 Independence Blvd.
Virginia Beach, VA 23455   757-464-9361
Fax: 757-460-7606

Summer reading programs, braille writer, magnifiers, closed-circuit T.V., large-print photocopier, cassette books and magazines, children's books on cassette, home visits and other reference materials on blindness and other handicaps.

Susan Head, Librarian

5169 Virginia State Library for the Visually and Physically Handicapped
1901 Roane Street
Richmond, VA 23222   804-367-0014

Summer reading programs, braille writer, magnifiers, closed-circuit T.V., large-print photocopier, cassette books and magazines, children's books on cassette, home visits and other reference materials on blindness and other handicaps.

Mary Ruth Halapatz, Librarian

Washington

5170 Washington Library for the Blind and Physically Handicapped
821 Lenora Street
Seattle, WA 98129   206-464-6930
Fax: 206-464-0247
e-mail: wtbbl@spl.lib.wa.us
www.spl.lib.wa.us

Summer reading programs, braille writer, magnifiers, closed-circuit T.V., large-print photocopier, cassette books and magazines, children's books on cassette, home visits and other reference materials on blindness and other handicaps.

Jan Ames, Librarian

West Virginia

5171 Cabell County Public Library
455 Ninth Street Plaza
Huntington, WV 25701   304-523-9451
Fax: 304-528-5701

Summer reading programs, braille writer, magnifiers, closed-circuit T.V., large-print photocopier, cassette books and magazines, children's books on cassette, home visits and other reference materials on blindness and other handicaps.

Suzanne Coldiron, Librarian

5172 Kanawha County Public Library
123 Capitol Street
Charleston, WV 25301   304-558-2323
Fax: 304-348-6530

Summer reading programs, braille writer, magnifiers, closed-circuit T.V., large-print photocopier, cassette books and magazines, children's books on cassette, home visits and other reference materials on blindness and other handicaps.

Dixie Smith, Librarian

5173 West Virginia Library Commission
1900 Kanawha Blvd. East
Charleston, WV 25305   304-340-3200
Fax: 304-558-4061
e-mail: fesenmf@mars.wrlc.wvnet.edu
www.wvlc.wvnet.edu

Summer reading programs, braille writer, magnifiers, closed-circuit T.V., large-print photocopier, cassette books and magazines, children's books on cassette, home visits and other reference materials on blindness and other handicaps.

Francis Fesenmainer, Librarian

5174 West Virginia School for the Blind
301 East Main Street
Romney, WV 26757   304-822-3521
Fax: 304-822-4896
e-mail: cjohn@access.mountain.net

Summer reading programs, braille writer, magnifiers, closed-circuit T.V., large-print photocopier, cassette books and magazines, children's books on cassette, home visits and other reference materials on blindness and other handicaps.

Cynthia Johnson, Librarian

Wisconsin

5175 Brown County Library
515 Pine Street
Green Bay, WI 54301   920-448-4400

Summer reading programs, braille writer, magnifiers, closed-circuit T.V., large-print photocopier, cassette books and magazines, children's books on cassette, home visits and other reference materials on blindness and other handicaps.

Angela Basten, Librarian

Research Centers

5176 Association for Research of Childhood Cancer
P.O. Box 251
Buffalo, NY 14225   716-681-4433

A non-profit organization staffed by volunteers and formed in 1971 by parents who had lost children to pediatric cancer. Chapter members raise funds by various projects in order to provide seed money to various pediatric research centers in order to find a cure and, ultimately, prevent the types of cancers that attack children.

5177 Division for Research (CEC-DR)
The Council for Exceptional Children
1920 Association Drive
Reston, VA 20191   703-620-3660
Fax: 703-264-9474
TTY: 703-264-9446
www.cec.spec.org

Devoted to the advancement of research related to the education of individuals with disabilities and or who are gifted. Members include university, public, and private school teachers, researchers, administrators, psychologists, speech/language clinicians, parents of children with special learning needs.

5178 National Alliance for Research on Schizophrenia & Depression
60 Cutter Mill Road Suite 404
Great Neck, NY 11021   516-829-0091
800-829-8289
www.mhsource.com/narsad

5179 National Eye Research Foundation
910 Skokie Boulevard
Northbrook, IL 60062

Devoted to the enhancement of care and study of eye related diseases.

Alaska

5180 Alaska Services for Enabling Technology
P.O. Box 6485
Sitka, AK 99835   907-747-3019
e-mail: asetseak@aol.com

Technology group of parents, consumers and professionals; provides resources to help children and adults who have disabilities gain access to the benefits of technology. Includes nationwide network of community-based assistive technology, resource centers, hands on consultants and product demonstrations.

California

5181 Computer Access Center
5901 Green Valley Circle, Suite 320
Culver City, CA 90230   310-338-1597
                              Fax: 310-338-9318
                          e-mail: cac@cac.org
                                  www.cac.org

Includes nationwide network of community-based assistive technology, resource centers, hands on consultants and product demonstrations.

5182 Team of Advocates for Special Kids
100 W Cerritos Avenue
Anaheim, CA 92805   714-533-8275
                         Fax: 714-533-2533
                     e-mail: taskca@aol.com

Technology group of parents, consumers and professionals; provides resources to help children and adults who have disabilities gain access to the benefits of technology. Includes nationwide network of community-based assistive technology, resource centers, hands on consultants and product demonstrations.

5183 University of California, San Francisco Dermatology Drug Research
515 Spruce
San Francisco, CA 94143   415-476-2001
                                Fax: 415-221-4751

Conducts clinical testing of new or existing pharmalogic agents used in the treatment of skin disorders.

John Koo, MD, Director

Utah

5184 Early Intervention Research Institute, Developmental Center
Utah State University

Logan, UT 84322   435-750-1172

5185 Primary Children's Medical Center
Graduate Parents
100 N Medical Drive
Salt Lake City, UT 84113   801-588-3899
                                 Fax: 801-588-3869
                         e-mail: PCSWAR2@jhc.com

Wyoming

5186 Parent and Information Center
5 N Lobban
Buffalo, WY 82834   307-684-2277
                          800-660-9742
                     Fax: 307-684-5314
             e-mail: tdawsonpic@vcn.com

Support network for parents of children with disabilities and/or chronic illness. Veteran parents offer support to parents who are just learning of their child's diagnosis. Offers support and insight into parenting a child with special needs, as well as referrals to trained veteran parents.

International

5187 Research Trust for Metabolic Diseases in Children
Goldengates Lodge Weston Rd., Crewe
Cheshire,
United Kingdom

Dedicated to providing the most up-to-date medical knowledge for the families and friends of people suffering from this and related diseases.

Audio Video

5188 Assisting Parents Through the Mourning Process
Hope, Inc.
55 East 100 North
Logan, UT 84321   435-752-9533
                        Fax: 435-752-9533

Describes the mourning process experienced by some parents of children with disabilities and ways in which the professional can help them through the process.

20 minutes

5189 CANCER
Rosen Publishing Group
29 East 21st St.
New York, NY 10010   212-777-3017
                            800-237-9932
                       Fax: 212-436-4643
           e-mail: rosenpub@tribeca.ios.com

Interviews with experts and cancer patients reveal the many types, causes, and treatments for cancer. Recommended for grades 7-12.

30 Minutes
ISBN: 0-823921-76-0

5190 Disability Awareness

Louise Welsh Schrank, author

Active Parenting Publishers
810 Franklin Court, Suite B
Marietta, GA 30067

800-825-0060
Fax: 770-429-0334
www.activeparenting.com

Helps viewers think about how they feel when confronted by people with disabilities. Close-captioned with study guide.

19 minutes

5191 Face First

Fanlight Productions
47 Halifax Street
Boston, MA 02131

617-469-4999
Fax: 617-469-3379
e-mail: fanlight@fanlight.com
www.fanlight.com

Profiles of several people born with facial deformities; they chronicle both physical pain and the pain of rejection, as well as the strengths that have enabled them to achieve successful adult lives.

29 minutes

5192 Heart to Heart

Blind Children's Center
4120 Marathon Street
Los Angeles, CA 90029

323-664-2153
Fax: 323-665-3828
e-mail: info@blindchildrenscenter.org
www.blindchildrenscenter.org

Parents of blind and partially sighted children talk about their feelings.

videotape

5193 It's Just Part of My Life

National Kidney Foundation
30 East 33rd Street
New York, NY 10016

212-889-2210
800-622-9010
Fax: 212-689-9261
www.kidney.org

A 15-minute program for adolescent dialysis patients and their families.

5194 LOVAAS Learning Videotapes

Dr. O. Ivar Lovaas, Director of UCLA Young Autism, author

8700 Shoal Creek Blvd
Austin, TX 78757

800-897-3202
Fax: 800-397-7633

Five videotapes which present valuable information on the content and execution of learning strategies for children with developmental disabilities. Tape 1-Getting Ready to Learn; 2-Early Language; 3-Basic Self-Help Skills, 4-Advanced Language; and 5-Expanding Your Child's World. You can purchase the complete set for $740.00 or separately as listed.

5195 Laughter Therapy

P.O. Box 827
Monterey, CA 93942

408-625-3788

These people can supply tapes of old Candid Camera movies to patients. Maintains a library of 50 topics.

5196 Lead Poisoning

Fanlight Productions
47 Halifax St
Boston, MA 02130

617-469-4999
Fax: 617-469-3379
e-mail: fanlight@fanlight.com
www.fanlight.com

The disastrous effects of environmental lead on both children and adults. Dartmouth Hitchcock Medical Center Series, The Doctor is In...

28 minutes

5197 Let's Eat

Blind Children's Center
4120 Marathon Street
Los Angeles, CA 90029

323-664-2153
Fax: 323-665-3828
e-mail: info@blindchildrenscenter.org
www.blindchildrenscenter.org

Teaches competent feeding skills to children with visual impairments.

videotape

5198 Meeting the Challenge: Parenting Children with Disabilities

Active Parenting Publishers
810 Franklin Court, Suite B
Marietta, GA 30067

800-825-0060
Fax: 770-429-0334
www.activeparenting.com

Award-winning video for parents of special-needs children. Other parents share their stories.

94 minutes

5199 No Fears, No Tears

Fanlight Productions
47 Halifax St
Boston, MA 02130

617-469-4999
Fax: 617-469-3379
e-mail: fanlight@fanlight.com
www.fanlight.com

Dr. Leora Kuttner explore the effects of children's pain management therapies. See original No Fears, No Tears - 13 Years Later.

27 minutes

5200 No Fears, No Tears - 13 Years Later
Fanlight Productions
47 Halifax St
Boston, MA 02130   617-469-4999
Fax: 617-469-3379
e-mail: fanlight@fanlight.com
www.fanlight.com

Dr. Leora Kuttner explore the effects of children's pain management therapies 13 years after use. See original No Fears, No Tears.

47 minutes

5201 Not Just a Cancer Patient

Jana Levenson Brenman & Tom Hill, author

Fanlight Productions
47 Halifax Street
Boston, MA 02130
800-937-4113
Fax: 617-524-8838
e-mail: fanlight@tiac.net
www.fanlight.com

Focuses on several articulate teenagers who are undergoing cancer treatment to help caregivers understand the needs and feelings of this population.

23 Minutes
ISBN: 1-572950-86-2

5202 See What I Feel

Alan P. Sloan, author

Britannica Film Co.
345 Fourth Street
San Francisco, CA 94107   415-227-9457

A blind child tells her friends about her trip to the zoo. Each experience was explained as a blind child would experience it. A teacher's guide comes with this video.

Films

5203 Stress Reduction Tapes, Stress Reduction Clinic
University Massachusetts Medical
P.O. Box 547
Lexington, MA 02173   508-856-2656
www.mindfulnesstapes.com

There are two tapes sold separately that are appropriate for preteens or adolescents. Tapes may be ordered from the website.

5204 We Can do it: Children Cope with Cancer
Ajn Company
555 West 57th Street
New York, NY 10019   212-582-8820
800-225-5256
Fax: 212-586-5462

Showes children techniques that will help them deal with their cancer treatment.

14 Minutes

5205 When Parents Can't Fix It
Fanlight Productions
47 Halifax St
Boston, MA 02130   617-469-4999
Fax: 617-469-3379
e-mail: fanlight@fanlight.com
www.fanlight.com

Looks at the stresses and rewards in the lives of five families who are raising children with disabilities. Offers a realistic look and different family strengths and coping styles.

58 minutes

Web Sites

5206 Adolescent Health On-Line
www.ama-assn.org

Information on adolescent health issues, including GAPS (Guidelines for Adolescent Preventive Services).

5207 American Board of Pediatrics
www.aap.org

5208 American College of Medical Genetics
www.faseb.org/genetics/acmg/

5209 American Society of Pediatric Neurosurgeons
www.aspn.org

5210 Americans with Disabilities Act Document Center
janweb.icdi.wvu.edu

5211 Archives of Pediatric and Adolescent Medicine
www.ama-assn.org

5212 Children's Health Information Network
www.ohsu.edu/cliniweb

A site providing web resources for children's health issues.

5213 Cliniweb
www.ohsu.edu/cliniweb

5214 Council for Exceptional Children
www.cec.sped.org

5215 Council of Regional Networks for Genetic Services: CORN

e-mail: lje@rw.ped.emory.edu

CORN brings together network representatives to facilitate communication and planning for genetic services, as well as to address national public health priorities in genetics.

5216 Easter Seals
www.easterseals.org

5217 European Society for Paediatric Urology
www.espu.org/

5218 GeneClinics: Medical Genetics Knowledge Base
www.geneclinics.org

Knowledge base of up-to-date information relating to testing the diagnosis, management, and counseling of those with inherited disorders.

5219 HealthWeb: Pediatrics
www.galter.nwu.edu/hw/ped

5220 International Foundation for Functional Gastrointestinal Disorders
www.iffgd.org

5221 KidsHealth at the AMA
www.ama-assn.org

Includes state-to-state guide to poison control centers, database of pediatricians and hospitals, basic-home care instructions and immunizations.

5222 LSUMC Family Medicine Patient Education
lib-sh.lsumc.edu

5223 MEDLINE from the National Library of Medicine
www.nlm.nih.gov

Database of medical information.

5224 MUMS: National Parent to Parent Network
www.waisman.wisc.edu/~rowley/mums/html

5225 MedWebplus: Pediatrics
www.medwebplus.com

Links to electronic publications, societies, patient information, databases in pediatrics.

5226 Medical Economics Company
www.medec.com

Full text for Non-Prescription Drugs and the PDR Guide to Drug Interactions.

5227 Medical Matrix: Pediatrics
www.medmatrix.org/SPages/Pediatric.asp

Peer-reviewed pediatric resources such as journals, news, text, practie guidlines and patient education.

5228 National Information Center for Children and Youth with Disabilities
www.nichcy.org

Offers answers on early intervention, special eduation, individualized education programs, and family, legal and adult transitional issues.

5229 National Institute on Disability and Rehabilitative Research (NIDRR)
www.ed.gov/offices/OSERS/NIDRR/

5230 National Library Service for the Blind and Physically Handicapped
lcweb.loc.gov/nls/nls.html

5231 National Organization for Rare Disorders Inc. (NORD)
www.nord_rdb.com

Committed to the identification, treatment and cure of rare disorders through programs of education, advocacy, research and service.

5232 Nuclear Medicine at Children's Hospital, Boston
nucmedweb.tch.harvard.edu

5233 Office of Special Education and Rehabilitative Services
www.ed.gov/offices/OSERS/

5234 Online Mendelian Inheritance in Man
www3.ncbi.nlm.nih.gov/Omim/searchomim.

Database of human genes and genetic disorders, complete with pictures, text, and referance information.

5235 PDR - Physicians' Desk Reference
www.pdr.net

5236 PEDINFO: an index of the Pediatric Internet
www.uab.edu/pedinfo

Collection of links to pediatric information maintained by the University of Alabama at Birmingham.

5237 Pediatric Database (Pedbase)
www.icondata.com/health/pedbase/files/

Discusses epidemiology, differential diagnosis (primary-genetic and secondary-nongenetic), pathogenesis, history, clinical features, investigations (imaging studies, serum, urine), and management (supportive).

5238 Pediatric Points of Interest
www.med.jhu.edu

Links to hospitals specializing in pediatrics, organizations, patient education materials, discussion lists, and journals.

5239 Pregnancy and Child Health Resource Center from Mayo Health O@sis
www.mayohealth.org

Covers the pediatric content of the much larger Mayo Health Oasis site, including: Stopping group B strep; Renewed effort to protect newborns; Playing it safe at Halloween; Children snoring.

5240 PubMed
www.ncbi.nlm.nih.gov/PubMed

Free links to participating online journals and other related databases.

5241 Rare Genetic Diseases in Children (NYU)
www.mcrcr2.med.nyu.edu

5242 Rare Genetic Diseases in Children: Disability Resources Directory
mcrcr2.med.nyu.edu

5243 Society for Adolescent Medicine
www3.uchc.edu/~sam

Discusses topics like Corporal Punishment in Schools, Eating Disorders, School-Based Health Clinics, includes meeting updates and society news activities.

5244 Southern Illinois University School of Medicine
www.siumed.edu/peds/teaching/patient/%20

Patient education material that links to cardiology teaching files and links to prescription drug information.

5245 TRIP Database
www.gwent.nhs.gov

Clinical guidelines, systematic reviews, and links to evidence-based medicine sites.

5246 TransWeb
1327 Jones Drive Suite 150
Ann Arbor, MI 48105   734-998-7314
Fax: 734-998-6710
www.transweb.org

Information about organ transplants, over the internet.

5247 WebMD Community Services
www.shn.net

Online consumer health information.

Books

5248 A Curriculum for Profoundly Handicapped Students
8700 Shoal Creek Blvd.
Austin, TX 78757
800-897-3202
Fax: 800-397-7633

This step-by-step guide describes how to assess and teach students with profound disabilities. It provides a sensible approach to pinpointing skills deficits and helping students master these skills. Detailed directions tell how to make and measure progress in the following basic areas: gross motor skills, fine motor skills, cognition skills, receptive communications skills, expressive communication skills, and social/affective skills.

388 pages Large Format
ISBN: 0-890794-47-2

5249 A Practical Parent's Handbook on Teaching Children with Learning Disabilities

Shelby Holley, author

Charles C. Thomas Publishing, Ltd.
2600 South First Street
Springfield, IL 62704   217-789-8980
800-258-8980
Fax: 217-789-9130
e-mail: books@ccthomas.com
www.ccthomas.com

Designed for the adult with no previous teaching experience so they may design and implement an effective remedial program. Second section provides simple objective tests that show what a child knows and what he/she needs to learn.

308 pages $41.95paperback
ISBN: 0-398059-03-9

5250 A Social Maturity Scale for Blind Preschool Children

Kathryn E. Maxfield, author

American Foundation for the Blind
11 Penn Plaza
New York, NY 10001   212-502-7600
800-232-5463
Fax: 212-502-7777
www.afb.org

An adaptation of the Vineland Social Maturity
Scale for use with children from infancy to 6
years of age.

57 pages Softcover
ISBN: 0-891280-59-6

5251 A Special Way to Care Friends of Karen
Box 217
Croton Falls, NY 10519

Free guide for those who wish to provide finan-
cial/emotional support for families of ill children. Discusses how to differentiate between
interference and advocacy. Explains how to organize, manage, and perpetuate a support fund.
Excellent resource.

**5252 Adaptive Play for Special Needs Children Strategies
to Enhance Communication**

Caroline Ramsey Musselwhite, author

8700 Shoal Creek Blvd.
Austin, TX 78757
800-897-3202
Fax: 800-397-7633

Adaptive play refers to play that has been altered in form, complexity, or intent to serve the
needs of children with disabilities. This book
summarizes recent advances in using play as a
learning tool, developing adaptive play materials, teaching specific skills through play, and
supporting the use of play in all settings.

249 pages Softcover
ISBN: 0-890793-03-4

**5253 Adolescent Drug Abuse: How to Spot it, Stop it and
Get Help for Your Family**

Nikki Babbit, Ph.D, author

O'Reilly and Associates, Inc.
101 Morris Street
Sebastopol, CA 95472
800-998-9938
Fax: 707-829-0104
e-mail: patientguides@oreilly.com
www.patientcenters.com

This book offers parents clear information, support and guidance by helping them understand
the disease model of drug abuse, and that its not
their fault, overcome family confusion, denial,
and excuses to getting help, find allies in the
community to help your child feel the appropriate consequences of his/her actions, know what
to look for in chemical assessment facilities and
see what kind of help can be given to your child
in treatment, listen to voices of dozens of parents and teens.

**5254 An Introduction to the Nature and Needs of Students
with Mild Disabilities**

Carroll J. Jones, author

Charles C. Thomas Publishing, Ltd.
2600 South First Street
Springfield, IL 62704   217-789-8980
800-258-8980
Fax: 217-789-9130
e-mail: books@ccthomas.com
www.ccthomas.com

Ideal source information for the special educator. Information on services in Europe/US, legislation and litigation.

300 pages $50.95paperback
ISBN: 0-398067-11-2

**5255 An Orientation and Mobility Primer for Families
and Young Children**

Bonnie Dodson-Burk, author

American Foundation for the Blind
11 Penn Plaza
New York, NY 10001   212-502-7600
800-232-5463
Fax: 212-502-7777
www.afb.org

Practical information for helping a child learn
about his or her environment right from the
start. Covers sensory training, concept development and orientation skills.

48 pages Softcover
ISBN: 0-891281-57-6

5256 Analysis of Human Genetic Linkage

Jurg Ott, author

Offers a concise introduction to human genetic linkage analysis and gene mapping. Provides mathematical and statistical foundations of linkage analysis for researchers and practitioners, as well as practical comments on available computer programs and websites. Includes a chapter on complex traits, such as diabetes, some cancers, and psychiatric conditions, an overview of nonparametric approaches to linkage and association analysis, and a chapter on two-locus inheritance.

405 pages
ISBN: 0-801861-40-3

5257 Art for All the Children: Approaches to Therapy for Children with Disabilities

Frances E. Anderson, author

Charles C. Thomas Publishing, Ltd.
2600 South First Street
Springfield, IL 62704   217-789-8980
                              800-258-8980
                         Fax: 217-789-9130
             e-mail: books@ccthomas.com
                       www.ccthomas.com

Second edition for art therapists in training and for in-service professionals in art therapy, art education and special education who have children with disabilities as part of their case/class load.

398 pages $48.95paperback
ISBN: 0-398057-97-4

5258 Art-Centered Education and Therapy for Children with Disabilities

Frances E. Anderson, author

Charles C. Thomas Publishing, Ltd.
2600 South First Street
Springfield, IL 62704   217-789-8980
                              800-258-8980
                         Fax: 217-789-9130
             e-mail: books@ccthomas.com
                       www.ccthomas.com

Explores the concept that we must live, learn and develop through art, emphasizing how art offers one of the most powerful ways to grow and develop socially, physically and emotionally as well as academically.

284 pages $35.95paperback
ISBN: 0-398058-96-2

5259 Assistive Technology for Children with Disabilities

Sharon Lesar Judge & H. Phil Parette, author

Brookline Books/Lumen Editions
P.O. Box 1047
Cambridge, MA 02238   617-868-0360
                              800-666-2665
                         Fax: 617-868-1772
          e-mail: brooklinebks@delphi.com
             www.people.delphi.com/brooklinebks

Explores the wide range of considerations involved in evaluating children's needs, selecting and prescribing devices, and training children, families, and teachers to use the technology.

Softcover
ISBN: 1-571290-51-6

5260 Baby Book for the Developmentally Challenged Child

Rene Matthews and Christina Haberman RN, author

Exceptional Parent Library
P.O. Box 1807
Englewood Cliffs, NJ 07632   201-947-6000
                                    800-535-1910
                               Fax: 201-947-9376
                 e-mail: eplibrary@aol.com
                       www.eplibrary.com

This baby book is for parents to write milestones for their developmentally challenged child. It incorporates the usual baby book features with very special sections covering any special needs.

48 pages Hardcover

5261 Battles, Hassles, Tantrums & Tears: Strategies for Coping

Susan Beekman, Jeanne Holmes, author

Active Parenting Publishers
810 Franklin Court, Suite B
Marietta, GA 30067
                              800-825-0060
                         Fax: 770-429-0334
                       www.activeparenting.com

Chock-full of field-tested tactics to help parents handle conflict creatively.

222 pages

5262 Behavioral Vision Approaches for Persons With Physical Disabilities

William Padula, author

Optometric Extension Program Foundation, Inc.
1921 East Carnegie Suite 3L
Santa Ana, CA 92705   949-250-8070
                         Fax: 949-250-8157

A discussion of thefffffffffffvaohfafhfhixcbcbdjor approach to providing directions for prescriptive and therapeutic services for the visually handicapped child or adult.

197 pages

5263 Blindness and Early Childhood Development

David H. Warren, author

American Foundation for the Blind
11 Penn Plaza
New York, NY 10001   212-502-7600
                            800-232-5463
                        Fax: 212-502-7777
                            www.afb.org

A review of current knowledge on motor and locomotor development, perceptual development, language and cognitive processes, and social, emotional and personality development. 2nd Edition

384 pages Softcover
ISBN: 0-891281-23-1

5264 Book on Special Children

P.O. Box 305
Congers, NY 10920   914-638-1236
                        Fax: 914-638-0842

Distributes books by mail to professionals and parents of handicapped children.

Irene Slovak

5265 Books About Disabilities, Special Needs Project

3463 State St, Ste 282
Santa Barbara, CA 93105   805-683-9633
                                800-333-6867

Special Needs Project offers many excellent books about physical and mental disabilities (particularly children's), hospitalization and general health, and other books about parenting. The list includes Computer Resources for Persons with Disabilities for parents looking for ways computers might assist their child with a disability.

Free Catalog

5266 Books on Special Children

Irene Slovac, author

P.O. Box 305
Congers, NY 10920   914-638-1236
                        Fax: 914-638-0842

Distributes books by mail to professionals and parents of handicapped children.

5267 Brothers, Sisters, and Special Needs

Debra H. Lobato, Ph.D., author

Brookes Publishing
P.O. Box 10624
Baltimore, MD 21285   410-337-9580
                            800-638-3775
                        Fax: 410-337-8539
                e-mail: custserv@pbrookes.com
                    www.brookespublishing.com

Information and activities for helping youg siblings of children with chronic illnesses and developmental disabilities.

224 pages Softcover

5268 Building the Healing Partnership: Parents, Professionals, and Children

Patricia T. Leff and Elaine H. Walizer, author

Brookline Books/Lumen Editions
P.O. Box 1047
Cambridge, MA 02238   617-868-0360
                            800-666-2665
                        Fax: 617-868-1772
                e-mail: brooklinebks@delphi.com
                www.people.delphi.com/brooklinebks

Successful programs understand that the disabled child's needs must be considered in the context of a family. This book was specifically written for practitioners who must work with families but have insufficient training in family systems assessment and intervention. It is a valuable blend of theory and practice with pointers for applying the principles.

Softcover
ISBN: 0-91479-63-8

5269 Building the Helping Partnership

Patricia Taner Leff and Elaine H. Walizer, author

Brookline Books/Lumen Editions
P.O. Box 1047
Cambridge, MA 02238   617-868-0360
                            800-666-2665
                        Fax: 617-868-1772
                e-mail: brooklinebks@delphi.com
                www.people.delphi.com/brooklinebks

Using powerful personal stories of both parents and professionals, this book conveys the day-to-day struggles and triumphs or caring for children with persisting medical needs. Presenting the perspectives of parents and health care professionals, this insightful book enhances mutual understanding and guides readers toward constructive communications.

310 pages Softcover
ISBN: 0-914797-60-3

5270 Can't Your Child See? A Guide for Parents and Professionals

Eileen P. Scott, James E. Jan, and Roger D.Freeman, author

8700 Shoal Creek Blvd.
Austin, TX 78757

800-897-3202
Fax: 800-397-7633

This third edition offers optimistic and practical information for helping children who are visually impaired reach their full potential. Parent counselors, teachers, day-care workers, physicians, nurses, psychologists, physiotherapists, other professionals, and parents will find the expanded information about the effects of visual impairment on normal development and suggestions for remediation useful.

279 pages Softcover
ISBN: 0-890796-04-1

5271 Cancervive

6500 Wilshire Blvd, Ste 500
Los Angeles, CA 90048   213-655-3758

This nonprofit organization that helps cancer survivors deal with the challenges of life after cancer. They offer support groups in some states, insurance information and assistance, and patient advocacy. They also publish a coloring book (kids age 3-6), a story/activity book (age 7-11), and a guide for teachers of children with cancer.

5272 Catalog of Prenatally Diagnosed Conditions

David D. Weaver, M.D., author

A catalog of detailed information on approximately 800 conditions that have been diagnosed prenatally. Includes the methods of detecting fetal abnormalities, the abnormal findings, and the published references in which the condition is reported. Conditions are grouped according to related disorders, using a numbering system based on that developed by Victor McKusick for Mendelian Inheritance in Man. The third edition contains approximately 200 new entries and 850 new references.

711 pages
ISBN: 0-801860-44-X

5273 Child Life in a Health Care Setting

Child Life Council
11820 Parklawn Drive #202
Rockville, MD 20852   301-881-7090
Fax: 301-881-7092
e-mail: clcstaff@childlife.org
www.childlife.org

Deborah Brouse, Executive Director

5274 Childhood Cancer Survivors: A Practical Guide to Your Future

Nancy Keene, Wendy Hobbie, and Kathy Ruccione, author

O'Reilly and Associates, Inc.
101 Morris Street
Sebastopol, CA 94572

800-998-9938
Fax: 707-829-0104
e-mail: patientsguide@oreilly.com
www.patientsguide.com

Long-term survivors of childhood cancer face a unique future. Some will encounter insurance and employment challenges, some will have emotional challenges, and some will have on-going health problems related to treatment. This book charts the territory for long-term suvivorship by covering follow-up schedules for health monitoring, emotional aspects including relationship challenges, employment and insurance, and medical late effects.

5275 Children and Trauma: A Guide for Parents and Professionals

Cynthia Monahon, author

Jossey-Bass
350 Sansome Street
San Francisco, CA 94104   415-433-1740
800-956-7739
Fax: 800-605-2665
www.josseybass.com

A clear and comprehensive guide to understanding the emotional aftermath of childhood crises. A must read for parents and other caregivers who live or work with children.

240 pages
ISBN: 0-787910-71-6

5276 Children with Disabilities

Mark L. Batshaw, author

Brookes Publishing
P.O. Box 10624
Baltimore, MD 21285   410-337-9580
800-638-3775
Fax: 410-337-8539
e-mail: custserv@pbrookes.com
www.brookespublishing.com

Extensive coverage of genetics, heredity, pre- and postnatal development, specific disabilities, family roles, and intervention. Features chapters on substance abuse, HIV, and AIDS. Down's Syndrome, fragile X syndrome, behavior managment, transitions to adulthood, and health care in the 21st century. Also reveals the causes of many conditions that can lead to developmental disabilities.

1997 960 pages Hardcover

5277 Children with Special Needs: A Resource Guide for Parents, and Educators

Karen L. Lungu, author

Charles C. Thomas Publishing, Ltd.
2600 South First Street
Springfield, IL 62704   217-789-8980
                              800-258-8980
                         Fax: 217-789-9130
          e-mail: books@ccthomas.com
                    www.ccthomas.com

Writing from her experience as a parent of a special needs child and her background of a therapist and educator, the author presents a most readable text of many helpful resources including state-by-state listings of support groups and private agencies. Special features include personal accounts from parents who have dealt with special needs issues.

234 pages $36.95 paper
ISBN: 0-398069-33-6

5278 Children with Visual Impairments: A Parents' Guide

M. Cay Holbrook, PhD, author

Woodbine House
6510 Bells Mill Road
Bethesda, MD 20817   301-468-8800
                            800-843-7323
                       Fax: 301-897-5838
     e-mail: info@woodbinehouse.com
               www.woodbinehouse.com

Provides parents with comforting advice and practical information on visual impairments. Describes the causes, diagnosis and treatment of visual impairments and discusses the effects it has upon a child's development, daily routines and family life.

375 pages Softcover
ISBN: 0-933149-36-0

5279 Chilhood Emergencies - What To Do, A Quick Reference Guide

The Marin Child Care Council, author

Bull Publishing Company
P.O. Box 208
Palo Alto, CA 94302   650-676-2855
                             800-676-2855
                        Fax: 650-327-3300
     e-mail: Bullpublishing@msn.com
                       www.bullpub.com

Handy flip-book provides quick and clear instructions for action in resonse to some of the most common childhood emergencies, including cuts and wounds, broken bones, abdominal pain, burns, toothaches, convulsion, abrasions, eye and ear injuries, bites (insect and animal), bleeding, choking, freezing and frostbite, seizures, and CPR.

44 pages
ISBN: 0-923521-33-X

5280 Communicating with Children: Suportive Interactions in Hospitals

Child Life Council
11820 Parklawn Drive #202
Rockville, MD 20852   301-881-7090
                        Fax: 301-881-7092
     e-mail: clcstaff@childlife.org
                    www.childlife.org

Deborah Brouse, Executive Director

5281 Communication Skills for Visually Impaired Learners

R.K. Harley, M.B. Truman, L.D. Sanford, author

Charles C. Thomas Publishing, Ltd.
2600 South First Street
Springfield, IL 62704   217-789-8980
                              800-258-8980
                         Fax: 217-789-9130
          e-mail: books@ccthomas.com
                    www.ccthomas.com

The plan of the book incorporates the latest research findings with the practical experiences learned in the classroom.

322 pages $49.95 paper
ISBN: 0-398066-92-2

5282 Concept Development for Visually Impaired Children: A Resource Guide

William T. Lydon, author

American Foundation for the Blind
11 Penn Plaza
New York, NY 10001   212-502-7600
                            800-232-5463
                       Fax: 212-502-7777
                            www.afb.org

A program for integrating such concepts as body imagery, gross motor movement, posture and tactile discrimination into the curriculum from kindergarten on.

80 pages Softcover
ISBN: 0-891280-18-9

5283 Conditional Love: Parents' Attitudes Toward Handicapped Children

Greenwood Publishing Group, Inc.
88 Post Road West, P.O. Box 5007
Westport, CT 06880   203-226-3571
                                          800-225-5800
                              Fax: 203-222-1502
          e-mail: custserv@greenwood.com
                      www.greenwood.com

Offers parents' information on understanding disabled children and mainstreaming them into their "normal" family life.

312 pages

5284 Coping Skills Interventions for Children and Adolescents

Susan G. Forman, author

Jossey-Bass
350 Sansome Street
San Francisco, CA 94104   415-433-1740
                                              800-956-7739
                                  Fax: 800-605-2665
                          www.josseybass.com

Provides a wide range of coping skills interventions for helping children learn to handle everyday stress and deal better academic, interpersonal, and physical demands.

215 pages
ISBN: 1-555424-93-7

5285 Coping in Young Children Early Interventions

Child Life Council
11820 Parklawn Drive #202
Rockville, MD 20852   301-881-7090
                                  Fax: 301-881-7092
            e-mail: clcstaff@childlife.org
                          www.childlife.org

Deborah Brouse, Executive Director

5286 Counseling Parents of Children with Chronic Illness or Disability

Hilton Davis, Ph.D., author

Brookes Publishing
P.O. Box 10624
Baltimore, MD 21285   410-337-9580
                                              800-638-3775
                                  Fax: 410-337-8539
            e-mail: custserv@pbrookes.com
                      www.brookespublishing.com

144 pages Softcover

5287 Creative Play Activities for Children with Disabilities

Lisa Rappaport Morris,MS and Linda Schultz, MS
Ed, author

Human Kinetics
P.O. Box 5076
Champaign, IL 61825
                                          800-747-4457
                              Fax: 217-351-2674
                  e-mail: emilyh@hkusa.com
                      www.humankinetics.com

Contains 250 games and activities designed to help children with all types of disabilities grow through play. Each chapter focuses on a particular 'world' or activity theme. Themes include exploring the wolrd of the senses, active games, building and creating, imaginative outdoor fun and water play, and group games and activities.

232 pages

5288 Deciphering the System: a Guide for Families of Young Disabled Children

Paula J. Beckman and Gayla Beckman Boyes, author

Brookline Books/Lumen Editions
P.O. Box 1047
Cambridge, MA 02238   617-868-0360
                                              800-666-2665
                                  Fax: 617-868-1772
            e-mail: brooklinebks@delphi.com
                  www.people.delphi.com/brooklinebks

This book helps parents of children with disabilities to understand the system that provides services to their child. Co-written by a professional and a parent, this book includes a glossary with professional jargons and an extensive list of resources.

208 pages Softcover

5289 Developing Personal Safety Skills in Children with Disabilities

Freda Briggs, M.A., author

Brookes Publishing
P.O. Box 10624
Baltimore, MD 21285   410-337-9580
                                              800-638-3775
                                  Fax: 410-337-8539
            e-mail: custserv@pbrookes.com
                      www.brookespublishing.com

A guide for teachers, parents, and caregivers, this volume explores the issue of personal safety for children with disabilities and offers strategies for empowering and protecting them at home and in school. Recognizing that children with disabilities need personal safety skills, offers, curriculum ideas and exercises, and advocates the development of self-esteem and assertiveness so that children can protect themselves.

220 pages Softcover

5290 Development of Social Skills by Blind and Visually Impaired Students

Sharon Zell Sacks, author

American Foundation for the Blind
11 Penn Plaza
New York, NY 10001   212-502-7600
                                    800-232-5463
                              Fax: 212-502-7777
                                    www.afb.org

Offers an examination of the social interactions of blind and visually impaired children in mainstreamed settings and the community that highlights the need to teach social interaction skills to children and provide them with support.

232 pages Softcover
ISBN: 0-891282-17-3

5291 Developmental Assessment for Students with Severe Disabilities (DASH-2)

Pro-Ed
8700 Shoal Creek Boulevard
Austin, TX 78757   512-451-3246
                                   800-897-3202
                              Fax: 512-451-8542
                                   www.proedinc.com

Concise information about individuals who are functioning between birth and 6-11 developmentally. It consists of five Pinpoint Scales, which assess performance in language, sensory-motor skills, activities of daily living, basic academic skills, and social-emotional skills. Sensitive to small changes in skill performance. Defined as task resistive, needing full assistance, needing partial assistance, needing minimal assistance or independent perform.

5292 Developmental Assessment of Young Children (DAYC)

Judith K. Voress, Taddy Maddox, author

Pro-Ed
8700 Shoal Creek Boulevard
Austin, TX 78757   512-451-3246
                                   800-897-3202
                              Fax: 512-451-8542
                                   www.proedinc.com

Test measures the five domains: cognition, communication, social-emotional development, physical development and adaptive behavior.

Complete Kits

5293 Developmental Disabilities in Infancy and Childhood

Brookes Publishing
P.O. Box 10624
Baltimore, MD 21285   410-337-9580
                                   800-638-3775
                              Fax: 410-337-8539
           e-mail: custserv@pbrookes.com
                   www.brookespublishing.com

This two volume set explores advances in assessment and treatment, retains a clinical focus, and incorporates recent developments in research and theory. Can be purchased individually or as a set (Vol. 1: Neurodevelopmental Diagnosis and Treatment; Vol. 2: The Spectrum of Developmental Disabilities).

Hardcover

5294 Diagnosis and Psychopharmacology of Childhood and Adolescent Disorders

J M Wiener, author

John Wiley & Sons, INC.
605 Third Avenue
New York, NY 10158   212-850-6000
                              Fax: 212-850-6088
                                   www.wiley.com

Marketed for pediatricians, child psychiatrists and other mental health workers in private practices and hospital settings.

519 pages
ISBN: 0-471617-57-1

5295 Directory of Camps for the Blind and Visually Impaired Children & Adults

American Foundation for the Blind
11 Penn Plaza
New York, NY 10001   212-502-7600
                                   800-232-5463
                              Fax: 212-502-7777
                                   www.afb.org

A guide to 200 sleepaway camps and day camps in the United States. Descriptions cover types of campers, age ranges, special activities offered, length of seasons and contact names.

34 pages Papberack
ISBN: 0-891281-59-2

5296 Directory of Child Life Programs

Child Life Council
11820 Parklawn Drive #202
Rockville, MD 20852   301-881-7090
                              Fax: 301-881-7092
           e-mail: clcstaff@childlife.org
                   www.childlife.org

Deborah Brouse, Executive Director

5297 Directory of Kidney and Urologic Diseases
Organization
2 Information Way
Bethesda, MD 20892   301-654-3810
Fax: 301-907-8906
e-mail: nddic@info.niddk.nih.gov
www.niddk.nih.gov

5298 Dying and Disabled Children: Dealing with the Loss
and Grief

Harold M. Dick, M.D., author

The Haworth Press, Inc.
10 Alice Street
Binghamton, NY 13904   607-722-5857
800-342-9678
Fax: 607-722-6362
e-mail: getinfo@haworthpressinc.com
www.haworthpressinc.com

In this sensitive and compassionate look at terminally ill and disabled children, professionals
from the medical community examine the
stresses faced by their parents and siblings.
They address the crucial element of communication in dealing with a child's serious illness.
Ethical decision making, learning to recognize
the child's suffering, and talking to children
about death are honestly and clearly discussed.

153 pages Hardcover

5299 Early Focus: Working with Young Blind and
Visually Impaired Children

Rona L. Pogrund, author

American Foundation for the Blind
11 Penn Plaza
New York, NY 10001   212-502-7600
800-232-5463
Fax: 212-502-7777
www.afb.org

Describes early intervention techniques used
with blind and visually impaired children and
stresses the benefits of family involvement and
transdisciplinary teamwork.

160 pages Softcover
ISBN: 0-891282-15-7

5300 Early Intervention
8700 Shoal Creek Blvd
Austin, TX 78757

800-897-3202
Fax: 800-397-7633

Based on a collaborative, transdisciplinary, community-based early intervention model for professionals developing programs for infants and
toddlers who are disabled or at risk and their
families, this text enables parents and professionals to advocate for and implement appropriate services.

394 pages
ISBN: 0-890796-21-1

5301 Empowerment Resource Centers
O'Reilly and Associates, Inc.
101 Morris Street
Sebastopol, CA 95472
800-998-9938
Fax: 707-829-0104
e-mail: patientguides@oreilly.com
www.patientcenters.com

Offers articles, comprehensive up-to-the-minute
health information, resources and references on
autism, bipolar disorders, childhood luekemia,
hydrocephalus, and childhood cancer. This information is free to print out as long as you retain copyright notice on the printouts.

5302 End-Stage Renal Disease: Choosing a Treatment
That's Right for You
2 Information Way
Bethesda, MD 20892   301-654-3810
Fax: 301-907-8906
e-mail: nddic@info.niddk.nih.gov
www.niddk.nih.gov

5303 Enhancing Self-Concepts and Acheivement of
Mildly Handicapped Students

Carroll J. Jones, author

Charles C. Thomas Publishing, Ltd.
2600 South First Street
Springfield, IL 62704   217-789-8980
800-258-8980
Fax: 217-789-9130
e-mail: books@ccthomas.com
www.ccthomas.com

This is a valuable review of what are current
best practices for understanding and interven-
ing on behalf of mildly handicapped learners
with emotionally fragile self-concepts.

294 pages $39.95 paper
ISBN: 0-398057-60-5

5304 Equals in Partnership: Basic Rights for Families of
Children with Blindness
N.A.P.V.I.
P.O. Box 317
Watertown, MA 02272
800-562-6265
Fax: 617-972-7444
e-mail: napvi@perkins.pvt.kiz.ma.us
www.spedex.com/napvi

5305 Essential Elements in Early Intervention: Visual Impairment, Multiple Disabilities
AFB Press/ American Foundation of the Blind
11 Penn Plaza Suite 300
New York, NY 10001　　　　212-502-7600
　　　　　　　　　　　　　800-232-3044
　　　　　　　　　　　Fax: 212-502-7774
　　　　　　　　　　　TDD: 212-502-7662
　　　　　e-mail: afborder@abdintl.com
　　　　　　　　　　　　　www.afb.org

This comprehensive resource provides a range of information on effective early intervention with young children who are visually impaired and have other disabilities. It contains valuable explanations of functional and clinical vision and hearing assessments, descriptions of evaluative and educational techniques, and useful suggestions for working with families and professional teams.

1996 503 pages
ISBN: 0-891283-05-6

Deborah Chen, Editor

5306 Exceptional Parent Library
S. Schwartz, Ph.D. and J.E. Heller Miller, M.Ed., author
Exceptional Parent Library
P.O. Box 1807
Englewood Cliffs, NJ 07632　　　201-947-6000
　　　　　　　　　　　　　800-535-1910
　　　　　　　　　　　Fax: 201-947-9376
　　　　　e-mail: eplibrary@aol.com
　　　　　　　　　　www.eplibrary.com

An updated and expanded how-to guide for using eveyday toys to develop communication skills in children with disabilities and make playtime a fun, educational experience.

5307 Family Book: For Parents
G. Allan Roeher Institute/York University
Kinsman Building, 4700 Keele Street
New York, Ontario,
Canada　　　　　　　　　416-661-9611
　　　　　　　　　　　Fax: 416-661-5701

What happens when you find out that your child has a mental handicap? What can you do to cope and what support can you expect? These are the kinds of questions assessed by this informative and useful text that aims to help parents and families of children with a handicap.

52 pages

5308 Family and ADPKD: A Guide for Children and Parents
Arlene B. Chapman, MD, & Lisa M.
Guay-Woodford, MD, author
Polycystic Kideny Research Foundation
4901 Main Street, Ste 200
Kansas City, MO 64112　　　816-931-2600
　　　　　　　　　　　　　800-753-2873
　　　　　　　　　　　Fax: 816-931-8655
　　　e-mail: pdkcure@pkrfoundaiton.org
　　　　　　　　　　www.kume.edu/pkrf/

This brand new book focuses on the questions most commonly asked by children and parents about ADPKD. It is divided into two sections: one for children and one for parents.

5309 Family-Centered Care for Children Needing Specialized Services
Child Life Council
11820 Parklawn Drive #202
Rockville, MD 20852　　　　301-881-7090
　　　　　　　　　　　Fax: 301-881-7092
　　　e-mail: clcstaff@childlife.org
　　　　　　　　　　www.childlife.org

Deborah Brouse, Executive Director

5310 Family-Centered Service Coordination: A Manual For Parents
Irene Zipper, C. Hinton, M. Weil, and K. Rounds, author
Brookline Books/Lumen Editions
P.O. Box 1047
Cambridge, MA 02238　　　　617-868-0360
　　　　　　　　　　　　　800-666-2665
　　　　　　　　　　　Fax: 617-868-1722
　　　e-mail: brooklinebks@delphi.com
　　　www.people.delphi.com/brooklinebks

A manual designed to orient and educate parents about issues of service coordination, to assist families in caring for an infant or toddler with developmental delays or disabilities.

34 pages Softcover

5311 Feeding and Nutrition for the Child with Special Needs
Marsha Dunn Klein, Tracy A. Delane, author
Pro-Ed
8700 Shoal Creek Boulevard
Austin, TX 78757　　　　　512-451-3246
　　　　　　　　　　　　　800-897-3202
　　　　　　　　　　　Fax: 512-451-8542
　　　　　　　　　　www.proedinc.com

A wide selection of uniquely integrated feeding and nutrition recommendations at your fingertips. Parent-friendly illustrated handouts.

5312 Feeding and Swallowing Disorders in Infancy

Lynn S. Wolf, Robin P. Glass, author

Pro-Ed
8700 Shoal Creek Boulevard
Austin, TX 78757   512-451-3246
                         800-897-3202
                    Fax: 512-451-8542
                    www.proedinc.com

This practical resource integrates information in the areas of sucking, swallowing, and breathing to aid in evaluation and treatment of infant ages birth to one year. Thorough and easy-to-understand with illustrations.

5313 First Steps

Blind Children's Center
4120 Marathon Street
Los Angeles, CA 90029   323-664-2153
                          Fax: 656-665-3828
          e-mail: info@blindchildrenscenter.org
                    www.blindchildrenscenter.org

A handbook for teaching young children who are visually impaired. Designed to assist students, professionals and parents working with children who are visually impaired.

203 pages

5314 For Teenagers: Visiting the Hospital

Child Life Council
11820 Parklawn Drive #202
Rockville, MD 20852   301-881-7090
                         Fax: 301-881-7092
          e-mail: clcstaff@childlife.org
                    www.childlife.org

Deborah Brouse, Executive Director

5315 From the Heart

J.D.B. Marsh, author

Exceptional Parent Library
P.O. Box 1807
Englewood Cliffs, NJ 07632   201-947-6000
                                800-535-1910
                           Fax: 201-947-9376
          e-mail: eplibrary@aol.com
                    www.eplibrary.com

Eye-opening narratives based on their parent support process, nine mothers explore the intense, sometimes painful terrain of raising a child with special needs.

5316 Get a Wiggle On

Sherry Reynor, author

American Alliance for Health, Phys. Ed. & Dance
1900 Association Drive
Reston, VA 22091   703-476-3400

Gives teachers and parents practical suggestions for helping blind and visually impaired infants grow and learn like other children.

80 pages
ISBN: 0-883140-77-2

5317 God's Special Children

K.J. Karren, author

Horizon Publishers
P.O. Box 490
Bountiful, UT 84011   801-295-9451

The book is divided into three sections. First: handicapped individuals share their own stories. Second, parents give useful insights. Third: professional guidance is offered concerning true challenges and encouragments of those individuals.

220 pages Hardcover

5318 Handbook of Consultation Services for Children

Zins, Kratochwill, Elliot, Editors, author

Jossey-Bass
350 Sansome Street
San Francisco, CA 94104   415-433-1740
                             800-956-7739
                        Fax: 800-605-2665
                        www.josseybass.com

Provides research foundations and practical information needed for joint problem-solving. Presents an overview of a variety of treatments.

464 pages
ISBN: 1-555425-48-8

5319 Handbook of Parent Training: Parents as Co-Therapists for Children's Behavior

James M. Briesmeister and Charles E. Schaefer, author

John Wiley & Sons, INC.
605 Third Avenue
New York, NY 10158   212-850-6000
                        Fax: 212-850-6088
                        www.wiley.com

A book written for professionals who work with troubled children. Therapists learn how to teach parents of troubled children effective skills so that they can better understand and communicate with them.

594 pages
ISBN: 0-471163-43-0

5320 Helping Baby Grow: Level 1 'Baby's First Year'

Active Parenting Publishers
810 Franklin Court, Suite B
Marietta, GA 30067

800-825-0060
Fax: 770-429-0334
www.activeparenting.com

Winner of the National Parenting Center Seal of Approval Award, this program encourages movement and sensory exploration with the adult as the facilitator in playful interactions.

0-12 months

5321 Helping Baby Grow: Level 2 'Baby's Second Year'

Active Parenting Publishers
810 Franklin Court, Suite B
Marietta, GA 30067

800-825-0060
Fax: 770-429-0334
www.activeparenting.com

Developmentally appropriate activities program for baby's second year.

12-24 months

5322 Helping Children Cope with Stress

Child Life Council
11820 Parklawn Drive #202
Rockville, MD 20852

301-881-7090
Fax: 301-881-7092
e-mail: clcstaff@childlife.org
www.childlife.org

Deborah Brouse, Executive Director

5323 Helping the Visually Impaired Child With Developmental Problems

Sally Rogow, author

Baker & Taylor, Int'l
1200 US Highway 22 East
Bridgewater, NJ 08807

908-429-4074
Fax: 908-429-4037
e-mail: intsale@bakertaylor.com

This book aims to explore the human consequences of severe visual problems combined with other handicaps.

216 pages Softcover
ISBN: 8-077290-27-

5324 History of Childhood and Disability

Philip Safford and Elizbeth Safford, author

Baker & Taylor, Int'l
1200 US Highway 22 East
Bridgewater, NJ 08807

908-429-4074
Fax: 908-429-4037
e-mail: intsale@bakertaylor.com

This book presents an interdisciplinary perspective on children considered exceptional and how services have evolved in reponse to their diverse neeeds.

1996 352 pages

5325 Hormonal Chaos

The Scientific and Social Origins of the Environmental Endocrine Hypothesis. Sheldon Krimsky traces the emergence of an unorthodox hypothesis that casts new suspicions on a broad range of modern industrial chemicals. At the heart of his story is the Environmental Endocrine Hypothesis, the assertion that a class of chemicals called endocrine disruptors are interfering with the normal functioning of hormones in animals and humans.

256 pages
ISBN: 0-801862-79-5

5326 How to Build Special Furniture and Equipment for Handicapped Children

Ruth B. Hofmann, author

Charles C. Thomas Publishing, Ltd.
2600 South First Street
Springfield, IL 62704

217-789-8980
800-258-8980
Fax: 217-789-9130
e-mail: books@ccthomas.com
www.ccthomas.com

100 pages
ISBN: 0-398008-54-X

5327 How to Get Your Kid to Eat... But Not Too Much

Ellyn Satter, RD, MS, MSSW, author

Bull Publishing Company
P.O. Box 208
Palo Alto, CA 94302

650-322-2855
800-676-2855
Fax: 650-327-3300
e-mail: Bullpublishing@msn.com
www.bullpub.com

What should a parent do with a child who wants to snack continuously? Or a young teen who has declared herself a vegetarian and refuses to eat any type of meat and only a few vegetables? Or a child claims he doesn't like what's been prepared, only to turn around and eat the exact same thing at a friend's house? Satter addresses these concerns and many others surrounding the relationship between parents, children, and food in a warm, friendly, and supportive way. A easy to read and helpful book.

408 pages
ISBN: 0-923521-83-9

Jim Bull, Publisher

5328 How to Handle a Hard-to-Handle Kid

C. Drew Edwards, PhD, author

Active Parenting Publishers
810 Franklin Court, Suite B
Marietta, GA 30067

800-825-0060
Fax: 770-429-0334
www.activeparenting.com

Some children are simply more challenging than others. Learn why this is true and how to use specific strategies to respond effectively.

216 pages

5329 Human Kinetics News

Joseph P. Winnick, EdD and Francis X. Short PED, author

1607 North Market St, P.O.Box 5076
Champaigne, IL 61825
217-351-5076
Fax: 217-351-2674
www.humankinetics.com

Human Kinetics is the first resource to offer educators a systematic process for developing fitness criteria for young students with special needs. Teachers no longer have to attempt to adapt standard fitness tests to fit the needs of children with disabilities. Guidebook for understanding and administering the test and interpreting the results to develop a health-related, criterion-referenced physical fitness test for youngsters ages 10 to 17 with disablties.

1998 155 pages Softcover
ISBN: 0-736000-21-6

Katherine Johnson, Promotions Department

5330 In Time and with Love

Marilyn Segal, Ph.D., author

Newmarket Press
18 East 48th Street
New York City, NY 10017
212-239-8040
Fax: 212-832-3629

For families and caregivers of preteen and handicapped children in their first three years - more than one hundred tips for adjusting and coping.

208 pages

5331 Infants, Children, and Adolescents

Child Life Council
11820 Parklawn Drive #202
Rockville, MD 20852
301-881-7090
Fax: 301-881-7092
e-mail: clcstaff@childlife.org
www.childlife.org

Deborah Brouse, Executive Director

5332 Internalizing Disorders in Children and Adoloscents

William H. Reynolds, author

John Wiley & Sons, INC.
605 Third Avenue
New York, NY 10158
212-850-6000
Fax: 212-850-6088
www.wiley.com

Marketed toward child psychologists, educational/school psychologists and pediatricians.

352 pages
ISBN: 0-471506-48-6

5333 Keys to Parenting a Child with a Learning Disability

Marilyn Segal, Ph.D., author

Newmarket Press
18 E. 48th Street
New York City, NY 10017
212-239-8040
Fax: 212-832-3629

For families and caregivers of preteen and handicapped children in their first three years - more than one hundred tips for adjusting and coping.

208 pages

General Resources/Books

5334 Legislative Handbook for Parents

E.E. Castillo, author

N.A.P.V.I.
P.O. Box 317
Watertown, MA 02272

800-562-6265
Fax: 617-972-7444
e-mail: napvi@perkins.pvt.kiz.ma.us
www.spedex.com/napvi

Written by parents for parents in dealing with Legislative Processes that ultimately affect their children's lives.

24 pages Softcover

5335 Little Children, Big Needs

D. Weinhouse, Ph.D. And M. Weinhouse, M.A., author

Exceptional Parent Library
P.O. Box 1807
Englewood Cliffs, NJ 07632

201-947-6000
800-535-1910
Fax: 201-947-9376
e-mail: eplibrary@aol.com
www.eplibrary.com

Contains candid interviews with fifty families of children with a wide variety of disabilities.

5336 Mainstreaming and the American Dream

Howard L. Nixon II, author

American Foundation for the Blind
11 Penn Avenue
New York, NY 10001

212-502-7600
800-232-5463
Fax: 212-502-7777
www.afb.org

Based on in-depth interviews with parents and professionals, this research monograph presents information on the needs and aspirations of parents of blind and visually impaired children.

256 pages Softcover
ISBN: 0-891281-91-6

5337 Mainstreaming the Visually Impaired Child

Michael D. Orlansky, author

N.A.P.V.I.
P.O. Box 317
Watertown, MA 02272

800-562-6265
Fax: 617-972-7444
e-mail: napvi@perkins.pvt.kiz.ma.us
www.spedex.com/napvi

A unique, informative guide for teachers and educational professionals that work with the visually impaired.

121 pages Softcover

5338 Meals Without Squeals - Child Care Feeding Guide & Cookbook

Christine Berman, MPH, RD, & Jacki Fromer, author

Bull Publishing Company
P.O. Box 208
Palo Alto, CA 94302

650-322-2855
800-676-2855
Fax: 650-327-3300
e-mail: Bullpublishing@msn.com
www.bullpub.com

Simple, straightforward information on children's growth, accompanied age-specific, child-tested recipes. Explains how common feeding problems can be solved and show ways to offer children positive experiences with food. Current information on children's nutritional needs, introduction to the Feed Guide Pyramid, plus how to read Nutritional facts on food labels, updated listings of educational and community nutritional resources and more.

288 pages
ISBN: 0-923521-39-9

5339 Misunderstood Child

Larry B. Silver, author

Gallery Bookshop
P.O. Box 270
Mendocino, CA 95460

707-937-2665

A guide for parents with learning disabled children.

224 pages Softcover

5340 Mobility Training for People with Disabilities

William Goodman, author

Children adn adults with mental, visual, physical, and hearing impairments can learn to travel.

144 pages

5341 More Alike Than Different: Blind and Visually Impaired Children

American Foundation for the Blind
11 Penn Plaza
New York, NY 10001

212-502-7600
800-232-5463
Fax: 212-502-7777
www.afb.org

858

Offers photographs of blind and visually impaired children around the world learning to read and write, travel independently and performing basic living skills. Covers the most recent technological advances and demonstrates the universality of educational needs and goals.

Papberback
ISBN: 0-891281-69-0

5342 Mothers Talk About Learning Disabilities

S. Schwartz, Ph.D. and J.E. Heller Miller, M.Ed., author

Gallery Bookshop
P.O. Box 270
Mendocino, CA 95460   707-937-2665

In this work, the mother of two learning disabled boys seeks to give mothers in similar circumstances encouragement, support, and everyday advice.

157 pages

5343 Movement and Allied Disorders in Childhood

M M Robertson and V Eapen, author

John Wiley & Sons, INC.
605 Third Avenue
New York, NY 10158   212-850-6000
Fax: 212-850-6088
www.wiley.com

This book examines various movement disorders in children including Tics, Tourette's Syndrome and Dystonia.

342 pages
ISBN: 0-471953-24-5

5344 Neurobiological Disorders in Children and Adolescents: New Directions

Jossey-Bass Publishers
350 Samsome Street
San Francisco, CA 94104   415-433-1740
800-956-7739
Fax: 800-605-2665
www.josseybass.com

1992 Softcover

5345 New Language of Toys

S. Schwartz, Ph.D. and J.E. Heller Miller, M.Ed., author

Exceptional Parent Library
P.O. Box 1807
Englewood Cliffs, NJ 07632   201-947-6000
800-535-1910
Fax: 201-947-9376
e-mail: eplibrary@aol.com
www.eplibrary.com

An updated and expanded how-to guide for using everyday toys to develop communication skills in children with disabilities and make playtime a fun educational experience.

5346 Normal Children Have Problems, Too

Stanley Turecki, MD, author

Active Parenting Publishers
810 Franklin Court, Suite B
Marietta, GA 30067
800-825-0060
Fax: 770-429-0334
www.activeparenting.com

Award winning book about how to successfully resolve problems such as poor self-image, sibling rivalry, sadness, fears, sleep problems, lying and more.

255 pages

5347 Organizing and Maintaining Support Groups for Parents of Children with Chronic Ill

Minna Newman Nathanson, author

19 Mantua Road
Mount Royal, NJ 08061   609-224-1742
Fax: 609-423-3420
e-mail: amkent@smarthub.com
www.aach.org

5348 Our Blind Children: Growing and Learning with Them

Berthold Lowenfeld, author

Charles C. Thomas Publishing, Ltd.
2600 South First Street
Springfield, IL 62704   217-789-8980
800-258-8980
Fax: 217-789-9130
e-mail: books@ccthomas.com
www.ccthomas.com

260 pages $27.95 paper
ISBN: 0-398022-00-3

5349 Parental Voice: Problems Faced by Parents of the Deaf-Blind

Robert Holzberg, Sara Walsh-Burton, author

Charles C. Thomas Publishing, Ltd.
2600 South First Street
Springfield, IL 62704   217-789-8980
800-258-8980
Fax: 217-789-9130
e-mail: books@ccthomas.com
www.ccthomas.com

Parents from differing backgrounds and cultures present their personal accounts of how they dealt with their handicapped child from birth through adulthood. After each story is an interpretation and commentary by an authority in the field of special education.

172 pages $28.95 paper
ISBN: 0-398065-53-5

5350 Parenting Preschoolers: Suggestions For Raising Young Blind Children

Kay Alicyn Ferrell, author

American Foundation for the Blind
11 Penn Plaza
New York, NY 10001
212-502-7600
800-232-5463
Fax: 212-502-7777
www.afb.org

Provides practical answers to questions most frequently asked by parents and gives advice on what to expect, how to adapt to a child's situation and what to look for in early education programs.

28 pages
ISBN: 0-891289-98-4

5351 Perkins Activity and Resource Guide: A Handbook for Teachers

Perkins School for the Blind, Publications
175 North Beacon Street
Watertown, MA 02172

This is a comprehensive, two volume guide with over 1,000 pages of activities, resources and instructional strategies for teachers and parents of students with visual and multiple disabilities.

5352 Popular Games and Activities for Blind, Visually Impaired & Disabled People

Peter Richards, author

American Foundation for the Blind
15 West 16th Street
New York, NY 1001
212-502-7600
800-232-5463
Fax: 212-502-7777
www.afb.org

A manual of easy-to-follow instructions for more than 50 games and activities for blind and visually impaired persons of all ages, their families, recreation leaders and health care professionals.

64 pages Large Print
ISBN: 0-959974-78-4

5353 Practical Pediatric Oncology

D'Angio, Sinniah, Meadows, Evans, Pritchard, author

John Wiley & Sons, Inc.
1 Wiley Drive
Somerset, NJ 08875
732-469-4400
Fax: 732-302-2300
e-mail: custserv@wiley.com
www.wiley.com

A guide for oncologists and pediatricians.

320 pages
ISBN: 0-471588-35-0

5354 Preparing Your Child for Repeated or Extended Hospitalizations

Child Life Council
11820 Parklawn Drive #202
Rockville, MD 20852
301-881-7090

5355 Preschool Learning Activities for the Visually Impaired Child

Illinois Department Of Education, author

N.A.P.V.I.
P.O. Box 317
Watertown, MA 02272
800-562-6265
Fax: 617-972-7444
e-mail: napvi@perkins.pvt.kiz.ma.us
www.spedex.com/napvi

This guide for parents offers games and activities to keep visually impaired children active during the preschool years.

91 pages Softcover

5356 Prescriptions for Children with Learning and Adjustment Problems

Charles C. Thomas Publishing, Ltd.
2600 South First Street
Springfield, IL 62704
217-789-8980
800-258-8980
Fax: 217-789-9130
e-mail: books@ccthomas.com
www.ccthomas.com

A Consultant's Desk Reference

1988 Hardcover

5357 Psychoeducational Assessment of Visually Impaired and Blind Students

Sharon Bradley-Johnson, author

Pro-Ed
8700 Shoal Creek Boulevard
Austin, TX 78758
512-451-3246
Fax: 512-451-8542

Professional reference book that addresses the problems specific to assessment of visually impaired and blind children. Of particular value to the practitioner are the extensive reviews of available tests, including ways to adapt those not designed for use with the visually handicapped.

140 pages Softcover
ISBN: 0-890791-08-2

5358 Psychologically Battered Child

Garbarino, Guttman, Seeley, author

Jossey-Bass
350 Sansome Street
San Francisco, CA 94104   415-433-1740
                                 800-956-7739
                          Fax: 800-605-2665
                          www.josseybass.com

Provides guidelines for those who identify and treat psychological maltreatment of children and adolescents and also cleary defines different types of maltreatment.

308 pages
ISBN: 1-555420-02-8

5359 Psychosocial Research on Pediatric Hospitalization and Health Care

Child Life Council
11820 Parklawn Drive #202
Rockville, MD 20852   301-881-7090
                      Fax: 301-881-7092
         e-mail: clcstaff@childlife.org
                      www.childlife.org

Deborah Brouse, Executive Director

5360 Reading and Learning Disability: A Nueropsychological Approach

Estelle L. Fryburg, author

Charles C. Thomas Publishing, Ltd.
2600 South First Street
Springfield, IL 62704   217-789-8980
                               800-258-8980
                        Fax: 217-789-9130
         e-mail: books@ccthomas.com
                        www.ccthomas.com

A practical guidebook for the education of the learning disabled and also as a text in graduate courses.

398 pages $64.95 paper
ISBN: 0-398067-44-9

5361 Resources for Family Centered Intervention for Infants, Toddlers, and Preschoolers

Hope, Inc.
55 East 100 North
Logan, UT 84321   435-752-9533
                   Fax: 435-752-9533

Describes children with vision impairment in terms of characteristics, needs, and parent concerns.

Two volumes

5362 Show Me How: A Manual for Parents of Preschool Blind Children

Mary Brennan, author

American Foundation for the Blind
11 Penn Plaza
New York, NY 10001   212-502-7600
                            800-232-5463
                     Fax: 212-502-7777
                            www.afb.org

A practical guide for parents, teachers and others who help preschool children attain age-related goals. Covers issues on playing precautions, appropriate toys and facilitating relationships with playmates.

56 pages Softcover
ISBN: 0-891281-13-4

5363 Since Owen, A Parent-to-Parent Guide for Care of the Disabled Child

Charles Callahan, author

Special Needs Project
3463 Strat Street, #282
Santa Barbara, CA 93105
                            800-333-6867

Against the background of his experience as the parent of a severely disabled young man, Callahan writes conscientiously to other parents.

486 pages

5364 Something's Wrong with My Child!

Harriet Wallace Rose, author

Charles C. Thomas Publishing, Ltd.
2600 South First Street
Springfield, IL 62704   217-789-8980
                               800-258-8980
                        Fax: 217-789-9130
         e-mail: books@ccthomas.com
                        www.ccthomas.com

A valuable resource in helping parents and professionals to better understand themselves in dealing with the emotionally charged subject of children with disabilities.

234 pages $33.95 paper
ISBN: 0-398068-98-4

5365 Special Child

Siegfried M. Pueschel, M.D., author

Brookes Publishing
P.O. Box 10624
Baltimore, MD 21285   410-337-9580
                          800-638-3775
                          Fax: 410-337-8539
              e-mail: custserv@pbrookes.com
                  www.brookespublishing.com

A Source Book for Parents of Children with Developmental Disabilities, 2nd Edition. This book includes specifics on detections, prognosis, and treatment of various conditions. It also provides detailed information on education, intervention, advocacy, financial planning, and medical and technological advances that may affect the lives of children with special needs.

464 pages Softcover

5366 Special Kind of Parenting

Julia Darnell, author

La Leche League International
P.O. Box 4079
Schaumburg, IL 60168   847-519-7730
                            Fax: 847-519-0035
                      www.laleche.league.org

Disabled children have special needs which challenge their parents' emotional and physical resources. This book guides parents through the problems and helps them discover their disabled child as an individual. The author covers both facts and feelings about handicap, parents' reactions to the initial diagnosis, the grieving process, and effects on the marriage and the rest of the family. They also provide suggestions for chooking the programs and professionals best suited.

172 pages Softcover

5367 Starting Points

Blind Children's Center
4120 Marathon Street
Los Angeles, CA 90029   323-664-2153
                            Fax: 323-665-3828
              e-mail: info@blindchildrenscenter.org
                  www.blindchildrenscenter.org

Basic information for the clasroom teacher of 3 to 8 year olds whose multiple disabilities include visual impairment.

160 pages

5368 Strategies for Working with Families of Young Children with Disabilities

Brookes Publishing
P.O. Box 10624
Baltimore, MD 21285   410-337-9580
                          800-638-3775
                          Fax: 410-337-8539
              e-mail: custserv@pbrookes.com
                  www.brookespublishing.com

This text offers useful techniques for collaborating with and supporting families whose youngest members either have a disability or are at risk for developing a disability. The authors address specific issues such as cultural diversity, transitions to new programs, and diagreements between families and professionals.

272 pages Softcover

5369 Student Teaching Guide for Blind And Visually Impaired College Students

Lou Alonso, author

American Foundation for the Blind
15 West 16th Street
New York, NY 10011   212-502-7600
                            800-232-5463
                          Fax: 212-502-7777
                            www.afb.org

A comprehensive resource designed to enable the student to enter the classroom of a university or college with confidence.

52 pages Large Print
ISBN: 0-891281-42-8

5370 Teaching Children About Food

Christine Berman, MPH, RD, & Jacki Fromer, author

Bull Publishing Company
P.O. Box 208
Palo Alto, CA 94302   650-322-2855
                            800-676-2855
                          Fax: 650-327-3300
              e-mail: Bullpublishing@msn.com
                    www.bullpub.com

Wriiten as a companion book to Meals Without Squeals, this book teaches parents and child care providers: cooking and gardening activities for children, tips to help children become smart consumers, ways to reach appreciation for cultural diversity regarding food choices and preparations, and an understanding of relationships between food and our environment.

96 pages
ISBN: 0-923521-15-1

5371 Teaching Developmentally Disabled Children

O. Ivar Lovaas, author

Pro-Ed
8700 Shoal Creek Boulevard
Austin, TX 78757   512-451-3246
800-897-3202
Fax: 512-451-8542
www.proedinc.com

Instructional program for teachers, nurses and parents that shows how to help developmentally disabled children function more normally at home, in school, and in the community.

250 pages Large Format
ISBN: 0-936104-78-3

5372 Teaching Students with Moderate/Severe Disabilities, including Autism

Elva Duran, author

Charles C. Thomas Publishing, Ltd.
2600 South First Street
Springfield, IL 62704   217-789-8980
800-258-8980
Fax: 217-789-9130
e-mail: books@ccthomas.com
www.ccthomas.com

A valuable resource guide to help teachers, parents and caregivers provide the best educational opportunities for students with moderate and severe disabilities. Added chapters on cross-cultural groups and second language learners.

416 pages $58.95 paper
ISBN: 0-398067-00-7

5373 Test Accommodations for Students With Disabilities

Edward Burns, author

Charles C. Thomas Publishing, Ltd.
2600 South First Street
Springfield, IL 62704   217-789-8980
800-258-8980
Fax: 217-789-9130
e-mail: books@ccthomas.com
www.ccthomas.com

Considers legal questions, theoretical issues, and pratical methods for meeting the assessment needs of students with disabilities and implementing valid test accomodations.

340 pages $49.95 paper
ISBN: 0-398068-44-5

5374 Therapies for Children

Charles E. Schaefer, Howard L. Millman, author

Jossey-Bass
350 Sansome Street
San Francisco, CA 94104   415-433-1740
800-956-7739
Fax: 800-605-2665
www.josseybass.com

Using a novel digest format, this handbook brings together current knowledge about child therapy. Over one hundred thirty-five different clinical techniques are concisely presented and a full range of behavior problems are presented.

524 pages
ISBN: 0-875893-37-6

5375 There's Something Wrong with My Child!

Harriet Wallace Rose, author

Charles C. Thomas Publishing, Ltd.
2600 South First Street
Springfield, IL 62704   217-789-8980
800-258-8980
Fax: 217-789-9130
e-mail: books@ccthomas.com
www.ccthomas.com

A straight forward presentation to help professionals and parents to better understand themselves in dealing with the emotionally charged subject of disabled children.

210 pages Softcover

5376 To a Different User

P. Clarke, author

Alliance for Parental Involvement in Education
P.O. Box 59
East Chatham, NY 12060

Parents of special needs children contributed to this book.

5377 Touch the Baby: Blind & Visually Impaired Children As Patients

Lois Harrell, author

American Foundation for the Blind
11 Penn Plaza
New York, NY 10001   212-502-7600
800-232-5463
Fax: 212-502-7777
www.afb.org

A how-to manual for health care professionals working in hospitals, clinics and doctors' offices. Teaches the special communication and touch-related techniques needed to prevent blind and visually impaired patients from withdrawing from healthcare workers and the outside world.

13 pages
ISBN: 0-891281-97-5

5378 Touchpoints: The Essential Reference

T. Berry Brazelton, M.D., author

Active Parenting Publishers
810 Franklin Court, Suite B
Marietta, GA 30067

800-825-0060
Fax: 770-429-0334
www.activeparenting.com

Provides sympathy and insight into the emotional, behavioral, cognitive and physical development of children birth through 6 years old.

0-6 years 569 pages

5379 Treating Adolescents

Jossey-Bass
350 Sansome Street
San Francisco, CA 94104

415-433-1740
800-956-7739
Fax: 800-605-2665
www.josseybass.com

An up-to-date summary of treatments for teen's issues: depression, eating disorders, anxiety, conduct and more.

442 pages
ISBN: 0-787902-06-3

Hans Steiner, Editor

5380 Treating School-Age Children

Jossey-Bass
350 Sansome Street
San Francisco, CA 94104

415-433-1740
800-956-7739
Fax: 800-605-2665
www.josseybass.com

Expert contributors provide the knowledge and tools needed for assessing and treating problems such as hyperactivity, depression, obsession, compulsions, phobias and more.

289 pages
ISBN: 0-787908-78-9

Hans Steiners, Editor

5381 Understanding Anemia

Ed Uthman, M.D., author

University Press of Mississippi
3825 Ridgewood Road
Jackson, MS 39211

601-432-6205
800-737-7788
Fax: 601-432-6217
e-mail: press@ihl.state.ms.us
www.upress.state.ms.us

Medicine for the lay reader, a book detailing causes and treatments of the various forms of anemia.

160 pages Hardcover
ISBN: 1-578060-38-9

5382 Understanding Birth Defects

Karen Gravelle, author

Franklin Watts c/o Grolier
90 Old Sherman Turnpike
Danbury, CT 06816

203-797-3500
800-621-1115
Fax: 203-797-3197
www.grolier.com

What birth defects are, their genetic and environmental origins and what can be done to help, plus the problems of low birth weight are discussed.

128 pages
ISBN: 0-531109-55-0

5383 Utilizing Switch Interfaces with Children Who Are Severely Physically Challenged

Carol Goossens' and Sharon Sapp Crain, author

8700 Shoal Creek Blvd.
Austin, TX 78757

800-897-3202
Fax: 800-397-7633

This clinical handbook is valuable to all professionals previously frustrated by their attempts to provide reliable switch access to children who are severely physically challenged. For these children, computer access is the key to unlocking their social, emotional, linguistic, and academic growth. Whether a child needs to use a switch to control an adapted battery-powered toy or to control a sophisticated talking computer, reliable access is a must.

316 pages Large Format
ISBN: 0-890795-16-9

5384 Visual Handicaps and Learning

Natalie Barraga, author

Pro-Ed
8700 Shoal Creek Boulevard
Austin, TX 78758

512-451-3246
Fax: 512-451-8542

This text covers a range of topics associated with visual impairment, from past practices to up-to-date research, and from legal responsibilities to personal beliefs, without losing sight of the individual child.

180 pages
ISBN: 0-890791-56-2

5385 Visually Handicapped Child In Your Class

Elizabeth K. Chapman, author

Paul H. Brookes Publishing Co.
P.O. Box 10624
Baltimore, MD 21285

800-638-3134

This book considers the theory and issues relating to the movement to integrate visually handicapped children into ordinary schools and offers practical suggestions to teachers to help such children participate fully in school life.

192 pages Softcover
ISBN: 0-304314-00-5

5386 We Need Not Walk Alone: After the Death of Compassionate Friends

P.O. Box 3696
Oak Brook, IL 60522

708-990-0010

Bereaved parents and siblings write about their grief in prose and poetry. $14.95

5387 When 'NO' Gets You Nowhere: Teaching Your Toddler and Child Self-Control

Mark L. Brenner, author

Active Parenting Publishers
810 Franklin Court, Suite B
Marietta, GA 30067

800-825-0060
Fax: 770-429-0334
www.activeparenting.com

With this book you will learn the seven proven steps for instilling self-control in toddlers and young children.

153 pages

5388 Your Child in the Hospital: A Practical Guide for Parents

Nancy Keene & Rachel Prentice, author

O'Reilly & Associates, INC.
101 Morris Street
Sebastopol, CA 95472

800-998-9938
Fax: 707-829-0104
e-mail: patientguides@oreilly.com
www.patientcenters.com

This book serves as an excellent guide to making your child's stay in the hospital as easy as possible. It includes such topics as dealing with doctors, coping with procedures and obtaining support from family and friends. The second edition features a journal to help open communication and give the child a measure of control over the experience.

176 pages
ISBN: I-565925-73-4

5389 Your Child, Your Family & ARPKD

Polycystic Kidney Research Foundation
4901 Main Street, Ste 200
Kansas City, MO 64112

816-931-2600
800-753-2873
Fax: 816-931-8655
e-mail: pdkcure@pkrfoundation.org
www.kumc.edu/pkr/

This second edition book focuses on the questions most commonly asked about ARPKD in order to help families understand more about the disease.

Children's Books

5390 An Alphabet About Kids with Cancer

Rita Berglund, author

Compassion Books
477 Hannah Branch Road
Burnsville, NC 28714

704-675-9670
Fax: 704-675-9687

This book manages to inspire and celebrate life while informing kids about feelings and treatment related to childhood cancer.

Hardcover

5391 Belonging

Deborah Kent, author

Dial Books
375 Hudson Street
New York, NY 10014

212-366-2000

Meg attended special schools for the blind until she was ready for high school. She decided that she wanted to go to a regular high school. She and her mother practiced her walks to school and studied the layout of the building prior to school starting, but had to adjust to the crowds and the pace of the new school.

200 pages Hardcover
ISBN: 0-803705-30-1

5392 Beside Me

William Latka, author

Leader Dog For The Blind
1964 Park Street, Regina
SK S4P 3G4, IT,   306-565-8211

Marion became blind as an adult. She was totally dependent on her parents to move around
and go places she wanted to be. Marion decided
to go to the leader-dog program and learn to use
a leader dog. Particularly she wanted the independence she would need to go to college.

5393 Cancer - Overview Series for Young Adults

Lucent Books
P.O. Box 289011
San Diego, CA 92198   619-485-7424
                                 Fax: 619-485-9549

Questions are answered for young adults on the
issues of cancer prevention and treatment.

1991
ISBN: 1-560061-25-1

5394 Don't Feel Sorry for Paul

Bernard Wolf, author

J.B. Lippincott
East Washington Square
Philadelphia, PA 19105   215-238-4200

Paul is seven but was born with deformities of
both hands and feet. Paul wears a prosthesis on
both feet so he can walk. He has a third prosthesis for his right hand with hooks to use as fingers.

94 pages Hardcover
ISBN: 0-397315-88-0

5395 Help Yourself: Tips for Teenagers With Cancer

National Cancer Institute
Bldg 31, Rm 10A24
Bethesda, MD 20892

                                 800-422-6237

This magazine-style booklet is designed to provide information and support adolescents with
cancer.

37 pages

5396 Hospital Days: Treatment Ways

National Cancer Institute
Bldg 31, Rm 10A24
Bethesda, MD 20892

                                 800-422-6237

Coloring book helping to orient children with
cancer to hospital and treatment procedures.

26 pages

5397 In the Hospital

Peter Alsop and Bill Harley, author

Compassion Books
477 Hannah Branch Road
Burnsville, NC 28714   704-675-9670
                                 Fax: 704-675-9687

Wonderful songs and entertaining stories dealing with being sick, being different, being scared
and finding strength and hope.

Audiotape/Book

5398 Kathy's Hats: A Story of Hope

Trudy Krisher, author

Albert Whitman & Company
6340 Oakton Street
Morton Grove, IL 60053   847-531-0033
                                 800-255-7675
                                 Fax: 847-531-0039

When Kathy turns nine she learns she has cancer. When she loses her hair due to the chemotherapy, she feels ugly and awkward. This is a
matter-of-fact book about a tough time and subject, and its calm adn respectable treatment well
serves a story that is indeed one of hope.

32 pages Hardcover
ISBN: 0-807541-16-8

5399 Kemo Shark

Kidscope, Inc.
3400 Peachtree Rd, Ste 703
Atlanta, GA 30326   404-233-3560
                                 www.kidscope.com

Color comic book designed to help children with
the psychological and physiological changes in a
family where a parent has cancer and chemotherapy.

5400 Living with Blindness

Steve Parker, author

Franklin Watts c/o Grolier
90 Old Sherman Turnpike
Danbury, CT 06816   203-797-3500
                                 800-621-1115
                                 Fax: 203-797-3197
                                 www.grolier.com

Shows how persons with visual impairments and
blindness can overcome their disability and lead
productive lives.

32 pages Grades 5-7
ISBN: 0-531108-43-0

5401 My Book for Kids with Cancer

Jason Gaes, author

Waterfront Books
98 Brookes Avenue
Burlington, VT 05401   802-658-7477

Frustrated because he couldn't find any books about kids who survived cancer, Jason decided to write his own.

32 pages

5402 One Day at a Time - Children Living with Leukemia

Thomal Bergman, author

Gareth Stevens,Inc
1555 North River Center Drive
Milwaukee, WI 53212   414-225-0333
                             Fax: 414-225-0377
                             www.gsinc.com

ISBN: 1-555329-13-6

5403 Out of the Corner of My Eye

Nicolette Ringgold, author

American Foundation for the Blind
11 Penn Plaza
New York, NY 10001   212-502-7600
                            800-232-5463
                            Fax: 212-502-7777
                            www.afb.org

A personal account of students' vision loss and subsequent adjustment that is full of practical advice and cheerful encouragement, told by an 87 year old retired college teacher who has maintained her independence and zest for life.

ISBN: 0-891281-93-2

5404 Phoenix Rising: How to Survive Your Life

Cynthia D. Grant, author

Atheneum Publishing
866 3rd Avenue
New York, NY 10022   212-614-1300

This story focuses on Jessie, a 17-year-old girl, who finds her sister's diary that she wrote during her treatment for cancer.

Grades 7-10

5405 Sammy's Mommy has Cancer: For Children Who Have a Loved One with Cancer

Sherry Kohlenberg, MHA, author

Gareth Stevens, Inc
1555 North River Drive
Milwaukee, WI 53212   414-225-0333
                             Fax: 414-225-0377
                             www.gsinc.com

32 pages

5406 Seeing-Children Living with Blindness

Thomas Bergman, author

Gareth Stevens
1555 North River Center Drive
Milwaukee, WI 53212   414-225-0333
                             800-341-3569
                             Fax: 414-225-0377

Go with Thomas to a special school for children who can't see, where you will meet Andrew, Kate, Jordan, Katherine, Peter and Kent. Read what they told Thomas about being blind, about daily life, their feelings, the funny and sad things.

ISBN: 1-555329-15-2

5407 Silver Kiss

Annette Klause, author

Delacorte
1540 Broadway
New York, NY 10103   212-354-6500

This moving tale describes the feelings of Zoe as her mother dies of cancer and her family attempts to shield her from seeing the slow decline in her mother.

Grades 8-12

5408 They Never Want to Tell You: Children Talk About Cancer

David Bearison, author

Harvard University Press
79 Gardner Street
Cambridge, MA 02138   617-495-2600

A comprehensive book that focuses on eight children who share their various experiences with cancer.

Grades 7-12

5409 Waiting for Johnny Miracle

Alice Hendricks Bach, author

Harper & Row
10 East 53rd Street
New York, NY 10022   212-207-7000

This powerful book focuses on Becky, a 17-year-old girl who must face the fear of cancer after being diagnosed with a malignant tumor. This book brings up the painful issues that come with the pain, treatment and death of cancer.

Grades 8-12

5410 When Eric's Mom Fought Cancer

Judith Vigna, author

Albert Whitman & Company
6340 Oakton Street
Morton Grove, IL 60053   847-581-0033
                                800-225-7675
                                Fax: 847-584-0039

This book is aimed to help children deal with illness in their homes.

Grades Pre-3
ISBN: 0-807588-83-0

5411 Why God Gave Me Pain

Shirley Holdren, author

Loyola University Press
3441 N. Ashland Avenue
Chicago, IL 60657   773-281-1818

Using a girl's diary entries, this book expounds on the side effects of cancer as well as the psychological ramifications of the debilitating disease.

5412 Working with Visually Impaired Young Students

Ellen Trief, author

Charles C. Thomas Publishing, Ltd.
2600 South First Street
Springfield, IL 62704   217-789-8980
                                800-258-8980
                                Fax: 217-789-9130
                                e-mail: books@ccthomas.com
                                www.ecthomas.com

Offers a curriculum model to early intervention programs providing services to visually impaired young children, from birth to age three. An extensive review of the literature is included along with measurable behavioral objectives for each developmental level.

1992 230 pages Papercover
ISBN: 0-398064-66-0

5413 You Seem Like a Regular Kid to Me

Anne Corn, author

American Foundation for the Blind
11 Penn Plaza
New York, NY 10001   212-502-7600
                                800-232-5463
                                Fax: 212-502-7777
                                www.afb.org

An interview with Jane, a blind child, tells other children what it's like to be blind. Jane explains how she gets around, takes care of herself, does her school work, spends her leisure time and even pays for things when she can't see money.

16 pages
ISBN: 0-891289-21-6

Magazines

5414 Childswork Childsplay
135 Dupont Street P.O. Box 760
Plainview, NY 11803
                                800-962-1141
                                Fax: 800-262-1886
                                www.childswork.com

Full of training tools for children of all ages.

63 pages

5415 Exceptional Parent Magazine
209 Harvard Street Suite 303
Brookline, MA 02146   617-730-5800
                                800-852-2884
                                Fax: 617-730-8742

Lex Frieden, Program Director

5416 Future Reflections
National Federation of the Blind
1800 Johnson Street
Baltimore, MD 21230   410-659-9314
                                Fax: 410-685-5653
                                e-mail: nfb@inmdiges.net
                                www.nfb.org

National magazine written specifically for parents and educators of blind children. Each issue addresses various topics important to blind children, their families and to school personnel.

Quarterly

5417 International Journal of Dermatology
International Society of Dermatology
200 1st Street SW
Rochester, MN 55905   507-284-3736

Focuses on information for dermatologists and the whole specialty of dermatology research and education.

10x Annually

5418 Journal of Visual Impairment and Blindness
American Foundation for the Blind
11 Penn Plaza
New York, NY 10001   212-502-7600
                           800-232-5463
                           Fax: 212-502-7777
                           www.afb.org

Published in braille, regular print and on cassette this journal contains a wide variety of subjects including rehabilitation, psychology, education, legislation, medicine, technology, employment, sensory aids and childhood development as they relate to visual impairments.

10X year

5419 Journal of the Academy of Dermatology
American Academy of Dermatology
930 N Meacham Road
Shaumburg, IL 60173   847-330-0230
                            Fax: 847-330-0050
                            www.aad.org

A scientific publication serving the clinical needs of the specialty and provides a wide selection of articles on various topics important to continuing medical education of Academy members and the international dermatologic community.

Monthly

5420 Reaching, Crawling, Walking - Let's Get Moving
Blind Children's Center
4120 Marathon Street
Los Angeles, CA 90029   323-664-2153
                              Fax: 323-665-3828
                e-mail: info@blindchildrenscenter.org
                        www.blindchildrenscenter.org

Orientation and mobility for visually impaired preschool children.

24 pages

5421 Seeing Candy
National Association for Visually Handicapped
22 West 21st Street, 6th Floor
New York, NY 10010   212-889-3141
                           Fax: 212-727-2931
                           e-mail: staff@navh.org
                           www.navh.org

This newsletter offers short stories, news, medical updates, assistive device information, poems, resources, crossword puzzles and more for the visually impaired.

Bi-Annually

5422 Tactic
Clovernook Home and School for the Blind
7000 Hamilton Avenue
Cincinnati, OH 45231   513-522-3860

Quarterly

Newsletters

5423 ABDC Newsletter
Association of Birth Defect Children
930 Woodcock Road, Suite 225
Orlando, FL 32803   407-245-7035
                          800-313-2223
                          Fax: 407-895-0824
                          e-mail: abdc@birthdefects.org
                          www.birthdefects.org

Offers updated information on the association activities, events and medical updates.

8 pages Quarterly

5424 Awareness
N.A.P.V.I.
P.O. Box 317
Watertown, MA 02272
                          800-562-6265
                          Fax: 617-972-7444
                          e-mail: napvi@perkins.pvt.kiz.ma.us
                          www.spedex.com/napvi

Newsletter offering regional news, sports and activities, conferences, camps, legislative updates, book reviews, audio reviews, professional question and answer column and more for the visually impaired and their families.

Quarterly

5425 Child Life Council Newsletter
Child Life Council
11820 Parklawn Drive, Suite 202
Rockville, MD 20852   301-881-7090
                            Fax: 301-881-7092
                            e-mail: clcstaff@childlife.org
                            www.childlife.org

The Child Life Council newsletter provides information to promote the well-being of children and families in health care settings. Newsletter is provided to members only.

12 pages quarterly

Diane Demarest, Editor

5426 Children's Hopes and Dreams
Wish Fulfillment Foundation
280 Route 46
Dover, NJ 07801   973-361-7366
                                           Fax: 973-361-6627
                            e-mail: chdfdover@juno.com
                  childrenscharities.org/childrens_wisheso

Dream Newsletter (describes dreams recently ful-
filled, events, request and info about programs)
available upon request; at no cost. 4 times per
year.

10,000 Members

5427 D.V.H. Quarterly
University of Arkansas at Little Rock
2801 S. University Ave.
Little Rock, AR 72204
                                 Fax: 501-663-3536

Offers information on upcoming events, conferences and workshops on and for visual disabilities. Book reviews, information on the newest
resources and technology, educational programs, want ads and more.

Quarterly

Bob Brasher, Editor

5428 Dermatology Focus
Dermatology Foundation
1560 Sherman Avenue
Evanston, IL 60201   847-328-2256

Includes membership activities, research articles
and lists recipients of foundation awards.

Quarterly

5429 Dermatology World
American Academy of Dermatology
930 N Meacham Road
Shaumburg, IL 60173   847-330-0230
                                           Fax: 847-330-0050
                                           www.aad.org

Offers Academy members information outside
the clinical realm. It carries news of government actions, reports of socioeconomic issues, so-
cietal trends and other events which impinge on
the practice of dermatology.

Monthly

5430 Developmental Disabilities Nurses Associations
228 Grimes Street, Suite 24
Eugene, OR 97402
                                           800-888-6733
                                           Fax: 541-485-7372
                            e-mail: ddnahq@aol.com
                                           www.ddna.org

Information on a specialty nursing organization
that certifies nurses in developmental disabilities.

Quarterly

C.A. Coleman-Bryson, Editor

5431 MAGIC Foundation for Children's Growth
1327 North Harlem Avenue
Oak Park, IL 60302   708-383-0808
                                           800-362-4423
                                           Fax: 708-383-0899
                                           TTY: 123-019-99
                  e-mail: mary@magicfoundation.org
                                 www.magicfoundation.org

Information on the support and education provided to families of children with growth related
disorders, including Growth Hormone Deficiency; Precocious Puberty; Congenital Adrenal
Hyperplasia; McCune Albright Syndrome; Congenital Hypothyroidism; Russell-Silver Syndrome; Tuners Syndrome; Sepo Optic Dysplasia.

36 pages Quarterly

Mary Andrews, Executive Director

**5432 National Library Service for the Blind & Physically
Handicapped**
Library of Congress Reference Section
1291 Taylor Street NW
Washington, DC 20542   202-707-5100
                                           800-424-8567
                                           Fax: 202-707-0712
                                           TTY: 202-707-0744
                                           TDD: 202-707-0744
                                           e-mail: nis@loc.gov
                                           www.loc.gov/nls

Provides information and advocacy resources
for families and professionals, including listings
of organizations focusing on more specific areas
of concern to families and young adults who
have disabilities. Administers a natural library
service that provides recorded and braille reading materials to eligible children and adults who
cannot read standard print.

12 pages Quarterly
ISSN: 1046-1663

Vicki Fitzpatrick, Editor

5433 PAL News
Federation for Children with Special Needs
1135 Tremont Street, Suite 420
Boston, MA 02116   617-482-2915
                                           800-331-0688
                                           Fax: 617-572-2094
                            e-mail: fcsninfo@fcsn.org
                                           www.fcsn.org

Offers information on medical and technological updates in the area of research on birth defects, support groups and family resources for persons with disabled children.

Quarterly

5434 Progress In Dermatology
Dermatology Foundation
1560 Sherman Avenue
Evanston, IL 60201   847-328-2256

Bulletin offering information on research reports and clinical trials.

Quarterly

5435 Talking Book Topics
National Library Services for the Blind
1291 Taylor Street NW
Washington, DC 20542   202-707-5100
                             Fax: 202-707-0712

Offers hundreds of listings of books, fiction and nonfiction, for adults and children on cassette. Also offers listings on foreign language books on cassette, talking magazines and reviews.

Bi-Monthly

Pamphlets

5436 ABDC Newsletter Volume Reprints
Association of Birth Defect Children
930 Woodcock Road, Suite 225
Orlando, FL 32803   407-245-7035
                          800-313-2223
                     Fax: 407-895-0824
         e-mail: abdc@birthdefects.org
                  www.birthdefects.org

Offers a variety of reprints from the ABCD newsletter on birth defects.

5437 About Children's Eyes
National Association for Visually Handicapped
22 West 21st Street, 6th Floor
New York, NY 10010   212-889-3141
                          Fax: 212-727-2931
                e-mail: staff@navh.org
                        www.navh.org

How to identify the child with a visual problem.

5438 About Children's Vision: A Guide For Parents
National Association for Visually Handicapped
22 West 21st Street, 6th Floor
New York, NY 10010   212-889-3141
                          Fax: 212-727-2931
                e-mail: staff@navh.org
                        www.navh.org

Offers a better understanding of the normal and possible abnormal development of a child's eyesight.

5439 Advanced Cancer: Living Each Day
National Cancer Institute
Bldg 31, Rm 10A24
Bethesda, MD 20892   800-422-6237

Booklet delving into all aspects of everyday living with cancer. Offers information on coping, how children react, facing the unknown, living wills, additional resources and making treatment decisions.

30 pages

5440 Alternative Ways To Take Insulin
2 Information Way
Bethesda, MD 20892   301-654-3810
                          Fax: 301-907-8906
         e-mail: nddic@info.niddk.nih.gov
                  www.niddk.nih.gov

5441 Amyloidosis and Kidney Disease
2 Information Way
Bethesda, MD 20892   301-654-3810
                          Fax: 301-907-8906
         e-mail: nddic@info.niddk.nih.gov
                  www.niddk.nih.gov

5442 Basic Family Library
Candlelighters' Childhood Cancer Foundation
7910 Woodmont Avenue, Ste 460
Bethesda, MD 20814   301-657-8401
                          800-366-2223

A bibliography of materials on childhood cancers, medical support, death abd bereavement and materials for children.

5443 Birth Defects: A Brighter Future
March of Dimes Resource Center
1275 Mamaroneck Avenue
White Plains, NY 10605   888-663-4637
                          Fax: 914-997-4763

5444 Camps for Children with Cancer and their Siblings
Candlelighters' Childhood Cancer Foundation
7910 Woodmont Avenue, Ste 460
Bethesda, MD 20814   301-657-8401
                          800-366-2223

A listing by state of day and overnight camp programs, children served and programs.

5445 Candlelighters Guide to Bone Marrow Transplants in Children
Candlelighters' Childhood Cancer Foundation
7910 Woodmont Avenue, Ste 460
Bethesda, MD 20814   301-657-8401
                           800-366-2223

For parents who are contemplating a BMT or harvest for their child or whose child is undergoing the procedure.

5446 Childhood Nephrotic Syndrome
2 Information Way
Bethesda, MD 20892   301-654-3810
                    Fax: 301-907-8906
           e-mail: nddic@info.niddk.nih.gov
                    www.niddk.nih.gov

5447 Children and Kidney Disease
American Kidney Fund
6110 Executive Blvd #1010
Rockville, MD 20852   301-881-3052
                             800-638-8299
                        Fax: 301-881-0898
                           www.kidney.org

5448 Dancing Cheek to Cheek
Blind Children's Center
4120 Marathon Street
Los Angeles, CA 90029   323-664-2153
                        Fax: 323-665-3828
       e-mail: info@blindchildrenscenter.org
              www.blindchildrenscenter.org

Discusses beginning social, play and language interactions.

33 pages

5449 Family Guide - Growth and Development of the Partially Seeing Child
National Association for Visually Handicapped
22 West 21st Street, 6th Floor
New York, NY 10010   212-889-3141
                        Fax: 212-727-2931
            e-mail: staff@navh.org
                    www.navh.org

Offers information for parents and guidelines in raising a partially seeing child.

5450 Financial Assistance and Insurance for People with Kidney Disease
2 Information Way
Bethesda, MD 20892   301-654-3810
                    Fax: 301-907-8906
           e-mail: nddic@info.niddk.nih.gov
                    www.niddk.nih.gov

5451 Financial Help for Diabetics Care
2 Information Way
Bethesda, MD 20892   301-654-3810
                    Fax: 301-907-8906
           e-mail: nddic@info.niddk.nih.gov
                    www.niddk.nih.gov

5452 Gastoparesis in Diabetes
2 Information Way
Bethesda, MD 20892   301-654-3810
                    Fax: 301-907-8906
           e-mail: nddic@info.niddk.nih.gov
                    www.niddk.nih.gov

5453 Glycemic Index and Diabetes
2 Information Way
Bethesda, MD 20892   301-654-3810
                    Fax: 301-907-8906
           e-mail: nddic@info.niddk.nih.gov
                    www.niddk.nih.gov

5454 Heart Disease, High Blood Pressure, Stroke and Diabetes
2 Information Way
Bethesda, MD 20892   301-654-3810
                    Fax: 301-907-8906
           e-mail: nddic@info.niddk.nih.gov
                    www.niddk.nih.gov

5455 Heart to Heart
Blind Children's Center
4120 Marathon Street
Los Angeles, CA 90029   213-664-2153
                        Fax: 213-665-3828
       e-mail: info@blindchildrenscenter.org
              www.blindchildrenscenter.org

Parents of blind and partially sighted children talk about their feelings.

12 pages

5456 Helping Children Cope While a Sibling Undergoes Bone Marrow Transplant
Eileen Manella, CSW, author

Bone Marrow Foundation
981 First Avenue, Ste 129
New York, NY 10022   212-838-3029
                  e-mail: thebmf@aol.com
                   www.bonemarrow.org

Discusses the wide array of emotions felt by the entire family as a child receives a bone marrow transplant.

5457 Hepatitis B: Your Child at Risk
American Liver Foundation
1425 Pompton Avenue
Cedar Grove, NJ 07009   973-857-2626
                               800-223-0179

5458 How to Find More About Your Child's Birth Defect Or Disability
Association for Birth Defect Children
930 Woodcock Road, Suite 225
Orlando, FL 32803   407-245-7035
800-313-2223
Fax: 407-895-0824
e-mail: abdc@birthdefects.org
www.birthdefects.org

An informational fact sheet that encourages parents who have a child with a birth defect or disability to become the expert on the child's disability with some suggestions on how to educate themselves.

5459 Hypoglycomia
2 Information Way
Bethesda, MD 20892   301-654-3810
Fax: 301-907-8906
e-mail: nddic@info.niddk.nih.gov
www.niddk.nih.gov

5460 Interstitial Cyctitis
Information Clearinghouse
1 Information Way
Bethesda, MD 20892   301-654-3820
Fax: 301-907-8906
e-mail: ndoc@info.niddk.nih.gov
www.niddk.nih.gov

5461 Joint and Bone Conditions Related to Diabetes
2 Information Way
Bethesda, MD 20892   301-654-3810
Fax: 301-907-8906
e-mail: nddic@info.niddk.nih.gov
www.niddk.nih.gov

5462 Kidney Disease and African Americans
2 Information Way
Bethesda, MD 20892   301-654-3810
Fax: 301-907-8906
e-mail: nddic@info.niddk.nih.gov
www.niddk.nih.gov

5463 Kidney Disease of Diabetes
Information Clearinghouse
1 Information Way
Bethesda, MD 20892   301-654-3820
Fax: 301-907-8906
e-mail: ndoc@info.niddk.nih.gov
www.niddk.nih.gov

5464 Learning Problems or Learning Disabilities
Consumer Information Center
Dept 509B
Pueblo, CO 81009

Free government publication that explains the differences between learning problems and disabilities. It contains a chart that shows language and reasoning skills to watch for at different ages.

5465 Learning to Play
Blind Children's Center
4120 Marathon Street
Los Angeles, CA 90029   323-664-2153
Fax: 323-665-3828
e-mail: info@blindchildrenscenter.org
www.blindchildrenscenter.org

Discusses how to present play activities to the visually impaired preschool child.

12 pages

5466 Let's Eat
Blind Children's Center
4120 Marathon Street
Los Angeles, CA 90029   213-664-2153
Fax: 213-665-3828
e-mail: info@blindchildrenscenter.org
www.blindchildrenscenter.org

Teaches competent feeding skills to children with visual impairments.

28 pages

5467 Liver Transplant Fund
American Liver Foundation
1425 Pompton Avenue
Cedar Grove, NJ 07009   973-857-2550
800-223-0179

5468 Liver Transplantation
American Liver Foundation
1425 Pompton Avenue
Cedar Grove, NJ 07009   973-857-2626
800-223-0179

5469 Looking for Diabetes Recipes and Cookbooks
2 Information Way
Bethesda, MD 20892   301-654-3810
Fax: 301-907-8906
e-mail: nddic@info.niddk.nih.gov
www.niddk.nih.gov

5470 Managing Your Child's Eating Problems During Cancer Treatment
National Cancer Institute
Bldg. 31, Rm 10A24
Bethesda, MD 20892
800-422-6237

Contains information about the importance of nutrition, side effects of cancer and its treatment.

32 pages

5471 Medullary Sponge Kidney
2 Information Way
Bethesda, MD 20892　　　　301-654-3810
　　　　　　　　　　　Fax: 301-907-8906
　　　　　e-mail: nddic@info.niddk.nih.gov
　　　　　　　　　　　www.niddk.nih.gov

5472 Move with Me
Blind Children's Center
4120 Marathon Street
Los Angeles, CA 90029　　　　323-664-2153
　　　　　　　　　　　Fax: 323-665-3828
　　　　e-mail: info@blindchildrenscenter.org
　　　　　　　www.blindchildrenscenter.org

A parent's guide to movement development for visually impaired babies.

12 pages

5473 NPF Benefits of Membership Pamphlets
National Psoriasis Foundation
6600 SW 92nd Avenue Suite 300
Portland, OR 97223　　　　503-244-7404
　　　　　　　　　　　800-723-9166
　　　　　　　　　　Fax: 503-245-0626
　　　　　e-mail: getinfo@npfusa.org
　　　　　　　　　　www.psoriasis.org

Offers all the pamphlets that are published through the foundation for members. Includes NPF 800 number and reply tear-off card.

5474 New Challenge: Responding to Families
Federation for Children with Special Needs
1135 Tremont Street, Suite 420
Boston, MA 02116　　　　617-482-2915
　　　　　　　　　　　800-331-0688
　　　　　　　　　　Fax: 617-572-2094
　　　　　e-mail: fcsninfo@fcsn.org
　　　　　　　　　　www.fcsn.org

Addresses the needs of children with emotional, behavioral and mental disorders and their families.

5475 Nutrition and Kidney Disease
2 Information Way
Bethesda, MD 20892　　　　301-654-3810
　　　　　　　　　　　Fax: 301-907-8906
　　　　　e-mail: nddic@info.niddk.nih.gov
　　　　　　　　　　www.niddk.nih.gov

5476 Pain, Pain Go Away: Helping Children with Pain
Pat McGrath, G. Allen Finley, & Judith Ritchie, author

Association for the Care of Children's Health
7910 Woodmont Ave., Ste. 300
Bethesda, MD 20814　　　　301-654-6549
　　　　　　　　　　　800-808-2224
　　　　　　　　　　Fax: 301-986-4553

This booklet teaches parents about pain in children. Topics inlcude: What is pain?; sources of pain; measuring pain; how the body reacts; pain management; cancer pain; burn pain; and other pain.

1993

5477 Preparing your Child for a Bone Marrow Transplant
Eileen Manella, CSW, author

Bone Marrow Foundation
981 First Ave, Ste. 129
New York, NY 10022　　　　212-838-3029
　　　　　　　　e-mail: thebmf@aol.com
　　　　　　　　　　www.bonemarrow.org

Discusses the wide array of emotions felt by the entire family as a child receives a bone marrow transplant.

5478 Proteinuria
2 Information Way
Bethesda, MD 20892　　　　301-654-3810
　　　　　　　　　　　Fax: 301-907-8906
　　　　　e-mail: nddic@info.niddk.nih.gov
　　　　　　　　　　www.niddk.nih.gov

5479 Psychosocial Issues of Growth Delayed Children
Human Growth Foundation
7777 Leesburg Pike Suite 202S
Falls Church, VA 22043　　　　703-883-1773
　　　　　　　　　　　800-451-6434

5480 Renal Tubular Acidosis
2 Information Way
Bethesda, MD 20892　　　　301-654-3810
　　　　　　　　　　　Fax: 301-907-8906
　　　　　e-mail: nddic@info.niddk.nih.gov
　　　　　　　　　　www.niddk.nih.gov

5481 Selecting a Program
Blind Children's Center
4120 Marathon Street
Los Angeles, CA 90029　　　　323-664-2153
　　　　　　　　　　　Fax: 323-665-3828
　　　　e-mail: info@blindchildrenscenter.org
　　　　　　　www.blindchildrenscenter.org

A guide for parents of infants and preschoolers with visual impairments.

28 pages

5482 Skin Problems and Diabetes
2 Information Way
Bethesda, MD 20892   301-654-3810
                           Fax: 301-907-8906
              e-mail: nddic@info.niddk.nih.gov
                           www.niddk.nih.gov

5483 Standing On My Own Two Feet
Blind Children's Center
4120 Marathon Street
Los Angeles, CA 90029   323-664-2153
                           Fax: 323-665-3828
         e-mail: info@blindchildrenscenter.org
                    www.blindchildrenscenter.org

A step-by-step guide to designing and constructing simple, individually tailored adaptive mobility devices for preschool-age children who are visually impaired.

36 pages

5484 Students with Cancer: A Resource for The Educator
National Cancer Institute
Bldg. 31, Rm 10A24
Bethesda, MD 20892
                           800-422-6237

Designed for teachers who have students with cancer in their classrooms or schools.

22 pages

5485 Talk to Me
Blind Children's Center
4120 Marathon Street
Los Angeles, CA 90029   323-664-2153
                           Fax: 323-665-3828
         e-mail: info@blindchildrenscenter.org
                    www.blindchidlrenscenter.org

A language guide for parents of deaf children.

11 pages

5486 Talk to Me II
Blind Children's Center
4120 Marathon Street
Los Angeles, CA 90029   323-664-2153
                           Fax: 323-665-3828
         e-mail: info@blindchildrenscenter.org
                    www.blindchidlrenscenter.org

A sequel to Talk To Me, available in English and Spanish.

15 pages

5487 Talking with Your Child About Cancer
National Cancer Institute
Bldg 31, Room 10A24
Bethesda, MD 20892
                           800-422-6237

Designed for the parent whose child has been diagnosed with cancer.

16 pages

5488 Travel and Diabetes
2 Information Way
Bethesda, MD 20892   301-654-3810
                           Fax: 301-907-8906
              e-mail: nddic@info.niddk.nih.gov
                           www.niddk.nih.gov

5489 Urethritis
2 Information Way
Bethesda, MD 20892   301-654-3810
                           Fax: 301-907-8906
              e-mail: nddic@info.niddk.nih.gov
                           www.niddk.nih.gov

5490 What Everyone Should Know About Leukemia
Leukemia and Lymphoma Society
                           800-955-4572

Written in easy-to-read terms with explanatory line drawings, this booklet explains leukemia, its symptoms, treatment and its probable causes.

16 pages

5491 When Someone In Your Family Has Cancer
National Cancer Institute
Bldg. 31, Rm 10A24
Bethesda, MD 20892
                           800-422-6237

Written for young people whose parent or sibling has cancer.

28 pages

5492 When Your Child Has a Life-Threatening Illness
Thomas Frantz, author

Association for the Care of Children's Health
8701 Hartsdale Avenue
Bethesda, MD 20817   301-493-5113

A concise, supportive booklet for parents. Sections include initial reactions, hope, communication, other children, impact on marriage, and single parent families.

1983

5493 Wish Fulfillment Organizations
Candlelighters' Childhood Cancer Foundation
7910 Woodmont Ave., Ste 460
Bethesda, MD 20814   301-657-8401
                           800-366-2223

A list of groups granting wishes of children with life-threatening, chronic or terminal illnesses, with criteria and contacts.

5494 Young People with Cancer: A Handbook For Parents
National Cancer Institute
Bldg. 31, Rm 10A24
Bethesda, MD 20892
                           800-422-6237

Discusses the most common types of childhood cancer, treatments, and side effects and issues that may arise when a child is diagnosed with cancer.

86 pages

5495 Your Kidneys and How They Work
Information Clearinghouse
1 Information Way
Bethesda, MD 20892   301-654-3820
                      Fax: 301-907-8906
                 e-mail: ndoc@info.niddk.nih.gov
                      www.niddk.nih.gov

Camps

5496 Camp Allen
56 Camp Allen Road
Bedford, NH 03110   603-622-8471

A summer camp for individuals with disabilities.

5497 Camp Courageous
P.O. Box 418
Monticello, IA 52310   319-465-5916

Over 3,500 disabled campers have attended this recreational and respite care facility. The camp is open 24 hours a day, 365 days a year and operates entirely on donations.

5498 Camp Fantastic
Special Love, Inc.
117 Youth Development Ct
Winchester, VA 22602   703-667-3774

Nonprofit organization that provides enriching programs for chidren with cancer. Including Camp Fantastic.

5499 Children's Assn. for Maxiumum Potential C.A.M.P.
P.O. Box 27086
San Antonio, TX 78227   210-671-2598

Overnight camping, day-care, respite and rehabilitation to children with severe medical, physical or mental disabilities. Large medical staff enables nationwide acceptnace of children with severe problems.

5500 VISIONS/Vacation Camp for the Blind
500 Greenwich Street, 3rd Floor
New York, NY 10013   212-625-1616
                           888-245-8333
                      Fax: 212-219-4078
                 e-mail: camp@visionvcb.org
                      www.visionvcb.org

Family programs at Vacation Camp for the Blind in Rockland County, NY for children who are blind, severely visually impaired or multi-handicapped. Parent or guardian must attend winter weekends and summer session.

Betsy Fabricant, Camp Director
Nancy D. Miller, Executive Director

DESCRIPTION

5501 CELLS AND TISSUES

The human body consists of literally trillions of atoms, molecules, and cells that are organized in several "structural levels."

- Atoms and molecules. Atoms of oxygen, sodium, nitrogen, and carbon, for example, are the infinitesimal "building blocks" of the most basic level of living matter of the body. Atoms link to one another to form molecules.

- Cells. These are the smallest structural units that are able to live independently. The human body has billions of cells that are functionally integrated to perform the complex, vital tasks necessary for sustaining life. Cells are organized in the following ways:

- Tissues. Bodily tissues are organizations of structurally similar, specialized cells that carry out a common function.

- Organs. The organs of the body are groupings of two or more different types of tissues incorporated into a functional, structural unit to perform certain, specialized functions.

- Bodily systems. These comprise the final level of structural organization within the body.

Bodily systems consist of several interdependent organs that work together to perform integrated functions.

Certain mechanisms enable cells of the body to conduct activities that are vital for ongoing growth and survival. These include the processes of metabolism and homeostasis.

Metabolism

Metabolism refers to all the physical and chemical processes occurring within the body's tissues, including catabolism and anabolism. Catabolism refers to the breakdown of large, complex substances into simpler, smaller substances, usually resulting in the release of energy. During anabolism, complex substances are built up from simpler substances, usually resulting in consumption of energy. The processes of respiration, circulation, digestion, and excretion, for example, collectively enable the body to pro-

vide those substances required for metabolism and remove the by-products or waste products of metabolism. Abnormal changes in genetic material (mutations) or inherited defective genes may cause inborn errors of metabolism, affecting the body's ability to function properly.

Homeostasis

Homeostasis refers to the processes by which the body maintains a balanced internal environment (equilibrium). In order to maintain homeostasis, the body requires oxygen, water, other nutrients, and regulated atmospheric pressure and body temperature, for example. Because disturbances from the external environment as well as cellular activity continually challenge internal equilibrium, the body has ongoing self-regulating systems (feedback systems) that induce the responses necessary to maintain or restore homeostasis. For example, abnormally decreased levels of oxygen in the blood are counteracted by increased breathing rates that restore normal blood oxygen levels.

Cells

Cells are extremely complex, containing several subcellular structures vital to life. Human cells vary greatly in size and shape and are adapted for their specific functions. However, most cells are similar in structure. They contain fluid material known as cytoplasm surrounded by a thin, outer membrane (plasma membrane). The plasma membrane separates the fluid and specialized structures (organelles) within each cell from the fluid that surrounds and bathes the cells of the body. The cytoplasm of most human cells contains a circular, membrane-bound structure known as the nucleus.

Plasma Membrane

The plasma membrane serves to keep cells intact. In addition, it regulates the entry of oxygen and certain vital nutrients into cells, enabling the passage of carbon dioxide and other waste materials out of cells. Certain protein molecules on the surface of the plasma membrane also bind with other protein molecules, activating particular cellular functions.

Cytoplasm

The cytoplasm is essentially the "living matter" of the cell, containing the fluid that comprises the cell's inner environment and the specialized parts known as organelles. The organelles include the following:

- Ribosomes are relatively tiny particles that function as

"protein factories." They produce proteins, which are large molecules consisting of combinations of certain chemical "building blocks" (amino acids). Proteins play an essential role in the body. Particular proteins serve as the source of "building materials" for certain tissues and organs of the body (e.g., muscle, skin, blood, etc.). Other protein compounds known as enzymes accelerate the rate of chemical reactions in the body. Proteins also play an essential role in the elimination of waste materials and have many other functions.

- The endoplasmic reticulum (ER) is a complex network of small tubular membranes arranged in complex folds. This network winds throughout the cytoplasm of a cell. Passageways within the endoplasmic reticulum transport proteins and other substances to different areas within a cell. Rough ER has a rough texture due to the presence of ribosomes attached to its outer surface. Carbohydrates fats, and certain types of proteins are manufactured within smooth ER.

- The Golgi apparatus, which is located near the nucleus, is a system of microscopic, stacked membranous sacs and spaces. Small "bubbles" or sacs (vesicles) from the smooth ER transport newly produced proteins to the Golgi apparatus, where they fuse with the Golgi sacs. The Golgi apparatus then processes and modifies the proteins and packages them into small vesicles. These vesicles break away and eventually fuse with the plasma membrane, at which point they break open and release their contents outside of the cell for transport to other cells.

- Centrioles are typically paired, rod-like structures that participate in cell division.

- Mitochondria are tiny organelles that have double membranes and sacs with inner, folded partitions. Known as the "power plants" of the cells, the mitochondria serve as the major source of cellular energy production due to their complex, ongoing chemical reactions.

- Lysosomes are the major digestive units of cells. Enzymes within lysosomes break down (digest) particles of nutrients as well as certain invading particles such as bacteria.

- Cilia are hair-like projections on the surfaces of certain cells that move together in a wave-like manner. For example, cilia within the mucous membranes of the respiratory tract (respiratory mucosa) propel mucus upward and out of the tract.

Nucleus

The nucleus regulates cellular activities by controlling the functions of the organelles and cell reproduction. It is surrounded by a nuclear envelope that encloses a cellular material within the nucleus known as nucleoplasm. Pores within the nuclear envelope's membranes enable the interior of the nucleus to "communicate" with the cell's cytoplasm. The nucleoplasm of the nucleus contains several structures including the nucleolus and chromatin.

The nucleolus regulates the formation of ribosomes within the nucleus. Ribosomes then move through the nuclear envelope to the cell's cytoplasm, where they engage in protein production.

Chromatin, the material within the nucleus from which chromosomes are created, consists of thread-like structures comprising protein and deoxyribonucleic acid (DNA). DNA is the carrier of the genetic code and is described as a "double helix" because of its relatively long, spiraling, ladder-like structure. It consists of strands of certain chemical groups that are linked by pairs of substances known as "bases." There are four types of bases including adenine, which always pairs with thymine, and the base cytosine, which always pairs with guanine. Therefore, the sequence of bases on one strand of the helix coincides with the sequence on the other strand, enabling DNA molecules to duplicate before cell division.

Chromosomes

During the division and reproduction of cells, DNA condenses and gradually forms into the rod-like structures known as chromosomes. The DNA of the chromosomes carries the genetic information that controls the ultimate growth, development, and functioning of the body and determines the expression of certain inherited traits, such as blood groups, various physical characteristics (e.g., hair color, eye color, height), etc.

The cell that is produced when an egg (ovum) is fertilized by a sperm is known as a zygote. With the first and each subsequent division of the zygote, chromosomes within the zygote's nucleus are duplicated. Therefore, in most cases, all cells in the human body contain the same chromosomal material. In rare cases, some individuals may have some cells that contain differences in certain genetic material (mosaicism) due to an error in cellular division.

The nuclei of cells (except for ova and sperm) normally contain 46 individual chromosomes, one of each pair from the mother and the other from the father. Chromosome pairs are numbered from 1 to 22 with a 23rd pair consisting of one X chromosome from the mother and an X or a Y chromosome from the father. Males have an X and a Y chromosome and females have two X chromosomes comprising the 23rd pair. Each chromosome has a long arm designated "q" and a short arm designated "p." Both arms are further divided into numbered bands. Every individual chromosome contains thousands of genes, which are the hereditary units that contain segments of DNA. Genes function within cells by regulating the production of proteins. The 46 human chromosomes collectively contain approximately 100,000 genes that, together, are referred to as the "human genome."

Chromosomal Disorders

In some cases, due to certain abnormalities during cellular division (meiosis or mitosis), individuals may have abnormalities in the structure or number of chromosomes in the nuclei of cells of the body. There may be extra or missing whole chromosomes or chromosomal material within all or some of the body's cells. Because chromosomes contain many genes, the range and severity of associated symptoms and physical findings may vary greatly, depending upon the exact nature and location of the chromosomal abnormality.

RNA

Genes, which are sections of DNA, regulate the production of certain proteins. Ribonucleic acid or RNA is essential in "decoding" the inherited instructions within genes. RNA is similar in structure to one strand of DNA, with some differences - e.g., replacement of the base thymine with uracil. During the formation of RNA, a strand of DNA "unwinds" and a duplicate copy of a gene sequence is created. This copy is known as messenger RNA or mRNA. The mRNA migrates from the nucleus to the cytoplasm, promoting protein production in the ribosomes and endoplasmic reticulum. The ribosomes use information within the mRNA molecule to translate chemical "building blocks" known as amino acids into a properly sequenced protein strand.

Cellular Reproduction: Mitosis

Most cells of the body are replicated or reproduced during a complex process known as mitosis. During mitosis, a single cell divides in order to form two "daughter cells" with chromosomes identical to those within the original cell. The process of mitosis enables the body to produce new cells, to replace cells that have been damaged or lost due to injury or disease, and to replace cells that have aged and no longer function efficiently.

Neoplasms: Benign or Malignant Tumors

Sometimes mitosis may become uncontrolled, resulting in the development of an abnormal mass of replicating cells known as a neoplasm. Such growths may be non-cancerous (benign tumors) or cancerous (malignant).

Cellular Reproduction: Meiosis

Reproductive cells in the male and female sex glands (gonads, including the testes and ovaries) carry out a different form of cell division known as meiosis. During mitosis, one cell division occurs, creating two daughter cells, each of which contains 46 chromosomes. Unlike mitosis, two cellular divisions occur during meiosis, resulting in four daughter cells, each of which contains half of the chromosomes (i.e., 23 chromosomes).

Genetic Mutations

During the processes of mitosis and meiosis, the chromosomes within an original cell and thus its genetic material (DNA) are replicated and passed along to its daughter cells. Sometimes, errors may occur during this replication process, resulting in small changes or mutations in genetic composition. Such genetic mutations are passed along with every subsequent division of the daughter cell. For example, a genetic mutation may occur during the production of a reproductive cell (ovum or sperm). If that cell is eventually involved in fertilization, the resultant zygote and all of its reproduced cells will contain the same genetic error. Thus, every cell of the developing embryo and fetus will contain the identical mutant gene.

Genes function within cells by directing the manufacture of a particular protein. Therefore, mutations of a particular gene may impair the appropriate production of its protein. The effects of a particular gene mutation depend upon the function of its protein within the body. Disorders that result due to such mutations are termed genetic disorders.

Genetic Disorders

Human traits are the result of the interaction of two genes, one received from the mother and one received from the father. There are typically two genes engaged in the regulation of a particular protein. If one such gene changes or mutates and "overrides" the instructions of the normal gene on the other chromosome, the abnormal gene is said to be dominant. If the mutated gene is not expressed and is "masked" by the normal gene on the other chromosome, the mutated gene is termed recessive. In such recessive cases, two copies of the mutated gene are required for possible expression of the disease trait.

Genetic disorders may be classified into unifactorial and multifactorial defects. Unifactorial genetic disorders result due to abnormalities of a single gene or gene pair. Such disorders may be autosomal or X-linked.

In autosomal dominant disorders, the presence of a single copy of the disease gene results in the disorder. The mutated gene "overrides" or dominates the other normal gene. An affected individual may have inherited the disease gene from one of his or her parents, or the disease may arise as a result of an abnormal change (mutation) that occurred randomly, for unknown reasons (sporadically). If an individual with an autosomal dominant disorder has children, the offspring have a 50 percent risk of inheriting the defective gene.

In autosomal recessive disorders, two copies of the same disease gene are necessary for an individual to potentially develop the disorder. If both parents carry a single copy of the disease gene, the offspring have a 25 percent risk of inheriting both disease genes and expressing the disorder. Fifty percent of their children risk being carriers, and 25 percent may receive both normal genes for that trait.

In X-linked disorders, the disease gene is located on the X chromosome. As discussed earlier, females have two X chromosomes, whereas males have one X chromosome from the mother and one Y chromosome from the father. In females, certain disease traits on the X chromosome may be "masked" by the presence of a normal gene on the other X chromosome. In other cases, certain disease traits may not be fully masked by the normal gene; as a result, some females who carry a single copy of such a disease gene (heterozygous carriers) may express some of the symptoms associated with the disorder. In such cases, heterozygous females often have more variable, less severe symptoms than affected males. Because males have only one X chromosome, if they inherit such a disease gene, they generally express the physical characteristics or other findings associated with the disease and are typically more severely affected than females. Males with X-linked disorders transmit the disease gene to their daughters but not to their sons.

Females with one copy of such a disease gene have a 50 percent risk of transmitting the gene to their daughters and their sons.

In multifactorial disorders, susceptibility to a disorder is determined by the interaction of several different genes, possibly in association with the involvement of certain environmental factors.

Tissues

As mentioned above, tissues are groups of structurally similar cells that perform a common function. Different tissues within the human body may vary greatly in terms of the size, shape, and specific functioning of their cells.

There are four main types of tissue in the human body including epithelial tissue, connective tissue, muscle tissue, and nervous tissue.

Epithelial tissue or epithelium covers the surfaces of the body, lines most of its hollow structures or cavities, and serves to provide protection and support. In addition, some epithelial tissues permit the absorption of certain nutrients (e.g., oxygen into the blood); help to protect the body against invading microorganisms; or produce and release certain secretions. The cells within epithelial tissue are tightly packed together and contain no blood vessels; however, blood vessels within underlying connective tissue provide epithelial cells with nutrients. Different types of epithelial tissue are categorized based upon cellular shape and thickness.

Connective Tissue

The purpose of connective tissue, the most widely distributed tissue of the body, is to bind together and, along with the skeleton, provide a supporting framework to bodily tissues and organs. The shape and arrangement of connective tissue cells and the intercellular substance between such cells differ depending upon the type of connective tissue. There are several major forms of connective tissue in the body including the following:

- Areolar tissue, which consists of cells embedded in webs of loosely arranged fibers, supports and provides form to most internal organs of the body.

- Adipose tissue, which consists of fat cells within a mesh of areolai tissue, serves to insulate the body against heat loss, protect and cushion certain areas of the body, and store fat as a future energy source.

- Fibrous connective tissue, which consists primarily of parallel rows of white collagen fibers, are the cords of strong, dense, flexible tissue that connect muscle to bone (tendons). Collagen is the major structural protein of the body.

- Bone, the hardest connective tissue of the body, provides a supportive framework, assists in movement, and houses bone marrow.

- Cartilage, which has the consistency of firm or gel-like plastic, helps to absorb shock and provides flexibility.

- Blood, which has a liquid matrix, has several functions including providing a defense against invading microorganisms, repairing damage to blood vessels and tissues through blood clotting, and transporting oxygen, vital nutrients, and waste products.

- Muscle tissue enables movement through muscle contraction and relaxation.

- The nervous tissue of the body includes specialized cells that ensure ongoing, rapid communication between structures of the body and the control of bodily functions necessary to maintain life. (For more information about muscle and nervous tissue, please refer to the sections entitled "The Muscular System" and "The Nervous System.")

DESCRIPTION

5502 BLOOD

The blood is a circulating tissue composed of fluid and other formed elements such as red blood cells, platelets, various white blood cells, etc. The study of the blood, its components, and blood-forming tissues is known as hematology. Blood is pumped by the heart through the body's arteries, veins, and capillaries. The noncellular, fluid portion of the blood is a pale, yellowish liquid known as plasma. The blood has several functions including:

- To serve as a transport system, carrying oxygen and other vital nutrients to bodily tissues and promoting the exchange and removal of carbon dioxide and other waste products from cells.

- To help provide a defense against invading microorganisms, foreign tissue cells, and certain abnormal cells.

- To help repair damage to blood vessels and tissues through the process of blood clotting.

Blood Plasma

Approximately half of the blood's volume consists of plasma. This liquid, noncellular portion of the blood is approximately 95 percent water. In addition, the blood plasma also contains dissolved sugars (e.g., glucose, etc.), fats, salts, vitamins and minerals, amino acids necessary for the production of cellular proteins, and chemical messengers (such as hormones) that regulate specific cellular activities. Plasma also contains certain plasma proteins including globulins (e.g., antibodies, which are produced in response to a particular foreign protein [antigen]); albumins, which play an important role in thickening the blood; and fibrinogen, a protein that is essential for blood clotting. In addition, certain waste products are dissolved in plasma and transported to the kidneys for excretion.

Formed Elements

The formed elements of the blood include red blood cells (erythrocytes), white blood cells (leukocytes), and platelets (thrombocytes). Red blood cells, platelets, and some white blood cells are produced in the bone marrow. However, most white blood cells are produced by lymphatic tissue (e.g., lymph nodes, spleen, thymus).

Red Blood Cells

The red blood cells (RBCs) are mostly rounded, double concave cells with thin centers and thicker edges. A cubic millimeter of blood contains approximately five million red blood cells. The relatively large surface area of the red blood cells allows them to absorb and release oxygen molecules, and their shape facilitates their movement through narrow blood vessels. As mentioned above, red blood cells are produced in the bone marrow, where the rate of their formation is regulated by erythropoietin, a hormone produced by the kidneys. They typically circulate in the blood for approximately four months, at which time they break apart and are removed from the blood by the liver.

The red blood cells perform several essential functions. For example, RBCs transport carbon dioxide from the body's cells to the lungs for release into the environment. Carbon dioxide is a harmful waste product that is generated by normal cellular activities. The red blood cells also carry hemoglobin, an essential protein that contains iron. This red pigmented protein chemically combines (binds) with oxygen, producing oxyhemoglobin, which enables the red blood cells to transport oxygen to cells.

The various blood groups, such as blood types A, B, AB, and 0, are classified based upon the presence or absence of certain antigens (or "marker proteins"). Antigens are proteins that stimulate the body to produce antibodies. The red blood cells may have two types of antigens: namely, A and/or B. The different A or B blood types are classified according to whether the red blood cells have both, one or the other, or neither antigen. In individuals with type B blood, for example, the body does not produce antibodies to inactivate or destroy the type B antigen; however, the blood plasma contains anti-A antibodies. In individuals with type A blood, the red blood cells contain type A antigen and the blood plasma has anti-B antibodies. In type 0 blood, the red blood cells contain neither type A nor type B antigens, whereas the blood plasma has both anti-A and anti-B antibodies. In contrast, in individuals with type AB blood, the red blood cells have both type A and type B antigens, and the blood plasma contains neither anti-A nor anti-B antibodies.

In approximately 85 percent of individuals, red blood cells also contain an antigen called Rh factor. Those with this antigen are said to have Rh-positive blood, whereas those without the antigen have Rh-negative blood.

White Blood Cells

White blood cells (WBCs) are larger than red blood cells; however, they are present in the blood in lower quantities. A cubic millimeter of blood contains approximately 7,500 white blood cells.

The white blood cells include two major categories: granular leukocytes, which have granules in the substance of the cell outside the nucleus (cytoplasm), and nongranular leukocytes. Granular leukocytes include neutrophils, eosinophils, and basophils, and nongranular leukocytes include lymphocytes and monocytes.

Neutrophils and monocytes, which are also known as phagocytes, are responsible for isolating, engulfing, and destroying microorganisms that have invaded the bloodstream. These cells engulf the microorganisms and digest them in a process known as phagocytosis.

Lymphocytes originate in the bone marrow and mature in lymphatic tissue. They become active immune cells in response to the presence of invading microorganisms. Lymphocytes known as B lymphocytes produce specific antibodies to inhibit certain microorganisms, whereas those known as T lymphocytes may actively destroy microorganisms or assist in the functions of the B lymphocytes. (For more information, see the sections entitled "The Lymphatic System" and "The Immune System.")

Eosinophils help protect the body from various irritants that may cause allergies and are able to participate in phagocytosis. In addition, white blood cells known as basophils also play a role in allergic reactions and secrete certain chemicals such as heparin, which assists in the prevention of clotting as the blood circulates through the blood vessels (intravascular clotting).

Although granular leukocytes may have a lifespan of only a few days, nongranular leukocytes may survive for over six months. In fact, in some cases, certain individual lymphocytes may remain in the bloodstream for years.

Platelets
Platelets, which are the smallest blood cells, are produced in the bone marrow by specialized cells known as megakaryocytes and typically survive for approximately nine days. A cubic millimeter of blood contains approximately 250,000 platelets.

Platelets usually circulate in the bloodstream in an inactive state. However, when a blood vessel wall is injured, platelets respond through a complex process by clumping at the injury site and sticking to one another. The platelets and damaged tissue cells also release certain chemicals that stimulate blood clotting (coagulation) factors in the blood plasma. Due to a series of complex reactions, long filaments of fibrin, a fibrous gel, are produced that capture circulating platelets, red blood cells, and white blood cells. Once the damaged blood vessel is "plugged," the filaments contract, forming a solid blood clot.

In some cases, blood clots may form in undamaged blood vessels, potentially blocking vital blood supply to certain tissues and organs. A stationary blood clot is called a thrombus. If a portion of such a clot dislodges and circulates in the bloodstream, it is known as an embolus. Healthy blood vessel walls secrete the chemical prostacyclin, which helps to prevent the unnecessary activation of platelets and clot formation.

DESCRIPTION

5503 CARDIOVASCULAR SYSTEM

The cardiovascular system, also known as the circulatory system, consists of the heart and the blood vessels. The functions of the cardiovascular system include the following:

- To maintain the continual flow of blood throughout the body, providing cells with oxygen and vital nutrients.

- To assist in the removal of carbon dioxide and other waste products from cells.

Anatomy

The heart, a hollow, muscular organ the approximate size and shape of a clenched fist, is an efficient pump that maintains the continuous flow of blood through the vessels to all areas of the body. It is located between the lungs in approximately the center of the chest, with its right margin located under the right side of the breastbone (sternum) and the remaining areas pointing toward the left. The "tip" or the lowest point of the heart, known as the apex, rests on the diaphragm and is situated beneath the left nipple.

The heart consists of four chambers and is divided into left and right sides by a thick, fibrous, and muscular central partition known as the septum. The upper chambers of the heart are known as atria, and the lower chambers are called ventricles. Each chamber is referred to by its location: i.e., the left and right atria and the left and right ventricles. The atria are smaller and have thinner walls than the ventricles. The walls of the chambers of the heart are composed of specialized cardiac muscle known as the myocardium, and their internal surfaces are lined with a thin layer of smooth membrane tissue called the endocardium.

Blood enters the heart through large blood vessels (veins) that open into the atria; therefore, the atria are sometimes referred to as the receiving chambers. Because blood is pumped out of the heart via large blood vessels (arteries) that emerge from the ventricles, these lower chambers may also be called the pumping chambers.

The heart and the roots of its major blood vessels are surrounded by a membrane (pericardium) that consists of two fibrous layers. The pericardium has a tough outer layer (fibrous pericardium) that surrounds the heart like a loose-fitting bag, providing space for the heart to beat. The inner layer (serous pericardium) consists of an innermost "sheet" (visceral layer) that is attached to the heart and an outermost layer (parietal layer) that lines the inside of the fibrous pericardium. A space between the inner layers contains a thin film of fluid that lubricates the opposing surfaces of the inner membranes, enabling the heart to beat without friction.

Cardiac Function

Contraction of the heart muscle is termed systole, whereas relaxation is known as diastole. The atria and ventricles beat in a precise rhythmic pattern. One cycle of this pattern is known as a heartbeat. As the atria contract, they force blood into the ventricles. Once the ventricles fill with blood, they contract, pumping blood out of the heart.

The pumping action of the heart also involves the heart valves at the entrance to and exit from the ventricles. These valves control and direct the flow of blood through the heart. Two heart valves separate the atria from the ventricles (atrioventricular valves), preventing the backward flow of blood into the atria during ventricular contraction. The valves include the mitral or bicuspid valve, situated between the left atrium and left ventricle, and the tricuspid valve, located between the right atrium and right ventricle. In addition, two heart valves (semilunar valves) are situated between the two ventricles and the large blood vessels that transport blood away from the heart during ventricular contractions. The aortic valve, located where the major artery of the body (aorta) arises from the base of the left ventricle, enables blood to flow from the left ventricle into the aorta while preventing the backward flow of blood into the ventricle. The pulmonary valve, situated where the pulmonary artery arises from the base of the right ventricle, enables blood to flow from the right ventricle to the lungs while preventing the backward flow of blood.

"Oxygen-poor" or deoxygenated blood that has circulated through the body enters the right side of the heart into the right atrium through two large veins (the superior and inferior vena cava). The blood is then directed across the tricuspid valve into the right ventricle. When the ventricle contracts, the tricuspid valve closes and blood is pumped across the pulmonary semilunar valve into the pulmonary artery and on to the lungs, where the exchange of oxygen and carbon dioxide occurs. Oxygen-rich blood is returned to the left atrium by way of four pulmonary veins and is directed across the mitral valve into the left ventricle. When the ventricle contracts, the mitral valve closes and blood is pumped across the aortic semilunar valve into the aorta for circulation to the body's tissues.

The heart muscle or myocardium requires an ongoing supply of oxygen and other nutrients to function efficiently; thus, the coronary circulation transports vital oxygen-rich (oxygenated) and nutrient-rich arterial blood to the heart muscle, returning deoxygenated, nutrient-poor blood back to the venous system. Blood is transported to the myocardium by way of the left and right coronary arteries, which are the first branches from the aorta. Once blood is circulated to the myocardium, supplying the heart with oxygen and other nutrients, it passes into the cardiac veins, which then empty into the coronary sinus and into the right atrium, along with the deoxygenated blood from the superior vena cava and the inferior vena cava.

Each heartbeat, also known as a cardiac cycle, consists of the contraction (systole) and relaxation (diastole) of the atria and ventricles. In order for the heart to pump efficiently, the different areas of the heart and the cardiac muscle fibers must work together in an exact sequence. Precise coordination is achieved through the transmission of electrical impulses originating from the heart's natural "pacemaker" (the sinoatrial node at the top of the right atrium). These signals are then relayed to the various areas of the heart via a complex system of fibers (atrioventricular node, bundle of His, and Purkinje fibers). The electrical transmissions are delivered with precision timing to various areas of the heart, resulting in a rhythmic beat.

The Blood Vessels

Blood vessels are like a system of complex tubing of different sizes through which blood flows to various parts of the body. Different types of blood vessels have different purposes. For example:

• Some vessels ensure the movement of blood from one part of the body to another.

• Other vessels (i.e., the capillaries) facilitate the exchange of certain nutrients and waste products between the blood and the fluid surrounding cells within bodily tissues.

Function

There are several types of blood vessels including arteries, arterioles, capillaries, venules, and veins. The arteries, which carry blood away from the heart, progressively subdivide into smaller and smaller vessels known as arterioles, which control blood flow into the minute vessels known as capillaries. The arterioles help to regulate proper arterial

blood distribution and pressure by constricting or expanding as necessary. The thin walls of microscopic capillaries facilitate the exchange of nutrients and waste products between the blood and tissue fluid surrounding the cells. For example, oxygen and glucose move from the blood in the capillaries to the fluid surrounding cells and then into the cells themselves; in contrast, carbon dioxide and other waste products move from the cells into the blood within the capillaries. The oxygen-poor blood then flows from the capillaries into the small blood vessels known as venules. The venules join with other venules and progressively increase in size, becoming larger veins that transport the blood toward the heart.

The systemic circulation also includes a specialized group of vessels known as the hepatic portal circulation, within which blood flow follows a somewhat different route. Veins from certain organs, such as the stomach, intestines, spleen, pancreas, and gall bladder, do not transport blood directly into the inferior vena cava but, rather, into the hepatic portal vein, which carries blood to veins, venules, and capillaries within the liver. Nutrients pass from the blood in the capillaries into liver cells where various toxic substances are filtered from the blood. Hepatic veins carry blood from the liver and rejoin the systemic circulation via the inferior vena cava.

Structure

Arteries and veins consist of three layers including an outermost layer (tunica adventitia), a middle layer of smooth muscle (involuntary muscle) tissue (tunica media), and an inner lining (tunica intima or endothelium). The middle layer of arteries is thicker than that of veins, enabling the arteries to withstand the pressure of ventricular contractions. In contrast, blood returning to the heart via the veins remains at a relatively low pressure. The passage of blood through the veins is assisted by involuntary muscle that compresses the walls of the veins; in addition, veins have one-way valves that prevent the backward flow of blood. Capillaries have extremely thin walls and cannot be seen by the naked eye. They consist of only one layer (tunica intima), enabling oxygen and certain wastes to easily pass through them.

Fetal Blood Circulation

Because the developing fetus must obtain nutrients and oxygen from the mother's blood, the fetal circulation differs somewhat from the circulation after birth. During pregnancy, blood vessels (umbilical arteries) carry fetal blood to the placenta, where oxygen and nutrients are exchanged between the fetal and maternal blood supply, and then return blood to the fetus via the umbilical vein. Two relatively small umbilical arteries carry deoxygenated blood to the placenta, whereas a larger umbilical vein carries oxygen-rich blood back to the fetus. The fetal circulation also includes vascular channels or openings (e.g., ductus venosus, ductus arteriosus, foramen ovale), enabling most of the oxygenated blood to bypass the liver and developing lungs, and be delivered to the heart and brain. In most cases, once an infant is born and the pulmonary circulation is established, these fetal vascular channels close and the umbilical blood vessels collapse soon after birth.

DESCRIPTION

5505 DERMATOLOGIC SYSTEM

The dermatologic system includes the skin, the largest organ of the body, and its derivatives, such as the skin glands, the hair, and the nails. The skin, the sheet-like, outermost covering of body tissue, has several vital functions:

- To serve as a sensory organ. The skin's millions of sensory nerve endings (receptors) serve as somatic sense organs, enabling the body to respond to pain, variations in temperature, pressure or touch sensations, and other important changes in the surrounding environment.

- To help protect the human body from the harmful effects of the sun, chemicals, invading microorganisms, injuries, fluid loss, and other hazards.

- To assist in normalizing the body's temperature through the regulation of blood flow close to the body's surface and sweat secretion. For example, when the body is too cold, blood vessels within the skin constrict to help conserve body heat. When the body is too hot, blood vessels within the inner layer of the skin (dermis) widen (dilate) and the sweat glands secrete perspiration to cool the body.

The skin comprises several tissue layers including a thin, outermost layer (epidermis); a thicker, inner layer (dermis); and a thick underlying layer of subcutaneous tissue, which is a loose layer of connective tissue and fat. The subcutaneous tissue helps to insulate the body from extremes in temperature, protects underlying tissues from injury, and serves as a stored energy source.

Epidermis

The epidermis, which serves as the protective outer layer of skin, is made up of tightly packed cells (epithelial cells) that are arranged in layers. The thickness of the epidermis is variable; for example, it is relatively thick on the palms of the hands, yet comparatively thin on the eyelids.

The outermost layer of the epidermis (stratum corneum epidermidis) consists of dead cells that create a tough, protective covering. As the dead cells are sloughed off, they are replaced by new cells that are produced by rapidly dividing cells within the innermost layer of the epidermis (stratum germinativum). As new cells rise upward through cellular layers (strata) and approach the surface, their cytoplasm -

i.e., the inner substance of cells other than the nucleus - is replaced by the tough protein keratin. In addition, specialized cells (melanocytes) within the deepest layer of the epidermis produce melanin, a pigment that gives coloration to the skin.

Dermis

The dermis, the innermost layer of skin, consists of connective tissue, lymph vessels, blood vessels, sensory nerve endings (skin receptors), and muscle fibers, as well as other specialized structures, including sweat glands, sebaceous glands, and hair follicles.

The uppermost portion of the dermis contains rows of peg-like projections (dermal papillae) that help bind together the dermal and epidermal layers (dermal-epidermal junction) and form the characteristic grooves and ridges (dermatoglyphic patterns) on the skin of the palms and tips of the fingers. Such ridges, which are unique to each individual, develop before birth.

The deeper portion of the dermis contains a network of fibers including those that provide the skin with the necessary toughness (collagen fibers) as well as elasticity and the ability to stretch (elastic fibers). The number of elastic fibers decreases with advancing age and the level of fat stored within the subcutaneous tissue is also reduced. Consequently, the skin loses its elasticity.

Skin Glands

The sweat glands within the dermis are classified according to their location and type of secretion. These glands include the eccrine and apocrine glands. The eccrine glands are the most widespread sweat glands in the body. Their function is to produce sweat or perspiration, which helps to eliminate certain waste products (e.g., uric acid, etc.) and maintain a constant body temperature.

The apocrine glands, larger glands that produce a thicker secretion than that of the eccrine glands, are primarily located under the arms (axillae) and around the genitals. Such glands begin to function during puberty.

The dermis also contains sebaceous glands, tiny glands that open into hair follicles. They produce an oily secretion known as sebum that helps to lubricate the hair and skin and protect the skin from drying. Sebum secretion increases during adolescence (due to increased levels of certain sex hormones); however, it decreases during later adulthood, contributing to skin wrinkling and cracking.

Hair

When epidermal cells grow into the dermis, a small tube called a hair follicle may be formed. The growth of a hair begins from a tiny cluster of cells (hair papilla) at the base of the follicle. New hair replaces any that has been cut or plucked, for example, as long as the hair papilla is alive. The hair itself is a thread-like structure consisting of dead cells filled with keratin. The root is that portion of the hair that remains hidden within the follicle, whereas the shaft is the visible portion of the hair. A particular hair color results from the amount and specific form of the pigment melanin that has been produced by melanocytes at the base of the hair follicle.

A few areas of the body are hairless, including the palms of the hands, the soles of the feet, and the lips. Most hair on the body is fine and barely visible, with the most visible hair typically including that on the scalp, the eyebrows, and the eyelashes. Coarse hair also typically develops under the arms and in the pubic area during puberty (i.e., in response to the secretion of certain hormones). In addition, most males also develop coarser hair in the facial area, on the trunk, and on the arms and legs.

Skin Receptors

The dermis also has sensory nerve endings (skin receptors) that function as sense organs (i.e., somatic sense organs), transmitting messages to the brain concerning temperature, touch, pressure, and pain. For example, Pacini's corpuscle receptors, which are located deep within the dermis, detect pressure and vibration on the surface of the skin. Meissner's corpuscle receptors, which are usually close to the skin's surface, detect light touch sensations.

Other skin receptors include those that detect other touch sensations, cold, heat, vibration, or pain. (For further information on somatic sense organs, please see the section entitled "The Sensory Organs.")

Nails

The nails are produced when epidermal cells on the ends of the fingers and toes fill with the tough protein keratin. The nail body is the visible portion of the nail, whereas the remainder of the nail, known as the nail root, is hidden by a fold of skin (cuticle). A portion of the nail body that is closest to the root has a white, crescent-shaped area called the lunula. Tissue underneath the nail, known as the nail bed, contains many blood vessels, causing it to appear pinkish in color.

DESCRIPTION

5505 DIGESTIVE SYSTEM

The digestive system consists of those organs that break down food into small chemical components that ultimately may be used by cells of the body for energy (metabolism), growth, and repair. It includes the alimentary canal or gastrointestinal (GI) tract, which is the long, hollow passageway through which food passes, as well as associated organs, such as glands whose secreted juices help to break down (digest) food. Organs that comprise the GI tract include the mouth, pharynx, esophagus, stomach, small intestine, large intestine, and anus. Associated organs include the tongue, teeth, gall bladder, and digestive glands, such as the salivary glands, pancreas, and liver.

Nutrients

The foods of an individual's diet primarily include water as well as other nutrients necessary for growth and development. These include proteins, which play an essential role in cell repair and replacement; vitamins; carbohydrates, which serve as the primary energy source and assist in the breakdown and metabolism of other nutrients; fats; and minerals. Most minerals and vitamins may be absorbed into the blood circulation from the digestive system with no change in structure. However, other nutrients must be broken down into smaller, simpler food molecules. Food is broken down (digested) through physical and chemical processes. Physical breakdown of food materials is performed by the chewing and grinding actions of the teeth, for example. The actions of certain digestive enzymes (i.e., substances that act as catalysts in the breakdown of proteins and other nutrients) as well as other substances (e.g., acids) chemically break down food as it travels through the GI tract. Thus, the nutrients are reduced into smaller (less complex) molecules that may be absorbed through the lining of the intestinal wall for distribution to body cells.

Layers of the GI Tract

The hollow internal space within the alimentary canal or GI tract is known as the lumen. The walls of the GI tract consist of four layers of tissue, including an outermost covering (serosa); the mucous membrane (mucosa), which produces the mucus that lines the canal; the submucosa, a layer of connective tissue beneath the mucosa; and underlying layers of muscle tissue (muscularis). Regular, rhythmic contractions of involuntary (smooth) muscle within these layers of underlying muscle tissue propel food through the GI tract in a process known as peristalsis.

Mouth

Digestion begins in the mouth. The roof of the mouth, known as the palate, has a hard, bony, front portion (hard palate) and a soft, fleshy area (soft palate) that consists primarily of muscle. The tongue, which forms most of the floor of the mouth, is a flexible, muscular organ that helps manipulate food during chewing. It also contains the microscopic chemical receptors (taste receptors) that produce the nerve impulses necessary for taste (taste buds).

The teeth, which assist in the chewing and grinding of food, are firmly attached to the upper and lower jaws. The gums (gingiva), which consist of a mucous membrane and supporting fibrous tissues, surround the teeth, serving as "shock absorbers" and keeping the teeth tightly set into the jaws. Enclosing the oral cavity are the cheeks and the upper and lower fleshy structures known as the lips. In addition, as with all of the GI tract, the mouth is lined by a mucous membrane. Saliva, a thin, watery fluid that is secreted by the salivary glands and the mucosa of the mouth, assists in the process of swallowing by moistening the oral mucosa, lubricating food, initiating the breakdown of certain food products through its digestive enzymes, and promoting the sense of taste.

Teeth

The teeth are essential for the chewing, tearing, and grinding of food (mastication) as it mixes with saliva.

Humans typically have two sets of teeth including the primary (deciduous) teeth and the permanent (secondary) teeth. There are usually 20 primary teeth that erupt between the ages of six months and two to three years. The primary teeth are gradually replaced by the permanent teeth beginning at about six years of age. Adults typically have 32 permanent teeth.

There are four major types of teeth that are classified based upon their shape and location:

- Incisors are chisel-shaped and have sharp edges for cutting during mastication. The incisors are the eight front teeth (i.e., four in the upper jaw and four in the lower jaw).

- Canines or cuspids are sharp, pointed teeth that tear or pierce food. The four canines (i.e., two in the upper jaw and two in the lower jaw) are situated next to the incisors.

• Premolars or bicuspids have large, flat surfaces with two grinding "cusps" to assist in the breakdown of food during mastication. The eight premolars are situated next to and in back of the canines. The primary teeth include no premolars.

• Molars or tricuspids also have large, flat surfaces, yet have three grinding "cusps." The 12 molars are located in back of the premolars. The primary teeth typically include only four molars in the upper jaw and four in the lower jaw.

The interior of each tooth contains living pulp, which includes connective tissue, sensory nerves, and blood and lymphatic vessels. The pulp is surrounded by the dental tissue known as dentin. In addition, each tooth is divided into a crown, neck, and root. The crown, the exposed portion of a tooth, is covered by enamel, the hardest tissue in the human body. The neck, which is the narrow portion of the tooth surrounded by the gums, and the root, which fits into the bony socket of the lower or upper jaw, are covered by the sensitive dental tissue cementum. A fibrous membrane (periodontal membrane) connects the cementum to the jaw and gums.

Salivary Glands

The salivary glands are the three pairs of glands that secrete saliva. Their secretions are released into ducts that empty into the mouth. Because the salivary glands release their secretions into ducts, they are exocrine glands. The salivary glands include the parotid, submandibular, and sublingual glands. The parotid glands, the largest of the salivary glands, are located below and in front of the ears at the angles of the jaws. Their ducts open inside the cheeks. The submandibular glands are located toward the back of the mouth, and their ducts open under the tongue. The ducts of the sublingual glands secrete saliva onto the floor of the mouth. Saliva contains digestive enzymes (salivary amylase) that initiate the chemical digestion of certain foods (e.g., carbohydrates).

Pharynx

The pharyx, also known as the throat, is a muscular tube lined with mucous membranes and is part of the digestive and respiratory systems. Food and fluids enter the throat from the mouth and exit via the esophagus. However, air normally enters the pharynx from the nasal cavities and exits via the larynx. (For more information, please see the section entitled "The Respiratory System.")

Esophagus

The esophagus is a muscular tube that transports food from the pharynx to the stomach. It is also lined with a mucous membrane. The upper portion of the esophagus is encircled by a ring-shaped muscle (sphincter) that opens to allow the passage of food products. A similar muscle (cardiac sphincter) is located where the esophagus joins the stomach. The walls of the esophagus contain strong, smooth muscle fibers whose rhythmic, wave-like contractions (peristalsis) propel food toward the stomach.

Stomach

The stomach is a hollow, pouch-like organ located in the upper portion of the abdominal cavity. It continues the breakdown of food that began in the mouth. Once food passes through the cardiac sphincter from the esophagus, it is contained in the stomach by contraction of the ring-shaped muscle at the end of the stomach (pyloric sphincter). The walls of the stomach consist of three layers of smooth muscle and are lined with mucous membrane containing specialized cells that secrete gastric juices. These juices contain hydrochloric acid and digestive enzumes (e.g., pepsin) that are necessary for the breakdown of proteins. Rhythmic contractions of the stomach's smooth muscle layers mix digesting food with gastric juices, forming a semi-liquid mixture known as chyme.

Once partially digested food has been mixed into chyme, relaxation of the pyloric sphincter and contractions of the stomach propel the chyme into the duodenum of the small intestine.

Small Intestine

The small intestine has three sections: the duodenum, jejunum, and ileum. The function of the small intestine is to continue the breakdown of food product as it travels through the GI tract and to promote the absorption of nutrients into the bloodstream. As rhythmic contractions of smooth muscles (peristalsis) propel food through the small intestine, digestive juices from the pancreas and bile from the liver are added to partially digested food within the duodenum. In addition, the mucous lining of the small intestine contains tiny glands that secrete intestinal digestive juice. Mucus, the enzymes within the intestinal digestive juice (e.g., maltase, sucrase, lactase, peptidase), and the secretions from the pancreas and liver serve to further break down food into smaller food molecules that may be more easily absorbed.

The mucosa of the small intestine is organized into several circular folds (plicae) covered with minute projections known as villi. Each villus contains finger-like lymphatic vessels (lacteals) that absorb fat-soluble nutrients (lipids) from the small intestine for transport to the blood circulation. Such fats are absorbed in the form of chyle, a cloudy, milky liquid containing products of digestion. The villi also contain blood capillaries that absorb certain products of digestion (e.g., amino acids, sugars).

Pancreas

The pancreas, an elongated gland located across the back of the abdomen, functions as both an exocrine and an endocrine gland. It primarily consists of exocrine tissue that secretes pancreatic juice into ducts entering the duodenum. Pancreatic juice is an essential digestive juice that contains enzymes (e.g., trypsin, lipase, amylase) necessary for the breakdown of proteins, fats, and carbohydrates. The pancreas also contains tiny clumps of endocrine cells (pancreatic islets) that secrete certain hormones directly into the bloodstream.

The exocrine cells of the pancreas secrete their enzymes into several ducts that combine to form the main pancreatic duct. This duct joins with the common bile duct, which conveys bile from the gall bladder, and then opens into the duodenum. Most of the digestive enzymes secreted by the exocrine cells are activated by enzymes within the duodenum. In addition, exocrine cells of the pancreas secrete sodium bicarbonate, a substance that neutralizes the hydrochloric acid within the stomach's gastric juice as it enters the duodenum.

Liver, Bile Ducts, and Gall Bladder

The liver, one of the largest organs of the body, is located within the upper right abdominal cavity. As part of the digestive system, the liver functions as an exocrine gland whose cells secrete the substance known as bile into a network of ducts (bile ducts). Bile, a liquid that consists of waste products, cholesterol, and bile salts, carries waste products from the liver and assists in the digestion and absorption of fats within the small intestine. The bile ducts transport bile from the liver to the gall bladder and on to the uppermost region of the small intestine (duodenum). The gall bladder, a small, muscular sac located under the liver, stores and concentrates bile from the liver. When chyme that contains fats (lipids) enters the duodenum from the stomach, the fats stimulate the secretion of a hormone (cholecystokinin) from the mucous membrane of the duodenum; in turn, the hormone stimulates contraction of the gall bladder, forcing bile into the small intestine.

The liver also has several additional essential functions in the body. These include regulating the blood levels of amino acids, the building blocks of proteins; helping to filter toxic substances from the blood; and producing certain proteins within the fluid portion of the blood (blood plasma). Such proteins include certain components that play a role in blood clotting (coagulation factors); particular blood proteins (complement system) that, when activated, destroy invading microorganisms; and the protein albumin, which helps to regulate the exchange of water between the bloodstream and bodily tissues. In addition, the liver produces cholesterol and certain proteins that transport fats in the bloodstream to cells throughout the body and processes hemoglobin for use of its iron content. Hemoglobin is the protein that enables red blood cells to transport large amounts of oxygen to cells.

Large Intestine

The large intestine is the organ that forms the lower portion of the GI tract. This organ, which has a larger diameter than the small intestine, consists of several areas. These include a pouch-like area (cecum); the ascending, transverse, descending, and sigmoid colons, the last of which descends into the pelvic area and terminates in the rectum; and the end of the rectum known as the anal canal, which terminates at the external opening known as the anus. In addition, the appendix, a small, tubular structure, hangs from the cecum. Because the appendix contains lymphatic tissue, it may play a small role in helping to protect the body against infection; however, it has no known role in the body's digestive system.

As food matter that has not been broken down or absorbed moves through the lower region of the small intestine (ileum), it passes into the large intestine through the ileocecal valve. Bacteria within the large intestine acts upon the undigested material, potentially resulting in the release and absorption of additional nutrients. Water, vitamins, fats, and minerals are absorbed into the bloodstream through the lining of the large intestine. Remaining undigested material is expelled through the rectum, anal canal, and anus as feces. Swelling (distension) of the rectum typically stimulates the desire to defecate, i.e., empty feces from the rectum. Two ring-shaped muscles (sphincters) usually remain contracted to keep the anus closed except during the process of defecation. The inner anal sphincter consists of involuntary (smooth) muscle, whereas the outer anal sphincter is composed of voluntary muscle.

DESCRIPTION

5506   ENDOCRINE SYSTEM

The term "endocrine system" is used to describe a group of specialized tissues, glands, and other structures that have the ability to produce (i.e., elaborate) and secrete certain complex chemical substances (hormones) into the bloodstream or lymphatic circulation. These hormones have specific effects on certain bodily functions. Hormones assist in regulating the body's growth; controlling the rate of chemical processes in the body (metabolism); promoting the maturation and function of reproductive organs and the development of secondary sexual characteristics (puberty); and regulating many other bodily activities. Endocrine glands secrete hormones directly into the bloodstream or lymphatic circulation for transport to particular tissues or organs. Each hormone molecule may eventually combine with (or bind to) a specific area (receptor) on the surface of a cell within its "target organ," triggering the appropriate response. In contrast, exocrine glands are "outwardly secreting glands" - i.e., they secrete certain substances into ducts for emptying into a particular cavity or onto a bodily surface. (For example, the salivary glands of the digestive system secrete saliva via ducts that empty into the mouth.)

The endocrine glands include the pituitary gland, gonads (ovaries and testes), thyroid gland, parathyroid glands, adrenal glands, pancreatic islets, thymus, pineal gland, and placenta.

Pituitary Gland

The pituitary gland, also known as the "master gland," is a relatively small structure located deep in a saddle-shaped cavity in the skull (sella turcica). The gland is connected to a region of the brain known as the hypothalamus by a stalk of nerve fibers (pituitary stalk). The hypothalamus controls the functioning of the pituitary gland through direct nerve stimulation as well as through the actions of certain nerve cells that secrete hormones (hormone-releasing and hormone-inhibiting factors) into the bloodstream for transport directly to the pituitary. Hormone-releasing factors cause the secretion of certain hormones by the pituitary gland, whereas hormone-inhibiting factors inhibit the production and release of such hormones.

The pituitary gland is divided into two main regions: i.e., the anterior pituitary gland (adenohypophysis) and the posterior pituitary gland (neurohypophysis). Each region is responsible for producing different hormones. The anterior

lobe of the pituitary gland produces the following hormones, most of which are considered tropic hormones, i.e., hormones that stimulate the growth of another endocrine gland and the secretion of its hormones.

- Prolactin stimulates the growth of the female breasts (mammary glands) during pregnancy and the secretion of milk by the mammary glands after birth.

- Growth hormone serves to stimulate body development.

- Melanocyte-stimulating hormone (MSH) controls the amount of dark brown or black pigment (melanin) produced by certain specialized skin cells (melanocytes).

- Thyroid-stimulating hormone (TSH) stimulates the production of thyroid hormones.

- Adrenocorticotropic hormone (ACTH) stimulates the growth of the outer regions of the adrenal glands (adrenal cortex) and their production of hormones.

- Follicle-stimulating hormone (FSH) and luteinizing hormone (LH), which are known as gonadotropins, stimulate the gonads, i.e., the sex glands (ovaries and testes) within which the reproductive cells (ova and sperm) are produced.

In addition, the posterior region of the pituitary gland releases two hormones:

- Antidiuretic hormone (ADH) decreases urine production by increasing the reabsorption of water from urine into the blood.

- Oxytocin stimulates powerful contractions of involuntary (smooth) muscle within the uterus during labor. This hormone also stimulates the secretion of milk (lactation) by the female mammary glands during breast-feeding.

Gonads

In females, the paired glands known as the ovaries produce the female sex cells (ova or eggs), and, in males, the paired structures called the testes produce the male sex cells (spermatozoa or sperm). Follicle-stimulating hormone (FSH) produced by the pituitary gland promotes the growth and maturation of the cavities in the ovaries (follicles) within which the ova develop and mature; in addition, it stimulates the ovarian follicles' production of the female hormone estrogen. In males, FSH promotes the growth and maturation and production of sperm by the long, coiled tubules (seminiferous tubules) that form the bulk of the testes. In addition, in females, luteinizing hormone (LH) produced by the pituitary gland stimulates the maturation of ovarian follicles and their eggs, the follicles' secretion of estrogen, and the monthly release of ova from the follicles (ovulation). LH stimulates the formation of glandular structures (corpus luteum) within the ruptured follicles that secrete the female hormones progesterone and estrogen. In males, LH stimulates the cells located between the seminiferous tubules in the testes to produce and secrete the male sex hormone testosterone. (For more information, please see the section entitled "Female and Male Reproductive Systems.")

Thyroid Gland

The horseshoe-shaped thyroid gland consists of two lobes on either side of the windpipe (trachea) that are joined by a narrow region of tissue (isthmus). Tissue within the thyroid gland consists of follicular cells and parafollicular cells. The follicular cells, which comprise most of the thyroid gland, secrete the thyroid hormones thyroxine (T_4) and triiodothyronine (T_3). Certain amounts of the thyroid hormones are stored as a semifluid material within the follicular cells, from which they are released into the bloodstream as required. The parafollicular cells secrete the hormone calcitonin.

Secretion of the thyroid hormones T_4 and T_3 is controlled by the pituitary gland. These hormones assist in regulation of the metabolic rate, i.e., chemical activities within cells that release energy from nutrients or consume energy to create certain substances. The thyroid hormones also play a vital role in the normal mental and physical development and growth of infants and children.

Release of the hormone calcitonin occurs independently of the pituitary gland and hypothalamus. This hormone – in coordination with parathyroid hormone released by the parathyroid glands - helps to regulate the concentrations of calcium in the body. Calcium is a mineral that is important for proper functioning of the cells, blood clotting, muscle contraction, nerve impulse transmission, and other vital functions. Most calcium in the body is stored in bones of the skeleton. Secretion of calcitonin inhibits the loss of bone (resorption).

Parathyroid Glands

The parathyroid glands are the two pairs of small, oval glands on the back of both lobes of the thyroid gland. These glands produce parathyroid hormone, which serves to increase levels of calcium in the blood. In contrast to secretion of calcitonin, release of parathyroid hormone stimulates the breakdown (resorption) of bone.

Adrenal Glands

The adrenal glands are small, triangular organs that curve over the top of each kidney. The outer region (adrenal cortex) and inner region (adrenal medulla) of the glands have different functions.

The secretion of hormones by the adrenal cortex is regulated by hormones produced by the pituitary gland (e.g., adrenocorticotropic hormone [ACTH]). The adrenal cortex consists of three distinct zones of cells. The outer zone secretes hormones known as mineralocorticoids that help to regulate the levels of certain mineral salts (e.g., sodium) in the blood. The main mineralocorticoid, known as aldosterone, assists in maintaining the delicate balance between sodium and potassium - ultimately helping to regulate blood pressure and blood volume.

The middle and inner zones of the adrenal cortex together secrete hormones known as glucocorticoids, such as hydrocortisone. Glucocorticoids help to regulate the body's use of carbohydrates, fats, and proteins; maintain normal blood pressure; produce certain anti-inflammatory effects; and decrease the production of certain white blood cells that produce antibodies (anti-allergic effect). The middle and inner zones of the adrenal cortex also secrete small amounts of sex hormones (androgens) that stimulate the development of male secondary sexual characteristics and the female sexual drive.

The adrenal medulla or inner region of the adrenal glands releases the hormones epinephrine and norepinephrine in response to nerve impulses from sympathetic nerve fibers. The release of such hormones into the bloodstream serves to increase the heart rate, widen the air passages of the lungs, and dilate blood vessels that supply the skeletal muscles of the body.

Pancreatic Islets

The pancreas, an elongated gland that is located across the back of the abdomen, is divided into a head, body, and tail. It primarily consists of exocrine tissue that secretes digestive enzymes necessary for the breakdown of proteins, fats, carbohydrates, and certain acids.

The endocrine tissue of the pancreas, known as pancreatic islets or islets of Langerhans, consists of tiny clumps of cells among the exocrine cells. The alpha cells of the pancreatic islets secrete glucagon, whereas the beta cells secrete insulin. Glucagon promotes a chemical process (glycogenolysis) during which glycogen, a carbohydrate that is stored in the liver, is broken down into glucose and released into the bloodstream. Insulin serves to regulate and stabilize blood glucose levels by promoting the movement of energy-rich glucose into the cells of the body. The secretion of glucagon increases blood glucose levels. In contrast, secretion of insulin decreases levels of glucose in the blood.

Thymus

The thymus, a small lymphoid organ located behind the breastbone (sternum) in the upper portion of the chest, consists of two lobes that join in front of the windpipe (trachea). This organ functions as an essential part of the immune system, beginning its functions at approximately the twelfth week of fetal development until puberty. The thymus serves as a source of certain white blood cells (lymphocytes) before birth. In addition, the organ secretes hormones (e.g., thymosin) that promote the development of specialized lymphocytes, known as T lymphocytes, which defend the body against certain microorganisms (i.e., during cell-mediated immunity.)

Pineal Gland

The pineal gland is a small, cone-shaped gland that is located deep in the brain. It secretes the hormone melatonin, which is thought to play a role in regulating puberty, ovarian cycles, mood, sleep, and the body's "internal clock" (e.g., 24-hour circadian cycle).

Placenta

The placenta, the organ that develops in the uterus during pregnancy, serves to connect the blood supplies of the mother and the developing fetus. It develops from the chorion, i.e., the outermost layer of cells from the fertilized egg (zygote). The placenta produces chorionic gonadotropin hormone, which stimulates the ovaries to produce the female sex hormones estrogen and progesterone. Both of these hormones are necessary for the functioning of the placenta during pregnancy.

DESCRIPTION

5507 IMMUNE SYSTEM

The body's immune system consists of specialized proteins, cells, and tissues that function to protect the body against:

- Invading microorganisms (e.g., bacteria, viruses, etc.) that may cause disease.

- Foreign tissue cells (such as those that may have been transplanted from a donor).

- Toxins (such as harmful chemicals).

- Cells that have become cancerous.

Nonspecific Immunity

Certain mechanisms provide the body with general protection from invading cells and toxins, maintaining "nonspecific immunity." For example, nonspecific immunity is provided by the presence of certain physical barriers that may prevent the entry of invading cells or toxins or expel them - as well as chemical barriers that may destroy invading cells or toxins. Such barriers include certain enzymes within the saliva of the mouth, tears, and sweat; the protective barrier of the skin; the cough reflex; hairs within the nose and the sneeze reflex; the presence of harmless bacteria within the intestines that help to control harmful microorganisms; and secretion of mucus by cells lining certain organs of the respiratory tract.

In addition, tissue injury results in an inflammatory response, which consists of a series of nonspecific immune reactions. During an inflammatory response - which produces characteristic swelling, discomfort, and redness - the blood vessels widen (dilate), increasing the blood supply and enabling certain white blood cells to move from the vessels to the site of injury. For example, invading microorganisms typically encounter white blood cells known as phagocytes, which contain the infection by engulfing and destroying the microbes (phagocytosis). Invading microorganisms may also encounter certain naturally produced substances, such as a group of blood proteins (complement system) that, when activated, serve to destroy such microbes, or interferons, proteins that are produced in response to viral infection.

Specific Immunity

Specific immunity consists of particular defenses against certain invading microorganisms or toxins and includes inborn and acquired immunity. From birth, individuals are immune to certain diseases that affect other animals (inborn immunity). Acquired immunity is obtained when certain protective proteins known as antibodies are passed to a developing fetus via the mother's placenta or to an infant via the mother's breast milk. Acquired immunity also results from casual exposure to certain disease-causing agents and immunization (stimulation of the immune system to provide protection against a particular disease, such as through vaccination).

Humoral or Cellular Immune Responses

Specific immunity, which relies on the actions of the white blood cells known as lymphocytes, includes the humoral- and cell-mediated immune responses.

Humoral Response

A humoral-mediated immune response, also known as an antibody-mediated response, primarily consists of the production of antibodies by cells called B lymphocytes or B cells. B lymphocytes initially arise from primitive cells in the bone marrow known as stem cells. Shortly before and after birth, certain stem cells develop into immature B cells. When immature B cells recognize a disease-causing agent as foreign (antigen), they develop into activated B cells. Activated B cells rapidly divide into two lines of cells (clones): plasma cells, which secrete large amounts of antibodies into the blood, and memory cells, which are stored within the lymph nodes until they are stimulated by the same antigen that prompted their formation. They then also develop into plasma cells, secreting antibodies into the blood in response to the recognized antigen.

When antibodies are secreted into the blood, they bind to their specific antigens (antibody-antigen complex), making the antigens or the cells on which they are located harmless. Phagocytes then engulf and destroy large numbers of such antibody-antigen complexes. The binding of antibodies and antigens may stimulate the complement system, thereby improving the efficiency of phagocytosis.

Cellular Response

Cell-mediated immunity defends the body against certain microorganisms and possibly cancerous cells through the actions of particular white blood cells known as T lymphocytes or T cells. These cells initially develop within the thymus before birth. They arise from stem cells that migrate from the bone marrow to the thymus, where their development is facilitated by certain hormones. Newly formed T cells then migrate from the thymus to other lymphatic tissues, primarily the lymph nodes.

There are two main types of T lymphocytes involved in cell-mediated immunity including the helper cells and killer cells. Helper cells assist in the recognition of certain antigens and help to activate killer cells. The killer cells bind to cells invaded by viruses or other microbes and destroy them. It is thought that killer cells may function similarly against cancerous cells or foreign tissue cells.

Allergies and Autoimmune Disease

In some cases, humoral- or cell-mediated immune responses may inappropriately occur against the body's own tissues. Such "autoimmunity" may result in hypersensitivity or autoimmune diseases. A hypersensitivity reaction is characterized by an excessive immune response to a substance that the body perceives as foreign (sensitizing antigen). For example, an allergic reaction is a hypersensitive response that occurs upon exposure to previously encountered, usually environmental substances (allergens), such as pollen, dust, or certain foods. Autoimmune diseases may be caused by the production of antibodies against the body's own cells (autoantibodies) and inappropriate cell-mediated immune responses against self antigens (autoantigens). One proposed theory suggests that certain viruses or bacteria may play some role in provoking an abnormal autoimmune reaction. For example, when a foreign protein from an invading bacterium or virus is very similar to one of the body's proteins, the immune system may be unable to distinguish between the invading and the "self" protein, potentially triggering an autoimmune response. It is not known what role genetic, hormonal, or other environmental factors may play in contributing to such a response. Autoimmune diseases may be localized, affecting a particular tissue, or may involve many tissues and organs of the body (systemic).

Infectious Diseases and Vaccination

The purpose of immunization is to induce immunity to provide protection against a certain disease. In response to a vaccine, the body's immune system produces certain immune defenses, such as antibodies or particular white blood cells, that should protect against infection upon exposure to the disease-causing organism.

There are two major types of vaccination. In passive vaccination, antibodies obtained from a donor who was previously exposed to the microorganism are introduced into the body, thereby providing short-term protection against the disease-causing organism. In active vaccination, noninfectious portions of bacteria or viruses are introduced into the body, stimulating the production of antibodies against the foreign protein, resulting in longer-term immunity.

Some vaccines are intended for the general population, particularly infants and young children, such as immunization against the infectious diseases diphtheria, pertussis, and tetanus (DPT); measles, mumps, and rubella; hepatitis B; and polio. The recommended ages for immunization may vary from case to case. A child's pediatrician can recommend an appropriate immunization schedule.

Other vaccines are available for individuals who are at risk for certain infectious diseases due to their work situations (e.g., health care workers); their living situations or age groups (e.g., students living in dormitories, elderly individuals in nursing homes); local outbreaks of dangerous infectious diseases; or travel in certain countries.

Some individuals should not receive certain vaccinations, such as people with deficient immune systems. In addition, particular vaccines should not be given to young children or pregnant women.

DESCRIPTION

5508 LYMPHATIC SYSTEM

The lymphatic system includes a network of vessels known as lymphatics that collect the fluid lymph from different areas of the body and drain this fluid into the bloodstream. The lymphatic system also functions as part of the immune system, which protects the body against invading microorganisms (such as bacteria and viruses) and other foreign tissue cells.

Lymph and Lymphatic Vessels

The blood and the cardiovascular system play an essential role in transporting oxygen and other vital nutrients to body cells as well as transporting carbon dioxide and other waste products away from the cells. Such nutrients and wastes are exchanged through the walls of the microscopic blood vessels known as capillaries. However, there are some substances, such as dissolved protein molecules and excessive fluids, that cannot be transported across the walls of the capillaries. Such substances return to the bloodstream via lymph, a thin, watery fluid that accumulates in minute spaces located between tissue cells.

Lymphatic fluid passes through a network of minute vessels (lymphatic capillaries) located within the tissue spaces. Lymphatic capillaries are microscopic in diameter and consist of a single layer of cells (endothelium). The cellular layer is porous, enabling dissolved protein molecules, other substances, and fluid to enter the lymphatic capillaries. Lymph moves in one direction through the capillaries and other vessels of the system with the assistance of valves within the vessels.

The lymphatic capillaries also include the lacteals, finger-like projections within the wall of the small intestine. The lacteals absorb fats from the intestine into the lymphatic system for transport to the blood circulation. Such fats are absorbed in the form of chyle, a cloudy, milky liquid containing fat-soluble products of digestion (lipids). Lymph that is moving through lymphatic capillaries passes into progressively larger lymphatic vessels known as lymph venules and lymph veins and then drains into the thoracic duct or the right lymphatic duct. The thoracic duct, which is the largest lymph vessel, collects lymph from most of the body. It is located in the abdominal area and contains a pouch-like cavity (cisterna chyli) that serves as a reservoir, storing lymph that is passing toward its entrance into the bloodstream. The right lymphatic duct collects lymph from the right upper quarter of the body, including the right arm as well as the right side of the neck, head, and chest. Both of the ducts drain lymph into the blood circulation via veins within the neck area.

Lymph Nodes

As lymph moves through the lymphatic system, it is filtered by a network of lymph nodes, small structures that are located along the course of the lymphatic vessels. The lymph nodes consist of a fibrous outer shell and an inner mass of lymphatic tissue. Lymph passes into these nodes via several small lymph vessels (afferent lymph vessels) and exits through a single, larger lymph vessel (efferent lymph vessel). Although there are some single nodes along the pathway of the lymphatic system, most nodes consist of clusters. Most lymph nodes are located in the neck, mouth, groin, and under the arms (axillae).

Lymph nodes store certain white blood cells (lymphocytes) and are thought to play a role in producing antibodies. Lymphocytes and antibodies are components of the immune system and play an essential role in fighting infection. In addition, the lymph nodes filter out microorganisms and other foreign bodies carried by the lymphatic fluid. Thus, the lymph nodes function as a potential barrier to the spread of infection and other diseases by trapping or destroying certain foreign substances before they are able to enter the bloodstream.

Additional Lymphoid Tissue Organs

In addition to the lymph nodes, the lymphatic system includes the lymphoid tissue organs known as the thymus, spleen, and tonsils.

Thymus

The thymus is a relatively small lymphoid tissue organ that is located behind the breastbone (sternum) in the upper portion of the chest. It consists of two lobes that join in front of the windpipe (trachea). The lymphoid tissue of each lobe consists of tightly packed lymphocytes in a framework of epithelial tissue. The thymus gradually enlarges until puberty and then begins to decrease in size. Its lymphoid and epithelial tissues are gradually replaced by fatty tissue.

The thymus plays an essential role in the immune system beginning at approximately the twelfth week of fetal development until puberty. It serves as a source of lymphocytes before birth and then promotes the development of certain special lymphocytes, known as T lymphocytes, through secretion of certain hormones (e.g., thymosin). T lymphocytes that develop in the thymus then migrate to the lymph nodes, spleen, tonsils, and other lymphatic tissues. (For more information on T lymphocytes, please see "The Immune System.")

Spleen

The spleen, the largest lymphoid tissue organ in the body, is a spongy, fist-sized organ located in the upper left portion of the abdomen behind the lower ribs. The lymphoid tissue of the spleen includes pulp-like masses of lymphocytes and other white blood cells (e.g., monocytes) that isolate, engulf, and kill invading microorganisms during a process known as phagocytosis. In addition, the spleen also contains red blood cells.

The functions of the spleen include removing microorganisms and other foreign substances from the blood through filtration and phagocytosis; functioning as a reservoir for blood that may be released and returned to the bloodstream as needed; and regulating the quality of circulating red blood cells. The spleen removes and destroys worn-out red blood cells approximately four months after their production. Red blood cells that are inappropriately shaped or otherwise defective may also be removed. During this process, the spleen retains the iron from within the red blood cells' hemoglobin for later use.

Tonsils

The tonsils are the masses of lymphoid tissue located under the mucous membranes at the back of the throat and in the mouth. These lymphoid organs, which serve as the front line against invading microorganisms, help to prevent infection in the oral and nasal cavities. The tonsils include the lingual tonsils near the base of the tongue, the palatine tonsils on either side of the throat, and the pharyngeal tonsils (also known as adenoids) located near the back (posterior) opening of the nasal cavity.

DESCRIPTION

5509　MUSCULAR SYSTEM

The muscles of the body, collectively referred to as the muscular system, consist of bundles of specialized cells that, unlike other cells, have the ability to contract and relax, resulting in movement of body parts and organs. There are two main types of muscles: namely, skeletal muscle and smooth muscle. In addition, the cardiac muscle is a highly specialized muscle that is sometimes referred to as a third muscle type.

Skeletal Muscle

The skeletal muscles, so named because they attach to bones of the skeleton, are the most prominent muscles in the body and typically contribute to approximately 40 to 45 percent of an individual's body weight. These muscles may also be referred to as striated ("cross striped") muscles or voluntary muscles because their movements are under voluntary control.

Each skeletal muscle consists of groups of thread-like muscle cells, known as muscle fibers, in a highly organized arrangement. Each muscle fiber is made up of slender, striated strands called myofibrils that, in turn, are composed of bunches of microscopic, thread-like structures known as myofilaments. The myofilaments contain minute fibers or threads of proteins known as myosin and actin. The interactions of these proteins are essential for muscle contraction. During voluntary movement, skeletal muscle contracts and the bone to which it is attached (via tendons) moves in response to the contraction.

Neuromuscular Activities and Voluntary Movement

The brain regulates voluntary movements of skeletal muscles by sending impulses to the nerve fibers that supply the muscle fibers (motor neurons). The area where nerve endings and muscle fibers join is known as the neuromuscular junction. When the brain sends such impulses, nerve endings release a specialized chemical (the neurotransmitter acetylcholine) that serves to stimulate the muscle fibers. A complex series of electrical and chemical processes is initiated resulting in muscle contraction.

When voluntary movements occur, there are coordinated contractions and simultaneous relaxations of several muscles. In other words, as several muscles contract, one muscle is primarily responsible for producing the particular movement (prime mover or agonist) and the others (syner-gists) contract in order to assist the prime mover in making the movement in question. While such muscles contract, other muscles known as antagonists simultaneously relax, producing movements that oppose those of the prime mover and synergists. Such coordination of skeletal muscle movements helps to ensure smooth rather than jerky motions.

In addition to producing movement, the skeletal muscles also function to maintain posture and to produce body heat. For example, skeletal muscles are typically maintained at a level of slight, continuous contraction (muscle tone). Such muscle tone helps the body to maintain proper posture - i.e., the specific positioning of body parts to support their optimum function, place the least strain on different areas of the body, and maintain proper weight distribution. In addition, muscle fiber contraction creates much of the heat that the body needs to maintain its proper temperature.

Smooth Muscle

Smooth muscle cells have a smooth appearance when viewed under a microscope, lacking the cross stripes (striations) of skeletal muscle cells. Rather, they consist of elongated, "spindle-shaped" cells that are typically organized parallel to one another. Also known as involuntary muscles since their movements are not under voluntary control, the smooth muscles help to regulate certain functional movements of internal organs. For example, in the process known as peristalsis, the rhythmic contractions of smooth muscle propel food forward through the digestive tract. Smooth muscle is also located within the blood vessel walls and several other areas of the body.

The actions of the smooth muscles are regulated by the autonomic nervous system, the portion of the nervous system that controls involuntary activities of blood vessels, organs, and other tissues and organ systems. Neurotransmitters released at nerve endings contribute to the series of events that leads to contraction of smooth muscles. As with the skeletal muscles, smooth muscle contractions rely upon the interactions between the myosin and actin filaments. In addition, smooth muscle cell activities may be affected by changes in the chemical composition of the fluid surrounding the cells as well as the release of certain hormones.

Cardiac Muscle

Cardiac muscle, also known as the myocardium, is a special type of striated muscle that is located only in the heart. Like the cells within the skeletal muscles, cardiac muscle cells also have cross striations. In addition, there are dark bands or disks (intercalated disks) at the junctures of adjacent cardiac fibers. These disks enable the fibers to contract as a unit, thereby ensuring the heart's efficiency in pumping blood throughout the circulatory system.

As with the smooth muscles, contraction of cardiac muscle is regulated by the autonomic nervous system. Cardiac muscle activities may also be affected by the release of specific hormones. Electrical impulses that stimulate a regulated, coordinated sequence of contractions originate from the heart's "pacemaker" (sinoatrial node), an area within the upper right chamber of the heart (right atrium).

DESCRIPTION

5510 NERVOUS SYSTEM

The nervous system is a complex network of structures that functions to:

- Obtain information about the body's internal environment and the external environment,

- Relay and analyze such "data."

- Initiate, integrate, and control appropriate responses to this information.

The nervous system includes the brain and spinal cord, known as the central nervous system; nerves that extend from the brain and spinal cord to all areas of the body, referred to as the peripheral nervous system; somatic sense organs, which are distributed in almost every area of the body but concentrated primarily in the skin; and special sensory organs, such as the eyes. In addition, the peripheral nervous system is further subdivided into the autonomic nervous system, which includes structures that regulate involuntary functions of the body.

Nervous System Cells

Cells of the nervous system ensure ongoing, rapid communications between different structures of the body and the control of bodily functions necessary to maintain life. There are two main types of cells within the nervous system:

- Nerve cells, also known as neurons, which conduct (transmit) impulses.

- Glia, which are the support cells of the neurons.

Neurons contain a cell body, one or more slender, branching projections (dendrites) that transmit impulses toward the cell body, and a slender extension (axon or nerve fiber) that carries nerve impulses away from the cell body. A whitish, fatty substance known as myelin forms a protective "wrapping" or insulating sheath around certain axons, serving as an electrical insulator and ensuring the efficient conduction of nerve impulses. There are three types of neurons:

- Sensory neurons (afferent neurons) carry impulses to the brain and spinal cord from all areas of the body.

- Motor neurons (efferent neurons) transmit impulses away from the brain and spinal cord to certain tissues (e.g., muscle or glandular tissues).

- Interneurons (connecting or central neurons) carry impulses from sensory neurons to motor neurons.

Glia hold together and protect neurons. The different types of glia include the following:

- Astrocytes are relatively large cells with thread-like projections. These "branches" connect with blood capillaries and neurons, holding them in proximity to one another. The walls of the capillaries and the projections of the astrocytes participate in the formation of the "blood-brain barrier," which functions to separate systemic blood circulation from the central nervous system. This barrier prevents or slows the passage of certain toxic substances or infectious agents from the blood to the central nervous system.

- Oligodendroglia produce myelin and hold together nerve fibers.

- Microglia are relatively small cells with slender projections. When brain tissue becomes inflamed, these cells migrate toward the affected tissue, surround invading microorganisms or waste products, and digest them (phagocytosis).

Nerves and Nerve Impulses

Nerves consist of one or more bundles of impulse-carrying fibers known as axons that extend from the brain and spinal cord to all areas of the body. Certain nerves transmit impulses from particular receptor organs to the brain and spinal cord (afferent impulses) or from the CNS to certain specialized tissues (efferent impulses). White matter within the central nervous system and peripheral nervous system consists of bundles of axons that are myelinated; in contrast, gray matter of the nervous system primarily includes neuron cell bodies, dendrites, and unmyelinated axons.

The pathways by which nerve impulses are transmitted by neurons are known as neuron pathways. Nerve signals are electrical impulses or waves of electrical disturbances that result due to complex electrochemical changes in a neuron's environment. Such nerve impulses travel from the axon of one neuron (presynaptic neuron) to the dendrite of another neuron (postsynaptic neuron). The junction between two neurons is known as a synapse. As an electrical impulse reaches a synapse, the presynaptic neuron's axon releases small numbers of chemical substances known as neurotransmitters, which bind to certain areas (receptors) of the postsynaptic neuron. Consequently, the electrical impulse is conducted across the synapse to the postsynaptic neuron's dendrite. Thus, neurotransmitters are the chemical substances that enable neurons to communicate with one another.

Central Nervous System

The central nervous system includes the brain and the spinal cord. Bones of the skull enclose the brain, and bones of the spinal column (vertebrae) surround the spinal cord. In addition, a three-layered membrane (meninges) provides additional protection for the brain and spinal cord. The tough, fibrous outermost layer is known as the dura mater. The delicate middle layer, called the arachnoid mater, is separated from the elastic innermost layer (pia mater) by a space (subarachnoid space) that contains cerebrospinal fluid (CSF). This fluid, which acts as a protective "shock absorber," flows through the cavity within the vertebrae containing the spinal cord (spinal canal), the four cavities of the brain (ventricles), and the subarachnoid space.

Brain

The brain controls and regulates the many functions of the central nervous system including muscle control and coordination, sensory reception and response, and speech production as well as elaboration of thought and emotions. It consists of several major regions including the brain stem, diencephalon, cerebellum, and cerebrum.

Brain Stem

The brain stem consists of three structures: the medulla oblongata, pons, and midbrain. All regions of the brain stem serve as "two-lane" conduction "highways," with motor fibers relaying impulses from the brain to the spinal cord, and sensory fibers conducting messages from the spinal cord to other areas of the brain.

The medulla oblongata, a thick extension of the spinal cord, is located above the large opening (foramen magnum) in the bone that forms the back of the skull (occipital bone). It primarily consists of white matter mixed with bits of gray matter (reticular formation). The medulla contains groups of nerve cells (nuclei) of the ninth, eleventh, and twelfth cranial nerves, thereby receiving and sending impulses involved in the sensation of taste and sending messages to

muscles involved in swallowing, speech, and movements of the neck, shoulders, and tongue, for example. This region of the brain stem also contains nuclei of the tenth cranial nerve (vagus nerve) and thus receives and relays information concerning the regulation of blood vessel diameter (thus affecting blood pressure), beating of the heart, breathing, and digestion.

The pons and the midbrain both also contain white matter mixed with bits of gray matter. The pons has bundles of nerve fibers that connect with the region of the brain known as the cerebellum. In addition, it contains nuclei of the fifth, sixth, seventh, and eighth cranial nerves, thus relaying messages involved in movement of the eyes, jaws, and muscles of facial expression as well as receiving and transmitting sensory impulses from the face and ears. The midbrain contains nuclei of the third and fourth cranial nerves and therefore relays messages to muscles involved in controlling the reactions of the pupils of the eyes as well as five of the six muscles that move the eyes.

Diencephalon

The diencephalon is the region of the brain located between the midbrain and the cerebrum. It includes the hypothalamus and the thalamus.

The hypothalamus, a relatively small area of the brain, is situated under the thalamus and above the pituitary gland. One of its functions is to regulate the sympathetic nervous system, a division of the autonomic nervous system. The sympathetic nervous system controls certain involuntary activities during times of stress, such as raising blood pressure, increasing the heart rate and the breathing rate, and widening (dilating) the pupils. The hypothalamus is also involved in regulating body temperature, appetite, moods and emotions (such as anger, fear, etc.), and the sleep cycle.

Sleep and the Brain

Sleep is a natural state characterized by reduced consciousness and metabolic activity. During sleep, the brain typically engages in two main cycles, known as REM (rapid eye movement) and NREM (nonrapid eye movement) sleep. NREM sleep, which makes up approximately 80 percent of sleep in adults (and about 50 percent of sleep in infants), consists of four progressively deeper stages of sleep characterized by slow, deep brain waves; muscle relaxation; and regular, reduced autonomic activities (e.g., slowed breathing and heart rate; lowered blood pressure; etc.). Episodes of REM sleep periodically alternate with NREM sleep. REM sleep, which is associated with dreaming, includes increased levels of brain activity, irregular autonomic activities, rapid eye movements, and involuntary muscle jerks. A complete sleep cycle is usually about 90 minutes. Most individuals experience approximately four or five sleep cycles each night. It is not completely understood why sleep is a necessity, although most scientists agree that the brain requires regular rest to ensure optimum functioning - and that dreaming may help the brain to sort, manipulate, and store information obtained during waking activities. Many different areas of the brain, including the hypothalamus, are thought to play a role in regulating sleep.

The hypothalamus also controls the functions of the pituitary gland, an endocrine gland also known as the "master gland." The hypothalamus is attached to the pituitary gland by a stalk of nerve fibers known as the pituitary stalk. It regulates the gland's activities through direct nerve stimulation as well as through the actions of certain nerve cells whose axons secrete chemicals (hormone-releasing and hormone-inhibiting factors) into the bloodstream for transport directly to the pituitary. Hormone-releasing factors cause the secretion of certain hormones by the pituitary gland, whereas hormone-inhibiting factors halt the production and release of such hormones.

The thalamus consists of two masses of gray matter located above the hypothalamus. The neurons within the thalamus relay impulses from sense organs of the body to the outer region of the cerebrum (cerebral cortex); transmit motor impulses from the cerebral cortex toward the spinal cord; associate certain sensations with emotions (e.g., unpleasant or pleasant feelings); and play a role in the body's state of responsiveness to sensory stimulation (arousal or alerting mechanisms).

Cerebellum

The cerebellum, a two-lobed, rounded region of the brain, has a "wrinkled" surface and is located under the back portion of the cerebrum and behind the brain stem. The surface (cortex) of the cerebellum contains parallel ridges that are separated by deep fissures. Three stalks of nerve fibers (peduncles) that arise from the inner side of each cerebellar hemisphere link to different areas of the brain stem. Messages between the cerebellum and other regions of the brain travel along these nerve stalks. Through messages transmitted via the brain stem, the cerebellum receives information concerning muscle contraction and relaxation and posture. The cerebellum works in conjunction with the basal ganglia and the thalamus, adjusting messages relayed

to muscle groups from a certain area of the cerebrum (motor cortex) in order to maintain normal postures, sustain balance, and produce smooth and coordinated movements.

Cerebrum

The cerebrum is the largest area of the brain and is responsible for voluntary movements, sensory perception, emotions, memory, and comprehensive thought. The cerebrum contains several ridges (gyri) and grooves (sulci or fissures) and one deep groove known as the longitudinal fissure that divides the cerebrum into two halves (cerebral hemispheres). The left cerebral hemisphere controls the right side of the body, whereas the right hemisphere controls the left side of the body due to crossing of nerve fibers in the medulla of the brain stem. A thick band of myelinated nerve fibers known as the corpus callosum joins the lower midportions of and carries messages between the cerebral hemispheres. In addition, each hemisphere contains a fluid-filled cavity known as a ventricle (first and second or lateral ventricles). These ventricles communicate with a third ventricle in the center of the brain, and a fourth ventricle is located between the brain stem and the cerebellum.

Two sulci divide each hemisphere into four lobes that are designated by the bones over them: i.e., frontal, temporal, parietal, and occipital lobes. The surface of the cerebrum, called the cerebral cortex, consists of a thin layer of gray matter, whereas most of the interior of the cerebrum contains bundles of myelinated nerve fibers (white matter) known as tracts. In addition, deep within the white matter of the cerebrum are paired nerve cell clusters of gray matter known as the basal ganglia. Their function includes assisting in the regulation of muscular actions as well as initiating and ceasing movements.

The cerebrum has various areas that are responsible for particular complex functions. These areas include the following:

- Sensory areas, which receive sensory information from somatic sense organs (e.g., in the skin, muscles, internal organs) and special sense organs (e.g., ears, eyes, etc.) and analyze and sort such information.

- Motor areas, which transmit messages that control muscles, resulting in movement.

- Association areas, which link sensory and motor areas, integrate information received from the various sense organs, and engage in memory storage, recall, recognition, decision making, judgment, comprehensive thought, and the experience of emotions.

Mental, Emotional, or Behavioral Disorders

Psychiatry is a branch of medicine that studies the cause, prevention, and treatment of emotional, mental, and behavioral disorders. There is evidence in the medical literature that these disorders may be the result of genetic factors (sporadic or inherited) or physiological abnormalities of the brain's biochemistry. Environmental factors may also play a role, or it is possible that these disorders are the result of a combination of many of these factors. There are different branches of psychiatry that reflect such different approaches including neuropsychiatry, a branch of medicine that specializes in psychiatric disease due to abnormalities of brain functioning, and social psychiatry, which studies the role that cultural and social factors may have on the development and progression of mental illness.

Spinal Cord

The spinal cord is housed inside a central canal within the spinal column and extends from the foramen magnum at the base of the skull to the bottom of the first vertebra of the lower back. It is a long, cylindrical structure of nerve tissue and is an extension of the medulla oblongata of the brain stem. As mentioned above, the spinal cord is enclosed and protected by a three-layered membrane (meninges) and is bathed by cerebrospinal fluid.

The inner core of the spinal cord consists of gray matter (i.e., primarily containing nerve cell bodies and dendrites). Its outer portion is composed of columns of white matter that contain bundles of myelinated nerve fibers (spinal tracts). These pathways transmit sensory impulses from the spinal cord to the brain (ascending tracts) and motor impulses from the brain to the spinal cord (descending tracts). Certain ascending tracts transmit impulses that produce sensations of temperature and pain, and certain descending tracts convey impulses that control specific voluntary movements.

Peripheral Nervous System

The peripheral nervous system refers to those nerves outside the central nervous system. This part of the nervous system establishes communications between the brain and spinal cord and outlying (peripheral) parts of the body, such as muscles, glands, and internal organs. Nerves of the peripheral nervous system include the cranial nerves and the spinal nerves.

The cranial nerves are the 12 nerve pairs that arise directly from the brain and emerge through various openings in the skull (foramen). The cranial nerve pairs:

- Carry sensory impulses to the brain that are analyzed, sorted, and integrated, resulting in vision, smell, taste, hearing, and/or balance.

- Transmit motor and/or sensory information to particular areas of the head and neck.

- Convey impulses to glands and organs, resulting in certain involuntary (autonomic) activities.

The cranial nerve pairs include the:

- First cranial nerves or olfactory nerves
- Second cranial nerves or optic nerves
- Third cranial nerves or oculomotor nerves
- Fourth cranial nerves or trochlear nerves
- Fifth cranial nerves or trigeminal nerves
- Sixth cranial nerves or abducens nerves
- Seventh cranial nerves or facial nerves
- Eighth cranial nerves or vestibulocochlear nerves
- Ninth cranial nerves or glossopharyngeal nerves
- Tenth cranial nerves or vagus nerves
- Eleventh cranial nerves or accessory nerves
- Twelfth cranial nerves or hypoglossal nerves

The spinal nerves are the 31 pairs of nerves that emerge from either side of the spinal cord through gaps between adjacent bones (vertebrae) in the spinal column. The nerves are assigned a specific letter and number based upon the level of the spinal column from which they emerge. Eight pairs of spinal nerves are attached to the cervical segments; 12 pairs to the thoracic segments; five pairs to the lumbar segments; five pairs to the sacrospinal segments; and one pair to the coccygeal segment. The designation "C2," for example, refers to the pair of spinal nerves attached to the second segment of the cervical region of the spinal cord. The spinal nerves that emerge from the spinal cord branch to form many of the nerves supplying the trunk and limbs. The function of the spinal nerves is to transmit sensory and motor impulses between the spinal cord to those areas of the body that are not supplied (innervated) by the cranial nerve pairs. More specifically, the sensory nerve fibers of the spinal nerves transmit impulses from sensory receptors in muscles, internal organs, and the skin to the spinal cord, whereas the motor nerve fibers convey motor impulses from the spinal cord to glands and muscles.

Autonomic Nervous System

The autonomic nervous system (ANS) is that portion of the peripheral nervous system responsible for regulation of the involuntary functioning of certain tissues and organs. The ANS includes specialized motor neurons that transmit impulses from the brain stem or the spinal cord to involuntary muscle tissue, cardiac muscle tissue, and specialized glandular cells that produce and secrete certain chemical substances (e.g., hormones, enzymes).

The autonomic nervous system includes two groups of motor neurons (preganglionic and postganglionic neurons) and a group of nerve cell bodies (ganglia) located between them. The cell bodies and dendrites of preganglionic neurons are located in gray matter of the brain stem or spinal cord, and their axons extend to a set of ganglia in the peripheral nervous system. Within the ganglia, the endings of preganglionic neuron axons join with cell bodies or dendrites of postganglionic neurons, which, in turn, convey nerve impulses from ganglia to smooth muscle, cardiac muscle, or glandular tissue. The tissues to which postganglionic neurons transmit impulses are known as visceral effectors.

The autonomic nervous system is further subdivided into the sympathetic and the parasympathetic nervous systems.

Sympathetic Nervous System

The sympathetic nervous system functions to prepare the body for an emergency. When the body is affected by stress, such as occurs during strong emotions (fear, anger) or exercise, sympathetic nerve impulses increase to many of the body's visceral effectors, resulting in what is sometimes called the "fight-or-flight response." During this response, the heart and breathing rates increase; the pupils of the eyes widen (dilate); and secretions of certain glands increase, while those of other glands decrease. In addition, most blood vessels constrict, resulting in raised blood pressure; blood vessels that supply skeletal muscle widen, supplying additional blood; and the digestive process slows due to a reduction in the rate of the wave-like contractions of smooth muscle within the GI tract.

Parasympathetic Nervous System

The parasympathetic nervous system controls most visceral nerve transmission under normal circumstances, thus slowing and steadying certain bodily activities. For example, impulses conducted by parasympathetic neurons tend to increase peristalsis, speeding the digestive process; slow the heart and breathing rates; contract the pupils; and stimulate the salivary glands.

Autonomic Nervous System Neurotransmitters

There are four distinct types of nerve fibers (axons) in the autonomic nervous system that release certain neurotransmitters (i.e., acetylcholine or norepinephrine). The sympathetic and parasympathetic nervous systems work somewhat, although not completely, in opposition to each other (antagonistic), since each division may inhibit certain visceral effectors and activate others.

DESCRIPTION

5511 FEMALE AND MALE REPRODUCTIVE SYSTEMS

The female reproductive system includes those organs that enable females to produce the specialized reproductive or sex cells (gametes) known as eggs (ova); engage in reproductive activity; provide nourishment to a fertilized ovum (zygote) during embryonic and fetal development; and give birth. The male reproductive system consists of those organs that enable males to produce and store the reproductive cells (gametes) known as sperm, engage in reproductive activity, and fertilize ova with sperm. The production and secretion of certain chemical substances (hormones) by glands of the endocrine system promote the maturation and normal functioning of reproductive organs and the development of secondary sexual characteristics (puberty) in males and females.

Female Reproductive System

The female reproductive system includes several organs, such as the ovaries, fallopian tubes, uterus, vagina, and vulva. With the exception of the vulva (external genitalia), the female reproductive organs are located within the pelvic cavity. In addition, the female breasts (mammary glands) are supportive glands of the female reproductive system.

Ovaries

The female reproductive cells are produced in the paired structures known as the ovaries. These small, egg-shaped glands contain cavities known as follicles in which the female sex cells develop and mature (oogenesis). As females reach puberty (i.e., which typically has an onset between approximately nine to 13 years of age), the follicles begin to release eggs (ovulation) on a regular monthly cycle. This cycle is regulated by female sex hormones (estrogen and progesterone) that are also secreted by the ovaries.

The hormone estrogen promotes the development of female secondary sexual characteristics and normal functioning of reproductive organs (i.e., puberty). It promotes the development and maturation of female reproductive organs; development of the breasts; development of female body contours caused by fat deposition in the breasts and hip area, for example; and initiation (menarche) and regulation of the menstrual cycle. The menstrual cycle is the recurring monthly cycle during which the mucous membrane lining of the uterus (endometrium) is shed; begins to regrow, becoming thick and supplied with blood; is maintained in

the uterus; and is again shed. The thickening of the endometrium is stimulated by the hormone progesterone in preparation for implantation of a fertilized egg (zygote). If such fertilization does not occur, progesterone and estrogen production decrease, causing the uterine lining and the unfertilized egg to be shed (menstruation). Progesterone also plays an essential role in the normal functioning of the placenta, the organ that nourishes the developing embryo and fetus during pregnancy.

Fallopian Tubes

A funnel-shaped duct, known as a fallopian tube, uterine tube, or oviduct, extends from each ovary to the uterus. Each tube ends in a structure shaped like a funnel whose edge has finger-like projections. When an egg is released from an ovary, it enters the fallopian tube with the assistance of the beating motions of these projections and microscopic hairs (cilia) on their surfaces. These motions help to propel the egg toward the uterus. In addition, the fallopian tubes serve as the passageways within which the male sex cells (sperm) move toward the ovaries.

Uterus

The uterus, a hollow, pear-shaped organ composed almost entirely of muscle (myometrium), is the organ within which a fertilized egg (zygote) becomes implanted and the developing embryo and fetus is nourished and grows during pregnancy. The organ consists of a lower narrow section known as the cervix and an upper portion called the body. The uterus usually lies in the pelvic cavity behind the bladder. However, during pregnancy, the uterus expands in size as the developing fetus grows and may eventually extend to the top of the abdominal cavity. During the end of pregnancy, strong uterine muscular contractions cause the cervix to open and widen (dilate) and expel the fetus through the vagina.

Other Components of the Female Reproductive System

The vagina is the muscular passage that connects the cervix and the external genitalia and is the portion of the female reproductive tract that opens to the exterior of the body. The vulva is the external, visible portion of the genitalia in females (external genitalia).

Breasts

The female breasts (mammary glands), which are supportive glands of the female reproductive system, produce milk to nourish infants after birth (lactation). The female breast consists of approximately 15 to 20 divisions or lobes embedded within fatty tissue. Each lobe is composed of smaller lobules of milk-secreting glandular cells that are organized in grape-like clusters (alveoli). The small ducts that drain the alveoli have their outlet within the nipple. The circular, colored (pigmented) area of skin surrounding the nipple is known as the areola. Due to secretion of the hormones progesterone and estrogen by the placenta and the ovaries during pregnancy, the milk-secreting glandular cells become active, causing the nipple to become enlarged. Before and after birth, the glands initially produce a thin, watery fluid (colostrum) containing antibodies and proteins that help to protect the newborn from certain infections. Another hormone known as prolactin is responsible for the secretion of milk.

Male Reproductive System

The male reproductive system also includes several organs, such as the testes, reproductive ducts, seminal vesicles, bulbourethral glands, prostate gland, and penis.

Testes

In males, the gonads, i.e., the sex glands within which the reproductive cells are produced, are the paired, oval-shaped structures known as the testes. The male sex cells produced by the testes, known as spermatozoa or sperm, are responsible for fertilizing the female ova. The testes are located in a pouch-like structure called the scrotum.

Each testis is surrounded by a tough, fibrous membrane (tunica albuginea) and contains a long, narrow, coiled structure known as a seminiferous tubule. Sperm develop within the walls of the tubules in a process known as spermatogenesis. In addition, cells located between the tubules produce the male sex hormone testosterone. This male hormone and certain hormones produced in the pituitary gland (gonadotropin hormones) are responsible for the development and production of sperm.

As males reach puberty (i.e., which typically has an onset between approximately 12 to 14 years of age), increased secretion of testosterone promotes muscle and bone growth, stimulates the development of male secondary sexual characteristics, and promotes the normal functioning of the reproductive organs. More specifically, it stimulates sperm production; the development and maturation of male reproductive organs (e.g., seminal vesicles, prostate gland); and the development of male characteristics (e.g., deepening of the voice due to enlargement of the larynx and the vocal cords, growth of facial and body hair, etc.).

Reproductive Ducts

Sperm develop within the walls of the seminiferous tubules of the testes and pass through several reproductive ducts: i.e., the epididymis, ductus (vas) deferens, ejaculatory duct, and urethra. The first of these is the epididymis, a tightly coiled tube that runs along the top and behind the testes. The ductus or vas deferens is the muscular, movable tube that enables sperm to pass from the testes and the epididymis. The ductus deferens joins the duct from the seminal vesicles to form the ejaculatory duct. This duct enables sperm to empty into the urethra, the tube that passes along the length of the penis and carries sperm to the exterior of the body. In males, the urethra also serves as the passageway through which urine is excreted from the body.

Other Components of the Male Reproductive System

Semen (seminal fluid) is a fluid consisting of sperm as well as the secretions of certain supportive sex glands of the male reproductive tract. Such glands include the seminal vesicles, the prostate gland, and the bulbourethral glands. Semen serves to protect sperm from the acidic environment within the female reproductive tract.

The seminal vesicles, a pair of pouch-like glands, produce the largest portion of the semen's volume. The secretions of the seminal vesicles contain the sugar fructose, which provides a source of energy promoting the mobility of the sperm. The prostate gland, the chestnut-shaped organ under the bladder and in front of the rectum, secretes a thin fluid that forms a portion of the semen's volume and helps sperm to maintain their mobility. The bulbourethral glands, also known as Cowper's glands, are two relatively small, pea-shaped organs located below the prostate gland. The glands produce mucus-like fluids that form a small portion of the semen's volume. In addition, such secretions help to lubricate the end of the urethra. The penis is the portion of the male genitalia through which semen and urine pass.

DESCRIPTION

5512 RESPIRATORY SYSTEM

The respiratory system, comprising the air passages from the nose, throat, bronchial tubes, and lungs, is responsible for filtering the air that enters the body, supplying oxygen to the body, and removing carbon dioxide from the blood. This process is known as respiration. Certain organs of the respiratory system also influence speech and help to produce the sense of smell (olfaction).

The organs of the respiratory system are often classified into the upper and lower respiratory tract. The upper respiratory tract, which consists of organs that are located outside the chest cavity (thorax), includes the nose, pharynx, and larynx. The organs within the lower respiratory tract are located primarily within the thorax and include the trachea, the bronchial tree, and the lungs. The term "pulmonary" refers to the lungs.

Nose

The nose functions as the uppermost portion of the respiratory tract. This hollow passage, which connects the nasal cavities and the upper portion of the throat (nasopharynx), serves to filter, warm, and moisten the air entering the respiratory tract. Mucous membranes (respiratory mucosa) covered by microscopic hairs (cilia) line the entire nasal passage, as well as most passageways of the respiratory tract. Located within the nasal mucosa are specialized nerve receptors necessary for the sense of smell. (For more information on the sense of smell, please see the section entitled "The Sensory Organs.")

During inspiration, air enters the respiratory tract through the nostrils (external nares). Small hairs within the nostrils trap foreign particles, such as dust, pollen, or microorganisms, thus protecting against infection and allergic responses. Filtered air passes into the nasal cavities, which have moist surfaces due to mucus production. The nasal cavities are divided by a structure made of cartilage (nasal septum). Bones surrounding the nose contain hollow, air-filled cavities (paranasal sinuses) that affect the resonance of sound (e.g., during speech). In addition, these mucous membrane-lined cavities, which drain into the nasal cavities, assist in producing mucus for the respiratory tract.

As air passes through the nasal cavities, it is warmed, humidified, and filtered by three thin, mucosa-covered structures (conchae). Mucus on the surface of the conchae

and other organs of the respiratory tract flows toward the nasopharynx due to the healing action of the cilia, which help to move trapped foreign particles out of the respiratory tract.

Pharynx

The pharynx, also known as the throat, is a muscular tube lined with mucous membranes. The throat is part of both the respiratory and digestive systems and is divided into three regions: an uppermost portion (nasopharynx) that serves as an air passage; an area of the throat behind the mouth (oropharynx) that is a passage for food and air; and a lower segment (laryngopharynx) that functions as a passage for food only. Air normally enters the pharynx from the nasal cavities (although it may sometimes enter through the mouth) and exits via the larynx. However, food enters the pharynx from the mouth and continues through the digestive system via the esophagus.

The eustachian or auditory tubes also open into the nasopharynx, connecting the middle ears and the throat. In addition, the masses of lymphoid tissue that serve as the "front line" against invading microorganisms (tonsils) are located under the mucous membranes at the back of the pharynx.

Larynx

The larynx, also known as the voice box, connects the pharynx with the trachea. It consists of several areas of fibrous, flexible connective tissue (cartilage) and is also lined with mucous membranes. The larynx is responsible for producing the voice and preventing food from entering the airway during swallowing.

The opening of the larynx is partially covered by a "lid-like" flap of cartilage known as the epiglottis. This structure normally remains open, maintaining the larynx as part of the airway. However, when swallowing occurs, the epiglottis closes, sealing off the opening of the larynx and preventing food from passing into the larynx and the trachea. In addition, two strong, fibrous sheets of tissue known as the vocal cords stretch across the interior of the larynx. Passage of air over the vocal cords results in vibrations that help to create speech.

Trachea

The trachea, also known as the windpipe, extends from the larynx to an area behind the upper breastbone (sternum), where it then divides to form the two bronchi. The windpipe is a tube-like structure composed of elastic and fibrous tissues, smooth (involuntary) muscle, and rings of cartilage that help to keep the trachea open (patent). As with other organs of the respiratory tract, the trachea is also lined with mucous membranes (respiratory mucosa) covered by microscopic hairs (cilia). The secreted mucus helps to trap tiny foreign particles remaining in the inhaled air of the trachea, and the beating action of the cilia propels the mucus upward toward the pharynx and out of the respiratory tract.

Bronchial Tree

Because the numerous air passages of the lungs resemble an upside-down, tree-like structure, the bronchi and their branching airways are known as the bronchial tree. The trachea branches to form the main bronchi (primary bronchi) of the left and right lungs. Both of the primary bronchi then branch into smaller bronchi (secondary bronchi). The bronchi walls consist of three layers including an outer layer of fibrous, dense tissue; a middle layer of smooth muscle; and an inner layer of mucous membranes. In addition, the walls of the primary and secondary bronchi, like the trachea, are kept open by rings of cartilage, allowing the passage of air.

The bronchi divide into progressively smaller airways that eventually branch into tiny passages known as bronchioles. The walls of the bronchioles include only smooth muscle. The bronchioles then branch into microscopic tubes known as alveolar ducts that lead to the alveolar sacs. The walls of the alveolar sacs consist of many microscopic, grape-like structures called alveoli. The alveoli lie in contact with microscopic blood vessels (capillaries). The exchange of oxygen and carbon dioxide takes place across the thin walls of the alveoli, i.e., oxygen moves from the alveoli to the blood while carbon dioxide moves from the blood to the alveoli.

Lungs

The lungs, which are spongy, elastic organs located in the chest cavity, are divided into lobes: the left lung has two lobes, whereas the right lung has three. The narrow, rounded, upper area of each lung is known as the apex, and the broad, concave, lower portion of each lung that rests on the diaphragm is referred to as the base. In addition, a thin, moist, two-layered membrane known as the pleura lines the outside of the lungs and the inside of the chest cavity. A small amount of fluid separates the two layers of the pleura, serving as a lubricant as the lungs contract and expand during respiration.

The act of breathing (pulmonary ventilation) consists of two phases: inspiration and expiration. During inspiration, the chest and lungs expand, and air is drawn into the lungs. During expiration, the chest and lungs contract and air is forced out of the lungs.

Pulmonary Circulation

Pulmonary circulation refers to the movement of blood through vessels between the heart and the lungs for the removal of carbon dioxide and the addition of oxygen (oxygenation) to the blood. When the right lower chamber of the heart (ventricle) contracts, "oxygen-poor" (deoxygenated) blood is pumped to the lungs via the pulmonary artery. From there, the blood flows through the capillaries that lie in contact with the air-filled alveoli. Oxygen moves across the thin walls of the alveoli into the blood, whereas carbon dioxide is transported by the blood to the alveoli. Carbon dioxide exits the lungs during expiration. Oxygenated blood is returned to the left upper chamber of the heart (atrium) via four pulmonary veins and is propelled into the left ventricle. When the left ventricle contracts, the blood is pumped into the major artery of the body (aorta) for circulation to the body's tissues. In addition, the blood that nourishes the lungs themselves is supplied by the bronchial arteries.

DESCRIPTION

5513   SENSORY ORGANS

Certain specialized components of the nervous system, known as sense organs, are able to recognize specific stimuli in the external environment that affect the body, such as light, sound, temperature, or pressure. When the specialized microscopic structures that comprise the sensory organs (sensory receptors) recognize certain stimuli, they produce nervous impulses that are sent to the brain, the spinal cord, or both. (For more information on the brain and spinal cord, please see the section entitled "The Nervous System.") The sense organs may be classified into two general categories: the somatic sense organs and the special sense organs.

Somatic Sense Organs

The somatic sense organs include microscopic sensory receptors distributed in almost every area of the body, including the skin (where most sensory receptors are concentrated), joints, muscles, blood vessel walls, and internal organs. Stimulation of sensory receptors may result in different sensations of touch, such as pain, changes in temperature, pressure, or vibration, or may provide information concerning the movement or positioning of certain areas of the body. Only a small percentage of the nerve impulses transmitted by these sensory receptors is consciously perceived - i.e., sent to a region in the outer surface of the brain known as the sensory cortex.

Special Sense Organs

Sensory receptors for the special senses of hearing, vision, smell, and taste, are collected in the special sense organs, including the eyes (i.e., in the retinas), the ears (within the hearing apparatus), the nose (smell receptors), and the tongue (taste receptors). Sensory information received by these special sense organs travels to the brain via the cranial nerves, the 12 nerve pairs that arise from the brain and emerge through various openings in the skull. Most sensory information is transmitted to the sensory cortex of the brain.

The Ears, Hearing, and Balance

The ear is the special sensory organ involved in hearing and balance. It consists of three major parts including:

- External ear
- Middle ear
- Inner ear

The External Ear

The external ear includes the visible portion of the ear (pinna or auricle) and the external auditory canal. The pinna consists of folds of cartilage and skin surrounding the opening of the auditory canal, which is the tube that extends into the lower cranium bone (temporal bone) and ends at the partition between the external and middle ear (eardrum or tympanic membrane). The skin of the auditory canal contains specialized glands (ceruminous glands) that produce cerumen, a waxy substance that traps dust and other foreign bodies. Sound waves pass through the auditory canal and strike the eardrum, causing it to vibrate.

The Middle Ear

The middle ear, a tiny cavity between the eardrum and the inner ear, contains three minute, movable bones (ossicles) that conduct sound to the inner ear. The names of the bones essentially describe their shapes: i.e., the malleus (hammer), incus (anvil), and stapes (stirrup). When the eardrum vibrates in response to sound waves, the vibrations are transmitted and amplified by the three ear bones. The stapes' movement against a membrane-covered opening to the inner ear results in movement of the fluid within the inner ear.

The eustachian or auditory tube connects the middle ear to the uppermost region of the throat (nasopharynx). Although the eustachian tube is usually closed at rest, it opens due to muscle contractions associated with swallowing or yawning. The eustachian tube is shorter in infants and young children than in older children and adults. As a result, when an upper respiratory tract infection occurs, infants and young children have an increased likelihood of experiencing the backward flow of secretions from the nasopharynx into the middle ear space and associated infection of the middle ear (otitis media).

The Inner Ear

The inner ear contains a maze of complex, winding passages (known as the labyrinth) deep within the temporal bone. The major parts of the inner ear include the organ of hearing, known as the cochlea, and the organ of balance, the semicircular canals.

The cochlea, a hollow, coiled passage that resembles a snail's shell, contains the organ of Corti and thick fluid. The organ of Corti has tiny cells with hair-like extensions projecting into the fluid. Vibrations transmitted to the inner ear cause the fluid and the hair-like extensions to vibrate.

As a result, the hair cells are stimulated to generate nerve impulses that are transmitted by the vestibulocochlear nerve (acoustic nerve or eighth cranial nerve) to the brain.

The three semicircular canals are fluid-filled tubes containing specialized hair cells that respond to movement of the fluid. When movements of the head cause fluid movement within a canal, the cells initiate nerve impulses to the brain via the vestibulocochlear nerve, resulting in necessary adjustments to maintain balance.

The Eyes and Vision

The eye is a specialized sensory organ that is actually part of the central nervous system. It focuses light waves to create an image on the nerve-rich membrane at the back of the eye (retina). The retina, in turn, converts the image into nerve impulses that are transmitted to the brain via the optic nerve (second cranial nerve).

Anatomy and Function of the Eye

The eye is embedded in pads of fat within the bony socket in the skull. Movements of the eye are regulated by a network of six muscles, each of which moves the eye in a particular direction or directions.

The outermost layer of the eye, known as the sclera, is a tough, fibrous tissue that includes the "white" of the eye and the cornea, which is the front, circular, transparent area that serves as the eye's primary lens. A flexible mucous membrane, the conjunctiva, covers the sclera and lines the eyelid; in addition, the conjunctiva contains several glands that secrete tears and mucus. The eyelid consists of a thin layer of skin over muscle that covers a thin plate of connective tissue (tarsal plate). The edge of the eyelid contains a row of strong protective hairs known as eyelashes as well as several glands (meibomian glands) that produce an oily secretion known as sebum. The combined actions of the tear-secreting and mucus-producing glands of the conjunctiva and the meibomian glands of the eyelid produce an essential tear film that protects the conjunctiva and cornea from damage due to drying. The eyelid spreads the tear film over the cornea during the blink reflex, helping to ensure clear vision. Moreover, the eyelid further protects the eye by closing quickly as an involuntary reaction (reflex action) to the approach of any foreign object.

The middle layer of the eye, known as the choroid, includes two involuntary muscles: the iris and the ciliary muscle. The iris, the pigmented area visible through the cornea, is a circular muscle with a hole in its center known as the pupil, which controls the amount of light entering the eye. When certain fibers in the iris contract, the pupil widens, allowing in additional light; in contrast, when other iris fibers contract, the pupil constricts, allowing in less light. The lens of the eye, which is behind the pupil, is held in place by the ciliary muscle, a circular muscle that changes the shape of the lens to make appropriate adjustments in focus. For example, the ciliary muscle contracts when the eye focuses on near objects and relaxes when the eye views distant objects.

The hollow main cavity of the eye is filled with fluids that help to ensure the proper shape of the eyeball and assist in bending light rays that fall on the retina. The fluids include the thin, watery fluid in front of the lens (aqueous humor) and the jelly-like fluid behind the lens (vitreous humor). The retina, the innermost layer of the eye, is a complex, nerve-rich membrane upon which images created by the cornea and the lens fall. More specifically, as light passes through the cornea, the pupil, the aqueous humor, the lens, and the vitreous humor, it is bent (refracted) so that it is properly focused on the retina, which contains millions of tiny nerve cells that respond to light (photoreceptors). Such nerve cells are named based upon their shapes: i.e., rods and cones. Rods are stimulated by dim light and are necessary for night vision. Cones are stimulated by brighter light and are the receptors for daytime vision. Three different types of cones respond to the colors red, blue, or green. The rods and cones convert images formed on the retina into nerve impulses that are transmitted by the optic nerve (second cranial nerve) to the brain.

The Nose and the Smell Receptors

In addition to serving as the uppermost region of the respiratory tract, the nose also functions as the special sensory organ involved in the sense of smell (olfaction). The chemical receptors necessary for olfaction are specialized nerve cell endings located in a small area of mucous membrane (nasal mucosa) lining the nasal cavities. The olfactory cells have specialized, microscopic hairs (cilia) that are stimulated by different chemicals. In response to such chemicals, the cilia generate nerve impulses that pass through the olfactory nerve (first cranial nerve) to the smell centers of the brain.

The Tongue and the Taste Receptors

The tongue is the muscular, flexible organ in the floor of the mouth. This organ - which also plays an essential role in producing speech, breaking down food during chewing (mastication), and swallowing - functions as a specialized sensory organ involved in taste.

There are approximately 10,000 microscopic chemical receptors known as taste buds that produce the nerve impulses required for taste. Although most are located on the tongue, there are also some taste buds on the roof of the mouth (palate) and the back of the throat. The taste buds surround the bases of nipple-shaped elevations (papillae) that cover the surface of the tongue and other tissues.

Specialized cells within the taste buds (gustatory cells) generate nerve impulses in response to dissolved chemicals within saliva. Most of these impulses pass through the facial nerve (seventh cranial nerve) and the glossopharyngeal nerve (ninth cranial nerve) to the taste center of the brain. Stimulation of the taste buds results in four types of taste sensations including sour, sweet, bitter, and salty. Other taste sensations or "flavors" result due to the combined stimulation of taste and olfactory receptors.

DESCRIPTION

5514 SKELETAL SYSTEM

The average human skeletal system consists of 206 bones, cartilage, and adjoining joints, tendons, and ligaments. The skeleton provides the body with a supportive, protective framework for attached muscles and underlying tissues and organs. The bones are living organs, enabling the human body to grow and adapt.

Major functions of the skeletal system:

- To provide a supporting framework for the softer tissues of the body.

- To facilitate movement. The skeleton serves as a firm, strong framework on which muscles can pull to move the different areas of the body.

- To protect and support delicate tissues and organs. For example, the skull surrounds and protects the brain, and the bones of the spinal column (vertebrae) surround and protect the spinal cord.

- To serve as a reservoir for calcium, a mineral that is essential for proper cellular functioning, transmission of nerve impulses, muscle contraction, heart (cardiac) functioning, blood clotting (coagulation), and other bodily processes. When blood calcium drops below normal levels (hypocalcemia), calcium is released into the blood stream from its storage in the bones; likewise, when blood calcium rises above normal levels (hypercalcemia), calcium is reabsorbed into the bones from the blood.

- To "house" bone marrow that produces blood cells. The red bone marrow, a soft mesh of fatty connective tissue within the cavities of some bones, contains developing red blood cells and white blood cells as well as megakaryocytes, the parent cells of platelets. Although red bone marrow is present in all bones during childhood, it is eventually replaced by yellow bone marrow in some bones by adolescence. Yellow marrow produces some white blood cells; however, it is less active than red marrow. By adulthood, red marrow is present only in certain bones, such as skull bones, collarbones (clavicles), shoulder blades (scapulae), vertebrae, breastbone (sternum), ribs, and hipbones.

Bones and Cartilage

Most bone surfaces are covered with periosteum, a tough, thick, fibrous membrane containing a network of nerves that supply (innervate) and blood vessels that nourish the underlying bone. The periosteum of younger bones is typically thick with a significant blood supply; however, as bones age, the periosteum gradually becomes thinner and has a reduction in blood supply. Beneath the periosteum is a dense, hard shell known as compact bone, which contains columns of bone cells (vascular haversian canals) that play an essential role in bone growth, nutrition, and repair. The compact bone surrounds spongy bone that is porous, containing spaces. The spaces within spongy bone and the cavities within hollow bones contain bone marrow.

In a developing embryo, most bones begin to form during approximately the fifth or sixth week of pregnancy. Initially, the skeleton primarily consists of cartilage, a fibrous connective tissue with a consistency of firm or gel-like plastic. During approximately the seventh or eighth week of embryonic development, the process of ossification begins, during which cartilage is gradually replaced by bone. The "remodeling" of a growing bone is possible due to the ongoing activity of bone-forming cells known as osteoblasts and bone-resorbing cells called osteoclasts. The combined activities of osteoblasts and osteoclasts gradually transform the cartilage skeleton into appropriately shaped, proportioned bones. In addition, ongoing activity of osteoblasts and osteoclasts enables bones to react to stress including injury by making necessary adaptations in density, size, and shape. When an infant is born, many bones of the skeleton still consist primarily of cartilage that will gradually develop into bone (ossify). Initially, the shafts (diaphyses) of the long bones are separated from the ends (epiphyses) by a layer of cartilage (epiphyseal plate), thereby enabling the bones to grow. Growth ceases when the cartilage between the shafts and the ends of bones is no longer present.

The human skeleton consists of four different types of bones that are primarily classified by their shape. Long bones are those whose length exceeds their thickness and breadth, such as the upper arm bone (humerus) and the thigh bone (femur). Short bones have dimensions that are essentially equal, such as the wrist (carpal) bones. Flat bones, which are actually bent or curved in most cases, include the bone of the forehead (frontal bone).

Irregular bones consist of those that may not be classified as long, short, or flat; such bones include the hipbones and the vertebrae.

In addition, the human skeleton is classified into two main divisions: the axial and the appendicular skeletons. The axial skeleton includes bones of the center (or axis) of the body, i.e., the skull, the unshaped bone supporting the muscles at the back of the tongue (hyoid bone), the three pairs of tiny bones in the middle ears that help to conduct sound (auditory ossicles), the breastbone (sternum), the ribs, and the spinal vertebrae. The appendicular skeleton consists of bones of the shoulder and pelvis (limb girdles) and attached limb bones including bones of the wrists, hands, arms, ankles, feet, and legs. There are 80 bones in the axial skeleton and 106 bones in the appendicular skeleton.

Joints

Bones within the skeleton are connected by different types of joints. There are three main types of joints including fixed joints that are firmly secured with fibrous tissue, such as joints between bones of the skull (sutures); joints that allow a small degree of movement, such as those between the central areas (bodies) of the vertebrae; and "mobile" joints that allow a large degree of movement in one, two, or, in some cases, many different directions. Most joints fall into the latter category, such as the hip and shoulder joints, which are considered "ball-and-socket" joints, i.e., the mobile joints that allow the widest range of movements. In mobile joints, the ends of the two joining bones are covered with a layer of cartilage that helps to reduce friction during movement. In addition, the spaces between the joints and bones are lined with a connective tissue membrane (synovial membrane) that secretes a thick fluid to lubricate the joints.

Ligaments and Tendons

Joints are supported by ligaments, tough, white fibrous bands of tissue that bind together the ends of bones and prevent overextended, excessive joint movements (hypermobility). In addition, the muscles that control the movements of joints are anchored to bone by tendons, which are strong, dense, flexible cords of connective tissue.

The Skull

The skull surrounds and protects the brain and serves as a firm point of attachment for the muscles of the head and neck. It consists of the facial skeleton as well as the bones that form the bony shell encasing the brain (cranium).

Fourteen bones form the facial skeleton including the jawbones, cheekbones, bones forming the eye sockets, and bones of the nasal bridge and cavity. The cranium consists of eight bones including bones forming the forehead (frontal bone); the bulging, upper sides of the cranium (the two parietal bones); the lower sides of the cranium (the two temporal bones); the central portion of the base of the cranium (sphenoid bone); the base of the cranium as well as the roof and most of the walls of the upper portion of the nasal cavity (ethmoid bone); and the back of the cranium (occipital bone).

All bones of the adult skull, with the exception of the lower jawbone (mandible), are fixed to one another by immovable fibrous joints (sutures). At birth, however, ossification of skull bones is incomplete; therefore, infants have membrane-covered gaps between bones of the skull where the bones have not fully fused. Such gaps, known as "soft spots" or fontanelles, are present under the front (anterior fontanelle) and back (posterior fontanelle) of the scalp at birth. The fontanelles allow compression of the skull during birth, thereby minimizing the risk that the bones may be broken during delivery. The anterior fontanelle, which is diamond-shaped and approximately one inch across, typically closes by the age of approximately 18 months. The posterior fontanelle is about one-quarter of an inch across and usually closes by approximately two months of age.

Many bones of the skull contain air-filled spaces or cavities (sinuses), such as those that open into the nose (paranasal sinuses). In addition, there are cavities in the lower sides of the cranium (temporal bones) that contain certain structures of the inner and middle ears. The skull also has several natural openings (foramen) that allow for the passage of particular blood vessels and nerves. Such blood vessels include those that transport blood to and from the brain (e.g., carotid arteries and jugular veins), and such nerves include the 12 nerve pairs that emerge from the brain and conduct impulses for such functions as smell; taste; sight; hearing; certain movements, such as those of the eyes, the tongue, the head, or the shoulders; etc. A large opening in the base of the skull (foramen magnum) is the passage through which the spinal cord becomes continuous with the lowest region of the brain (medulla oblongata).

The Vertebrae

The spine or vertebral column consists of 33 bones known as vertebrae, including seven cervical vertebrae, 12 thoracic vertebrae, five lumbar vertebrae, five fused bones forming a large triangular bone (sacrum) in the lower spine, and, in the lowest segments of the spinal column, four rudimentary bones making up the coccyx. Together, the sacrum and the coccyx form the back of the pelvis. The cervical vertebrae comprise the skeleton of the neck, whereas the thoracic vertebrae form the spinal column of the upper back. The lumbar vertebrae comprise the vertebral column of the lower back superior to the sacrum.

There are several curves in the vertebral column that serve to increase its strength, enabling the spine to support the weight of the body. In addition, such curves provide the body with balance, making standing and walking possible. The spinal column in adults has four curves: i.e., the small of the back and the neck curve inward (lumbar and cervical curves) and the thoracic and the lowermost vertebrae curve outward (thoracic and sacral curves). In newborns, however, the spinal column has one continuous convex curve. As infants develop the ability to support their head and move it independently, the neck (cervical region) develops a concave curve; as they begin to stand and walk, the lower back (lumbar region of the spinal column) also develops a concave curve.

DESCRIPTION

5515 URINARY SYSTEM

The urinary system, which consists of the two kidneys, the ureters, the bladder, and the urethra, filters waste products from the blood, returns essential nutrients back into the blood, and produces and excretes urine.

The Kidneys

The kidneys, which are located at the back of the abdominal cavity, are situated on either side of the spinal column above the waistline. The right kidney lies beneath the liver. The left kidney, which is usually slightly higher than the right, is located below the spleen.

The primary functions of the kidneys are to regulate the delicate balance of electrolytes including sodium and potassium; control the acid-base balance of the body (i.e., ensuring that the blood and other bodily fluids are neither too acidic nor too alkaline); and filter soluble wastes from the blood and eliminate these waste products. More specifically, the purpose of the kidneys includes the following:

- To filter certain waste products (e.g., urea, ammonia) and excessive sodium and water from the blood.

- To reabsorb particular substances and return them to the blood.

- To regulate the levels of certain substances in the blood and maintain the appropriate balance between water and salt content in the body (i.e., by filtration, reabsorption, and secretion).

- To regulate blood pressure and the production and release of red blood cells. For example, cells of the juxtaglomerular apparatus of the kidneys secrete a hormone (renin) that results in the constriction of blood vessels, thereby raising blood pressure. In addition, the kidneys produce erythropoietin, a hormone that assists in stimulating and regulating the production and release of red blood cells (erythrocytes) from the bone marrow. An increase in the number of circulating red blood cells boosts the body's capacity to carry oxygen to its tissues and organs.

Urine Production and Excretion

The kidneys each contain approximately one million nephrons, the filtering units of the kidneys. Each nephron consists of two primary components, the renal corpuscle and the renal tubule, both of which are further divided into additional regions.

The top of each nephron consists of a cup-shaped structure known as Bowman's capsule. Within Bowman's capsule is a network of tiny capillaries known as a glomerulus. Together, the two structures are known as the renal corpuscle. As blood flows through the kidneys, the fluid portion of the blood is filtered by minute pores in the blood vessels of the glomerulus and the inner layer of Bowman's capsule. The fluid then moves into the region between the inner and outer layers of Bowman's capsule and enters into the first portion of the renal tubule (proximal convoluted tubule), where most filtered substances (e.g., most of the water, glucose, and sodium) are reabsorbed into the blood via capillaries around the tubules (peritubular capillaries). Next, as fluid moves into the loop of Henle, sodium and other electrolytes are pumped out. As the fluid passes through the next portion of the renal tubule (distal convoluted tubule), additional sodium is removed in exchange for potassium. Diluted fluid from distal convoluted tubules then passes into a collecting tubule, where fluid may continue to pass through the urinary tract as diluted urine or be returned to the blood to ensure appropriate water content in the body.

Urine then drains from the collecting tubules into central collecting areas (renal pelvis) of each kidney, which are the upper portions of the ureters. The ureters are narrow muscular tubes lined by mucous membranes. Contractions of the ureters' muscular walls move small quantities of urine into the bladder, a hollow organ that gradually expands as the volume of urine increases. As the bladder nears its capacity, nerve signals are transmitted to the brain to signal that urination is necessary. When urination occurs, the circular muscle (sphincter) between the bladder and the urethra opens, allowing urine to pass out of the body. Contractions of the bladder create pressure that forces urine into the urethra and out its external opening (urinary meatus).

DESCRIPTION

5516 PRENATAL AND POSTNATAL GROWTH AND DEVELOPMENT

Human growth and development may be encompassed in two broad categories: namely, prenatal growth and postnatal growth.

Prenatal Growth

The prenatal period, which means the "period before birth," begins when the male reproductive cell (sperm) fertilizes the female reproductive cell (egg or ovum). The fertilized egg (zygote) is a single cell containing all the genetic information (DNA) necessary for the growth and development of a human being. Half of the genetic information (in the form of 23 chromosomes) comes from the egg and half is from the sperm (for a total of 46 chromosomes).

As the zygote begins to travel down the mother's fallopian tube, its single cell immediately begins to divide (in the process called mitosis). (Please see the section entitled "Cells and Tissues" for more information.) In approximately three days, the zygote has become a solid mass of cells known as a morula. About a week to 10 days after fertilization, what has become a hollow, cellular "ball" (blastocyst) becomes implanted in the lining of the mother's uterus. During the zygote's journey to the uterus for implantation, the ovum supplies nutrients necessary for development of the embryo. The "embryonic phase" of development extends from fertilization until the end of the eighth week of pregnancy (gestation).

As the blastocyst continues to develop, its walls form an outer layer of membranes (chorion) that surrounds and protects the embryo. In addition, an inner layer of membranes (amnion) forms the amniotic sac, the fluid-filled sac within which the embryo grows and develops and is protected.

The chorion develops into the placenta, the organ attached to the lining of the uterus that serves to connect the blood supplies of the mother and the developing embryo, enabling the exchange of vital nutrients (including oxygen) and waste products. Blood from the embryo flows through a cord-like structure (umbilical cord) to the placenta and passes into tiny, finger-like blood vessels (chorionic fingers/villi) surrounded by maternal blood. The umbilical cord contains three blood vessels: two umbilical arteries that carry oxygen-poor (deoxygenated) blood and a larger umbilical vein that carries oxygen-rich (oxygenated) blood.

Teratogens and Birth Defects

A thin layer of tissue separates the developing embryo's blood from the mother's blood, thus providing protection from certain harmful substances that may circulate in the mother's bloodstream. However, in some cases, particular substances, such as certain infectious agents or drugs (teratogens), may cross this barrier, potentially interfering with prenatal growth and causing developmental abnormalities. The specific abnormalities that may result depend upon a number of factors, including the stage of development during which such exposure occurred, certain genetic influences, the specific teratogen in question, and other environmental factors. Birth defects are abnormalities that are apparent at birth (congenital) or early infancy. Such malformations may occur due to prenatal exposure to teratogens, genetic factors, or a combination of both (multifactorial).

As mentioned above, the embryonic stage of development takes place from fertilization until the end of the eighth week of gestation. The fetal stage of development extends from the ninth week of gestation until birth. Pregnancy is usually approximately 39 weeks in duration and is divided into three phases known as trimesters, each of which is about three months in length.

By approximately the third week of gestation, the head of the developing embryo begins to form and the region that will later become the brain and spinal cord (neural crest) starts to develop. At about four weeks, "buds" of tissue have begun to form that will later develop into certain organs (e.g., liver, lungs, pancreas, etc.) and into the arms, hands, legs, and feet (limb buds); the neural tube continues to develop; and rudimentary eyes form. By approximately five weeks, all internal organs have begun to develop, the jaws form, and the limb buds continue to grow. And by six weeks, the nose, mouth, and ears are beginning to develop and fingers and toes are becoming apparent.

Early during the first trimester, the growing embryo develops three layers of cells known as primary germ layers: an inner layer (endoderm), a middle layer (mesoderm), and an outer layer (ectoderm). Specific tissues and organs develop from each of these layers. For example, the lining of the lungs, gastrointestinal tract, and thyroid arise from the endoderm; the dermis of the skin, the muscles, most bones, the kidneys, and the circulatory system arise from the mesoderm; and the facial bones, the brain and spinal cord, the sensory organs such as the eyes and ears, and the epidermis of the skin arise from the ectoderm. By approximately the fourth month of gestation, the internal organs and organ systems are formed and almost mature. Growth and development continues until approximately nine months' gestation, when birth typically occurs.

Labor and Birth

Birth is the process during which the fetus moves from the uterus down through the cervix and passes out through the vagina. During the end of pregnancy, the uterus begins to contract in preparation for birth. The process known as labor begins when contractions become regular and occur at progressively shorter intervals. In addition, strong uterine muscular contractions cause the cervix to open and widen (dilate), and the membranes surrounding the amniotic fluid rupture, resulting in the release of the amniotic fluid through the vagina ("breaking of the waters"). The process of labor includes the following stages:

- First stage, which begins with the onset of contractions and ends with full dilation of the cervix.

- Second stage, during which the baby exits through the vagina.

- Third stage, during which the placenta is expelled through the vagina.

Postnatal Growth and Development

The postnatal period, which means "the period after birth," begins at birth and extends until death. The most rapid rate of growth during one's development occurs prenatally during embryonic and fetal development. Although the rate of growth decreases after birth, it remains high during childhood, particularly during the first year of life. Individuals also experience a "growth spurt" at the onset of puberty that progresses until their adult height is obtained.

During the first five months of life, infants grow approximately 30 percent in height and their weight usually doubles. By the age of one year, their height has increased by about 50 percent from birth and their weight has typically tripled. Height and weight are carefully measured and recorded during regular visits to pediatricians to ensure that growth is progressing at a predictable, steady rate. Physicians use measurements known as percentiles to compare the height and weight of infants who are of the same age. If an infant is said to be at the "fiftieth percentile" for weight, 50 percent of infants weigh more and 50 percent weigh less. If an infant is at the "tenth percentile" for

height, 90 percent of infants have a higher height and 10 percent have a lower height. When assessing growth and development, physicians consider the actual percentile as well as changes in percentiles between visits.

Between birth and adolescence, the relative proportions of the head, limbs, and trunk change dramatically. For example, an infant's head tends to be about one-quarter of the height of the body; however, an adult's head is approximately one-eighth that of the height of the body. In addition, from childhood to adulthood, the trunk tends to become proportionally shorter and the legs proportionally longer.

Different organs have varying rates of growth. For example, the human brain is about one-quarter of its adult size at birth. The brain grows primarily during the first year of life and is typically three-quarters of its adult size by the age of one year. In contrast, the small lymphoid organ known as the thymus gradually enlarges until puberty, at which time it begins to decrease in size (involution).

Developmental Milestones

Infants and children develop mental, physical, and behavioral skills in certain stages known as developmental milestones. Although the particular rate of development may vary from child to child, most children typically acquire such skills at certain ages. The development of these skills depends upon a number of factors including the following:

Genetic factors, e.g., certain developmental patterns, such as developing the ability to speak earlier than otherwise expected, may be present in particular families.

Physical factors, e.g., visual or hearing impairment may interfere with the ability to learn certain skills, potentially necessitating the use of special supportive techniques or services to ensure that children have the best chance to reach their developmental potential.

Environmental factors, e.g., appropriate levels of stimulation are important in helping children to develop certain skills, such as receiving regular verbal stimulation to promote language development.

When infants are born, they primarily communicate any needs (e.g., hunger, thirst, etc.) by crying. In addition, certain essential reflex reactions are typically present at birth. For example, when any objects touch newborns' lips, they usually respond by sucking (sucking reflex). When a side of the mouth is touched, newborns typically move their head toward that side, enabling them to locate the mother's nipple for breast-feeding (rooting reflex). And when newborns are startled, they stretch their arms and legs forward and out and extend their fingers (startle or Moro's reflex). These reflex reactions gradually fade as infants develop muscle strength and the ability to conduct and coordinate certain voluntary movements. For example, hand-eye coordination skills include watching objects, developing the ability to focus, tracking moving objects, and forming an association between seeing and performing certain actions by focusing on hand movements.

Development is typically assessed by evaluating the acquisition of skills in the areas of vision and fine movement, hearing and speech, locomotion, and social behavior. The following is a description of developmental milestones that are generally acquired during the first year of life:

By approximately one month of age, infants are usually able to:

- Focus on faces
- Bring their hands toward the face (e.g., mouth, eyes)
- Look at objects directly in front of them
- Turn toward familiar voices and respond to other sounds
- Move their heads from side to side while lying on their stomachs

At about three months, infants are usually able to:

- Track objects that move approximately 180 degrees
- Grasp objects placed in their hands
- Smile at familiar voices (e.g., mother's or father's)
- Make sounds that begin to resemble speech
- Raise their heads 45 degrees when lying on their stomachs
- Bear weight on their legs with support
- Spontaneously smile

At approximately five months, infants are usually able to:

- Reach for objects
- Listen carefully to certain voices
- Hold their heads steady while upright
- Roll from the stomach to the back

At about six months, infants are usually able to:

- Reach out for and move objects from one hand to another
- Turn their heads to locate sounds
- Laugh, make certain vowel sounds, and babble to toys
- Roll from back to front and vice versa
- Sit with support

At the age of nine months, infants are usually able to:

- Look for toys that have been hidden
- Grasp for toys that are out of reach
- Manipulate objects with both hands
- Listen to and comprehend certain sounds
- Occasionally utter strings of syllables (e.g., "mama" or "dada")
- Attempt to crawl, sit without support, and pull themselves to a sitting or standing position
- Step on alternative feet with support

By 12 months of age, infants are usually able to:

- Grasp and release objects
- Say several words
- Respond when they hear their names
- Wave good-bye
- Move from their stomachs to a sitting position
- Crawl on their hands and knees
- Walk by holding furniture
- Walk without support for a few steps or with one hand held

Glossary

A Concise Guide to Medical Terminology

This Guide is designed to help the reader decipher some unfamiliar terms used in the disorder descriptions. It is helpful to divide medical terms into their basic elements: prefix, root, and suffix. Following these examples are more than 200 commonly used medical prefixes, roots, and suffixes.

→ **Example 1:** The medical term *microcephaly* is a combination of "micr(o)," meaning small, and "cephal(o)," which means head. Therefore, microcephaly denotes an abnormally small head. In contrast, "macr(o)" means large. Thus, *macrocephaly* indicates an unusually large head.

→ **Example 2:** The word *polydactyly* includes "poly," meaning much or many, and "dactyl," which refers to fingers or toes. Thus, the medical term polydactyly means the presence of extra fingers or toes. Accordingly, because "brachy" means short, the word *brachydactyly* indicates abnormally short fingers or toes.

→ **Example 3:** The term *myositis* is a combination of "my(o)," which denotes muscle, and "itis," meaning inflammation. Therefore, myositis means muscle inflammation. When "cardi(o)," meaning heart, is added, forming the term *myocarditis*, the meaning becomes inflammation of heart muscle.

Medical Prefixes, Roots, and Suffixes

a-	absence of, without		**cerebr(o)-**	brain
ab-	away from		**cervic-**	neck
acou-	hear		**chole-**	bile
aden(o)-	gland		**chondr(o)-**	cartilage
-algia	pain		**circum-**	around
andr(o)-	man		**contra.**	against, counter
angi(o)-	vessel		**cost(o)-**	rib
ankyl(o)-	bent, crooked		**crani(o)-**	skull
ante-	before		**cry(o)-**	cold
anti-	against, counter		**crypt(o)-**	conceal, hide
artexi(o)-	artery		**cyan(o)-**	blue
arthr(o)-	joint		**cyst(o)-**	bladder
auri-	ear		**cyt(o)-**	cell
aut(o)-	self		**dactyl-**	digit, finger or toe
bacteri(o)-	bacteria		**de-**	away from, down
bio-	life		**dent(o)-**	tooth
blast(o)-	bud, early embryonic budding		**dermat(o)-**	skin
blephar(o)-	eyelid		**di-**	two
brachi(o)-	arm		**dia-**	apart, through
brachy-	short		**dipl(o)-**	double
brady-	slow		**dors(o)-**	back
bronch(o)-	bronchi		**dys-**	abnormal, bad
bucc(o)-	cheek		**-emia**	blood
carcin(o)-	cancer		**en-**	in, on
cardi(o)-	heart		**end(o)-**	inside, within
-cele	hernia, protrusion, tumor		**enter(o)-**	intestine
cent-	one hundred		**epi-**	above, upon
centr(o)-	center		**erythr(o)-**	red
cephal(o)-	head		**eso-**	inside, within

esthesi(o)-	feel, perceive	mamm(o)-	breast
eu-	normal, well	mast(o)-	breast
ex-	away from, outside	medi-	middle
extra-	beyond, in addition, outside of	mega-	great, large
flav(o)-	yellow	megal(o)-	great, large
galact(o)-	milk	melan(o)-	black
gastr(o)-	stomach	mening(o)-	membrane
gen(o)-	gene or reproduction	mes(o)-	middle
gloss(o)-	tongue	meta-	after, beyond
glyc(o)-	sweet	metr(o)-	uterus
gnath(o)-	jaw	micr(o)-	small
.gram	draw, record, write	mill-	one thousand
graph(o)-	record, write	mon(o)-	only, single, sole
gynec(o)-	woman	morph(o)-	form, shape, structure
hemat(o)-	blood	myel(o)-	marrow
hemi-	half	my(o)-	muscle
hepat(o)-	liver	myx(o)-	mucus
hex-	six	narc(o)-	stupor
hidr(o)-	sweat	nas(o)-	nose
hist(o)-	tissue	necr(o)-	corpse, death
hom(o)-	common, same	nephr(o)-	kidney
hydr(o)-	water	neur(o)-	nerve
hyper-	above, beyond, excessive	nos(o)-	disease
hypn(o)-	sleep	ocul(o)-	eye
hyp(o)-	below, deficient, low	odont(o)-	tooth
hyster(o)-	uterus	-odyn(o)-	distress, pain
iatr(o)-	physician	olig(o)-	deficient, few, little
idi(o)-	distinct, separate	-oma	neoplasm, tumor
ili(o)-	intestines	omphal(o)-	navel
inter-	among, between	onc(o)-	mass, tumor
intra-	inside, within	onych(o)-	nail
ischi(o)-	hip	oo-	egg
-itis	inflammation	ophthalm(o)-	eye
kary(o)-	nucleus	oro-	mouth
kilo-	one thousand	orchi(o)-	testicle
kinet(o)-	move	osse(o)-	bone
labio-	lips	oste(o)-	bone
lact(o)-	milk	ot(o)-	ear
lapar(o)-	flank, loin	ovari(o)-	ovary
laryng(o)-	larynx	oxy-	sharp
latero-	side	pachy-	thick
leuc(o)-	white	para-	beside, beyond, resembling
leuk(o)-	white	path(o)-	disease
lien(o)-	spleen	ped(o)-	child
lingu(o)-	tongue	penia-	abnormal reduction, deficient
lip(o)-	fat	pent(a)-	five
lith(o)-	stone	per-	throughout
lymph(o)-	lymph, water	pen-	around
macr(o)-	large	phag(o)-	consume, eat
mal-	abnormal, bad	pharmaco-	drug, medicine
malac(o)-	soft	pharyng(o)-	throat

phleb(o)-	vein		**sial(o)-**	saliva
phon(o)-	sound		**somat(o)-**	body
phot(o)-	light		**spasm(o)-**	spasm
pil(o)-	hair		**spermat(o)-**	seed
-plasia	development, formation		**splen(o)-**	spleen
platy-	broad, flat		**spondyl(o)-**	vertebra
pleur(o)-	rib, side		**spor(o)-**	spore
-pnea	breathing		**steat(o)-**	fat
pneumat(o)-	air, breathing		**sten(o)-**	compressed, narrow
pneum(o)-	air, breath, lung		**stomat(o)-**	mouth, opening
pod(o)-	foot		**sub-**	below, near under
poly-	many, much		**super-**	above, beyond, excessive
post-	after, behind		**syn-**	together, with
pre-	before, in front of		**tachy-**	fast, rapid
pro-	before, in front of		**tel(o)-**	end
proct(o)-	rectum		**tetra-**	four
pseud(o)-	false		**therm(o)-**	heat
psych(o)-	mind		**thorac(o)-**	chest
pulmon(o)-	lung		**thromb(o)-**	clot
pyel(o)-	pelvis		**-tome**	instrument for cutting
pyr(o)-	fire, heat		**tox(o)-**	poison
quadri-	four		**traumat(o)-**	wound
rachi(o)-	spine		**tri-**	three
re-	again, back		**trich(o)-**	hair
ren(o)-	kidneys		**troph(o)-**	food, nourishment
retr(o)-	backward, behind		**-uria**	urine
rheo-	flow		**vas(o)-**	vessel
rhin(o)-	nose		**vertebr(o)-**	vertebrae
sangui-	blood		**vesic(o)-**	bladder or blister
sarc(o)-	flesh		**xanth(o)-**	yellow
scler(o)-	hard		**xer(o)-**	dry
-scope	instrument for examining		**zyg(o)-**	junction, union
semi-	half			

Guidelines for Obtaining Additional Information and Resources

Many parents and caregivers are interested in obtaining information regarding *physicians* who specialize in certain pediatric disorders, accredited *hospitals, approved drugs or medical devices* for certain pediatric conditions, or current *clinical trials* that are investigating possible new therapies for particular diseases. In addition, some individuals may wish to have access to medical journal articles and other medical literature that may be available on their child's disorder, disease, or condition. Following are several tips that may be shared with parents and caregivers in their efforts to obtain such information and resources.

➜ **Disease-Specific Resources:** Many of the disease-specific resources in this *Directory* maintain listings of physicians who are experts in a particular pediatric disorder. They may also offer information on accredited hospitals with appropriate specialty departments. In addition, many may provide information on standard therapies for certain pediatric conditions and ongoing clinical trials that are investigating possible new therapies. Some of these organizations, such as certain national voluntary health associations (NVHAs) or support groups, function as patient registries, working closely with expert physicians, researchers, and university medical centers specializing in specific pediatric disorders.

➜ **Online "Physician Finder" Services:** Several professional medical associations provide searchable databases on the Internet as a public service for individuals who wish to obtain information on physicians.

Example: The *American Medical Association (AMA) Physician Select* database provides information on licensed physicians in the United States, including credential data that has been verified by medical schools, residency training programs, certifying and licensing boards, and accrediting agencies. AMA Physician Select enables online visitors to search for physicians by name, medical specialty, or geographic location. This online service is located at <http://www.ama-assn.org/aps/amahg.htm>.

Example: The *American Board of Medical Specialties® (ABMS) Public Education Program* offers an online physician locator and information service known as the *CertifiedDoctor Verification Service*. This service, which lists all physicians certified by ABMS Member Boards, allows online visitors to verify board certification status, specialty, and location of physicians who are certified by one or more of the ABMS Member Boards. The ABMS also provides the *Certified/Doctor Locator Service,* which lists physicians certified by ABMS Member Boards who have subscribed to the service. Such listings include board certification(s), address, telephone number, and hospital affiliation(s). These online services may be accessed at <http://www.certifieddoctor.org/>.

Example: The U.S. federal government has an online service known as *healthfinder®* that serves as a Web portal or directory for those who are interested in locating current, high quality health information and resources on the Internet. The area of the site entitled "Smart Choices: Choosing Quality Care" provides additional Web resources and medical professional associations that may be helpful in locating physicians. The healthfinder® site is located at <http://www.healthfinder.gov>.

→ **Hospital Accreditation:** Individuals who are interested in learning about a particular medical facility's accreditation status may consider contacting the *Joint Commission on Accreditation of Healthcare Organizations (JCAHO)*. JCAHO is the United States' leading health care quality evaluator and accredits approximately 18,000 health care facilities, organizations, and programs. Accreditation by JCAHO is recognized as a "Seal of Approval," indicating that the hospital meets certain standards of performance and is committed to meeting state-of-the-art performance expectations. JCAHO offers an online service known as *Quality Check*™ that enables online visitors to obtain information about an organization's accreditation, such as how it was rated during its most recent evaluation or performed in particular areas. This service is located at <http://wwwjcaho.org/acr_info/hosp.htm>. Callers may also receive information concerning a hospital's accreditation status by calling the Joint Commission, Customer Service at (630) 792-5800.

→ **Hospital Public Information Lines and Web Sites:** Many hospitals are creating and strongly promoting special public information lines. Such help lines are often publicized within local or regional newspapers and in the introductory sections of local phone books. In addition, many hospitals are creating Web sites that: offer information on their services and programs; link to sites offered by different departments or facilities; discuss ongoing research; provide searchable physician directories; publish newsletters, various reports, press releases, and other materials; and offer a variety of additional information. These Web sites may be located by visiting various search engines and using the name of the facility as a search term. (For more information, see *Search Engines* below.)

→ **Academic Hospitals:** If children have been diagnosed with a chronic, difficult-to-treat, or relatively uncommon disorder or if they remain undiagnosed after visits to several primary care or specialist pediatricians, parents or other caregivers may wish to consider taking their children to a major academic medical center. Generally, such teaching hospitals use state-of-the-art testing techniques, have comprehensive evaluation centers, and follow multidisciplinary approaches to diagnosis and treatment. In addition, such centers are often affiliated with medical schools where clinical research is conducted.

→ **Food and Drug Administration:** Individuals who are interested in learning more about approved drug therapies or medical devices for certain pediatric disorders may wish to contact the *Food and Drug Administration (FDA)*. The FDA is the U.S. agency that enforces federal regulations to prevent the sale and distribution of dangerous or impure substances, such as unsafe foods, impure cosmetics, or unsafe or ineffective drugs or medical devices. For example, according to the FDA Modernization Act of 1997, one of the agency's primary objectives is "to promote the public health by promptly and efficiently reviewing clinical research and taking appropriate action on the marketing of regulated products in a timely manner." The agency is a branch of the U.S. Department of Health and Human Services. The FDA's Web site provides: FAQs (Frequently Asked Questions) areas; Consumer Drug Information Sheets; information on new and generic drug approvals, medical device product approvals, and drug labeling changes; health advisories; and access to MedWatch, the FDA's Medical Products Reporting Program. MedWatch enables consumers and health care professionals to report adverse reactions to approved medical products directly to the FDA and/or the manufacturers. The primary purpose of MedWatch is to ensure the rapid identification of potential health hazards associated with approved medical products and the prompt communication of safety information to the health care and medical communities. The FDA's Web site is located at <http://www.fda.gov>. The agency's address follows:

FDA (HFE-88)
5600 Fishers Lane
Rockville, MD 20857
Toll-free: (888) INFO-FDA or (888) 463-6332

→ **Clinical Research:** A clinical protocol is a scientific study that evaluates the safety or effectiveness (efficacy) of a particular drug therapy or medical device in humans. Clinical studies enable researchers and physicians to determine new and more effective ways to prevent, diagnose, manage, and treat disease. Medications and treatments that are found to be safe and effective during laboratory and animal testing must then prove safe and effective in humans before they are approved for use by the general public. Participation in clinical studies may only occur if individuals volunteer and are fully informed and understanding of both the potential benefits and risks of such participation ("informed consent"). Participants may voluntarily leave a clinical study at any time.

Research on new drugs, which are known as *investigational new drugs* or *INDS,* is conducted in three phases:

➤ *Phase I Study* - The main objective of a Phase I study is to establish the *safety* of the investigational new drug. Such studies:

  • may take several months
  • typically involve a relatively small number of participants who are healthy volunteers
  • are designed to evaluate the IND's biologic activities in the human body (e.g., absorption, metabolism, etc.) and its potential side effects as drug dosages are raised

➤ *Phase II Study* - The purpose of a Phase II study is to establish the *safety and efficacy* of the investigational new drug in treating a specific disease. Such studies:

  • may take from several months to a few years
  • may include a relatively small number or up to several hundred patients
  • usually involve randomized, double-blind trials. During such studies, one group of participants receives the drug (experimental group) and the other group is given a harmless, unmedicated substance (placebo) or a standard, well-established therapy (control group). The information concerning which patients are included in which group is hidden from both the patients and the researchers.

➤ *Phase III Study* - The purpose of a Phase III study is to evaluate the overall *safety, efficacy, possible adverse effects, and benefits* of the investigational new drug in a large number of patients and to compare such therapy with the use of well-established treatments or with an untreated disease course. Such studies:

  • may last for several years
  • may involve hundreds or thousands of patients
  • may include research teams from multiple national or international clinical centers
  • typically involve randomized, double-blind trials

If an investigational new drug successfully completes Phase III studies, the drug's sponsor may request FDA approval for marketing to the public, which is known as a *New Drug Approval* (NDA). In some cases, additional clinical research may be conducted:

➤ *Phase IV Study* - The purpose of a Phase IV study may be to:

- monitor the drug's long-term efficacy
- compare the drug with other medications that have been available for longer periods

As mentioned above, disease-specific organizations and registries, support groups, and online services may serve as essential sources of information concerning clinical studies for a particular disease. There are also several additional, more general resources that promote and provide information on clinical trials:

Example: The *Warren Grant Magnuson Clinical Center,* which is part of the National Institutes of Health (NIH), is a federally funded biomedical research hospital. The Clinical Center was designed to support studies conducted by the NIH. Only individuals with conditions or disorders under NIH investigation are admitted for treament, and all patients must be referred by their physicians. The Clinical Center's Web site includes a clinical research database that enables online visitors to search for current research studies by certain predefined parameters, such as primary disease category, or specific diagnosis, symptom, sign, or other keywords. The Clinical Center's Web site is located at <http://www.cc.nih.gov/> and its Protocol Database may be accessed at <http://clinicalstudies.info.nih.gov/>. The Clinical Center's address follows:

Department of Health and Human Services
Public Health Service
National Institutes of Health (NIH)
Warren G. Magnuson Clinical Center
Patient Recruitment and Referral Center
10 Cloister Court-Building 61
Bethesda, MD 20892
Toll-free: (800) 411-1222
E-mail: prrc@cc.nih.gov

Example: *CenterWatch, Inc.* provides a *Clinical Trials Listing Service*™ on its Web site for patients and research professionals. The site provides listings of over 7,000 national and international clinical trials that are searchable by geographic region and therapeutic area. Interested individuals may also sign up for CenterWatch's confidential *Patient Notification Service,* which provides notification via e-mail of future clinical trial postings in a certain therapeutic area. CenterWatch's Clinical Trials Service also provides: a listing of NIH-funded clinical research programs that are currently being conducted at the NIH's Warren Grant Magnuson Clinical Center; a general explanation of clinical trials, profiles of clinical research centers; listings of medications recently approved by the FDA; and linkage to health-related sites for patients and patient advocates. The Clinical Trials Listing Service™ is located at <http://www.centerwatch.com>. CenterWatch's address follows:

CenterWatch, Inc.
581 Boylston Street
Boston, MA 02116
Phone: (617) 247-2327
Fax: (617) 247-2535
E-Mail: cntrwatch@aol.com

Example: The *National Cancer Institute (NCI)* offers an online service known as *CancerNet*™ that provides information for patients and family members, health professionals, and researchers. The site offers: information on current clinical trials; summaries on cancer prevention, screening, treatment, and supportive care; cancer fact sheets; and linkage to the *Physician Data Query* or *PDQ*® *Cancer Information Service,* the NCI's cancer database. PDQ contains a registry of open and closed cancer clinical trials as well as directories of organizations, physicians, and genetic counselors who provide cancer care. CancerNet™ also provides access to *cancerTrials*™*,* a clinical trials information center, and *CANCERLIT*®*,* a bibliographic database. CancerNet™ is located at <http://cancernet.nci.nih.gov/>. The NCI also offers a Cancer Information Service (CIS) for callers Monday through Friday from 9 a.m. to 4:30 p.m., Eastern Standard Time. The CIS may be reached at (800) 422-6237. Individuals with hearing impairment who have TTY equipment may call (800) 332-8615.

Example: *OncoLink* is an online resource on the Internet that is affiliated with the University of Pennsylvania Medical Center and the University of Pennsylvania Cancer Center. The site provides: information on cancer clinical trials; symptom management; personal experiences and psychosocial support; cancer causes, prevention, and screening; FAQs (frequently asked questions); financial issues for cancer patients; and additional topics. The site is located at <http://www.oncolink.upenn.edu>.

Search Engines. If individuals are interested in locating a particular organization's Web site but do not have its address or wish to determine what online services may be available in a certain subject area, Internet search engines are an essential resource. Search engines enable online visitors to conduct general or targeted searches for information within their areas of interest and appropriate to their needs. In addition to searching for and providing direct linkage to certain Web sites, many search engines enable users to search for e-mail discussion groups (listservs), UseNet newsgroups, FAQs (frequently asked questions), or other tools. Following is a sample listing of some of the search engines available on the Web:

➢ **Achoo:** <http://www.achoo.com>
➢ **Altavista:** <http://www.altavista.com>
➢ **DejaNews** (for Newsgroups and forum topics): <http://www.deja.com>
➢ **Dogpile:** <http://www.dogpile.com>
➢ **Excite:** <http://www.excite.com>
➢ **HotBot:** <http://www.hotbot.com>
➢ **Lycos:** <http://www.lycos.com>
➢ **Metacrawler:** <http://www.metacrawler.com>
➢ **Snap.com:** <http://www.snap.com>
➢ **Yahoo:** <http://www.yahoo.com>

General Medical and Professional Association Sites: Some individuals may be interested in visiting medical sites that offer general information on disease and health issues. In addition, many professional medical associations and societies have Web sites that provide access to patient and professional information, press releases, journals, clinical updates, and other areas that may be helpful to those interested in pediatric disorder topics. Following is a brief listing of such sites:

- ➤ **American Academy of Family Physicians:** <http://www.aafp.org/>
- ➤ **American Academy of Pediatrics:** <http://www.aap.org/>
- ➤ **American Medical Association:** <http://www.arna-assn.org/>
- ➤ **HealthAtoZ:** <http://www.HealthAtoZ.com>
- ➤ **HealthGate:** <http://www.healthgate.com/>
- ➤ **iVillage (BetterHealth):** <http://www.betterhealth.com>
- ➤ **John Hopkins Health Information:** <http://www.intelihealth.com/IH/ihtIH>
- ➤ **Mayo Clinic Health Oasis:** <http://www.mayohealth.org/>
- ➤ **Medical Matrix:** <http://www.medmatrix.org/index.asp>
- ➤ **Medscape:** <http://www.medscape.com>
- ➤ **US Pharmacopeia** (information on medications): <http://www.usp.org/>

Medical Journal Articles. Individuals who are interested in accessing abstracts summarizing medical journal articles may visit the National Library of Medicine's (NLM's) *PubMed.* The PubMed search service provides free access to the approximately nine million medical journal citations within NLM's *MEDLINE.* MEDLINE is essentially the online version of *Index Medicus,* a monthly subject/author guide to articles in thousands of medical journals. Online visitors to PubMed may conduct searches for medical journal citations and abstracts by journal title and date, author, and topic. In addition to providing access to selected journal abstracts, PubMed offers links to participating online journals and enables registered users to order full-text articles for a fee. (If individuals are interested in accessing other medical journal sites, such online journals may often be located by using various search engines.) PubMed may be accessed at <http://www.ncbi.nlm.nih.gov/PubMed/>. In addition, several general medical sites provide access to PubMed and enable users to order full-text journal articles for a fee.

Online Mendelian Inheritance in Man (OMIM). Individuals who wish to access comprehensive and timely medical information on genetic disorders may be interested in visiting OMIM™ or *Online Mendelian Inheritance in Man,* a database of genetic disorders and human genes. This searchable database, which is written and edited by Dr. Victor A. McKusick and colleagues at Johns Hopkins University and other locations, was developed for the Web by the National Center for Biotechnology Information (NCBI). OMIM™ contains entries on genetic diseases, clinical synopses, links to relevant MEDLINE citations, and more. OMIM™ is located at <http://www3.ncbi.nlm.nih.gov/omim/>.

INDEXES:

Entry Index
Geographic Index
Subject Index

American Skin Association, 914, 2277, 2724, 2728, 4112
American Sled Hockey Association, 4398
American Sleep Apnea Association, 153
American Sleep Disorders Association, 2947
American Social Health Association, 2458, 3028
American Society for Deaf Children, 1927
American Society for Reproductive Disorders, 4246
American Society of Pediatric Neurosurgeons, 5209
American Society of Reproductive Medical Fertility Fact Sheet, 4280
American Speech, Language, Hearing Association, 1928
American Speech-Language-Hearing Association, 3802
American Wheelchair Table Tennis Association, 4399
Americans with Disabilities Act, 3700
Americans with Disabilities Act Document Center, 5210
Amniotic Band Syndrome, 94
Amplification for Children with Auditory Deficits, 2036
Amyloidosis and Kidney Disease, 5441
An Alphabet About Kids with Cancer, 5390
An Association for Persons with Mental and Developmental Disabilities, 3120
An Early Prader-Willi Syndrome Diagnosis & How to Make it Easier on Parents, 3400
An Introduction to Cystic Fibrosis for Patients and Families, 1408
An Introduction to Your Child Who Has Cerebral Palsy, 964
An Introduction to the Nature and Needs of Students with Mild Disabilities, 5254
An Orientation and Mobility Primer for Families and Young Children, 5255
Anal Fissure, 2595
Analgesic Rebound Headaches - Fact Sheet, 2883
Analysis of Human Genetic Linkage, 5256
Anemia of Sarcoidosis, 3562
Anencephaly, 107
Anencephaly Support Foundation, 108
Angels in the Sun Brain Tumor Support Group, 708
Angiokeratomas, 114
Aniridia, 117
Aniridia Network, 120
Aniridia Web Site, 121
Ankylosing Spondylitis, 123, 133
Ann Whitehill Down Syndrome Program, 1522
Anodontia, 134
Anorectal Malformations, 142
Answering Your Questions About Spina Bifida, 3937
Answers to Some Commonly Asked Questions, 4285
Anxiety & Depression In Adults & Children, 1443
Anxiety Disorders Association of America, 1425, 3189, 3284
Anxiety Disorders Institute, 3285
Anxiety Panic Internet Resource, 3296
Anxiety and Phobia Treatment Center, 3286
Anxiety and Phobia Workbook, 3302
Anyone Can Have a Bleeding Problem, 2437
Aortic Valve Stenosis, 144
Apnea Identification Program, 4020
Apnea of Prematurity, 152
Apparent Life-Threatening Event and Sudden Infant Death Syndrome, 4058
Appendicitis, 2596
Approaching Equality, 2037
Archives of Pediatric and Adolescent Medicine, 5211
Archway, Inc, 4719
Arizona Ataxia Support Group National Ataxia Foundation, 279
Arizona Chapter of Crohn's & Colitis Foundation of America, 1203
Arizona Early Intervention Program Department of Economic Security, 4605
Arizona Hearing Resources, 1975
Arizona Sleep Disorders Center, 2959
Arizona Technology Access Program Institute for Human Development, 4606

Arkansas Children's Program, 2281
Arkansas Cystic Fibrosis Center, 1298
Arkansas Department of Health - SIDS Information & Counseling Program, 4001
Arkansas Disability Coalition, 4614
Arkansas Easter Seals Technology Resource Center, 5003
Arkansas Regional Library for the Blind and Physically Handicapped, 5004
Arkansas Rehabilitation Research and Training Center for Deaf Persons, 1976
Arkenstone, Inc, 4400
Arlington County Department of Libraries, 5162
Armond U. Mascia CF Center, 1360
Arnold-Chiari Family Network, 159
Arnold-Chiari Malformation, 158
Around the Clock, 407
Art Projects for the Mentally Retarded Child, 2848
Art for All the Children: Approaches to Therapy for Children with Disabilities, 5257
Art-Centered Education and Therapy for Children with Disabilities, 5258
Artery, 2425
Arthritis, 2708
Arthritis Foundation, 126, 1022, 2698
Arthritis Information: Children, 2713
Arthritis Society, 2699
Arthritis in Children, 2714
Arthritis in Children and La Artritis Infantojuvenil, 2715
Arthritis in Children: Resources for Children, Parents and Teachers, 2716
Arthrogryposis Multiplex Congenita, 163
Arthrogryposis Support Group, 168
Article Reprint Exchange, 2438
Ask the Doctor: Depression, 1444
Aspects of Autism - Biological Research, 534
Asperger Syndrome, 174
Asperger Syndrome: A Guide for Educators and Parents, 181
Assessment and Management of Mainstreamed Hearing-Impaired Children, 2038
Assessment of Hearing Impaired People, 2039
Assisstive Technology Training & Services, 4709
Assistance Technology Project, 4826
Assisting Parents Through the Mourning Process, 5188
Assistive Media, 77
Assistive Technologies of Alaska, 4602
Assistive Technology Access Partnership, 4927
Assistive Technology Alliance DSHS/DVR, 4972
Assistive Technology Center Simi Valley Hospital, 5010
Assistive Technology Collaborative, 4850
Assistive Technology Partnership, 4843
Assistive Technology Project, 4676, 4713, 4720, 4933, 4962
Assistive Technology Project, Human Resources, Voc. and Rehab. Services, 4888
Assistive Technology Services Network, 4765
Assistive Technology System, 4967
Assistive Technology Training & Information Center (ATTIC), 5060
Assistive Technology Training and Information Center, 4735
Assistive Technology for Children with Disabilities, 5259
Assistive Technology for Kansas Project, 4759
Association for Children and Adults with Learning Disabilities, Inc., 1596
Association for Children with Down Syndrome, 1507
Association for Children with Hand or Arm Deficiency (REACH), 102, 2769
Association for Education & Rehabilitation of the Blind & Visually Impaired, 1131, 4401
Association for Neuro-Metabolic Disorders, 3952
Association for Neuro-Metabolic Disorders, 2756, 2809, 2896, 3271, 4096
Association for Persons with Mental and Developmental Disabilities, 1030, 1119, 3102, 3241, 3784
Association for Persons with Severe Handicaps, 4402

B

C

G

H

J

M

N

O

P

Presbyterian-University Hospital, Pulmonary Sleep Evaluation Center, 3005
Preschool Education Programs for Children with Autism, 577
Preschool Learning Activities for the Visually Impaired Child, 5355
Preschool Programs - Division of Special Populations, 4773
Prescription Parents, 1096
Prescriptions for Children with Learning and Adjustment Problems, 5356
President's Committee on Employment of People with Disabilities, 4571
President's Committee on Mental Retardation, 4570
Presidential Proclamation - National Sarcoidosis Awareness Day, 3576
Preuss Foundation, 674
Preventing Antisocial Behavior Interventions, 1129
Preventing Epilepsy, 3747
Prevention Initiatives State Department of Education, 4671
Prevention Initiatives, Early Childhood Initiative, State Dept. of Education, 4672
Prevention Resource Guide: Pregnant Postpartum Women and Their Infants, 1744
Primary Biliary Cirrhosis, 2636
Primary Brain Cancer Support Group Lutheran Hospital, 737
Primary Children's Medical Center, 5185
Primary Sclerosing Cholangitis, 2637
A Primer of Brain Tumors, 869
Prince George's County Memorial Library Talking Book Center, 5093
Princeton University, Cutaneous Communication Laboratory, 1988
Procedure Coding for Hemophilia Treatment, 2417
Proctitis, 2638
Professional Assistance Center for Education (PACE), 5053
Programs for Exceptional Children, 4936
Progress In Dermatology, 5434
Project Empower, 4824
Project Image, 2725
Project PODER, 4950
Project PROMPT, 4774
Project Special Care, 4750
Project Start, 4825
Protein C Deficiency, 3426
Proteinuria, 5478
Prozac Nation: Young & Depressed in America, A Memoir, 1461
Psoriasis, 3428, 3437
Psoriasis Help Group, 3435
Psoriasis Newsletter, 3441
Psoriasis Research, 3444
Psoriasis Research Institute, 3431
Psoriasis on Specific Skin Sites, 3445
Psoriasis,, 3438
Psoriasis: Common Questions & Their Answers, 3446
Psoriasis: How it Makes You Feel, 3447
Psoriasis: Questions and Anwers, 3439
Psoriatic Arthritis, 3448
Psych Central, 1053, 3111, 3129, 3197, 3252, 3794
Psychiatric Medicine & Prader-Willi Syndrome, 3416
Psychoeducational Assessment of Hearing- Impaired Students, 2156
Psychoeducational Assessment of Hearing-Impaired Students, 2155
Psychoeducational Assessment of Visually Impaired and Blind Students, 5357
Psychoeducational Profile — Revised Vol.1, 578
Psychological Aspects of Narcolepsy, 3022
Psychological Factors in Sarcoidosis, 3577
Psychological Trauma, 3305
Psychologically Battered Child, 5358
Psychoses and Pervasive Development Disorders in Childhood and Adolescence, 1060

Psychosocial Aspects of Muscular Dystrophy and Allied Diseases - Coping, 2930
Psychosocial Issues of Growth Delayed Children, 5479
Psychosocial Research on Pediatric Hospitalization and Health Care, 5359
Psychotherapy of Severe and Mild Depression, 1462
Ptosis, 3455
PubMed, 5240
Public Health Services of Louisiana, 4016
Publications From the National Information Center on Deafness, 2268
Puget Sound Blood Center, 2403
Pull-Through Network, 2473
Pull-Thru Network, 143
Pull-thru Network News, 2480
Pulmonary Hypertension, Primary, 3464
Pulmonary Hypertention Association, 3467
Pulmonary Sarcoidosis: Evaluation with High Resolution, 3578
Pulmonary Sarcoidosis: What We Are Learning, 3579
Pulmonary Valve Stenosis, 3470
Putting on the Brakes, 468
Pyloric Stenosis, 3475

Q

Q and A: Hepatitis B Prevention, 1086
Quad Cities Brain Tumor Support Group, 739
Quality Life Concepts, 4842
Quest Magazine, 2935
Questions & Answers About Depression & Its Treatment, 1463
Questions & Answers About Diet and Nutrition, 1278
Questions Most Often Asked the NSF, 3644
Questions and Answers About Complications, 1279
Questions and Answers About Crohn's Disease & Ulcerative Colitis, 1280
Questions and Answers About Emotional Factors in Ileitis and Colitis, 1281
Questions and Answers on Hearing Loss, 2269

R

R.F. Stolinsky Research Laboratories, 1810
RP Messenger, 3510
RSV Center, 3492
Radiation Therapy of Brain Tumors Part I: A Basic Guide, 890
Radiation Therapy of Brain Tumors Part II: Background and Research Guide, 891
Rainbow Connection, 4644
Raising Your Hearing-Impaired Child, 2157
Raising a Child with Diabetes a Guide for Parents, 2664
Raising a Child with Spina Bifida: An Introduction, 3932
Raleigh Area Brain Tumor Support Group, 801
Rapid Gastric Emptying (Dumping Syndrome), 2639
Rare Genetic Diseases in Children, 1779, 1796, 2456, 4334
Rare Genetic Diseases in Children (NYU), 113, 162, 1652, 2502, 2542, 2734, 2748, 2789, 5241
Rare Genetic Diseases in Children: Disability Resources Directory, 5242
Raynaud's & Scleroderma Association, 3592
ReHab Net, 1900
Reach: the Association for Children with Hand or Arm Deficiency, 1759, 1764
Reaching Harmony: Native American Family Support, Inc., 4612
Reaching the Autistic Child A Parent Training Program, 579
Reaching, Crawling, Walking - Let's Get Moving, 5420
Reading Between the Lips, 2214
Reading and Deafness, 2158
Reading and Learning Disability: A Nueropsychological Approach, 5360
Realities in Coping with Progressive Neuromuscular Diseases, 2931

Turner's Syndrome Society of Southeastern Wisconsin, 4263, 4279
Turner's Syndrome Society of Southwestern Ohio, 4270
Turner's Syndrome Society of West Illinios, 4264
Twenty Years At Hull House, 3630
22Q and You Center, 1488
25 Ways to Promote Spoken Language in Your Child with a Hearing Loss, 2245
Tyler for Life Foundation, 1780, 2503, 2735
Type A Behavior, 3256

U

UAB Cystic Fibrosis Center/Children's Hospital, 1302
UCD Northern Central California Hemophilia Program, 2344
UCLA, 3174
UCSD Comprehensive Hemophilia Treatment Center, 2345
UK O.I. Foundation, 3217
UK Osteogenesis Imperfecta Foundation, 3222
UNC CF Center, 1366
US Blind Golfers Association, 4700
US Disabled Ski Team, 4959
US Rowing Assocation, 4751
US Wheelchair Weightlifting Association, 4926
USA Deaf Sports Federation, 1972
USC - Neonatology Research Units, 4052
UTMB, 3235
Ulcerative Colitis, 2642, 4287
Ulster County Social Services, 4887
Ultimate Stranger: The Autistic Child, 589
Understanding Anemia, 5381
Understanding Asthma, 246
Understanding Attention Deficit Disorder, 414
Understanding Autism, 527
Understanding Birth Defects, 5382
Understanding Brain Tumors: Glioblastoma Multiforme, 893
Understanding Childhood Obesity, 3176
Understanding Cystic Fibrosis, 1403
Understanding Dental Health, 1423
Understanding Depression, 1469
Understanding Down Syndrome, 1584
Understanding Ear Infections, 2194
Understanding Gestational Diabetes, 2678
Understanding Hemophilia: A Young Person's Guide, 2420
Understanding Herpes, 2467, 3036
Understanding Hyperactivity, 490
Understanding Juvenile Rheumatoid Arthritis, 2706
Understanding Narcolepsy, 3025
Understanding Panic Disorder, 1482
Understanding Scoliosis, 3615
Understanding Seizure Disorders, 3696
Understanding Sickle Cell Disease, 3780
Understanding Your Teenager's Depression, 1470
Understanding and Coping with Your Child's Brain Tumor, 894
Understanding and Treating Children with Autism, 590
Understanding the Nature of Autism, 591
United Cerebral Palsy Association, 950
United Cerebral Palsy Research and Educational Foundation, 954
United Leukodystrophy Foundation, 2758
United Liver Association, 618
United Liver Foundation, 2732, 3040
United Ostomy Association, 2475
United Ostomy Association Hotline, 4292
United States Cerebral Palsy Athletic Association, 951
Univ. of Texas - Southwestern Med. Ctr. at Dallas - Clinical Ctr. for Liver Disease, 620
University Affiliated Program, School of Medicine, 4940
University Alabama Birmingham, 2827
University Graz, Austria, 4188
University Medical Center Hemophilia Program, 2368

University Students with Autism and Asperger's Syndrome Web Site, 180, 532
University Treatment Center of University Hospitals of Cleveland, 2381
University of Adelaide Hydrocephalus Department, 2543
University of Alabama Speech and Hearing Center, 1974
University of California, Irvine Brain Imaging Center, 1886
University of California, Northern Comprehensive Sickle Cell Center, 3767
University of California, San Francisco Dermatology Drug Research, 858, 1887, 3207, 3211, 5183
University of Chicago, 614, 1077
University of Chicago Children's Hospital, Department of Pediatrics, 1330
University of Chicago, Temporal Bone Laboratory for Ear Research, 1993
University of Cincinnati College of Medicine/Division of Pediatrics, 1372
University of Colorado, Boulder Communication Disorders Clinic, 3804
University of Connecticut Health Center, 1315
University of Florida, 4189
University of Florida Hemophilia Treatment Center, 2349
University of Illinois At Chicago Consultation Clinic for Epilepsy, 3680
University of Illinois at Chicago, Craniofacial Center, 5058
University of Iowa, 1157, 3043
University of Iowa Birth Defects and Genetic Disorders Unit, 5066
University of Iowa Hospitals & Clinics, 1325
University of Kansas Center for Research on Learning, 5073
University of Maine, Conley Speech and Hearing Center, 1983
University of Miami, Mailman Center For Child Development, 5029
University of Michigan, 2567
University of Michigan Hemophilia Center, 2362
University of Michigan, Communicative Disorders Clinic, 3807
University of Michigan, Cystic Fibrosis Center, 1347
University of Michigan, Kresge Hearing Research Institute, 1994
University of Minnesota, 3462
University of Minnesota Comprehensive Hemophilia Center, 2365
University of Minnesota Cystic Fibrosis Center, 1348
University of Mississippi Medical Center, 1349
University of Missouri-Columbia Cystic Fibrosis Center, 1352
University of Nebraska at Omaha Pediatric Pulmonary/Cystic Fibrosis Center, 1354
University of Nebraska, Lincoln Barkley Memorial Center, 1987
University of Nevada, Reno Speech And Language Pathology Department, 3808
University of North Carolina at Chapel Hill, Division of Speech & Hearing, 518, 3814
University of Oklahoma Cystic Fibrosis Center, 1373
University of Oklahoma, Speech & Hearing Center, 3818
University of Ottawa, 900
University of Pennsylvania, Depression Research Unit, 1435
University of Pittsburg Medical Center, 3423
University of Pittsburgh Cystic Fibrosis Center/Children's Hospital, 1377
University of South Alabama Cystic Fibrosis Center, 1301
University of Southern California Comprehensive Sickle Cell Center, 3768
University of Tennessee Hemophilia Clinic, 2395
University of Tennessee, Center For Neuroscience, 3687
University of Texas Health Science Center at Houston - Speech & Hearing, 3822
University of Texas Medical Branch at Galveston, Clinical Research Center, 3018
University of Texas Sleep/Wake Disorders Center, 3011
University of Texas at Dallas, Callier Center for Communication Disorders, 3823, 3839

Z

Alabama

ARC of Morgan County, 4592
Alabama Chapter of Asthma and Allergy Foundation of America, 191
Alabama Chapter of Crohn's & Colitis Foundation of America, 1202
Alabama Chapter of the National Hemophilia Foundation, 2296
Alabama Institute for the Deaf & Blind, 4593
Birmingham Support Group National Ataxia Foundation, 278
Brain Injury Association of Alabama, 1830
Bureau of Family Health Services Alabama Department of Public Health, 3998
Civitan International Research Center, 1992
Down Syndrome Clinic, Children's Hospital of Alabama, 1516
Early Intervention Program, 4594
Friends for Life Auburn United Methodist Church, 4595
Greater Kansas City Chapter of Asthma and Allergy Foundation of America, 195
Hemophilia Clinic - Childrens' Rehabilitation Service, 2337
Knollwoodpark Hospital Sleep Disorders Center, 2958
Magic Moments c/o Children's Hospital of Alabama, 4596
Mobile Association for the Blind, 4999
Mobile Hemophilia Clinic, 2338
PWSA of Alabama, 3348
Pediatric Brain Tumor Support Group, 678
Special Education Action Committee Huntsville Outreach Office, 4597
Special Education Action Committee, Inc., 4598
Special Education Services, 4599
Spina Bifida Association of Alabama, 3847
Statewide Technology Access & Response System for Alabamians with Disabilities, 4600
UAB Cystic Fibrosis Center/Children's Hospital, 1302
University of Alabama Speech and Hearing Center, 1974
University of South Alabama Cystic Fibrosis Center, 1301

Alaska

Alaska Department of Education, 4601
Alaska Services for Enabling Technology, 5180
Assistive Technologies of Alaska, 4602
Brain Injury Association of Alaska, 1831
Maternal, Child & Family Health, Early Intervention/Infant Learning Program, 4603
PARENTS, Inc., 4604
SIDS Information & Counseling Program Alaska Department of Health, 3999
Turner's Syndrome Society of Alaska, 4250

Arizona

Arizona Ataxia Support Group National Ataxia Foundation, 279

Arizona Chapter of Crohn's & Colitis Foundation of America, 1203
Arizona Early Intervention Program Department of Economic Security, 4605
Arizona Hearing Resources, 1975
Arizona Sleep Disorders Center, 2959
Arizona Technology Access Program Institute for Human Development, 4606
Bell's Palsy Research Foundation, 610
Blake Foundation Children's Achievement Center, 4607
Brain Injury Association of Arizona, 1832
Center for Neurodevelopmental Studies, 521
Cystic Fibrosis Center - Phoenix Children's Hospital, 1303
Division of Special Education State Department of Education, 4608
Educational Services for the Visually Impaired, 5000
Foundation for Children with Down Syndrome, 1517
Mountain States Regional Hemophilia Center, 2339
National Association for Parents of the Visually Impaired, 4609
Office of Maternal & Child Health Arizona Department of Health, 4000
PWSA of Arizona, 3349
Pilot Parent Partnerships, 4610
Pilot Parents of Southern Arizona, 4611
Reaching Harmony: Native American Family Support, Inc., 4612
Southwest Human Development, 4613
Special Needs Center/Phoenix Public Library, 5001
Spina Bifida Association of Arizona, 3848
St. Joseph's Hemophilia Center, 2340
Technology Access Center of Tucson, 5002
Tucson Cystic Fibrosis Center, 1300
Turner's Syndrome Society of Arizona, 4251

Arkansas

Arkansas Cystic Fibrosis Center, 1298
Arkansas Department of Health - SIDS Information & Counseling Program, 4001
Arkansas Disability Coalition, 4614
Arkansas Easter Seals Technology Resource Center, 5003
Arkansas Regional Library for the Blind and Physically Handicapped, 5004
Arkansas Rehabilitation Research and Training Center for Deaf Persons, 1976
Brain Injury Association of Arkansas, 1833
CLOC Regional Library, 5005
Crowley Ridge Regional Library, 5006
DD Services, Department of Human Services, 4615
FOCUS, Inc., 4616
Fort Smith Library for the Blind and Handicapped, 5007
Hemophilia Center of Arkansas, 2341
Increasing Capabilities Access Network, 4617
Northwest Ozarks Regional Library for the Blind and Handicapped, 5008
PWSA of Arkansas, 3350
Parent to Parent Arc of Arkansas, 4618

Research and Training Center for Persons Who Are Deaf or Hard of Hearing, 1977
Special Education Section State Department of Education, 4619
Spina Bifida Association of Arkansas, 3852

California

American Action Fund for Blind Children and Adults, 5009
Assistive Technology Center Simi Valley Hospital, 5010
Bereavement Group for Children, 4620
Blind Children's Center, 5011
Braille Institute Desert Center, 5012
Braille Institute Sight Center, 5013
Braille Institute Youth Center, 5014
Brain Injury Association of California, 1834
Brain Tumor Patient & Family Support Group, 679
Brain Tumor Support Group at Newport Beach, 711
Brain Tumor Support Group at San Diego, 712
Brain Tumor Support Group at San Luis Obispo, 713
Brain Tumor Support Group at Santa Monica, 714
Brain Tumor Support Program Cedars-Sanai Neurosurgical Inst. & Wellness Community, 680
Brian Wesley Ray Cystic Fibrosis Center, 1304
CARE Family Resource Center, 4621
California Assistive Technology System, 4622
California SIDS Program, 4002
Carolyn Kordich Family Resource Center, 4623
Center for Accessible Technology, 5015
Central California Chapter of the National Hemophilia Foundation, 2297
Central California Support Group National Ataxia Foundation, 280
Challenged Family Resource Center, 4624
Children Living with Illness, 681
Children's Hospital - Pediatric Pulmonary Center, 1305
Children's Hospital Medical Center of Northern California, 1518
Children's Hospital of Los Angeles, 1306
Clearinghouse for Specialized Media and Technology, 5016
Comfort Connection Family Resource Center, 4625
Computer Access Center, 5181
Cooley's Anemia Foundation-California, 4132
Costa Mesa Support Group National Ataxia Foundation, 281
Cystic Fibrosis Center, 1307
Cystic Fibrosis Center, University of California at San Francisco, 1308
Cystic Fibrosis and Pediatric Pulmonary Center, 1309
Cystic Fibrosis and Pediatric Respiratory Diseases Center, 1310
Early Intervention Program Department of Developmental Services, 4626
Early Start Family Resource Network, 4627
Epilepsy Foundation of Northern California, 3664

Exceptional Family Resource Center, 4628
Exceptional Family Support, Education and Advocacy Center, 4629
Exceptional Parents, 4630
Families Caring for Families, 4631
Family First Program Alpha Resource Center, 4632
Family Focus Resource Center, 4633
Family Resource Center, 4634
Foundation for Glaucoma Research, 1150
Fresno Brain Tumor Support Group, 682
Greater Bay Area Chapter Crohn's and Colitis Foundation, 1204
Greater Los Angeles Chapter of Crohn's & Colitis Foundation of America, 1205
H.E.A.R.T.S. Connection Family Resource Center, 4635
Harbor Regional Center Family and Professional Resource Center, 4636
Hear Center, 1978
Hemophilia Association of San Diego County, 2298
Hemophilia Comprehensive Care Center at The Children's Hospital of L.A., 2342
Hydrocephalus Parent Support Group, 2517
Hydrocephalus Support Group of Southern California, 2518
Inland Empire Brain Tumor Support Group, 683
Loma Linda University Sleep Disorders Clinic, 2960
Long Beach Chapter of Crohn's & Colitis Foundation of America, 1206
Los Angeles Ataxia Support Group National Ataxia Foundation, 282
Lymphoma Research Foundation of America, 3149
MATRIX: Parent Network and Family Resource Center, 4637
Matrix Family Resource Center of the North Bay, 4638
Mercy Sleep Laboratory, 3013
Miller Children's Hospital Pediatric Pulmonary/Cystic Fibrosis Cent, 1311
Narthern California Support Group National Ataxia Foundation, 283
Neuroscience Institute Brain Tumor Support Group, 684
New Beginnings - The Blind Children's Center, 5017
Northern California Chapter of Asthma and Allergy Foundation of America, 192
Northern California Chapter of the National Hemophilia Foundation, 2299
Northridge Hospital: Leavey Cancer Center, 685
Orange County Chapter of Crohn's & Colitis Foundation of America, 1207
Orange County Support Group National Ataxia Foundation, 284
Orthopaedic Biomechanics Laboratory, 953
Orthopaedic Hospital's Hemophilia Treatment Center, 2343
PWS Foundation of California, 3351
PWS Foundation of California (Solana Beach), 3352
PWSA of California, 3353
Pacific Southwest Regional Genetics Group, 285
Palo Alto Brain Tumor Support Group, 686

Parent Helping Parents of San Francisco, 4639
Parents Helping Parents of San Francisco, 4640
Parents Helping Parents of Santa Clara, 4641
Peaks and Valleys Family Resource Center, 4642
Pediatric Disabilities Clinic, Down Syndrome Clinic, 1519
Peninsula Support & Education Group for Parents of Children with Brain Tumors, 687
Phase One, 4643
Psoriasis Research Institute, 3431
Rainbow Connection, 4644
Sacramento Area Brain Tumor Support Group, 688
Sacramento Area Hydrocephalus Group, 2519
Sacramento Center for Assistive Technology, 5018
Sacramento Valley Chapter of Crohn's & Colitis Foundation of America, 1208
San Diego Chapter of Crohn's & Colitis Foundation of America, 1209
San Diego Cystic Fibrosis and Pediatric Pulmonary Disease Center, 1312
San Diego Support Group National Ataxia Foundation, 286
San Francisco Brain Tumor Support Group, 689
San Francisco Public Library for the Blind and Print Handicapped, 5019
San Gabriel/Pomona Parents' Place, 4645
Santa Barbara Brain Tumor Support Group, 690
Santa Cruz County Brain Tumor Support Group, 691
Santa Rosa Brain Tumor Support Group, 692
Scleroderma Research Foundation, 3595
Scripps Clinic Sleep Disorders Center, 2961
Sickle Cell Disease Foundation of California, 3762
Sleep Disorders Center at California Pacific Medical Center, 2962
South Bay Brain Tumor Support Group, 693
South Central Los Angeles Regional Center for Devlopmentally Disabled Persons, Inc, 4646
Southern California Chapter of Asthma and Allergy Foundation of America, 193
Southern California Neuropsychiatric Institute, 1885
Southern California Pediatric Brain Tumor Network, 694
Special Connections Family Resource Ctr., 4647
Special Education Division State Department of Education, 4648
Spina Bifida Association of Bay Area, 3849
Spina Bifida Association of East Bay, 3853
Spina Bifida Association of Greater Rialto, 3854
Spina Bifida Association of Greater San Diego, 3855
Spina Bifida Association of Oakdale California, 3850
Spina Bifida Association of Sacramento Valley, 3856
Spina Bifida Association of Stanford, 3857

Spina Bifida Association of the Central Coast, 3851
Stanford CF Center, 1313
Stanford University Center for Narcolepsy, 2963
Starlight Children's Foundation, 4649
Support Group for Caregivers of Brain Tumor Patients, 695
Support Group for Parents of Children with Brain Tumors, 696
Support for Families of Children with Disabilities, 4650
Team Advocates for Special Kids, Anaheim, 4652
Team Advocates for Special Kids, San Diego, 4651
Team of Advocates for Special Kids, 5182
Technology Access Center, 5020
Turner's Syndrome Society of Bay Area, 4252
UCD Northern Central California Hemophilia Program, 2344
UCSD Comprehensive Hemophilia Treatment Center, 2345
USC - Neonatology Research Units, 4052
University of California, Irvine Brain Imaging Center, 1886
University of California, Northern Comprehensive Sickle Cell Center, 3767
University of California, San Francisco, 3207
University of California, San Francisco Brain Tumor Research Center, 858
University of California, San Francisco Dermatology Drug Research, 5183
University of California, San Francisco Laboratory for Neurotrauma, 1887
University of Southern California Comprehensive Sickle Cell Center, 3768
Variety Audio, Inc., 5021
Vital Options, 697
Warmline Family Resource Center, 4653
Wellness Community San Francisco/East Bay, 698
West Los Angeles Brain Tumor Support Group, 699
Wish Upon a Star, 4654

Colorado

Brain Injury Association of Colorado, 1835
Brain Tumor Patient Family Group, 700
Brain Tumor Patient/Family Group, 701
Brain Tumor Resource and Vital Encouragement, 702
Brain Tumor Support Group, 703
Colorado Assistive Technology Program, 4655
Colorado Consortium of Intensive Care Nurseries United Parents (UP), 4656
Colorado SIDS Program, 4003
Delta/Montrose Parent to Parent, 4657
Denver Children's Hospital, 1314
Denver Colorado Support Group National Ataxia Foundation, 287
Denver Early Childhood Connections, 4658
Disability Connection and RAFT, Larimer County's Early Childhood Connection, 4659
Effective Parent Project, Inc, 4660
El Groupo Vida, 4661

Help Parent Spport Group Hope &
Education for Loving Parents, 4662
Hemophilia Society of Colorado, 2300
Little People of America Front Range
Chapter, 4663
Mile High Down Syndrome Association,
4664
Mountain States Regional Genetics
Services Network, 289
NNFF of Colorado, 3049
National Jewish Medical & Research
Center Denver, 205
Northern Colorado Area Support Group
National Ataxia Foundation, 290
Oasis, Inc, 4665
PEAK Parent Center, Inc., 4666
PWSA of Colorado, 3354
Parent Support Group of Littleton &
Auora, 4667
Parents Encouraging Parents, 4668
Parents Supporting Parents of Eagle
County, 4669
Parents Supporting Parents of Garfield
and Pitkin County, 4670
Pike's Peak Area Support Group National
Ataxia Foundation, 291
Prevention Initiatives State Department of
Education, 4671
Prevention Initiatives, Early Childhood
Initiative, State Dept. of Education, 4672
R.F. Stolinsky Research Laboratories,
1810
Resources for Young Children and
Families, Inc, 4673
Rocky Mountain Chapter of Crohn's &
Colitis Foundation of America, 1210
Speech, Language, & Hearing Center
University of Colorado, 4674
Spina Bifida Association of Colorado, 3858
Turner's Syndrome Society of Rocky
Mountain, 4253
University of Colorado, Boulder
Communication Disorders Clinic, 3804
Wilderness on Wheels Foundation, 4675

Connecticut

Assistive Technology Project, 4676
BMT Family Support Network, 38
Brain Injury Association of Connecticut,
1836
Brain Tumor Support Group, 704
CPAC, 4677
Central Connecticut Chapter of Crohn's
& Colitis Foundation of America, 1211
Chapel Haven, Inc., 5022
Connecticut Area Support Group
National Ataxia Foundation, 292
Connecticut Brain Tumor Support Group
(Adult), 705
Department of Mental Retardation, 4678
Division of Child & Family Studies, 4679
Gaylord Rehab and Sleep Center, 2964
NNFF of Connecticut, 3050
Northern Connecticut Chapter of Crohn's
& Colitis Foundation of America, 1212
PWSA of Connecticut, 3355
PWSA of Connecticut (North Haven), 3356
Parent to Parent Network of Connecticut
the Family Center, 4680
SIDS Program Connecticut Department of
Health, 4004

Spina Bifida Association of Connecticut,
3861
State Department of Education, 4681
Terri Gotthelf Lupus Research Institute,
4084
Tourette Syndrome Clinic, 4175
Turner's Syndrome Society of
Connecticut, 4254
University of Connecticut Health Center,
1315
Yale Hemophilia Center, 2346
Yale University Cystic Fibrosis Research
Center, 1316
Yale University, Behavioral Medicine
Clinic, 1437
Yale University, Ribicoff Research
Facilities, 1438

Delaware

Brain Injury Association of Delaware, 1837
Delaware Assisstive Technology Initiative,
4682
Delaware Division of Libraries for the
Blind and Physically Handicapped, 5023
Department of Public Instruction, 4683
Division of Management Services
Department of Health & Social
Services, 4684
PWSA of Delaware, 3357
Parent Information Center of Delaware,
4685
Parent Information Center of Delaware,
Inc, 4686
Pediatric Brain Tumor Support Group,
706
SIDS Information & Counseling - Division
Of Public Health, 4005
Sarcoidosis Support Group - Delaware,
3541
Spina Bifida Association of Delaware, 3862

District of Columbia

Advocates for Justice and Education, 4687
Brain Research Center, 855
DC Arc, 4688
DC-EIP Services, 4689
District of Columbia Public Library/
Librarian for the Deaf Community, 1979
Division of Community Health Nursing,
4006
Gallaudet University, Center for Auditory
and Speech Sciences, 1980
Gallaudet University, Cued Speech Team,
3829
Georgetown University Child
Development Center, 4690
Georgetown University Child
Development Center, 5024
Georgetown University Sleep Disorders
Center, 2965
Giddings School Special Education
Division, 4691
Hemophilia Treatment Center at
Children's National Medical Center,
2347
Howard University Center for Sickle Cell
Disease, 3769
Metropolitan D.C. Cystic Fibrosis Center,
1317
National Brain Research Association, 857
Partnership for Assistive Technology, 4692

Sarcoidosis Support Group - Washington
DC, 3542
Scottish Rite Center for Childhood
Language Disorders, 3805
United Cerebral Palsy Research and
Educational Foundation, 954
Volta Bureau Library, 1981
Washington DC Metropolitan Area
Support Group, 707

Florida

Alliance for Assistive Service and
Technology (FAAST), 4693
Angels in the Sun Brain Tumor Support
Group, 708
Brain Injury Association of Florida, 1838
Brain Tumor Support Group, 709
Brain Tumor Support Group at Miami,
710
Brain Tumor Support Group at St
Petersburg, 715
Brain Tumor Support Group at St.
Petersburg, 716
Brain Tumor Support Group at Tampa,
717
Broward County Support Group National
Ataxia Foundation, 293
CF & Pediatric Pulmonary Disease
Center, 1318
Cancer Support Group for Children, 718
Center for Independence Technology and
Education, (CITE), 5025
Children's Medical Services Program
Florida SIDS Program, 4007
Children's Wish Foundation, 4694
Clearwater, FL Support Group National
Ataxia Foundation, 294
Collier, Hendy, and Glades Counties
Epilepsy Foundations of Florida, 3665
Comprehensive Pediatric Hemophilia
Center, 2348
Cystic Fibrosis Center - All Children's
Hospital, 1320
Cystic Fibrosis Center Orlando Regional
Medical Center, 1319
Early Intervention Unit, Division of
Children's Medical Services, 4695
Epilepsy Association of Big Bend, 3666
Epilepsy Foundation of South Florida,
3667
Epilepsy Services of North Central
Florida, 3668
Epilepsy Services of Northeast Florida,
3669
Epilepsy Services of West Central Florida,
3670
Family Network on Disabilities, 4696
Florida Chapter of Asthma and Allergy
Foundation of America, 194
Florida Chapter of the National
Hemophilia Foundation, 2301
Florida Cystic Fibrosis, 1299
Florida Department of Education, 4697
Florida Division of Blind Services, 5026
Florida Ophthalmic Institute, 1149
Florida's Collaboration for Young
Children and their Families Head State,
4698
Gold Coast Chapter of Crohn's & Colitis
Foundation of America, 1213
Jacksonville Public Library, 5027
Lee County Epilepsy Foundations of
Florida, 3671

Mid-Illinois Talking Book Center, 5049

NNFF of Illinois, 3055

National Association for Parents of the Visually Impaired, 4726

National Center for Latinos with Disabilities, 4727

National Eye Research Foundation, 5179

National Library of Dermatologic Teaching Slides, 5050

Next Steps - Parents Reaching Parents, 4728

North Central Region Helen Keller National Center, 4729

Northern Illinois Center for Adaptive Technology, 5051

Office of Community Health and Prevention Bureau of Early Intervention, DHR, 4730

PWSA of Illinois, 3363

PWSA of Illinois Group, 3364

Parent to Parent Network, 4731

Parents Alliance Employment Project, 5052

Parents of Children with Brain Tumors (PCBT), 733

Professional Assistance Center for Education (PACE), 5053

Region V Office Program Consultants For Maternal and Child Health, 4011

Regional Comprehensive Hemophilia Center of Central and Northern Illinois, 2351

Saint Francis Medical Center Specialty Clinics, CF Center, 1329

Sarcoidosis Support Group - Illinois, 3543

Scoliosis Research Society, 3608

Shawnee Library System, 5054

Shriners Hospital for Children, 3606

Southern IL Child and Family Connections, 4732

Southern, IL Support Group National Ataxia Foundation, 302

Spina Bifida Association of Illinois, 3870

State Board of Education Department of Special Education, 4733

Sulzberger Institute for Dermatologic Education, 5055

Talking Book Center of North West Illinois, 5056

Technical Aids & Assistance for the Disabled Center, 5057

University of Chicago Children's Hospital, Department of Pediatrics, 1330

University of Chicago, Temporal Bone Laboratory for Ear Research, 1993

University of Illinois At Chicago Consultation Clinic for Epilepsy, 3680

University of Illinois at Chicago, Craniofacial Center, 5058

Indiana

ATTAIN: Assistive Technology Through Action in Indiana, 4734

Allen County Public Library, 5059

Ann Whitehill Down Syndrome Program, 1522

Assistive Technology Training & Information Center (ATTIC), 5060

Assistive Technology Training and Information Center, 4735

Bartholomew County Public Library, 5061

Brain Injury Association of Indiana, 1843

Brain Tumor Support Group, 734

Brain Tumor Support Group at Indianapolis, 735

Brain Tumor Support Group of Indiana, 736

Central Indiana Support Group National Ataxia Foundation, 303

Cystic Fibrosis and Chronic Pulmonary Disease Clinic, 1331

Division of Special Education Department of Education, 4736

Down Syndrome Association of Central Indiana, 4737

Down Syndrome Association of NWI, 4738

Down Syndrome Support Association of Southern Indiana (DSSASI), 4739

Elkhart Public Library, 5062

Family Resource Center of Southeast Indiana, 4740

First Direction, 4741

First Steps, 4742

First Steps for Families, 4743

First Steps, Early Interventions, New Horizons Rehabilitation, 4744

Future Choices, 4745

Hemophilia Foundation of Indiana, 2305

IN*SOURCE, 4746

Indiana Chapter of Crohn's & Colitis Foundation of America, 1217

Indiana Parent Information Network (IPIN), 4747

Indiana Resource Center for Autism, 511

Indiana State Board of Health - SIDS Project, 4012

Indiana University Cystic Fibrosis Center, 1332

Knox County Advocates, 4748

Methodist Hospital Sleep Center, 2966

MidWest Medical Center - Sleep Disorders Center, 2967

NE Indiana Cerebellar Ataxia Support Group, 304

NEO Fight, 4749

NNFF of Indiana, 3056

Northwest Indiana Subregional Library for Blind and Physically Handicapped, 5063

PWSA of Indiana, 3365

Primary Brain Cancer Support Group Lutheran Hospital, 737

Project Special Care, 4750

Riley Hemophilia and Thrombophilia Center, 2352

Sleep Alertness Center, Lafayette Home Hospital, 2968

Sleep Disorders Center, Good Samaritan Hospital, 2969

Sleep/Wake Disorders Center, Community Hospitals of Indianapolis, 2970

Special Services Division - Indiana State Library, 5064

Spina Bifida Association of Central Indiana, 3871

Spina Bifida Association of Northeast Indiana, 3872

Spina Bifida Association of Northern Indiana, 3873

US Rowing Assocation, 4751

Iowa

ARC of East Central Iowa Pilot Parents, 4752

Blank Children's Hospital Cystic Fibrosis Center, 1324

Brain Injury Association of Iowa, 1844

Bureau of Childern, Family, and Community Services, 4753

Camp Courageous, 5497

Down Syndrome Clinic, Child & Young Adult Clinic, 1523

Eastern Iowa Chapter of Crohn's & Colitis Foundation of America, 1218

Family Educator Connection Program, 4754

Great Plains Genetic Service Network, 305

Great Plains Regional Hemophilia Center, 2353

Iowa Chapter of Crohn's & Colitis Foundation of America, 1219

Iowa Program for Assistive Technology, 4755

Iowa SIDS Program, 4013

Iowa Support Group National Ataxia Foundation, 288

Iowa's System of EI Services, 4756

Library Commission for the Blind, 5065

NNFF of Iowa, 3057

Neurological Center of Iowa, 738

PWSA of Iowa, 3366

Parent Educator Connection, 4757

Parent Educator Connection Program Resource Center for Issues in Special Ed, 4758

Quad Cities Brain Tumor Support Group, 739

Sioux County Iowa Chapter National Ataxia Foundation, 306

Spina Bifida Association of Iowa, 3874

Turner's Syndrome Society of Iowa/New Found Friends, 4257

University of Iowa Birth Defects and Genetic Disorders Unit, 5066

University of Iowa Hospitals & Clinics, 1325

Kansas

Assistive Technology for Kansas Project, 4759

CKLS Headquarters, 5067

Child & Family Center, 1123

Department of Health & Environment, 4760

Families Together, Inc., 4761

Families Together/Parent to Parent of KS, 4762

Great Plains Region Helen Keller National Center, 4763

Greater Kansas City Chapter of Crohn's & Colitis Foundation of America, 1220

Headstrong Brain Tumor Support Group, 740

Kansas Department of Health & Environment Bureau of Family Health, 4014

Kansas State Library, 5068

Kansas University Medical Center, Cystic Fibrosis Center, 1333

Manhattan Public Library, 5069

PWSA of Kansas, 3367

Prenatal Diagnostic and Genetic Center, 5070

South Central Kansas Library System, 5071

Special Education Administration State Department of Education, 4764
Spina Bifida Association of Kansas, 3875
St. Joseph Medical Center Cystic Fibrosis Care and Teaching Center, 1334
Technology Resource Solutions for People, 5072
University of Kansas Center for Research on Learning, 5073
Wesley Medical Research Institutes, 5074
Wichita Public Library, 5075

Kentucky

Assistive Technology Services Network, 4765
Bluegrass Technology Center, 5076
Brain Injury Association of Kentucky, 1845
Cincinnati Ohio Area Support Group National Ataxia Foundation, 308
College of Education - Western Kentucky University, 4766
Cystic Fibrosis Center, Kentucky University, 1335
Division of Preschool Services, 4767
EnTech: Enabling Technologies of Kentuckiana, 5077
Infant-Toddler Program, Division of Mental Retardation, 4768
Kentuckian Hemophilia Foundation, 2306
Kentucky Brain Tumor Support Group, 741
Kentucky Chapter of Crohn's & Colitis Foundation of America, 1221
Kentucky Department of Human Resources Bureau of Health Services, 4015
Kentucky Library for the Blind and Physically Handicapped, 5078
Kosair Children's CF Center, 1336
Louisville Free Public Library, 5079
NNFF of Kentucky, 3058
Northern Kentucky Talking Book Library, 5080
PWSA of Kentucky, 3368
Special Parent Involvement Network, 4769
Spina Bifida Association of Kentucky, 3876
Turner's Syndrome Society of Kentucky, 4258
Western Kentucky Assistive Technology Consortion, 5081

Louisiana

Brain Injury Association of Louisiana, 1846
Cystic Fibrosis & Pediatric Pulmonary Center, 1337
Division of Special Populations, 4770
E-NAF (Electric NAF) Support Group National Ataxia Foundation, 309
Families Helping Families of Greater New Orleans, 4771
Greater New Orleans Brain Tumor Support Group, 742
Louisiana Assistive Technology Access Network, 4772
Louisiana Chapter National Ataxia Foundation, 310
Louisiana Chapter of Crohn's & Colitis Foundation of America, 1222

Louisiana Chapter of the National Hemophilia Foundation, 2307
Louisiana Comprehensive Hemophilia Care Center, 2354
Louisiana State Library, 5082
Louisiana State University Genetics Section of Pediatrics, 5083
PWSA of Region Gulf Coast (Louisiana, Mississippi), 3369
Preschool Programs - Division of Special Populations, 4773
Project PROMPT, 4774
Public Health Services of Louisiana, 4016
Spina Bifida Association of Greater New Orleans, 3877
Tulane University Cystic Fibrosis Center, 1338
Turner's Syndrome Society of Gulf Coast, 4259

Maine

Bangor Public Library, 5084
Brain Injury Association of Maine, 1847
Brain Tumor Support Group, 743
Brain Tumor Support Group of Maine, 744
Brain Tumor Support Grp of Maine, 745
CDC Lincoln County, 4775
Cary Library, 5085
Central Maine Cystic Fibrosis Center, 1339
Child Department Services, 4776
Child Department Services, Department of Education, 4777
Children's Dream Factory of Maine, 4778
Consumer Information and Technology Training Exchange (Maine CITE), 4779
Department of Human Services, 4017
Eastern Maine Medical Center, Cystic Fibrosis Clinical Center, 1340
Jackson Laboratory, 1808
Lewiston Public Library, 5086
Maine Medical Center, Cystic Fibrosis Center, 1341
Maine State Library, 5087
Maine Support Groups National Ataxia Foundation, 311
New England Regional Genetics Group, 312
New England Regional Genetics Group, 5088
Portland Public Library, 5089
Sleep Laboratory, Maine Medical Center, 3015
Special Needs Parent Info Network, 4780
University of Maine, Conley Speech and Hearing Center, 1983
Waterville Public Library, 5090
York County Parent Awareness. Inc, 4781

Maryland

ARC Family Connection Parent to Parent Program, 4782
Baltimore Headache Institute, 2869
Brain Injury Association of Maryland, 1848
Brain Tumor Support Group of Maryland, 746
Captioned Films/Videos, 1984
Chesapeake Chapter National Ataxia Foundation, 313

Department of Pediatrics, University of Maryland, 1524
Developmental Pediatrics School of Medicine, University of Maryland, 4783
International Center for Skeletal Dysplasia, 1807
International Center for Skeletal Dysplasia, 4356
Johns Hopkins Department of Orthopaedics Surgery, 3605
Johns Hopkins University Sleep Disorders Center, 2971
Kennedy Krieger Institute, Down Syndrome Clinic, 1525
Learning Independence Through Computers, 5091
Little People's Research, 7
MD Infant/Toddler/Preschool Services, 4785
MD Infant/Toddler/Preschool Services Division, 4784
Maryland Chapter of Crohn's & Colitis Foundation of America, 1223
Maryland Infant and Toddlers Program Family Support Network, 4786
Maryland SIDS Information & Counseling Program, 4018
Maryland State Library for the Blind and Physically Handicapped, 5092
Maryland-Greater Washington, DC Chapter of Asthma and Allergy Foundation of America, 196
Mt. Washington Pediatric Clinic, 1526
NNFF of Maryland - Mid-Atlantic Region, 3059
National Hemophilia Foundation, Maryland Chapter, 2308
National Institute of Dental Research, 2802
National Organization of Parents of Blind Children, 4787
PWSA of Maryland & Metro Washington DC Inc, 3370
Parents Place of Maryland, Inc., 4788
Parents of Children with Down Syndrome ARC of Montgomery County, 1527
Partners in Intensive Care, Inc., 4789
Patient Recruitment & Public Liaison Office Clinical Center, 4328
Prince George's County Memorial Library Talking Book Center, 5093
Schizophrenia Research Branch: Division of Clinical and Treatment Research, 1044
Spina Bifida Association of Chesapeake-Polomac, 3878
Spina Bifida Association of Maryland, 3879
Spina Bifida Association of the Eastern Shore, 3880
Technology Assistance Program Maryland Rehab Center, 4790
Turner's Syndrome Society of Maryland, 4260

Massachusetts

Affiliated Children's Arthritis Centers of New England, 2701
Berkshire Center, 5094
Boston Area Support Group National Ataxia Foundation, 314
Boston Hemophilia Center, 2355
Boston Sickle Cell Center, 3771

Boston University Aphasia Research Center, 1888

Braille and Talking Book Library Perkins School for the Blind, 5095

Brain Center Brain Tumor Support Group, 747

Brain Injury Association of Massachusetts, 1849

Brain Tissue Resource Center, 854

Brain Tumor Support Group, 748

Brain Tumor Support Group at Ann Arbor, 758

Brain Tumor Support Group at Burlington, 749

Brain Tumor Support Group at Hampden, 750

Brain Tumor Support Group at Worcester University of Massachusetts Medical Ctr., 751

Bureau of Early Childhood Programs, 4791

Caption Center, 1985

Carroll Center for the Blind, 5096

Center for Interdisciplinary Research on Immunologic Diseases, 204

Center for Sleep Diagnostics, 2972

Children's Happiness Foundation, 4792

Children's Hospital, Cystic Fibrosis Center, 1342

Cooley's Anemia Foundation - Massachusetts Chapter, 4134

Developmental Evaluation Center, 1705

Down Syndrome Program - Children's Hospital Boston, 1528

Early Intervention Services, 4793

Eaton-Peabody Laboratory of Auditory Physiology, 1986

Educational Development Center, Inc (EDC), 4794

Families Coping with Mental Illness, 1042

Family Ties MA Dept. of Public Health, 4795

Federation for Children with Special Needs, 4796

Federation for Children with Special Needs, 4797

Greater Boston Parent to Parent, 4798

Headstrong, 752

Hemophilia Center of the New England Medical Center, 2356

Hydrocephalus Support Group, 2520

Long Term Survivors Support Group, 753

Marshfield, MA Support Group National Ataxia Foundation, 315

Massachusetts Assistive Technology Partnership, 4799

Massachusetts Center for SIDS, 4019

Massachusetts General Hospital Support Group for Brain Tumor Patients & Family, 754

Massachusetts, New England Hemophilia Association, 2309

NNFF of Massachusetts, 3060

National Training Center for Professional AIDS Education, 1704

Neurological Support Group of St. Luke's Hospital, 755

New England Chapter of Asthma and Allergy Foundation of America, 197

New England Chapter of Crohn's & Colitis Foundation of America, 1224

New England Region Helen Keller National Center, 4800

New England Support Group National Ataxia Foundation, 316

PWSA of Massachusetts, 3371

PWSA of Region New England, 3372

Parent Education/Support Group, 756

Sleep Disorders Unit, Beth Israel Hospital, 2973

Spina Bifida Association of Massachusetts, 3881

Talking Book Library at Worcester Public Library, 5097

Turner's Syndrome Society of New England, 4261

Michigan

Apnea Identification Program, 4020

Barbara Ann Karmanos Cancer Institute, 757

Brain Injury Association of Michigan, 1889

Brain Injury Association of Michigan, 1916

Brain Tumor Support Group, 769

Brain Tumor Support Group at Detroit, 759

Brain Tumor Support Group at Grand Rapids, 760

Brain Tumor Support Group for Patients & Families - U. of Michigan Medical Ctr, 761

Burger School for the Autistic, 512

CAUSE, 4801

Cystic Fibrosis Care, Teaching & Resource Center, 1343

Cystic Fibrosis Center/Pediatric Pulmonary and Sleep Medicine, 1344

Detroit Michigan Ataxia Support Group National Ataxia Foundation, 317

Early on Michigan, 4802

East Lansing Cystic Fibrosis Center, 1345

Eastern Michigan Hemophilia Center, 2357

Family Support Network of Michigan Parent Participation Program-MDCH, 4803

Frederick Douglas Branch for Specialized Services and Physically Handicapped, 5098

Glaucoma Laser Trabeculoplasty Study, 1151

Grand Rapids Chapter of Crohn's & Colitis Foundation of America, 1225

Greater Grand Rapids Pediatric Hemophilia Program, 2358

Hemophilia Foundation of Michigan, 2310

Hemophilia Treatment Center at Munson Medical Center, 2359

Hydrocephalus Support Group - Michigan, 2521

Kalamazoo Center for Medical Studies, 1346

Kent County Library for the Blind and Physically Handicapped, 5099

Library of Michigan Service for the Blind, 5100

Livingston County CMH Services, 4804

Macomb Library for the Blind and Physically Handicapped, 5101

Michigan Chapter of Allergy and Asthma Foundation of America, 198

Michigan Chapter of Crohn's & Colitis Foundation of America, 1226

Michigan Hemophilia Foundation, 2311

Michigan State University Hemophilia Comprehensive Care Clinic, 2360

Michigan's Assistive Technology Resource, 5102

Mideastern Michigan Library Co-op, 5103

Muskegon County Library for the Blind, 5104

NNFF of Michigan, 3061

Northland Library Cooperative, 5105

Office of Special Education, 4805

PWSA of Michigan, 3373

Parents are Experts, 4806

Regional Hemophilia Treatment Center, 2361

Rehabilitation Institute of Michigan, 1890

Seeking Techniques Advancing Research in Shunts (STARS), 2530

Sleep Disorders Center of Henry Ford Hospital, 2974

Spectrum Brain Tumor Support Group, 762

Spina Bifida Association of Grand Rapids, 3882

Spina Bifida Association of Southeastern Michigan, 3883

Spina Bifida Association of Upper Peninsula Michigan, 3884

Spina Bifida and Hydrocephalus Association of Southwestern Michigan, 3885

TECH 2000 Project Michigan Disability Rights Coalition, 4807

Turner's Syndrome Society of Southeastern Michigan, 4263

University of Michigan Hemophilia Center, 2362

University of Michigan, Communicative Disorders Clinic, 3807

University of Michigan, Cystic Fibrosis Center, 1347

University of Michigan, Kresge Hearing Research Institute, 1994

Upper Peninsula Library for the Blind, 5106

Washtenaw County Library, 5107

Wayne County Regional Library for the Blind & Physically Handicapped, 5108

Wayne State University Comprehensive Sickle Cell Center, 3772

Wayne State University, Guardjian-Lesser Biomechanics Laboratory, 1891

West Michigan Cancer Center Support Group, 763

West Michigan Regional Hemophilia Center, 2363

Minnesota

ARC Suburban, 4808

Brain Injury Association of Minnesota, 1850

Brain Tumor Support Group at Duluth, 764

Brain Tumor Support Group at Robbinside, 765

Brain Tumor Support Group at St. Paul Minnesota Neurology Specialists, 766

Brain Tumor Support Group for Benign Tumors - Minneapolis Neuroscience Inst., 767

Brain Tumor Support Group for Malignant Tumors, Minneapolis Neuroscience Inst., 768

Chicago County, MN Support Group National Ataxia Foundation, 318

Department of Children, Family, & Learning, 4809
Down Syndrome Clinic of Minneapolis Children's Medical Center, 1529
Family to Family Network ARC of Hennepin County, 4810
Hemophilia Foundation of Minnesota and the Dakotas, 2312
Interagency Early Intervention Project, 4811
KDWB Variety Family Center, 5109
Mayo Clinic and Foundation, 2918
Mayo Comprehensive Hemophilia Center, 2364
Minneapolis, MN Support Group National Ataxia Foundation, 319
Minnesota Library for the Blind & Physically Handicapped, 5110
Minnesota Sudden Infant Death Center, 4021
Minnesota-Dakotas Chapter of Crohn's & Colitis Foundation of America, 1227
National Resource Library on Youth With Disabilities, 5111
PACER Center, Inc., 5112
PACER Computer Resource Center, 4812
PWSA of Minnesota, 3374
Parents for Parents, 4813
Pilot Parents in Anoka and Ramsey Counties, 4814
Pilot Parents of Northeast Minnesota, 4815
STAR Program, 4816
Southwestern Minnesota Support Group National Ataxia Foundation, 321
Spina Bifida Association of Minnesota, 3886
Star Center for Family Health, 5113
Turner's Syndrome Society of Minnesota, 4262
University of Minnesota Comprehensive Hemophilia Center, 2365
University of Minnesota Cystic Fibrosis Center, 1348
Vinland Center, 4817
Voyageur Outward Bound School, 4818
Wilderness Inquiry, 4819
Windmill Project, 4820

Mississippi

Brain Injury Association of Mississippi, 1851
First Steps Program, 4821
Mississippi Chapter National Ataxia Foundation, 322
Mississippi Chapter of Crohn's & Colitis Foundation of America, 1228
Mississippi Hemophilia Foundation, 2313
Mississippi Library Commission, 5114
Mississippi State Department of Health and Child Health Services, 4022
Office of Special Education, 4822
Parent Partners, 4823
Project Empower, 4824
Project Start, 4825
Spina Bifida Association of Mississippi, 3887
University of Mississippi Medical Center, 1349

Missouri

AMOR - A Cancer Support Group for Patients & Their Families, 770
Assistance Technology Project, 4826
Brain Cancer Support Group Mid-America Cancer Center, 771
Brain Injury Association of Kansas & Greater Kansas City, 1852
Brain Injury Association of Kansas and Greater Kansas City, 1853
Brain Injury Association of Missouri, 1854
Brain Tumor Support Group, 772
Brain Tumor Support Network of St. Louis, 773
Central Area, Missouri Support Group National Ataxia Foundation, 323
Central Institute for the Deaf, 1995
Central Missouri Area Support Group National Ataxia Foundation, 325
Children's Mercy Hospital, Down Syndrome Clinic, 1530
Children's Mercy Hospital, University of Missouri, 1350
Children's Therapy Center, 4827
Cystic Fibrosis, Pediatric Pulmonary and Pediatric Gastrointestinal Center, 1351
Department of Elementary and Secondary Education, 4828
Disabilities Advocacy & Support Network, 4829
Down Syndrome Medical Clinic, 1531
Family Resource Network, 4830
Judevine Center for Autism, 513
Kansas City Support Group National Ataxia Foundation, 326
Kansas City, MO Support Group National Ataxia Foundation, 307
Midwest Sleep Diagnostics, 2975
Missouri Illinois Regional Hemophilia Comprehensive Treatment Center, 2366
Missouri Parents Act, 4831
NNFF of Missouri, 3062
National Hemophilia Foundation, Heart of America Chapter, 2314
PWSA of Missouri, 3375
Parent Act, 4832
Pediatric Brain Tumor Support Network, 774
Positive Parenting Partners United Services, 4833
Positive Solutions for Life Challenges, 4834
Region VII Office Program Consultants For Maternal and Child Health, 4023
Spina Bifida Association of Greater St. Louis, 3888
Springfield, MO Area Support Group National Ataxia Foundation, 327
St. Louis Chapter of Asthma and Allergy Foundation of America, 199
St. Louis Chapter of Crohn's & Colitis Foundation of America, 1229
St. Louis, MO Support Group National Ataxia Foundation, 324
Technology Access Center, 5115
Turner's Syndrome Society of West Illinios, 4264
University of Missouri-Columbia Cystic Fibrosis Center, 1352
Washington University Cystic Fibrosis Center, 1353
Whitney Library for the Blind - Assemblies of God, 5116
Wishing Well Foundation, 4835

Wolfner Memorial Library for the Blind, 5117

Montana

Brain Injury Association of Montana, 1855
Brain Tumor Support Group, 775
CO-TEACH/Division of Educational Research and Service, 4836
Developmental Disabilities Program, 4837
Division of Special Education, 4838
MonTECH, 4839
Montana Department of Health & Environmental Sciences, 4024
Montana State Library, 5118
Parents Let's Unite for Kids, 4840
Parents, Let's Unite for Kids, 4841
Quality Life Concepts, 4842

Nebraska

Assistive Technology Partnership, 4843
Boys Town National Research Hospital, 3828
Boys Town National Research Hospital, 3838
Brain Injury Association of Nebraska, 1856
Center for Hearing Loss in Children, 1996
Individual and Family Support Arc of Lincoln & Lancaster County, 4844
Nebraska Chapter of the National Hemophilia Foundation, 2315
Nebraska Library Commission Talking Book and Braille Service, 5119
Nebraska Parents Center, 4845
Nebraska Regional Hemophilia Center, 2367
Nebraska SIDS Foundation, 4025
North Platte Public Library, 5120
Omaha, NE Support Group National Ataxia Foundation, 328
PWSA of Nebraska, 3376
Parent Assistance Network, 4846
Parent Support Group, 4847
Parents Encouraging Parents, 4848
Special Education Office State Department of Education, 4849
Spina Bifida Association of Nebraska, 3889
University of Nebraska at Omaha Pediatric Pulmonary/Cystic Fibrosis Center, 1354
University of Nebraska, Lincoln Barkley Memorial Center, 1987

Nevada

Assistive Technology Collaborative, 4850
Brain Injury Association of Nevada, 1857
Brain Injury Association of Northern Nevada, 1858
Children's Lung Specialists, 1355
Early Intervention Services Division of Child & Family Services, 4851
Educational Equity, Special Education Branch, 4852
Las Vegas-Clark County Library District, 5121
NNFF of Nevada, 3063
Nevada Parent Network, 4853
Nevada Parents Encouraging Parents (PEP), 4854

Nevada State Division of Health, Maternal & Child Health, 4026

Nevada State Library and Archives, 5122

PWSA of Nevada, 3377

Turner's Syndrome Society of Nevada, 4265

University Medical Center Hemophilia Program, 2368

University of Nevada, Reno Speech And Language Pathology Department, 3808

New Hampshire

Brain Injury Association of New Hampshire, 1859

Brain Tumor Support Group, 776

Bureau of Early Learning, 4855

Camp Allen, 5496

Cystic Fibrosis Care and Teaching Center, 1356

Dartmouth Center for Genetics & Child Development, 1532

Dartmouth Hitchcock Hemophilia Center, 2369

Dartmouth-Hitchcock Sleep Disorders Center Dartmouth Medical Center, 2976

Division of Special Education, 4856

Family Center Early Supports & Services, 4857

High Hopes Foundation of New Hampshire Inc, 4858

NNFF of Northern New England, 3064

New Hampshire SIDS Program, 4027

New Hampshire State Library, 5123

Parent Information Center, 4859

Parent to Parent of New Hampshire, 4860

Portsmouth Regional Home, 777

Sleep/Wake Disorders Center, Hampstead Hospital, 2977

Technology Partnership Project Institute on Disability/UAP, 4861

Turner's Syndrome Society of Northern New England, 4266

New Jersey

Belmar, New Jersey Support Group National Ataxia Foundation, 329

Brain Injury Association of New Jersey, 1860

Brain Tumor Support Group, 778

Brain Tumor Support Group at Livingston, 779

Brain Tumor Support Group at North Plainfield, Muhlenberg Regional Med. Cnt, 780

Brain Tumor Support Group at Plainfield Muhlenberg Reg. Med. Cntr., Neuroscience, 781

Brain Tumor Support Group of Monmouth County, 782

Center for Enabling Technology, 5124

Cooley's Anemia Foundation - New Jersey Chapter, 4135

Division of Student Services, 4862

Early Intervention Program, 4863

Epilepsy Foundation of New Jersey, 3674

Epliepsy Foundation New Jersey, 3675

Fairlawn, NJ Support Group National Ataxia Foundation, 330

Family Support Center of New Jersey, 4864

Foundation for Children with Down Syndrome, 1533

Greater New Jersey Chapter of Crohn's & Colitis Foundation of America, 1230

Hydrocephalus Parents Support Group, 2522

Monmouth Medical Center, Cystic Fibrosis & Pediatric Pulmonary Center, 1357

NNFF of New Jersey, 3065

Nadeene Brunini Comprehensive Hemophilia Care Center, 2370

National Alliance for Autism Research, 522

New Jersey Center for Outreach and Services for the Autism Community(COSAC), 514

New Jersey Department of Health - Child Health Program, 4028

New Jersey Institute of Technology Center For Biomedical Engineering, 1809

New Jersey Library for the Blind and Physically Handicapped, 5125

New Jersey Medical School Department of Pediatrics, 1358

New Jersey Statewide Parent to Parent, 4865

PWSA of New Jersey, 3378

Princeton University, Cutaneous Communication Laboratory, 1988

S.E. Pennsylvania Chapter of Asthma and Allergy Foundation of America, 201

Sarcoidosis Support Group - Central New Jersey, 3544

Sarcoidosis Support Group - New Jersey, 3545

Sleep Disorders Center, Newark Beth Israel Medical Center, 2978

Spina Bifida Association of Bergen and Passaic Counties, 3890

Spina Bifida Association of New Jersey, 3891

Statewide Parent Advocacy Network, 4866

Technology Assistive Resource Program, 4867

Turner's Syndrome Society of New Jersey, 4267

New Mexico

Brain Injury Association of New Mexico, 1861

EPICS Project SW Communication Resources, 4868

Long Term Services Division, 4869

NM Alliance for the Neurologically Impaired, 783

New Mexico Chapter of Crohn's & Colitis Foundation of America, 1231

New Mexico SIDS Information & Counseling Program, 4029

New Mexico State Library for the Blind And Physically Handicapped, 5126

Parents Reaching Out, 4870

Parents Reaching Out (PRO), 4871

Region 5 of the National Association for Parents of the Visually Impaired, 4872

Special Education Unit, 4873

Spina Bifida Association of New Mexico, 3892

Technology Assistance Program, 4874

Ted R. Montoya Hemophilia Program, 2371

New York

Adult & Pediatric Hemophilia Clinics SUNY Health Sciences Center, 2372

Advocacy Center, 4875

Advocates for Children of New York, 4876

Albany Medical College Pediatric Pulmonary & Cystic Fibrosis Center, 1359

Albany New York Regional Comprehensive Hemophilia Center, 2373

Armond U. Mascia CF Center, 1360

Association for Research of Childhood Cancer, 5176

Brady Institute, 1892

Brain Injury Association of New York, 1862

Brain Trauma Foundation, 1881

Brain Tumor Support Group, 784

Brain Tumor Support Group at Manhattan, 785

Brain Tumor Support Group at Schenectady, 786

Brain Tumor Support Group of CNY, 787

Brain Tumor Support Grp., 788

Brainstormers, 789

Brooklyn College of City University of New York - Speech & Hearing Center, 3809

CF & Pediatric Pulmonary Care Center, 1361

CF, Pediatric Pulmonary & GI Center, 1362

Capital District Chapter of Crohn's & Colitis Foundation of America, 1232

Capital Regional Sleep-Wake Disorders Center, 2979

Center for Sleep Medicine of the Mount Sinai Medical Center, 2980

Childhood Survivors of Cancer, 790

Children's Clinical Research Center, 1703

Children's Lung and Cystic Fibrosis Center, 1363

City University of New York Center for Research in Speech and Hearing, 3810

Columbia Presbyterian Medical Center, 2919

Columbia Presbyterian Medical Center Sleep Disorders Center, 2981

Columbia University Clinical Research Center for Muscular Dystrophy, 2920

Columbia University Comprehensive Sickle Cell Center, 3773

Cooley's Anemia Foundation - Rochester, 4136

Cooley's Anemia Foundation - Staten Island, 4137

Cooley's Anemia Foundation - Suffolk Chapter Office, 4138

Cooley's Anemia Foundation - Westchester, 4139

Cooley's Anemia Foundation-Buffalo, 4140

Cooley's Anemia Foundation-Queens, 4141

Crohn's & Colitis Foundation of America, Inc. (CCFA), 1263

Dana Alliance for Brain Initiatives, 1882

Developmental Evaluation Clinic, 1534

Early Intervention Program, 4877

Epilepsy Foundation of Long Island, 3676

Fairfield/Westchester Chapter of Crohn's & Colitis Foundation of America, 1234

Friends of Karen, 4878

Goodays Brain Tumor Support Group, 791

Greater New York Chapter of Crohn's & Colitis Foundation of America, 1235

Helen Keller International, 5127

Helen Keller National Center, 5128

Hemophilia Center of Western New York, 2316

Hemophilia Center of Western New York, 2374

Institute for Basic Research In Developmental Disabilities, 5129

Institute for Basic Research in Developmental Disabilities, 515

International Center for Hearing and Speech Research, 3811

JGB Cassette Library International, 5130

Keren-Or, Inc., 5131

Laboratory of Dermatology Research, 5132

Long Island Adult Brain Tumor Support Group - Nassau Chapter, 792

Long Island Brain Tumor Support Group, 793

Long Island Chapter of Crohn's & Colitis Foundation of America, 1236

Marty Lyons Foundation, Inc., 4879

Mary M. Gooley Hemophilia Center of the National Hemophilia Foundation, 2317

NHF Camp Directory, 2451

NNFF of New York/New Jersey, 3066

Nassau Library System, 5133

National Alliance for Research on Schizophrenia & Depression, 639

National Alliance for Research on Schizophrenia & Depression, 1041

National Alliance for Research on Schizophrenia & Depression, 1043

National Alliance for Research on Schizophrenia & Depression, 5178

National Center for the Study of Wilson's Disease, Inc, 4347

National Cued Speech Association, 3812

National Headquarters of Crohn' & Colitis Foundation of America, 1237

National Leukemia Research Association,Inc, 41

Neurology Research Center, 3681

New York Chapter of Asthma and Allergy Foundation of America, 200

New York City Area Support Group National Ataxia Foundation, 331

New York City Information & Counseling Program for SIDS, 4030

New York Department of Education, 4880

New York Foundation for Otologic Research, 1997

New York State Talking Book & Braille Library, 5134

New York University, 2921

New York University Medical Center Auxillary of Tisch Hospital, 2523

PWSA of New York, 3379

PWSA of New York Alliance, 3380

Parent Network Center, 4881

Parent to Parent of New York State, 4882

Parents Caring and Sharing, 39

Pediatric Pulmonary Center, 1364

People Treated for Brain Tumors and their Caregivers, 794

People Treated for Brian Tumors and Their Caregivers, 795

Rehabilitation, Research & Training Center For Persons with TBI, 1883

Resources for Children with Special Needs, 4883

Rochester Chapter of Crohn's & Colitis Foundation of America, 1238

Rockefeller University Laboratory for Investigative Dermatology, 5135

SLE Foundation, Inc., 4083

SUNY Health Science Center at Brooklyn Sickle Cell Center, 3774

Schizophrenic Biologic Research Center, 1045

Schneider Children's Hospital of Long Island, 1365

Sickle Cell Disease Foundation of Greater New York, 3765

Sinergia/Metropolitan Parent Center, 4884

Sleep Center, Community General Hospital, 2982

Sleep Disorders Center of Rochester, St. Mary's Hospital, 2983

Sleep Disorders Center of Western New York Millard Fillmore Hospital, 2984

Sleep Disorders Center, University Hospital, 2985

Sleep-Wake Disorders Center, Montefiore Sleep Disorders Center, 2986

Sleep-Wake Disorders Center, New York Presbyterian Hospital, 2987

Southern Tier Chapter of Crohn's & Colitis Foundation of America, 1239

Southern Tier Hemophilia Center, 2375

Spina Bifida Association of Albany/Capital District, 3893

Spina Bifida Association of Greater Rochester, 3894

Spina Bifida Association of Nassau County, 3895

Spina Bifida Association of Western New York, 3896

Spina Bifida Association of the Niagara Frontier, 3897

St. Joseph's Hospital Health Center Sleep Laboratory, 2988

St. Mary's Healthcare System for Children, 4885

State University College at Fredonia Youngerman Center, 3813

State University College at Plattsburgh Auditory Research Laboratory, 1998

State University of New York Health Sciences Center, 516

Support for Parents of Children with Brain Tumors, 796

Syracuse University, Institute for Sensory Research, 1999

TRIAD Project Advocates for Persons with Disabilities, 4886

Techspress Resource Center for Independent Living, 5136

Teddi Project, 4699

Turner's Syndrome Society of Long Island and New York City, 4268

Ulster County Social Services, 4887

Upper Hudson Valley Chapter of National Hemophilia Foundation, 2318

VISIONS/Vacation Camp for the Blind, 5500

Wallace Memorial Library, 1989

Western New York Area Support Group National Ataxia Foundation, 332

Western New York Chapter of Crohn's & Colitis Foundation of America, 1240

Western New York Chapter of Crohn's & Colitis Foundation of America, 1241

Winthrop-University Hospital Sleep Disorders Center, 2989

Yeshiva University, Institute of Communication Disorders, 2000

North Carolina

Assistive Technology Project, Human Resources, Voc. and Rehab. Services, 4888

Autism Society of North Carolina, 517

Bowman Grey School of Medicine - Hemophilia Diagnostic Center, 2376

Brain Injury Association of North Carolina, 1863

Brain Tumor Support Group, 797

Carolina Computer Access Center Metro School, 5137

Charlotte Brain Tumor Support Group, 798

Comprehensive Hemophilia Diagnostic and Treatment Center, 2377

Duke Brain Tumor Support Group, 799

Duke Pediatric Brain Tumor Family Support Program, 800

Duke University Comprehensive Sickle Cell Center, 3775

Duke University Epilepsy Research Center, 3682

Duke University, Center for the Advanced Study of Epilepsy, 3683

ECAC, Inc., 4889

Exceptional Children Division, 4890

Family Support Network of North Carolina, 4891

Hemophilia Foundation of North Carolina, 2319

North Carolina Chapter of Crohn's & Colitis Foundation of America, 1242

North Carolina Library for the Blind, 5138

North Carolina SIDS Information and Counseling Program, 4031

PWSA of North Carolina, 3381

Partnerships for Inclusion, 4892

Pediatric Rheumatoid Clinic, 2702

Raleigh Area Brain Tumor Support Group, 801

Rockingham County Schools, 4893

Sickle Cell Disease Association of the Piedmont, 3766

Spina Bifida Association Lipomysiomeningcele Family Support, 3898

Spina Bifida Association of North Carolina, 3899

Turner's Syndrome Society of North Carolina, 4269

UNC CF Center, 1366

University of North Carolina at Chapel Hill, Brain Research Center, 518

University of North Carolina at Chapel Hill, Division of Speech & Hearing, 3814

Wake Forest University Comprehensive Epilepsy Program, 3684

Winston-Salem, NC Support Groups National Ataxia Foundation, 333

North Dakota

Children's Hospital Merit Care Down Syndrome Service, 1535

Developmental Disabilities Unit, 4894

Interagency Program Assistive
Technology, 4895

Native American Family Network System
Arrowhead Shopping Center, 4896

North Dakota Comprehensive Hemophilia
Center, 2378

North Dakota SIDS Management
Program, 4032

PWSA of North Dakota, 3382

Special Education Division, 4897

St. Alexius Medical Center/CF Center,
1367

Ohio

American Council of Blind Parents, 5139

Bethesda Oak Hospital, Sleep Disorders
Center, 2990

Blick Clinic for Developmental
Disabilities, 5140

Brain Tumor Support Group, 802

Bureau of EI Services, 4898

Case Western Research University, Bolton
Brush Growth Study Center, 1806

Case Western Reserve University Applied
Neural Control Laboratory, 3685

Case Western Reserve University Cystic
Fibrosis Center, 1368

Celebrating Families of Children &
Adults with Special Needs, 4899

Center for Research in Sleep Disorders,
3016

Center for Sleep & Wake Disorders,
Miami Valley Hospital, 2991

Central Ohio Brain Tumor Support
Group, 803

Central Ohio Chapter of Crohn's &
Colitis Foundation of America, 1243

Central Ohio Chapter of the National
Hemophilia Foundation, 2320

Child Advocacy Center, 4900

Children's Hospital Hemophilia
Treatment Center, 2379

Children's Hospital Research Foundation,
3530

Cincinnati Center for Developmental
Disorders, 1536

Cleveland Brain Tumor Patient Network -
Adult and Pediatric, 804

Cleveland Clinic Foundation, Sleep
Disorders Center, 2992

Cleveland Hearing and Speech Center,
3815

Cleveland Public Library, 5141

Clinical Genetics - Down Syndrome
Children's Hospital, 1537

Clinical Research Center, Pediatrics, 619

Clinical Research Center, Pediatrics, 3531

Columbus Children's Hospital, Cystic
Fibrosis Center, 1369

Comprehensive Sickle Cell Center, 3776

Division of Early Childhood Education,
4901

Down Syndrome Clinic, Department of
Pediatrics, 1538

Down Syndrome Clinic, Rainbow Babies
and Children's Hospital, 1539

East Central Regional Office, 4902

Family Information Network, 4903

Greater Cincinnati Chapter of Crohn's &
Colitis Foundation of America, 1244

Kent State University, Speech and
Hearing Clinic, 3816

Kettering Medical Center, Sleep Disorders
Center, 2993

Lewis H. Walker, M.D., CF Center, 1370

Miami Valley Downs Syndrome
Association, 4904

NNFF of Ohio, 3067

Neuro-Oncology Support Group, 805

Northeastern Illinois Chapter of Crohn's
& Colitis Foundation of America, 1245

Northeastern Ohio Chapter of Crohn's &
Colitis Foundation of America, 1246

Northern Ohio Chapter of the National
Hemophilia Foundation, 2321

Northwest Ohio Hemophilia Association,
2322

Northwest Ohio Hemophilia Treatment
Center, 2380

Northwest Ohio Sleep Disorders Center,
2994

OCECD, 4905

Ohio Brain Injury Association, 1864

Ohio Protection and Advocacy
Organization, 4906

Ohio Regional Library for the Blind and
Physically Handicapped, 5142

Ohio Sleep Medicine Institute, 2995

Ohio State University Hospitals, Sleep
Disorders Center, 2996

Ohio Support Group National Ataxia
Foundation, 334

Ohio University School of Hearing and
Speech Sciences, 3817

Operation Liftoff of Ohio, 4907

PWSA of Ohio, 3383

Parent Project for Muscular Dystrophy
Research, Inc, 2922

Pediatric Pulmonary Center, 1371

Perinatal and Infant Health Unit - SIDS
Information and Counseling Program,
4033

Society for Rehabilitation, 4908

Southwest Ohio Brain Tumor Support
Group Brain Tumor Support Group,
806

Southwestern Ohio Chapter of the
National Hemophilia Foundation, 2323

Spina Bifida Association of Canton, 3900

Spina Bifida Association of Central Ohio,
3901

Spina Bifida Association of Cincinnati,
3902

Spina Bifida Association of Cleveland,
3903

Spina Bifida Association of Greater
Dayton, 3904

Spina Bifida Association of Northwest
Ohio, 3905

Spina Bifida Association of Tri-County
Ohio, 3906

St. Vincent Medical Center, Sleep
Disorders Center, 2997

Support Group for Parents of Children
with a Brain Tumor, 807

Technology Resource Center, 5143

Train Ohio Super Computer Center, 4909

Turner's Syndrome Society of
Southwestern Ohio, 4270

University Treatment Center of University
Hospitals of Cleveland, 2381

University of Cincinnati College of
Medicine/Division of Pediatrics, 1372

West Central Ohio Hemophilia Center,
2382

Youngstown Hemophilia Center, 2383

Oklahoma

Brain Injury Association of Oklahoma,
1865

NNFF of Oklahoma, 3068

North Central Oklahoma Support Group
National Ataxia Foundation, 335

Oklahoma ABLE Tech Wellness Center,
4910

Oklahoma Chapter of Crohn's & Colitis
Foundation of America, 1247

Oklahoma Chapter of the National
Hemophilia Foundation, 2324

Oklahoma Comprehensive Hemophilia
Diagnostic Treatment Center, 2384

Oklahoma Library for the Blind &
Physically Handicapped, 5144

Oklahoma State Department of Health -
Maternal and Child Health Services,
4034

PWSA of Oklahoma, 3384

Parents Reaching Out in Oklahoma, 4911

Special Education Office, 4912

Spina Bifida Association of Oklahoma,
3907

Tulsa City-County Library System, 5145

Turner's Syndrome Society of Oklahoma,
4271

University of Oklahoma Cystic Fibrosis
Center, 1373

University of Oklahoma, Speech &
Hearing Center, 3818

Oregon

Brain Injury Association of Oregon, 1866

Brain Tumor Support Group, 808

Early Childhood CARES Program, 4913

Early Intervention Programs, 4914

Hemophilia Foundation of Oregon, 2325

NNFF of Oregon - Patient Information
and Support Only, 3069

Oregon Cope Project, 4915

Oregon Health Sciences University
Research Center, 2001

Oregon State Library, Talking Book and
Braille Services, 5146

PWSA of Oregon, 3385

Pacific Northwest Regional Genetics
Group, 336

Regional Resource Center on Deafness,
1990

SIDS Resource of Oregon, 4035

Special Education Programs, 4916

Technology Access for Life Needs Project,
4917

Willamette Valley Ataxia Support Group
National Ataxia Foundation, 337

Pennsylvania

Albert Einstein Medical Center
Hemophilia Program, 2385

Braim Tumor Support Group of the
Lehigh Valley, 809

Brain Injury Association of Eastern
Pennsylvania, 1867

Brain Injury Association of Western
Pennsylvania, 1868

Brain Tumor Family Support Group, 810

Brain Tumor Support Group, 811

Brain Tumor Support Group at Bradford,
812

Turner's Syndrome Society of South
Carolina, 4274

South Dakota

DakotaLink, 4937
NNFF of South Dakota - Northern Plains,
3073
Office of Special Education, 4938
Sioux Falls Hemophilia Treatment Center,
2392
Sioux Valley Hospital, South Dakota
Cystic Fibrosis Center, 1380
South Dakota Department of Health, 4039
South Dakota Parent Connection, 4939
South Dakota State Library, 5153
University Affiliated Program, School of
Medicine, 4940

Tennessee

Bill Wilkerson Center, 2003
Brain Injury Association of Tennessee,
1871
Center for Early Childhood, 4941
East Tennessee Chapter of Crohn's &
Colitis Foundation of America, 1254
East Tennessee Comprehensive
Hemophilia Center, 2393
East Tennessee Technology Access Center,
5154
First Regional Hemophilia Center, 2394
Memphis Cystic Fibrosis Center, 1381
Memphis State University, Center for the
Communicatively Impaired, 3820
NNFF of Tennessee, 3074
Nashville Brain Tumor Support Group,
827
Office of Special Education, State
Department of Education, 4942
Office of Special Education, State Dept of
Education, 4943
PWSA of Tennessee, 3388
Regional Brain Tumor Support Group,
828
STEP, 4944
Sarcoidosis Research Institute, 3549
Spina Bifida Association of
Mid-Tennessee, 3916
St. Jude Children's Research Hospital,
5155
TN Hemo & Bleeding Disorders
Foundation, 2330
Technology Access Center of Middle
Tennessee, 4945
Tennessee SIDS Program, 4040
University of Tennessee Hemophilia
Clinic, 2395
University of Tennessee, Center For
Neuroscience, 3687
Vanderbilt Comprehensive Hemophilia
Center, 2396
West Tennessee Chapter of Crohn's &
Colitis Foundation of America, 1255
West Tennessee Special Technology
Access, 5156

Texas

Baylor College of Medicine, 2924
Baylor College of Medicine Birth Defects
Center, 5157

Baylor College of Medicine Epilepsy
Research Center, 3688
Baylor College of Medicine, Sleep
Disorder and Research Center, 3017
Brain Injury Association of Texas, 1872
Brain Tumor Support Group at Austin,
829
Brain Tumor Support Group at Dallas,
830
Brain Tumor Support Group at Plano, 831
Brain Tumor Support Group for Families
of Children with Brain and Spinal
Tumors, 832
CF Center, Pulmonary Section, 1382
Children's Assn. for Maxiumum Potential
C.A.M.P., 5499
Cook-Ft. Worth Medical Center, CF
Center, 1383
Cooley's Anemia Foundation - Texas, 4142
Cystic Fibrosis Care, Teaching and
Research Center, 1384
Cystic Fibrosis-Lung Disease Center
Santa Rosa Children's Hospital, 1385
Down Syndrome Clinic - Texas, 1544
Golden Triangle Area Support Group
National Ataxia Foundation, 343
Grassroads Consortium, 4946
Gulf States Hemophilia Diagnostic and
Treatment Center, 2397
HOPE (Helping Oncology Parents
Endure) Brain Tumor Foundation of
the Southwest, 833
Harris County Health Department, 4041
Houston Area Brain Tumor Network, 834
Houston Area Brain Tumor Support
Network, 835
Houston Ear Research Foundation, 2004
Houston-Gulf Coast/South Texas Chapter
of Crohn's & Colitis Foundation of
America, 1256
Hydrocephalus Association of North
Texas, 2526
Lone Star Chapter of the National
Hemophilia Foundation, 2331
National Phenylketonuria (PKU)
Foundation, 3276
North Texas Chapter of Allergy and
Allergy Foundation of America, 202
North Texas Chapter of Crohn's & Colitis
Foundation of America, 1258
North Texas Comprehensive Pediatric
Hemophilia Center, 2398
North Texas Support Group National
Ataxia Foundation, 344
Office of the Dean, University of Texas at
Austin, 4947
PWSA of Texas, 3389
Parent Case Management, 4948
Partners Resource Network, 4949
Pediatric Sickle Cell Disease Program
University of Texas Southwestern
Medical, 3777
Project PODER, 4950
Rehabilitation, Research and Training
Center in Traumatic Brain Injuries,
1884
San Antonio Support Group National
Ataxia Foundation, 345
Shirvers Cancer Center Brain Tumor
Support Group, 836
Shirvers Cancer Center Brain Tumor
Support Group, 837
Sleep Disorders Center for Children, 3009
Sleep Medicine Associates of Texas, 3010

South Central Region Helen Keller
National Center, 4951
South Texas Comprehensive Hemophilia
Center - Santa Rosa Health Corp., 2399
Special Education Programs, 4952
Spina Bifida Association of Austin, 3917
Spina Bifida Association of Dallas, 3918
Spina Bifida Association of Texas, 3919
Spina Bifida Association of Texas, Gulf
Coast, 3920
Spina Bifida Association of Texas/Alamo
Area Support Group, 3921
Texas Assistive Technology Partnership,
4953
Texas Interagency Council on Early
Childhood Intervention, 4954
Texas Regional Genetics Network, 346
Texas State Library, 5158
Texas Tech University Speech-Language-
Hearing Clinic, 3821
Tri-Services Military CF Center, 1386
Turner's Syndrome Society of Houston,
4275
Univ. of Texas - Southwestern Med. Ctr.
at Dallas - Clinical Ctr. for Liver
Disease, 620
University of Texas Health Science Center
at Houston - Speech & Hearing, 3822
University of Texas Medical Branch at
Galveston, Clinical Research Center,
3018
University of Texas Sleep/Wake Disorders
Center, 3011
University of Texas at Dallas, Callier
Center for Communication Disorders,
3823
University of Texas at Dallas, Callier
Center for Communication Disorders,
3839
University of Texas, Mental Health
Clinical Research Center, 1436
We've Just Begun to Live Brain Tumor
Support Group, 838
West Texas Brain Tumor Support Group,
839

Utah

Brain Injury Association of Utah, 1873
Computer Center for Citizens with
Disabilities, 4956
Early Intervention Program, 4957
Early Intervention Research Institute,
Developmental Center, 5184
NNFF of Utah, 3075
National Hemophilia Foundation, Utah
Chapter, 2332
PWSA of Utah, 3390
PWSA of Utah (Orem), 3391
Peer-Led Brain Tumor Support Group,
840
Primary Children's Medical Center, 5185
Special Education Services Unit, 4958
Spina Bifida Association of Utah, 3922
Turner's Syndrome Society of Salt Lake
City, 4276
US Disabled Ski Team, 4959
University of Utah, 2925
University of Utah Intermountain Cystic
Fibrosis Center, 1387
Utah Center for Assistive Technology, 4960
Utah Department of Health, 4042
Utah Parent Center, 4961

Utah State Library Commission, 5159
Utah Support Group National Ataxia Foundation, 347

Vermont

Assistive Technology Project, 4962
Brain Injury Association of Vermont, 1874
Center on Disabilities and Community Inclusion, 4963
Family, Infant, and Toddler Project, 4964
Medical Center Hospital of Vermont, 1388
Special Education Unit, 4965
Vermont Department of Health - SIDS Information and Counseling Program, 4043
Vermont Department of Libraries, 5160
Vermont Parent Information Center, 4966
Vermont Regional Hemophilia Center, 2400

Virginia

Alexandria Library Talking Book Service, 5161
Arlington County Department of Libraries, 5162
Assistive Technology System, 4967
Brain Injury Association of Virginia, 1875
Brain Tumor Support Group, 841
CF Center/University of Virginia School of Medicine, 1389
Camp Fantastic, 5498
Cystic Fibrosis Program of the Medical College of Virginia, 1390
Division for Research (CEC-DR), 5177
Division on Visual Impairments, 5163
Eastern Virginia Medical Center, 1391
Fairfax County Public Library, 5164
Greater Washington, D.C. Chapter of Crohn's & Colitis Foundation of America, 1259
Hampton Roads Chapter of Crohn's & Colitis Foundation of America, 1260
Hampton Subregional Library for the Blind, 5165
Hemophilia Association of the Capital Area, 2333
Hemophilia Treatment Center of Tidewater Virginia, 2401
Infant & Toddler Program, 4968
National Sudden Infant Death Syndrome Research Center, 4051
Newport News Public Library System, 5166
Office of Special Education, State Dept of Education, 4969
PWSA of Virginia, 3392
Parent Education Advocacy Training Center, 4970
Roanoke City Public Library System, 5167
Sarcoidosis Self-Help Group - Virginia, 3546
Speech Simulation Research Foundation, 3824
Spina Bifida Association of the National Capital Area, 3923
Tidewater Center for Technology Access, 4971
Turner's Syndrome Society of National Capitol Area, 4277
University of Virginia Communication Disorders Program, 1991

University of Virginia Hemophilia Treatment Center, 2402
Virginia Beach Public Library, 5168
Virginia Commonwealth University, Rehab Research and Training Center, 1895
Virginia SIDS Program - Virginia Department of Health, 4044
Virginia State Library for the Visually and Physically Handicapped, 5169

Washington

Adult Brain Tumor Support Group, 842
Assistive Technology Alliance DSHS/DVR, 4972
Brain Injury Association of Washington, 1876
Brain Tumor Support Group University of Washington Medical Center, 843
Brain Tumor Support Group at Seattle, 844
Epilepsy Association of Washington, 3679
Hemophilia Foundation of Washington, 2334
Hydrocephalus Support Group of Seattle, 2527
Infant Toddler Early Intervention Program, 4973
NNFF of Washington, 3076
NW Sarcoidosis Support Group, 3547
Northwest Hospital Brain Tumor Group Support Hotline, 846
Northwest Hospital Brain Tumor Support Group, 845
Northwestern Region Helen Keller National Center, 4974
Office of the Superintendent of Public Instruction, 4975
PWSA of Region Northwest, 3393
PWSA of Washington, 3394
Pacific NW Support Group, 3548
Puget Sound Blood Center, 2403
Region X Office Program Consultants for Maternal and Child Health, 4045
Rotary Wishing Well, Inc., 4976
Seattle, WA Area Support Group National Ataxia Foundation, 348
Spina Bifida Association of Evergreen, 3924
Turner's Syndrome Society of Inland Northwest, 4278
University of Washington - the Model Preschool Center for Children, 1545
University of Washington CF Center, 1392
University of Washington Department of Speech & Hearing Sciences, 3825
University of Washington Speech and Hearing Clinic, 3826
Washington Library for the Blind and Physically Handicapped, 5170
Washington PAVE, 4977
Washington State Chapter of Asthma and Allergy Foundation of America, 203
Washington State Chapter of Crohn's & Colitis Foundation of America, 1261
Wishing Star Foundation, 4978

West Virginia

Autism Services Center, 519
Autism Training Center, 520

Brain Injury Association of West Virginia, 1877
Cabell County Public Library, 5171
Early Intervention Program, 4979
Hemophilia Center of West Virginia, 2404
Huntington Area Hemophilia Association, 2405
Kanawha County Public Library, 5172
Office of Special Education Administration, 4980
PWSA of West Virginia, 3395
Southern West Virginia Brain Tumor Support Group, 847
West Virginia Assistive Technology System, 4981
West Virginia Chapter, 2335
West Virginia Department of Health and Human Services, 4046
West Virginia Library Commission, 5173
West Virginia Parent Training and Information, 4982
West Virginia School for the Blind, 5174
West Virginia University Mountain State Cystic Fibrosis Center, 1393

Wisconsin

American Red Cross Hemophilia Center, 2406
Birth to 3 Program, 4983
Brain Injury Association of Wisconsin, 1878
Brain Tumor Support Group, 848
Brain Tumor Support Group at Milwaukee, 849
Brain Tumor Support Group at Wauwatosa Froederdt Memorial Lutheran Hospital, 850
Brain Tuor Support Group at Milwaupee, 851
Brown County Library, 5175
Counseling and Research Center for SIDS, 4047
Development and Training Center, 4984
Division of Community Services, 4985
Early Childhood Handicapped Prgrams, 4986
Eau Claire Hemophilia Center, 2407
Fox Valley Hydrocephalus Support Group, 2528
GLaRGG BLuRBB, 349
Great Lakes Hemophilia Foundation, 2336
Gundersen Clinic Comprehensive Hemophilia Treatment Center, 2408
Hematology Treatment Center of the Great Lakes Hemophilia Foundation, 2409
Information Centers for Lithium, Bipolar Disorders Treatment & Obsessive Compuls, 638
International Bone Marrow Transplant Registry Medical College of Wisconsin, 40
International Scoliosis Research Center, 3607
John Sierzant Brain Tumor Support Group, 852
LODAT (Living One Day at a Time) Brain Tumor Support Group, 853
Lithium Infomation Center, 3185
Madison, WI Area Support Group National Ataxia Foundation, 350
Medical College of Wisconsin Cystic Fibrosis Center, 1394

NNFF of Wisconsin, 3077
Northeastern Wisconsin Hemophilia
  Center, 2410
Obsessive-Compulsive Information
  Center, 3186
PWSA of Wisconsin, 3396
PWSA of Wisconsin - Madison, 3397
Parent Education Project of Wisconsin,
  Inc, 4987
Spina Bifida Association of Northeastern
  Wisconsin, 3925
Spina Bifida Association of Northern
  Wisconsin, 3926
Spina Bifida Association of Southeastern
  Wisconsin, 3927
Spina Bifida Association of Wisconsin,
  3928
Spina Bifida Association of the Greater
  Fox Valley, 3929
Thurday's Child, 4988
Turner's Syndrome Society of
  Southeastern Wisconsin, 4279
University of Wisconsin - Madison
  Neuropsychology Laboratory, 3689
University of Wisconsin, Auditory
  Physiology Center, 3827
University of Wisconsin-Madison Cystic
  Fibrosis/Pulmonary Center, 1395
WisTech, 4989
Wisconsin Chapter of Crohn's & Colitis
  Foundation of America, 1262

Wyoming

Brain Injury Association of Wyoming,
  1879
Division of Developmental Disabilities,
  4990
NNFF of Wyoming, 3078
Parent Information Center, 4991
Parent and Information Center, 5186
Special Education Unit, 4992
Wyoming Department of Health, 4048
Wyoming's New Options in Technology
  (WYNOT), 4993

Canada

Canada Support Group National Ataxia
  Foundation, 351
Children's Wish Foundation of Canada,
  4995
Easter Seal of Canada, 4996
Lymphoma Research Foundation Canada,
  3148
Sleep Disorders Centre of Metropolitan
  Toronto, 3012
South Central Ontario National Ataxia
  Foundation, 352

United Kingdom

Arthrogryposis Support Group, 168
Research Trust for Metabolic Diseases in
  Children, 90
Research Trust for Metabolic Diseases in
  Children, 2759
Research Trust for Metabolic Diseases in
  Children, 2898
Research Trust for Metabolic Diseases in
  Children, 3277
Research Trust for Metabolic Diseases in
  Children, 4101

Research Trust for Metabolic Diseases in
  Children, 5187